WORK REWORK REWORK REWORK REWORK REWORK
Printed at: Sat Sep 26 19:30:13 2026 on device cbhp04-90

Batch 51850CB00018B

51850CBX00295BA	9783036574875	Radiation Damage in Biomolecules and Cells				
CASE	6.69X9.61	398	<O>	1.25	MATTE	(1)
51850CBX00296BA	9783038422747	Selected Papers from 6th Annual Conference				
CASE	6.69X9.61	398	<O>	1.25	MATTE	(1)
51850CBX00297BA	9783725877997	Artificial Intelligence in Participatory Enviro				
CASE	6.69X9.61	396	<N>	1.1875	MATTE	(1)
51850CBX00298BA	9783725854776	Enabling Strategies and Policies toward a Sus				
CASE	6.69X9.61	396	<N>	1.1875	MATTE	(1)
51850CBX00299BA	9783036598376	Implementing the 3Rs in Laboratory Animal				
CASE	6.69X9.61	396	<N>	1.1875	MATTE	(1)
51850CBX00300BA	9783036519135	Indoor Positioning and Navigation				
CASE	6.69X9.61	396	<N>	1.1875	MATTE	(1)
51850CBX00301BA	9783725845828	New Advances in Distributed Computing an				
CASE	6.69X9.61	396	<N>	1.1875	MATTE	(1)
51850CBX00312BA	9783725802548	Chitosan, Chitosan Derivatives and Their Ap				
CASE	6.69X9.61	388	<N>	1.1875	MATTE	(1)
51850CBX00319BA	9783036599137	Energy, Electrical and Power Engineering 2				
CASE	6.69X9.61	386	<N>	1.1875	MATTE	(1)
51850CBX00320BA	9783725853533	Mechanical Properties and Engineering Appli				
CASE	6.69X9.61	386	<N>	1.1875	MATTE	(1)
51850CBX00329BA	9783036552408	Bio and Synthetic Based Polymer Composite				
CASE	6.69X9.61	382	<N>	1.1875	MATTE	(1)
51850CBX00332BA	9783036576022	Image and Video Processing and Recognition				
CASE	6.69X9.61	382	<N>	1.1875	MATTE	(1)
51850CBX00344BA	9783725854134	Cellular and Molecular Mechanisms in Gyn				
CASE	6.69X9.61	376	<N>	1.1875	MATTE	(1)
51850CBX00349BA	9783725817436	Environmental Exposure, Biomonitoring and				
CASE	6.69X9.61	374	<N>	1.1875	MATTE	(1)
51850CBX00368BA	9783036589664	Energy-Efficient Communication Networks a				
CASE	6.69X9.61	368	<M>	1.125	MATTE	(1)
51850CBX00372BA	9783725856992	Surface Engineering and Mechanical Properti				
CASE	6.69X9.61	368	<M>	1.125	MATTE	(1)
51850CBX00376BA	9783725871742	Advanced Research in Flexible Risers and P				
CASE	6.69X9.61	364	<M>	1.125	MATTE	(1)
51850CBX00379BA	9783725856619	Inclusive Smart Cities				
CASE	6.69X9.61	364	<M>	1.125	MATTE	(1)
51850CBX00385BA	9783725870288	Fractional Differential Equations, Inclusions				
CASE	6.69X9.61	362	<M>	1.125	MATTE	(1)

REWORK REWORK REWORK REWORK REWORK REWORK

Printed at: Sat Sep 26 19:30:13 2026 on device cbhp04-90

Batch 51850CB00018B

51850CBX00413BA	9783725855759	Numerical and Evolutionary Optimization 20
CASE	6.69X9.61	354 <M> 1.125 MATTE (1)
51850CBX00415BA	9783036575902	Plant Cell Wall Proteins and Development
CASE	6.69X9.61	354 <M> 1.125 MATTE (1)
51850CBX00419BA	9783725811007	Bioelectronics & Wearable Devices: Sensing
CASE	6.69X9.61	352 <M> 1.125 MATTE (1)
51850CBX00423BA	9783036567815	Frontiers in Protein Structure Research
CASE	6.69X9.61	352 <M> 1.125 MATTE (1)
51850CBX00427BA	9783036573274	Pathogenesis of Pregnancy-Related Complica
CASE	6.69X9.61	352 <M> 1.125 MATTE (1)
51850CBX00437BA	9783725818259	Digital Image Processing: Advanced Technol
CASE	6.69X9.61	348 <L> 1.0625 MATTE (1)
51850CBX00466BA	9783725879274	Nature-Based Solutions-2nd Edition
CASE	6.69X9.61	342 <L> 1.0625 MATTE (1)
51850CBX00493BA	9783036572642	Bio-Inspired Smart Machines: Structure, Mec
CASE	6.69X9.61	336 <L> 1.0625 MATTE (1)
51850CBX00495BA	9783036563800	Monitoring and Modelling of Geological Dis
CASE	6.69X9.61	336 <L> 1.0625 MATTE (1)
51850CBX00510BA	9783725850914	Urban Resilience and Heritage Management
CASE	6.69X9.61	334 <L> 1.0625 MATTE (1)
51850CBX00679BA	9783036573694	Heat Transfer and Heat Recovery Systems
CASE	6.69X9.61	300 <J> 0.9375 MATTE (1)
51850CBX00682BA	9783036515083	Molecular Basis of Apomixis in Plants
CASE	6.69X9.61	300 <J> 0.9375 MATTE (1)
51850CBX00683BA	9783039363346	Nanomaterials to Enhance Food Quality, Saf
CASE	6.69X9.61	300 <J> 0.9375 MATTE (1)
51850CBX00684BA	9783036554419	Numerical Modeling in Civil and Mining Ge
CASE	6.69X9.61	300 <J> 0.9375 MATTE (1)
51850CBX00685BA	9783725877492	Plant Extracts as Functional Food Ingredients
CASE	6.69X9.61	300 <J> 0.9375 MATTE (1)
51850CBX00750BA	9783725878154	Design and Synthesis of Bioactive Compou
CASE	6.69X9.61	290 <J> 0.9375 MATTE (1)
51850CBX00766BA	9783725867387	Industrial CFD and Fluid Modelling in Engi
CASE	6.69X9.61	288 <J> 0.9375 MATTE (1)
51850CBX00767BA	9783036538846	Land Perspectives: People, Tenure, Planning,
CASE	6.69X9.61	288 <J> 0.9375 MATTE (1)
51850CBX00780BA	9783036581774	Multifunctional Application of Biopolymers
CASE	6.69X9.61	286 <J> 0.9375 MATTE (1)

WORK REWORK REWORK REWORK REWORK REWORK

Printed at: Sat Sep 26 19:30:13 2026 on device cbhp04-90

Batch 51850CB00018B

51850CBX00790BA CASE	9783725869947 6.69X9.61	Advances in Environmental Hydraulics 284 <J> 0.9375 MATTE (1)
51850CBX00793BA CASE	9783725849116 6.69X9.61	Data-Driven Intelligent Modeling and Optim 284 <J> 0.9375 MATTE (1)
51850CBX00806BA CASE	9783036580500 6.69X9.61	Causal Inference for Heterogeneous Data an 282 <J> 0.9375 MATTE (1)
51850CBX00821BA CASE	9783725864065 6.69X9.61	Bioactive Compounds and Functional Foods i 280 <I> 0.875 MATTE (1)
51850CBX00841BA CASE	9783725850877 6.69X9.61	Contact Line Dynamics and Droplet Spreadi 278 <I> 0.875 MATTE (1)
51850CBX00845BA CASE	9783036580135 6.69X9.61	Health Properties of Plant Bioactive Compou 278 <I> 0.875 MATTE (1)
51850CBX00872BA CASE	9783725849017 6.69X9.61	Algorithms for Games AI 274 <I> 0.875 MATTE (1)
51850CBX00886BA CASE	9783725871766 6.69X9.61	Sustainable Applications for Machine Learni 274 <I> 0.875 MATTE (1)
51850CBX00890BA CASE	9783036595214 6.69X9.61	Energy Saving, Storage and Carbon Emissio 272 <I> 0.875 MATTE (1)
51850CBX00896BA CASE	9783725876877 6.69X9.61	Numerical Analysis and Applied Mathemati 272 <I> 0.875 MATTE (1)
51850CBX00971BA CASE	9783725847556 6.69X9.61	Research on River Engineering 264 <I> 0.875 MATTE (1)
51850CBX00972BA CASE	9783725863488 6.69X9.61	Resilient Cities and Land Take Effective Man 264 <I> 0.875 MATTE (1)
51850CBX00973BA CASE	9783725854615 6.69X9.61	Sensors for Machine Condition Monitoring, 264 <I> 0.875 MATTE (1)
51850CBX00974BA CASE	9783725868728 6.69X9.61	Skin Anti-Aging Strategies 264 <I> 0.875 MATTE (1)
51850CBX00975BA CASE	9783036592466 6.69X9.61	The 3rd International Conference on Advanc 264 <I> 0.875 MATTE (1)
51850CBX01622BA CASE	9783725808052 6.69X9.61	Mining Innovation 218 <G> 0.75 MATTE (1)
51850CBX01650BA CASE	9783036574455 6.69X9.61	Impacts of Molecular Structure on Nucleic A 216 <G> 0.75 MATTE (1)
51850CBX01652BA CASE	9783725854790 6.69X9.61	Molecular Structure, Electronic and Vibratio 216 <G> 0.75 MATTE (1)
51850CBX01653BA CASE	9783036556413 6.69X9.61	Natural Products: Therapeutic Properties and 216 <G> 0.75 MATTE (1)

REWORK REWORK REWORK REWORK REWORK REWORK

Printed at: Sat Sep 26 19:30:13 2026 on device cbhp04-90

Batch 51850CB00018B

51850CBX01811BA CASE	9783725803477 6.69X9.61	Honoring Prof. Dr. Valentin A. Stonik for His 206 <F> 0.6875 MATTE (1)
51850CBX01817BA CASE	9783036507408 6.69X9.61	Paediatric Formulation: Design and Develop 206 <F> 0.6875 MATTE (1)
51850CBX01860BA CASE	9783036589459 6.69X9.61	Innovative Materials and Processes for Rem 204 <F> 0.6875 MATTE (1)
51850CBX01875BA CASE	9783725847259 6.69X9.61	Bio-Inspired Soft Robotics: Design, Fabricat 202 <F> 0.6875 MATTE (1)
51850CBX01889BA CASE	9783036583679 6.69X9.61	Magnetic Materials, Thin Films and Nanostru 202 <F> 0.6875 MATTE (1)
51850CBX01924BA CASE	9783036568683 6.69X9.61	Insect Microbiome and Immunity 200 <F> 0.6875 MATTE (1)
51850CBX01946BA CASE	9783036584164 6.69X9.61	Applications of Artificial Intelligence in New 198 <F> 0.6875 MATTE (1)
51850CBX01954BA CASE	9783725817207 6.69X9.61	Laser Additive Manufacturing: Design, Mate 198 <F> 0.6875 MATTE (1)
51850CBX01956BA CASE	9783725876631 6.69X9.61	Natural Active Compounds from Foods: Appl 198 <F> 0.6875 MATTE (1)
51850CBX01957BA CASE	9783725850235 6.69X9.61	New Methods and Applications for UAVs 198 <F> 0.6875 MATTE (1)
51850CBX01960BA CASE	9783036569338 6.69X9.61	Probiotics and Antimicrobial Effect 198 <F> 0.6875 MATTE (1)
51850CBX01964BA CASE	9783725858033 6.69X9.61	Recent Advances in Understanding Systemic 198 <F> 0.6875 MATTE (1)
51850CBX01968BA CASE	9783725844722 6.69X9.61	State-of-the-Art Environmental Microbiolog 198 <F> 0.6875 MATTE (1)
51850CBX01981BA CASE	9783036597065 6.69X9.61	Advancements in Soil and Sustainable Agric 196 <F> 0.6875 MATTE (1)
51850CBX02008BA CASE	9783725876754 6.69X9.61	Plant Protein Processing: Technological Inno 196 <F> 0.6875 MATTE (1)
51850CBX02049BA CASE	9783036566238 6.69X9.61	State-of-the-Art Avian Viruses Research in 194 <F> 0.6875 MATTE (1)
51850CBX02056BA CASE	9783725873364 6.69X9.61	Advanced Electrocatalysis Materials Design: 192 <F> 0.6875 MATTE (1)

The Impact of the COVID-19 Emergency on the Quality of Life of the General Population

The Impact of the COVID-19 Emergency on the Quality of Life of the General Population

Editor

Michele Roccella

MDPI • Basel • Beijing • Wuhan • Barcelona • Belgrade • Manchester • Tokyo • Cluj • Tianjin

Editor
Michele Roccella
University of Paler
Italy

Editorial Office
MDPI
St. Alban-Anlage 66
4052 Basel, Switzerland

This is a reprint of articles from the Special Issue published online in the open access journal *Journal of Clinical Medicine* (ISSN 2077-0383) (available at: https://www.mdpi.com/journal/jcm/special_issues/COVID-19_psychology).

For citation purposes, cite each article independently as indicated on the article page online and as indicated below:

LastName, A.A.; LastName, B.B.; LastName, C.C. Article Title. *Journal Name* **Year**, *Volume Number*, Page Range.

ISBN 978-3-0365-3639-2 (Hbk)
ISBN 978-3-0365-3640-8 (PDF)

Contents

About the Editor xiii

Michele Roccella, Gioacchino Lavanco and Luigi Vetri
The New COVID-19 Related Psychological Distress Pandemic
Reprinted from: *J. Clin. Med.* **2022**, *11*, 237, doi:10.3390/jcm11010237 1

Giuseppe Forte, Francesca Favieri, Renata Tambelli and Maria Casagrande
The Enemy Which Sealed the World: Effects of COVID-19 Diffusion on the Psychological State of the Italian Population
Reprinted from: *J. Clin. Med.* **2020**, *9*, 1802, doi:10.3390/jcm9061802 3

Antonio Narzisi
Phase 2 and Later of COVID-19 Lockdown: Is it Possible to Perform Remote Diagnosis and Intervention for Autism Spectrum Disorder? An Online-Mediated Approach
Reprinted from: *J. Clin. Med.* **2020**, *9*, 1850, doi:10.3390/jcm9061850 17

Shanny Sade, Eyal Sheiner, Tamar Wainstock, Narkis Hermon, Shimrit Yaniv Salem, Tamar Kosef, Talya Lanxner Battat, Sharon Oron and Gali Pariente
Risk for Depressive Symptoms among Hospitalized Women in High-Risk Pregnancy Units during the COVID-19 Pandemic
Reprinted from: *J. Clin. Med.* **2020**, *9*, 2449, doi:10.3390/jcm9082449 29

Julian Maciaszek, Marta Ciulkowicz, Blazej Misiak, Dorota Szczesniak, Dorota Luc, Tomasz Wieczorek, Karolina Fila-Witecka, Pawel Gawlowski and Joanna Rymaszewska
Mental Health of Medical and Non-Medical Professionals during the Peak of the COVID-19 Pandemic: A Cross-Sectional Nationwide Study
Reprinted from: *J. Clin. Med.* **2020**, *9*, 2527, doi:10.3390/jcm9082527 41

Mohammad Nami, Bharathi S. Gadad, Li Chong, Usman Ghumman, Amogh Misra, Shrikanth S. Gadad, Dharmendra Kumar, George Perry, Samuel J. K. Abraham and K. S. Rao
The Interrelation of Neurological and Psychological Symptoms of COVID-19: Risks and Remedies
Reprinted from: *J. Clin. Med.* **2020**, *9*, 2624, doi:10.3390/jcm9082624 53

Agata Fiumara, Giuseppina Lanzafame, Alessia Arena, Annamaria Sapuppo, Federica Raudino, Andrea Praticò, Piero Pavone and Rita Barone
COVID-19 Pandemic Outbreak and its Psychological Impact on Patients with Rare Lysosomal Diseases
Reprinted from: *J. Clin. Med.* **2020**, *9*, 2716, doi:10.3390/jcm9092716 65

Antonio Vena, Marco Berruti, Andrea Adessi, Pietro Blumetti, Michele Brignole, Renato Colognato, Germano Gaggioli, Daniele Roberto Giacobbe, Luisa Bracci-Laudiero, Laura Magnasco, Alessio Signori, Lucia Taramasso, Marco Varelli, Nicoletta Vendola, Lorenzo Ball, Chiara Robba, Denise Battaglini, Iole Brunetti, Paolo Pelosi and Matteo Bassetti
Prevalence of Antibodies to SARS-CoV-2 in Italian Adults and Associated Risk Factors
Reprinted from: *J. Clin. Med.* **2020**, *9*, 2780, doi:10.3390/jcm9092780 73

Paweł Wańkowicz, Aleksandra Szylińska and Iwona Rotter
Evaluation of Mental Health Factors among People with Systemic Lupus Erythematosus during the SARS-CoV-2 Pandemic
Reprinted from: *J. Clin. Med.* **2020**, *9*, 2872, doi:10.3390/jcm9092872 83

Juliana Alvares Duarte Bonini Campos, Bianca Gonzalez Martins, Lucas Arrais Campos, João Marôco, Rayya Ahmed Saadiq and Rodrigo Ruano
Early Psychological Impact of the COVID-19 Pandemic in Brazil: A National Survey
Reprinted from: *J. Clin. Med.* **2020**, *9*, 2976, doi:10.3390/jcm9092976 . . . . **91**

José Ángel Martínez-López, Cristina Lázaro-Pérez, José Gómez-Galán and María del Mar Fernández-Martínez
Psychological Impact of COVID-19 Emergency on Health Professionals: Burnout Incidence at the Most Critical Period in Spain
Reprinted from: *J. Clin. Med.* **2020**, *9*, 3029, doi:10.3390/jcm9093029 . . . . **105**

Pietro Smirni, Gioacchino Lavanco and Daniela Smirni
Anxiety in Older Adolescents at the Time of COVID-19
Reprinted from: *J. Clin. Med.* **2020**, *9*, 3064, doi:10.3390/jcm9103064 . . . . **123**

Dariusz Krok and Beata Zarzycka
Risk Perception of COVID-19, Meaning-Based Resources and Psychological Well-Being amongst Healthcare Personnel: The Mediating Role of Coping
Reprinted from: *J. Clin. Med.* **2020**, *9*, 3225, doi:10.3390/jcm9103225 . . . . **133**

Silvia San Román-Mata, Félix Zurita-Ortega, Pilar Puertas-Molero, Georgian Badicu and Gabriel González-Valero
A Predictive Study of Resilience and Its Relationship with Academic and Work Dimensions during the COVID-19 Pandemic
Reprinted from: *J. Clin. Med.* **2020**, *9*, 3258, doi:10.3390/jcm9103258 . . . . **149**

Luca Flesia, Merylin Monaro, Cristina Mazza, Valentina Fietta, Elena Colicino, Barbara Segatto and Paolo Roma
Predicting Perceived Stress Related to the Covid-19 Outbreak through Stable Psychological Traits and Machine Learning Models
Reprinted from: *J. Clin. Med.* **2020**, *9*, 3350, doi:10.3390/jcm9103350 . . . . **161**

Tom Burke, Anna Berry, Laura K. Taylor, Owen Stafford, Eddie Murphy, Mark Shevlin, Louise McHugh and Alan Carr
Increased Psychological Distress during COVID-19 and Quarantine in Ireland: A National Survey
Reprinted from: *J. Clin. Med.* **2020**, *9*, 3481, doi:10.3390/jcm9113481 . . . . **179**

Aleksandra M. Rogowska, Iuliia Pavlova, Cezary Kuśnierz, Dominika Ochnik, Ivanna Bodnar and Petro Petrytsa
Does Physical Activity Matter for the Mental Health of University Students during the COVID-19 Pandemic?
Reprinted from: *J. Clin. Med.* **2020**, *9*, 3494, doi:10.3390/jcm9113494 . . . . **195**

Rubén Nieto, Rebeca Pardo, Beatriz Sora, Albert Feliu-Soler and Juan V. Luciano
Impact of COVID-19 Lockdown Measures on Spanish People with Chronic Pain: An Online Study Survey
Reprinted from: *J. Clin. Med.* **2020**, *9*, 3558, doi:10.3390/jcm9113558 . . . . **215**

Jerónimo J. González-Bernal, Mirian Santamaría-Peláez, Josefa González-Santos, Paula Rodríguez-Fernández, Benito León del Barco and Raúl Soto-Cámara
Relationship of Forced Social Distancing and Home Confinement Derived from the COVID-19 Pandemic with the Occupational Balance of the Spanish Population
Reprinted from: *J. Clin. Med.* **2020**, *9*, 3606, doi:10.3390/jcm9113606 . . . . **231**

Stefanie Jung, Jonas Kneer and Tillmann H.C. Krüger
Mental Health, Sense of Coherence, and Interpersonal Violence during the COVID-19 Pandemic Lockdown in Germany
Reprinted from: *J. Clin. Med.* **2020**, *9*, 3708, doi:10.3390/jcm9113708 . . . . **241**

Jessica Burrai, Paolo Roma, Benedetta Barchielli, Silvia Biondi, Pierluigi Cordellieri, Angelo Fraschetti, Alessia Pizzimenti, Cristina Mazza, Stefano Ferracuti and Anna Maria Giannini
Psychological and Emotional Impact of Patients Living in Psychiatric Treatment Communities during Covid-19 Lockdown in Italy
Reprinted from: *J. Clin. Med.* **2020**, *9*, 3787, doi:10.3390/jcm9113787 . . . . **253**

Yohanes Andy Rias, Yafi Sabila Rosyad, Roselyn Chipojola, Bayu Satria Wiratama, Cikra Ikhda Safitri, Shuen Fu Weng, Chyn Yng Yang and Hsiu Ting Tsai
Effects of Spirituality, Knowledge, Attitudes, and Practices toward Anxiety Regarding COVID-19 among the General Population in INDONESIA: A Cross-Sectional Study
Reprinted from: *J. Clin. Med.* **2020**, *9*, 3798, doi:10.3390/jcm9123798 . . . . **263**

Emanuela Mari, Angelo Fraschetti, Giulia Lausi, Alessandra Pizzo, Michela Baldi, Elena Paoli, Anna Maria Giannini and Francesco Avallone
Forced Cohabitation during Coronavirus Lockdown in Italy: A Study on Coping, Stress and Emotions among Different Family Patterns
Reprinted from: *J. Clin. Med.* **2020**, *9*, 3906, doi:10.3390/jcm9123906 . . . . **279**

Giovanni Bruno, Anna Panzeri, Umberto Granziol, Fabio Alivernini, Andrea Chirico, Federica Galli, Fabio Lucidi, Andrea Spoto, Giulio Vidotto and Marco Bertamini
The Italian COVID-19 Psychological Research Consortium (IT C19PRC): General Overview and Replication of the UK Study
Reprinted from: *J. Clin. Med.* **2021**, *10*, 52, doi:10.3390/jcm10010052 . . . . **297**

Maria Stella Epifanio, Federica Andrei, Giacomo Mancini, Francesca Agostini, Marco Andrea Piombo, Vittoria Spicuzza, Martina Riolo, Gioacchino Lavanco, Elena Trombini and Sabina La Grutta
The Impact of COVID-19 Pandemic and Lockdown Measures on Quality of Life among Italian General Population
Reprinted from: *J. Clin. Med.* **2021**, *10*, 289, doi:10.3390/jcm10020289 . . . . **315**

María del Carmen Pérez-Fuentes, Iván Herrera-Peco, María del Mar Molero Jurado, Nieves Fátima Oropesa and José Jesús Gázquez Linares
Predictors of Threat from COVID-19: A Cross-Sectional Study in the Spanish Population
Reprinted from: *J. Clin. Med.* **2021**, *10*, 692, doi:10.3390/jcm10040692 . . . . **335**

Masar Gjaka, Kaltrina Feka, Antonino Bianco, Faton Tishukaj, Valerio Giustino, Anna Maria Parroco, Antonio Palma and Giuseppe Battaglia
The Effect of COVID-19 Lockdown Measures on Physical Activity Levels and Sedentary Behaviour in a Relatively Young Population Living in Kosovo
Reprinted from: *J. Clin. Med.* **2021**, *10*, 763, doi:10.3390/jcm10040763 . . . . **345**

Adina Turcu-Stiolica, Maria Bogdan, Mihaela-Simona Subtirelu, Andreea-Daniela Meca, Adriana-Elena Taerel, Irina Iaru, Maria Kamusheva and Guenka Petrova
Influence of COVID-19 on Health-Related Quality of Life and the Perception of Being Vaccinated to Prevent COVID-19: An Approach for Community Pharmacists from Romania and Bulgaria
Reprinted from: *J. Clin. Med.* **2021**, *10*, 864, doi:10.3390/jcm10040864 . . . . **361**

Dariusz Juchnowicz, Jacek Baj, Alicja Forma, Kaja Karakuła, Elżbieta Sitarz, Jacek Bogucki and Hanna Karakula-Juchnowicz
The Outbreak of SARS-CoV-2 Pandemic and the Well-Being of Polish Students: The Risk Factors of the Emotional Distress during COVID-19 Lockdown
Reprinted from: *J. Clin. Med.* **2021**, *10*, 944, doi:10.3390/jcm10050944 . . . . **373**

Paweł Wańkowicz, Aleksandra Szylińska and Iwona Rotter
The Impact of the COVID-19 Pandemic on Psychological Health and Insomnia among People with Chronic Diseases
Reprinted from: *J. Clin. Med.* **2021**, *10*, 1206, doi:10.3390/jcm10061206 . . . . **395**

Eliasz Kańtoch and Anna Kańtoch
Cardiovascular and Pre-Frailty Risk Assessment during Shelter-In-Place Measures Based on Multimodal Biomarkers Collected from Smart Telemedical Wearables
Reprinted from: *J. Clin. Med.* **2021**, *10*, 1997, doi:10.3390/jcm10091997 . . . . **403**

Keun-Mi Lee, Hae-Jin Ko, Geon Ho Lee, A-Sol Kim and Dong-Wook Lee
A Well-Structured Follow-Up Program is Required after Recovery from Coronavirus Disease 2019 (COVID-19); Release from Quarantine is Not the End of Treatment
Reprinted from: *J. Clin. Med.* **2021**, *10*, 2329, doi:10.3390/jcm10112329 . . . . **423**

Magdalena Iorga, Raluca Iurcov and Lavinia-Maria Pop
The Relationship between Fear of Infection and Insomnia among Dentists from Oradea Metropolitan Area during the Outbreak of Sars-CoV-2 Pandemic
Reprinted from: *J. Clin. Med.* **2021**, *10*, 2494, doi:10.3390/jcm10112494 . . . . **435**

Víctor-María López-Ramos, Benito León-del-Barco, Santiago Mendo-Lázaro and María-Isabel Polo-del-Río
Coping Strategies by University Students in Response to COVID-19: Differences between Community and Clinical Groups
Reprinted from: *J. Clin. Med.* **2021**, *10*, 2499, doi:10.3390/jcm10112499 . . . . **451**

Dominika Ochnik, Aleksandra M. Rogowska, Cezary Kuśnierz, Monika Jakubiak, Astrid Schütz, Marco J. Held, Ana Arzenšek, Joy Benatov, Rony Berger, Elena V. Korchagina, Iuliia Pavlova, Ivana Blažková, Zdeňka Konečná, Imran Aslan, Orhan Çınar, Yonni Angel Cuero-Acosta and Magdalena Wierzbik-Strońska
A Comparison of Depression and Anxiety among University Students in Nine Countries during the COVID-19 Pandemic
Reprinted from: *J. Clin. Med.* **2021**, *10*, 2882, doi:10.3390/ jcm10132882 . . . . **465**

Magdalena Kludacz-Alessandri, Renata Walczak, Liliana Hawrysz and Piotr Korneta
The Quality of Medical Care in the Conditions of the COVID-19 Pandemic, with Particular Emphasis on the Access to Primary Healthcare and the Effectiveness of Treatment in Poland
Reprinted from: *J. Clin. Med.* **2021**, *10*, 3502, doi:10.3390/jcm10163502 . . . . **487**

Silvana Miceli, Barbara Caci, Michele Roccella, Luigi Vetri, Giuseppe Quatrosi and Maurizio Cardaci
Do Mental Health and Vitality Mediate the Relationship between Perceived Control over Time and Fear of COVID-19? A Survey in an Italian Sample
Reprinted from: *J. Clin. Med.* **2021**, *10*, 3516, doi:10.3390/jcm10163516 . . . . **509**

Mateusz Cybulski, Urszula Cwalina, Dorota Sadowska and Elżbieta Krajewska-Kułak
The Assessment of the Severity of COVID-19-Related Anxiety Symptoms in Participants of the University of the Third Age in Poland: A Cross-Sectional Study among Internet Survey Respondents
Reprinted from: *J. Clin. Med.* **2021**, *10*, 3862, doi:10.3390/jcm10173862 . . . . **521**

Magdalena Gebska, Łukasz Kołodziej, Bartosz Dalewski, Łukasz Pałka and Ewa Sobolewsk
The Influence of the COVID-19 Pandemic on the Stress Levels and Occurrence of Stomatoghnatic System Disorders (SSDs) among Physiotherapy Students in Poland
Reprinted from: *J. Clin. Med.* **2021**, *10*, 3872, doi:10.3390/jcm10173872 . . . . **533**

Francesca Pisano, Giulia Torromino, Daniela Brachi, Agnese Quadrini, Chiara Incoccia and Paola Marangolo
A Standardized Prospective Memory Evaluation of the Effects of COVID-19 Confinement on Young Students
Reprinted from: *J. Clin. Med.* **2021**, *10*, 3919, doi:10.3390/jcm10173919 . . . . **547**

Ghaydaa A. Shehata, Romany Gabra, Sara Eltellawy, Mohamed Elsayed, Dina Elsayed Gaber and Hatem A. Elshabrawy
Assessment of Anxiety, Depression, Attitude, and Coping Strategies of the Egyptian Population during the COVID-19 Pandemic
Reprinted from: *J. Clin. Med.* **2021**, *10*, 3989, doi:10.3390/jcm10173989 . . . . **561**

Aleksandra Maria Rogowska, Cezary Kuśnierz and Dominika Ochnik
Changes in Stress, Coping Styles, and Life Satisfaction between the First and Second Waves of the COVID-19 Pandemic: A Longitudinal Cross-Lagged Study in a Sample of University Students
Reprinted from: *J. Clin. Med.* **2021**, *10*, 4025, doi:10.3390/jcm10174025 . . . . **571**

Siddarth Agrawal, Sebastian Makuch, Mateusz Dróżdż, Bartłomiej Strzelec, Małgorzata Sobieszczańska and Grzegorz Mazur
The Impact of the COVID-19 Emergency on Life Activities and Delivery of Healthcare Services in the Elderly Population
Reprinted from: *J. Clin. Med.* **2021**, *10*, 4089, doi:10.3390/jcm10184089 . . . . **593**

Concetta Polizzi, Sofia Burgio, Gioacchino Lavanco and Marianna Alesi
Parental Distress and Perception of Children's Executive Functioning after the First COVID-19 Lockdown in Italy
Reprinted from: *J. Clin. Med.* **2021**, *10*, 4170, doi:10.3390/jcm10184170 . . . . **613**

Anna Pokryszko-Dragan, Justyna Chojdak-Łukasiewicz, Ewa Gruszka, Marcin Pawłowski, Tomasz Pawłowski, Anna Rudkowska-Mytych, Joanna Rymaszewska and Sławomir Budrewicz
Burden of COVID-19 Pandemic Perceived by Polish Patients with Multiple Sclerosis
Reprinted from: *J. Clin. Med.* **2021**, *10*, 4215, doi:10.3390/jcm10184215 . . . . **631**

Fátima Frade, Lia Jacobsohn, Juan Gómez-Salgado, Rosário Martins, Regina Allande-Cussó, Carlos Ruiz-Frutos and João Frade
Impact on the Mental and Physical Health of the Portuguese Population during the COVID-19 Confinement
Reprinted from: *J. Clin. Med.* **2021**, *10*, 4464, doi:10.3390/jcm10194464 . . . . **645**

Karolina Filipska, Monika Biercewicz, Adam Wiśniewski, Renata Jabłońska, Agnieszka Królikowska, Emilia Główczewska-Siedlecka, Kornelia Kedziora-Kornatowska and Robert Ślusarz
High Rate of Elder Abuse in the Time of COVID-19—A Cross Sectional Study of Geriatric and Neurology Clinic Patients
Reprinted from: *J. Clin. Med.* **2021**, *10*, 4532, doi:10.3390/jcm10194532 . . . . **659**

Shaghayegh Modaberi, Esmaeel Saemi, Peter A. Federolf and Steven van Andel
A Systematic Review on Detraining Effects after Balance and Fall Prevention Interventions
Reprinted from: *J. Clin. Med.* **2021**, *10*, 4656, doi:10.3390/jcm10204656 . . . . **671**

Magdalena Gebska, Bartosz Dalewski, Łukasz Pałka, Łukasz Kołodziej and Ewa Sobolewska
Type D Personality and Stomatognathic System Disorders in Physiotherapy Students during the COVID-19 Pandemic
Reprinted from: *J. Clin. Med.* **2021**, *10*, 4892, doi:10.3390/jcm10214892 . . . . **683**

Carlos Ruiz-Frutos, Diemen Delgado-García, Mónica Ortega-Moreno, Daniel Duclos-Bastías, Dánica Escobar-Gómez, Juan Jesús García-Iglesias and Juan Gómez-Salgado
Factors Related to Psychological Distress during the First Stage of the COVID-19 Pandemic on the Chilean Population
Reprinted from: *J. Clin. Med.* **2021**, *10*, 5137, doi:10.3390/jcm10215137 . . . . **695**

Fernando Espina-López, Emilia Moreno-Sánchez, Francisco-Javier Gago-Valiente, Jesús Sáez-Padilla, Vanesa Salado-Navarro and María-de-los-Ángeles Merino-Godoy
Psychological Discomfort in Nursing Degree Students as a Consequence of the COVID-19 Pandemic
Reprinted from: *J. Clin. Med.* **2021**, *10*, 5467, doi:10.3390/jcm10235467 . . . . **711**

Kinga Janik, Urszula Cwalina, Grażyna Iwanowicz-Palus and Mateusz Cybulski
An Assessment of the Level of COVID-19 Anxiety among Pregnant Women in Poland: A Cross-Sectional Study
Reprinted from: *J. Clin. Med.* **2021**, *10*, 5869, doi:10.3390/jcm10245869 . . . . **723**

Aleksandra Maria Rogowska, Cezary Kuśnierz and Dominika Ochnik
Correction: Rogowska et al. Changes in Stress, Coping Styles, and Life Satisfaction between the First and Second Waves of the COVID-19 Pandemic: A Longitudinal Cross-Lagged Study in a Sample of University Students. *J. Clin. Med.* 2021, *10*, 4025
Reprinted from: *J. Clin. Med.* **2022**, *11*, 276, doi:10.3390/jcm11010276 . . . . **733**

Angela Browne, Owen Stafford, Anna Berry, Eddie Murphy, Laura K. Taylor, Mark Shevlin, Louise McHugh, Alan Carr and Tom Burke
Psychological Flexibility Mediates Wellbeing for People with Adverse Childhood Experiences during COVID-19
Reprinted from: *J. Clin. Med.* **2022**, *11*, 377, doi:10.3390/jcm11020377 . . . . **735**

Tina Vilovic, Josko Bozic, Sanja Zuzic Furlan, Marino Vilovic, Marko Kumric, Dinko Martinovic, Doris Rusic, Marko Rada and Marion Tomicic
Mental Health Well-Being and Attitudes on Mental Health Disorders among Family Physicians during COVID-19 Pandemic: A Connection with Resilience and Healthy Lifestyle
Reprinted from: *J. Clin. Med.* **2022**, *11*, 438, doi:10.3390/jcm11020438 . . . . **749**

Manuela Bacanoiu, Mircea Danoiu, Mihnea Marin, Mihai Robert Rusu and Ligia Rusu
New Recovery Strategies in Motor and Cognitive Functions, before, during and after Home-Confinement COVID-19, for Healthy Adults and Patients with Neurodegenerative Diseases: Review
Reprinted from: *J. Clin. Med.* **2022**, *11*, 597, doi:10.3390/jcm11030597 . . . . **767**

Katerina Papanikolaou, Vassiliki Ntre, Ioanna-Maria Gertsou, Evdokia Tagkouli, Chara Tzavara, Artemios Pehlivanidis and Gerasimos Kolaitis
Parenting Children with Autism Spectrum Disorder during Crises: Differential Responses between the Financial and the COVID-19 Pandemic Crisis
Reprinted from: *J. Clin. Med.* **2022**, *11*, 1264, doi:10.3390/jcm11051264 . . . . **793**

About the Editor

Michele Roccella holds a Degree in Medicine and Surgery and a Specialization in Child Neuropsychiatry at the University of Palermo (Italy). He obtained the title of PhD in Neuropsychopathology of Learning Processes in Developmental Age at the Second University of Naples (Italy). He holds the Diploma Interuniversitaire de Myologie des Universitès Aiax-Marseille II et Paris VI Pierre et Marie Curie (France). He is currently Associate Professor of Child Neuropsychiatry at the Department of Psychological, Pedagogical, Physical Exercise and Training at the University of Palermo. Since November 2019, he has been Director of the School of Specialization in Child Neuropsychiatry at the Department of Promotion of Maternal-Child Health, of Internal and Specialized Medicine of Excellence "G. D'Alessandro" (PROMISE) of the University of Palermo (Italy). He is the author of several monographs and over 500 publications in national and international journals. He has been awarded several prizes and awards, including that of the Russian Academy of Sciences in Moscow (Russia). Research activities and interests: neurodevelopmental disorders; gender dysphoria; the study of neuropsychological functions in children with epilepsy and in chromosomal–genetic syndromes.

Journal of
Clinical Medicine

MDPI

Editorial

The New COVID-19 Related Psychological Distress Pandemic

Michele Roccella [1], Gioacchino Lavanco [1] and Luigi Vetri [2,*]

1 Department of Psychology, Educational Science and Human Movement, University of Palermo, 90128 Palermo, Italy; michele.roccella@unipa.it (M.R.); comunicazioni@gioacchinolavanco.it (G.L.)
2 Oasi Research Institute-IRCCS, Via Conte Ruggero 73, 94018 Troina, Italy
* Correspondence: lvetri@oasi.en.it

Although a few years have passed since the beginning of the COVID-19 pandemic, a large body of scientific literature is already present on the impact that the worldwide spread of the virus has had on people's quality of life.

The studies conducted on previous decade's epidemics, such as SARS, MERS and the H1N1 flu, as well as the research conducted the day after other types of catastrophes, have shown us the possible psychopathological implications linked to unexpected and massive events, which threaten the health and safety of individuals and undermine the stability of communities.

A total of 50 studies, 48 research articles and 2 reviews, included in the Special Issue "The Impact of the COVID-19 Emergency on the Quality of Life of the General population", fully reflect the complexity and the psychological and health implications caused by the unprecedented health, economic and social emergency provoked by the pandemic spread of the SARS-CoV-2 virus.

The interesting research included in the Special Issue essentially concern three macro-areas.

The first area of interest includes the analysis of the neuropsychological implications determined by the COVID-19 pandemic. These studies already clearly showed that the effects of the rapid spread of an epidemic go well beyond the morbidity and mortality of the infected people, strongly affecting various areas of the entire population's daily life, with inevitable repercussions on mental health [1–5].

The second macro-area analyzed by the studies of this Special Issue concerns the health measures necessary to face the coronavirus emergency, in particular in relation to prevention, treatment, and subsequent follow-up measures. In this phase of coexistence with COVID-19, the territory and its resources represent the crucial place for controlling the epidemic but, at the same time, also the place where new opportunities can be found for prevention and health promotion interventions [6–10].

The third macro-area of interest regarded the effects of the COVID-19 pandemic on the management and evolution of other diseases. Unfortunately, fear is becoming a reality. In an attempt to limit the damage caused by COVID-19, the right to health and care of people with other serious diseases is further jeopardized [11–15].

The outbreak of COVID-19 evidenced the vulnerability of the health system and of the patients with chronic or rare diseases; it also highlighted their needs in terms of access to care, adhesion to a therapy schedule, and home care.

The COVID-19 pandemic represents a catastrophe of global dimensions, the first traumatic event on a global scale in the most recent history of humanity. Although the degree of individual exposure to a traumatic event such as this is extremely variable because of different environmental, personal and professional factors, it can be considered in some ways an "in vivo experiment" in the psychopathology of the masses; heterogeneous for geographical, economic and cultural reasons, the world population is exposed in an extreme and persistent way to the same trauma in a short time.

In summary, the articles in this Special Issue reiterate how the unprecedented health, economic and social emergency that our society is experiencing is causing an increase in

Citation: Roccella, M.; Lavanco, G.; Vetri, L. The New COVID-19 Related Psychological Distress Pandemic. *J. Clin. Med.* **2022**, *11*, 237. https://doi.org/10.3390/jcm11010237

Received: 21 December 2021
Accepted: 28 December 2021
Published: 2 January 2022

mental distress in subjects with a pre-existing psychiatric pathology, particularly in health workers, but also in the general population. In particular, the prevalence of symptoms of anxiety, depression, and post-traumatic stress disorder is clearly increasing in the general population, and the scientific community is called to give answers in order to avoid the current viral pandemic turning into a psychological distress pandemic.

Author Contributions: Conceptualization and writing—original draft preparation, G.L., M.R. and L.V.; writing—review and editing, M.R. and L.V. All authors have read and agreed to the published version of the manuscript.

Funding: This research received no external funding.

Conflicts of Interest: The authors declare no conflict of interest.

References

1. Miceli, S.; Caci, B.; Roccella, M.; Vetri, L.; Quatrosi, G.; Cardaci, M. Do Mental Health and Vitality Mediate the Relationship between Perceived Control over Time and Fear of COVID-19? A Survey in an Italian Sample. *J. Clin. Med.* **2021**, *10*, 3516. [CrossRef] [PubMed]
2. Smirni, P.; Lavanco, G.; Smirni, D. Anxiety in Older Adolescents at the Time of COVID-19. *J. Clin. Med.* **2020**, *9*, 3064. [CrossRef] [PubMed]
3. Gębska, M.; Kołodziej, Ł.; Dalewski, B.; Pałka, Ł.; Sobolewska, E. The Influence of the COVID-19 Pandemic on the Stress Levels and Occurrence of Stomatoghnatic System Disorders (SSDs) among Physiotherapy Students in Poland. *J. Clin. Med.* **2021**, *10*, 3872. [CrossRef] [PubMed]
4. Burke, T.; Berry, A.; Taylor, L.K.; Stafford, O.; Murphy, E.; Shevlin, M.; McHugh, L.; Carr, A. Increased psychological distress during COVID-19 and quarantine in Ireland: A national survey. *J. Clin. Med.* **2020**, *9*, 3481. [CrossRef] [PubMed]
5. Flesia, L.; Monaro, M.; Mazza, C.; Fietta, V.; Colicino, E.; Segatto, B.; Roma, P. Predicting perceived stress related to the COVID-19 outbreak through stable psychological traits and machine learning models. *J. Clin. Med.* **2020**, *9*, 3350. [CrossRef] [PubMed]
6. Narzisi, A. Phase 2 and later of COVID-19 lockdown: Is it possible to perform remote diagnosis and intervention for autism spectrum disorder? An online-mediated approach. *J. Clin. Med.* **2020**, *9*, 1850. [CrossRef] [PubMed]
7. Rogowska, A.M.; Pavlova, I.; Kuśnierz, C.; Ochnik, D.; Bodnar, I.; Petrytsa, P. Does physical activity matter for the mental health of university students during the COVID-19 pandemic? *J. Clin. Med.* **2020**, *9*, 3494. [CrossRef] [PubMed]
8. Kludacz-Alessandri, M.; Walczak, R.; Hawrysz, L.; Korneta, P. The Quality of Medical Care in the Conditions of the COVID-19 Pandemic, with Particular Emphasis on the Access to Primary Healthcare and the Effectiveness of Treatment in Poland. *J. Clin. Med.* **2021**, *10*, 3502. [CrossRef] [PubMed]
9. Lee, K.-M.; Ko, H.-J.; Lee, G.H.; Kim, A.; Lee, D.-W. A Well-Structured Follow-Up Program is Required after Recovery from Coronavirus Disease 2019 (COVID-19); Release from Quarantine is Not the End of Treatment. *J. Clin. Med.* **2021**, *10*, 2329. [CrossRef] [PubMed]
10. Modaberi, S.; Saemi, E.; Federolf, P.A.; van Andel, S. A systematic review on detraining effects after balance and fall prevention interventions. *J. Clin. Med.* **2021**, *10*, 4656. [CrossRef] [PubMed]
11. Wańkowicz, P.; Szylińska, A.; Rotter, I. Evaluation of mental health factors among people with systemic lupus erythematosus during the SARS-CoV-2 pandemic. *J. Clin. Med.* **2020**, *9*, 2872. [CrossRef] [PubMed]
12. Nieto, R.; Pardo, R.; Sora, B.; Feliu-Soler, A.; Luciano, J.V. Impact of COVID-19 lockdown measures on Spanish people with chronic pain: An online study survey. *J. Clin. Med.* **2020**, *9*, 3558. [CrossRef] [PubMed]
13. Pokryszko-Dragan, A.; Chojdak-Łukasiewicz, J.; Gruszka, E.; Pawłowski, M.; Pawłowski, T.; Rudkowska-Mytych, A.; Rymaszewska, J.; Budrewicz, S. Burden of COVID-19 Pandemic Perceived by Polish Patients with Multiple Sclerosis. *J. Clin. Med.* **2021**, *10*, 4215. [CrossRef] [PubMed]
14. Filipska, K.; Biercewicz, M.; Wiśniewski, A.; Jabłońska, R.; Królikowska, A.; Główczewska-Siedlecka, E.; Kędziora-Kornatowska, K.; Ślusarz, R. High Rate of Elder Abuse in the Time of COVID-19—A Cross Sectional Study of Geriatric and Neurology Clinic Patients. *J. Clin. Med.* **2021**, *10*, 4532. [CrossRef] [PubMed]
15. Maciaszek, J.; Ciulkowicz, M.; Misiak, B.; Szczesniak, D.; Luc, D.; Wieczorek, T.; Fila-Witecka, K.; Gawlowski, P.; Rymaszewska, J. Mental health of medical and non-medical professionals during the peak of the COVID-19 pandemic: A cross-sectional nationwide study. *J. Clin. Med.* **2020**, *9*, 2527. [CrossRef] [PubMed]

Journal of
Clinical Medicine

MDPI

Article

The Enemy Which Sealed the World: Effects of COVID-19 Diffusion on the Psychological State of the Italian Population

Giuseppe Forte [1,*], Francesca Favieri [1], Renata Tambelli [2] and Maria Casagrande [2,*]

[1] Department of Psychology, "Sapienza" University of Rome, 00185 Rome, Italy; francesca.favieri@uniroma1.it

[2] Department of Dynamic and Clinical Psychology, "Sapienza" University of Rome, 00185 Rome, Italy; renata.tambelli@uniroma1.it

* Correspondence: g.forte@uniroma1.it (G.F.); maria.casagrande@uniroma1.it (M.C.)

Received: 5 May 2020; Accepted: 8 June 2020; Published: 10 June 2020

Abstract: Background: Starting from the first months of 2020, worldwide population has been facing the COVID-19 pandemic. Many nations, including Italy, took extreme actions to reduce the diffusion of the virus, profoundly changing lifestyles. The Italians have been faced with both the fear of contracting the infection and the consequences of enforcing social distancing. This study was aimed to understand the psychological impact of the COVID-19 outbreak and the psychopathological outcomes related to the first phase of this emergency. Methods: The study included 2291 respondents. An online survey collected information on socio-demographic variables, history of direct or indirect contact with COVID-19, and additional information concerning the COVID-19 emergency. Moreover, psychopathological symptoms such as anxiety, mood alterations and post-traumatic symptomatology were assessed. Results: The results revealed that respectively 31.38%, 37.19% and 27.72% of respondents reported levels of general psychopathological symptomatology, anxiety, and PTSD symptoms over the cut-off scores. Furthermore, a significant worsening of mood has emerged. Being a female or under the age of 50 years, having had direct contact with people infected by the COVID-19, and experiencing uncertainty about the risk of contagion represent risk factors for psychological distress. Conclusions: Our findings indicate that the first weeks of the COVID-19 pandemic appear to impact not only on physical health but also on psychological well-being. Although these results need to be considered with caution being based on self-reported data collected at the beginning of this emergency, they should be used as a starting point for further studies aimed to develop interventions to minimize both the brief and long-term psychological consequences of the COVID-19 pandemic.

Keywords: COVID-19; pandemic; anxiety; psychopathological symptomatology; mood; post-traumatic stress disorder (PTSD); emergency

---

1. Introduction

In December 2019, an outbreak of pneumonia associated with a new coronavirus (i.e., severe acute respiratory syndrome due to coronavirus 2 (SARS-CoV-2)) was reported in Wuhan, China. In the following weeks, the infection attracted worldwide attention for its rapid and exponential diffusion across different countries around the world. On 12 February 2020, WHO named it Coronavirus Disease 2019 (COVID-19) [1].

At the beginning of April 2020, COVID-19 has infected more than one and a half million people, causing over 80,000 deaths in 204 countries [1]. This viral infection spread quickly, becoming unstoppable, and forcing the WHO to declare it a pandemic [1]. Although the containment measures implemented in China have been successful in the reduction of new cases by more than 90%, this trend was not reported in other countries, including Italy. According to the Italian Institute of Health, Italy, until 8 April 2020, has had 139,442 confirmed cases of infection and 17,699 deaths, becoming one of the countries with the highest rate of death due to the COVID-19 outbreak [2]. On 8 March 2020, the Italian Government adopted extraordinary measures to limit viral transmission, minimizing contacts with people infected by the virus. The Italian population has been subjected to a period of forced social distancing, with restricted movements. It is the first time in Italy that such restrictive measures have been taken to contain the spread of infection. These actions had a high impact on the Italian lifestyles (e.g., working, education, social interactions). However, there are worldwide precedents for these measures. For example, during the 2003 outbreak of severe acute respiratory syndrome (SARS) in China and Canada, or during the 2014 Ebola occurrence in Africa [3], quarantine and social distancing rules were also imposed.

Recent reviews suggest that the psychological impact of quarantine and social distancing is wide-ranging, substantial, and can be long-lasting, including anxiety and mood disorders, psychological distress and post-traumatic stress disorder, sleep disturbance, and other psychopathological conditions [3,4]. Accordingly, as reported by previous studies on the COVID-19 emergency in China [5–9], we aimed to investigate the psychological status of the Italian people in the early stages of the COVID-19 outbreak, trying to define the reaction of the Italians to the government's measures of enforced social distancing in this extraordinary situation. Specifically, we focused our attention on the level of anxiety, mood, and other psychopathological symptoms as indicators of general distress in the current conditions. We also tried to identify possible differences in the Italian territorial areas (North, Central and South Italy) as a consequence of the heterogeneous diffusion of the contagion that has seen North Italy as the central core of the emergency, with the highest number of infections and deaths due to COVID-19.

Moreover, we tried to evaluate mood changes by comparing participants' self-perception of mood before and after the spread of the infection.

2. Methods

2.1. Study Design and Participants

A web-based cross-sectional survey, implemented using the Kobo Toolbox platform and broadcasted through mainstream social-media (such as Facebook, Twitter, Instagram, Telegram), was used to collect data among the Italian speaking population. In our opinion, this procedure represents the best data collection strategy in the present phase of forced social distancing, and it leads to reaching the largest number of people. The survey was carried out from 18 March 2020 to 31 March 2020. A brief presentation informed the participants about the aims of the study, and electronic informed consent was requested from each participant before starting the investigation. The survey took approximately 30 min to complete. When the participants' responses to the survey lasted less than 5 min or more than 60 min, data were excluded to ensure a standard quality of questionnaires. Participation was entirely voluntary and free of charge. To guarantee anonymity, no personal data, which could allow the identification of participants, was collected. For the current research, being at least 18 years old was the only inclusion criterion employed.

After a short demographic questionnaire, the participants answered questions that assessed knowledge and perceptions related to the spread of COVID-19 and the government measures adopted to contain it. Finally, Italian versions of standardized questionnaires were administered to assess psychological dimensions. This study was conducted in accordance with the Declaration of Helsinki and was approved by the Ethics Committee of the Department of Dynamic and Clinical Psychology of the "Sapienza" University of Rome (protocol number: 0000266). Participants could withdraw from the study at any time without providing any justification, and the data were not saved. Only the questionnaire data that had a complete set of answers were considered. Ninety-eight per cent of the total respondents (2291 out of 2332 people) who started the questionnaires completed the entire survey, and the related data were considered for statistical analyses.

The main demographic characteristics of the sample are shown in Table 1.

Table 1. Demographic characteristics of the sample and their distribution in the Italian territorial areas.

	Overall Sample (*n* = 2.291)	North Italy (*n* = 541)	Central Italy (*n* = 574)	South Italy (*n* = 1.176)
Gender, *n* (%)				
Male	580 (25.3)	107 (18.4)	121 (20.9)	352 (60.7)
Female	1708 (74.6)	434 (25.4)	451 (26.4)	823 (48.2)
Other	3 (0.1)	-	2 (66.7)	1 (33.3)
Age, *n* (%)				
18–29 years old	1571 (68.6)	342 (21.8)	374 (23.8)	855 (54.4)
30–49 years old	485 (21.2)	156 (32.2)	130 (26.8)	199 (41.0)
>50 years old	235 (10.3)	43 (18.3)	70 (29.8)	122 (51.9)
Education, *n* (%)				
Until middle School	99 (4.4)	22 (22.2)	18 (18.2)	59 (59.6)
High School	1136 (49.6)	265 (23.3)	242 (21.3)	629 (55.4)
Undergraduate				
Health care	246 (10.7)	49 (19.9)	80 (32.5)	117 (47.6)
Other	660 (28.8)	174 (26.4)	165 (25.0)	321 (48.6)
Post-graduated				
Health care	63 (2.7)	10 (15.9)	28 (44.4)	25 (39.7)
Other	87 (3.8)	21 (24.1)	41 (47.1)	25 (28.7)
Occupation, *n* (%)				
Student	1073 (46.8)	207 (19.3)	272 (25.3)	594 (55.4)
Employed	688 (30.0)	227 (33.0)	162 (23.5)	299 (43.5)
Unemployed	279 (12.2)	52 (18.6)	61 (21.9)	166 (59.5)
Self-Employed	222 (9.7)	50 (22.5)	64 (28.9)	108 (48.6)
Retired	29 (1.3)	5 (17.2)	15 (51.7)	9 (31.1)
Number of inhabitants in own city, *n* (%)				
<2.000	124 (5.4)	28 (22.6)	17 (13.7)	79 (63.7)
2.000–10.000	453 (19.8)	130 (28.7)	81 (17.9)	242 (53.4)
10.000–100.000	937 (40.9)	199 (21.2)	174 (18.6)	564 (60.2)
>100.000	777 (33.9)	184 (23.7)	302 (38.9)	291 (37.5)
Quarantine Experience, *n* (%)				
Alone	234 (10.2)	74 (31.6)	59 (25.2)	101 (43.2)
Others	2.057 (89.8)	467 (22.7)	515 (25.0)	1.075 (52.3)
Infection by the virus				
Yes	9 (0.4)	2 (22.2)	2 (22.2)	5 (55.6)
No	1707 (74.5)	374 (21.6)	409 (23.6)	951 (54.8)
Do not know	575 (25.1)	192 (33.4)	163 (28.4)	220 (38.3)
Direct contact with people infected by COVID-19				
Yes	40 (1.7)	28 (70.0)	6 (15.0)	6 (15.0)
No	1441 (62.9)	274 (19.0)	337 (23.4)	830 (58.6)
Do not know	810 (35.4)	239 (29.5)	231 (28.5)	340 (42.0)
Knowledge of people infected by COVID-19				
Yes	550 (24.0)	237 (43.1)	126 (22.9)	187 (30.4)
No	1741 (76.0)	304 (17.5)	448 (25.7)	989 (56.8)
Knowledge of people in ICU due to COVID-19				
Yes	177 (7.7)	87 (49.2)	39 (22.0)	51 (28.8)
No	2114 (92.3)	454 (21.5)	535 (25.3)	1.125 (53.2)
Knowledge of people died due to COVID-19				
Yes	112 (4.9)	66 (58.9)	21 (18.8)	25 (22.3)
No	2179 (95.1)	475 (21.8)	553 (25.4)	1151 (58.2)

2.2. Ethical Standards

The authors assert that all procedures contributing to this work comply with the ethical standards of the relevant national and institutional committees on human experimentation and with the Helsinki Declaration of 1975, as revised in 2008.

3. Outcomes

3.1. Demographic Questionnaire and COVID Related Information

The first session of this questionnaire required information about gender, age, education and occupation, city, and region of origin. The second section aimed to evaluate personal knowledge about COVID-19 diffusion, individual perception of the situation, and lifestyle changes related to government restrictions.

3.2. Symptom Checklist-90 (SCL-90)

The SCL-90 [10] (Italian Version: 11) is a 90-items questionnaire aimed to assess psychological distress and symptomatology. The items are rated on a five-point Likert scale, ranging from 'not at all' (0) to 'extremely' (4). Ten primary symptom dimensions are measured: Somatization, Obsessive-Compulsive, Interpersonal Sensitivity, Depression, Anxiety, Anger-Hostility, Phobic Anxiety, Paranoid Ideation, Psychoticism, and Sleep Disturbance. A Global Severity Index provides measures of overall psychological distress. Higher scores in each dimension indicate greater distress and psychopathological symptomatology. A cut-off score of 0.90 was selected to define higher psychopathological symptomatology, in line with previous studies on the general Italian population [11,12]. The internal consistency in the participants of the present study was $\alpha = 0.97$.

3.3. State-Trait Anxiety Inventory (STAI-Y)

The STAI measures state and trait anxiety [13] (Italian Version: 14). The questionnaire includes 40 items. Twenty items refer to state anxiety (STAI-S) and evaluate how participants feel about anxiety "right now, at this moment"; 20 items refer to trait anxiety (STAI-T) and assess how people "generally feel" about anxiety. The items are rated on a four-point Likert scale, ranging from 1 (not at all) to 4 (very much so). In both the State and Trait anxiety scales, higher scores indicate greater anxiety levels. A cut-off point of 55 was used to define higher state anxiety, according to Kvaal et al. [14]. Although this study was interested in assessing state anxiety, trait anxiety was also measured to check whether the anxious state could be explained by a high anxious trait of the Italian population. The internal consistency of STAI in the sample of this study was adequate ($\alpha = 0.60$).

3.4. Mood Scales

Fifteen mood aspects (insecurity, helplessness, sadness, fear, anger, frustration, stress, anxiety, depression, boredom, serenity, happiness, preoccupation, tranquility, energy) both positive and negative were assessed to examine the emotional impact of the current situation. In these evaluations, the participant was required to refer to two different periods. The first was December, preceding the outbreak of the contagion (December 2019); the second period referred to the last week. The mood scales required a response on a 10-point Likert scale [15], from 0 (not at all) to 10 (very much). The use of mood scales has mainly been adopted to analyse the self-reported conditions of individual mood [16–18]. The items on the Mood Scales presented high internal consistency ($\alpha = 0.75$).

3.5. Impact of Event Scale- Revised(IES-R)

The IES-R is a self-report measure designed to assess PTSD symptomatology according to the Diagnostic and Statistical Manual of Mental Disorders—Fourth version (DSM-IV) criteria for PTSD. The questionnaire requires the indication of the magnitude of distress on specific dimensions (e.g., recurring dreams, feelings of anger and irritability) related to specific life events (i.e., the current COVID-19 emergency) referring to the last seven days [19] (Italian Version: 20). The three subscales measure Avoidance (the tendency to avoid thoughts or reminders about the incident), Intrusion (difficulty in staying asleep, dissociative experiences similar to flashbacks), and Hyperarousal (irritated feeling, angry, difficulty in sleep onset). The IES-R requires a response on a 5-point Likert-scale, from 0 (not at all) to 4 (extremely). The score on an IES-R subscale is the mean of the scores of the items of that cluster. The IES-R also gives an overall score (IES-R total that is the sum of the scores of the three subscales). The cut-off of 33 was adopted to indicate a high risk of PTSD symptomatology [20,21]. In the present sample, the IES-R presented high internal consistency ($\alpha = 0.95$).

3.6. Statistical Analysis

Descriptive analyses were conducted to describe demographic characteristics, and COVID-19 related aspects in the Italian population, considering the different Italian territorial areas. Student's t-test was performed to compare our data on anxiety, general psychological symptomatology, and PTSD symptomatology with data from the general Italian population, reported by previous studies. Specifically, our data on anxiety were compared with those reported by Corno et al. [22], SCL-90 outcomes were compared with the data given by Holi et al. [12], and PTSD indices were compared with the results of Ashbaugh et al. [23].

Analyses of Variance (ANOVAs) were performed to explore the potential difference in the impact of COVID-19 in the Italian territorial areas. The differences between North Italy, Central Italy, and South Italy were reported for State and Trait Anxiety, psychopathological symptomatology (Somatization, Obsessive-Compulsive, Interpersonal Sensitivity, Depression, Anxiety, Anger-Hostility, Phobic Anxiety, Paranoid Ideation, Psychoticism, and Sleep Disturbance), and PTSD symptomatology (IES-R). Furthermore, within-subjects ANOVA designs were adopted to compare the respondents' self-reporting mood before and during the COVID-19 emergency.

Logistic regressions were performed to explore the influence of demographic factors and experiences which were COVID-19 related in determining risk for state anxiety (STAI), psychopathological symptoms (SCL-90), and PTSD symptomatology (IES-R).

All data were analyzed using Statistical Package for Social Sciences (SPSS) version 24.0 and Statistica 10.0 (StatSoft.inc., Tulsa, OK, USA). p-values of less than 0.05 were considered statistically significant. To better control the results for the multiple comparison analyses, the Bonferroni correction was adopted; in these cases, an adjusted p-value of less than 0.01 was considered statistically significant.

4. Results

The characteristics of the respondents are shown in Table 1.

Two thousand two hundred ninety-one individuals completed the questionnaires, 580 (25.3%) were males, and 1708 (74.6%) were females; the mean age of the participants was 30.0 years (SD: 11.5 years; age range: 18–89). The most represented age range was 18–29 years (68.6%). Most of the participants (1136; 49.6%) received a high school education and were students (1073; 46.8%) or employees (688; 30.0%). The respondents' current locations were sorted considering territorial area: North (23.6%), Central (25.1%), and South (51.3%) of Italy. Most of the participants live in urban areas (937; 40.9%) with a number of inhabitants between 10,000 and 100,000.

Among all respondents, only 9 (0.4%) were infected by the COVID-19, and 40 (1.7%) were sure that they had had close contacts with individuals suspected of COVID-19 infection (see Table 1). Of the overall sample, 112 respondents (4.9%) and 177 (7.7%) respectively knew people dead and patients in intensive care units (ICU) because of COVID-19 infection.

Comparisons of state and trait anxiety, psychopathological symptomatology, and post-traumatic symptomatology during the COVID-19 epidemic were made with data from the general population.

The comparisons of psychological outcomes during the COVID-19 epidemic in the Italian population with data from the general population are presented in Table 2.

Table 2. Mean and SD of state and trait anxiety (STAI), psychopathological symptomatology (SCL-90) and post-traumatic symptomatology (IES) outcomes of the responders and comparison with data from the general population.

	Respondents' Data	General Population's Data	t Student	p
Anxiety (STAI)				
State of Anxiety	Males: 44.28 (11.98) Females: 52.62 (12.06)	Males: 39.03 (10.00) Females: 44.32 (12.75)	t Males: 4.49 t Females: 9.64	p Males: <0.0001 p Females: <0.0001
Trait of Anxiety	Males: 40.12 (10.80) Females: 44.41 (11.15)	Males: 39.82 (7.62) Females: 45.30 (9.42)	t Males: <1 t Females: 1.44	p Males: 0.77 p Females: 0.25
Psychopathological Symptomatology (SCL-90)				
Somatization	0.71 (0.71)	0.67 (0.55)	<1	0.32
Obsessive-Compulsive	0.91 (0.78)	0.82 (0.57)	2.04	<0.05
Interpersonal Sensitivity	0.58 (0.64)	0.74 (0.55)	4.36	<0.0001
Depression	1.01 (0.81)	0.73 (0.55)	6.14	<0.0001
Anxiety	0.86 (0.75)	0.53 (0.49)	7.83	<0.0001
Anger-Hostility	0.65 (0.65)	0.58 (0.53)	1.89	<0.05
Phobic Anxiety	0.58 (0.70)	0.24 (0.39)	8.71	<0.0001
Paranoid Ideation	0.57 (0.62)	0.53 (0.58)	1.11	0.26
Psychoticism	0.44 (0.53)	0.31 (0.48)	4.25	<0.0001
Sleep Disturbance	0.37 (0.36)	-	-	-
Global Index Severity	0.74 (0.59)	0.60 (0.44)	4.18	<0.0001
Post-Traumatic Stress Disorder Screening (IES)				
PTSD Total	22.39 (18.08)	20.6 (19.4)	2.42	<0.05

Considering SCL-90 indices, depression ($t = 6.14$; $p < 0.0001$), anxiety ($t = 7.83$; $p < 0.0001$), anger-hostility ($t = 1.89$; $p < 0.05$), phobic anxiety ($t = 9.71$; $p < 0.0001$), psychoticism ($t = 4.25$; $p < 0.0001$), and global severity index ($t = 4.18$; $p < 0.0001$) significantly differ from Holy's data [12], indicating greater psychopathological symptomatology in our sample.

Considering STAI indices, state anxiety appears to be higher in our sample compared to data reported by Corno et al. [22] in an Italian sample that considered the levels of anxiety separately in both males and females (males: $t = 4.49$; $p < 0.0001$; females: $t = 9.64$; $p < 0.0001$), while no significant differences were present considering trait anxiety.

Finally, PTSD related symptomatology assessed by the IES-R resulted higher in our sample compared to the data reported by Ashbaugh et al. [23] ($t = 2.41$; $p < 0.05$) (see Table 2).

4.1. The Difference in Psychological Outcomes between North, Central, and South Italy

Table 3 reports the differences in psychological outcomes, considering the three territorial areas of Italy.

Table 3. Mean and SD of state and trait anxiety (STAI), psychopathological symptomatology (SCL-90) and post-traumatic stress symptomatology (IES-R) outcomes in the different Italian territorial areas, and ANOVA's results.

	Overall Sample	North Italy	Central Italy	South Italy	F	p
Anxiety (STAI)						
State of Anxiety	50.51 (12.53)	51.58 (12.72)	50.10 (11.77)	50.21 (12.47)	2.62	0.07
Trait of Anxiety	43.32 (11.21)	43.76 (11.4)	43.40 (10.53)	43.08 (11.15)	<1	0.50
Psychopathological Symptomatology (SCL-90)						
Somatization	0.71 (0.71)	0.73 (0.74)	0.72 (0.69)	0.70 (0.71)	<1	0.68
Obsessive-Compulsive	0.91 (0.78)	0.90 (0.80)	0.88 (0.73)	0.92 (0.79)	<1	0.58

Table 3. *Cont.*

	Overall Sample	North Italy	Central Italy	South Italy	F	p
Interpersonal Sensitivity	0.58 (0.64)	0.60 (0.64)	0.55 (0.62)	0.58 (0.66)	<1	0.37
Depression	1.01 (0.81)	1.08 (0.83)	1.01 (0.78)	0.98 (0.82)	2.52	0.08
Anxiety	0.86 (0.75)	0.91 (0.80)	0.84 (0.72)	0.84 (0.75)	1.90	0.15
Anger-Hostility	0.65 (0.65)	0.59 (0.59)	0.65 (0.69)	0.66 (0.64)	2.40	0.10
Phobic Anxiety	0.58 (0.70)	0.59 (0.69)	0.58 (0.71)	0.59 (0.71)	<1	0.90
Paranoid Ideation	0.57 (0.62)	0.54 (0.62)	0.55 (0.62)	0.60 (0.68)	2.10	0.12
Psychoticism	0.44 (0.53)	0.43 (0.50)	0.43 (0.51)	0.43 (0.55)	<1	0.74
Sleep Disturbance	0.37 (0.36)	0.41 (0.38)	0.38 (0.36)	0.35 (0.35)	4.55	<0.01
Global Severity Index	0.74 (0.59)	0.76 (0.59)	0.73 (0.56)	0.74 (0.61)	<1	0.66
Post-Traumatic Stress Disorder Screening (IES-R)						
Intrusion	1.01 (0.91)	1.0 (0.92)	1.03 (0.91)	0.98 (0.90)	1.04	0.35
Avoidance	1.05 (0.83)	1.07 (0.81)	1.05 (0.80)	1.05 (0.85)	<1	0.91
Hyperarousal	0.97 (0.93)	0.99 (0.91)	1.00 (0.91)	0.9 (0.94)	<1	0.57
Total Subscales	3.04 (2.48)	3.11 (2.45)	3.08 (2.43)	2.99 (2.51)	<1	0.61
PTSD Total	22.39 (18.08)	22.91 (17.88)	22.62 (17.72)	22.04 (18.37)	<1	0.61

Considering psychopathological symptomatology assessed by the SCL-90, significant differences were reported only in the sleep disturbance subscale ($F_{2,2288} = 4.55$; $p < 0.01$; $p\eta^2 = 0.004$). People from North Italy reported higher sleep disturbances compared to people from South Italy ($p < 0.003$). However, no other significant differences were observed (see Table 3).

ANOVAs on STAI subscales did not highlight significant differences between individuals from North, Central, and South Italy.

Finally, considering PTSD, no significant differences were reported in IES-R subscales (see Table 3).

4.2. The Impact of the COVID-19 Emergency on Self-Reported Mood

The results on the difference in subjective mood before and during the COVID-19 epidemic are shown in Table 4 and Figure 1. The analyses confirmed for all dimensions a perceived worsening of mood by the respondents.

Table 4. Mean and SD of self-reported mood before and during COVID-19 emergency, and ANOVA results.

	Mood before the COVID-19 Emergency	Mood during the COVID-19 Emergency	$F_{(1,2290)}$	p	$p\eta^2$
Insecurity	3.31 (2.81)	6.86 (2.62)	2584.89	<0.0001	0.53
Helplessness	3.26 (3.18)	7.43 (2.68)	3018.68	<0.0001	0.57
Sadness	3.06 (2.76)	6.24 (2.72)	2128.68	<0.0001	0.48
Fear	2.38 (2.64)	6.48 (2.74)	3869.14	<0.0001	0.63
Anger	2.59 (2.80)	5.03 (3.29)	1071.69	<0.0001	0.32
Frustration	2.63 (2.81)	5.30 (3.24)	1380.20	<0.0001	0.38
Stress	4.72 (2.91)	5.78 (3.06)	191.53	<0.0001	0.08
Anxiety	4.14 (3.03)	6.07 (3.04)	856.91	<0.0001	0.27
Depression	1.92 (2.55)	3.49 (3.18)	731.68	<0.0001	0.24
Boredom	2.05 (2.51)	5.33 (3.29)	2052.99	<0.0001	0.47
Preoccupation	3.79 (2.72)	7.36 (2.37)	2994.75	<0.0001	0.57
Tranquility	5.95 (2.43)	3.53 (2.42)	1506.60	<0.0001	0.40
Energy	6.47 (2.39)	4.42 (2.59)	1152.18	<0.0001	0.33
Serenity	6.20 (2.40)	3.81 (2.29)	1639.44	<0.0001	0.42
Happiness	6.20 (2.49)	3.67 (2.33)	1992.88	<0.0001	0.47

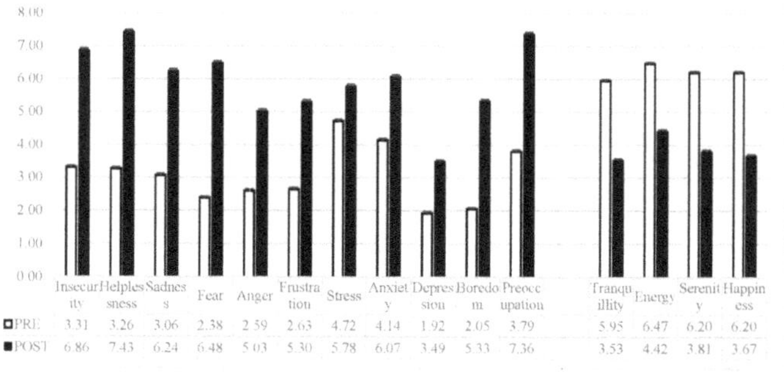

Figure 1. Means and standard errors of self-reported mood before and during the COVID-19 emergency.

4.3. *Prevalence and Risk Factors of Psychological Distress during the COVID-19 Pandemic*

Figure 2 shows the prevalence of psychopathological symptomatology, state of anxiety, and PTSD, stratified by gender, age, territorial areas, knowledge of people affected by COVID-19, and loneliness in social distancing experience.

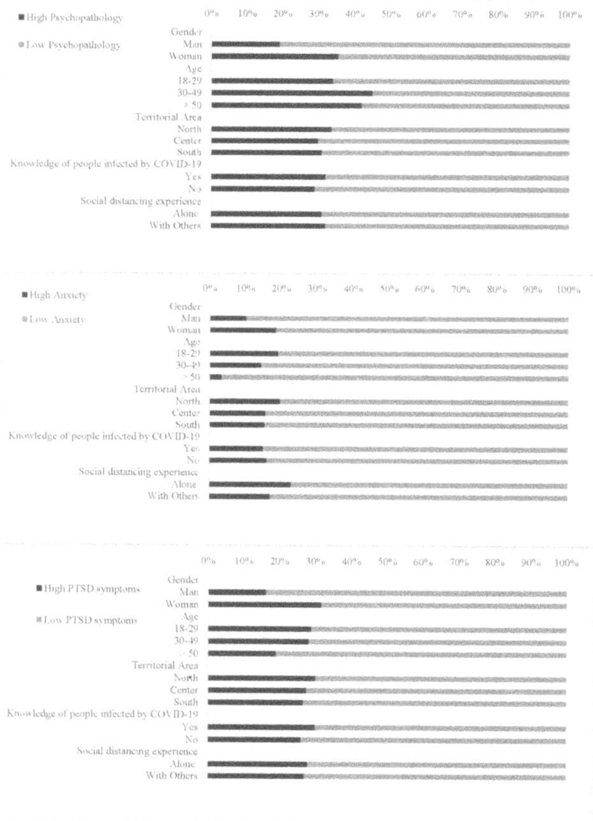

Figure 2. The prevalence of psychopathological symptomatology, state of anxiety, and PTSD, stratified by gender, age, territorial areas, knowledge of people affected by COVID-19, and loneliness in social distancing experience.

The prevalence of psychopathological symptomatology was 31.38% for the SCL-90, 37.19% for state anxiety assessed by the STAI, and 27.72% for PTSD symptomatology assessed with the IES-R.

Logistic regressions showed that the risk of developing psychopathological symptomatology was higher in females (OR = 2.32; 95% CI = 1.85–2.92), in people younger than 50 years (OR > 1.68), in individuals that felt uncertainty about the possibility of contracting the COVID-19 infection (OR = 1.29; 95% CI = 1.06–1.58) or about the possibility to have direct contact with people infected by COVID-19 (OR = 1.33; 95% CI = 1.10–1.59) and in people who knew infected people (OR = 1.25; 95% CI = 1.02–1.53) or people who died due toi COVID-19 (OR = 1.62; 95% CI = 1.10–2.39). The risk of developing anxiety was higher in females (OR = 3.10; 95% CI = 2.47–3.89), in individuals younger than 50 years (OR > 1.47), in undergraduates (OR =1.68; 95% CI = 1.05–2.68), in postgraduates in health care professions (OR = 3.00; 95% CI = 1.22–7.39), and in people uncertain regarding the possibility of being infected by COVID-19 (OR = 1.29; 95% CI = 1.06–1.56) or in persons uncertain about the possibility of having had direct contact with people infected by COVID-19 (OR = 1.30; 95% CI = 1.09–1.55). Higher risk of PTSD symptomatology was associated with females (OR = 2.39; 95% CI = 1.88–3.05); being aged between 18 and 49 years (OR > 1.66); having uncertainty regarding the possibility of contracting the infection (OR = 1.22; 95% CI = 0.99–1.50); the possibility of having had direct contact with people infected by COVID-19 (OR = 1.32; 95% CI = 1.09–1.59); having known infected people (OR = 1.34; 95% CI = 1.09–1.66) o4 people hospitalized in ICU (OR = 1.45; 95% CI = 1.00–2.00) or who had died due to COVID-19 (OR = 1.88; 95% CI = 1.28–2.77) (See Table 5).

Table 5. Results of logistic regression analyses.

	High Psychopathology			High Anxiety Symptoms			High PTSD		
Prevalence in the overall sample, *n* (%)	719 (31.38)			852 (37.19)			635 (27.72)		
	B	OR (95% CI)	*p*	B	OR (95% CI)	*p*	B	OR (95% CI)	*p*
Gender, *n* (%)									
Male		Reference			Reference			Reference	
Female	0.84	2.32 (1.85–2.92)	<0.0001	1.13	3.10 (2.47–3.89)	<0.0001	0.87	2.39 (1.88–3.05)	<0.0001
Age, *n* (%)									
18–29 years old	0.74	2.10 (1.50–2.95)	<0.0001	0.38	1.47 (1.09–1.98)	<0.01	0.54	1.71 (1.21–2.41)	<0.01
30–49 years old	0.52	1.68 (1.16–2.46)	<0.01	0.52	1.68 (1.20–2.35)	<0.01	0.51	1.66 (1.14–2.43)	<0.01
>50 years old		Reference			Reference			Reference	
Education, *n* (%)									
Until middle School		Reference			Reference			Reference	
High School	0.25	1.28 (0.81–2.02)	0.29	0.52	1.67 (1.07–2.67)	<0.05	0.14	1.15 (0.71–1.85)	0.57
Undergraduate									
Other	0.16	1.18 (0.74–1.88)	0.50	0.52	1.68 (1.05–2.68)	<0.05	0.36	1.43 (0.88–2.33)	0.15
Health Care	−0.07	0.93 (0.55–1.57)	0.78	0.21	1.24 (0.74–2.08)	0.42	−0.13	0.88 (0.51–1.52)	0.65
Post-graduated									
Other	0.13	1.14 (0.61–2.14)	0.68	0.54	1.71 (0.92–3.17)	0.10	0.45	1.56 (0.82–2.96)	0.17
Health Care	−10.00	0.37 (0.16–0.87)	<0.05	0.07	1.07 (0.53–2.16)	0.86	0.06	1.06 (0.51–2.21)	0.87
Occupation, *n* (%)									
Student		Reference			Reference			Reference	
Employed	−0.41	0.67 (0.54–0.82)	<0.0001	−0.13	0.88 (0.72–1.07)	0.20	−0.17	0.85 (0.68–1.05)	0.13
Unemployed	−0.08	0.92 (0.70- 1.21)	0.55	0.20	1.22 (0.93–1.59)	0.15	0.03	1.03 (0.77–1.38)	0.83
Self-Employed	−0.38	0.68 (0.49–0.94)	<0.05	−0.16	0.85 (0.63–1.15)	0.30	−0.20	0.82 (0.59–1.15)	0.25
Retired	−0.96	0.38 (0.15–1.01)	<0.05	−0.15	0.86 (0.40–1.87)	0.71	−0.25	0.78 (0.33–1.84)	0.56
Territorial Area									
North Italy	0.12	1.13 (0.91–1.40)	0.28	0.14	1.15 (0.94–1.42)	0.19	0.17	1.18 (0.95–1.48)	0.14
Central Italy	−0.05	0.95 (0.77–1.18)	0.65	0.03	1.03 (0.84–1.27)	0.77	0.04	1.04 (0.83–1.31)	0.72
South Italy		Reference			Reference			Reference	
Number of inhabitants, *n* (%)									
<2.000		Reference			Reference			Reference	
2.000–10.000	0.34	1.40 (0.91–2.17)	0.13	0.27	1.31 (0.87–1.96)	0.20	−0.07	0.93 (0.60–1.46)	0.76

Table 5. *Cont.*

	High Psychopathology			High Anxiety Symptoms			High PTSD		
10.000–100.000	0.13	1.14 (0.75–1.73)	0.54	−0.06	0.94 (0.64–1.39)	0.76	0.04	1.04 (0.70–1.59)	0.84
>100.000	0.09	1.09 (0.72–1.66)	0.69	−0.18	0.83 (0.56–1.23)	0.36	0.03	1.03 (0.68–1.58)	0.88
Quarantine Experience, *n* (%)									
Alone	0.03	0.97 (0.72–1.30)	0.83	−0.27	0.76 (0.57–1.02)	0.06	0.003	1.00 (0.74–1.36)	0.98
Others		Reference			Reference			Reference	
Infection by the virus									
Yes	−0.41	0.67 (0.14–3.22)	0.61	0.82	2.26 (0.60–8.45)	0.23	−1.07	0.34 (0.04–2.74)	0.31
Do not Know	0.26	1.29 (1.06–1.58)	<0.01	0.25	1.29 (1.06–1.56)	<0.01	0.20	1.22 (0.99–1.50)	0.06
No		Reference			Reference			Reference	
Direct contact with people infected by COVID-19									
Yes	0.16	1.17 (0.60–2.29)	0.65	0.32	1.38 (0.73–2.60)	0.32	0.22	1.24 (0.62–2.47)	0.54
Do not Know	0.28	1.33 (1.10–1.59)	<0.01	0.26	1.30 (1.09–1.55)	<0.01	0.27	1.32 (1.09–1.59)	<0.01
No		Reference			Reference			Reference	
Knowledge of people infected by COVID-19									
Yes	0.22	1.25 (1.02–1.53)	<0.05	0.06	1.06 (0.87–1.29)	0.58	0.30	1.34 (1.09–1.66)	<0.01
No		Reference			Reference			Reference	
Knowledge of people in ICU for COVID-19									
Yes	0.23	1.26 (0.92–1.74)	0.16	0.04	0.95 (0.69–1.31)	0.77	0.37	1.45 (1.00–2.00)	<0.05
No		Reference			Reference			Reference	
Knowledge of people died for COVID-19									
Yes	0.48	1.62 (1.10–2.39)	<0.01	0.21	1.23 (0.84–1.81)	0.28	0.63	1.88 (1.28–2.77)	<0.001
No		Reference			Reference			Reference	

5. Discussion

Sudden outbreak events always pose huge challenges to the countries where they occur, impacting not only on physical health but also on social and mental well-being. From this perspective, the COVID-19 pandemic will have long-term consequences, influencing international and national public health policies.

This study is part of a series of works aimed at investigating the characteristics and the psychological effects of the COVID-19 pandemic and the restrictive measures adopted by the Italian Government during the early and more severe stages of the COVID-19 outbreak [24,25]. Since the outbreak of the COVID-19 epidemic, the Italian Government imposed a lockdown in North Italy, expanding it nationwide following the exponential diffusion of the pandemic from the Northern territorial areas to both the Central and South areas. These severe limitations included the request for both people infected by the virus and healthy citizens to isolate themselves at home, prohibiting all other than indispensable activities, and making it mandatory to wear surgical masks to enter public places. Our data were collected near the infection peak (between the end of March and the beginning of April 2020) [2], and they provide an accurate snapshot of Italians' perception of this emergency.

This study delivers further information to add to the findings reported on the Chinese population that was the first to be severely affected by COVID-19 [5–8,26], indicating that the effects of this pandemic on the psychopathological conditions are similar in the Italian and Chinese populations. In both countries younger age, student status, female gender and direct contact with COVID-19 infection are associated with a greater psychological impact of the emergency, involving many psychopathological dimensions (e.g., anxiety, distress, sleep disturbance) [5–9,26].

One of the aims of the study was to analyse the psychological impact of the COVID-19 outbreak in the different Italian territorial areas. North Italy was the first area in Italy infected by the COVID-19 and in which social distancing was imposed. It continues to have the highest prevalence of contagion and deaths, with a heavy burden on the public health system. Accordingly, we expected an impact of these conditions on the psychological well-being and mental health of its inhabitants. However, although respondents from North Italy reported more sleep disturbances and a relatively higher state of anxiety compared to those from Central and South Italy, no other differences were observed in psychopathological symptoms and PTSD risk [23]. These results would seem to underline that psychological status is not only influenced by the direct effects of a justifiable fear of contagion but also by the indirect consequences of the COVID-19 outbreak such as the restrictive measures, that equally influenced people of all the Italian regions, generating a similar psychological pattern. This assumption would be confirmed by the comparison of our results with data from the general Italian population. The differences in the selection of the sample do not allow a generalizability of these results. Most of the psychological symptoms assessed by the SCL-90 subscales are significantly higher in our sample compared to data from the general population. Only somatization and paranoid ideation resulted in being not significantly different from data on the general population. These last findings do not agree with recent data on the Chinese population [27], and they could appear incongruous because medical emergencies might induce higher somatization and intrusive and threatening thoughts. However, these results concord with those found during the SARS epidemic [28].

The high prevalence of anxiety evidenced in our sample highlights that the COVID-19 pandemic has increased alert levels and generated a high level of state anxiety in the population, confirming results of previous studies on SARS, Influenza A virus subtype H1N1 [29–31], and COVID-19 [6–8].

In our sample, 27.72% of the respondents presented PTSD symptomatology, and risk of PTSD higher than that reported in the general population, at least as regards the symptoms evaluated with the IES-R questionnaire [23]. This result should be interpreted with caution because it referred to the first weeks of the emergency when people could perceive the rapid spread of the virus and the extraordinary measures adopted by the Government as sudden stressors, and it is known that sudden stressors affect the daily lives of individuals drastically. On the other hand, this first Italian perception of the current situation would seem to give a photograph of the real impact of the COVID-19 outbreak on mental health.

Another interesting result concerns the impact of the pandemic on mood. Respondents perceived a significant change in their mood, with a sensitive decrease of positive mood (e.g., happiness, serenity) and a high increase of negative mood (e.g., sadness, preoccupation, boredom) after the COVID-19 spread and the consequent social distancing measures. From a clinical point of view, this result could suggest a possible risk of mood disorders, such as depression, as long-term consequences of a pandemic [32]. However, it must be underlined that these data are not obtained prospectively, and the causal relationship cannot be confirmed. Self-reported moods are subject to memory distortions and bias, and they should be taken with caution.

Overall, the results highlighted high levels of anxiety, psychopathological symptoms and PTSD symptoms in Italian respondents during the first critical phase of the spread of the COVID-19 pandemic and of the Government measures taken to contain it.

However, the results of the present study also suggested which people are most vulnerable to the psychological consequences of the COVID-19 outbreak. This unexpected situation seems to have had a higher impact on females and people under 50 years. Moreover, to have had direct contact with people infected by the virus, and to know people more or less severely infected by the COVID-19 (i.e., people hospitalized in an intensive care unit or people dying as consequences of COVID-19 infection) emerged as other relevant risk factors for psychological well-being. All these characteristics would make people more vulnerable to developing anxiety, psychopathological symptoms, and PTSD-related symptoms, confirming results observed in previous studies [8,33]. These risk factors may depend on different aspects of the COVID-19 pandemic. The high psychopathological risk related to direct experience with the COVID-19 infection could depend on the fear of contagion, while being younger could be a risk factor due to the sense of constraint caused by social distancing and the other measures taken by the Italian Government [3].

Our study reports that COVID-19 infected 0.4% of the sample. This result is higher than the data on the general Italian population (0.22%), updated on the 30 March 2020 [2], but it indicates the high rate of healthy individuals in the sample. Both this consideration and the data on risk factors would confirm that, even without real exposure to the COVID-19 and an actual infection, fighting against an invisible enemy could affect mental health. Uncertainty, fear about infection and social consequences of a pandemic could be triggers for psychopathological symptoms, and they should be considered in further studies.

Although some psychological characteristics are linked to medical conditions [34–37], psychological consequences of at-risk people are often overlooked during an epidemic emergency as reported for SARS and H1N1 [29,30,33]. Once again, the importance of not disregarding mental health and intervening during and after the pandemic emergency in the most affected psychological dimensions appear relevant in a long-term perspective.

This study gives a picture of the psychological well-being of the Italian population at the beginning of the COVID-19 emergency. However, some limitations must be considered. Despite the large sample size, it is not possible to overcome the limitation of a cross-sectional study, which does not allow us to determine a causal relationship between the variables. Also, the use of an online survey presents other limitations. Selection bias of participant recruitment is a consequence of this methodological choice. This bias is expressed by some characteristics of our sample, such as the higher number of respondents younger than 30 years, and the high number of females and people from South Italy. Another limit related to the online survey can be associated with convenience sampling that may have induced the collection of responses primarily from people who feel strongly about the considered issue. These limitations reduce the representativeness of our findings and may have influenced the results of the study. Therefore, they must be considered. However, the adoption of an online survey was the best solution in this emergency in which social distancing measures limit data collection.

In conclusion, a global response is desperately needed to prepare health systems to face the new challenge of the COVID-19 outbreak. Despite the underlined limitations, these preliminary findings, in line with the results of previous studies, evidenced that the diffusion of this pandemic can be related to anxiety, changes in mood, high psychopathological symptomatology, and could be associated with the development of PTSD. Moreover, similarly to the results of other studies on the COVID-19 pandemic, these findings should be considered preliminary, but they can be useful to predispose interventions aimed at improving the psychological conditions of the population. Generally, there is still a lack of relevant research on psychological aspects during the COVID-19 epidemic. It would be essential to analyse further psychological dimensions related to the COVID-19 outcomes, such as lifestyle changes, fear, and perception of the emergency, to assess their role in influencing the psychological status of the Italian population.

We hope that these preliminary data can be useful to other researchers in analysing the impact of the infection and social isolation due to COVID-19 diffusion. It is our desire that COVID-19 be defeated but also that the research on this topic grows so that we can start thinking about the mental health of those involved in this severe emergency.

Author Contributions: Conceptualization, G.F., M.C., F.F., R.T.; Methodology, G.F., M.C., F.F.; Formal Analysis, G.F., F.F.; Investigation, G.F., M.C., F.F., R.T.; Resources, M.C., R.T.; Data Curation, F.F., G.F.; Writing—Original Draft Preparation, M.C., F.F., G.F.; Writing—Review & Editing, M.C., G.F., F.F., R.T.; Supervision, M.C., R.T. All authors have read and agreed to the published version of the manuscript.

Funding: This research received no specific grant from any funding agency, commercial or not-for-profit sectors.

Acknowledgments: There is no funding support for this survey. We would like to thank Gianluca Pistore and all the people who helped in the data collection by sharing our survey on various social media.

Conflicts of Interest: The authors declare no conflict of interest.

References

1. World Health Organization. Coronavirus Disease (COVID-2019) Situation Reports. Available online: https://www.who.int/emergencies/diseases/novel-coronavirus-2019/situation-reports/ (accessed on 8 April 2020).
2. Istituto Superiore di Sanità. Epicentro. Coronavirus. Available online: https://www.epicentro.iss.it/coronavirus/ (accessed on 8 April 2020).

3. Brooks, S.K.; Webster, R.K.; Smith, L.E. The psychological impact of quarantine and how to reduce it: Rapid review of the evidence. *Lancet* **2020**, *395*, 912–920. [CrossRef]
4. Hossain, M.M.; Sultana, A.; Purohit, N. Mental health outcomes of quarantine and isolation for infection prevention: A systematic umbrella review of the global evidence. *Epidemiol. Health* **2020**, e2020038. Available online: https://papers.ssrn.com/sol3/papers.cfm?abstract_id=3561265 (accessed on 8 April 2020). [CrossRef]
5. Yu, H.; Li, M.; Li, Z.; Xiang, W.; Yuan, Y.; Liu, Y.; Li, Z.; Xiong, Z. Coping Style, Social Support and Psychological Distress in the General Chinese Population in the Early Stages of the COVID-2019 Epidemic. *SSRN Electron. J.* **2020**. [CrossRef]
6. Cao, W.; Fang, Z.; Hou, G.; Han, M.; Xu, X.; Dong, J.; Zheng, J. The psychological impact of the COVID-19 epidemic on college students in China. *Psychiatry Res. Neuroimaging* **2020**, *287*, 112934. [CrossRef] [PubMed]
7. Sun, L.; Sun, Z.; Wu, L.; Zhu, Z.; Zhang, F.; Shang, Z.; Jia, Y.; Gu, J.; Zhou, Y.; Wang, Y.; et al. Prevalence and Risk Factors of Acute Posttraumatic Stress Symptoms during the COVID-19 Outbreak in Wuhan, China. *MedRxiv* **2020**. [CrossRef]
8. Huang, Y.; Zhao, N. Generalized anxiety disorder, depressive symptoms and sleep quality during COVID-19 epidemic in China: A web-based cross-sectional survey. *Psychiatry Res.* **2020**, *288*, 112954. [CrossRef]
9. Lai, J.; Ma, S.; Wang, Y.; Cai, Z.; Hu, J.; Wei, N.; Wu, J.; Du, H.; Chen, T.; Li, R.; et al. Factors Associated With Mental Health Outcomes Among Health Care Workers Exposed to Coronavirus Disease 2019. *JAMA Netw. Open* **2020**, *3*, e203976. [CrossRef]
10. Derogatis, L.R.; Cleary, P.A. Confirmation of the dimensional structure of the SCL-90: A study in construct validation. *J. Clin. Psychiatry* **1977**, *33*, 981–989. [CrossRef]
11. Cassano, G.B.; Conti, L.; Levine, J. SCL-90. In *Repertorio Delle Scale di Valutazione in Psichiatria*; SEE: Firenze, Italy, 1999; pp. 325–332.
12. Holi, M.M.; Marttunen, M.; Aalberg, V. Comparison of the GHQ-36, the GHQ-12 and the SCL-90 as psychiatric screening instruments in the Finnish population. *Nord. J. Psychiatry* **2003**, *57*, 233–238. [CrossRef]
13. Spielberger, C.D.; Gorsuch, R.L.; Lushene, R.; Vagg, P.R.; Jacobs, G.A. *Manual for the State-Trait Anxiety Scale*; Consulting Psychologists: Palo Alto, CA, USA, 1983.
14. Kvaal, K.; Ulstein, I.; Nordhus, I.H.; Engedal, K. The Spielberger State-Trait Anxiety Inventory (STAI): The state scale in detecting mental disorders in geriatric patients. *Int. J. Geriatr. Psychiatry* **2005**, *20*, 629–634. [CrossRef] [PubMed]
15. Pedrabissi, L.; Santinello, M. *Verifica Della Validità Dello STAI forma Y di Spielberger*; Giunti Organizzazioni Speciali: Firenze, Italy, 1989.
16. Louangrath, P. Reliability and Validity of Survey Scales. *Intern. J. Res. Method Soc. Sci.* **2018**, *4*, 50–62.
17. Curcio, G.; Casagrande, M.; Bertini, M. Sleepiness: Evaluating and quantifying methods. *Int. J. Psychophysiol.* **2001**, *41*, 251–263. [CrossRef]
18. Hasson, D.; Arnetz, B.B. Validation and findings comparing VAS vs. Likert scales for psychosocial measurements. *Int. Electron. J. Health Educ.* **2005**, *8*, 178–192.
19. Weiss, D.S.; Marmar, C.R. The impact of event scale—Revised. In *Assessing Psychological Trauma and PTSD*; Wilson, J.P., Keane, T.M., Eds.; Guilford Press: New York, NY, USA, 1997; pp. 399–411.
20. Pietrantonio, F.; De Gennaro, L.; Di Paolo, M.C.; Solano, L. The Impact of Event Scale: Validation of an Italian version. *J. Psychosom. Res.* **2003**, *5*, 389–393. [CrossRef]
21. Creamer, M.; Bell, R.; Failla, S. Psychometric properties of the Impact of Event Scale—Revised. *Behav. Res. Ther.* **2003**, *41*, 1489–1496. [CrossRef] [PubMed]
22. Corno, G.; Molinari, G.; Baños, R. Assessing positive and negative experiences: Validation of a new measure of well-being in an Italian population. *Riv. Psichiatr.* **2016**, *51*, 110–115. [PubMed]
23. Ashbaugh, A.R.; Houle-Johnson, S.; Herbert, C.; El-Hage, W.; Brunet, A. Psychometric Validation of the English and French Versions of the Posttraumatic Stress Disorder Checklist for DSM-5 (PCL-5). *PLoS ONE* **2016**, *11*, e0161645. [CrossRef] [PubMed]
24. Favieri, F.; Forte, G.; Tambelli, R.; Casagrande, M. The Italians in the Time of Coronavirus: Psychosocial Aspects of Unexpected COVID-19 Pandemic. *SSRN Electron. J.* **2020**. [CrossRef]

25. Casagrande, M.; Favieri, F.; Tambelli, R.; Forte, G. The enemy who sealed the world: Effects quarantine due to the COVID-19 on sleep quality, anxiety, and psychological distress in the Italian population. *Sleep Med.* **2020**. Available online: https://www.sciencedirect.com/science/article/pii/S1389945720302136 (accessed on 12 May 2020).
26. Wang, C.; Pan, R.; Wan, X.; Tan, Y.; Xu, L.; Ho, C.S.; Ho, R.C.M. Immediate Psychological Responses and Associated Factors during the Initial Stage of the 2019 Coronavirus Disease (COVID-19) Epidemic among the General Population in China. *Int. J. Environ. Res. Public Health* **2020**, *17*, 1729. [CrossRef] [PubMed]
27. Tian, F.; Li, H.; Tian, S.; Yang, J.; Shao, J.; Tian, C. Psychological symptoms of ordinary Chinese citizens based on SCL-90 during the level I emergency response to COVID-19. *Psychiatry Res. Neuroimaging* **2020**, *288*, 112992. [CrossRef]
28. Chen, C.-S.; Wu, H.-Y.; Yang, P.; Yen, C.-F. Psychological Distress of Nurses in Taiwan Who Worked During the Outbreak of SARS. *Psychiatr. Serv.* **2005**, *56*, 76–79. [CrossRef] [PubMed]
29. Hall, R.C.; Hall, R.C.; Chapman, M.J. The 1995 Kikwit Ebola outbreak: Lessons hospitals and physicians can apply to future viral epidemics. *Gen. Hosp. Psychiatry* **2008**, *30*, 446–452. [CrossRef] [PubMed]
30. Rubin, G.J.; Potts, H.; Michie, S. The impact of communications about swine flu (influenza A H1N1v) on public responses to the outbreak: Results from 36 national telephone surveys in the UK. *Health Technol. Assess.* **2010**, *14*, 183–266. [CrossRef] [PubMed]
31. Van Bortel, T.; Basnayake, A.; Wurie, F.; Jambai, M.; Koroma, A.S.; Muana, A.T.; Hann, K.; Eaton, J.; Martin, S.; Nellums, L.B. Psychosocial effects of an Ebola outbreak at individual, community and international levels. *Bull. World Health Organ.* **2016**, *94*, 210–214. [CrossRef] [PubMed]
32. Keita, A.K.; the PostEboGui Study Group; Taverne, B.; Savané, S.S.; March, L.; Doukoure, M.; Sow, M.S.; Touré, A.; Etard, J.F.; Barry, M. Depressive symptoms among survivors of Ebola virus disease in Conakry (Guinea): Preliminary results of the PostEboGui cohort. *BMC Psychiatry* **2017**, *17*, 1–9. [CrossRef]
33. Su, T.-P.; Lien, T.-C.; Yang, C.-Y.; Su, Y.L.; Wang, J.-H.; Tsai, S.-L.; Yin, J.-C. Prevalence of psychiatric morbidity and psychological adaptation of the nurses in a structured SARS caring unit during outbreak: A prospective and periodic assessment study in Taiwan. *J. Psychiatr. Res.* **2007**, *41*, 119–130. [CrossRef]
34. Casagrande, M.; Mingarelli, A.; Guarino, A.; Favieri, F.; Boncompagni, I.; Germanò, R.; Germanò, G.; Forte, G. Alexithymia: A facet of uncontrolled hypertension. *Int. J. Psychophysiol.* **2019**, *146*, 180–189. [CrossRef] [PubMed]
35. Casagrande, M.; Boncompagni, I.; Mingarelli, A.; Favieri, F.; Forte, G.; Germanò, R.; Germanò, G.; Guarino, A. Coping styles in individuals with hypertension of varying severity. *Stress Health* **2019**, *35*, 560–568. [CrossRef] [PubMed]
36. Casagrande, M.; Boncompagni, I.; Forte, G.; Guarino, A.; Favieri, F. Emotion and overeating behavior: Effects of alexithymia and emotional regulation on overweight and obesity. *Eat. Weight. Disord.* **2019**, 1–13. [CrossRef]
37. Casagrande, M.; Favieri, F.; Guarino, A.; Di Pace, E.; Langher, V.; Germanò, G.; Forte, G. The Night Effect of Anger: Relationship with Nocturnal Blood Pressure Dipping. *Int. J. Environ. Res. Public Health* **2020**, *17*, 2705. [CrossRef]

Journal of
Clinical Medicine

MDPI

Article

Phase 2 and Later of COVID-19 Lockdown: Is it Possible to Perform Remote Diagnosis and Intervention for Autism Spectrum Disorder? An Online-Mediated Approach

Antonio Narzisi

IRCCS Stella Maris Foundation, 56018 Pisa, Italy; antonio.narzisi@fsm.unipi.it

Received: 24 May 2020; Accepted: 11 June 2020; Published: 13 June 2020

Abstract: COVID-19 is still in phase 2. The lockdown has been significantly reduced compared to phase 1. The centers and institutions that deal with the diagnosis and intervention of children with autism spectrum disorder (ASD) require rapid functional adaptation to respond to patients' needs. The possibility of using technology to activate and manage diagnostic (preliminary diagnosis) and intervention processes should be explored. Two developed telemedicine working models for diagnosis and intervention, including synchronous and asynchronous transmissions, are presented. They are proposals not yet supported by the data. The diagnosis step is composed by two different and consecutives phases: (A) pre-specialistic consultation (PSC) and (B) specialistic assessment. The intervention step implemented well-recognized evidence-based models for preschoolers, school-aged, and older children in an online format. Parents' support is also included. The described working models have the purpose of carrying out preliminary specialistic answers to the families without aiming to replace preferable in-person assessment. Based on previous research findings, the telemedicine approach is accepted by parents, increases their sense of competence, increases the parent intervention adhesion, and improves the social communication competencies for children with ASD. In conclusion, the presented working models must be considered partial responses to the current emergency status and at the same time as possible integrations into traditional approaches.

Keywords: autism; COVID-19; children; diagnosis; intervention; parents; remote

---

1. Introduction

COVID-19 is still in phase 2. The lockdown has been significantly reduced compared to phase 1. However, extreme attention and caution must be paid when carrying out daily activities. Gatherings must be avoided, and the safety distance must be maintained. For this reason, it is necessary to partially reorganize workplaces, where the presence of many people could represent a risk of contagion. Among these workplaces, the centers and institutions that deal with the diagnosis and intervention of children require rapid functional adaptation. Traditional methods for carrying out diagnostic assessments and intervention sessions will be able to resume at full capacity in phase 3 and later. So, in this bridging phase, we must think of new and agile ways to give at least an initial response to the clinical needs of families and patients [1]. Among the infant disorders, it is well recognized that autism spectrum disorder (ASD) has an elevated incidence, higher than 1/100 [2,3], and the requests for evaluation are many. Usually, the diagnosis of ASD involves a very close contact between the specialist and the children, especially when they are at preschool age. It could also be difficult and/or counterproductive to invite a child with ASD to wear certain safety devices (e.g., masks) during the diagnostic assessments. For this type of reason, it is necessary to think of a functional alternative between postponing the evaluation (in phase 3 or later) and/or making the child, family, and specialists run a high risk of contagion. At this time, the possibility of using technology to activate and manage diagnostic (or better, a preliminary diagnosis) and intervention processes in the field of ASD should be explored and tested.

In the field of ASD diagnosis, few studies have deepened the use of telemedicine. However, previous studies confirm the practicability, accuracy, and clinical efficacy of the telemedicine-based assessment of ASD for preschoolers and school-aged children [4,5]. Recent research contributions have shown the parents' ability to gather clinically relevant videos of child behavior in the home setting and to share significant developmental history information, as well as the diagnosticians' skill to detect appropriate behavioral examples in the videos to meet the diagnostic criteria for ASD [6,7].

Recently, Sutantio and colleagues [8] showed that a telemedicine methodology using a protocol-guided video recording evaluation has significant validity compared with direct assessment (DA) for diagnosing ASD.

In a pilot work, Juarez and colleagues [4] showed that a large portion (75%) of children with ASD may be accurately identified through the remote adoption of standardized assessment practices (reaching a sensitivity of 78.95%), and many parents and providers recognized the clinical value of the practice.

In a fascinating study, Fusaro and colleagues [9] tried to enlarge the concept and practicability of home video analysis by applying an Autism Diagnostic Observation Schedule (ADOS) [10] item, not the complete assessment, to ASD. Particularly, they tested the practicability of answering the ADOS module 1 item when viewing brief (10 min) formless videos to discriminate videos including children with ASD from videos of children who have no signs of ASD [9]. The results showed high classification accuracy (96.8% with 94.1% sensitivity and 100% specificity) and inter-rater reliability (88%) and together demonstrate that the ADOS module 1 item can be used on formless videos to effectively distinguish behavioral differences among children with and without ASD. Although not all items on the ADOS were expected to be pertinent to the formless videos, authors did find that most of the items could be applied. Items regarding vocalization, the use of words or phrases, unusual eye contact, responsive social smile, and repetitive interests or behaviors were the most recurrent behaviors shown in analyzed videos [9]. In conclusion, the authors demonstrated the potential for the video-based detection of ASD applying standard diagnostic items to ASD in short, formless home videos and further suggested that at least a portion of the effort associated with the detection and monitoring of ASD may be mobilized and moved outside of traditional clinical settings [9].

Unlike diagnosis, there is an increasing bulk of studies supporting the usefulness of telemedicine for intervention [11,12]. In 2018, Bearss and colleagues [13] carried out a feasibility pilot study of parent training with preschoolers with ASD using a telemedicine approach. The findings of their study were very promising; in fact, 93% of parents completed intervention, with almost 100% of sessions frequented (91.6%). Therapists reached 98% fidelity to the intervention guidelines and 93% of expected outcome measures were collected. Furthermore, 78.6% of children were evaluated as much/very much improved. Parent training through telemedicine was suitable to parents and the intervention could be carried out reliably by therapists. Among the studies in this area, it is important to report the randomized trial that compared telemedicine parent training in the Early Start Denver Model (P-ESDM) with a community intervention. Telemedicine training facilitated higher parent fidelity gains and program satisfaction for more of the P-ESDM than the community group at the end of the 12-week training period and at follow-up. The children's social communication skills improved for both groups regardless of parent fidelity [14]. Even if results of this type need to be further studied, deepened, and better understood, they seem to recommend the feasibility of telemedicine training with an enriched parent intervention procedure and satisfaction from the program.

The main aim of this paper is to share telemedicine working models for preliminary diagnosis and intervention that we started to adopt at CETRA. CETRA is a highly specialized center for autism spectrum disorders (accredited by the Italian National Health Service) sited in Pisa, Italy. It offers in-person diagnosis and clinical intervention services, including evidence-based parent-mediated intervention. The in-person working model of CETRA involves the use of video feedback with parents during the intervention (inspired by the PACT model of Green and colleagues [15]) and the analysis of the videos used during the diagnostic process. Additional clinical offerings include support groups for parents, training for therapists, and research both in the area of diagnosis and intervention. Since the beginning of the COVID-19 period, most of the clinical activities have been remotely reorganized, developing a working model in telemedicine.

2. Material and Methods

2.1. A Telemedicine Working Model for Diagnosis

The developed telemedicine working model for diagnosis is composed of two different and consecutives phases: (A) pre-specialistic consultation (PSC) and (B) specialistic assessment (SA) (see Figure 1).

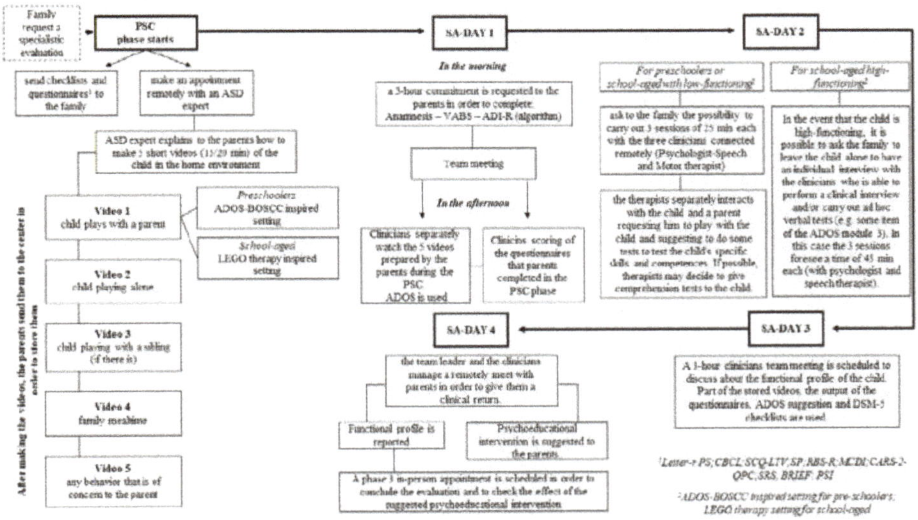

Figure 1. Working model for (preliminary) diagnosis. PSC: pre-specialistic consultation; SA: specialistic assessment; ASD: Autism Spectrum Disorder; ADOS-BOSCC: Autism Diagnostic Observation Schedule-Brief Observation of Social Communication Change; VABS: Vineland Adaptive Behaviour Scales; ADI-R: Autism Diagnostic Interview-Revised; DSM-5: Diagnostic and Statistical Manual of Mental Disorders-5.

2.1.1. Pre-Specialistic Consultation (PSC)

The pre-specialistic consultation (PSC) phase starts when the family calls the reservation center to request a specialist evaluation. The receptionist, after having recorded the patient and family data, (1) sends the 11 questionnaires and checklists below to the family and (2) makes an appointment remotely (online Zoom platform or similar) with an expert psychologist in the field of the diagnosis of ASD.

2.1.2. Questionnaire and Checklists

We use 11 questionnaires and checklists of which we have consolidated expertise:

(1) The Leiter–R parent social–emotional rating scales [16] provides the parent's perception of the child's cognitive/social functioning and emotion regulation.

(2) The Behavior Rating Inventory of Executive Function Preschool Version (BRIEF-P) [17] offers the possibility of a structured assessment of the executive functioning at preschool age, maximizing the opportunity to detect deficiencies and difficulties and to intervene promptly.

(3) The Behavior Rating Inventory of Executive Function 2, (BRIEF-2) [18] is a set of questionnaires for parents of school-aged children designed to evaluate executive function from multiple perspectives.

(4) The Child Behavior Check List (CBCL) [19] is a parent-report measure designed to record the problem behaviors of boys and girls. Each item describes a specific behavior and the parent is asked to rate its frequency on a three-point Likert scale. The scoring gives a summary profile including a DSM-oriented scale.

(5) The MacArthur Communicative Development Inventory (MCDI) [20] includes word comprehension, word expression, and gestures. Because the children could be older than those in the normative groups, raw data will be used instead of standard scores.

(6) The Questionnaire for Parents or Caregivers (CARS2-QPC) [21] is a parent report measure; the areas covered by the CARS2-QPC include the individual's early development, social, emotional, and communication skills, repetitive behaviors, play and routines, and unusual sensory interests.

(7) The Repetitive Behavior Scale—Revised (RBS-r) [22] is a developed questionnaire that captures the following factors of RRB: ritualistic/sameness behavior, stereotypic behavior, self-injurious behavior, compulsive behavior, and restricted interests.

(8) The Social Communication Questionnaire (SCQ)–Life Time Form (SCQ-LT) [23] is filled out by parents to evaluate children's communication, social, and relational skills. SCQ has established high comparative agreement with the Autism Diagnostic Interview—Revised™. The Lifetime Form focuses on the child's entire developmental history.

(9) The Sensory Profile (SP) [24] evaluates the child's sensory processing patterns in the context of home, school, and community-based activities. Parents indicate their perception of the frequency with which their child exhibits atypical behaviors in response to sensory stimulation. The SP evaluates tactile, visual/auditory, taste/smell, and movement sensitivity, auditory filtering, low energy/weakness, and sensation seeking [25].

(10) The Social Responsiveness Scale (SRS) [26] is a quick scale of evaluation of mutual social behavior, communication, and repetitive and stereotyped behaviors characteristic of autism spectrum disorders in children between four and 18 years of age.

(11) The Parenting Stress Index 4 [27] is focused on the clinical identification of specific problems and strengths in relation to the child, the parent, and the family system.

2.1.3. Meeting with an Expert Psychologist in the Field of the Diagnosis of ASD

During the remote meeting the psychologist explains to the parents how to make some short videos of the child in the home environment.

At the end of the meeting, the psychologist sends to the family a brochure summarizing all the explained procedures to make videos. The PSC phase is distinguished by the age group of the children.

For preschoolers, the psychologist advises a parent to produce 15–20 min of the following five videos:

(a) The child playing with a parent (ADOS-BOSCC inspired setting [28]), 15 min.

A brief child–parent free play interaction aimed at observing the behavioral profile of the child. Parents are asked to place toys on the floor. Parents are instructed to play as usual, without making any additional demands on their child.

(b) The child playing alone (ADOS-2 free play inspired setting [10]), 15 min.

Parents are asked to place toys on the floor and on a small table (or a shelf). The request made to parents is to video record the child while he/she is playing with the toys that he/she spontaneously chooses from those proposed. The goal of this video is to observe the functional and symbolic use of objects, the sensory characteristics, the presence of restricted and repetitive behaviors, the presence of gergophasia, and the child's ability to vary the play activity.

(c) The child playing with a sibling (if there is one), 15 min.

The (b) and (c) scenarios provide opportunities for the child to show typical social interaction skills and play. The setting is the same as video (b). In this case, the goal of the video is to observe the quality of social interaction with another child (in this case familiar). We are interested in observing social openings, the response to shared attention, the response to names, the child's ability to draw attention, the quality of the social response, and the verbal and non-verbal communication skills.

(d) Family mealtime, 15 min.

The preferred setting for this video is that of breakfast, lunch, snack time, or dinner. The goal of this video is to observe the oral–motor skills and the presence of food selectivity [29]. This type of observation is very important both from the behavioral point of view and for ad hoc suggestions from the speech therapist.

(e) Any behavior that worries parents, 15 min;

The setting of this video is not minimally structured. The goal is to obtain a video recording that describes a specific behavior that has attracted the parents' concern.

The points from (b) to (e) are inspired by Nazneen's work [6,7].

For school-aged children, the videos and their duration are the same, except with regard video (a).

For these boys and girls, for video (a), it was decided to record their interaction with a parent in a setting similar to that of LEGO therapy [30]. The parent is asked to build a LEGO set (or other construction, or another game) together with the child. Through this, the therapist can remotely observe the child's social skills, such as turn taking, problem solving, collaboration, and social communication.

For both preschoolers and school-aged children, all videos should have been made on different days in order to have a wider view of the child's behavior.

The five videos and the questionnaires/checklists were sent via internet to the Diagnostic Autism Team at least 1 week before the start of phase B (specialistic assessment).

In the PSC phase, the family can request technical help from the psychologist at any time if doubts or uncertainties arise about how to prepare the videos. Overall, about 3 h were scheduled to complete the PSC phase.

2.2. Specialistic Assessment (SA)

The specialistic assessment phase requires a four-day commitment from the family.

During the first day, a 3 h commitment is requested from the parents (preferably in the morning). During this time, the psychologist carries out the anamnesis of the child (1 h) and administers the ADI-R algorithm [31] (1 h) and the Vineland/VABS [32–34] to the parent (1 h).

The Autism Diagnostic Interview—Revised (ADI-R) [31] is an interview aimed at obtaining a complete range of information for assessing autism spectrum disorders.

ADI-R is aimed at parents or educators of subjects from early childhood to adulthood with a mental age above 2 years. It focuses on the systematic and standardized observation of behaviors that are rarely found in non-clinical subjects, and mainly on the three areas of functioning: (1) language and communication, (2) mutual social interaction, and (3) stereotyped behaviors and restricted interests. The ADI-R is divided into an interview protocol and five algorithms, which can be used at various ages for diagnosis or intervention.

The Vineland Adaptive Behavior Scale—II Edition (VABS-II) [32] is a parent interview; it assesses adaptive behavior (AB). Specifically, VABS-II has the aim of measuring the AB in the domains of communication, daily living skills, socialization, and motor skills. The evaluation of AB is necessary for the diagnosis of intellectual disability disorder and, in accordance with the DSM-5, for the evaluation of the severity level of autistic disorder.

After anamnesis, ADI-R, and VABS-II administration, a team meeting (1 h) is scheduled to update everyone on the information received from the psychologist during the online meeting with the parents. After the meeting, the team, separately, watches the five videos prepared by the parents during the PSC phase and they finalize the scoring of the questionnaires that the parents completed in the PSC phase.

All clinicians watch the videos, although the global clinical evaluation of the five videos is performed by an expert clinical practitioner that is ADOS-2 certified, both for clinical and research use [10].

The ADOS-2 is widely considered a gold standard and is one of the most common behavioral instruments used to aid in the diagnosis of ASD [10]. It allows a semi-structured and standardized assessment of communication, social interaction, play, and restricted and repetitive behaviors, through a series of activities that directly elicit behaviors related to a diagnosis of autism spectrum disorder. Through the observation and coding of these behaviors, it is possible to obtain useful information for diagnosis, intervention planning, and insertion in educational contexts. The diagnostic algorithm consists of two domains, social affect and restricted, repetitive behaviors, combined into one score to which thresholds are applied [3,35]. As suggested by Fusaro and colleagues [9], the modules of the ADOS are used for the global clinical scoring of the five videos.

Following Fusaro and colleague's indications, the code is applied if the video resolutely depicts a behavior and/or contains opportunities for the child to show the inquired behavior, otherwise the behavioral item is coded as not applicable (N/A) [9]. We calculate the ADOS-2 algorithm and then the videos are marked ASD when the score is > 7 (for module 1) and > 8 (for module 2). The ADOS modules 3 and 4 are administered in a remote connection with the patient and not in the analysis of asynchronous videos [36].

During the second day we ask to the family about the possibility of carrying out three remote sessions of 25 min each with the three clinicians. In the sessions, the clinicians interact with the child and a parent.

If the child is preschool aged, we ask the parent, in advance, to prepare a setting that is ADOS-BOSCC inspired [28]. If instead the child is older and not autonomous, we ask the parent to interact with him/her in a LEGO therapy-inspired setting [30].

In the three sessions, a psychologist, a speech therapist, and a psychomotor specialist interact, separately, with the parent, requesting him/her to play with the child and suggest some tests to check the child's specific skills and competences. If possible, the clinicians may decide to give comprehension tests to the child. In the event that the child is high-functioning, it is possible to ask the family to leave the child alone to have an individual interview with the clinicians, who are able to perform a clinical interview and/or carry out ad hoc verbal tests (e.g., some items of ADOS module 3). In this case, the three sessions last for 45 min each (with psychologist and speech therapist separately).

During the third day, a 3 h team meeting is scheduled to discuss the functional profile of the child. Part of the stored videos and the output of the questionnaires and checklists are used. A checklist with Diagnostic and Statistical Manual (DSM-5) [37] criteria is used to help diagnose ASD. The family remains available for any questions from the therapists. The DSM-5 checklist includes a symptomatic dyad: (A) persistent deficits in social communication and social interaction across multiple contexts and (B) restricted, repetitive patterns of behavior, interests, or activities, which are made up of specific sub-criteria. Each of these categories includes from three to four sub-criteria. Criterion A is further divided into three sub-criteria: A1 (problems with social initiation and response), A2 (problems with nonverbal communication), and A3 (problems with social awareness and insight, as well as with the broader concept of social relationships). Criterion B is divided into four sub-criteria, including B1 (atypical speech, movements, and play), B2 (rituals and resistance to change), B3 (preoccupations with objects or topics) and B4 (atypical sensory behaviors). The DSM-5 contains specific examples and symptoms for each point [8,37].

The final preliminary diagnosis (ASD or non-ASD) is based on clinical judgement supported by the DSM-5 total checklist score, parent interviews, questionnaires/checklists, and through the analysis of both the five videos recorded by the parents (asynchronous transmission) on which the ADOS module is applied by an experienced psychologist and the direct observation of the child in live video conferencing (synchronous transmission).

During the fourth day, the team leader, together with clinicians, manage a remote meeting with the parents in order to give them clinical feedback about the functional profile and the preliminary diagnosis of their child. During the meeting, individualized psychoeducational advice is provided to parents. Overall, about 13 h are scheduled to complete the SA phase (9 h for evaluations and 4 h for meetings).

3. A Telemedicine Working Model for Intervention

The telemedicine working model for intervention that has been developed was aimed at both preschoolers and older children (see Figure 2).

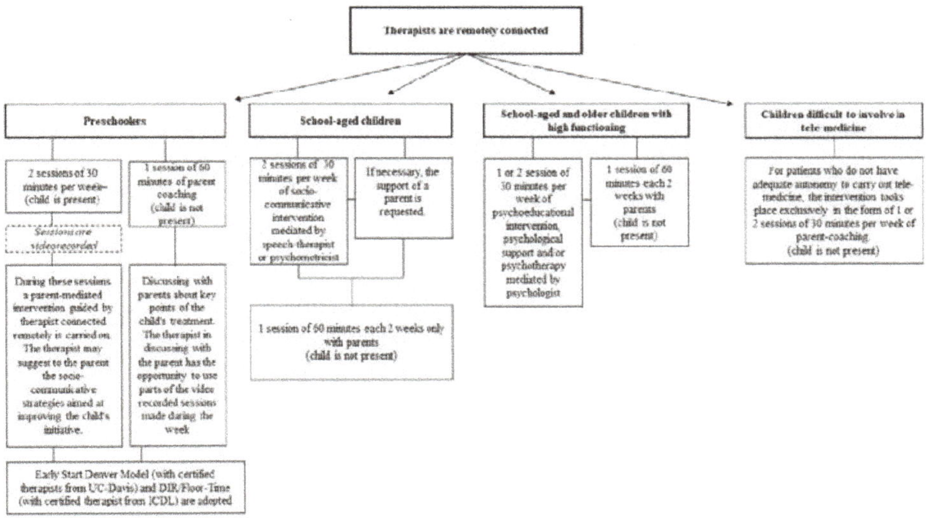

Figure 2. Working model for intervention.

For preschoolers, two sessions of 30 min each per week are expected. During these sessions, a parent-mediated remote intervention, guided by therapist, is carried out. The therapist may suggest to the parents the socio-communicative strategies aimed at improving the child's initiative. The two sessions (with parent–child and therapist remotely connected) are video recorded. During the week, another session of 60 min (remotely) is added to the two described before with the purpose of discussing with the parents the key points of the child's intervention (without the child). The therapist, in the discussion with the parents, can use parts of the recorded sessions made during the week.

For the preschoolers, the adopted intervention models are the so-called Naturalistic Developmental Behavioral Interventions (NDBI) [38]. The NDBI are evidence-based intervention models; they are based both on behavioral learning and on developmental sciences. The Early Start Denver Model [39,40] (with certified therapists from University of California (UC)-Davis) and DIR/Floor-Time [41] (with certified therapist from Interdisciplinary Council on Development and Learning (ICDL)) are remotely implemented. Remote parenting coaching, to provide parents/caregivers with tools and strategies to teach and engage their child through play and everyday routines, such as mealtimes, bathing, and dressing, is provided [42].

Therapists are supervised by an experienced psychologist in the field of early intervention.

For school-aged children, two 30 min online speech and communication therapy sessions are suggested per week. If necessary, the support of a parent is requested. The efficacy of speech and communication therapy delivered via telemedicine has been well documented [43]. During speech and communication therapy, the therapist and child are remotely connected, and they can interact in real time through audio and video with images and learning materials [43]. One session of 60 min every two weeks with parents is provided (without the child) to share the child's improvements and difficulties, as well as to suggest practical advice for the parents to perform at home.

For high-functioning children, it is established to continue the psychoeducational interventions, psychological support, and psychotherapy; however, the duration was modified to 30 min a week instead the original 60 min of in-person therapy. The high psychiatric vulnerability and/or comorbidity of children with ASD is widely documented. Among them, anxiety disorder is one of the most reported [44]. Psychiatric comorbidities could contribute to a depletion of development, especially in adolescence. The alert state caused by the COVID-19 pandemic could be a difficult event to mentalize for children with ASD. For this reason, if the children were engaged in psychotherapy before the COVID-19 alert, it is important that they continue the therapy in online video or audio mode with the same weekly appointments. Continuing therapy could reduce anxiety, control mood, and offer children a private space to talk to a specialist [1].

One session of 60 min every two weeks with parents is also provided (without the child).

For patients who do not have the adequate autonomy to carry out online therapy, the intervention takes place exclusively in the form of one or two 30 min sessions a week for remote parent coaching.

During remote parent coaching, parents are invited to (1) share a home video (10–15 min) with therapists related to the child's behavior during structured sessions in a home setting or during free play and (2) discuss with therapists individualized strategies and methods of intervention for their child.

4. Conclusions

Our telemedicine working models represent a union between synchronous transmission (i.e., live video conferencing as two-way video and audio interactions between the therapists and parents/child for interviews and other behavioral observation of the child) and asynchronous transmission (i.e., "store and forward" transmissions of recorded video, data, and questionnaires/checklists) [45].

Telemedicine should not totally take the place of in-person clinical services; however, in this moment, it could be required to provide answers to families who are concerned about the health of their children with ASD. The described working model for diagnosis has the purpose of carrying out a preliminary assessment which does not have the purpose of replacing preferable in-person assessment. The described working model for diagnosis may not be suitable for all families, and in some cases, it could be even contraindicated (i.e., low confidence with technology). For some of them, it is difficult to perform a remote evaluation. Therefore, in some cases, the in-person evaluation cannot be replaced even partially by the remote one. However, for other children, this working model for diagnosis can provide useful indications and suggest the start of an individualized intervention. It is our decision that all the children who carry out the remote evaluation with telemedicine have an in-person appointment when phase 3 of the lockdown begins, in order to conclude the evaluation and to check the effect of the suggested psychoeducational intervention. The presented working model represents a scheme which obviously can be flexible; therefore, it is possible, in some cases, to increase the number of expected days to complete the evaluation. The presented working model for diagnosis could permit clinicians to look at otherwise inaccessible children's behaviors in their natural setting, and to observe parent–child reciprocity [7]. The proposed working model for diagnosis makes it possible for parents to register videos in their home, during their daily activities, which permits the capture of natural expressions of child behavior that are broadly recognized as essential to a precise and comprehensive assessment [6]. The background of the presented working model for diagnosis is based on previous studies that showed that a telemedicine procedure could be adequate for acquiring children's diagnostic profiles in a way that parents report as easy and acceptable [4]. Currently, the clinical judgment of the professional must establish the adequacy of telemedicine on a case-by-case basis.

The described working model for intervention with ASD children is not exhaustive and it needs to be tried out; however, it is supported from preliminary research findings in this field [14,46]. The telemedicine approach is accepted by parents [13], increases their sense of competence [47], increases the parent intervention accuracy, and improves the socio-communicative competencies of children with ASD [41,48].

Because of distancing and lockdowns, a functional use of telemedicine is pivotal. Clinical services are moving to digitalization and remote approaches to respond current patients' needs [49,50]. During COVID-19 phase 2 and later, telemedicine and in-person diagnosis and intervention must alternate.

In the future, even when the COVID-19 alert expires, telemedicine can play an essential role in speeding up the autism diagnosis process. Because of the high number of evaluation requests for ASD, there are very long waiting lists. The systematic increase in telemedicine, together with traditional assessment in-person procedures will significantly decrease the needed times for a diagnostic indication. Early diagnosis is crucial to help a child with ASD, since early identification can significantly improve the child's developmental trajectory. Moreover, research has shown that young children who receive the early intervention can have higher chances of demonstrating significant gains in functioning than children diagnosed later.

In conclusion, the presented working models for preliminary diagnosis and intervention must be considered as both a partial response to the current emergency status and, at the same time, as a possible integration into traditional approaches.

Author Contributions: Conceptualization, methodology and writing draft, A.N. The author has read and agreed to the published version of the manuscript.

Funding: This research received no funds.

Acknowledgments: I would like to thank the parents and children I meet every day in my work.

Conflicts of Interest: No conflict of interest is reported.

References

1. Narzisi, A. Handle the Autism Spectrum Condition during Coronavirus (COVID-19) Stay at Home period: Ten Tips for Helping Parents and Caregivers of Young Children. *Brain Sci.* **2020**, *1*, 10.
2. Maenner, M.J.; Shaw, K.A.; Baio, J.; Washington, A.; Patrick, M.; DiRienzo, M.; Christensen, D.L.; Wiggins, L.D.; Pettygrove, S.; Andrews, J.G.; et al. Prevalence of Autism Spectrum Disorder Among Children Aged 8 Years—Autism and Developmental Disabilities Monitoring Network, 11 Sites, United States, 2016. *Mmwr Surveill. Summ.* **2020**, *69*, 1–12. [CrossRef] [PubMed]
3. Narzisi, A.; Posada, M.; Barbieri, F.; Chericoni, N.; Ciuffolini, D.; Pinzino, M.; Romano, R.; Scattoni, M.L.; Tancredi, R.; Calderoni, S.; et al. Prevalence of Autism Spectrum Disorder in a large Italian catchment area, a school-based population study within the ASDEU project. *Epidemiol. Psychiatr. Sci.* **2018**, *29*, e5. [CrossRef] [PubMed]
4. Juárez, A.P.; Weitlauf, A.S.; Nicholson, A.; Pasternak, A.; Broderick, N.; Hine, J.; Stainbook, J.A.; Warren, Z. Early Identification of ASD through Telemedicine: Potential Value for Underserved Populations. *J. Autism Dev. Disord.* **2018**, *48*, 2601–2610. [CrossRef] [PubMed]
5. Sutherland, R.; Trembath, D.; Hodge, M.A.; Rose, V.; Roberts, J. Telehealth and autism: Are telehealth language assessments reliable and feasible for children with autism? *Int. J. Lang. Commun. Disord.* **2019**, *54*, 281–291. [CrossRef]
6. Smith, C.; Rozga, A.; Matthews, N.; Oberleitner, R.; Nazneen, N.; Abowd, G. Investigating the accuracy of a novel telehealth diagnostic approach for Autism Spectrum Disorder. *Psychol Assess.* **2017**, *29*, 245–252. [CrossRef]

7. Nazneen, N.; Rozga, A.; Smith, C.; Oberleitner, R.; Abowd, G.; Arriaga, R. A Novel System for Supporting Autism Diagnosis Using Home Videos: Iterative Development and Evaluation of System Design. *J. Mir Mhealth Uhealth.* **2015**, *3*, e68. [CrossRef]
8. Sutantio, J.D.; Pusponegoro, H.D.; Sekartini, R. Validity of Telemedicine for Diagnosing Autism Spectrum Disorder: Protocol-Guided Video Recording Evaluation. *Telemed. E-Health* **2020**. [CrossRef]
9. Fusaro, V.A.; Daniels, J.; Duda, M.; DeLuca, T.F.; D'Angelo, O.; Tamburello, J.; Maniscalco, J.; Wall, D.P. The Potential of Accelerating Early Detection of Autism through Content Analysis of YouTube Videos. *PLoS ONE* **2014**, *9*, e93533. [CrossRef]
10. Lord, C.; Luyster, R.; Gotham, K.; Guthrie, W. (ADOS-2) Manual (Part II): Toddler Module. In *Autism Diagnostic Observation Schedule*, 2nd ed.; Western Psychological Services: Torrence, CA, USA, 2012.
11. Johnsson, G.; Kerslake, R.; Crook, S. Delivering allied health services to regional and remote participants on the autism spectrum via video-conferencing technology: Lessons learned. *Rural Remote Health.* **2019**, *19*, 5358. [CrossRef]
12. Carter, A.S.; Messinger, D.S.; Stone, W.L.; Celimli, S.; Nahmias, A.S.; Yoder, P. Randomized controlled trial of Hanen's 'More Than Words' in toddlers with early autism symptoms. *Child Psychol. Psychiatry* **2011**, *52*, 741–752. [CrossRef] [PubMed]
13. Bearss, K.; Burrell, T.L.; Challa, S.A.; Postorino, V.; Gillespie, S.E.; Crooks, C.; Scahill, L. Feasibility of Parent Training via Telehealth for Children with Autism Spectrum Disorder and Disruptive Behavior: A Demonstration Pilot. *J. Autism Dev. Disord.* **2018**, *48*, 1020–1030. [CrossRef] [PubMed]
14. Vismara, L.; McCormick, C.; Wagner, A.; Monlux, K.; Nadhan, A.; Young, G. Telehealth Parent Training in the Early Start Denver Model: Results From a Randomized Controlled Study. *Focus Autism Other Dev. Disabil.* **2018**, *33*, 2. [CrossRef]
15. Green, J.; Charman, T.; McConachie, H.; Aldred, C.; Slonims, V.; Howlin, P.; Le Couteur, A.; Leadbitter, K.; Hudry, K.; Byford, S.; et al. Parent-mediated communication-focused treatment in children with autism (PACT): A randomised controlled trial. *Lancet* **2010**, *19*, 2152–2160. [CrossRef]
16. Roid, G.L. Leiter international performance scale-revised: Examiner's manual. In *Leiter International Performance Scale-Revised*; Roid, G.H., Miller, L.J., Eds.; Stoelting: Wood Dale, IL, USA, 1997.
17. Greene, J.A.; Trujillo, S.; Isquith, P.K.; Gioia, G.A.; Espy, K.A. *Enhanced Interpretation of the Behavior Rating Inventory of Executive Function–Preschool Version (BRIEF-P) (White Paper)*; PAR: Lutz, FL, USA, 2019.
18. Gioia, G.A.; Isquith, P.K.; Guy, S.C.; Kenworthy, L. *Behavior Rating Inventory of Executive Function®(BRIEF®2)*, 2nd, ed.; PAR Inc.: Lutz, FL, USA, 2015.
19. Achenbach, T.M.; Rescorla, L. *Manual for the ASEBA Preschool Forms and Profile*; Univeristy of Vermont: Burlington, VT, USA, 2000.
20. Fenson, L.; Pethick, S.; Renda, C.; Cox, J.L.; Dale, P.S.; Reznick, J.S. Short-form versions of the MacArthur Communicative Developmental Inventories. *Appl. Psycholinguist.* **2000**, *21*, 95–116. [CrossRef]
21. Schopler, E.; Van Bourgondien, M.E.; Wellman, G.J.; Love, S.R. *Childhood Autism Rating Scale*, 2nd ed.; Western Psychological Services: Los Angeles, CA, USA, 2010.
22. Lam, K.S.; Aman, M.G. The Repetitive Behavior Scale-Revised: Independent validation in individuals with autism spectrum disorders. *J. Autism Dev. Disord.* **2007**, *37*, 855–866. [CrossRef] [PubMed]
23. Rutter, M.; Bailey, A.; Lord, C. *Social Communication Questionnaire (SCQ) Manual*; Western Psychological Services: Los Angeles, CA, USA, 2000.
24. Dunn, W. *Sensory Profile*; Harcourt Assessment: San Antonio, TX, USA, 1999.
25. James, K.; Lucy, J.; Millera, L.J.; Schaaf, R.; Nielsene, D.M.; Schoena, S.A. Phenotypes within sensory modulation dysfunction. *Compr. Psychiatry* **2011**, *52*, 715–724. [CrossRef] [PubMed]
26. Constantino, J.; Gruber, J. *Social Responsiveness Scale (SRS) Manual*; Western Psychological Services: Los Angeles, CA, USA, 2005.
27. Abidin, R.R. *Parenting Stress Index*, 4th ed.; PAR: Lutz, FL, USA, 2012.
28. Grzadzinski, R.; Carr, T.; Colombi, C.; McGuire, K.; Dufek, S.; Pickles, A.; Lord, C. Measuring Changes in Social Communication Behaviors: Preliminary Development of the Brief Observation of Social Communication Change (BOSCC). *J. Autism Dev. Disord.* **2016**, *46*, 2464–2479. [CrossRef]

29. Ausderau, K.K.; St John, B.; Kwaterski, K.N.; Nieuwenhuis, B.; Bradley, E. Parents' Strategies to Support Mealtime Participation of Their Children With Autism Spectrum Disorder. *Am. J. Occup. Ther.* **2019**, *73*, 7301205070p1–7301205070p10. [CrossRef]
30. Peckett, H.; MacCallum, F.; Knibbs, J. Maternal experience of Lego Therapy in families with children with autism spectrum conditions: What is the impact on family relationships? *Autism* **2016**, *20*, 879–887. [CrossRef]
31. Lord, C.; Rutter, M.; Le Couteur, A. Autism Diagnostic Interview-Revised: A revised version of a diagnostic interview for caregivers of individuals with possible pervasive developmental disorders. *J. Autism Dev. Disord.* **1994**, *24*, 659–685. [CrossRef] [PubMed]
32. Sparrow, S.S.; Balla, D.A.; Cicchetti, D.V.; Doll, E.D. *Vineland-II: Vineland Adaptive Behavior Scales: Survey Forms Manual*; American Guidance Service: Circle Pines, MN, USA, 2005.
33. Balboni, G.; Tasso, A.; Muratori, F.; Cubelli, R. The Vineland-II in preschool children with Autism Spectrum Disorders: An item content category analysis. *J. Autism Dev. Disord.* **2016**, *46*, 42–52. [CrossRef] [PubMed]
34. Balboni, G.; Belacchi, C.; Bonichini, S.; Coscarelli, A. *Vineland-II. Vineland Adaptive Behavior Scales Second Edition Survey Interview Form*; Giunti OS Organizzazioni Speciali: Firenze, Italy, 2016.
35. Gotham, K.; Risi, S.; Pickles, A.; Lord, C. The Autism Diagnostic Observation Schedule: Revised Algorithms for Improved Diagnostic Validity. *J. Autism Dev. Disord.* **2007**, *37*, 613–627. [CrossRef] [PubMed]
36. Schutte, J.L.; McCue, M.P.; Parmanto, B.; McGonigle, J.; Handen, B.; Lewis, A.; Pulantara, I.W.; Saptono, A. Usability and Reliability of a Remotely Administered Adult Autism Assessment, the Autism Diagnostic Observation Schedule (ADOS) Module 4. *Telemed J. E Health* **2015**, *21*, 176–184. [CrossRef] [PubMed]
37. APA. *Diagnostic and Statistical Manual of Mental Disorders*, 5th ed.; Psychiatric Association: Washington, DC, USA, 2013.
38. Schreibman, L.; Dawson, G.; Stahmer, A.C.; Landa, R.; Rogers, S.J.; McGee, G.G.; Kasari, C.; Ingersoll, B.; Kaiser, A.P.; Bruinsma, Y.; et al. Naturalistic Developmental Behavioral Interventions: Empirically Validated Treatments for Autism Spectrum Disorder. *J. Autism Dev. Disord.* **2015**, *45*, 2411–2428. [CrossRef]
39. Dawson, G.; Rogers, S.; Munson, J.; Smith, M.; Winter, J.; Greenson, J.; Donaldson, A.; Varley, J. Randomized, controlled trial of an intervention for toddlers with autism: The Early Start Denver Model. *Pediatrics* **2010**, *125*, e17–e23. [CrossRef]
40. Colombi, C.; Narzisi, A.; Ruta, L.; Cigala, V.; Gagliano, A.; Pioggia, G.; Siracusano, R.; Rogers, S.J.; Muratori, F.; Prima Pietra Team. Implementation of the Early Start Denver Model in an Italian community. *Autism* **2018**, *22*, 126–133. [CrossRef]
41. Greenspan, S.I.; Wieder, S.; Simons, R. *The Child with Special Needs: Encouraging Intellectual and Emotional Growth*; Addison-Wesley/Addison Wesley Longman: Boston, MA, USA, 1998.
42. Rogers, S.J.; Dawson, G.; Vismara, L.A. *An Early Start for Your Child with Autism: Using Everyday Activities to Help Kids Connect, Communicate, and Learn*; Guilford Press: New York, NY, USA, 2012.
43. Towey, M.P. Speech Telepractice: Installing a Speech Therapy Upgrade for the 21st Century. *Int. J. Telerehabilitation* **2012**, *4*, 73–78. [CrossRef]
44. Lai, M.C.; Kassee, C.; Besney, R.; Bonato, S.; Hull, L.; Mandy, W.; Szatmari, P.; Ameis, S.H. Prevalence of co-occurring mental health diagnoses in the autism population: A systematic review and meta-analysis. *Lancet Psychiatry* **2019**, *6*, 819–829. [CrossRef]
45. CASP. The Council of Autism. *Organizational Guidelines and Standards.* Available online: www.casproviders.org (accessed on 21 May 2020).
46. Parsons, D.; Cordier, R.; Vaz, S.; Lee, H.C. Parent-Mediated Intervention Training Delivered Remotely for Children With Autism Spectrum Disorder Living Outside of Urban Areas: Systematic Review. *J. Med. Internet Res.* **2017**, *14*, e198. [CrossRef]
47. Hepburn, S.L.; Blakeley-Smith, A.; Wolff, B.; Reaven, J.A. Telehealth delivery of cognitive-behavioral intervention to youth with autism spectrum disorder and anxiety: A pilot study. *Autism* **2016**, *20*, 207–218. [CrossRef] [PubMed]
48. Ingersoll, B.; Berger, N.I. Parent Engagement with a Telehealth-Based Parent-Mediated Intervention Program for Children with Autism Spectrum Disorders: Predictors of Program Use and Parent Outcomes. *J. Med. Internet Res.* **2015**, *6*, e227. [CrossRef] [PubMed]

49. Townsend, E.; Nielsen, E.; Allister, R.; Cassidy, S.A. Key ethical questions for research during the COVID-19 pandemic. *Lancet Psychiatry* **2020**, *7*, 381–383. [CrossRef]
50. Stainbrook, J.A.; Weitlauf, A.S.; Juárez, A.P.; Taylor, J.L.; Hine, J.; Broderick, N.; Nicholson, A.; Zachary, W. Measuring the service system impact of a novel telediagnostic service program for young children with autism spectrum disorder. *Autism* **2019**, *23*, 1051–1056. [CrossRef]

Journal of
Clinical Medicine

MDPI

Article

Risk for Depressive Symptoms among Hospitalized Women in High-Risk Pregnancy Units during the COVID-19 Pandemic

Shanny Sade [1,*], Eyal Sheiner [1], Tamar Wainstock [2], Narkis Hermon [1], Shimrit Yaniv Salem [1], Tamar Kosef [3], Talya Lanxner Battat [1], Sharon Oron [1] and Gali Pariente [1]

1 Department of Obstetrics and Gynecology, Soroka University Medical Center, Ben-Gurion University of the Negev, Beer-Sheva 8457108, Israel; sheiner@bgu.ac.il (E.S.); nicky.narkis@gmail.com (N.H.); Yanivshi@bgu.ac.il (S.Y.S.); talyalan@gmail.com (T.L.B.); sharonmelamed1@gmail.com (S.O.); galipa@bgu.ac.il (G.P.)
2 Department of Public Health, Faculty of Health Sciences, Ben-Gurion University of the Negev, Beer-Sheva 8457108, Israel; wainstoc@bgu.ac.il
3 Department of psychiatry, Soroka University Medical Center, Ben-Gurion University of the Negev, Beer-Sheva 8457108, Israel; tamar.kosef@gmail.com
* Correspondence: shanny.ogen@gmail.com; Tel.: +972-544-664-110

Received: 23 June 2020; Accepted: 29 July 2020; Published: 31 July 2020

Abstract: Objective: Higher rates of mental disorders, specifically depression, were found among affected people in previous epidemiological studies taken after disasters. The aim of the current study was to assess risk for depression among pregnant women hospitalized during the "coronavirus disease 2019" (COVID-19) pandemic, as compared to women hospitalized before the COVID-19 pandemic. Study design: A cross-sectional study was performed among women hospitalized in the high-risk pregnancy units of the Soroka University Medical Center (SUMC). All participating women completed the Edinburgh Postnatal Depression Scale (EPDS), and the results were compared between women hospitalized during the COVID-19 strict isolation period (19 March 2020 and 26 May 2020) and women hospitalized before the COVID-19 pandemic. Multivariable logistic regression models were constructed to control for potential confounders. Results: Women hospitalized during the COVID-19 strict isolation period (n = 84) had a comparable risk of having a high (>10) EPDS score as compared to women hospitalized before the COVID-19 pandemic (n = 279; 25.0% vs. 29.0%, p = 0.498). These results remained similar in the multivariable logistic regression model, while controlling for maternal age, ethnicity and known mood disorder (adjusted odds ratio (OR) 1.0, 95% CI 0.52–1.93, p = 0.985). Conclusion: Women hospitalized at the high-risk pregnancy unit during the COVID-19 strict isolation period were not at increased risk for depression, as compared to women hospitalized before the COVID-19 pandemic.

Keywords: COVID-19; depression; EPDS; pandemic; pregnancy

---

1. Introduction

The "coronavirus disease" (COVID-19) caused by Severe Acute Respiratory Syndrome Coronavirus 2 (SARS-COV-2), was first isolated in January 2020, after a series of respiratory infections of unknown etiology were detected in China [1,2].

SARS-COV-2 was first diagnosed in Israel on 21 February 2020, among Israelis returning from abroad or from those who came in contact with infected tourists. According to the World Health Organization (WHO) report from June, 823,813 cases have been diagnosed in Israel since then [3]. At the onset of the study, 19 March, there were 529 cases of COVID-19 in Israel, with daily change of 23.89% from the previous day. In comparison, in Italy at the same day there were 41,035 cases, with a daily rise of 14.9%, and in Spain, 3431 cases, with a daily rise of 35.19% [3]. The Israeli Ministry of Health recommended soon after that all citizens returning from Eastern countries, and later on, from all other countries, stay in quarantine for two weeks following their return, in order to minimize the contagion. Not long after, on 12 March, preschools, schools and higher education closed, public transportation was halted and social isolation was implemented. Since March 2020, using satellite information and cellular phone location, the Israeli Ministry of Health sent automated text messages to individuals identified as being close to positively diagnosed citizens, informing them that they should stay in quarantine and contact a health care provider in the case that any symptom develops.

Previous epidemiological studies were taken in order to assess the effect of a pandemic on the mental health of affected people. During the 2003 (Severe Acute Respiratory syndrome (SARS) pandemic, studies have demonstrated depression, anxiety, panic attack, psychotic symptoms, delirium and even suicidal ideations among the pandemic survivors [4]. The survivors also experienced psychological effects of physical symptoms, such as anxiety and insomnia regarding fever and dysphoria due to nausea [5].

Likewise, the sudden outbreak of COVID-19, the unpredictability of the situation, quarantine for indefinite periods, myths and misinformation about the epidemic, the unavailability of vaccine and the overflow of information on social media have affected the public social health [4,6], and even provoked extreme behavior like suicidal ideations [7].

The onset of depression is reported to peak during childbearing years and is approximately twice more common in women than in men [8]. Pregnancy and postpartum period are vulnerable times for onset or relapse of mental illness, with depression and anxiety being the most common psychiatric disorders [9]. Studies have demonstrated serious concerns of depressive symptoms during pregnancy, in terms of maternal morbidity and adverse neonatal outcomes [10]. Pregnant women hospitalized in a high-risk pregnancy unit are described to have fair risk for depression, varying from 27–44% [11–13].

With little existing published data, focusing on depression among pregnant women hospitalized during the COVID-19 pandemic, and in light of its potential adverse effect on both the mother and the infant, we aimed to assess the incidence of depression among women hospitalized in the high-risk units during the COVID-19 strict isolation period, as compared with the incidence of depression among women hospitalized in the high-risk units before the COVID-19 pandemic.

2. Materials and Methods

2.1. Population and Setting

The study recruited women hospitalized in high-risk units in the Soroka University Medical Center (SUMC). Recruitment and data collection were done during the COVID-19 pandemic strict isolation period, between 19 March 2020 and 26 May 2020. Women who were hospitalized in the high-risk pregnancy units before the COVID-19 pandemic (between November 2016 and April 2017) served as the comparison group. The comparison group was composed of women who were recruited for previous study performed in the same high-risk pregnancy units [11]. High risk pregnancy was defined according to the Israeli Ministry of Health statement regarding criteria for high-risk pregnancy. These include maternal chronic illness (such as cardiac disease, pulmonary disease, hypertension, diabetes), obstetric and gynecological history (such as recurrent pregnancy loss, congenital abnormalities, intrauterine fetal death), and other conditions, such as multiple gestation, suspected intrauterine growth retardation, suspected macrosomia and more [14]. SUMC, located in southern Israel, is the largest country birth center, with more than 17, 000 births a year. The study was approved by the SUMC IRB Committee (IRB approval # 0079-20-SOR).

2.2. Study Design

A cross-sectional study was performed; women hospitalized in the high-risk pregnancy units during the COVID-19 pandemic were compared to historic unexposed group hospitalized at the same units, before the COVID-19 pandemic. Each woman participated at a single time-point. Every day, during the time frame of the study, the research team handed out self-reported questionnaires to all women who met the inclusion criteria, in the high-risk pregnancy unit, following an oral and written explanation on the study course and purpose. All hospitalized women were approached, regardless of hospitalization length or indication. Each woman from both the exposed and the comparison group, answered questions regarding her socioeconomic state, medical background, obstetrical history, current pregnancy course, and completed the Edinburgh Postnatal Depression Scale (EPDS) questionnaire. Both the exposed group and the comparison group fulfilled the questionnaires prospectively at the hospital. This screening test, established by Cox et al. in 1987 [15], was developed for diagnosing pregnant and postpartum women who are at high risk for depression. This questionnaire is widely used, based on the American College of Obstetrics and Gynecology (ACOG) recommendations [16]. According to the Israeli Ministry of Health statement from January 2014, a score of 10 and above on the EPDS indicates a high risk for depression in a pregnant woman, and requires further assessment and treatment by a mental health specialist [17]. This cutoff score has been recommended by the developers of the scale [15], and has previously been used in several other studies, as indicating a risk for both antenatal and postpartum depression [13]. The questionnaire consists of 10 self-completed questions regarding mood in the past week. The scores in each question are summed, and a final score of <10 is defined as low risk for depression. A score of ≥ 10 defines a person at risk for depression [15]. Background variables assessed included maternal demographic, medical and obstetrical data. Data were collected in a cross-sectional format, at two time points. Data regarding the comparison group were collected as part of a previous prospective study that was taken in the same high-risk units [11]. The group of women which served as the "unexposed" group was available from an historic study [11], and so the sample size of this group was fixed. As soon as the COVID-19 spread to Israel, and following the strict isolation regulation, the study team began to recruit women to participate in this study (following IRB approval of the study protocol). Since the isolation has gradually released, its effect could no longer be studied, and 90 women were recruited in the relevant period. Based on a priori assumptions, the given sample size would have enabled us to detect a difference of (OR = 2.17) between the study groups in the risk for EPDS ≥ 10. When planning the study, a greater difference in EPDS ≥ 10 was expected between the groups (odds ratio > 2). This big difference was not detected between the groups, however the strict isolation period has discontinued, and therefore recruitment stopped. Since recruitment timing was critical for the studied question, a power analysis was performed based on the give sample and the detected differences.

2.3. Definitions

Mood disorder was defined as any psychiatric diagnoses mentioned in the computerized data of each woman.

Chronic illness included diabetes mellitus, hypertension, gastrointestinal disorders, cardiac disorders, respiratory disorders, rheumatic disorders and thyroid disorders.

Positive suicidal ideation was defined as any positive answer to question number 10 ('The thought of harming myself has occurred to me') in the EDPS questionnaire.

2.4. Statistical Analysis

Statistical analysis was performed using SPSS version 23.0, IBM SPSS statistics for Windows, version 23.0. Armonk, NY: IBM Corp. Comparison of continuous variables was performed using Student's *t*-test and Chi-square test was used to examine differences in the distribution of categorical variables. Multivariable logistic regression models were constructed to examine the association between the independent and dependent variables, while adjusting for confounding factors based on the univariate analysis, as well as clinically important variables, including maternal age, ethnicity and known mood disorder.

The strategy for model building was as follows: background characteristics were compared between the study groups (exposed and unexposed women). Variables associated with the exposure (i.e., were different between the study groups) were suspected as confounding variables, and they were tested in the multivariable models, to determine whether they are also associated with the outcome variable, and are therefore possibly confounding the association between the exposure and the outcome. A suspected confounding variable included the having a history of mood disorders. Maternal age and ethnicity are both variables with clinical significance. Ethnicity in our study population represents social, cultural, educational and religious differences between the groups, which have been known to affect EPDS scores [18,19].

3. Results

A total of 369 women were included in the study: 90 women who were hospitalized in the high-risk pregnancy units during the COVID-19 pandemic strict isolation period, and 279 women before the COVID-19 pandemic. The response rate of the study was 93.33%; 90 women were included in the study, 6 refused to complete the questionnaire.

EPDS questionnaires with missing data on ≥1 questions were excluded from the analysis of the total EPDS score (of EPDS ≥ 10), but were included in the comparison of responses to question 10, if this was not missing. A total of 19 questionnaires were excluded.

Table 1 summarizes maternal demographic and obstetric features of both groups. Mean maternal age was comparable between the groups, as was ethnicity and gravidity. Likewise, no significant differences were noted between the groups, in terms of fertility treatments, chronic illnesses, body mass index (BMI), bad obstetric history and indication for current hospitalization, such as suspected intra-uterine growth restriction. Rates of mood disorders were lower among pregnant women hospitalized during the COVID-19 pandemic, compared to pregnant women hospitalized before the COVID-19 pandemic.

Table 1. Demographic and obstetric characteristics of the study population.

Characteristic		Hospitalization during the "Coronavirus Disease" (Coronavirus Disease 2019 (COVID-19)) Pandemic n = 84 (%)	Hospitalization before the COVID-19 Pandemic n = 279 (%)	p Value
Maternal age, years	<20	2.4	4.3	0.444
	20–35	79.8	82.4	
	>35	17.9	13.3	
Gestational age at hospitalization, weeks (mean + SD)		33.7 ± 5.1	34.0 ± 4.8	0.771
Ethnicity	Jewish	50.0	61.2	0.071
	Bedouins	50.0	38.8	
Marital status	Married	90.4	92.8	0.460
	Other	9.6	7.2	
Gravidity	1	28.6	26.2	0.153
	2–4	42.9	53.8	
	5≤	28.6	20.1	

Table 1. *Cont.*

Characteristic		Hospitalization during the "Coronavirus Disease" (Coronavirus Disease 2019 (COVID-19)) Pandemic *n* = 84 (%)	Hospitalization before the COVID-19 Pandemic *n* = 279 (%)	*p* Value
Parity	1	34.5	34.8	0.116
	2–4	46.4	54.5	
	5≤	19.0	10.8	
Fertility treatments		10.7	9.5	0.738
Diabetes mellitus		11.4	9.5	0.625
Past abortions		38.6	38.8	0.972
* body mass index (BMI)	<20	0.0	1.1	0.567
	20–24.99	18.8	24.9	
	25–29.99	43.5	40.5	
	>30	37.7	33.5	
Mood disorder		10.7	20.8	0.037
Chronic illness		22.6	17.7	0.311
Premature rapture of membranes		4.8	4.7	0.969
Suspected intra-uterine growth restriction		9.5	7.5	0.554
Past intra-uterine fetal death		4.8	7.6	0.388
Past neonatal death		2.4	2.8	0.857
Past pre-eclampsia		8.5	6.2	0.494
Past congenital abnormalities		4.8	6.0	0.676

* Missing value: BMI: *n* = 25.

Table 2 describes the scores of the self-completed EDPS questions. No significant differences were noted between the two groups in any of the questions.

Table 2. Scores of the EDPS questions, among women hospitalized in the high-risk pregnancy units during and before the COVID-19 pandemic.

EDPS Question		Hospitalization during the COVID-19 Pandemic *n* = 84 (%)	Hospitalization before the COVID-19 Pandemic *n* = 279 (%)	*p* Value
1- I have been able to laugh and see the funny side of things	0- As much as I always could	57.5	68.5	0.068
	1- Not quite so much now	35.0	21.5	
	2- Definitely not so much now	5.0	4.3	
	3- Not at all	2.5	5.7	
2- I have looked forward with enjoyment to things	0- As much as I ever did	57.0	65.3	0.552
	1- Rather less than I used to	27.8	23.5	
	2- Definitely less than I used to	10.1	6.9	
	3- Hardly at all	5.1	4.3	
3- I have blamed myself unnecessarily when things went wrong	0- Yes, most of the time	8.5	8.0	0.533
	1- Yes, some of the time	14.6	17.4	
	2- Not very often	22.0	28.3	
	3- No, never	54.9	46.4	

Table 2. *Cont.*

EDPS Question		Hospitalization during the COVID-19 Pandemic $n = 84$ (%)	Hospitalization before the COVID-19 Pandemic $n = 279$ (%)	p Value
4- I have been anxious or worried for no good reason	0- No, not at all	43.9	44.4	0.717
	1- Hardly ever	24.4	19.5	
	2- Yes, sometimes	23.2	28.2	
	3- Yes, very often	8.5	7.9	
5- I have felt scared or panicky for no good reason	0- Yes, quite a lot	1.2	6.5	0.250
	1- Yes, sometimes	18.5	14.0	
	2- No, not much	23.5	23.7	
	3- No, not at all	56.8	55.8	
6- Things have been getting on top of me	0- Yes, most of the time I haven't been able to cope at all	9.0	9.3	0.964
	1- Yes, sometimes I haven't been coping as well as usual	25.6	27.2	
	2- No, most of the time I have coped quite well	29.5	26.5	
	3- No, I have been coping as well as ever	35.9	36.9	
7- I have been so unhappy that I have had difficulty sleeping	0- Yes, most of the time	7.5	7.2	0.886
	1- Yes, sometimes	13.8	15.1	
	2- Not very often	22.5	18.6	
	3- No, not at all	56.3	59.1	
8- I have felt sad or miserable	0- Yes, most of the time	11.3	8.7	0.813
	1- Yes, quite often	10.0	11.8	
	2- Not very often	28.7	27.2	
	3- No, not at all	50.0	52.7	
9- I have been so unhappy that I have been crying	0- Yes, most of the time	3.7	6.8	0.356
	1- Yes, quite often	13.6	9.4	
	2- Only occasionally	27.2	21.9	
	3- No, never	55.6	61.9	
10- The thought of harming myself has occurred to me	0- Yes, quite often	0.0	0.7	0.387
	1- Sometimes	3.7	2.2	
	2- Hardly ever	4.9	2.2	
	3- Never	91.4	95.0	

Maternal depression risk, as assessed by the total EPDS score, is presented in Table 3. Women hospitalized during the COVID-19 pandemic had a comparable risk of having depression, expressed by a high (≥10) EPDS score, compared to women hospitalized before the COVID-19 pandemic (25.0% vs. 29.0%, $p = 0.498$). Rates of positive suicidal ideations (according to question number 10 in the EPDS questionnaire) were comparable between the groups (8.6% vs. 5.0%, $p = 0.221$).

Table 3. Edinburgh Postnatal Depression Scale (EPDS) results among women hospitalized in the high-risk pregnancy units, during and before the COVID-19 pandemic.

	Hospitalization during the COVID-19 Pandemic $n = 84$ (%)	Hospitalization before the COVID-19 Pandemic $n = 279$ (%)	p Value
Total EPDS score ≥ 10	25.0	29.0	0.498
Suicidal ideations (according to question number 10 in EPDS questionnaire)	8.6	5.0	0.221

Using a multivariable logistic regression model, controlling for maternal age, ethnicity and known mood disorder, women hospitalized during the COVID-19 pandemic had a comparable risk for depression, as compared to women hospitalized before the COVID-19 pandemic (adjusted OR 1.0, 95% CI 0.52–1.93, $p = 0.985$, Table 4). Another multivariable logistic regression model, controlling for maternal age, showed that women hospitalized during the COVID-19 pandemic had a comparable risk for suicidal ideation as compared to women hospitalized before the COVID-19 pandemic (adjusted OR 1.8, 95% CI 0.71–4.85, $p = 0.203$, Table 4).

Table 4. Multivariable logistic regression model for the association between timing of hospitalization and EDPS score ≥ 10.

	Model 1 EDPS Score > 10		
	Adjusted (Odds Ratio (OR))	**95% {Confidence Interval (CI)}**	***p* Value**
Hospitalization during the COVID-19 pandemic (vs. hospitalization before the COVID-19 pandemic)	1.0	0.52–1.93	0.985
Maternal age (years)	1.0	0.94–1.05	0.916
Ethnicity (Jewish vs. Bedouin)	0.3	0.21–0.66	0.001
Mood disorder	6.1	3.30–11.59	<0.001
	Model 2 Suicidal Ideation		
	Adjusted OR	**95% CI**	***p* Value**
Hospitalization during the COVID-19 pandemic (vs. hospitalization before the COVID-19 pandemic)	1.8	0.71–4.85	0.203
Maternal age (years)	0.8	0.81–0.97	0.009

4. Discussion

4.1. Principal Findings

Our study demonstrated a comparable risk for depression among women hospitalized in high-risk pregnancy units during the COVID-19 pandemic, compared to those hospitalized before the pandemic.

4.2. Results

Existing literature has demonstrated linkage between disaster exposure and mental health [20]. Studies showed that people exposed to natural disasters, including hurricanes, floods and earthquakes or specific collective traumatic events such as wars, may have series threat to mental health, with those who had higher exposure having greater rates of mental disorder [20,21]. Adverse mental health outcomes include particularly post-traumatic stress disorder, depression, or anxiety, including major depressive disorder and generalized anxiety disorder. In addition, health-related problems, such as somatic complaints, sleep disturbances, and substance abuse were reported among survivors of collective disasters [20–22].

Women are more vulnerable to disaster-related psychopathology than men [23–25]. Female gender has generally been associated with reduced resilience after disaster, but greater post-traumatic growth. After the Madrid train bombing, women reported more post-traumatic growth and positive changes, but also more negative changes and associated depression and anxiety [25].

Pregnant and post-partum women may be vulnerable to post-disaster psychopathology, and their mental health is of particular concern, because of their special role in taking care of their children and families [25]. Unplanned pregnancy, being multiparous and a poor marital relationship were associated with worse pregnancy mental health [23], while having support from the partner and family were protective [26,27]. Nevertheless, in our population, marital status was comparable between the groups.

Few studies, conducted world-wide following disasters, investigated the psychiatric morbidity of pregnant and post-partum women in the disaster areas. Khatry et al. examined the influence of the 2015 Nepal earthquake on pregnant women at the time. By using the EDPS score, they assessed clinically-significant symptoms of antenatal common mental disorders, their risks and protective factors. They found that pregnant women who experienced the earthquake had higher risk for clinically significant mental disorders. Women with greater vulnerability were those who lack intimate partner relationship, had prior pregnancy losses and who lack income-generating work [26].

Chang et al. examined the influence of Taiwan 921 earthquake on mental health in a group of women from Pu-LI, a town a few kilometers from the epicenter, who were pregnant during or immediately after the major earthquake disaster. The prevalence of minor psychiatric morbidity found was high, 29.2% of all women examined, with a positive correlation to post-traumatic stress disorder. A risk factor for psychiatric morbidity was spouse causality [27].

On the contrary, overall rates of depression and posttraumatic stress disorder were not significantly higher among groups of postpartum women from southern Louisiana who were pregnant during or shortly after the Hurricane Katrina [23]. In their next study, the authors demonstrated that, not only were the pregnant and post-partum women more resilient to the consequences of the disaster, they also grew and perceived benefits after the disaster [25].

Engel et al. investigated the consequences of the destruction of the World Trade Center on 11 September 2001 on the health of pregnant women and their fetuses. They enrolled women who were pregnant and living or working within close proximity to the disaster. They found that post-traumatic stress symptomatology and moderate depression were associated with long gestational duration [24].

As can be seen in other related studies, poor marital relationship was associated with worse pregnancy mental health [23], while having support from the partner and family were protective [25,27]. Our study failed to find such as association. This may be explained by the size of the cohort, or by the fact that our study assessed risk for depression by the EDPS questionnaire and not a diagnosis of depression. Results may have been different if we would have repeated the study few of months after delivery.

While most of the previous studies investigated post- disaster depression, our study investigated risk for depression during the COVID-19 pandemic. Mounder et al. investigated mental health response among health care workers during the first 4 weeks of the SARS outbreak in Toronto, Canada. The authors found that the most prominent emotional effects were fear, loneliness, boredom, anger, and worry about the effect of quarantine and contagion; they experienced the psychological effect of physical symptoms [5].

4.3. Clinical Implications

Our study demonstrated comparable rates of depression among women hospitalized in the high-risk pregnancy units during and before the COVID-19 pandemic. There are several possible explanations for this association. First, as was noted previously, many people, and especially pregnant and postpartum women, are resilient after terrible events, and may experience various forms of benefits [25]. Posttraumatic benefit relates to posttraumatic growth going beyond baseline to an improved state of functioning after trauma. Such growth is described as changed priorities, having a greater appreciation of life, an increased sense of strength, self-reliance, expressiveness, compassion, and improved relationships. Second, Harville et al. determined that greater experience of the disaster was associated with less resilience [25]. Resilience is the ability to overcome difficulties and stressors, and does not mean being completely unaffected by terrible events or not having limited periods of mental health problems. It is heavily influence by how closely the disaster personally affected them. Our study population did not have any patients with a proven infection with SARS-COV-2, which may be related to the pandemic self-experience of the women and their mental consequences enrolled in our study. The same group also demonstrated that mental health problems following forces on the general population might be even lower in post-partum women, possibly because of more social support and nurturing after difficult circumstances [23]. This may also explain the comparable rates of depression between the study groups. Bonnano et al. examined the prevalence of resilience among a large group of New York area residents during the six months following the 11 September terrorist attack, demonstrated that even among the groups with the most pernicious levels of exposure and highest rates of post-traumatic stress disorder, the proportion that were resilient never dropped below one third [28]. This may explain our findings of comparable depression rates between women during and before the pandemic, with a substantial percentage of the exposed women who demonstrated resilience. Finally, the EDPS questionnaire is a rather screening then diagnostic test, hence false negative results may occur. In addition, depression may evolve months after filling the questionnaire.

4.4. Strength and Limitations

Strengths of the study include the use of standardized mental health instrument and a systematic recruitment of an unselected population. However, our study has limitations. First, the sample size limits the generalizability of our data. Missing data can affect the value of patient reported outcome and the precision of the estimated change in the results, which may introduce a bias. Nevertheless, in our study, the only covariate that presented missing data was BMI, with a rate of less than 5% missing data. In addition, we have no data on trends over longer periods of hospitalization. Third, EDPS is not a diagnostic tool but a screening tool, hence, we may have a false negative result, and women with actual depression may not be diagnosed and get the social and psychiatric aid that they deserve. Another limitation of our study relates to the possible seasonality effects on the studied association, since exposed and unexposed were recruited in different season, due to the COVID-19 exposure window. Another limitation of the study is the wide range of the gestational week of the women participating in the study as depressive symptoms score may vary during gestation. Nevertheless, in our study, no difference was demonstrated between the groups in mean gestational age. Information regarding the extent of medication use in these women was unavailable, including psychotropics or other unmeasured confounders that were not accounted for.

Leading theories about the emergence of depression emphasize that depression often occurs following repeated stressors or feelings of hopelessness, but the study window is limited and occurs at the onset of the pandemic. It may not be enough time for depression to develop. Nevertheless, the study's main purpose was to assess risk for depression, rather than depression itself. As our study occurred at the onset of the pandemic, more studies should be taken in the future during later outbreaks of the COVID-19 pandemic, as leading theories about the emergence of depression emphasize that depression often occurs following repeated stressors or feelings of hopelessness.

Our study participants (both exposed and unexposed) were already hospitalized in high-risk pregnancy units. Therefore, it is possible that their own medical issues would take precedence over the stress of the pandemic, which could account for why there are no group differences. Hence, the results of the current study are not generalized to all pregnant women, as some of them may be experiencing heightened depressive symptoms during this pandemic.

4.5. Conclusions

In conclusion, our study found that women hospitalized in the high-risk pregnancy units during the COVID-19 pandemic have comparable risk for depression compared to the comparison group of high-risk pregnant women not hospitalized during the pandemic. More studies should be done in order to shed some more light on the association between hospitalization in the high-risk pregnancy units during the COVID-19 pandemic and depression, as well as to assess the prevalence of other mental disorders among this population during the COVID-19 pandemic.

Author Contributions: Conceptualization, E.S., G.P., S.Y.S. and T.K.; methodology, E.S.; software, T.W.; validation, E.S., G.P. and T.W.; formal analysis, T.W.; investigation, S.S.; resources, S.S., N.H., S.O., T.L.B.; data curation, S.S., E.S., G.P. and T.W.; writing—original draft preparation, S.S.; writing—review and editing, G.P., E.S. and T.W.;

visualization, S.S.; supervision, E.S.; project administration, E.S.; funding acquisition, none. All authors have read and agreed to the published version of the manuscript.

Funding: No source of financial support for the research.

Conflicts of Interest: The authors report no conflict of interest.

References

1. Borges do Nascimento, I.J.; Cacic, N.; Abdulazeem, H.M.; von Groote, T.C.; Jayarajah, U.; Weerasekara, I.; Esfahani, M.A.; Civile, V.T.; Marusic, A.; Jeroncic, A.; et al. Novel Coronavirus infection (COVID-19) in humans: A scoping review and meta-analysis. *J. Clin. Med.* **2020**, *9*, 941. [CrossRef] [PubMed]
2. Available online: https://www.who.int/docs/default-source/coronaviruse/situation-reports/20200121-sitrep-1-2019-ncov.pdf?sfvrsn=20a99c10_4 (accessed on 9 June 2020).
3. Available online: https://covid19.who.int/region/euro/country/il (accessed on 23 June 2020).
4. Ahmed, M.Z.; Ahmed, O.; Aibao, Z.; Hanbin, S.; Siyu, L.; Ahmad, A. Epidemic of COVID-19 in China and associated psychological problems. *Asian J. Psychiatry* **2020**, *51*, 102092. [CrossRef] [PubMed]
5. Maunder, R.; Hunter, J.; Vincent, L.; Bennett, J.; Peladeau, N.; Leszcz, M.; Sadavoy, J.; Verhaeghe, L.M.; Steinberg, R.; Mazzulli, T. The immediate psychological and occupational impact of the 2003 SARS outbreak in a teaching hospital. *CMAJ* **2003**, *168*, 1245–1251.
6. Nguyen, H.C.; Nguyen, M.H.; Do, B.N.; Tran, C.Q.; Nguyen, T.T.; Pham, K.M.; Pham, L.V.; Tran, K.V.; Duong, T.T.; Tran, T.V.; et al. People with suspected COVID-19 symptoms were more likely depressed and had lower health-related quality of life: The potential benefit of health literacy. *J. Clin. Med.* **2020**, *9*, 965. [CrossRef]
7. Goyal, K.; Chauhan, P.; Chhikara, K.; Gupta, P.; Singh, M.P. Fear of COVID 2019: First suicidal case in India. *Asian J. Psychiatry* **2020**, *49*, 101989. [CrossRef] [PubMed]
8. Yedid Sion, M.; Harlev, A.; Weintraub, A.Y.; Sergienko, R.; Sheiner, E. Is antenatal depression associated with adverse obstetric and perinatal outcomes? *J. Matern. Fetal Neonatal Med.* **2016**, *29*, 863–867. [CrossRef]
9. Biaggi, A.; Conroy, S.; Pawlby, S.; Pariante, C.M. Identifying the women at risk of antenatal anxiety and depression: A systematic review. *J. Affect Disord.* **2016**, *191*, 62–77. [CrossRef]
10. Howard, L.M.; Molyneaux, E.; Dennis, C.L.; Rochat, T.; Stein, A.; Milgrom, J. Non-psychotic mental disorders in the perinatal period. *Lancet* **2014**, *384*, 1775–1778. [CrossRef]
11. Hermon, N.; Wainstock, T.; Sheiner, E.; Golan, A.; Walfisch, A. Impact of maternal depression on perinatal outcomes in hospitalized women-a prospective study. *Arch. Women's Ment. Health* **2019**, *22*, 85–91. [CrossRef]
12. Brandon, A.R.; Trivedi, M.H.; Hynan, L.S.; Miltenberger, P.D.; Labat, D.B.; Rifkin, J.B.; Stringer, C.A. Prenatal depression in women hospitalized for obstetric risk. *J. Clin. Psychiatry* **2008**, *69*, 635–643. [CrossRef]
13. Byatt, N.; Hicks-Courant, K.; Davidson, A.; Levesque, R.; Mick, E.; Allison, J.; Simas, T.A. Depression and anxiety among high-risk obstetric inpatients. *Gen. Hosp. Psychiatry* **2014**, *36*, 644–649. [CrossRef] [PubMed]
14. Available online: https://www.health.gov.il/hozer/mk15_2011.pdf (accessed on 23 June 2020).
15. Cox, J.L.; Holden, J.M.; Sagovsky, R. Detection of postnatal depression. Development of the 10-item Edinburgh Postnatal Depression Scale. *Br. J. Psychiatry* **1987**, *150*, 782–786. [CrossRef] [PubMed]
16. ACOG Committee Opinion No. 757: Screening for perinatal depression. *Obstet. Gynecol.* **2018**, *132*, e208–e212. [CrossRef] [PubMed]
17. Available online: https://www.health.gov.il/hozer/bz03_2014.pdf (accessed on 23 June 2020).
18. Abu-Ganem, S.; Sheiner, E.; Sherf, M.; Wiznitzer, A.; Sergienko, R.; Shoham-Vardi, I. Lack of prenatal care in a traditional community: Trends and perinatal outcome. *Arch. Gynecol. Obstet.* **2012**, *285*, 1237–1242. [CrossRef] [PubMed]
19. Sheiner, E.; Shoham-Vardi, I.; Weitzman, D.; Gohar, J.; Carmi, R. Decisions regarding pregnancy termination among Bedouin couples referred to third level ultrasound clinic. *Eur. J. Obstet. Gynecol. Reprod. Biol.* **1998**, *76*, 141–146. [CrossRef]
20. Fergusson, D.M.; Horwood, L.J.; Boden, J.M.; Mulder, R.T. Impact of a major disaster on the mental health of a well-studied cohort. *JAMA Psychiatry* **2014**, *71*, 1025–1031. [CrossRef]
21. Perkonigg, A.; Kessler, R.C.; Storz, S.; Wittchen, H.U. Traumatic events and post-traumatic stress disorder in the community: Prevalence, risk factors and comorbidity. *Acta Psychiatr. Scand.* **2000**, *101*, 46–59. [CrossRef]

22. Foa, E.B.; Stein, D.J.; McFarlane, A.C. Symptomatology and psychopathology of mental health problems after disaster. *J. Clin. Psychiatry* **2006**, *67*, 15–25.
23. Harville, E.W.; Xiong, X.; Pridjian, G.; Elkind-Hirsch, K.; Buekens, P. Postpartum mental health after Hurricane Katrina: A cohort study. *BMC Pregnancy Childbirth* **2009**, *9*, 21. [CrossRef]
24. Engel, S.M.; Berkowitz, G.S.; Wolff, M.S.; Yehuda, R. Psychological trauma associated with the World Trade Center attacks and its effect on pregnancy outcome. *Paediatr. Perinat. Epidemiol.* **2005**, *19*, 334–341. [CrossRef]
25. Harville, E.W.; Xiong, X.; Buekens, P.; Pridjian, G.; Elkind-Hirsch, K. Resilience after Hurricane Katrina among pregnant and postpartum women. *Women's Health Issues* **2010**, *20*, 20–27. [CrossRef] [PubMed]
26. Khatri, G.K.; Tran, T.D.; Baral, S.; Fisher, J. Effect of the 2015 Nepal Earthquakes on symptoms of common mental disorders among women who are pregnant. *J. Affect. Disord.* **2018**, *228*, 238–247. [CrossRef] [PubMed]
27. Hoffma, S.; Hatch, M.C. Stress, social support and pregnancy outcome: Reassessment based on recent research. *Paediatr. Perinat. Epidemiol.* **1996**, *10*, 380–405. [CrossRef] [PubMed]
28. Bonanno, G.A.; Galea, S.; Bucciarelli, A.; Vlahov, D. Psychological resilience after disaster: New York City in the aftermath of the September 11th terrorist attack. *Psychol. Sci.* **2006**, *17*, 181–186. [CrossRef]

Journal of
Clinical Medicine

MDPI

Article

Mental Health of Medical and Non-Medical Professionals during the Peak of the COVID-19 Pandemic: A Cross-Sectional Nationwide Study

Julian Maciaszek [1], Marta Ciulkowicz [1], Blazej Misiak [2], Dorota Szczesniak [1,*], Dorota Luc [3], Tomasz Wieczorek [1], Karolina Fila-Witecka [1], Pawel Gawlowski [4] and Joanna Rymaszewska [1]

1. Department of Psychiatry, Wroclaw Medical University, Pasteura 10 Str., 50-367 Wroclaw, Poland; julian.maciaszek@umed.wroc.pl (J.M.); marta.ciulkowicz@student.umed.wroc.pl (M.C.); tomasz.wieczorek@student.umed.wroc.pl (T.W.); karolina.fila-witecka@student.umed.wroc.pl (K.F.-W.); joanna.rymaszewska@umed.wroc.pl (J.R.)
2. Department of Genetics, Wroclaw Medical University, Marcinkowskiego 1 Str., 50-368 Wroclaw, Poland; blazej.misiak@umed.wroc.pl
3. Practice of Family Doctors M.V. Domanscy, E. Gepperta 13 Str., 50-072 Wroclaw, Poland; dorota.luc@gmail.com
4. Department of Emergency Medical Service, Wroclaw Medical University, Parkowa 34 Str., 51-616 Wroclaw, Poland; pawel.gawlowski@umed.wroc.pl

* Correspondence: dorota.szczesniak@umed.wroc.pl; Tel.: +48-71-784-16-00

Received: 11 July 2020; Accepted: 3 August 2020; Published: 5 August 2020

Abstract: Background: The study aimed to compare psychopathological expressions during the COVID-19 (novel coronavirus disease 2019) pandemic, as declared on March 11th 2020 by the World Health Organization, with respect to which institutional variables might distinguish the impact of COVID-19 in medical and non-medical professionals. Methods: A cross-sectional study was performed nationwide between 16th March and the 26th April 2020 in Poland. A total of 2039 respondents representing all healthcare providers (59.8%) as well as other professionals filled in the sociodemographic section, the General Health Questionnaire-28 and the author's questionnaire with questions related to exposure to severe acute respiratory syndrome coronavirus 2 (SARS-CoV-2) infection, the availability of protective measures, quarantine, change of working hours and place of employment during the pandemic, as well as feelings associated with the state of the pandemic. Results: Medical professionals more often presented with relevant psychopathological symptoms (GHQ-28 (General Health Questionnaire-28) total score >24) than the non-medical group (60.8% vs. 48.0%, respectively) such as anxiety, insomnia and somatic symptoms even after adjustment for potential confounding factors. Male sex, older age and appropriate protective equipment were associated with significantly lower GHQ-28 total scores in medical professionals, whereas among non-medical professionals, male sex was associated with significantly lower GHQ-28 total scores. Conclusions: Somatic and anxiety symptoms as well as insomnia are more prevalent among medical staff than workers in other professions. Targeting the determinants of these differences should be included in interventions aimed at restoring psychological well-being in this specific population. Apparently, there are present gender differences in psychological responses that are independent of profession.

Keywords: SARS-CoV-2; psychiatry; infectious disease; healthcare personnel; psychopathological symptoms

1. Introduction

The novel coronavirus disease 2019 (COVID-19) was identified in Wuhan, China, in December 2019 and attributed to severe acute respiratory syndrome coronavirus 2 (SARS-CoV-2) infection. Subsequently, a rapid transmission of COVID-19 occurred across China and affected other countries. Although epidemics of infectious diseases have always had their place in history, this time, globalization has facilitated the spread of SARS-CoV-2, causing a pandemic, which was announced on March 11, 2020, by the World Health Organization (WHO). In addition, the WHO has estimated the COVID-19 mortality rate to be 3.4% [1]. Epidemiological studies have provided further evidence that the mortality rate increases with age and is associated with comorbid physical health impairments, especially those related to the cardiovascular system. Although the pandemic has largely changed research priorities, specific treatments and vaccines are not available yet [2]. Consequently, the COVID-19 outbreak has emerged as a global medical, social and economic threat.

Apart from the direct consequences of COVID-19, it has been identified that the pandemic might have a great impact on mental health through various mechanisms. Firstly, it has been found that SARS-CoV-2 can impact the central nervous system, leading to acute psychiatric manifestations [3]. Secondly, social isolation and quarantine may trigger a number of maladaptive responses manifesting as post-traumatic stress symptoms, anxiety, fear, anger and confusion [4]. There is also evidence that quarantine conditions might have long-term effects on mental health [5]. It has been shown that individuals affected by the pandemic are struggling with the fear of uncertainty, death, loss of job, drastic changes of lifestyle, stigmatization, isolation, separation from family and beloved persons, disruption of the usual routine of life and grief [6]. The impact of the COVID-19 pandemic is also largely associated with the ongoing economic crisis, the loss of jobs and reduced revenues [7].

The severe psychological and physical impact on medical staff in terms of mental health outcomes has already been identified during previous epidemics [8–10]. Emerging evidence also indicates that medical staff might be particularly vulnerable to the negative effects of the COVID-19 pandemic [11]. Indeed, medical professionals standing on the front lines have direct contact with patients suspected of being infected. Consequently, many medical professionals became infected and some of them died [12]. In light of the growing mortality related to SARS-CoV-2 infection, long working time, a high level of uncertainty in the management of infected patients, healthcare workers are reporting increasing levels of anxiety associated with numerous clinical activities and present with symptoms of depression [13]. Although it has been observed that psychopathological expressions among medical professionals may differ from those observed in the general population, studies in this field have been performed with small samples and there is still a lack of nationwide studies [14]. In addition, several mechanisms underlying the specificity of psychopathological expressions among medical professionals need to be taken into consideration. These include various individual factors (e.g., age, sex and the presence of children) and institutional factors (e.g., the length of service, changes to working time and the availability of personal protective equipment).

Taking into account the limitations of previous studies and a number of research gaps, we aimed to compare psychopathological expressions during the COVID-19 pandemic in medical and non-medical professionals on the basis of a nationwide survey. Furthermore, we tested the hypothesis that there are various individual and institutional determinants of these responses that might distinguish the impact of COVID-19 on the psychological responses among two groups of professionals.

2. Materials and Methods

2.1. Participants

Data were collected through an online survey administered between 16th March 2020 and the 26th April 2020 in Poland. The study was initiated 12 days after the first case of SARS-CoV-2 infection had been detected in Poland and covered the period of a rapid increase in the incidence of COVID-19 with subsequent social restrictions [15]. Participants over the age of 18 years were invited to participate in the survey that was distributed through social media and email addresses. The study was addressed to representatives of all medical professions as well as professions not related to healthcare. Participants representing the medical profession groups included doctors, nurses, paramedics, allied healthcare workers (pharmacists, physiotherapists, occupational therapists, and psychologists), technicians and administrators. Data analysis was limited to completed questionnaires. The study was approved by the Ethics Committee at the Wroclaw Medical University (Poland), and all participants provided written informed consent. The study was performed in accordance with the principles of the Declaration of Helsinki.

2.2. Measures

The survey consisted of three sections: the sociodemographic section, the author's questionnaire and the General Health Questionnaire-28 (GHQ-28). The sociodemographic questionnaire recorded data on general demographic characteristics such as age, sex, place of residence, marital status, education and profession. The author's questionnaire was based on questions related to exposure to SARS-CoV-2 infection, the availability of protective measures, quarantine, change of working hours and the place of employment during the pandemic, as well as feelings associated with the state of the pandemic.

The GHQ-28 is a 28-item questionnaire used to identify minor psychiatric disorders in the general population, divided into four subscales. These are somatic symptoms (items 1, 3, 4, 8, 12, 14 and 16), anxiety and insomnia (items 2, 7, 9, 13, 15, 17 and 18), social dysfunction (items 5, 10, 11, 25, 26, 27 and 28) and severe depression (items 6, 19, 20, 21, 22, 23 and 24) [16]. The GHQ-28 items are based on the 4-point Likert scale (0—not at all, 1—no more than usual, 2—rather more than usual, and 3—much more than usual). The total score ranges between 0 and 84, where higher scores refer to higher levels of distress. The cut-off for clinical relevance was set at 24 points as described elsewhere [17].

2.3. Study Outcomes

To evaluate the primary outcome variables, we measured the severity of psychopathological symptoms reported by the healthcare professionals and representatives of other professions during the survey administration period. Additionally, in order to obtain the secondary outcome variables, we investigated the association between individual and institutional factors and psychopathological outcomes assessed through the GHQ-28 score.

2.4. Statistical Analyses

The Mann-Whitney U test (for continuous variables) and chi-square or Fisher's exact test (for qualitative variables) were used to compare groups. Due to multiple comparisons, the Bonferroni correction was applied to the level of significance. Taking into account 32 bivariate comparisons, the level of significance was finally set at 0.0016. Significant between-group differences in the levels of psychopathology after the Bonferroni correction were further tested using the analysis of co-variance (ANCOVA). The analysis of co-variance (ANCOVA) was performed to investigate the differences in the levels of psychopathological manifestations between medical and non-medical professionals after co-varying for potential confounding factors. Additionally, a linear regression model was prepared with the backward stepwise selection algorithm based on the Akaike information criteria. The model included continuous variables such as age and length of service and qualitative variables such as gender, protection against infection, major changes in private life, fear for personal health, fear for the health of loved ones, impact of media reports on mental state, frustration, loneliness because of isolation, anger, use of alcohol and nicotine and contact with COVID-19 without protective measures. The results of the ANCOVA and linear regression analysis were considered significant if the p-value was less than 0.05. All analyses were performed in R R Core Team (version 3.5.3, 2019, https://www.r-project.org/).

3. Results

3.1. Participants

The general characteristics of the sample are presented in Table 1. Out of 2039 participants, 1216 (59.6%) individuals represented medical professions while 823 (40.4%) pursued non-medical occupations. The vast majority of respondents, regardless of career, were women (80.0% among medical professionals and 74.4% among non-medical professionals). Data were collected from respondents representing all administrative regions in Poland, and the majority of them (63.2%) represented very big cities (>300,000 inhabitants). The medical professionals included physicians (47.3%), nurses (16.5%), pharmacists (7.3%), laboratory diagnosticians (5.9%), dentists (5.3%), paramedics (4.9%), clinical psychologists or psychotherapists (3.5%), physiotherapists (3.3%), midwives (2%), secretaries or medical recorders (1.4%), occupational medical technicians (1.4%), dental assistants (0.7%), care assistants (0.4%), medical interns (0.1%) and occupational therapists (0.1%). The non-medical professionals included administrative staff and accountants (16.6%), teachers and lecturers (14.3%), service and trade workers (12.4%), Information Technology employees (11.7%), engineers and other highly qualified employees (9.7%), entrepreneurs (3.5%), people in managerial positions (3.4), manual workers (2.4%), scientists (1.9%), journalists (1.6%), social workers (1.3%), non-clinical psychologists or psychotherapists (1.3%), technical workers (1.2%), employees of uniformed services (0.5%) and others (18.2%). The number of females was significantly higher among the medical professionals. This group of participants was more likely to report an urban place of residence, caring for a disabled person, major changes in private life, working on a shift schedule, contact with a COVID-19 patient without personal protective equipment, contact with COVID-19 patients at work, work experience of death due to COVID-19 and too few employees compared to the workload. They were also less likely to report having children, work location change during the pandemic and appropriate protection against infection. Finally, medical professionals had significantly higher weekly working time and length of service.

Table 1. General characteristics of medical professionals and individuals representing non-medical professionals.

	Medical Professionals, n = 1216	Non-Medical Professionals, n = 823	p-Value
Sex, females	973 (80.0%)	612 (74.4%)	0.003
Age, years	39.23 (12.26)	40.4 (13.24)	0.093
Urban place of residence	1177 (96.79%)	756(91.86%)	<0.001
In relationship or married	934 (76.8%)	619 (75.2%)	0.437
Having children	622 (51.2%)	468 (56.9%)	0.013
Caring for a disabled person	219 (18.1%)	100 (12.2%)	<0.001
Major changes in private life	229 (24.1%)	115(18%)	0.011
Working time (hours per week)	44.89 (14.27)	39.15 (11.18)	<0.001
Length of service (years)	14.59 (12.53)	18.84 (11.94)	<0.001
Work location change during the COVID-19 pandemic	359 (29.9%)	418 (62.1%)	<0.001
Increase in working time	218 (19.7%)	157 (25.7%)	0.041
Work in a shift system	507 (42.4%)	56 (8.4%)	<0.001
Contact with the COVID-19 patient without personal protective equipment	207 (17%)	41 (5%)	<0.001
Confirmed COVID-19 infection	12 (1%)	3 (0.4%)	0.121
Contact with the COVID-19 patients at work	289 (24.1%)	9 (1.3%)	<0.001
Work experience of death due to COVID-19	41 (3.4%)	7 (1%)	0.003
Appropriate protection against infection	356 (29.7%)	522 (77.9%)	<0.001
Too few employees compared to the workload	798 (66.4%)	236 (35.5%)	<0.001

COVID-19, novel coronavirus disease 2019. Data expressed as n (%) or mean (SD).

3.2. Psychopathological Outcomes

Medical professionals more often met the criterion for the presence of relevant psychopathological symptoms (a GHQ-28 total score > 24) than the non-medical group (60.8% vs. 48.0%, respectively). Moreover, they had also significantly higher GHQ-28 scores (all subscales and the total score) than the other participants (Table 2). The observed statistical power for detecting between-group differences in the GHQ-28 scores was as follows: 64.8% for severe depression, 100% for somatic symptoms, 100% for anxiety and insomnia, 64.5% for social dysfunction and 100% for the GHQ-28 total score. The ANCOVA revealed a significant effect of group (medical vs. non-medical professionals) on the level of somatic symptoms, anxiety and insomnia as well as the GHQ-28 total score after co-varying for the effects of potential confounding factors (Table 3). There were significant independent effects of sex in all the ANCOVA models. The effect of age appeared to be significant in the ANCOVA model testing that included the GHQ-28 total score, the anxiety and insomnia domain and the depression domain as a dependent variable. In turn, the effect of having children was independently negatively associated with the depression score, while the reports of caring for a disabled person were significantly associated with the GHQ-28 score for somatic symptoms. There was also a significant and independent effect of shift work on the score for the somatic symptoms domain. Finally, the effect of group appeared to be non-significant in the ANCOVA models that included the GHQ-28 scores for social dysfunction and depression.

Table 2. Measures of psychopathology in medical professionals and individuals representing non-medical professions.

	Medical Professionals, n =1216	Non-Medical Professions, n =823	p-Value
GHQ-28—total score	29.7 (14.9)	26.1 (14.8)	<0.001
GHQ-28—positive scoring	739 (60.8%)	395(48.0%)	< 0.001
GHQ-28—somatic symptoms	7.7 (4.6)	6.5 (4.5)	<0.001
GHQ-28—anxiety and insomnia	10.0 (5.4)	8.2 (5.3)	<0.001
GHQ-28—social dysfunction	8.5 (3.5)	8.2 (3.5)	0.037
GHQ-28—severe depression	3.5 (3.9)	3.2 (3.9)	0.036
The use of sedatives	177(14.8%)	85 (12.7%)	0.234
Fear for personal health	679 (55.9%)	328 (39.9%)	<0.001
Fear for the health of loved ones	714 (58.7%)	426 (51.8%)	<0.001
Worsening of mental health due to media reports	811 (66.7%)	482 (58.5%)	<0.001
Frustration	990 (81.4%)	612 (74.4%)	<0.001
Loneliness because of isolation	754 (62%)	501 (60.9%)	0.138
Anger	919 (75.6%)	521 (63.3%)	<0.001
Increased alcohol or nicotine intake	305 (25.1%)	145 (17.6%)	0.002

GHQ-28, General Health Questionnaire-28. Data expressed as n (%) or mean (SD).

Table 3. Psychopathological expressions in medical and non-medical professionals after adjustment for potential confounding factors.

	GHQ-28 Total Score		GHQ-28 Somatic Symptoms		GHQ-28 Anxiety and Insomnia	
	F	p	F	p	F	p
Medical/non-medical profession	13.877	<0.001	12.678	<0.001	25.988	<0.001
Sex	77.337	<0.001	88.272	<0.001	93.801	<0.001
Age	6.438	0.011	3.757	0.053	5.383	0.020
Place of residence	0.675	0.411	2.720	0.099	0.666	0.415
Children	0.983	0.322	0.006	0.939	0.040	0.841
Caring for a disabled person	3.396	0.066	4.448	0.035	2.515	0.113
Change in working time	1.406	0.236	1.003	0.317	0.613	0.434
Shift work	3.225	0.073	5.279	0.022	3.122	0.077

Significant effects ($p < 0.05$) are marked in bold.

3.3. Determinants of Psychopathological Outcomes in Medical and Non-Medical Professionals

The results of the linear regression analysis testing for the factors related to the GHQ-28 total scores in the medical and non-medical professionals are shown in Table 4. Male sex, older age and appropriate protection against infection were associated with significantly lower GHQ-28 total scores in medical professionals. In turn, fear for the health of loved ones was associated with significantly higher GHQ-28 total scores in this group of participants. Among both groups, major changes in private life, fear for personal health, following media reports, frustration, loneliness, anger and increased use of alcohol and nicotine were also significantly associated with higher GHQ-28 total scores. In non-medical professionals, contact with a COVID-19 patient without personal protection equipment was correlated with significantly higher GHQ-28 total scores. Male sex was associated with significantly lower GHQ-28 total scores in participants involved in non-medical professions.

Table 4. Factors related to the GHQ-28 total scores in medical and non-medical professionals (results of linear regression analysis).

Group of Participants	Variable	Beta	*p*-Value	VIF	95% CI
Medical professionals	male sex	−4.789	<0.000	1.11	−6.520–3.058
	age	−0.047	0.022	1.93	−0.121–0.028
	urban place of residence	2.266	0.239	1.03	−1.507–6.039
	in relationship or married	−0.196	0.816	1.12	−1.851–1.459
	having children	−0.812	0.375	1.84	−2.607–0.983
	caring for a disabled person	1.379	0.136	1.12	−0.435–3.193
	professional inactivity	0.428	0.861	1.08	−4.365–5.220
	contact with COVID-19 without protective measures	0.798	0.395	1.11	−1.042–2.639
	confirmed SARS-CoV-2 infection	3.995	0.256	1.08	−2.908–10.397
	confirmed SARS-CoV-2 infection among family or friends	−1.561	0.235	1.07	−4.142–1.019
	death due to COVID-19 among family or friends	−0.429	0.929	1.02	−9.857–8.998
	contact with people with COVID-19 at work	1.075	0.202	1.14	−0.578–2.727
	experience of death from COVID-19 in the workplace	0.716	0.712	1.10	−3.092–4.524
	appropriate protection against infection	−1.742	0.029	1.18	−3.309–0.174
	major changes in private life	2.916	<0.000	1.10	1.284–4.547
	fear for my health	6.290	<0.000	1.46	4.681–7.899
	fear for the health of loved ones	2.926	<0.000	1.41	1.332–4.521
	media reports worsen mental state	3.224	<0.000	1.48	1.522–4.927
	frustration	4.251	<0.000	1.46	2.202–6.299
	loneliness because of isolation	2.841	<0.000	1.24	1.323–4.359
	anger	2.708	0.003	1.32	0.927–4.489
	increased alcohol of nicotine intake	6.127	<0.000	1.08	4.549–7.706
Non-medical professions	male sex	−2.583	0.018	1.11	−4.718–0.448
	age	0.070	0.146	1.45	−0.025–0.164
	urban place of residence	−1.297	0.468	1.02	−4.804–2.210
	in relationship or married	−1.509	0.209	1.20	−3.866–0.849
	having children	−0.928	0.453	1.70	−3.359–1.502
	caring for a disabled person	−1.555	0.263	1.09	−4.281–1.171
	professional inactivity	−5.106	0.142	1.11	−11.935–1.722
	contact with COVID-19 without protective measures	4.637	0.029	1.10	0.472–8.802
	confirmed SARS-CoV-2 infection	12.555	0.150	1.09	−4.554–29.663
	confirmed SARS-CoV-2 infection among family or friends	1.149	0.574	1.10	−2.859–5.157
	death due to COVID-19 among family or friends	1.682	0.760	1.08	−9.128–12.491
	contact with people with COVID-19 at work	−0.755	0.852	1.04	−8.677–7.167
	experience of death from COVID-19 in the workplace	−8.593	0.063	1.06	−17.658–0.473
	appropriate protection against infection	−0.136	0.906	1.10	−2.404–2.131
	major changes in private life	4.014	0.003	1.18	1.381–6.646
	fear for my health	7.371	<0.000	1.58	5.075–9.666
	fear for the health of loved ones	1.250	0.245	1.38	-0.862–3.362
	media reports worsen mental state	3.827	0.001	1.40	1.667–5.988
	frustration	5.088	0.000	1.47	2.586–7.591
	loneliness because of isolation	3.673	0.001	1.33	1.552–5.794
	anger	3.454	0.001	1.27	1.350–5.557
	increased alcohol of nicotine intake	5.324	0.000	1.04	3.016–7.632

SARS-CoV-2, Severe acute respiratory syndrome coronavirus 2.

4. Discussion

Our study indicates the occurrence of maladaptive psychological responses to the COVID-19 pandemic among medical workers in comparison to that in people performing other professions in Poland. The findings from this survey imply that healthcare professionals present with higher levels of psychopathological symptoms in terms of anxiety, insomnia and somatic symptoms than those representing other professions, even after adjustment for potential confounding factors.

To our knowledge, this is the first study comparing medical and non-medical professionals in terms of psychopathological manifestation during the COVID-19 pandemic. Over 60% of medical professionals and 48% of individuals working in non-medical professions from the study sample presented clinically relevant psychopathological symptoms. These findings are similar to those reported by a recent population-based study in China that reported symptoms of depression, anxiety, distress and insomnia in 34.0–71.5% of medical workers [18]. Similarly, another study reported that 63% of medical workers in Wuhan, China, demonstrated various psychopathological symptoms [19]. However, a lower prevalence of psychopathological symptoms compared to in our study was observed by the authors of the recent cross-sectional survey study based on over 4000 healthcare workers from Wuhan in which 39.1% of the study participants had psychological distress [20]. Lai et al. suggested that nurses, women, frontline medical workers and those working in Wuhan, China, were more likely to report various psychopathological symptoms [18], which is consistent with our findings in the relation to female sex. The vast majority of our results confirm observations from Asian countries during the initial stages of the COVID-19 pandemic [2,21]. Recently, there have been only a few reports defining the role of factors affecting the development of psychiatric symptoms in the pandemic [19,22–24]. However, there is still a lack of research identifying institutional and individual risk and protective factors affecting the mental health of healthcare workers and other citizens during the pandemic.

This study emphasizes that one of the most important institutional factors that affects mental health is the provision to medical workers of a sense of security in the workplace. The results point to the importance of appropriate protection against infection as the main mental-health-related factor during the pandemic that affects all the domains. This is in accordance with recent studies related to medical staff, which identify access to personal protective equipment as an independent predictor of a lower level of mental distress [25,26] as well as one of the main concerns of healthcare workers [20]. It seems that these results are not revealing; however, at the same time, our findings show that the vast majority of staff deem the institution's activities in providing security to be insufficient. This is likely not unique to Poland, as recent studies have also found a lack of personal protective equipment being reported by medical health workers across other countries [27–29]. Furthermore, the present study highlights that the sense of security could be considered from different perspectives. Both groups of medical and non-medical professionals revealed anxiety about the state of their health. This is consistent with the cross-sectional study performed in China in which the authors suggested the fear of being infected to be a risk factor for mental distress [30]. However, this study highlights another important factor, which is the fear for loved ones, that was visible only among medical professions. Medical workers remain with an internal dilemma related, on the one hand, to a sense of loyalty to the profession and their patients and, on the other hand, to the responsibility for their families [31]. This is confirmed by the recent study from Wuhan in which the authors demonstrated that the majority of healthcare workers were concerned about the infection of family members [20]. This kind of long-lasting internal emotional tension might be manifested in psychopathological symptoms among most medical workers during a pandemic, which has already been observed in 2003 during the outbreak of severe acute respiratory syndrome (SARS) [32] and in 2014–2015 during the Ebola outbreak [33]. Despite the discussed fear regarding the infection of family members among medical professionals on the one hand, we emphasized the protective effect of having children on the development of depressive symptoms and, on the other hand, the relationship between care for an elderly person and the severity of psychopathological symptoms. From an individual-level perspective, this study indicates that men were less prone to the presence of psychopathological symptoms. In our study, male sex appeared to be negatively associated with total GHQ-28 scores, which was observed among both medical and non-medical professionals. These reports are similar to the results of recent studies performed in China in which being female was considered a significant risk factor for the development of severe depressive and anxiety symptoms, and distress [18,22].

We emphasized that following media reports was a risk factor for developing psychopathological symptoms among both groups. Our results correspond with another Wuhan online survey study [34] where spending over 2 h checking COVID-19-related information via social media was correlated with anxiety and depressive symptoms. The issue of the impact of excessive searching for COVID-19 news on mental health is particularly up to date according to recent studies, which confirm that the pandemic affected the content searched on the internet [35,36].

We observed that medical professionals more often than other respondents suffered from somatic symptoms as well as anxiety and insomnia. A higher prevalence of somatic symptoms during stressful situations, such as work in outbreak conditions, can be considered a physiological reaction caused by increased activity of the autonomic nervous system. Although a short-term hyperactivity of the sympathetic nervous system does not lead to any serious health-related consequences, the prolonged hyperactivity of the stress-related hypothalamic-pituitary-adrenal axis might lead to fatigue, depression, and other health-related outcomes [37–39]. As demonstrated by studies on previous outbreaks [40,41], some of the medical workers during the SARS-CoV-2 pandemic may be at risk for post-traumatic stress disorder, which also appears to be connected with prolonged hypothalamic–pituitary–adrenal (HPA) axis overactivity [42,43]. From a psychodynamic perspective, prolonged emotional tension can lead medical workers to channel difficult emotional experiences into somatic symptoms and insomnia, which are easier for them to accept than developing depressive symptoms that may lead to an occupational dysfunction and could be understood as the effect of defense mechanisms.

There are some limitations of this study that need to be discussed. Firstly, we did not record the initial number of individuals approached for participation and the reasons for non-participation were not recorded. Therefore, the representativeness of the sample is limited. Another point is that the assessment of psychopathological symptoms was limited to the use of GHQ-28, and thus, we were not able to record specific diagnoses. It should also be noted that our survey was not administered longitudinally. In this regard, the temporal patterns of psychopathological expressions were not addressed. Another limitation is response bias due to the online form of the questionnaire distribution.

In summary, our study provides evidence that medical professionals are more vulnerable to developing anxiety, insomnia and somatic symptoms in response to the pandemic. In addition, thedeterminants of psychopathological expressions in these two groups differ in terms of age, care for an elderly or disabled person, contact with COVID-19 at work and contact with COVID-19 without protection measures. Apparently, there are present gender differences in psychological responses that are independent of the profession.

Nevertheless, these findings create grounds for personalizing interventions that aim to restore psychological wellbeing in medical and non-medical professionals as well as emphasizing key factors affecting the greater susceptibility for a negative psychological response during the pandemic, some of which are modifiable.

Author Contributions: Conceptualization, J.M. and M.C.; methodology, B.M. and D.S.; software, B.M.; validation, D.S. and J.R.; formal analysis, J.R.; investigation, J.M., M.C., B.M., D.S. and J.R.; resources, M.C., D.L., K.F.-W., T.W. and P.G.; data curation, B.M.; writing—original draft preparation, J.M., D.S. and B.M.; writing—review and editing, J.R., D.S. and B.M.; visualization, K.F.-W. and P.G.; supervision, J.R.; project administration, J.R.; funding acquisition, J.R. All authors have read and agreed to the published version of the manuscript.

Funding: This research was funded by Wroclaw Medical University, grant number ST.C230.18.014 and the article processing charge was financed from the funds granted by the Ministry of Science and Higher Education in the „Regional Initiative of Excellence" programme for the years 2019–2022, project number 016/RID/2018/19.

Acknowledgments: This study was supported by the Wroclaw Medical University grant (No. ST.C230.18.014).

Conflicts of Interest: The authors declare no conflict of interest. The funders had no role in the design of the study; in the collection, analyses, or interpretation of data; in the writing of the manuscript; or in the decision to publish the results.

References

1. World Health Organization. WHO Director-General's Opening Remarks at the Media Briefing on COVID-19. 3 March 2020. Available online: https://www.who.int/dg/speeches/detail/who-director-general-s-opening-remarks-at-the-media-briefing-on-covid-19---3-march-2020 (accessed on 17 May 2020).
2. Zhang, C.; Yang, L.; Liu, S.; Ma, S.; Wang, Y.; Cai, Z.; Du, H.; Li, R.; Kang, L.; Su, M.; et al. Survey of Insomnia and Related Social Psychological Factors Among Medical Staff Involved in the 2019 Novel Coronavirus Disease Outbreak. *Front. Psychiatry* **2020**, *11*, 306. [CrossRef] [PubMed]
3. Troyer, E.A.; Kohn, J.N.; Hong, S. Are we facing a crashing wave of neuropsychiatric sequelae of COVID-19? Neuropsychiatric symptoms and potential immunologic mechanisms. *Brain Behav. Immun.* **2020**, *87*, 34–39. [CrossRef] [PubMed]
4. Brooks, S.K.; Webster, R.K.; Smith, L.E.; Woodland, L. The psychological impact of quarantine and how to reduce it: Rapid review of the evidence. *Lancet* **2020**, *395*, 912–920. [CrossRef]
5. Lei, L.; Huang, X.; Zhang, S.; Yang, J.; Yang, L.; Xu, M. Comparison of Prevalence and Associated Factors of Anxiety and Depression Among People Affected by versus People Unaffected by Quarantine During the COVID-19 Epidemic in Southwestern China. *Med. Sci. Monit.* **2020**, *26*, e924609. [CrossRef] [PubMed]
6. Schwerdtle, P.; Morphet, J.; Hall, H. A scoping review of mentorship of health personnel to improve the quality of health care in low and middle-income countries. *Glob. Health* **2017**, *13*, 77. [CrossRef]
7. Nicola, M.; Alsafi, Z.; Sohrabi, C.; Kerwan, A.; Al-Jabir, A.; Iosifidis, C.; Agha, M.; Agha, R. The socio-economic implications of the coronavirus pandemic (COVID-19): A review. *Int. J. Surg.* **2020**, *78*, 185–193. [CrossRef]
8. Straus, S.E.; Wilson, K.; Rambaldini, G.; Rath, D.; Lin, Y.; Gold, W. Severe acute respiratory syndrome and its impact on professionalism: Qualitative study of physicians' behaviour during an emerging healthcare crisis. *BMJ* **2004**, *29*, 83. [CrossRef]
9. Lin, C.Y.; Peng, Y.C.; Wu, Y.H.; Chang, J.; Chan, C.H.; Yang, D.Y. The psychological effect of severe acute respiratory syndrome on emergency department staff. *Emerg. Med. J.* **2007**, *24*, 12–17. [CrossRef]
10. Goulia, P.; Mantas, C.; Dimitroula, D.; Mantis, D.; Hyphantis, T. General hospital staff worries, perceived sufficiency of information and associated psychological distress during the A/H1N1 influenza pandemic. *BMC Infect. Dis.* **2010**, *10*, 322. [CrossRef]
11. Williamson, V.; Murphy, D.; Greenberg, N. COVID-19 and experiences of moral injury in front-line key workers. *Occup. Med.* **2020**, kqaa052. [CrossRef]
12. Wu, J.T.; Leung, K.; Bushman, M.; Kishore, N.; Niehus, R.; De Salazar, P.M.; Cowling, B.J.; Lipsitch, M.; Leung, G.M. Estimating clinical severity of COVID-19 from the transmission dynamics in Wuhan, China. *Nat. Med.* **2020**, *26*, 506–510. [CrossRef] [PubMed]
13. Neto, M.L.R.; Almeida, H.G.; Esmeraldo, J.D.; Nobre, C.B.; Pinheiro, W.R.; De Oliveira, C.R.T.; Sousa, I.D.C.; Lima, O.M.M.L.; Lima, N.N.R.; Moreira, M.M.; et al. When health professionals look death in the eye: The mental health of professionals who deal daily with the 2019 coronavirus outbreak. *Psychiatry Res.* **2020**, *288*, 112972. [CrossRef] [PubMed]
14. Neto, M.L.R.; Almeida, H.G.; Esmeraldo, J.D.; Nobre, C.B.; Pinheiro, W.R.; De Oliveira, C.R.T.; Sousa, I.D.C.; Lima, O.M.M.L.; Lima, N.N.R.; Moreira, M.M.; et al. Multidisciplinary research priorities for the COVID-19 pandemic: A call for action for mental health science. *Lancet Psychiatry* **2020**, *7*, 547–560. [CrossRef]
15. Pinkas, J.; Jankowski, M.; Szumowski, Ł.; Lusawa, A.; Zgliczyński, W.S.; Raciborski, F. Public Health Interventions to Mitigate Early Spread of SARS-CoV-2 in Poland. *Med. Sci. Monit.* **2020**, *26*, e924730. [CrossRef] [PubMed]
16. Goldberg, D.; Hillier, V.F. A scaled version of the General Health Questionnaire. *Psychol. Med.* **1979**, *9*, 139–145. [CrossRef] [PubMed]
17. Makowska, Z.; Merecz, D. Polish adaptation of David Goldberg's general health questionnaire: GHQ-12, GHQ-28. In *Mental Health Evaluation Based on D. Goldberg's Questionnaires*, 1st ed.; Nofer Institute of Occupational Medicine: Lodz, Poland, 2002.
18. Lai, J.; Ma, S.; Wang, Y.; Cai, Z.; Hu, J.; Wei, N. Factors Associated with Mental Health Outcomes Among Health Care Workers Exposed to Coronavirus Disease 2019. *JAMA Netw. Open* **2020**, *3*, e203976. [CrossRef]

19. Kang, L.; Ma, S.; Chen, M.; Yang, J.; Wang, Y.; Li, R.; Yao, L.; Bai, H.; Cai, Z.; Yang, B.X.; et al. Impact on mental health and perceptions of psychological care among medical and nursing staff in Wuhan during the 2019 novel coronavirus disease outbreak: A cross-sectional study. *Brain Behav. Immun.* **2020**, *87*, 11–17. [CrossRef]
20. Rangachari, P.L.; Woods, J. Preserving Organizational Resilience, Patient Safety, and Staff Retention during COVID-19 Requires a Holistic Consideration of the Psychological Safety of Healthcare Workers. *Int. J. Environ. Res. Public Health* **2020**, *17*, 4267. [CrossRef]
21. Tan, B.Y.; Chew, N.W.; Lee, G.K.; Jing, M.; Goh, Y.; Yeo, L.L.; Zhang, K.; Chin, H.-K.; Ahmad, A.; Khan, F.A.; et al. Psychological Impact of the COVID-19 Pandemic on Health Care Workers in Singapore. *Ann. Intern. Med.* **2020**, *20*, 1083. [CrossRef]
22. Wang, C.; Pan, R.; Wan, X.; Tan, Y.; Xu, L.; Ho, C.S.; Ho, R.C. Immediate Psychological Responses and Associated Factors During the Initial Stage of the 2019 Coronavirus Disease (COVID-19) Epidemic Among the General Population in China. *Int. J. Environ. Res. Public Health* **2020**, *17*, 1729. [CrossRef]
23. Li, Z.; Ge, J.; Yang, M.; Feng, J.; Qiao, M.; Jiang, R.; Bi, J.; Zhan, G.; Xu, X.; Wang, L.; et al. Vicarious traumatization in the general public, members, and non-members of medical teams aiding in COVID-19 control. *Brain Behav. Immun.* **2020**, *88*, 916–919. [CrossRef] [PubMed]
24. Sasangohar, F.; Jones, S.L.; Masud, F.N.; Vahidy, F.S.; Kash, B.A. Provider Burnout and Fatigue during the COVID-19 Pandemic: Lessons Learned from a High-Volume Intensive Care Unit. *Anesth. Analg.* **2020**, *131*, 106–111. [CrossRef] [PubMed]
25. Zhang, S.X.; Liu, J.; Jahanshahi, A.A.; Nawaser, K.; Yousefi, A.; Li, J.; Sun, S. At the height of the storm: Healthcare staff's health conditions and job satisfaction and their associated predictors during the epidemic peak of COVID-19. *Brain Behav. Immun.* **2020**, *87*, 144–146. [CrossRef] [PubMed]
26. Amerio, A.; Bianchi, D.; Santi, F.; Costantini, L.; Odone, A.; Signorelli, C.; Costanza, A.; Serafini, G.; Amore, M.; Aguglia, A. Covid-19 pandemic impact on mental health: A web-based cross-sectional survey on a sample of Italian general practitioners. *Acta Biomed.* **2020**, *91*, 83–88. [CrossRef]
27. Raurell-Torredà, M.; Martínez-Estalella, G.; Frade-Mera, M.J.; Carrasco Rodríguez-Rey, L.F.; Romero de San Pío, E. Reflections Arising From the COVID-19 Pandemic. *Enferm. Intensiva* **2020**, *31*, 90–93. [CrossRef] [PubMed]
28. Ranney, M.L.; Griffeth, V.; Jha, A.K. Critical Supply Shortages—The Need for Ventilators and Personal Protective Equipment during the Covid-19 Pandemic. *N. Engl. J. Med.* **2020**, *382*, e41. [CrossRef] [PubMed]
29. Delgado, D.; Quintana, F.W.; Perez, G.; Liprandi, A.S.; Ponte-Negretti, C.; Mendoza, I.; Baranchuk, A. Personal Safety during the COVID-19 Pandemic: Realities and Perspectives of Healthcare Workers in Latin America. *Int. J. Environ. Res. Public Health* **2020**, *17*, 2798. [CrossRef]
30. Lu, W.; Wang, H.; Lin, Y.; Li, L. Psychological status of medical work force during the COVID-19 pandemic: A cross-sectionalstudy. *Psychiatry Res.* **2020**, *288*, 112936. [CrossRef]
31. Walton, M.; Murray, E.; Christian, M.D. Mental health care for medical staff and affiliated healthcare workers during the COVID-19 pandemic. *Eur. Heart J. Acute Cardiovasc. Care* **2020**, *9*, 241–247. [CrossRef]
32. Maunder, R.G.; Lancee, W.J.; Balderson, K.E.; Bennett, J.P.; Borgundvaag, B.; Evans, S.; Fernandes, C.M.; Goldbloom, D.S.; Gupta, M.; Hunter, J.J.; et al. Long-term psychological and occupational effects of providing hospital healthcare during SARS outbreak. *Emerg. Infect. Dis.* **2006**, *12*, 1924–1932. [CrossRef]
33. Ji, D.; Ji, Y.-J.; Duan, X.-Z.; Li, W.-G.; Sun, Z.-Q.; Song, X.-A.; Meng, Y.-H.; Tang, H.-M.; Chu, F.; Niu, X.-X.; et al. Prevalence of psychological symptoms among Ebola survivors and health care workers during the 2014-2015 Ebola outbreak in Sierra Leone: A cross-sectional study. *Oncotarget* **2017**, *8*, 12784–12791. [CrossRef] [PubMed]
34. Ni, M.Y.; Yang, L.; Leung, C.M.C.; Li, N.; Yao, X.I.; Wang, Y.; Leung, G.; Cowling, B.J.; Liao, Q.; Da Silva, E.; et al. Mental Health, Risk Factors, and Social Media Use During the COVID-19 Epidemic and Cordon Sanitaire among the Community and Health Professionals in Wuhan, China: Cross-Sectional Survey. *JMIR Ment. Health* **2020**, *7*, e19009. [CrossRef] [PubMed]
35. Effenberger, M.; Kronbichler, A.; Shin, J.I.; Mayer, G.; Tilg, H.; Perco, P. Association of the COVID-19 pandemic with Internet Search Volumes: A Google TrendsTM Analysis. *Int. J. Infect. Dis.* **2020**, *95*, 192–197. [CrossRef]
36. Misiak, B.; Szcześniak, D.; Koczanowicz, L.; Rymaszewska, J. The COVID-19 outbreak and Google searches: Is it really the time to worry about global mental health? *Brain Behav. Immun.* **2020**, *87*, 126–127. [CrossRef] [PubMed]

37. Adam, E.K.; Quinn, M.E.; Tavernier, R.; McQuillan, M.T.; Dahlke, K.A.; Gilbert, K.E. Diurnal cortisol slopes and mental and physical health outcomes: A systematic review and meta-analysis. *Psychoneuroendocrinology* **2017**, *83*, 25–41. [CrossRef] [PubMed]
38. Stetler, C.; Miller, G.E. Depression and hypothalamic-pituitary-adrenal activation: A quantitative summary of four decades of research. *Psychosom. Med.* **2011**, *73*, 114–126. [CrossRef]
39. Juruena, M.F.; Eror, F.; Cleare, A.J.; Young, A.H. The Role of Early Life Stress in HPA Axis and Anxiety. *Adv. Exp. Med. Biol.* **2020**, *1191*, 141–153. [CrossRef]
40. Wu, K.K.; Chan, S.K.; Ma, T.M. Posttraumatic stress, anxiety, and depression in survivors of severe acute respiratory syndrome (SARS). *J. Trauma. Stress* **2005**, *18*, 39–42. [CrossRef]
41. Jalloh, M.F.; Li, W.; Bunnell, R.E.; Ethier, K.A.; O'Leary, A.; Hageman, K.M.; Sengeh, P.; Jalloh, M.B.; Morgan, O.; Hersey, S.; et al. Impact of Ebola experiences and risk perceptions on mental health in Sierra Leone, July 2015. *BMJ Glob. Health* **2018**, *3*, e000471. [CrossRef]
42. Klaassens, E.R.; Giltay, E.J.; Cuijpers, P.; Zitman, F.G. Adulthood trauma and HPA-axis functioning in healthy subjects and PTSD patients: A meta-analysis. *Psychoneuroendocrinology* **2019**, *37*, 317–331. [CrossRef]
43. Schumacher, S.; Niemeyer, H.; Engel, S.; Cwik, J.C.; Laufer, S.; Klusmann, H.; Knaevelsrud, C. HPA axis regulation in posttraumatic stress disorder: A meta-analysis focusing on potential moderators. *Neurosci. Biobehav. Rev.* **2019**, *100*, 35–57. [CrossRef] [PubMed]

Journal of
Clinical Medicine

MDPI

Review

The Interrelation of Neurological and Psychological Symptoms of COVID-19: Risks and Remedies

Mohammad Nami [1,2,3,4,5,*,†], Bharathi S. Gadad [6,*,†], Li Chong [7,8,9], Usman Ghumman [6], Amogh Misra [10], Shrikanth S. Gadad [11,12,13], Dharmendra Kumar [14], George Perry [15], Samuel J. K. Abraham [16] and K. S. Rao [1,*]

1 Neuroscience Center, Instituto de Investigaciones Científicas y Servicios de Alta Tecnología (INDICASAT AIP), City of Knowledge 084301103, Panama
2 Department of Neuroscience, School of Advanced Medical Sciences and Technologies, Shiraz University of Medical Sciences, Shiraz 71348-14336, Iran
3 Dana Brain Health Institute, Iranian Neuroscience Society-Fars Chapter, Shiraz 71364-76172, Iran
4 Academy of Health, Senses Cultural Foundation, Sacramento, CA 66006, USA
5 Department of Cognitive Neuroscience, Institute for Cognitive Science Studies (ICSS), Pardis, Tehran 1658344575, Iran
6 Department of Psychiatry, Paul L. Foster School of Medicine, Texas Tech University Health Sciences Center at El Paso, El Paso, TX 79905, USA
7 Beijing Zhongke Jianlan Biotechnology Co., Ltd., Beijing 100101, China; chongli@moon.ibp.ac.cn
8 Zhongke Jianlan International Medical Research Institute, Melbourne, Victoria 3000-3999, Australia
9 Institute of Biophysics, Chinese Academy of Sciences, Beijing 100101, China
10 Department of Biochemistry, University of Texas, Austin, TX 78712, USA; kjr5n2009@gmail.com
11 Center of Emphasis in Cancer, Department of Molecular and Translational Medicine, Paul L. Foster School of Medicine, Texas Tech University Health Sciences Center El Paso, El Paso, TX 79905, USA; shrikanth.gadad@ttuhsc.edu
12 Department of Molecular and Translational Medicine, Paul L. Foster School of Medicine, Texas Tech University Health Sciences Center El Paso, El Paso, TX 79905, USA
13 Graduate School of Biomedical Sciences, Texas Tech University Health Sciences Center El Paso, El Paso, TX 79905, USA
14 Greater Heights Holistic Psychiatry, Houston, TX 77008, USA; Drkumar.dharmendra@gmail.com
15 Semmes Foundation Distinguished University Chair in Neurobiology, The University of Texas, San Antonio, TX 78249, USA; george.perry@utsa.edu
16 School of Medicine, Yamanashi University, Chuo 409-3898, Japan; drsam@nichimail.jp
* Correspondence: torabnami@sums.ac.ir (M.N.); bharathi.gadad@ttuhsc.edu (B.S.G.); jrao@indicasat.org.pa (K.S.R.)
† Both share equal first authorship.

Received: 29 June 2020; Accepted: 3 August 2020; Published: 13 August 2020

Abstract: COVID-19 has catastrophically affected the world's panoramic view of human well-being in terms of healthcare and management. With the increase in the number of cases worldwide, neurological symptoms and psychological illnesses from COVID-19 have increasingly upsurged. Mental health illness and affective disorders, including depression, obsessive-compulsive disorder, anxiety, phobia, and panic disorders, are highly impacted due to social distress. The COVID-19 pandemic not only affected people with pre-existing mental and affective illnesses, but also healthy individuals with anxiety, worrying, and panic symptoms, and fear conditioning. In addditon, the novel coronavirus is known to impact the central nervous system in the brain, resulting in severe and certain long-lasting neurological issues. Owing to the significance of neurological and psychological events, the present perspective has been an attempt to disseminate the impact of COVID-19 on neural injury through inflammation, and its interrelation with psychological symptoms. In this current review, we synthesize the literature to highlight the critical associations between SARS-CoV-2 infection and the nervous system, and mental health illness, and discuss potential mechanisms of neural injury through psycho-neuroimmunity.

Keywords: mental health; COVID-19; neurological; psychological; inflammation

1. Introduction

The current world has changed in all shapes since the emergence of the novel coronavirus. COVID-19 is a deadly virus and is also extremely contagious. The rapidly emerging COVID-19 pandemic has been taking a toll not only on overall health but also on the mental health of the general public, and especially those with previous history or episodes of mental illness [1]. A significant fraction of stress arises from the experience of monitoring ourselves or being monitored by others for the possible signs and symptoms of the disease [2]. Meanwhile, much of the mental health issues related to the COVID-19 pandemic stem from accumulating worries and concerns related to continued isolation, financial insecurity, contamination, and less-likelihood in returning to normality. Of note, the current state of health emergency has forced millions of people to stay socially distant from friends, family, colleagues, and even from their pets. Summing this up with the exponential fear, worrisome daily news, and fearful updates as well as the looming indefinite future, the rate of anxiety and stress- and fear-related disorders and depression seem to be on a steep rise. This is partly because we face a global issue, and as such, a global coalition is required to battle against COVID-19 [3].

In the latest pandemic time, it has become apparent that neurological and psychological involvement in COVID-19 are increasingly rising in the patient population. A subset of COVID patients is affected by neurological events such as headache, dizziness, or cerebrovascular symptoms [4–7]. The latest reports have also shown a sudden onset of anosmia and ageusia as an early sign of SARS-CoV-2 infection, suggesting that early neurological involvement might be highly relevant [4,5,7]. Currently, long-term neurological complications from COVID-19 infection are of great concern. Besides, the overarching issue is the situation of the socio-economic crisis and psychological distress rapidly occurring worldwide. Although social activities have been restricted in most countries, almost all movements were prohibited due to quarantine, leading to many psychological problems. The most critical consequences of the COVID-19 epidemic are of increased mental health issues, including stress, anxiety, and panic symptoms, and depression that has emerged increasingly [6,8]. The most common psychological symptoms are generalized fear and pervasive community anxiety, typically associated with disease outbreaks, with the escalation of new cases leading to increased anxiety and panic symptoms [6,8]. Overall, in this present review, we synthesize the literature to highlight the significant associations between SARS-CoV-2 infection and the nervous system, and mental health illness, and discuss potential mechanisms of neural injury through psychoneuroimmunity. Awareness of the possible psychoneurological manifestations in COVID-19 patients is of utmost importance for the management of potentially life-threatening and long-lasting psycho-neurological complications.

2. Key Challenges

The strong conditioned fear and anxiety about a disease potentially lead to often-overwhelming emotional dysregulation and mood changes both in adults and children [3]. Evidence has supported the notion that stress-related disorders not only leave an impact on overall mental health but also leverage neurocognitive predicaments. Indeed, stress is regarded as a significant yet under-appreciated factor in neurodegenerative diseases [9]. The critical challenge is that how we may cope with such growing anxiety differs in people based on their mental health background and the community or support system they live in [10].

The increased number of COVID-19 patients and shortage of staff and limited number of social interactions with physicians or healthcare professionals [11] led to a decline in face-to-face consultations and an increase in telemedicine. This, in turn, has caused elevations in stress levels, especially in individuals with severe mental health problems [12]. Moreover, because of COVID-19, all the elective surgical procedures have been postponed or canceled. They have caused immense stress in people that were scheduled for elective surgical procedures and those who require face-to-face consultations [13]. Some people including

(1) older adults or those with a chronic health problem, (2) children and adolescents, (3) those who help with COVID-19 such as first-line physicians and healthcare professionals, and (4) individuals with underlying mental health issues, affective disorders, and substance abusers are expected to experience and may reveal more substantial distressing worries in the present crisis [14].

The above can, in turn, alter one's affective health, cognitive fitness, sleeping, and eating patterns whereby maladaptive motivational structures such as the use of alcohol, smoking, and substance abuse tend to develop. As for the people with pre-existing mental illness, awareness about emerging or worsening symptoms becomes crucial. Individuals' reciprocal care and support and the significance of family function in today's crisis not only help people cope better with such anxiety but also make communities stronger against the COVID-19 physical and mental health burden [15–17]. Apart from all the recommended self-care measures for mental health and stress management, which we will briefly summarize here, the below points may also be of value where applicable. Such advice would include: (1) following the local public healthcare providers' advice and refraining from ill-advised comments, (2) seeking mental health services online or teletherapy where applicable and possible, (3) requesting prescription refills for the next 90 days supply in case one is taking particular medicines and adherence to medication therapy where needed, and (4) raising awareness on self-care particularly in people of a higher risk profile [18]. This would per se increase the risk and subsequent worry that the disease would spread faster and take a higher toll.

3. Geographical Distribution of COVID-19

Globally, more than 16 million confirmed cases of COVID-19 have been reported. By 28 June 2020, so far, the number of cases stands at 10,243,859 cases with 504,410 deaths and 5,553,495 recovered worldwide; the United States has topped the list among all the countries in the world with total cases 2,596,537; 128,152 deaths; 1,081,437 recovered; 1,386,948 confirmed cases; and 15,816 are in critical condition (courtesy: www.worldometers.info/coronavirus) (Figure 1). With the increase in the number of cases in the United States and worldwide, the active cases in the United States have surpassed the numbers recovered, which is an alarming situation that needs to be addressed. The number of cases and deaths data were accessed from the WHO and CDC until 28 June 2020. However, the case fatality rate is low for SARS-CoV2 (3–4%) in comparison with SARS-CoV (9.6%), case fatality source: https://www.worldometers.info/coronavirus/coronavirus-death-rate/ Also the death rate compared to active confirmed cases is low. To succumb to the current situation, strict rules and regulations from the CDC must be followed to reduce the number of cases. However, with these numbers of cases reported, it is unclear how many of the COVID-19 subjects have secondary complications with neurological or psychosocial or mental health issues. It is also the need of the hour to screen for other illnesses that have been impacted by COVID-19.

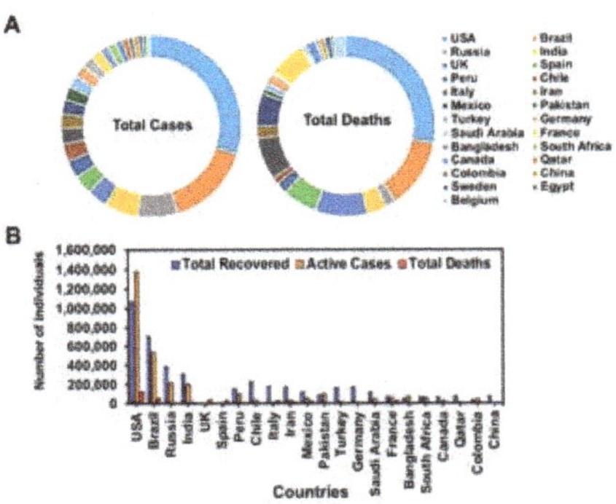

Figure 1. Total number of COVID-19 cases worldwide (25 countries on the list). Total confirmed cases and total deaths based on the countries (**A**), graphical representation of total recovered active cases, and fatalities based on the top 25 countries (**B**).

4. Psychological and Neurological Symptoms of COVID-19

The major psychological symptoms among people include signs of anxiety, panic attacks, depression, and suicide [19,20]. To elaborate, the symptoms include persistent worrying or feeling overwhelmed by emotions; restlessness and irritability; sleep problems like insomnia or excessive sleeping; sweating, trembling, shortness of breath, or a sense of choking; and lack of interest, significant weight loss/gain, feelings of worthlessness or excessive guilt, and repeated thoughts of death or suicide [6,19,20]. In the latest report from Ellul et al. (2020), it was observed that in patients with COVID-19 with a neurological or psychiatric disease reported for over three weeks, the majority of them had an altered mental status, which included encephalopathy, with a neuropsychiatric diagnosis, including psychosis, neurocognitive syndrome, and affective disorders [7]. Notably, patients had a cerebrovascular event, ischemic strokes, intracerebral hemorrhages, CNS vasculitis, and other cerebrovascular events [6,7]. Hence, it is highly essential to understand the underlying biological mechanism on how these psychoneurological events are affected by COVID-19.

5. Psychological Impact from COVID-19

In recent times, the COVID-19 pandemic has immensely led to an epidemiological and psychological crisis. With the increase in the days of lockdown worldwide, living in isolation, changes in our daily lives, job loss, financial hardship, and death of loved ones have tremendously impacted on the potential to affect mental health-related issues [19,20]. During the time of social distancing, psychological symptoms and mental health issues have increased around the world.

In a recent review published in Lancet recently by Brooks et al. (2020), a study comparing post-traumatic stress symptoms in both parents and children quarantined vs. not quarantined found that the mean post-traumatic stress scores were 4-fold higher in children who had been isolated than in those who were not isolated [21]. A total of 28% (27 of 98) of parents quarantined in this study reported revealed symptoms of a trauma-related mental health disorder. All other quantitative studies were based on survey data, and reported a high prevalence of signs of psychological distress and disease [21]. So far, the studies published in the literature are high in general psychological symptoms, emotional disturbance, depression, stress, low mood, irritability, insomnia, post-traumatic stress symptoms, anger, and emotional exhaustion [21].

A study conducted by Pappa et al. (2020) was based on the protocols registered on PROSPERO which is based on the data pooled using random-effects meta-analyses to study the prevalence of specific mood-related issues [20]. The PROSPERO study was conducted on healthcare professionals [20], where a total number of 33,062 participants with 13 studies were included for the meta-analyses. In 12 studies, anxiety was assessed with a prevalence rate of 32%, and major depression in 10 studies with an incidence rate of 22.8% [20,22,23]. Further, female healthcare professionals revealed higher rates of mental health-related symptoms compared to male healthcare workers. Furthermore, insomnia prevalence was estimated at 38.9%, suggesting that sleep disturbances were observed to be a significant issue [20,22,23]. Based on these pieces of evidence, healthcare professionals and others are experiencing mental health issues, including sleep disturbances, during this outbreak. Hence, it is highly essential to launch new ways of interventions through counseling, social interactions, and psychotherapy through "telemedicine" under these uncertain pandemic conditions.

6. Neurological Effects of COVID-19

Though the consequences of COVID-19 have led to mental health issues, the brain biotypes and brain or the neural taxonomy are likewise affected. Even though COVID-19 mainly affects the respiratory system, recent studies have shown its direct involvement in the central nervous system (C.N.S.). A study done in Wuhan, China showed that almost around 40% of COVID-19 patients experienced neurological symptoms. These were further divided into C.N.S. symptoms, peripheral nervous system (PNS) signs, and musculoskeletal symptoms. COVID-19 patients with mild neurological symptoms complained of headache and dizziness, and more severe patients suffered from acute cerebrovascular diseases and consciousness impairment [24].

Additionally, reports have indicated olfactory and taste disorders in patients with COVID-19 [25]. COVID-19 is currently found to be affecting the neuroendocrine-immune system and heavily suppressing it [26]. The neuroendocrine-immune system has been said to be involved in stress and coping strategies. This might be one of the reasons for having excessive stress. Another reason for elevated amounts of stress might be because periods of isolation and lack of social contact have been linked to causing high psychological distress and stress-related disorders [27]. Older patients with underlying conditions have been reported with more severe neurological symptoms [24]. Of note, COVID-19 patients in Beijing Ditan Hospital were found to have the presence of SARS-CoV-2 in their cerebrospinal fluid, which was confirmed by genome sequencing, which led to the presentation of viral encephalitis [28].

The mechanism of action of COVID-19 and its neurological effects are currently under study. The C.N.S. is protected from viruses with its multilayer barriers and its immune response system. However, different viruses can affect the brain through a variety of mechanisms. Some proposed mechanisms by which the virus can cause infection include direct brain injury, hypoxic damage, upregulated angiotensin-converting enzyme 2 (ACE-2) receptors, and immune insufficiency, which can lead to toxic, infectious encephalopathy, viral encephalitis, and even acute cerebrovascular disease [28]. The viruses have been found to cause direct brain injury through different mechanisms [29] including via blood circulation where the virus is released into the blood, causing an increase in the penetrability of the blood–brain barrier that leads to the virus entering the brain which causes encephalitis [30]. Some viruses can also direct damage to the brain by involving the sensory or motor nerve endings [31].

It has been proposed that coronavirus causes its neurological symptoms via hypoxia. Since the virus primarily causes respiratory symptoms including shortness of breath and lack of oxygen in the lungs and consequent anaerobic metabolism in the brain, this can lead to brain injury displayed by brain swelling, interstitial edema, or cerebral vasodilation, etc. [32,33]. Thus, hypoxia resulting from COVID-19 infection can result in neurological symptoms. COVID-19 also has the potential to cause hyperinflammation through cytokine storm syndrome [34]. A retrospective study on 150 COVID-19 patients, which was carried out in Wuhan, China, revealed a significant increase in ferritin levels as well as IL-6 levels. Such findings were shown to be positively correlated with the fatality rates in these patients. This would point towards the role of inflammation in multiple COVID-19 symptoms, including its often-devastating neurological issues [35]. Previously, in a mice model, coronavirus was shown to potentially infect nasal cells from where it gets transported to the olfactory bulb before affecting the brain. The removal of the olfactory bulb caused a delay in the transmission of the virus to the mice's brain [32,33]. Recently in Italy, a study reported that in COVID-19 cases, self-reported olfactory and taste disorders were found [25]. Despite such findings in the acute phase, long-term effects have yet to be studied. Another potential mechanism of COVID-19 causing brain injury is thought to be through ACE-2. ACE-2 receptors have been found in glial cells and neurons, which are a potential target of COVID-19. The attachment of the virus to these receptors facilitates the entry of the virus to the brain and resultant brain injury [36].

There is a crashing wave of neuropsychiatric sequelae of COVID-19. The major issues addressed related to COVID-19 are the neuropsychiatric symptoms and understanding the underlying immunological mechanisms. According to Julie Helms et al. (2020), 8 of the 58 COVID-19 patients (14%) admitted in the intensive care unit showed neurological and neuromuscular blockade [37]. Further, RT-PCR assays on the nasopharyngeal samples on all 58 patients revealed from subjects who were positive for acute respiratory syndrome COV2-SARS that seven developed ischemic attack, epilepsy, and mild cognitive impairment [37]. Further, since the impact of COVID-19 and mental health issues has recently been raised worldwide, it is essential to understand whether the rate or the association of suicidality has changed. It would, therefore, be interesting to follow the psychoneuroimmunology of COVID-19 subjects about the extent of mental health issues and the presence of suicidality. As one could speculate, the virus might lead to the immune response in vulnerable subtypes of the mood disorder population, as it was recently observed in cytomegalovirus [38].

7. Psychoneuroimmunity of COVID-19

One of the strong hypotheses on COVID19 and neuro-psychoimmunology is the strong interlink between changes in the cytokines and interleukins across the immune system [38]. Further studies have demonstrated the lack of naïve T cells, an increase in the senescent population of T lymphocytes, and shortening of telomeres in major depression [39]. A plausible approach to explore the association between the virus and the immune system function in major depression and other mood-related disorders is to check their immune response to the antigenic substance injected, such as endotoxin. The outbreak of a viral infection would be a great challenge, yet an opportunity to investigate the significance of an acute immune challenge on different domains of the psychopathology of mood disorders.

A study published in JAMA Neurology by Ling Mao et al. (2020) found that among 214 COVID-19 patients with a mean age of 52.7 [15.5] years, 126 patients had a non-severe infection, while 88 patients developed severe illness based on the respiratory infections [24]. Moreover, out of 214, 78 patients had neurological manifestations. Compared to non-severe infections, the severe ones were all from the elderly population and had underlying medical conditions, especially hypertension. COVID-19 patients with more severe infection had neurologic conditions such as acute cerebrovascular diseases, impaired consciousness, and musculoskeletal symptoms [24]. Furthermore, they observed that COVID-19 patients with severe infection had higher D-dimer levels compared to non-severe infection patients, suggesting the reason behind an increased risk for cardiovascular diseases [24]. Besides, patients with musculoskeletal symptoms were found to have elevated creatine kinase levels (400 U/L), and higher creatine kinase and lactate dehydrogenase levels than those without such symptoms [24]. Additionally, three patients had higher neutrophil counts, lower lymphocyte counts, higher C-reactive protein, and higher-D-dimer levels. The COVID-19 patients who already developed musculoskeletal symptoms also had multiorgan damage, including severe liver damage with increased lactate dehydrogenase, alanine aminotransferase, aspartate aminotransferase, blood urea nitrogen, and creatinine levels [24]. Hence, the infection-mediated immune response might have possibly caused abnormalities in the CNS. secondary to the upsurged interleukins. Patients with severe mental illness are bound to neglect the prevention of infection due to cognitive decline. The reduced physical activity due to the anxiety, fear of infection, and negative symptoms further leads to dysfunctional immunity [40]. However, patients free from COVID-19 infection are also psychologically impacted by the COVID-19 pandemic. Psychiatric morbidity is a paramount concern, as the virus may affect the CNS and provoke systemic inflammation [41]. A recent paper by Conti et al. (2020) reported that COVID-19 infection triggers the release of pro-inflammatory cytokines, including interleukin (I.L.)-1b and IL-6. SARS-COV2 is neurotropic and hence can invade nervous tissues and impede immune-functioning macrophages, microglia, or astrocytes in the CNS [42]. A neurotropic virus might activate microglial cells and induce a pro-inflammatory state [17]. The serum level of Interleukin-6, an essential member of the cytokine storm, is positively correlated with the severity of COVID-2019 symptoms [41]. Additionally, experiments have confirmed that primary glial cells cultured in vitro secrete a large number of inflammatory factors such as IL-6, IL-12, IL-15, and tumor necrosis factor-alpha (TNF-α) after being infected with CoV [32]. Furthermore, the hyperactivation of immune cells in the brain would eventually result in chronic inflammation and brain damage [28].

Bo Diao et al. reviewed the counts of total T cells, CD4+, CD8+ T-cell subsets, and serum cytokine concentrations retrospectively from 522 in-patients from two hospitals in Wuhan as well as 40 healthy controls [43]. Moreover, they further checked the expression of T-cell exhaustion markers programmed death-1 (PD-1), and T-cell immunoglobulin and mucin-domain containing-3 (Tim-3) were measured by flow cytometry in the peripheral blood of 14 COVID-19 cases. Based on their investigation, the T-cell count was found to be significantly reduced in COVID-19 patients, and the surviving T-cells were functionally exhausted [43]. Patients who were not at the ICU had a total T-cells, CD8+ T-cells, and CD4+ T-cells count lower than 800/μL, 300/μL, and 400/μL, respectively. This has mandated a continued aggressive intervention even in the immediate absence of more severe symptoms to prevent further deterioration in their condition [43]. There are also reports from the post-mortem pathology of COVID-19 patients who died in the U.S., showing the infiltration of CD-8+ T-cells within the alveoli [29].

Given the above, the cytokine storm created by an imbalance between CD-4+ and CD-8+ T-cells might be the plausible cause of acute respiratory distress syndrome in COVID-19 patients. Figure 2 depicts the viral and host factors that influence the pathogenesis of SARS-CoV-2. Physical and biopsychosocial and psychoneurooimmune effects impacted by the virus can be improved by a healthy lifestyle, exercise, a balanced diet, staying connected with family and loved ones using telecommunication or internet, and maintaining quality sleep. Hence, in a nutshell, it is highly imperative to build psychosocial resilience to enhance psychoneuroimmunity against the virus [40].

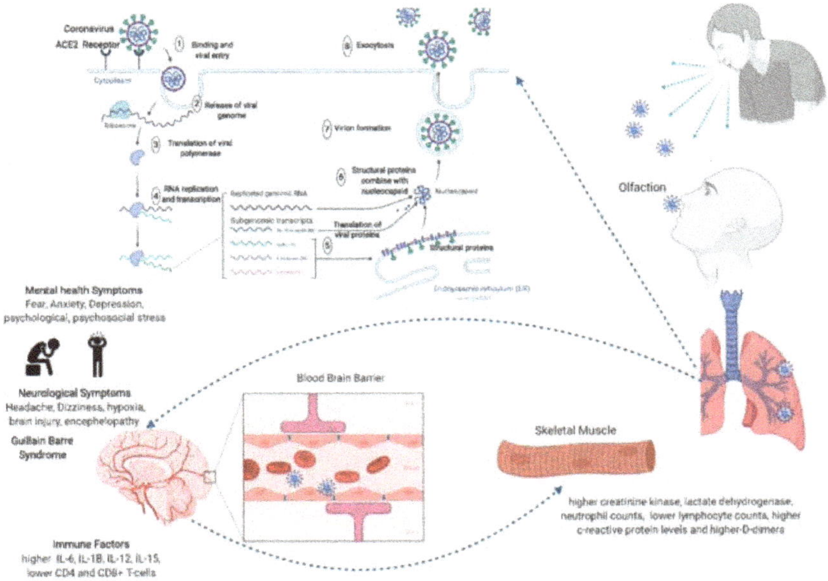

Figure 2. Putative mechanisms underlying neurobiological and psychological events of COVID-19 and their effect on mental health-related issues through psychoneuroimmunity. Virus–host interactions affect viral entry and replication—left panel: viral factor. SARS-CoV-2 is an enveloped positive single-stranded R.N.A. coronavirus. Two-thirds of viral R.N.A. is located in the first open reading frame that encodes 16 non-structure proteins. Host factors (right panel) can also influence susceptibility to infection and disease progression. COV2 enters the brain through olfaction, and since the virus is known to cross the blood–brain barrier, it can cause neurological symptoms like Guillain–Barré syndrome and mental health issues, including fear and anxiety for recovery. All these events are regulated by the cytokines and interleukins within the immune system.

So far, clinical observations have substantiated that patients with COVD-19 may portray a variety of neurological signs and symptoms. Milder symptoms include headache and nausea, while in more severe cases, fatal encephalitis may develop. Meanwhile, older patients and those with underlying conditions are at higher risk for developing neurological symptoms. Of note, anosmia and ageusia are now known to be common early symptoms which people need to be aware of. The long-term effects of COVID-19 are yet to be researched. Therefore, only more long-term research will answer whether these neurological deficits are reversible, recurring, or permanent.

8. Advisable Remedies

A. **Change in lifestyle and coping to overcome psychological distress:** In today's unprecedented health-related crisis, there are many tips and advice aimed to bring mental relief to people It is important to acknowledge the anxiety as feelings, considerations, and reactions; exercise as a classic anxiety reduction strategy; staying physically distant but not socially distant; maintaining sleeping habits; and that meditative practice and a healthy diet might boost the immune system [44]. This will eventually improve a patient's social and occupational functioning. Providing proper instructions and educating about the importance of mental health and the use of different modalities, including lifestyle changes, counseling, and psychotropic medications, can be beneficial. However, most people are trying to cope well, but it is highly important to identify early those individuals who are at risk for psychological morbidities such as younger individuals; addressing the emotional psychological and psychosocial responses in a timely manner; and establishing enhancing social support networks that can buffer against distress to combat negative psychological responses.

B. **Psycho-education, training, and counseling:** The mental healthcare system should be persistent in providing necessary psychosocial treatments. This can happen only through obstinate uninterrupted ambulatory care by protecting the psychiatrists, psychiatry, psychosocial healthcare workers, and staff. Patients should be well informed on how and where to seek help for COVID-19 infection and their mental illness relentlessly. Over and above, stress management measures such as mindfulness meditative training, relaxation techniques, yoga, praying, and similar practices will assist the mindful presence with the power of silence. With regards to meditation, in a recent paper, a unique protocol was proposed to conquer worry in the age of COVID-19, offering some geometric meditation techniques, along with a link to a video clip file dedicated to each method available free for public use [45]. We are already working on developing and validating an android-based smartphone app in three languages (Persian, English, and Spanish) aiming to assist users in conquering their distressing worries in today's life.

With everything that has changed with society as a result of the pandemic, there is a great need to develop more "wellness groups" to healthcare workers who are working tirelessly to treat patients during the current pandemic. These groups have also sparked a lot of conversation around where future needs may arise, as COVID-19 will undoubtedly be a large issue for the next 12–18 months. These groups and resources could also be adapted for other "frontline" essential workers, such as those in the food industry and delivery, as they may also experience similar stressors as healthcare workers. When one is responding to COVID-19 and is quarantined, mental predicaments become much harder. Even upon the release from quarantine, one might experience mixed feelings, including intense fear about his/her own and loved ones' health. Further, other symptoms such as sadness and irritation because a friend or loved one might have contracted COVID-19 can be frustrating. Other emotional and mental changes often result from the guilt of not being able to interact with other people, complete tasks, and take duties during the quarantine period. Furthermore, the financial and social burden of the issue adds to the mental health burden of the disease [1]. In such an instance, one needs to take time for himself/herself and his/her family to recover from responding to the pandemic. It would also be advised that individuals take a break from media coverage of COVID-19 and seek community assistance instead [1].

9. Conclusions

While the mechanisms behind the COVID-19 disease burden are being studied, it is now clear that patients suffering from diseases may develop a variety of psychoneurological signs and symptoms. As the numbers of COVID-19 cases continue to rise worldwide, there is an increasing number of studies that have reported psychoneurological symptoms, with the latest reports suggesting that COVID-19 patients suffer from Guillain–Barré syndrome and other long-lasting neurological complications. Studies published mainly from China and France have also reported the significance of neurological and mental health disorders in COVID-19 patients. According to these reports, up to 36% of patients have demonstrated psychoneurological symptoms. As such, the neurological and subsequent neuropsychiatric burden of the disease would require even further attention in our today's clinical practice against the virus. COVID-19 can potentially affect anyone, regardless of age, gender, and ethnicity.

Meanwhile, when someone has had mental traumas or experienced mental or long-term physical illness, or when an elderly finds himself/herself more vulnerable to the effects of coronavirus, the distressing worry turns to be off the chart. Thus, one needs to develop skills and awareness instead of making assumptions while acknowledging stress and managing it. This pandemic will be expected to continue reshaping the patient–physician relationship with the emergence of telemedicine. The pandemic would also continue to reinforce the global healthcare system to avoid further unpreparedness for similar crises. Over and above, public awareness campaigns and academic efforts need to be synergized to help people refrain from judging who is responsible for the virus spread instead of assisting them with how to stay mentally and physically safe by adequately following the outbreak updates from trusted resources. Increased screening of mental health symptoms during primary care or other medical specialty visits, and offering mental health services with the slightest degree of suspicion, can decrease the mental health burden.

In most cases, the COVID-19 related stress in a person without significant past psychiatric history can be diagnosed as an adjustment disorder. Adjustment disorder can be treated with counseling and minimal use of psychotropic medications. On the other hand, patients with pre-existing or chronic psychiatric illnesses may decompensate due to increased stress related to COVID-19. This patient population may benefit from more frequent mental healthcare visits, even if this can be provided via telemedicine. Increased visits with their mental health provider can ensure medication compliance and early detection of any relapse of their psychiatric symptoms. In specific cases, the physician may consider more liberal but very brief use of anxiety and sleep medications. The decision to use medication should be based upon the most recent evidence-based guidelines.

An accumulating body of recent evidence proposes that anxiety, depressive, and psychotic symptoms are all likely to worsen during extreme COVID-induced stress and social disruption. Moreover, patients will be at increased risk of relapse or recurrence of affective and psychotic illness. As such, it will be important when deciding on the best management plan (non-pharmacological/pharmacological) to consider all the relevant factors, including risk to self and others. It is important to understand the difference between short- and long-term use of psychotropic medications, and also to clarify the myths related to the addiction potential of all psychotropic medications. Although many psychiatric medicines are tightly regulated and prescribed only for long-term mental illnesses, it may be necessary for the governments to ease up prescription refill regulations. Teletherapy and online consultations with e-prescriptions would allow ease of access to the prescribed medications without referring to the mental healthcare provider in person. Perhaps in many occurrences, designated pharmacies might collect e-prescriptions plus the related contact info of the patients for home-delivery medicines. Notwithstanding the above, possible untoward or side-effects of such medication need to be noted. In other words, upon treatment with commonly prescribed psychotropic drugs, careful consideration should be given to whether now is the best time to commence, withdraw, or change patients from antidepressant, anxiolytic, or antipsychotic medications. For instance, in patients who receive ongoing treatment with benzodiazepines, the potential for tolerance and dependence needs to be considered. With regards to lithium carbonate, the optimal dosing should be governed by blood levels. Likewise, when prescribing or refilling clozapine, blood tests to monitor possible or probable neutropenia should be advised.

Author Contributions: Writing—original draft preparation, K.S.R., M.N., B.S.G., G.P.; writing—review and editing, K.S.R., B.S.G., S.S.G., U.G., A.M., D.K., L.C., S.J.K.A.; visualization, K.S.R., M.N., B.S.G., G.P., S.S.G., S.J.K.A., D.K., L.C. All authors have read and agreed to the published version of the manuscript.

Funding: KS Rao is thankful to the National Science system (S.N.I.) of SENACYT, and COVID19 Rapid Grant number 077 of SENACYT, the Republic of Panama for the support.

Acknowledgments: S.S.G. is a CPRIT (Cancer Prevention and Research Institute of Texas) scholar in cancer research, and also funded by a grant from CPRIT (RR170020). The figure illustration was created using the Biorender online tool. B.S.G. is supported by The Brain Behavior Research Foundation (NARSAD) grant and Mc. Kee Foundation grant.

Conflicts of Interest: The authors declare no conflict of interest.

References

1. Duan, L.; Zhu, G. Psychological interventions for people affected by the COVID-19 epidemic. *Lancet Psychiatry* **2020**, *7*, 300–302. [CrossRef]
2. Zautra, A.J. *Emotions, Stress and Health*; Oxford University Press: Oxford, UK, 2006.
3. Wong, A.H.K.; Pittig, A. Costly avoidance triggered by categorical fear generalization. *Behav. Res. Ther.* **2020**, *129*, 103606. [CrossRef] [PubMed]
4. Aghagoli, G.; Marin, B.G.; Katchur, N.J.; Chaves-Sell, F.; Asaad, W.F.; Murphy, S.A. Neurological Involvement in COVID-19 and Potential Mechanisms: A Review. *Neurocrit. Care* **2020**. [CrossRef] [PubMed]
5. Karadas, O.; Ozturk, B.; Sonkaya, A.R. A prospective clinical study of detailed neurological manifestations in patients with COVID-19. *Neurol. Sci.* **2020**, *41*, 1991–1995. [CrossRef]
6. Varatharaj, A.; Thomas, N.; Ellul, M.A.; Davies, N.W.S.; Pollak, T.A.; Tenorio, E.L.; Sultan, M.; Easton, A.; Breen, G.; Zandi, M.; et al. Neurological and neuropsychiatric complications of COVID-19 in 153 patients: A UK-wide surveillance study. *Lancet Psychiatry* **2020**. [CrossRef]
7. Ellul, M.A.; Benjamin, L.; Singh, B.; Lant, S.; Michael, B.D.; Easton, A.; Kneen, R.; Defres, S.; Sejvar, J.; Solomon, T. Neurological associations of COVID-19. *Lancet Neurol.* **2020**. [CrossRef]
8. Serafini, G.; Parmigiani, B.; Amerio, A.; Aguglia, A.; Sher, L.; Amore, M. The psychological impact of COVID-19 on the mental health in the general population. *QJM* **2020**. [CrossRef]
9. Machado, A.; Herrera, A.J.; de Pablos, R.M.; Espinosa-Oliva, A.M.; Sarmiento, M.; Ayala, A.; Venero, J.L.; Santiago, M.; Villaran, R.F.; Delgado-Cortes, M.J.; et al. Chronic stress as a risk factor for Alzheimer's disease. *Rev. Neurosci.* **2014**, *25*, 785–804. [CrossRef]
10. Ho, C.S.; Chee, C.Y.; Ho, R.C. Mental Health Strategies to Combat the Psychological Impact of COVID-19 Beyond Paranoia and Panic. *Ann. Acad. Med. Singap.* **2020**, *49*, 155–160.
11. Shi, Y.; Wang, J.; Yang, Y.; Wang, Z.; Wang, G.; Hashimoto, K.; Zhang, K.; Liu, H. Knowledge and attitudes of medical staff in Chinese psychiatric hospitals regarding COVID-19. *Brain Behav. Immun. Health* **2020**, *4*, 100064. [CrossRef]
12. Fatke, B.; Holzle, P.; Frank, A.; Forstl, H. COVID-19 Crisis: Early Observations on a Pandemic's Psychiatric Problems. *Dtsch. Med. Wochenschr.* **2020**. [CrossRef]
13. Shao, Y.; Shao, Y.; Fei, J.M. Psychiatry hospital management facing COVID-19: From medical staff to patients. *Brain Behav. Immun.* **2020**. [CrossRef] [PubMed]
14. Canady, V.A. Mental health groups providing support education in wake of COVID-19. *Ment. Health Wkly.* **2020**, *20*, 1–3. [CrossRef]
15. Chen, Q.; Liang, M.; Li, Y.; Guo, J.; Fei, D.; Wang, L.; He, L.; Sheng, C.; Cai, Y.; Li, X.; et al. Mental health care for medical staff in China during the COVID-19 outbreak. *Lancet Psychiatry* **2020**, *7*, e15–e16. [CrossRef]
16. Yang, Y.; Li, W.; Zhang, Q.; Zhang, L.; Cheung, T.; Xiang, Y.T. Mental health services for older adults in China during the COVID-19 outbreak. *Lancet Psychiatry* **2020**, *7*, e19. [CrossRef]
17. Li, W.; Yang, Y.; Liu, Z.H.; Zhao, Y.J.; Zhang, Q.; Zhang, L.; Cheung, T.; Xiang, Y.T. Progression of Mental Health Services during the COVID-19 Outbreak in China. *Int. J. Biol. Sci.* **2020**, *16*, 1732–1738. [CrossRef]
18. Xiang, Y.T.; Yang, Y.; Li, W.; Zhang, L.; Zhang, Q.; Cheung, T.; Ng, C.H. Timely mental health care for the 2019 novel coronavirus outbreak is urgently needed. *Lancet Psychiatry* **2020**, *7*, 228–229. [CrossRef]
19. Greenberg, N.; Brooks, S.K.; Wessely, S.; Tracy, D.K. How might the NHS protect the mental health of health-care workers after the COVID-19 crisis? *Lancet Psychiatry* **2020**. [CrossRef]
20. Pappa, S.; Ntella, V.; Giannakas, T.; Giannakoulis, V.G.; Papoutsi, E.; Katsaounou, P. Prevalence of depression, anxiety, and insomnia among healthcare workers during the COVID-19 pandemic: A systematic review and meta-analysis. *Brain Behav. Immun.* **2020**. [CrossRef]

21. Brooks, S.K.; Webster, R.K.; Smith, L.E.; Woodland, L.; Wessely, S.; Greenberg, N.; Rubin, G.J. The psychological impact of quarantine and how to reduce it: Rapid review of the evidence. *Lancet* **2020**, *395*, 912–920. [CrossRef]
22. Blake, H.; Bermingham, F.; Johnson, G.; Tabner, A. Mitigating the Psychological Impact of COVID-19 on Healthcare Workers: A Digital Learning Package. *Int. J. Environ. Res. Public Health* **2020**, *17*, 2997. [CrossRef] [PubMed]
23. Vachon, H.; Rintala, A.; Viechtbauer, W.; Myin-Germeys, I. Data quality and feasibility of the Experience Sampling Method across the spectrum of severe psychiatric disorders: A protocol for a systematic review and meta-analysis. *Syst. Rev.* **2018**, *7*, 7. [CrossRef] [PubMed]
24. Mao, L.; Jin, H.; Wang, M.; Hu, Y.; Chen, S.; He, Q.; Chang, J.; Hong, C.; Zhou, Y.; Wang, D.; et al. Neurologic Manifestations of Hospitalized Patients with Coronavirus Disease 2019 in Wuhan, China. *JAMA Neurol.* **2020**. [CrossRef]
25. Giacomelli, A.; Pezzati, L.; Conti, F.; Bernacchia, D.; Siano, M.; Oreni, L.; Rusconi, S.; Gervasoni, C.; Ridolfo, A.L.; Rizzardini, G.; et al. Self-reported olfactory and taste disorders in SARS-CoV-2 patients: A cross-sectional study. *Clin. Infect. Dis.* **2020**. [CrossRef] [PubMed]
26. Cao, X. COVID-19: Immunopathology and its implications for therapy. *Nat. Rev. Immunol.* **2020**, *20*, 269–270. [CrossRef] [PubMed]
27. Yang, J.; Tong, J.; Meng, F.; Feng, Q.; Ma, H.; Shi, C.; Yuan, J.; Yang, S.; Liu, L.; Xu, L.; et al. Characteristics and challenges of psychological first aid in China during the COVID-19 outbreak. *Brain Behav. Immun.* **2020**. [CrossRef] [PubMed]
28. Wu, Y.; Xu, X.; Chen, Z.; Duan, J.; Hashimoto, K.; Yang, L.; Liu, C.; Yang, C. Nervous system involvement after infection with COVID-19 and other coronaviruses. *Brain Behav. Immun.* **2020**. [CrossRef]
29. Koyuncu, O.O.; Hogue, I.B.; Enquist, L.W. Virus infections in the nervous system. *Cell Host Microbe* **2013**, *13*, 379–393. [CrossRef]
30. Unni, S.K.; Ruzek, D.; Chhatbar, C.; Mishra, R.; Johri, M.K.; Singh, S.K. Japanese encephalitis virus: From genome to infectome. *Microbes Infect.* **2011**, *13*, 312–321. [CrossRef]
31. Swanson, P.A., 2nd; McGavern, D.B. Viral diseases of the central nervous system. *Curr. Opin. Virol.* **2015**, *11*, 44–54. [CrossRef]
32. Bohmwald, K.; Galvez, N.M.S.; Rios, M.; Kalergis, A.M. Neurologic Alterations Due to Respiratory Virus Infections. *Front. Cell. Neurosci.* **2018**, *12*, 386. [CrossRef] [PubMed]
33. Guo, Y.R.; Cao, Q.D.; Hong, Z.S.; Tan, Y.Y.; Chen, S.D.; Jin, H.J.; Tan, K.S.; Wang, D.Y.; Yan, Y. The origin, transmission and clinical therapies on coronavirus disease 2019 (COVID-19) outbreak-an update on the status. *Mil. Med. Res.* **2020**, *7*, 11. [CrossRef] [PubMed]
34. Mehta, P.; McAuley, D.F.; Brown, M.; Sanchez, E.; Tattersall, R.S.; Manson, J.J.; HLH Across Speciality Collaboration, UK. COVID-19: Consider cytokine storm syndromes and immunosuppression. *Lancet* **2020**, *395*, 1033–1034. [CrossRef]
35. Huang, C.; Wang, Y.; Li, X.; Ren, L.; Zhao, J.; Hu, Y.; Zhang, L.; Fan, G.; Xu, J.; Gu, X.; et al. Clinical features of patients infected with 2019 novel coronavirus in Wuhan, China. *Lancet* **2020**, *395*, 497–506. [CrossRef]
36. Baig, A.M.; Khaleeq, A.; Ali, U.; Syeda, H. Evidence of the COVID-19 Virus Targeting the CNS: Tissue Distribution, Host-Virus Interaction, and Proposed Neurotropic Mechanisms. *ACS Chem. Neurosci.* **2020**, *11*, 995–998. [CrossRef] [PubMed]
37. Helms, J.; Kremer, S.; Merdji, H.; Clere-Jehl, R.; Schenck, M.; Kummerlen, C.; Collange, O.; Boulay, C.; Fafi-Kremer, S.; Ohana, M.; et al. Neurologic Features in Severe SARS-CoV-2 Infection. *N. Engl. J. Med.* **2020**. [CrossRef]
38. Brietzke, E.; Magee, T.; Freire, R.C.R.; Gomes, F.A.; Milev, R. Three Insights on Psychoneuroimmunology of Mood Disorders to Be Taken from the Covid-19 Pandemic. *Brain Behav. Immun. Health* **2020**. [CrossRef]
39. Holmes, E.A.; O'Connor, R.C.; Perry, V.H.; Tracey, I.; Wessely, S.; Arseneault, L.; Ballard, C.; Christensen, H.; Cohen Silver, R.; Everall, I.; et al. Multidisciplinary research priorities for the COVID-19 pandemic: A call for action for mental health science. *Lancet Psychiatry* **2020**. [CrossRef]
40. Kim, S.W.; Su, K.P. Using psychoneuroimmunity against COVID-19. *Brain Behav. Immun.* **2020**. [CrossRef]
41. Wan, S.; Yi, Q.; Fan, S.; Lv, J.; Zhang, X.; Guo, L.; Lang, C.; Xiao, Q.; Xiao, K.; Yi, Z.; et al. Relationships among lymphocyte subsets, cytokines, and the pulmonary inflammation index in coronavirus (COVID-19) infected patients. *Br. J. Haematol.* **2020**, *189*, 428–437. [CrossRef]

42. Conti, P.; Gallenga, C.E.; Tete, G.; Caraffa, A.; Ronconi, G.; Younes, A.; Toniato, E.; Ross, R.; Kritas, S.K. How to reduce the likelihood of coronavirus-19 (CoV-19 or SARS-CoV-2) infection and lung inflammation mediated by IL-1. *J. Biol. Regul. Homeost. Agents* **2020**, *34*. [CrossRef]
43. Bo Diao, C.W.; Tan, Y.; Chen, X.; Liu, Y.; Ning, L.; Chen, L.; Li, M.; Liu, Y.; Wang, G.; Yuan, Z.; et al. Reduction and Functional Exhaustion of T Cells in Patients with Coronavirus Disease 2019 (COVID-19). *Front. Immunol.* **2020**, *11*, 1–7. [CrossRef]
44. Del Rio, C.; Malani, P.N. COVID-19-New Insights on a Rapidly Changing Epidemic. *JAMA* **2020**. [CrossRef] [PubMed]
45. Nazaraghaei, F.; Nami, M. Conquering Worry Using the Brain-Based Geometric Meditative Approach in the Age of COVID-19. *J. Clin. Med.* **2020**, *1*, 1–7.

Journal of
Clinical Medicine

MDPI

Article

COVID-19 Pandemic Outbreak and its Psychological Impact on Patients with Rare Lysosomal Diseases

Agata Fiumara [1,*], Giuseppina Lanzafame [1], Alessia Arena [1], Annamaria Sapuppo [1], Federica Raudino [1], Andrea Praticò [1], Piero Pavone [1] and Rita Barone [2]

1 Regional Referral Centre for Inborn Errors Metabolism, Pediatric Clinic, Department of Clinical and Experimental Medicine, University of Catania, 95123 Catania, Italy; giusylanz@virgilio.it (G.L.); alessia.arena@gmail.com (A.A.); annamaria.pan@hotmail.it (A.S.); federica.raudino@tiscali.it (F.R.); andrea.pratico@unict.it (A.P.); ppavone@unict.it (P.P.)

2 Child Neuropsychiatry, Department of Clinical and Experimental Medicine, University of Catania, 95123 Catania, Italy; rbarone@unict.it

* Correspondence: fiumara@policlinico.unict.it

Received: 6 August 2020; Accepted: 19 August 2020; Published: 22 August 2020

Abstract: Background: Lysosomal storage disorders (LSDs) are rare, chronic, progressive multisystem diseases implying severe medical issues and psychological burden. Some of these disorders are susceptible to a treatment, which is administered weekly or every other week, in a hospital. During the COVID-19 (Corona Virus Disease 2019) pandemic lockdown, patients with LSDs on enzyme replacement therapy (ERT) missed their scheduled access to the Day Hospital to get their treatment. Methods: Based on the feeling that our patients were experiencing profound distress, we designed a structured telephone interview with the aim to evaluate how, and to which extent, the pandemic outbreak was changing their behavior and feelings about their chronic disease, the impact on therapies, and future expectations. The same interview was administered to an age-matched control group. Results: All interviewed people experienced an increase of anxiety, worries, and uncertainty fostered by incessant media updates. Moreover, a striking similarity emerged between the groups regarding forced home reclusion and the profound feeling to be excluded by normal life, well-known to those affected by a chronic rare disease. Conclusions: Although no statistically significant difference was found compared to controls, we felt that the reactions were qualitatively different, underlining the fragility and isolation of such patients.

Keywords: COVID-19 pandemic; ERT; lysosomal storage disease; psychological impact

---

1. Introduction

Since March 2020, the dramatic outbreak of Corona Virus Disease 2019 (COVID-19) in Italy has changed our lifestyle as individuals, physicians, and patients. Despite the evidence of minor involvement of children [1], pediatric units also had to deal with healthcare crises.

As a Referral Centre for Inborn Errors of Metabolism (IEM), we had to face an unexpected restriction concerning daily normal activity with lowering of programmed admissions for diagnosis and follow-up visits. Our concern was especially directed to those patients with lysosomal storage disorders (LSDs), which are rare, chronic, progressive, multisystem diseases associated with serious medical issues, physical disability, and psychological burden [2]. In the last decade, some of the LSDs became treatable by pharmacological therapy, such as intravenous (iv) enzyme replacement therapy (ERT) and oral substrate reduction therapy (SRT), or chaperones. During the COVID-19 alert, patients with LSDs, under regular treatment with ERT, failed their usual compliant behavior, missing scheduled infusions. Based on the feeling that our patients were experiencing profound distress, we designed a structured interview [3,4] with the aim to evaluate how, and to which extent, the COVID-19 pandemic was changing our patients' behavior and feelings about their chronic disease, the impact on therapies, and their future expectations. We emphasize the importance to investigate attitudes and behavior with respect to health treatment, especially among people with rare diseases, such as patients with LSD. They represent a group with increased vulnerabilities to COVID-19; thus, we felt the need to attempt any possible solution that would let them maintain treatment protocols and minimize disease progression.

2. Methods

2.1. Study Design and Participants

At our Regional Referral Centre for Metabolic diseases, Pediatric Clinic, Department of Clinical and Experimental Medicine, patients with different types of IEM are followed. At the time of the study, 33 of them were affected by a treatable LSD and thus were regularly admitted to the Day Hospital with a personal schedule of ERT (weekly or every other week) or followed-up every 3–6 months because of treatment at home.

In this study, we included 15/33 patients who accepted to undergo our interview. There were 9 females and 6 males with age ranging from 3 to 40 years. Seven of them were younger than 12 years.

Ten (66%) had Pompe disease (PD; 2 early infantile type (EOPD) and 8 late-onset type (LOPD)). The sample also included 2 patients with Mucopolysaccharidosis type IV (MPS IV), 2 pediatric patients with Gaucher disease, and 1 adult subject with Fabry disease. All participants were receiving iv ERT (alglucosidase alfa, elosulfase alfa, imiglucerase, or agalsidase beta, according to their disease). At the beginning of COVID-19 emergency, study patients with Gaucher disease or Fabry disease were on home therapy.

An ad hoc structured interview was developed and administered by phone and when possible by video calls (Table 1) during the third week of lockdown. The interview investigated personal feelings, familial relationship, degree of faith in others, and future perspectives and was inspired and developed in light of this extraordinary, life-threatening event. Quantitative data were obtained from dichotomous questions (Yes/No) used for a clear distinction of respondents' opinions.

According to the age, we got direct information from 8 subjects, while for 7 pediatric patients, the parents were asked to respond to the interview. A psychologist (GL) from the Centre contacted the patients or their caregivers to assess how the COVID-19 emergency modified the daily life of patients and their family, which changes were due to the resulting Government restrictions, how these were felt, and if any change had occurred with the personal therapy schedule. Moreover, we gathered information about the mood of the patients, their families, and social relationships, the need for psychological support, and their expectations for the future. Since we thought and developed the interview in light of this extraordinary event, the tool could not have been previously validated. To overcome this issue, a group of healthy volunteers was carefully selected for comparison. The control group included 15 healthy subjects matching one-to-one with the patient and caregiver sample, in terms of age, social condition, instruction level, and family composition.

Table 1. Structured interview (topic guide).

Name (Initials)
Sex
Age
School degree
Profession
Marital status
Diagnosis
Age at onset
Age at diagnosis
Age at start of ERT
Number of members in the family unit
How do you live family relationships?
How have they changed?
Which is your perception of the "Other"
How do you spend your time? Any changes because of pandemic?
Changes in daily routine
Changes in Hospital routine for therapy?
What do you think about the current situation?
What this pandemic is teaching you?
Which is your prevailing emotion at the moment?
How do you live the current situation?
Confident/not confident in others
Confident/not confident about web news or official news
Defense mechanisms/coping strategies
What is your vision on the future prospects of health and work?

2.2. *Statistical Analyses*

Data were presented as absolute frequencies and/or percentages for categorical variables. A comparison of proportions between groups was conducted by Chi square test with Yates' correction. Differences with $p \leq 0.05$ were considered to be significant. Data were analyzed using the SPSS software, v. 23. (*SPS*, Bologna, Italy)

3. Results

3.1. *Familial Relationships*

Relations with family members appeared to be felt positively in 54% of patients stating that, being at home, they were closer and linked to each other in a co-working and beloved environment. On the contrary, before the lockdown, family members were less involved; moreover, the use of video calls and socials allowed contact with less frequently seen relatives and increased reciprocal affection and the feeling to be part of the same family. In the control group, a positive evaluation was found only in 30%, although they also stated to have rediscovered human values and lost values.

A negative feeling was reported by 33% of our patients: they described intolerance, impatience, discomfort, distress, constriction, and impairment of contact with close relatives, if not by video calls. In contrast, 60% of the control group described a negative feeling of familial interrelationship because of isolation, uncertainty, fear, difficulties in handling children, and anxiety for older relatives with whom it was hard to communicate.

A small percentage of investigated patients (13%) and 10% of the control group denied significant changes, stating that they were used to this aloneness and isolation.

As a whole, no significant differences were observed in the rate of subjects experiencing positive, negative, or unchanged familial relationships between groups ($X^2(2, N = 25) = 1.7, p = 0.413$).

3.2. Social Relationships

Patients revealed a strong inclination to feel "others" negatively (87%), as other people were considered to be disrespectful, self-oriented, or dangerous and were to be avoided. Thus, relationships were commonly seen as characterized by lack of empathy, indifference, and detachment. In the control group, we also found a clear tendency to perceive other people negatively (80%). However, in the control group, the image of "others" was that of insecure, frightened, suspicious, avoidant, and elusive people, although considered only slightly inaccessible and deserving of being turned away.

A small percentage (6%) of our patients, on the contrary, stressed the empathic attitude toward others who were then sharing the common fragility state. In the control group, 20% reported social relations positively stating how useful it was to protect each other by avoiding contact and discovering new ways of social interaction even with neighbors. Only 7% of patients stated that they did not feel significant changes. The proportion of participants who experienced social relationships as dangerous or positive was not significantly different between groups ($X^2(1, N = 25) = 0.7, p = 0.068$).

3.3. Daily Routine changes

No significant differences between groups were observed in the rate of participants experiencing negative or positive reactions to modified daily activities ($X^2(1, N = 25) = 0.3, p = 0.802$).

Sixty percent of patients described boring moments, monotony, weakness, and stress for web lessons, limitation of normal activities, prohibitions in moving to familial places and seeing relatives, and the need for repetitive hand hygiene procedures. Likewise, the majority of control subjects (80%) demonstrated a negative reaction regarding the monotony of daily life, which was felt as difficulty in commitment to following rules, in the need for space and temporal organization, and in the occurrence of sleep–awake rhythm problems.

On the contrary, 20% of patients stated that they felt more relaxed and helped by the family dedicating more time to them. In addition, 20% of controls felt the changes positively, having more free time for themselves and for their domestic activities. Among patients, 20% felt that there were no changes in their daily routine.

3.4. Personal Feeling and Emotional Reactions

Mostly negative feelings were encountered in our patients' sample; 67% experienced fear, distress, anger, frustration, impotence, negative mood, and feeling of neglection; and 33% showed ambivalent emotions, with co-existence of astonishment, confusion, doubt, curiosity, and uncertainty alongside the need to protect their beloved ones.

Seventy percent of controls manifested aloneness, anxiety, concern, fear of the unknown, fear of contamination, sharing difficulties, pessimism, mood depression, sadness, and feeling of being in a surreal condition. On the contrary, 20% had a positive mood characterized by adaption, respect, positive dependence, and ability to find incitements and new energies; the remaining 10% showed ambivalent aspects with a hard and pessimistic approach, despite a feeling of well-being. In sum, the proportion of subjects suffering negative or positive feelings was not significantly different in the two groups ($X^2(1, N = 25) = 0.2, p = 0.902$).

3.5. Relationships with Authorities

Patients with LSDs expressed their belief in state, regional, and hospital Institutions in 67% of cases; 20% declared to be not confident; and 13% were uncertain because of discordant news and lack to timely assured protection devices. Similar results were obtained in the control group with 70% manifesting faith, 20% manifesting diffidence and the feeling to be abandoned, and 10% showing an uncertainty to judge about the emergency-handling strategies ($X^2(1, N = 25) = 0.1, p = 0.986$).

3.6. Psychological Defence Mechanisms

Defense mechanisms adopted by patients and controls during the COVID-19 emergency were analyzed: both groups tried to use mature psychological defenses (33% versus 36%, respectively) or denied any concern (11% of patients versus 7% of controls); annihilation was encountered in 11% of patients and 15% of controls; a tendency to discredit others was present in 11% of patients and 14% of controls; some of the patients (17%) activated distressing and pacifying actions; this was also seen in 7% of controls. A small percentage of patients (11%) showed a passive mood, demonstrating lack of affective interactions.

Almost half of the patients thought that, from this experience, they learnt something positive (47%) such as the real meaning of relationships, gratitude, and the ability to accept and respect others and to identify priorities. This feeling was even stronger in the control group (70%), stating that some positive aspects were coming from the actual situation as the discovery and enforcement of community spirit, sense of belonging to the same community and nation, values of life, solidarity, and the ability to face hard tasks and overcome limits gave a look inside themselves. Twenty percent of patients stated that they were living this experience in a negative way, learning disillusion, frustration, and resignation to death; 10% of controls lived this dramatic situation as subverting daily routine and forcing to reschedule life; 33% of patients stated that there was nothing to learn by this situation, but to just wait for improvement; and 20% of controls were not able to cope with the actual moment. The proportion of subjects who reported to have learnt positively or negatively from this experience did not differ between the groups ($X^2(1, N = 25) = 1.3, p = 0.5118$).

3.7. Future Perception

Almost half of the patients (53%) manifested negative anticipations, forecasting more preventive precautions, difficulties, limitations, and discomfort than those that had already suffered because of the disease, thus passing to resignation and unavoidable acceptance. Such a negative future perception was present in 50% of the control group, forecasting a sad, stressing, and financially hard future, with consequences on work and relationships. Nevertheless, 34% of patients had a positive vision of the future, including the opportunity to come back to normal life, due to a profound faith in scientific research. Fifty percent of controls prefigured the return to normal daily life, although with unavoidable changes in physical relationship and environment. Among the patients' group, 13% had a passive, static attitude without changes in future perspectives. No significant differences were observed between groups ($X^2(1, N = 25) = 1.3, p = 0.5118$).

3.8. Therapy Changes

Most patients (60%) refused to regularly come to the Hospital for their therapies because they feared that they would be infected. The remaining 40% respected their scheduled infusion in the Hospital, although they expressed their fear to be infected and thus showed a strict adhesion to hygiene procedures. All patients asked to be treated at home, except for a child that was severely affected with Pompe disease, whose parents felt safer coming to Day Hospital , but accurately checked the personnel health state. The fear of contamination was also observed in patients who had already been treated with home therapy as they were scared to allow people to come home.

4. Discussion

The Italian Government's emergency declaration on 9 March, 2020, drastically changed our lives. Every action, behavior, or even gesture was filtered by the COVID-19 alert. "Stay at home" was mandatory for all people, except for medical doctors, all health operators, and patients needing urgent medical care (www.salute.gov.it).

This study emerged from the observation of different reactions in patients with lysosomal disorders dealing with pandemic outbreak. LSDs are genetic, multisystem diseases [2]. To date, some of the rare

LSDs are susceptible to ERT, which has been shown to at least delay progression, allowing a better quality of life in terms of disabilities. Although, we offered a regular and COVID19-controlled service for these patients, who deserved to be regularly treated despite the emergency period, we observed that patients and their parents were extremely scared and worried about coming to the Hospital, fearing a higher risk for COVID contamination. Thus far, most of them missed their scheduled ERT. Conversely, those patients who had already been treated with home therapy refused treatment by the dedicated team because they felt that this could represent a potential source of the infection.

In this regard, Sechi et al. (2020) analyzed data collected by a questionnaire from 102 patients on ERT therapy for LSDs in Italy [5]. They found that almost 50% of patients who were receiving therapy at a hospital (61.8%) had disruptions, especially for personal feelings (fear of infection).

In the present study, we analyzed behavioral and emotional profiles of our patients with LSDs during the pandemic, compared to healthy controls. For this reason, a structured interview was created and administered online by a trained psychologist, already known to all patients as working in the Centre. Since we thought and developed the interview in light of this extraordinary event, the tool could not have been previously validated. The interview was made during the first week of lockdown, when both patients and controls were experiencing the same uncertainty resulting from the special situation. This study certainly may have some limits due to the small sample size, but this is the rule dealing with patients with rare diseases who are referred to a single center. Although no significant quantitative differences were observed in the type of response between clinical and control groups, there were some qualitative differences between the two groups in all investigated areas.

In general, all people forced to stay at home and freeze their jobs and who were far from common relationships, but too close to the familial nucleus members, experienced an increase in anxiety, worries, and uncertainty fostered by incessant media updates on virus lethality and virulence, underlining its invisible presence in our environment and in our lives.

Nevertheless, peculiar differences emerged in social relations and perception of "others". The clinical group, always accustomed to dealing with diversity, exclusion, and unawareness of others with respect to their lives of illness, perceived "others" mostly in a negative way, as dangerous, disrespectful, and not empathetic and to be avoided. The control group, although having the same negative perception, experienced "others" as frightened, insecure, suspicious, and elusive.

In the clinical group, daily routine was marked from the issues of illness and its treatment, while for the control group, main problems were related to difficulty in maintaining, according to an orderly sequence, rules, spaces, times, and sleep–wake rhythm.

On the other hand, it is singular that, in the percentage of positive representation of the routine changes, subjects in the clinical group believed that the positive element was the opportunity of a better relationship with family members, while among controls, positive elements relied on the possibility of being alone and doing something for themselves.

Data about future perception evidenced that, while the control group directed its attention to a future focused on economic, social, and environmental issues, patients prefigured a future always oriented by their critical situation being aware of their limits, in terms of treatment opportunities and life expectation.

We focused on the COVID-19 pandemic effects on medical care and health status of patients with LSDs. The real risk of contagion once again highlighted the vulnerability of patients with chronic rare diseases such as LSDs, the difficulty of coping with his or her defenses, and the need to trust and rely on others. In this case, the subjects preferred to refuse treatment, the only chance to improve their condition. They gathered all their defenses and tried to put in place all the resources and strategies available, such as resist and wait, for example, for home treatment, rather than face unarmed an unknown, enigmatic, and dangerous "enemy".

In our sample, a striking similarity emerged between the two groups, equally forced to stay at home and experience the same profound feeling to be excluded (Isolation and Inclusion, *The Lancet Psychiatry* 2020) [6] by normal life. The pandemic, which represented a scary event, suddenly occurring in the daily life, destabilizing, and giving rise to uncertainty, had the same impact as a diagnosis of a chronic rare disease.

The control group experienced the feeling to be involved in a mutual fight against a common enemy, thus enhancing brotherhood with others. The patients with lysosomal disorders and their families felt that COVID-19 opened the curtains, revealing their human condition of chronic exclusion and impairing their liberty to go out, walk, meet others, love, and breath without fear of death as all the others normally do. Especially the mothers of our patients reacted with strength and determination, feeling that other people can know understand their withdrawn lives to assist their sons. They could now teach others how to face isolation with dignity, aware of fragility, as they usually do: "I can't help from sadly smiling when my neighbors complain because their children are sad as they cannot go outside ... don't say it to me, please, my child and I do not go out since he was born and he is 4 years old. Now we are all the same, all confined at home ... you are not different from us, you also are vulnerable, now we all fear death".

The outbreak of COVID-19 evidenced the vulnerability of the patients with such rare diseases and their needs in terms of adhesion to the therapy schedule. Thus far, a special license for home therapy was approved by AIFA (Agenzia Italiana del Farmaco (Italian Medicines Agency), DET. 341/2020), including those drugs prescribed and dispensed only at hospitals. This determination allowed home treatment for most of our patients. The COVID-19 emergency revealed LSD patients' strength in terms of improved relationships, such as adhesion to the patients' group, family members, and community and their observance of imposed rules and precepts, trust in authority and doctors, and hope for improvement.

Author Contributions: Conceptualization, A.F. and G.L.; Data curation, G.L., A.A., A.S. and F.R.; Formal analysis, A.S. and R.B.; Investigation, G.L.; Methodology, G.L.; Supervision, A.A.; Validation, P.P.; Writing – review & editing, A.F., A.P. and R.B. All authors have read and agreed to the published version of the manuscript.

Funding: This research received no external funding.

Acknowledgments: The authors wish to thank the patients, their families, Battista Mangani, and Nefri Basile for their collaboration. The family association "Bacodirame" is deeply acknowledged for financing the University Research Grant for the Psychologist.

Conflicts of Interest: The authors declare no conflict of interest.

References

1. Ludvigsson, J.F. Systematic review of COVID-19 in children shows milder cases and a better prognosis than adults. *Acta Paediatr.* **2020**, *109*, 1088–1095. [CrossRef] [PubMed]
2. Platt, F.M.; D' Azzo, A.; Davidson, B.L.; Neufeld, E.F.; Tifft, C.J. Lysosomal storage diseases. *Nat. Rev. Dis. Prim.* **2018**, *4*, 27. [CrossRef] [PubMed]
3. Dyer, C. *Research in Psychology: A Practical Guide to Research Methods and Statistics*, 2nd ed.; Wiley Blackwell: Hoboken, NJ, USA, 2006.
4. Brooks, F.B.; Rubin, H.J.; Rubin, I.S. Qualitative Interviewing: The Art of Hearing Data. *Mod. Lang. J.* **1996**, *80*, 555. [CrossRef]
5. Sechi, A.; Macor, D.; Valent, S.; Da Riol, R.M.; Zanatta, M.; Spinelli, A.; Bianchi, K.; Bertossi, N.; Dardis, A.; Valent, F.; et al. Impact of COVID-19 related healthcare crisis on treatments for patients with lysosomal storage disorders, the first Italian experience. *Mol. Genet. Metab.* **2020**, *130*, 170–171. [CrossRef] [PubMed]
6. Isolation and Inclusion. *Lancet Psychiatr.* 2020, 7, p. 371. Available online: https://www.thelancet.com/journals/lanpsy/article/PIIS2215-0366(20)30156-5/fulltext (accessed on 21 August 2020). [CrossRef]

Journal of
Clinical Medicine

MDPI

Article

Prevalence of Antibodies to SARS-CoV-2 in Italian Adults and Associated Risk Factors

Antonio Vena [1], Marco Berruti [1,2], Andrea Adessi [3], Pietro Blumetti [4], Michele Brignole [5,6], Renato Colognato [4], Germano Gaggioli [7], Daniele Roberto Giacobbe [1], Luisa Bracci-Laudiero [8,9], Laura Magnasco [1], Alessio Signori [10], Lucia Taramasso [1], Marco Varelli [11], Nicoletta Vendola [12], Lorenzo Ball [13,14], Chiara Robba [14], Denise Battaglini [14], Iole Brunetti [14], Paolo Pelosi [13,14] and Matteo Bassetti [1,2,*]

1. Infectious Diseases Unit, San Martino Policlinico Hospital—IRCCS for Oncology and Neurosciences, 16132 Genoa, Italy; anton.vena@gmail.com (A.V.); marco.berruti1@gmail.com (M.B.); daniele.roberto.giacobbe@gmail.com (D.R.G.); lmagnasco90@gmail.com (L.M.); taramasso.lucia@gmail.com (L.T.)
2. Department of Health Sciences (DISSAL), University of Genoa, 16132 Genoa, Italy
3. Onilab Milano, 20123 Milano, Italy; adessi@onilab.it
4. Medical Center srl, Sesto Calende, 21018 Varese, Italy; Pietro.blumetti@medicalcentersrl.it (P.B.); renato.colognato@gmail.com (R.C.)
5. Department of Cardiology, Arrhytmology Centre and Syncope Unit, Ospedale del Tigullio, 16033 Lavagna, Italy; mbrignole@outlook.it
6. IRCCS Istituto Auxologico Italiano, Faint and Fall Programme, Ospedale San Luca, 20149 Milano, Italy
7. Division of Cardiology, Ospedale Villa Scassi, 16149 Genova, Italy; gaggioligermano@gmail.com
8. Institute of Translational Pharmacology, Consiglio Nazionale Delle Ricerche (CNR), 00185 Rome, Italy; luisa.braccilaudiero@ift.cnr.it
9. Division of Rheumatology and Immuno-Rheumatology Research Laboratories, Bambino Gesù Children's Hospital, 00165 Rome, Italy
10. Section of Biostatistics, Department of Health Sciences, University of Genova, 16132 Genova, Italy; alessio.signori.unige@gmail.com
11. Diagnostic Institute Varelli, Clinical Analysis, 80126 Napoli, Italy; marco.varelli@istitutovarelli.it
12. Division of Obstetrics and Gynecology, Sant'Andrea Hospital, 13100 Vercelli, Italy; vendola.n@yahoo.com
13. Department of Surgical Sciences and Integrated Diagnostics, University of Genoa, 16132 Genoa, Italy; lorenzo.loryball@gmail.com (L.B.); ppelosi@hotmail.com (P.P.)
14. Anesthesia and Intensive Care, San Martino Policlinico Hospital, IRCCS for Oncology and Neurosciences, 16132 Genoa, Italy; kiarobba@gmail.com (C.R.); battaglini.denise@gmail.com (D.B.); brunettimed@gmail.com (I.B.)

* Correspondence: matteo.bassetti@unige.it; Tel.: +39-010-555-4658; Fax: +39-010-555-6712

Received: 29 June 2020; Accepted: 18 August 2020; Published: 27 August 2020

Abstract: We aimed to assess the prevalence of and factors associated with anti- severe acute respiratory syndrome coronavirus-2 (SARS-CoV-2) positivity in a large population of adult volunteers from five administrative departments of the Liguria and Lombardia regions. A total of 3609 individuals were included in this analysis. Participants were tested for anti-SARS-CoV-2 antibodies [Immunoglobulin G (IgG) and M (IgM) class antibodies] at three private laboratories (Istituto Diganostico Varelli, Medical Center, and Casa della Salute di Genova). Demographic data, occupational or private exposure to SARS-CoV-2-infected patients, and prior medical history consistent with SARS-CoV-2 infection were collected according to a preplanned analysis. The overall seroprevalence of anti-SARS-CoV-2 antibodies (IgG and/or IgM) was 11.0% [398/3609; confidence interval (CI) 10.0%–12.1%]. Seroprevalence was higher in female inmates than in male inmates (12.5% vs. 9.2%, respectively, $p = 0.002$), with the highest rate observed among adults aged >55 years (13.2%). A generalized estimating equations model showed that the main risk factors associated with SARS-CoV-2 seroprevalence were the following: an occupational exposure to the virus [Odd ratio (OR) = 2.36; 95% CI 1.59–3.50, $p = 0.001$], being a long-term care facility resident (OR = 4.53; 95% CI 3.19–6.45, $p = 0.001$), and reporting previous symptoms of influenza-like illness (OR = 4.86; 95% CI 3.75–6.30, $p = 0.001$) or loss of sense of smell or taste (OR = 41.00; 95% CI 18.94–88.71, $p = 0.001$). In conclusion, we found a high prevalence (11.0%) of SARS-CoV-2 infection that is significantly associated with residing in long-term care facilities or occupational exposure to the virus. These findings warrant further investigation into SARS-CoV-2 antibody prevalence among the Italian population.

Keywords: SARS-CoV-2; COVID-19; antibodies; serological test

1. Introduction

In Italy, the first case of pandemic severe acute respiratory syndrome coronavirus-2 (SARS-CoV-2) infection was reported on 20 February, 2020. Since then, the number of cases increased rapidly in the north of the country, with the Lombardia and Liguria regions being heavily affected by the infection [1]. By the end of April 2020, approximately 85,000 laboratory confirmed cases -of SARS-CoV-2 infection were reported in this geographical area of the country [2]. However, these data included only a fraction of the real number of SARS-CoV-2 infections, since not all infected patients were symptomatic [3–5], required hospitalizations, or provided specimens for laboratory testing. The extent to which surveillance data reflect the true burden of the disease can also be affected by changes in laboratory testing recommendation [1]. Serology can represent a key element to overcoming these limits and to better understanding the infection statistics at a population level. The primary outcome of this study was to estimate the prevalence of SARS-CoV-2 antibodies. The secondary outcome was to evaluate possible factors associated with anti-SARS-CoV-2 positivity in a large population of individuals from five administrative departments of the Liguria and Lombardia regions.

2. Experimental Methods

This was an observational study designed to evaluate the prevalence and factors associated with SARS-CoV-2 infections among voluntary, unpaid individuals tested for SARS-CoV-2 antibodies in three private institutions (Istituto Diagnostico Varelli, Medical Center, and Casa della Salute di Genova) during March and April 2020. These institutions altogether include approximately 5,784,974 inhabitants living in five administrative departments (Milano, Varese, Pavia, Genova and Savona) of the Liguria and Lombardia regions. Each laboratory process, about 500,000 samples per year, offers a comprehensive range of tests including clinical biochemistry, serology, and genetic analysis.

2.1. Participants

We included non-hospitalized participants (aged > 18 years) who voluntarily tested for SARS-CoV-2 antibodies in an outpatient setting. After providing informed consent, a sample of venous blood was collected from each participant, all of whom also completed a questionnaire on potential risk factors for developing SARS-CoV-2 infection. Recorded data included age, sex. and occupational or private exposure to SARS-CoV-2 infected patients. In addition, information regarding stays at a long-term care facilities or prior medical history consistent with SARS-CoV-2 infection (influenza-like illness defined according to WHO criteria [6] or loss of smell or taste) within the previous month, were also collected.

2.2. Endpoint

The primary goal was to assess the prevalence of SARS-CoV-2 antibodies [either Immunoglobulin M (IgM) and G (IgG)] positivity among the study population. The secondary goal was to investigate the association between positive tests and demographics (age and sex), occupational and private contact with SARS-CoV-2 infected patients, living in long-term care facilities, and prior symptoms consistent with SARS-CoV-2 infection.

2.3. Detection of Infection

Blood samples were analyzed for serological detection at each participating laboratory by trained staff, unaware of the clinical details of the tested patients. The first laboratory (Istituto Diagnostico Varelli) used a chemiluminescent quantitative immunoassay detecting antibodies against nucleocapsid protein and spike protein (the MaglumiTM 2019) [7]. According to the manufacturer's recommendations, samples were considered positive above a threshold of 1.1 AU/mL for IgM and IgG. This cut-off resulted in clinical sensitivities/specificities of 78.6%/97.5% and 91.2%/97.3% for IgM and IgG, respectively [7,8]. The second laboratory (Medical Center) applied a rapid chromatographic immunoassay for the qualitative detection of IgG and IgM antibody against spike protein (Realy tech® 2019 nCOV/COVID-19 IgG/IgM Rapid Test Device). The manufacturer's reported a clinical sensitivity of 92% for IgM; 96% for IgG; and a specificity of 100% for IgM and IgG. The third laboratory (Casa della salute di Genova) assessed anti-SARS-CoV-2 antibodies using a commercially available point-of-care lateral flow immunoassay (Biosynex® Covid-19 BSS, Fribourg, Switzerland) that can simultaneously detect IgM and IgG in human blood, with an overall sensitivity of 88.7% and specificity of 90.6% [9]. This qualitative test detected antibodies against nucleocapsid and spike proteins. All laboratories used internal procedures to validate the diagnostic performance of serological tests. In all cases, the results showed values of sensitivity and specificity consistent with those reported by each manufacturer.

2.4. Statistical Analysis

All statistics were analyzed using SPSS software. Prevalence of anti-SARS-CoV-2 antibodies (IgM or IgG) was calculated and the exact binomial distribution was used to calculate 95% confidence intervals (CIs). The association between positive SARS-CoV-2 antibodies and study variables was estimated in two steps. First, a general linear univariate analysis was performed using a Chi-squared test. The second step used a generalized estimating equation (GEE) model to consider laboratory provenience, with SARS-CoV-2 seropositivity used as a dependent variable. Only differences with a p-values < 0.05 were considered statistically significant.

2.5. Ethical Consideration

The study protocol was approved by the Ethics Committee of Liguria Region (PI Prof. Matteo Bassetti-N. CER Liguria 381/2020-id 10770).

3. Results

3.1. Participant Demographics and Exposures

Between 1 March and 30 April 2020, 3609 individuals agreed to participate in the study. The mean number of screened individuals per administrative department was 721 (52–1430), representing 12 people per 100,000 inhabitants. The patients' demographics are outlined in Table 1.

Overall, 55.6% (2007/3609) were women and 44.4% were men (1602/3609). The median age was 51 years [interquartile range (IQR) 41–63], with the age group >55 years being most represented (41.4%; n = 1493/3609) and the 18–34 years group being the least represented (15.4%; n = 556/3609). All patients lived in the Lombardia and Liguria regions in the administrative departments of Varese (39.6%; n = 1430/3609), Pavia (24.1%; n = 871/3,609), Milano (21.2%; n = 764/3609), Genova (13.6%; n = 492/3609,) and Savona (1.4%; n = 52/3609;). Approximately 5.7% of the individuals (n = 207/3609) lived in a long-term care facility, whereas 5.0% (n = 179/3609) reported an occupational exposure to infected patients. When asked about recent medical history, 11.8% (n = 427/3609) reported symptoms consistent with influenza-like illness and 0.97% (n = 35/3609) reported loss of smell or taste within the previous month.

Table 1. Clinical characteristics of the study population.

Characteristics	N = 3609 (%)
Sex	
Female	2007 (55.6)
Male	1602 (44.4)
Age groups (Years)	
18–35	556 (15.4)
36–45	631 (17.4)
46–55	929 (25.7)
>55	1493 (41.4)
Region	
Lombardia	3065 (84.9)
Liguria	544 (15.1)
Administrative department	
Varese	1430 (39.6)
Pavia	871 (24.1)
Milano	764 (21.2)
Genova	492 (13.6)
Savona	52 (1.4)
Resident in a long-term care facility	207 (5.7)

3.2. Prevalence of Sars-CoV-2 Antibodies

Of the 3609 individuals included in the study population, 398 tested anti-SARS-CoV-2 positive [11.0% (CI 10.0%–12.1%)]. Seroprevalence was higher among women vs. men (12.5% vs. 9.2%, p = 0.002) and varied with age. The rate was highest among adults aged >55 years (13.2%), followed by adults aged 18–35 years (11.9%). As for geographical distribution, the highest prevalence of anti-Sars-COV-2 positivity was reported in the administrative departments of Savona (Figure 1). Table 2 shows estimated prevalence according to the three different laboratories.

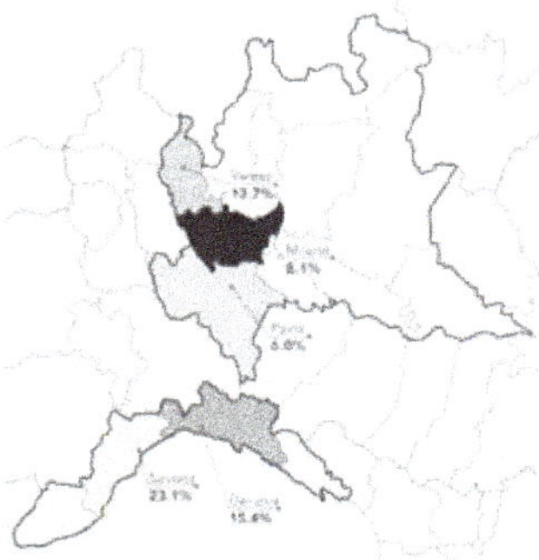

Figure 1. Serologically-confirmed cases of SARS-CoV-2 in the general Italian population from 1 March to 30 April 2020. Red and blue lines represent the boarders of the Lombardia and Liguria regions, respectively. Percentages show the number of positive samples per number tested in each administrative department.

3.3. Factors Associated with Anti-Sars-CoV-2 Antibodies Positivity

Several factors showed an association with anti-SARS-CoV-2 antibodies positivity with univariable analysis (Table 3). The variables that showed a p-value < 0.10 were also included in the GEE model (Table 4). The model showed that the main risk factors associated to SARS-CoV-2 seroprevalence were the following: occupational exposure to the virus (OR = 2.36; 95% CI 1.59–3.50, p = 0.001), living in a long-term care facility (OR = 4.53; 95% CI 3.19–6.45, p = 0.001), and reporting previous symptoms of influenza-like illness (OR = 4.86; 95% CI 3.75–6.30, p = 0.001) or loss of sense of smell or taste (OR = 41.00; 95% CI 18.94–88.71, p = 0.001).

Table 2. Prevalence of SARS-CoV-2 IgM and IgG antibodies according to the three different laboratories.

	n (%)	Sars-CoV-2 IgG+ or IgM (95% Confidence Interval)
Medical Center	1885 (52.2)	11.5% (10.1%–13.0%)
Istituto Diagnostico Varelli	1180 (32.7)	8.0% (6.5%–9.7%)
Casa della salute di Genova	544 (15.1)	16.2% (13.2%–19.5%)

Table 3. Prevalence of Sars-CoV-2 IgM and IgG antibodies and univariate analysis of factors potentially associated with infection (*n* = 3609).

Characteristics	Tested	SARS-CoV-2 IgG+ or IgM+	Univariate Analysis		
	N	n (%)	OR	95% CI	*p*-Value
		Sex			
Female	2007	251 (12.5)	1.36	1.12–1.65	0.002
Male	1602	147 (9.2)	Ref	Ref	Ref
		Age group (Years)			
18–35	556	66 (11.9)	1.10	0.83–1.46	0.50
36–45	631	45 (7.1)	0.57	0.41–0.79	0.001
46–55	929	90 (9.7)	0.82	0.64–1.05	0.24
>55	1493	197 (13.2)	1.44	1.17–1.78	0.001
		Living in a long-term care facility			
No	3402	312 (9.2)	Ref	Ref	Ref
Yes	207	86 (41.5)	7.56	5.58–10.23	0.001
		Occupational exposure			
No	3430	363 (10.6)	Ref	Ref	Ref
Yes	178	35 (19.7)	2.60	1.76–3.88	0.001
		Private Exposure			
No	3469	376 (10.8)	Ref	Ref	Ref
Yes	140	21 (15.0)	1.45	0.90–2.36	0.12
		Occurrence of Symptoms in the previous month			
No symptoms	3147	226 (7.2)	Ref	Ref	Ref
Influenza-like illness	427	427 (34.2)	6.71	5.27–8.54	0.001
Loss of sense or taste	35	26 (74.3)	37.33	17.28–80.64	0.001

CI Confidence Interval; OR Odd ratio; Ref Reference.

Table 4. Results of the generalized estimating equations model of risk factors associated with SARS-CoV-2 seroprevalence.

Characteristics	OR	95% CI	*p*-Value
Male sex	0.79	0.63–1.01	0.06
Age 36–45	1.40	0.99–1.93	0.06
Age > 55	1.17	0.88–1.55	0.27
Living in a long-term care facility	4.53	3.19–6.45	0.001
Occupational exposure	2.36	1.59–3.50	0.001
Prior history of influenza-like illness	4.86	3.75–6.30	0.001
Prior history of loss of sense or taste	41.00	18.94–88.71	0.001

CI Confidence Interval; OR Odd ratio.

4. Discussion

In the present observational study performed on a large sample of subject in northern Italy, we found the following: (1) the overall seroprevalence of anti-SARS-CoV-2 antibodies (IgG and/or IgM) was 11.0%; (2) occupational exposure to the virus, long-term care facility residency, as well as previous symptoms of influenza-like illness or loss of sense of smell or taste were independently associated with anti-SARS-CoV-2 positivity.

To the best of our knowledge, this is one of the first reports that attempts to describe the prevalence of coronavirus disease and to evaluate the potential circulation of SARS-CoV-2 in North Italy. The findings of our study showed that in a definite geographical area of Italy, approximately 630,000 people might have developed antibodies (11.0% of 5,784,974 inhabitants). This figure is significantly higher than the number of molecular-confirmed SARS-CoV-2 infections (~32,600 cases in the five administrative departments) reported by the Protezione Civile and the Italian National Institute of Health as of 30 April 2020 [2]. The high observed seroprevalence is consistent with recent studies (Table 5) performed in other heavily affected areas of Europe: 9.7% in Geneva, Switzerland [10] and 10.0% in Madrid, Spain [11,12].

Table 5. Summary of articles published in the literature reporting data regarding prevalence of SARS-CoV-2 antibodies in the general population.

Author	Country; Area	Number of Participants	Prevalence of Anti-SARS-CoV-2 Antibodies
Petersen M.S. [13]	Faroe Islands; Nationwide study	1075	0.6%
Biggs H. [14]	U.S.; two metropolitan Atlanta counties	696	2.5%
Menachemi N. [15]	U.S; Indiana	3658	2.79%
Fischer B. [16]	Germany; three federal states	3186	0.91%
Pollan M. [11]	Spain; Nationwide study	61,075	5.0%
Havers F. [17]	U.S; 10 sites	16,025	From 1.0% (San Francisco) to 6.9% (New York City)
Amorim Filho L. [18]	Brazil; Rio de Janeiro	2857	4.0%
Percivalle E. [19]	Italy; Lodi area	390	23.0%
Soriano V. [12]	Spain, Madrid	674	13.8%
Stringhini S. [10]	Switzerland, Geneve	2766	9.7%
Sood N. [20]	U.S., Los Angeles	1702	4.3%

Living in a long-term care facility was the strongest predictors of SARS-CoV-2 infection and was reported by 21.6% of anti-SARS-CoV-2-positive participants (n = 86/398). This connection was not unexpected [21–23], since long-term care facilities often have limited or no infection control programs [24,25] and are usually congregative settings where elderly people have greater exposure to infected patients in the case of respiratory outbreaks [26–28]. Therefore, our results emphasized the importance of implementing strategic bundles for infections prevention in long-term care facilities [29]. In this regard, educational interventions on healthcare providers' knowledge, as well as active surveillance of suspected cases and implementation of barrier precautions, were shown to play a vital role in limiting the spread of other respiratory outbreaks [26–28].

Reporting an occupational exposure to the virus also emerged as an independent factor associated with SARS-CoV-2 infection and was reported by 8.7% of anti-SARS-CoV-2-positive participants (n = 35/398). However, approximately two-thirds of anti-SARS-CoV-2-positive participants did not report any apparent risk depicting the widespread circulation of the virus in the Italian community, where it has become endemic.

As for clinical symptoms, we found that the prevalence of SARS-CoV-2 antibodies depends on the type of clinical manifestation reported by the patient, being particularly high in people who reported loss of smell or taste [30,31]. Interestingly, 8.6% of participants (n = 277/3224) who did not report any symptoms presented antibodies positivity. This finding suggests that non-apparent infection is relatively common in a healthy, active population, thus supporting the hypothesis that, as is true for other coronavirus infections [32], SARS-CoV-2 infection might also be asymptomatic or pauci-symptomatic and resolves spontaneously without any complications in many cases.

In our opinion, the findings of our study could have several implications for pandemic management. Because the real number of patients with SARS-CoV-2 infection is significantly higher than the PCR-confirmed cases, stringent lockdown strategies might possibly be re-implemented only when the intensive care units' capacities to handle emergencies are overwhelmed. Since a large proportion of patients with SARS-CoV-2 infection are asymptomatic, contract tracing methods to limit the spread of the infection could be particularly challenging. Thus, screening strategies beyond a symptoms-driven approach will be necessary for Italy (e.g., use of mobile applications) to identify enough infected persons to reach SARS-CoV-2 elimination targets [33]; our data could also be useful for vaccine design and implementation.

There are several limitations that should be discussed. Firstly, we do did have any information regarding previous SARS-CoV-2 molecular testing among those patients who tested positive. Accordingly, we cannot provide valuable estimates of antibody prevalence in people positive and negative in PCR testing. Secondly, we analyzed serum samples from patients who voluntarily decided to be tested. Therefore, the clinical characteristics of the sample might differ from those of the general Italian population. Thirdly, geographical prevalence of anti-SARS-CoV-2 antibodies might have been influenced by the type of serological tests used. However, the diagnostic performances of each test are similar to each other; in addition, the highest percentage of infected patients in the Liguria region agrees with recent evidence, suggesting the presence of anti-SARS-CoV-2 antibodies among blood donors from Savona and Genova since December 2019 (unpublished data reported by the Ligurian regional health authority ALISA). Fourthly, all tests we used are non-FDA approved and are yet to be validated. Therefore, prevalence estimates could change once new information on the accuracy of tests are available. Fifthly, the interpretation of the test is still under discussion, because even patients with confirmed SARS-CoV-2 infections have low or non-detectable antibodies titles several weeks after acute infection [34]. Lastly, based on the specificities of testing kits, we cannot exclude that some participants had false positive results due to past or present infection with other viruses, including non-SARS-CoV-2 coronavirus strains [35]. In addition, antibody response may be impaired in elderly, immuno-compromised or immunosuppressed participants, and may produce false negative serology test results [36].

5. Conclusions

In conclusion, the results of the present study demonstrate that infection rates based on surveillance data considerably underestimated the infection rates during the SARS-CoV-2 virus pandemic in Italy. The seroprevalence was much higher among people living in long-term care facilities or those with occupational exposure. In our opinion, these findings warrant further investigation into SARS-CoV-2 antibody prevalence among the Italian population.

Author Contributions: Conceptualization, M.B. (Marco Berruti) and M.B. (Matteo Bassetti); A.V.; methodology, A.V.; software, A.A.; P.B.; M.B. (Matteo Bassetti); R.C.; G.G.; D.R.G.; formal analysis, A.V. M.B. (Matteo Bassetti); investigation, A.A.; P.B.; M.B. (Matteo Bassetti); R.C.; G.G.; L.B.-L.; M.V.; N.V.; resources, A.A.; P.B.; M.B. (Michele Brignole); R.C.; G.G.; L.B.-L.; M.V.; N.V.; data curation, A.A.; P.B.; M.B. (Michele Brignole).; R.C.; G.G.; L.B.-L.; M.V.; N.V.; A.V.; writing—original draft preparation, A.V.; M.B. (Matteo Bassetti); writing—review and editing, A.V. P.P.; M.B. (Matteo Bassetti); L.T.; L.M.; I.B.; L.B.; C.R.; D.B. visualization, A.S.; supervision, M.B. (Matteo Bassetti); P.P.; funding acquisition A.A.; P.B.; M.B. (Michele Brignole); R.C.; G.G.; L.B.-L.; M.V.; N.V. All authors have read and agreed to the published version of the manuscript.

Funding: This research received no external funding.

Conflicts of Interest: Outside the submitted work, M.B. (Matteo Bassetti) has participated in advisory boards and/or received speaker honoraria from Achaogen, Angelini, Astellas, Bayer, Basilea, BioMeérieux, Cidara, Gilead, Menarini, MSD, Nabriva, Paratek, Pfizer, Roche, Melinta, Shionogi, Tetraphase, VenatoRx, and Vifor and has received study grants from Angelini, Basilea, Astellas, Shionogi, Cidara, Melinta, Gilead, Pfizer, and MSD. Outside the submitted work, D.R.G. reports honoraria from Stepstone Pharma GmbH and unconditional grants from MSD Italia and Correvio Italia. The authors declare no conflict of interest.

References

1. Onder, G.; Rezza, G.; Brusaferro, S. Case-Fatality Rate and Characteristics of Patients Dying in Relation to COVID-19 in Italy. *JAMA* **2020**, *323*, 1775–1776. [CrossRef]
2. Available online: http://www.salute.gov.it/portale/nuovocoronavirus/ (accessed on 30 April 2020).
3. Bassetti, M.; Vena, A.; Giacobbe, D.R. The novel Chinese coronavirus (2019-nCoV) infections: Challenges for fighting the storm. *Eur. J. Clin. Investig.* **2020**, *50*, e13209. [CrossRef]

4. Kim, G.U.; Kim, M.J.; Ra, S.H.; Lee, J.; Bae, S.; Jung, J.; Kim, S.-H. Clinical characteristics of asymptomatic and symptomatic patients with mild COVID-19. *Clin. Microbiol. Infect.* **2020**, *26*, 948.e1–948.e3. [CrossRef] [PubMed]
5. Mizumoto, K.; Kagaya, K.; Zarebski, A.; Chowell, G. Estimating the asymptomatic proportion of coronavirus disease 2019 (COVID-19) cases on board the Diamond Princess cruise ship, Yokohama, Japan, 2020. *Eurosurveillance* **2020**, *25*, 2000180. [CrossRef] [PubMed]
6. Thursky, K.; Cordova, S.P.; Smith, D.; Kelly, H. Working towards a simple case definition for influenza surveillance. *J. Clin. Virol.* **2003**, *27*, 170–179. [CrossRef]
7. Lippi, G.; Salvagno, G.L.; Pegoraro, M.; Militello, V.; Caloi, C.; Peretti, A.; Gaino, S.; Bassi, A.; Bovo, C.; Cascio, G.L. Assessment of immune response to SARS-CoV-2 with fully automated MAGLUMI 2019-nCoV IgG and IgM chemiluminescence immunoassays. *Clin. Chem. Lab. Med.* **2020**, *58*. [CrossRef]
8. Padoan, A.; Cosma, C.; Sciacovelli, L.; Faggian, D.; Plebani, M. Analytical performances of a chemiluminescence immunoassay for SARS-CoV-2 IgM/IgG and antibody kinetics. *Clin. Chem. Lab. Med.* **2020**, *58*. [CrossRef]
9. Li, Z.; Yi, Y.; Luo, X.; Xiong, N.; Liu, Y.; Li, S.; Sun, R.; Wang, Y.; Hu, B.; Chen, W.; et al. Development and clinical application of a rapid IgM-IgG combined antibody test for SARS-CoV-2 infection diagnosis. *J. Med. Virol.* **2020**, *92*. [CrossRef]
10. Stringhini, S.; Wisniak, A.; Piumatti, G.; Azman, A.S.; Lauer, S.A.; Baysson, H.; De Ridder, D.; Petrovic, D.; Schrempft, S.; Marcus, K.; et al. Seroprevalence of anti-SARS-CoV-2 IgG antibodies in Geneva, Switzerland (SEROCoV-POP): A population-based study. *Lancet* **2020**, *396*, 313–319. [CrossRef]
11. Pollan, M.; Perez-Gomez, B.; Pastor-Barriuso, R.; Oteo, J.; Hernan, M.A.; Perez-Olmeda, M.; Sanmartín, J.L.; Fernández-García, A.; Cruz, I.; De Larrea, N.F.; et al. Prevalence of SARS-CoV-2 in Spain (ENE-COVID): A nationwide, population-based seroepidemiological study. *Lancet* **2020**. [CrossRef]
12. Soriano, V.; Meirino, R.; Corral, O.; Guallar, M.P. SARS-CoV-2 antibodies in adults in Madrid, Spain. *Clin. Infect. Dis.* **2020**. [CrossRef]
13. Petersen, M.S.; Strom, M.; Christiansen, D.H.; Fjallsbak, J.P.; Eliasen, E.H.; Johansen, M.; Veyhe, A.S.; Kristiansen, M.F.; Gaini, S.; Møller, L.F.; et al. Seroprevalence of SARS-CoV-2-Specific Antibodies, Faroe Islands. *Emerg. Infect. Dis.* **2020**, *26*. [CrossRef]
14. Biggs, H.M.; Harris, J.B.; Breakwell, L.; Dahlgren, F.S.; Abedi, G.R.; Szablewski, C.M.; Drobeniuc, J.; Bustamante, N.D.; Almendares, O.; Schnall, A.H.; et al. Estimated Community Seroprevalence of SARS-CoV-2 Antibodies—Two Georgia Counties, 28 April–3 May 2020. *MMWR Morb. Mortal. Wkly. Rep.* **2020**, *69*, 965–970. [CrossRef] [PubMed]
15. Menachemi, N.; Yiannoutsos, C.T.; Dixon, B.E.; Duszynski, T.J.; Fadel, W.F.; Wools-Kaloustian, K.K.; Needleman, N.U.; Box, K.; Caine, V.; Norwood, C.; et al. Population Point Prevalence of SARS-CoV-2 Infection Based on a Statewide Random Sample—Indiana, 25–29 April 2020. *MMWR Morb. Mortal. Wkly. Rep.* **2020**, *69*, 960–964. [CrossRef] [PubMed]
16. Fischer, B.; Knabbe, C.; Vollmer, T. SARS-CoV-2 IgG seroprevalence in blood donors located in three different federal states, Germany, March to June 2020. *Eurosurveillance* **2020**, *25*, 2001285. [CrossRef] [PubMed]
17. Havers, F.P.; Reed, C.; Lim, T.; Montgomery, J.M.; Klena, J.D.; Hall, A.J.; Fry, A.M.; Cannon, D.L.; Chiang, C.-F.; Gibbons, A.; et al. Seroprevalence of Antibodies to SARS-CoV-2 in 10 Sites in the United States, 23 March–12 May 2020. *JAMA Intern. Med.* **2020**. [CrossRef]
18. Amorim Filho, L.; Szwarcwald, C.L.; Mateos, S.O.G.; Leon, A.; Medronho, R.A.; Veloso, V.G.; Lopes, J.I.F.; De Moraes Sobrino Porto, L.C.; Chieppe, A.; Werneck, G.L. Seroprevalence of anti-SARS-CoV-2 among blood donors in Rio de Janeiro, Brazil. *Rev. Saude Publica* **2020**, *54*, 69.
19. Percivalle, E.; Cambie, G.; Cassaniti, I.; Nepita, E.V.; Maserati, R.; Ferrari, A.; Di Martino, R.; Isernia, P.; Mojoli, F.; Bruno, R.; et al. Prevalence of SARS-CoV-2 specific neutralising antibodies in blood donors from the Lodi Red Zone in Lombardy, Italy, as at 06 April 2020. *Eurosurveillance* **2020**, *25*, 2001031. [CrossRef]
20. Sood, N.; Simon, P.; Ebner, P.; Eichner, D.; Reynolds, J.; Bendavid, E.; Bhattacharya, J. Seroprevalence of SARS-CoV-2-Specific Antibodies Among Adults in Los Angeles County, California, on 10–11 April 2020. *JAMA* **2020**, *323*, 2425–2427. [CrossRef]
21. Tan, L.F.; Seetharaman, S. Preventing the Spread of COVID-19 to Nursing Homes: Experience from a Singapore Geriatric Centre. *J. Am. Geriatr. Soc.* **2020**, *68*, 942. [CrossRef]

22. Abrams, H.R.; Loomer, L.; Gandhi, A. Grabowski DCCharacteristics of, U.S. Nursing Homes with COVID-19 Cases. *J. Am. Geriatr. Soc.* **2020**, *68*. [CrossRef] [PubMed]
23. McMichael, T.M.; Currie, D.W.; Clark, S.; Pogosjans, S.; Kay, M.; Schwartz, N.G.; Lewis, J.; Baer, A.; Kawakami, V.; Lukoff, M.D.; et al. Epidemiology of Covid-19 in a Long-Term Care Facility in King County, Washington. *N. Engl. J. Med.* **2020**, *382*, 2005–2011. [CrossRef]
24. Stone, P.W.; Herzig, C.T.; Pogorzelska-Maziarz, M.; Carter, E.; Bjarnadottir, R.I.; Semeraro, P.K.; Cohen, C.C.; Travers, J.; Schweon, S. Understanding infection prevention and control in nursing homes: A qualitative study. *Geriatr. Nurs.* **2015**, *36*, 267–272. [CrossRef] [PubMed]
25. Herzig, C.T.; Stone, P.W.; Castle, N.; Pogorzelska-Maziarz, M.; Larson, E.L.; Dick, A.W. Infection Prevention and Control Programs in US Nursing Homes: Results of a National Survey. *J. Am. Med. Dir. Assoc.* **2016**, *17*, 85–88. [CrossRef]
26. Pena, S.A.; Davis, S.S.; Lu, X.; Sakthivel, S.K.K.; Peret, T.C.T.; Rose, E.B.; Smelser, C.; Schneider, E.; Stone, N.D.; Watson, J. Severe Respiratory Illness Associated with Human Metapneumovirus in Nursing Home, New Mexico, USA. *Emerg. Infect. Dis.* **2019**, *25*, 383–384. [CrossRef]
27. Ursic, T.; Miksic, N.G.; Lusa, L.; Strle, F.; Petrovec, M. Viral respiratory infections in a nursing home: A six-month prospective study. *BMC Infect. Dis.* **2016**, *16*, 637. [CrossRef]
28. Seynaeve, D.; Augusseau-Riviere, B.; Couturier, P.; Morel-Baccard, C.; Landelle, C.; Bosson, J.L.; Gavazzi, G.; Mallaret, M.-R. Outbreak of Human Metapneumovirus in a Nursing Home: A Clinical Perspective. *J. Am. Med. Dir. Assoc.* **2020**, *21*, 104–109.e1. [CrossRef] [PubMed]
29. Montoya, A.; Cassone, M.; Mody, L. Infections in Nursing Homes: Epidemiology and Prevention Programs. *Clin. Geriatr. Med.* **2016**, *32*, 585–607. [CrossRef]
30. De Maria, A.; Varese, P.; Dentone, C.; Barisione, E.; Bassetti, M. High prevalence of olfactory and taste disorder during SARS-CoV-2 infection in outpatients. *J. Med. Virol.* **2020**. [CrossRef]
31. Butowt, R.; Bilinska, K. SARS-CoV-2: Olfaction, Brain Infection, and the Urgent Need for Clinical Samples Allowing Earlier Virus Detection. *ACS Chem. Neurosci.* **2020**, *11*, 1200–1203. [CrossRef]
32. Al-Tawfiq, J.A. Asymptomatic coronavirus infection: MERS-CoV and SARS-CoV-2 (COVID-19). *Travel Med. Infect. Dis.* **2020**, *35*, 101608. [CrossRef] [PubMed]
33. Iacobucci, G. Sixty seconds on the contact tracing app. *BMJ* **2020**, *369*, m1818. [CrossRef] [PubMed]
34. Wu, F.; Wang, A.; Liu, M.; Wang, Q.; Chen, J.; Xia, S.; Ling, Y.; Zhang, Y.; Xun, J.; Lu, L.; et al. Neutralizing antibody responses to SARS-CoV-2 in a COVID-19 recovered patient cohort and their implications. *medRxiv* 2020. [CrossRef]
35. Fang, B.; Meng, Q.H. The laboratory's role in combating COVID-19. *Crit. Rev. Clin. Lab. Sci.* **2020**, *57*, 400–414. [CrossRef] [PubMed]
36. Ghaffari, A.; Meurant, R.; Ardakani, A. COVID-19 Serological Tests: How Well Do They Actually Perform? *Diagnostics* **2020**, *10*, 453. [CrossRef] [PubMed]

Journal of
Clinical Medicine

MDPI

Article

Evaluation of Mental Health Factors among People with Systemic Lupus Erythematosus during the SARS-CoV-2 Pandemic

Paweł Wańkowicz *, Aleksandra Szylińska and Iwona Rotter

Department of Medical Rehabilitation and Clinical Physiotherapy, Pomeranian Medical University in Szczecin, Żołnierska 48, 71-210 Szczecin, Poland; aleksandra.szylinska@gmail.com (A.S.); iwrot@wp.pl (I.R.)
* Correspondence: pawel.wankowicz@pum.edu.pl; Tel.: +48-(91)-4800914

Received: 17 August 2020; Accepted: 3 September 2020; Published: 5 September 2020

Abstract: There are considerable psychological and psychiatric consequences of the pandemic. Researchers have started to take into account the real or perceived sense of social threats that may be expressed, such as anxiety, depression, and sleep disorders. However, analyses on pandemic-related anxiety, depression, and sleep disorders mostly rarely addresses the situation of people with autoimmune diseases. Therefore, the aim of this study was to assess the mental health factors among people with systemic lupus erythematosus by quantifying the severity of anxiety, depression, and sleep disorders during the SARS-CoV-2 pandemic. In total, 723 people took part in the study. The study group consisted of 134 individuals with a systemic lupus erythematosus. The control group consisted of 589 people without systemic lupus erythematosus. The regression adjusted by age, gender, and diagnosis of other chronic diseases showed individuals with systemic lupus erythematosus were at a much higher risk of elevated symptoms of anxiety on the GAD-7 scale (OR = 3.683; $p < 0.001$), depression on the PHQ-9 scale (OR = 4.183; $p < 0.001$), and sleep disorders on the Insomnia Severity Index (ISI) scale (OR = 6.781; $p < 0.001$). Therefore, the mental health of patients with systemic lupus erythematosus in the times of the SARS-CoV-2 pandemic is not only an extremely important medical problem but also a social one and must require special attention.

Keywords: SARS-CoV-2; COVID-19; SLE; GAD-7; PHQ-9; ISI

1. Introduction

The entire world is currently trying to cope with the global pandemic of a new coronavirus. This was first observed in the city of Wuhan in China at the end of 2019, when cases of new atypical pneumonia were discovered [1]. The International Committee on Virus Taxonomy called this type of coronavirus SARS-CoV-2 due to its similarity to a virus causing severe acute respiratory syndrome (SARS) [2]. The disease caused by the new virus is commonly referred to as COVID-19 and has a higher mortality rate than that for influenza and, unlike SARS, is far more contagious [3]. To date, SARS-CoV-2 has killed 750,000 people and over 21 million have been infected, causing a global pandemic which has posed a serious challenge to medical care systems worldwide. In Poland, there have been 55,000 confirmed cases and 1800 deaths.

Based on available information and clinical knowledge, the Center for Disease Control and Prevention (CDC) announced that the majority of SARS-CoV-2 infections are asymptomatic or oligosymptomatic except for the elderly and people of all ages with chronic diseases, who may experience severe symptoms of COVID-19 [4]. Depending on the report, chronic diseases occur in up to 50% of patients infected with SARS-CoV-2 and mortality rates in this group are significantly higher than in the average population. During the recent coronaviral epidemics, i.e., SARS and MERS, it was also observed that in the majority of people with chronic diseases, the symptoms were more severe and often led to death due to multi-organ failure [5].

The chronic diseases listed by the CDC as those that can lead to a severe course of COVID-19 include many conditions that can cause immunosuppression, e.g., autoimmune diseases, which are becoming increasingly common although their exact causes are largely unknown. This group of chronic diseases is associated with the dysfunction of the immune system and consists of an undirected reaction against one's own cells, tissues, and organs [6,7]. This reaction results from a complex interaction between environmental and genetic factors. In the United States alone, autoimmune diseases affect more than 25 million people and their incidence is constantly increasing. Despite global progress in the diagnosis of these diseases, it is still difficult to identify them at the preclinical stage.

There are also considerable psychological and psychiatric consequences of the pandemic, and, in general, other adverse epidemiological conditions created by the industrialized world. Researchers have started to take into account the real or perceived sense of social threats, fear, and uncertainty that may be expressed as anxiety, depression, and sleep disorders [8–12]. However, analyses on pandemic-related anxiety mostly concern health care workers, rarely addressing the situation of other groups, e.g., people with systemic lupus erythematosus (SLE) [13]. The current outbreak of SARS-CoV-2 infection has led to global changes in many dimensions of daily lives. Ubiquitous information about the number of deaths, new diseases, diseases predisposing one to a severe and unfavorable course of SARS-CoV-2 infection, lack of targeted treatment, social isolation, change of existing habits, long-term quarantine, and a limited or total lack of access to goods or medical support causes a huge mental burden by generating emotional stress, elevated anxiety, and sleep disturbances. Sleep disturbances, depression, and anxiety are commonly reported in SLE patients. However, their prevalence varies from study to study [6,14,15]. Therefore, the aim of this study was to assess the mental health factors among people with SLE by quantifying the severity of anxiety, depression, and sleep disorders during the SARS-CoV-2 pandemic.

2. Materials and Methods

This cross-sectional study was conducted in the Western Pomerania region in Poland from 3 May 2020 to 17 May 2020. The study area was showing an incidence at 6/100.00 and prevalence at 31/100.00 during this period. This study included 6 hospitals with clinics or wards that diagnosed or hospitalized COVID-19 patients. In total, 723 people took part in the study. The study group consisted of 134 individuals with SLE. The control group consisted of 589 people without SLE. Each of the survey participants gave their informed consent by taking part in the survey. The participants could stop the survey at any time. The survey was anonymous and ensured the full confidentiality of information.

In this study, we focused on the symptoms of anxiety, depression, and sleep disorders in all participants using the 7-item Generalized Anxiety Disorder scale (GAD-7; range 0–21; no anxiety ≤ 4, anxiety > 4) [16] to assess the severity of anxiety, the 9-item Patient Health Questionnaire (PHQ-9; range 0–27; no depression ≤ 4, depression >4) [17–22] to assess the severity of depression symptoms, and the 7-item Insomnia Severity Index (ISI; range 0–28; no insomnia ≤ 8, insomnia > 8) to assess the severity of sleep disorder symptoms [23–26]. Cut-off points for anxiety, depression, and insomnia were established in accordance with the literature. Participants with scores below the cut-off points were characterized as showing no symptoms, while those who obtained scores above the cut-off points were characterized as showing symptoms.

Each participant gave basic demographic data, including their gender (male or female) and age. Data on coexisting diseases such as diabetes mellitus, hypertension, heart failure, coronary heart disease, chronic obstructive pulmonary disease, and dyslipidemia were also collected from each participant. Each participant was also asked about tobacco smoking.

The Pomeranian Medical University Ethics Committee approved the study protocol (KB-0012/26/04/2020/Z) which conformed to the ethical guidelines of the Declaration of Helsinki.

Statistical Analysis

A licensed Statistica 13.0 program (StatSoft, Tulsa, OK, USA) was used for statistical analysis. The assessment of normal distribution was performed using the Shapiro–Wilk test. The analysis of quantitative data was performed using the Mann–Whitney U test. For the analysis of qualitative data, the X^2 test was used; if the subgroup size was small, the Yates correction was applied. The evaluation of the relationship between the analyzed parameters was performed using univariable logistic regression model analysis and was adjusted for potentially distorting data (age, gender, diagnosed hypertension, diabetes mellitus, dyslipidemia, and cigarette smoking). Statistical significance was set at a $p \leq 0.05$.

3. Results

3.1. Comparison of Coexisting Diseases and Basic Demographic Data between the Group of People with Systemic Lupus Erythematosus and People without a Diagnosis of Systemic Lupus Erythematosus

Individuals without a diagnosis of systemic lupus erythematosus significantly more often smoked cigarettes and were more likely to suffer from hypertension ($p < 0.001$, $p = 0.003$, respectively). On the other hand, people with systemic lupus erythematosus were significantly more often female and younger ($p < 0.001$, $p < 0.001$, respectively). A case comparison is presented in Table 1.

Table 1. Comparison of selected parameters in patients with and without systemic lupus erythematosus.

		Control (n = 589)	SLE (n = 134)	P
Sex	female	275 (46.69)	119 (88.81)	<0.001
	male	314 (53.31)	15 (11.19)	
Age [years], mean ± SD; Me		39.71 ± 7.07; 39.00	38.34 ± 5.62; 38.00	<0.001
Do you have hypertension? (n, %)	No	487 (82.68)	125 (93.28)	0.003
	Yes	102 (17.32)	9 (6.72)	
Do you have diabetes mellitus? (n, %)	No	574 (97.45)	133 (99.25)	0.340
	Yes	15 (2.55)	1 (0.75)	
Do you have coronary heart disease? (n, %)	No	588 (99.83)	133 (99.25)	0.814
	Yes	1 (0.17)	1 (0.75)	
Are you suffering from heart failure? (n, %)	No	587 (99.66)	134 (100.00)	0.814
	Yes	2 (0.34)	0 (0.00)	
Do you have dyslipidemia? (n, %)	No	470 (79.80)	115 (85.82)	0.139
	Yes	119 (20.20)	19 (14.18)	
Do you have the chronic obstructive pulmonary disease? (n, %)	No	586 (99.49)	134 (100.00)	0.934
	Yes	3 (0.51)	0 (0.00)	
Do you smoke cigarettes? (n, %)	No	329 (55.86)	130 (97.01)	<0.001
	Yes	260 (44.14)	4 (2.99)	

Abbreviations: p—statistical significance, n—number of patients, Me—median, SD—standard deviation.

3.2. Comparison of Mental Health and Sleep Factors between the Group of People with Systemic Lupus Erythematosus and People without a Diagnosis of Systemic Lupus Erythematosus

The survey involved 723 respondents. In total, 507 participants (70.1%) suffered from anxiety according to the GAD-7 score (>4 points). In total, 586 participants (81%) showed depressive symptoms on the PHQ-9 scale (>4 points). In total, 514 (71.1%) participants had insomnia according to the score of the ISI scale (>8 points). People with SLE were significantly more often had symptoms of anxiety, depression and sleep disorders compared to those without SLE ($p < 0.001$, $p < 0.001$, $p < 0.001$ respectively). These individuals with SLE also significantly more often demonstrated higher scores on all three scales (GAD-7, PHQ-9, and ISI) compared to those without SLE ($p < 0.001$, $p < 0.001$, $p < 0.001$ respectively). A case comparison is presented in Table 2.

Table 2. Comparison of the severity of anxiety, depression, and sleep disorders in patients with and without systemic lupus erythematosus during the SARS-CoV-2 pandemic.

		Control (n = 589)	SLE (n = 134)	P
GAD-7	Mean ± SD; Me	6.56±4.06; 6.00	19.66±1.10; 20.00	<0.001
	≤4	216 (36.67)	0 (0.00)	<0.001
	>4	373 (63.33)	134 (100.00)	
PHQ-9	Mean ± SD; Me	8.65 ± 4.27; 9.00	20.61 ± 2.01; 21.00	<0.001
	≤ 4	137 (23.26)	0 (0.00)	<0.001
	>4	452 (76.74)	134 (100.00)	
ISI	Mean ± SD; Me	10.18 ± 4.96; 11.00	22.66 ± 2.30; 23.00	<0.001
	≤ 8	209 (35.48)	0 (0.00)	<0.001
	>8	380 (64.52)	134 (100.00)	

Abbreviations: GAD-7—Generalized Anxiety Disorder scale; PHQ-9—Patient Health Questionnaire, ISI—Insomnia Severity Index, p—statistical significance, n—number of patients, Me—median, SD—standard deviation.

3.3. Comparison of Mental Health and Sleep Factors after Adjustment for Covariates

Due to the low frequency of occurrence, the analysis did not take into account coronary heart diseases, heart failure, and chronic obstructive pulmonary disease.

The analysis of the univariable logistic regression model showed that a diagnosis of SLE was associated with a much higher risk of elevated anxiety on the GAD-7 scale (OR = 3.443; $p < 0.001$), depression on the PHQ-9 scale (OR = 4.095; $p < 0.001$), and sleep disorders on the ISI scale (OR = 5.032; $p < 0.001$). After the results were adjusted by age, gender, and diagnosis of the following diseases: hypertension, diabetes mellitus, dyslipidemia, and cigarette smoking, the increased risk of anxiety on the GAD-7 scale (OR = 3.683; $p < 0.001$), depression on the PHQ-9 scale (OR = 4.183; $p < 0.001$), and sleep disorders on the ISI scale (OR = 6.781; $p < 0.001$) were confirmed. The results are presented in Table 3.

Table 3. Logistic regression model of the severity of mental health disorders in patients with and without systemic lupus erythematosus.

	SLE (No Adjusted)			p	SLE (Adjusted by Potentially Distorting)			p
	OR	Cl −95%	Cl +95%		OR	Cl −95%	Cl +95%	
GAD7	3.443	2.409	4.921	<0.001	3.683	2.271	5.974	<0.001
PHQ-9	4.095	2.786	6.020	<0.001	4.183	2.544	6.878	<0.001
ISI	5.032	3.184	7.954	<0.001	6.781	2.968	15.492	<0.001

Abbreviations: GAD-7—Generalized Anxiety Disorder scale; PHQ-9—Patient Health Questionnaire, ISI—Insomnia Severity Index, p—statistical significance, OR—odds ratio, CI—confidence interval. Notes: Potentially distorting data (age, gender, diagnosed hypertension, diabetes mellitus, dyslipidemia and cigarette smoking).

4. Discussion

When searching medical databases, we did not find any other study that compared mental health factors during the SARS-CoV-2 pandemic between people with and without SLE.

The current outbreak of SARS-CoV-2 infection has led to global changes in many dimensions of our daily lives. Ubiquitous information about the number of deaths, new diseases, diseases predisposing one to a severe and unfavorable course of SARS-CoV-2 infection, lack of targeted treatment, social isolation, change of existing habits, long-term quarantine, and a limited or total lack of access to goods or medical support does not only raise public health concerns but also causes a huge mental burden by generating emotional stress and elevated anxiety. It is widely assumed that the pandemic has aggravated depression, anxiety, and related sleep disorders.

In this study, a significant number of participants experienced symptoms of anxiety, depression, and insomnia, with a 100% prevalence of these symptoms in the group of people with SLE—this is different from the frequency of these disorders in other studies [8,12,27,28]. This may be due to the fact that our study was conducted in Europe where an infection problem on such a scale has not occurred for nearly 100 years, while the aforementioned studies were conducted in Asia where epidemics have been more frequent. This has meant that the institutions responsible for organizing the protection of public safety in China, Hong-Kong, and Taiwan have well-prepared procedures, well-trained service personnel, as well as an entire industry that is capable of adapting to the goal of fighting a pandemic. These differences may also arise from the different tools used to assess depression, anxiety, or sleep disorders and from the differences in the project design itself.

Epidemiological data provide evidence of a steady increase in autoimmune diseases over the last decade. It has long been known that autoimmune diseases show clear gender differences [29], with many more women contracting these diseases than men [30]. The effect of age varies, depending on the disease. According to the study by Fairwather et al., the majority of autoimmune diseases manifest themselves before the age of 50 and are characterized by acute cellular pathology, whereas those manifesting after 50 are characterized by chronic inflammation and fibrosis [31]. These findings concerning age and gender are consistent with the findings of this study, in which people with a diagnosed SLE were significantly younger and more frequently female compared to people without the SLE.

In recent years, many studies have been conducted on the relationship between anxiety, depression, and sleep disorders in patients with chronic diseases. It has been observed that patients with chronic diseases often exhibit mental disorders [32]. In the study conducted by Polukandrioti et al., it was noted that at least 20% of patients with coronary artery disease showed symptoms of anxiety and depression [33]. Other studies confirmed the same relationship in patients with chronic neurological diseases, chronic pain, kidney diseases, and respiratory diseases [34–39].

The most important discovery of our study is the fact that despite the significantly more frequent occurrences of chronic diseases in the group of people without a diagnosis of SLE, it was the group of patients with SLE that showed elevated symptoms of anxiety, depression, and sleep disorders ($p < 0.001$, $p < 0.001$, $p < 0.001$, respectively). These individuals, when the results were adjusted for age, gender, chronic diseases, and smoking, showed more than a 3.6 fold increase in the risk of anxiety symptoms, a more than 4.1 fold increase in the severity of depression symptoms, and more than a 6.7 fold increase in the severity of sleep disorders. An autoimmune disease in itself is a source of many stress factors, including reduced activity and fulfillment of social roles at home and work, financial difficulties related to reduced income and high costs of medical care, changes in external appearance resulting, among others, from complications of the applied immunosuppressive treatment, loss of independence, and impaired interpersonal relations [40]. Even slight intensification of the influence of everyday stress factors in people with autoimmune diseases may intensify the symptoms of the disease, i.e., adversely affecting the time of remission [41].

This is why patients with a diagnosis of SLE, even after adjusting for those differences in co-occurring conditions have more severity anxiety, depression, and sleep disorders, as confirmed by our study.

Our study had several limitations. First of all, it lacked longitudinal observations in people included in this study. Secondly, the number of respondents was limited. Thirdly, it was impossible to determine a correlation between the presence of anxiety, depression, insomnia, and a specific type of other autoimmune disease. Fourthly potential selection bias in who participated in the survey. This means that a longitudinal, multi-center study with a greater number of respondents is required.

5. Conclusions

In patients with a diagnosed SLE in the era of SARS-CoV-2 there is a higher risk of exacerbation of anxiety, depression, and sleep disorders than in patients with other chronic diseases. It is precisely these people, in a state of mental decompensation, who require informational support, medical support, stress reduction, and rest. Therefore, the mental health of patients with SLE in the times of the SARS-CoV-2 pandemic is not only an extremely important medical problem but also a social one and must require special attention.

Author Contributions: P.W. designed the study, included respondents in the study, collected the data, analyzed the data, participated in the drafting of the manuscript. A.S. included respondents in the study, collected the data, analyzed the data, participated in the drafting of the manuscript. I.R. included respondents in the study, collected the data, analyzed the data, participated in the drafting of the manuscript. All the authors edited, read and agreed to the published version of the manuscript.

Funding: This research received no grant from any funding agency in the public, commercial, or not-for-profit sectors.

Conflicts of Interest: The authors declares that there is no conflict of interest.

References

1. Li, Q.; Guan, X.; Wu, P.; Wang, X.; Zhou, L.; Tong, Y.; Ren, R.; Med, M.; Leung, K.S.M.; Lau, E.H.Y. Early Transmission Dynamics in Wuhan, China, of Novel Coronavirus-Infected Pneumonia. *N. Engl. J. Med.* **2020**, *382*, 1199–1207. [CrossRef] [PubMed]
2. Coronaviridae Study Group of the International Committee on Taxonomy of Viruses. The species Severe acute respiratory syndrome-related coronavirus: Classifying 2019-nCoV and naming it SARS-CoV-2. *Nat. Microbiol.* **2020**, *5*, 536–544. [CrossRef]
3. Yang, Y.; Peng, F.; Wang, R.; Guan, K.; Jiang, T.; Xu, G.; Sun, J.; Chang, C. The deadly coronaviruses: The 2003 SARS pandemic and the 2020 novel coronavirus epidemic in China. *J. Autoimmun.* **2020**, *109*, 102434. [CrossRef] [PubMed]
4. CDC. *Coronavirus Disease 2019 (COVID-19)*; US Department of Health and Human Services CDC: Atlanta, GA, USA, 2020. Available online: https://www.cdc.gov/coronavirus/2019-ncov/index.html (accessed on 15 August 2020).
5. Yang, Y.-M.; Hsu, C.-Y.; Lai, C.-C.; Yen, M.-F.; Wikramaratna, P.S.; Chen, H.-H.; Wang, T.-H. Impact of Comorbidity on Fatality Rate of Patients with Middle East Respiratory Syndrome. *Sci. Rep.* **2017**, *7*, 11307. [CrossRef] [PubMed]
6. Wańkowicz, P.; Bobrowska-Snarska, D.; Nowacki, P.; Brzosko, M. Clinical manifestations of neuropsychiatric systemic lupus erythematosus: A single-center study from West Pomerania Province in Poland. *Pol. Arch. Intern. Med.* **2020**, *130*, 82–84. [PubMed]
7. Wańkowicz, P.; Nowacki, P.; Brzosko, M.; Bobrowska-Snarska, D. An overlapping case of Bickerstaff brainstem encephalitis and acute motor axonal neuropathy variant of Guillain-Barre syndrome associated with Systemic Lupus Erythematosus. *Pol. Arch. Intern. Med.* **2018**, *129*, 50–51. [CrossRef] [PubMed]
8. Lai, J.; Ma, S.; Wang, Y.; Cai, Z.; Hu, J.; Wei, N.; Wu, J.; Du, H.; Chen, T.; Li, R.; et al. Factors Associated With Mental Health Outcomes Among Health Care Workers Exposed to Coronavirus Disease 2019. *JAMA Netw. Open* **2020**, *3*, e203976. [CrossRef] [PubMed]
9. Chen, Q.; Liang, M.; Li, Y.; Guo, J.; Fei, D.; Wang, L.; He, L.; Sheng, C.; Cai, Y.; Li, X.; et al. Mental health care for medical staff in China during the COVID-19 outbreak. *Lancet Psychiatry* **2020**, *7*, e15–e16. [CrossRef]
10. Bao, Y.; Sun, Y.; Meng, S.; Shi, J.; Lu, L. 2019-nCoV epidemic: Address mental health care to empower society. *Lancet* **2020**, *395*, e37–e38. [CrossRef]
11. Bohlken, J.; Schömig, F.; Lemke, M.R.; Pumberger, M.; Riedel-Heller, S.G. COVID-19 Pandemic: Stress Exposure of Healthcare Workers [COVID-19 Pandemic: Stress Experience of Healthcare Workers—A Short Current Review]. *Psychiatry Pract.* **2020**, *47*, 190–197.
12. Zhang, C.; Yang, L.; Liu, S.; Ma, S.; Wang, Y.; Cai, Z.; Du, H.; Li, R.; Kang, L.; Su, M.; et al. Survey of Insomnia and Related Social Psychological Factors Among Medical Staff Involved in the 2019 Novel Coronavirus Disease Outbreak. *Front. Psychiatry* **2020**, *11*, 306. [CrossRef] [PubMed]

13. Wańkowicz, P.; Szylińska, A.; Rotter, I. Assessment of Mental Health Factors among Health Professionals Depending on Their Contact with COVID-19 Patients. *Int. J. Environ. Res. Public Health* **2020**, *17*, 5849. [CrossRef] [PubMed]
14. Young, K.; Munroe, M.E.; Harley, J.B.; Guthridge, J.M.; Kamen, D.L.; Gilkensen, G.S.; Weisman, M.H.; Karp, D.R.; Wallace, D.J.; James, J.A.; et al. Less than 7 hours of sleep per night is associated with transitioning to systemic lupus erythematosus. *Lupus* **2018**, *27*, 1524–1531. [CrossRef] [PubMed]
15. Zhang, L.; Fu, T.; Yin, R.; Zhang, Q.; Shen, B. Prevalence of depression and anxiety in systemic lupus erythematosus: A systematic review and meta-analysis. *BMC Psychiatry* **2017**, *17*, 70. [CrossRef] [PubMed]
16. Spitzer, R.L.; Kroenke, K.; Williams, J.B.W.; Löwe, B. A Brief Measure for Assessing Generalized Anxiety Disorder. *Arch. Intern. Med.* **2006**, *166*, 1092–1097. [CrossRef]
17. Spitzer, R.L. Utility of a new procedure for diagnosing mental disorders in primary care. The PRIME-MD 1000 study. *JAMA* **1994**, *272*, 1749–1756. [CrossRef]
18. Spitzer, R.L.; Kroenke, K.; Williams, J.B.W.; Patient Health Questionnaire Primary Care Study Group. Validation and Utility of a Self-report Version of PRIME-MDThe PHQ Primary Care Study. *JAMA* **1999**, *282*, 1737–1744. [CrossRef]
19. Spitzer, R.L.; Williams, J.B.W.; Kroenke, K.; Hornyak, R.; McMurray, J. Validity and utility of the Patient Health Questionnaire in assessment of 3000 obstetrics-gynecologic patients. *Am. J. Obstet. Gynecol.* **2000**, *183*, 759–769. [CrossRef]
20. Kroenke, K.; Spitzer, R.L.; Williams, J.B.W. The PHQ-9: Validity of a brief depression severity measure. *J. Gen. Intern. Med.* **2001**, *16*, 606–613. [CrossRef]
21. Kroenke, K.; Spitzer, R.L. The PHQ-9: A New Depression Diagnostic and Severity Measure. *Psychiatr. Ann.* **2002**, *32*, 509–515. [CrossRef]
22. Löwe, B.; Unützer, J.; Callahan, C.M.; Perkins, A.J.; Kroenke, K. Monitoring depression treatment outcomes with the Patient Health Questionnaire-9. *Med. Care* **2004**, *42*, 1194–1201. [PubMed]
23. Morin, C.M. *Insomnia: Psychological Assessment and Management*; Guilford Press: New York, NY, USA, 1993.
24. Bastien, C. Validation of the Insomnia Severity Index as an outcome measure for insomnia research. *Sleep Med.* **2001**, *2*, 297–307. [CrossRef]
25. Yang, M.; Morin, C.M.; Schaefer, K.; Wallenstein, G.V. Interpreting score differences in the Insomnia Severity Index: Using health-related outcomes to define the minimally important difference. *Curr. Med. Res. Opin.* **2009**, *25*, 2487–2494. [CrossRef] [PubMed]
26. Morin, C.M.; Belleville, G.; Bélanger, L.; Ivers, H. The Insomnia Severity Index: Psychometric Indicators to Detect Insomnia Cases and Evaluate Treatment Response. *Sleep* **2011**, *34*, 601–608. [CrossRef]
27. Lee, S.; Chan, L.Y.; Chau, A.M.; Kwok, K.P.; Kleinman, A. The experience of SARS-related stigma at Amoy Gardens. *Soc. Sci. Med.* **2005**, *61*, 2038–2046. [CrossRef] [PubMed]
28. Su, T.-P.; Lien, T.-C.; Yang, C.-Y.; Su, Y.L.; Wang, J.-H.; Tsai, S.-L.; Yin, J.-C. Prevalence of psychiatric morbidity and psychological adaptation of the nurses in a structured SARS caring unit during outbreak: A prospective and periodic assessment study in Taiwan. *J. Psychiatr. Res.* **2007**, *41*, 119–130. [CrossRef]
29. Ngo, S.T.; Steyn, F.J.; McCombe, P.A. Gender differences in autoimmune disease. *Front. Neuroendocr.* **2014**, *35*, 347–369. [CrossRef]
30. Pollard, K.M. Gender differences in autoimmunity associated with exposure to environmental factors. *J. Autoimmun.* **2012**, *38*, J177–J186. [CrossRef]
31. Fairweather, D.; Frisancho-Kiss, S.; Rose, N.R. Sex Differences in Autoimmune Disease from a Pathological Perspective. *Am. J. Pathol.* **2008**, *173*, 600–609. [CrossRef]
32. Koyanagi, A.; Garin, N.; Olaya, B.; Ayuso-Mateos, J.L.; Chatterji, S.; Leonardi, M.; Koskinen, S.; Tobiasz-Adamczyk, B.; Haro, J.M. Correction: Chronic Conditions and Sleep Problems among Adults Aged 50 years or over in Nine Countries: A Multi-Country Study. *PLoS ONE* **2015**, *10*, e0138261. [CrossRef]
33. Polikandrioti, M.; Goudevenos, I.; Michalis, L.; Patsilinakos, S.; Nikolaou, V.; Olympios, C.; Dilanas, C.; Votteas, V.; Zompolos, S.; Elisaf, M. The effects of anxiety and depression on the needs of patients hospitalized with coronary disease. *Arch. Hell. Med.* **2012**, *29*, 33–43.
34. Gerontoukou, E.-I.; Michaelidoy, S.; Rekleiti, M.; Saridi, M.; Souliotis, K. Investigation of Anxiety and Depression in Patients with Chronic Diseases. *Heal. Psychol. Res.* **2015**, *3*, 2123. [CrossRef] [PubMed]

35. Janowski, K.; Kurpas, D.; Kusz, J.; Mroczek, B.; Jedynak, T. Health-Related Behavior, Profile of Health Locus of Control and Acceptance of Illness in Patients Suffering from Chronic Somatic Diseases. *PLoS ONE* **2013**, *8*, e63920. [CrossRef]
36. Voinov, B.; Richie, W.D.; Bailey, R.K. Depression and Chronic Diseases. *Prim. Care Companion CNS Disord.* **2013**, *15*. [CrossRef] [PubMed]
37. Wong, W.S.; Chen, P.P.; Yap, J.; Mak, K.H.; Tam, B.K.H.; Fielding, R. Chronic Pain and Psychiatric Morbidity: A Comparison between Patients Attending Specialist Orthopedics Clinic and Multidisciplinary Pain Clinic. *Pain Med.* **2011**, *12*, 246–259. [CrossRef]
38. Theofilou, P. Quality of life and mental health in hemodialysis and peritoneal dialysis patients: The role of health beliefs. *Int. Urol. Nephrol.* **2011**, *44*, 245–253. [CrossRef]
39. Yohannes, A.M.; Willgoss, T.G.; Baldwin, R.C.; Connolly, M.J. Depression and anxiety in chronic heart failure and chronic obstructive pulmonary disease: Prevalence, relevance, clinical implications and management principles. *Int. J. Geriatr. Psychiatry* **2010**, *25*, 1209–1221. [CrossRef]
40. Liang, M.H.; Rogers, M.; Larson, M.; Eaton, H.M.; Murawski, B.J.; Taylor, J.E.; Swafford, J.; Schur, P.H. The psychosocial impact of systemic lupus erythematosus and rheumatoid arthritis. *Arthritis Rheum.* **1984**, *27*, 13–19. [CrossRef]
41. Michelsen, B.; Kristianslund, E.K.; Sexton, J.; Hammer, H.B.; Fagerli, K.M.; Lie, E.; Wierød, A.; Kalstad, S.; Rødevand, E.; Krøll, F.; et al. Do depression and anxiety reduce the likelihood of remission in rheumatoid arthritis and psoriatic arthritis? Data from the prospective multicentre NOR-DMARD study. *Ann. Rheum. Dis.* **2017**, *76*, 1906–1910. [CrossRef]

Journal of
Clinical Medicine

MDPI

Article

Early Psychological Impact of the COVID-19 Pandemic in Brazil: A National Survey

Juliana Alvares Duarte Bonini Campos [1], Bianca Gonzalez Martins [1], Lucas Arrais Campos [2], João Marôco [3], Rayya Ahmed Saadiq [4] and Rodrigo Ruano [5,*]

1 School of Pharmaceutical Sciences, São Paulo State University (UNESP), Campus Araraquara, São Paulo 14800-903, Brazil; juliana.campos@unesp.br (J.A.D.B.C.); bia.g.martins@unesp.br (B.G.M.)
2 School of Dentistry, São Paulo State University (UNESP), Campus Araraquara, São Paulo 14801-903, Brazil; lucas.campos@unesp.br
3 William James Center for Research (WJCR), University Institute of Psychological, Social, and Life Sciences (ISPA), 1100-304 Lisbon, Portugal; jpmaroco@ispa.pt
4 Mayo Clinic College of Medicine General Interne Medicine and International Medicine, Mayo Clinic, Rochester, MN 55905, USA; Saadiq.Rayya@mayo.edu
5 Division of Maternal-Fetal Medicine, Department of Obstetrics and Gynecology, Mayo Clinic, Rochester, MN 55905, USA
* Correspondence: ruano.rodrigo@mayo.edu or rodrigoruano@hotmail.com; Tel.: +507-284-0210

Received: 27 August 2020; Accepted: 12 September 2020; Published: 15 September 2020

Abstract: Background: Isolation measures used to contain epidemics generate social interaction restrictions and impose changes in routines of the public that increase negative psychological outcomes. Anxiety and depression are the most common symptoms. Objective: To evaluate the mental health of the Brazilian population during the SARs-CoV-2 pandemic and its relationship with demographic and health characteristics. Methods: Adults from all Brazilian States participated (n = 12,196; women: 69.8%, mean age = 35.2 years). The Depression, Anxiety and Stress Scale, and the Impact of Event Scale–revised were used (online survey). Data validity and reliability were verified by confirmatory factor analysis and ordinal alpha coefficient. The probability of presenting psychological symptoms was calculated by multiple logistic regression and odds ratio (OR) (0 = without symptoms, 1 = with mild, moderate, and severe levels of symptoms). Results: High prevalence of depression (61.3%), anxiety (44.2%), stress (50.8%), and psychological impact (54.9%) due to the isolation experienced from the pandemic was found. Younger individuals (OR = 1.58–3.58), those that felt unsafe (OR = 1.75–2.92), with a previous diagnosis of mental health (OR = 1.72–2.64) and/or had general health problems before the pandemic (OR = 1.17–1.51), who noticed changes in their mental state due to the pandemic context (OR = 2.53–9.07), and excessively exposed to the news (OR = 1.19–2.18) were at increased risk of developing symptoms. Women (OR = 1.35–1.65) and those with lower economic status (OR = 1.38–2.69) were more likely to develop psychological symptoms. Lower educational levels increased the likelihood of depressive (OR = 1.03–1.34) and intrusive symptoms (OR = 1.09–1.51). *Conclusions*: The pandemic and related factors can have a high impact on the mental health of the population. Demographic characteristics can influence the occurrence of psychological symptoms.

Keywords: pandemic; COVID-19; mental health; quarantine

1. Introduction

Isolation and quarantine measures (used or experienced) during epidemics generate separation and restriction of human movement, imposing drastic changes in routine and the need for adaptation at a time of great physical, social, economic and psychological vulnerability. Despite all the efforts towards containing the spread of the disease, isolation and quarantine measures come with psychological costs to individuals and, therefore, some care and attention related to mental health must be provided [1–7]. The World Health Organization declared the new coronavirus disease (COVID-19) a pandemic on 11 March 2020. At the end of that month, due to the rapid increase of cases (or infections), Brazil declared a mandatory quarantine, excluding essential service workers.

The psychological consequences of quarantine and isolation measures have already been identified in previous epidemics such as SARS [8–11], Ebola [12,13], and H1N1 [14,15]. So far, most of the scientific information on the impact of the SARs-CoV-2 pandemic on mental health has been presented as letters to editors or brief reports from experts due to the ongoing nature of the pandemic and little data is available. The existing documents indicate that the current quarantine and mass social isolation can have concerning psychological effects [3,5–7,16]. As of July 2020, there were few published epidemiological studies focusing on the Chinese population, with some assessing the effects of the disease from a clinical point of view, including mental health in patients who contracted the disease [17,18] and the mental health effects on frontline healthcare workers highlighting their vulnerable situation [19,20]. Only four studies evaluated the mental health conditions on the general population—three from China and one from Brazil.

Gao et al. [21] investigated 4827 Chinese adults and reported a high prevalence of depression (48.3%), anxiety (22.6%), and concomitant depression and anxiety (19.4%). Wang et al. [22] reported that 16.5% of the 1210 Chinese respondents had symptoms of moderate to severe depression, 28.8% had severe anxiety, and 8.1% had moderate to severe stress levels. Figueiras et al. [23] carried out a study with 1460 Brazilian adults and reported that women, younger people, and those with less education had higher levels of depression and anxiety. The authors also describe behaviors of individuals during quarantine and their relationship to depression, anxiety, and stress symptoms. However, none of these studies evaluated a nationwide population. To date, only one nation-wide study has been carried out in China by Qiu et al. [24] with 52,730 participants from 36 provinces that found that peri-traumatic stress was related to sex, age, educational level, region of residence, local health structure, and being a migrant worker. Nevertheless, some areas of that large country were not included in the study.

The literature on COVID-19 is increasing in an exponential rate. Scientists around the world have been making efforts to understand the pandemic from different aspects. However, everyone has the same challenge, which is to provide quality responses as quickly as possible to the population. Science is being carried out in real time. In early September 2020, four more studies involving a general population sample (one Italian study [25], one Israeli [26], one from the United States [27] and one from United Kingdom [28]) were published with mental health data in the pandemic. Moccia et al. [25] conducted a study with 500 adults in the initial phase of the outbreak of SARs-CoV-2 in Italy (April). Of the participants, 62.0% reported not having psychological distress due to the pandemic, 19.4% had mild distress and 18.6% had moderate or severe, with women being the most affected. Individuals with cyclothymic, depressive and anxious temperaments were more likely to have moderate or severe psychological distress. Palgi et al. [26] conducted a study with 1059 adults to evaluate symptoms of depression and anxiety related to the SARs-CoV-2 pandemic in Israel. Most of the participants were women and had a high level of education. The youngest were more vulnerable to depressive and anxious symptoms and there was no relationship between these symptoms and the existence of pre-existing chronic diseases. Loneliness caused by isolation measures was the most prominent risk factor for the development of depressive and anxious symptoms.

Bruin [27] investigated the relationship between age and perceptions of risk, anxiety and depression during the pandemic in the United States. Data collection was carried out in March and 6,666 North American adults participated (52% women with an age range from 18 to 100 years [mean = 48.6; standard deviation = 16.6]). Older individuals had a greater perception of the risk of dying if they were infected with SARs-CoV-2, greater awareness that being in isolation reduces the risk of contagion and were less likely to have depression and anxiety.

To date, the UK study [28] appears to be the only longitudinal study that assessed changes in mental health in adults before and during the pandemic lockdown. The authors used data from the UK Household Longitudinal Study (UKHLS) which started in 2014, with surveys carried out at the beginning (for example, 1 January 2014) and at the end of two years (for example, 31 December 2015) with annual overlap. 15,376 individuals over the age of 16 from Wales, Scotland, Northern Ireland, and region of England participated. The mental distress increased from 18.9% (in 2018–2019) to 27.3% one month after the lockdown (April 2020). The current mean score for non-specific mental distress in the population was above expectations considering the estimated trend from 2014 to 2018. This increase was significantly higher among younger people, women, those with lower economic status and people living with children.

In a few days, new studies have been published with regards to the mental health impact during the COVID-19 pandemic. Among the recent studies, there is a systematic review/meta-analysis published by Salari et al. [29] that included 17 studies from 10 different countries. Among the most common psychological symptoms related to epidemics are post-traumatic stress [14], anxiety, and depression [1,4,6,22], which can be found during the isolation/quarantine period and can outlast the epidemic. Brooks et al. [1] highlight that this is due to the presence of specific stressors including the duration of the quarantine, fear of being infected, frustration and anger for the loss of the normal routine and reduction of physical and social contact, inadequate supply of food, water or accommodation, and confusing or inadequate information coming mainly from government and public agencies. Among the post-pandemic stressors, financial difficulties and social stigma towards infected individuals and health care workers are mentioned.

With a pandemic scenario, all individuals, to a greater or lesser degree, will depend on their mental resources to cope with the lifestyle changes, fears, and uncertainties. As the SARS-Cov2 pandemic, combined with the political and economic impact, imposes a new and distressing context, the monitoring of the population's mental health may contribute to establish individual or collective strategies of support, guidance, prevention, and intervention to minimize mental trauma during and after the pandemic. Still, Sani et al. [16] emphasize that the identification of possible predictors for the psychological impact of the pandemic on populations can be relevant for the elaboration of more targeted and resolute intervention plans.

This nationwide study was carried out to assess aspects related to the mental health of the Brazilian population during the coronavirus pandemic. The prevalence of depression, anxiety and stress symptoms and their relationship with demographic and context-related characteristics was verified.

We hypothesized that the prevalence of psychological symptoms is high in Brazil in view of sanitary, economic and political insecurity. We also hypothesized that younger people, women, people with previously diagnosed mental disorders and those most exposed to pandemic news are more likely to develop symptoms of depression, anxiety and stress and be psychologically impacted.

2. Methods

2.1. Study Design and Sample

This was a cross-sectional observational study. Data were collected online using Google Forms with the links to the form sent by email, WhatsApp, or social networks. Brazilian individuals over 18 years of age were able to participate. The minimum sample size was estimated using $\alpha = 5\%$, $p = 5\%$ (prevalence of mortality from COVID-19), $\varepsilon = 10\%$, and a loss rate of 25%. Thus, the minimum sample size was estimated at 9734. The sample was stratified by states to ensure a representation of all Brazilian States and the Federal District.

Information was collected on sex, age, state, monthly family income (1: below 240.00 USD; 2: between 240.00 USD and 383.00 USD; 3: between 384.00 USD and 1,652.00 USD; 4: between 1653.00 USD and 2153.00 USD; 5: above 2154.00 USD; 1 USD = 5.23 BRL; Available from: www.bcb.gov.br; Accessed 21 July 2020), number of people residing with the participant, time (minutes) spent per day watching or reading the news related to the pandemic, and education level (1: complete elementary

I school, 2: complete elementary II school, 3: complete high school, 4: complete higher education and 5: complete graduate school). Further information was obtained on the mental health and general health problems diagnosed before the pandemic, mental health status during the pandemic, knowing someone who tested positive for COVID-19, considering COVID-19 as dangerous or not, sense of safe, and the opinion if the news about this viral pandemic is confusion. Information regarding the absence or presence of mental health problems was obtained by asking the participant if he had already received a medical diagnosis related to mental health disorders at some point before the pandemic. Regarding general health, the information was obtained in the same way, but, asking about medical diagnosis related to health in general. In addition, the participants were asked if they noticed any changes in their mental health status after the pandemic began, felt safe or unsafe in view of the pandemic scenario, believed the coronavirus was dangerous or not and if they considered the news transmitted about the pandemic confusing or adequate/clarifying.

Respondents also completed the Depression, Anxiety and Stress Scale (DASS-21) [30,31] and the Impact of Event Scale-revised (IES-R) [32]. The time frame for psychological impact was considered the period since the beginning of the pandemic in Brazil (11 March 2020).

2.2. Procedures and Ethical Aspects

For data collection, a non-probabilistic snowball sampling method was used. The first contacts took place on 18 May 2020, with professors from different higher education institutions in Brazil using e-mails available on the institutions' websites. Invitations were also sent the official email addresses of the Slums Association (Central Única das Favelas (CUFA)) and seven non-governmental organizations (NGOs) in the country. The selected institutions were among the ten largest in the country and involved individuals of varying socioeconomic levels. To expand the sample, invitees were asked to pass on the survey link to their personal contacts. The researchers provided guidelines for distributing the link via email, WhatsApp, or social media. Data collection ended on 25 June 2020.

In Brazil, on 11 March 2020, social isolation measures began to be established. Six days later (March 17) the first death due to COVID-19 was confirmed, which contributed to the maintenance of the quarantine that lasted approximately until the beginning of July. After this period, there was a relaxation of social isolation, with a gradual reopening of trade and a recovery of the economy. During the 39-day period of data collection, the Brazilian Ministry of Health reported 973,894 cases of Covid-19 with 38,179 deaths due to the disease. At the beginning of the collection (May 18th) there were 254,220 cases and 16,792 deaths and on the last day of the collection (June 25th) there were 1,228,114 cases and 54,971 deaths due to COVID-19 reported in Brazil. During the data collection period, the highest number of COVID-19 deaths in 24 h in the country (n = 1.473) was reached on 4 June and the highest number of new cases in 24 h (n = 54.771) was observed on the 19th of June.

All subjects gave their informed consent for inclusion before they participated in the study. The study was conducted in accordance with the Declaration of Helsinki, and the protocol was approved by the National Research Ethics Commission of the Ministry of Health (CONEP) (C.A.A.E. 30604220.4.0000.0008).

2.3. Measuring Instruments

Symptoms of depression, anxiety, and stress were assessed using the Portuguese version of the DASS-21 [30,31]. The scale consists of 21 items distributed in three factors with a 4-point Likert-type response scale from 0 to 3 (0: did not apply to me at all, 1: some of the time, 2: a good part of time, 3: most of the time). The scores were calculated by adding the items' response of each subscale and the participants were classified using the cutoff points proposed by Lovibond & Lovibond [33], multiplying the sum of the responses by two (Depression: Normal—0 to 9, Mild—10 to 13, Moderate—14 to 20, Severe—21 to 27, and Extremely severe ≥ 28; Anxiety: Normal—0 to 7, Mild—8 to 9, Moderate—10 to 14, Severe—15 to 19, and Extremely severe ≥ 20; Stress: Normal—0 to 14, Mild—15 to 18, Moderate—19 to 25, Severe—26 to 33, and Extremely severe ≥ 34).

The degree of psychological impact related to the pandemic was identified using the Portuguese version of the IES-R [32]. The IES-R is composed of 22 items distributed in three factors (avoidance, intrusion, and hyperarousal) with a Likert-type response scale of 5 points (0—not at all, 1—slightly, 2—moderately, 3—very and 4—extremely). IES-R calculated by the sum of responses to all items on the scale) and the recommendation by Wang et al. [22] (Normal—0 to 23; Mild—24 to 32; Moderate—33 to 36; Severe—≥37) were proposed to estimate the prevalence of psychological impact and its degree of involvement. Next, the cutoff points were transposed, considering the corresponding percentiles, for each factor of the scale so that one can also estimate the prevalence and the degree of involvement for the three factors of the IES-R separately (Avoidance and Intrusion: Normal—0 to 8; Mild—9 to 11; Moderate—12 to 13; Severe—≥14; Hyperstimulation: Normal—0 to 6; Mild—7 to 8; Moderate—9 to 10; Severe—≥11).

2.4. Data Validity and Reliability Indicators

Confirmatory factor analysis (AFC) was performed with the weighted least squares means and variance adjusted (WLSMV). The fit of the theoretical models to the data was assessed using the Comparative Fit Index (CFI), Tucker-Lewis Index (TLI), and Root Mean Square Error of Approximation (RMSEA) with a 90% confidence interval. The fit was considered adequate if CFI and TLI ≥ 0.90, and RMSEA ≤ 0.10 [34]. The factor loadings (λ) of the items were considered adequate if $\lambda \geq 0.50$. Reliability was analyzed by the alpha ordinal coefficient (α) (adequate reliability: $\alpha \geq 0.70$). The analyses were conducted for the total sample (Brazil) and for each region of the country in order to identify possible model fit problems due to cultural differences. The MPLUS 7.2 program (Muthén and Muthén, Los Angeles, CA, USA) was used. The data were found to be valid and reliable and parameters are shown in Table 1.

Table 1. Psychometric parameters for fit of the models to the samples of the instruments used (Depression, Anxiety and Stress Scale (DASS-21), and Impact of Event Scale-revised, (IES-R)).

Instrument	Sample	n	Confirmatory Factor Analysis *				
			λ	CFI	TLI	RMSEA (90% CI)	α
DASS-21	Brazil	12,196	0.54–0.92	0.978	0.975	0.065 (0.064–0.066)	0.892–0.947
	Midwest	1026	0.52–0.92	0.973	0.970	0.068 (0.064–0.072)	0.879–0.944
	Northeast	3804	0.53–0.91	0.977	0.974	0.066 (0.064–0.067)	0.890–0.947
	North	1191	0.52–0.91	0.974	0.971	0.070 (0.066–0.074)	0.887–0.945
	Southeast	4677	0.55–0.93	0.980	0.977	0.064 (0.062–0.066)	0.896–0.949
	South	1498	0.55–0.93	0.981	0.978	0.059 (0.056–0.063)	0.892–0.941
IES-R †	Brazil	12,196	0.51–0.89	0.964	0.960	0.072 (0.071–0.073)	0.879–0.927
	Midwest	1026	0.53–0.89	0.968	0.964	0.067 (0.063–0.071)	0.883–0.928
	Northeast	3804	0.52–0.89	0.965	0.961	0.072 (0.070–0.074)	0.878–0.928
	North	1191	0.53–0.88	0.965	0.960	0.069 (0.065–0.072)	0.883–0.926
	Southeast	4677	0.50–0.89	0.964	0.959	0.073 (0.071–0.075)	0.877–0.926
	South	1498	0.50–0.89	0.963	0.958	0.072 (0.069–0.075)	0.871–0.924

* Comparative Fit Index (CFI), Tucker-Lewis Index (TLI), and Root Mean Square Error of Approximation (RMSEA) with a 90% confidence interval; † With fit refinement.

2.5. Statistical Analysis

Descriptive statistics were performed according to states. Then, an ordinal hierarchical model was developed to verify if the states' variable affected the results. Two levels were considered, the individual and state subgroup. At the individual level, the level of impact by depression, anxiety, and stress and the psychological impact (avoidance, intrusion and hyperarousal) were considered as dependent variables. Sex, age, education, monthly income, previous mental and general health problems, sense of safety, number of people living with the participant, time of exposure to the news, frequency of socialization, knowing someone who tested positive for COVID-19, and change in mental health status after the start of the pandemic were independent variables. To verify the cluster effect, the intraclass correlation coefficient (ICC) was used.

The prevalence of psychological symptoms were calculated according to sex (reference category (rc) = male), age group (rc: ≥ 55 years), number of people living with the participant, economic level (rc: < 240.00 USD), education level (rc: complete graduate school), sense of security in relation to the pandemic (rc: unsafe), previous health problems (rc: no), frequency of socialization (rc: equal to or greater than usual), prior mental illness (rc: absent), change in mental state due to the pandemic (rc: no), knowing someone who tested positive for COVID-19 (rc: no), time spent with the news (rc: < 60 min). A multiple logistic regression model was constructed and odds ratio (OR) per point and 95% confidence interval were calculated. The dependent variables (psychological symptoms) were grouped into absent (normal category = 0) and present (symptom present in some level of impact); time spent with the news was categorized according to 25th, 50th, and 75th percentiles (1: < 60 min; 2: 60–90 min; 3: 90–150 min; 4: ≥ 150 min) and age by the 25th, 50th, 75th and 90th percentiles (1: < 24; 2: 24–33; 3: 33–43; 4: 43–55; 5: ≥ 55 years). The significance level was 5%. The analyses were performed using the IBM SPSS Statistics v.22 software (IBM Corp, Armonk, NY, USA).

3. Results

A total of 13,584 people completed the questionnaires, but 95 were excluded for not meeting the inclusion criteria (61 were < 18 years of age and 34 were non-Brazilians). 1388 participants did not complete all items of the scales (DASS-21 and IER-S) and were excluded. Thus, the loss rate (considering individuals who did not respond to all the questions) was 10.2%, being below the expected from the sample size of the initial study (25%).

Of the included participants, 8.7% reported having an average monthly family income below 240.00 USD, 11.6% between 240.00 USD and 383.00 USD, 38.0% between 384.00 USD and 1652.00 USD, 16.1% between 1653.00 USD and 2153.00 USD, and 25.0% above 2154.00 USD. Regarding education, 50.1% had completed graduate studies, 20.7% had completed higher education, 28.8% had completed high school, and 0.4% had completed middle school. All Brazilian states were adequately represented (Table 2): 38.3% (n = 4677) were from the Southeast, 31.2% (n = 3804) from the Northeast, 12.3% (n = 1498) from the South, 9.8% (n = 1191) from the North, and 8.4% (n = 1026) from the Midwest.

There was a greater prevalence of women (69.8%) and younger people (50% < 33 years old and 10% ≥ 55 years) in the sample. The prevalence of previous mental health ranged from 20 to 43.1%. 81.5 to 95.2% of participants reported the appearance of some mental health symptom and 58.1 to 75.0% reported changes in their mental health status after the onset of the pandemic. Among individuals who had no previous medical diagnosis related to mental disorders (n = 8178), 85.5% reported the appearance of symptoms of psychological impairment after the start of the pandemic. Among individuals with a medical diagnosis of mental disorder, 96.2% reported new symptoms after the start of the pandemic. Considering the total sample, approximately 88.8% had some new symptoms after the start of the pandemic. A large number of people reported knowing someone who had tested positive for COVID-19 (68.8%) and most believed the coronavirus is a serious condition (97.9%) and felt unsafe about the current pandemic scenario (84.4%). Approximately one-third of participants found the broadcasted news confusing and the average time spent per day with news related to the pandemic was 125.2 (standard deviation = 128.9) min.

A cluster effect by states was not observed in the data, i.e., data variance due to the state of residence was very small (ICC for Depression = 0.050, Anxiety = 0.055, Stress = 0.054, Psychological impact related to the event = 0.025, Avoidance = 0.013, Intrusion = 0.017, Hyperarousal = 0.025). Thus, the subsequent analyzes will be presented for the whole of Brazil (n = 12,196).

Table 2. Population (*N*) according to the State and minimum sample size estimated (*n*), final sample size (*n′*), and demographic characteristics.

Abbreviation, State, Region	N *	n	n′	Mean (SD; min/max)		%							
				Age in Years	Number of People in the Residence	Women	COVID-19 Seriousness	Previous Mental Problem	Mental Symptom during Pandemic	Change in Mental Health during Pandemic	Know COVID-19 Positive People	Feeling Unsafe	News is Confusing
AC—Acre (North)	881,935	41	46	37.7 (8.3; 18/60)	3.0 (1.2; 1–6)	50.0	97.8	20.0	93.5	67.4	95.7	91.3	32.6
AL—Alagoas (Northeast)	3,337,357	155	199	35.6 (12.2; 18/70)	3.3 (1.5; 1/13)	60.6	100.0	24.0	88.4	66.8	91.0	89.4	30.7
AM—Amazonas (North)	4,144,597	192	201	38.2 (13.1; 18/69)	3.4 (1.7; 1/15)	62.5	97.5	25.6	87.6	65.7	96.5	81.6	34.8
AP—Amapá (North)	845,731	39	69	37.6 (11.5; 18/65)	3.3 (1.7; 1/10)	68.1	100.0	26.9	91.3	73.9	98.6	89.9	29.0
BA—Bahia (Northeast)	14,873,064	689	723	36.8 (12.3; 18/80)	3.0 (1.5; 1/15)	70.7	99.0	31.6	90.7	66.5	73.6	86.3	34.6
CE—Ceará (Northeast)	9,132,078	423	430	34.7 (12.3; 18/70)	3.5 (1.5; 1/10)	68.6	97.0	25.0	91.1	72.6	89.1	85.3	29.3
DF—Distrito Federal (Midwest)	3,015,268	140	256	35.3 (13.1; 18/73)	3.22 (1.3; 1/7)	72.7	98.4	43.1	89.1	75.0	68.8	86.3	39.5
ES—Espírito Santo (Southeast)	4,018,650	186	199	30.0 (10.5; 18/70)	3.3 (1.4; 1/9)	80.4	98.0	32.7	88.9	71.9	68.8	83.4	36.2
GO—Goiás (Midwest)	7,018,354	325	374	33.8 (11.9; 18/66)	3.3 (1.4; 1/10)	77.3	96.5	35.3	89.0	67.9	57.8	84.0	46.5
MA—Maranhão (Northeast)	7,075,181	328	1196	29.5 (10.4; 18/67)	3.8 (1.7;1/10)	65.4	98.2	24.3	89.7	68.5	94.1	84.1	36.4
MG—Minas Gerais (Southeast)	21,168,791	980	1006	33.8 (12.5; 18/72)	3.2 (1.3; 1/9)	71.3	98.8	35.2	89.8	67.2	44.5	84.7	37.1
MS—Mato Grosso do Sul (Midwest)	2,778,986	129	230	35.4 (11.2; 18/66)	3.0 (1.3; 1/7)	57.8	96.5	30.5	86.0	64.3	40.4	84.3	33.2
MT—Mato Grosso (Midwest)	3,484,466	161	166	33.0 (11.1; 18/62)	3.2 (1.5; 1/10)	63.9	92.2	31.3	84.3	58.4	46.4	81.3	36.6
PA—Pará (North)	8,602,865	398	442	35.3 (12.4; 18/94)	3.5 (1.6; 1/11)	67.6	98.2	23.7	93.4	71.7	97.7	86.0	37.8
PB—Paraíba (Northeast)	4,018,127	186	186	38.3 (11.7; 18/70)	3.2 (1.6; 1/11)	65.6	98.4	24.9	89.8	67.7	86.6	81.2	34.9
PE—Pernambuco (Northeast)	9,557,071	443	429	37.0 (12.1; 18/78)	3.3 (1.6;1/15)	63.9	98.6	24.6	90.1	64.3	88.6	85.8	34.3
PI—Piauí (Nordeste)	3,273,227	152	222	35.7 (10.6; 18/66)	3.6 (1.5; 1/8)	68.0	99.5	30.6	89.6	68.9	82.9	88.3	29.9
PR—Paraná (South)	11,433,957	530	536	39.3 (12.9; 18/72)	3.0 (1.3; 1/10)	71.5	95.9	36.7	88.8	64.4	50.6	81.5	35.0
RJ—Rio de Janeiro (Southeast)	17,264,943	800	868	38.3 (13.5; 18/78)	3.0 (1.4; 1/13)	69.7	98.2	30.2	88.4	62.7	88.5	85.3	34.2
RN—Rio Grande do Norte (Northeast)	3,506,853	162	167	29.0 (9.5; 18/64)	3.8 (1.6; 1/9)	66.5	98.2	29.9	95.2	70.1	74.9	80.8	31.1
RO—Rondônia (Norte)	1,777,225	82	124	37.1 (11.7; 19/69)	3.4 (1.8;1/10)	71.0	98.4	24.6	81.5	58.1	82.3	88.7	38.7
RR—Roraima (North)	605,761	28	239	28.3 (10.7; 18/68)	3.9 (1.9; 1/15)	67.8	97.9	30.6	89.5	74.9	81.2	87.0	36.8
RS—Rio Grande do Sul (South)	11,377,239	527	582	38.5 (14.0; 18/72)	2.8 (1.2; 1/8)	75.6	97.8	35.2	87.6	65.8	41.4	80.8	30.2
SC—Santa Catarina (South)	7,164,788	332	380	35.0 (12.8; 18/68)	2.9 (1.3; 1/10)	65.8	97.6	33.2	86.5	68.9	47.6	84.7	39.3
SE—Sergipe (Northeast)	2,298,696	106	252	31.2 (10.4; 18/64)	3.5 (1.6; 1/11)	70.2	99.6	26.7	90.4	68.3	77.4	88.8	37.7
SP—São Paulo (Southeast)	45,919,049	2127	2604	36.5 (14.8; 18/82)	3.1 (1.4; 1/10)	73.4	97.7	34.5	87.6	64.6	55.1	83.5	40.4
TO—Tocantins (North)	1,572,866	73	70	38.2 (10.3; 20/64)	3.0 (1.5; 1/8)	67.1	95.7	38.6	84.3	71.4	61.4	81.4	41.4
Total	210,147,125	9734	12,196	35.2 (13.0;18/94)	3.2 (1.50; 1/15)	69.8	97.9	31.2	88.9	66.8	68.8	84.4	36.5

* Brazilian Geography and Statistics Institute—IBGE: State population.

Table 3 shows the prevalence of depressive symptoms, anxiety, stress and the psychological impact due to the pandemic according to the level of symptoms.

Table 3. Prevalence (%) of symptoms of depression, anxiety and stress and the psychological impact due to the pandemic according to level of symptoms in Brazilian adults (n = 12,196).

		Level (%)			
Instrument	**Factor**	**Normal**	**Mild**	**Moderate**	**Severe or Extremely Severe**
DASS-21	Depression	38.7	14.5	21.8	25.0
	Anxiety	55.8	8.5	19.2	16.5
	Stress	49.2	15.5	16.9	18.4
IES-R	Psychological impact	45.1	19.7	7.2	28.0
	Avoidance	40.2	18.0	10.9	30.9
	Intrusion	53.2	14.3	7.1	25.3
	Hyperarousal	49.9	12.4	10.0	27.7

A high prevalence of depression, anxiety, stress, and psychological impact due to the pandemic was found in the population, especially at moderate and severe levels.

The occurrence of psychological symptoms according to demographic and pandemic-related characteristics is shown in Table 4. Younger people, those feeling unsafe in regards to the pandemic, with a previous mental health problem, who reported a change in their mental state, and who reported following the news to the greatest extent excessively follow the news had a higher risk of developing psychological symptoms. Women were more likely to develop psychological symptoms than men, except for depressive symptoms. The lower the economic level, the higher the chance of symptoms, except for stress. Lower education levels increased the likelihood of depressive and intrusive symptoms. The presence of previous health problems increased the chance of developing symptoms, with the exception of avoidance.

Table 4. Odds ratio (OR) with 95% confidence interval (95% CI) for psychological symptoms (0 = Absent/1 = Present) according to characteristics of interest.

	Symptom OR (IC 95%)						
Characteristic	**Depression**	**Anxiety**	**Stress**	**Psychological Impact-General**	**Avoidance**	**Intrusion**	**Hyperarousal**
Sex Male/Female *	1.10 (0.99–1.22)	1.40 † (1.26–1.54)	1.651 (1.49–1.83)	1.50 † (1.36–1.66)	1.57 † (1.43–1.72)	1.35 † (1.22–1.49)	1.40 † (1.26–1.55)
Age (≥55 years *) < 24	2.98 † (2.38–3.74)	1.78 † (1.42–2.23)	3.58 † (2.82–4.53)	2.52 † (2.02–3.14)	1.75 † (1.43–2.14)	1.58 † (1.27–1.97)	3.03 † (2.40–3.81)
24–33	2.05 † (1.72–2.45)	1.47 † (1.21–1.78)	2.56 † (2.10–3.12)	1.76 † (1.47–2.10)	1.27 † (1.08–1.49)	1.41 † (1.18–1.70)	2.18 † (1.80–2.64)
33–43	1.49 † (1.26–1.76)	1.21 (1.00–1.46)	1.93 † (1.59–2.34)	1.27 † (1.07–1.51)	1.00 (0.86–1.17)	1.06 (0.89–1.27)	1.54 † (1.28–1.85)
43–55	1.13 (0.95–1.35)	1.09 (0.90–1.33)	1.29 † (1.05–1.58)	1.12 (0.94–1.35)	0.92 (0.78–1.07)	0.99 (0.82–1.19)	1.24 (1.01–1.50)
N people in the residence	0.96 (0.92–0.99)	1.06 (1.03–1.10)	1.02 (0.98–1.05)	1.02 (0.99–1.05)	1.01 (0.98–1.04)	1.00 (0.97–1.03)	1.04 (1.01–1.08)
Economic level ‡ (>2154.00 USD *) < 240.00 USD	1.68 † (1.34–2.90)	2.69 † (2.20–3.28)	1.18 (0.96–1.46)	1.92 † (1.56–2.37)	1.38 † (1.14–1.67)	1.82 † (1.49–2.22)	1.91 † (1.55–2.36)
Between 240.00 USD and 383.00 USD	1.70 † (1.40–2.06)	2.47 † (2.07–2.95)	1.25 (1.03–1.50)	1.66 † (1.39–1.99)	1.55 † (1.31–1.84)	1.44 † (1.21–1.71)	1.60 † (1.33–1.92)
Between 384.00 USD and 1652.00 USD	1.37 † (1.20–1.55)	1.72 † (1.52–1.96)	1.08 (0.95–1.23)	1.42 † (1.26–1.61)	1.29 † (1.15–1.45)	1.26 † (1.12–1.43)	1.28 † (1.12–1.45)
Between 1653.00 USD and 2153.00 USD	1.13 (0.98–1.29)	1.31 † (1.13–1.51)	1.12 (0.97–1.30)	1.17 † (1.01–1.34)	1.22 † (1.07–1.38)	1.09 (0.94–1.25)	1.17 (1.01–1.36)
Education (completed graduate studies *) Up to Completed High School	1.55 † (1.30–1.84)	1.12 (0.96–1.32)	1.15 (0.97–1.36)	1.12 (0.95–1.32)	1.04 (0.89–1.21)	1.29 † (1.09–1.51)	1.13 (0.95–1.33)
Completed Higher Education	1.17 † (1.03–1.34)	1.02 (0.90–1.16)	0.99 (0.86–1.13)	1.02 (0.90–1.16)	1.01 (0.90–1.14)	1.05 (0.93–1.19)	1.00 (0.88–1.14)
Feel Unsafe/Safe *	2.52 † (2.22–2.87)	2.16 † (1.87–2.50)	2.70 † (2.33–3.13)	2.48 † (2.17–2.84)	1.75 † (1.56–1.97)	2.92 † (2.52–3.38)	2.67 † (2.31–3.09)
Health problems Yes/No *	1.17 † (1.05–1.30)	1.51 † (1.36–1.67)	1.31 † (1.18–1.47)	1.34 † (1.21–1.49)	1.08 (0.98–1.19)	1.42 † (1.28–1.57)	1.44 † (1.30–1.61)
Socialization Lower/equal or higher than usual *	1.14 (1.00–1.29)	1.08 (0.96–1.23)	0.99 (0.87–1.12)	1.03 (0.91–1.17)	0.99 (0.89–.11)	1.03 (0.91–1.17)	1.02 (0.90–1.16)
Previous mental disorder Yes/No *	2.38 † (2.14–2.65)	2.64 † (2.39–2.91)	2.58 † (2.32–2.87)	2.41 † (2.18–2.67)	1.72 † (1.56–1.89)	2.42 † (2.19–2.66)	2.57 † (2.32–2.85)
Mental health change due to pandemic Yes/No *	4.99 † (4.52–5.50)	5.19 † (4.65–5.80)	9.07 † (8.10–10.15)	5.06 † (4.58–5.59)	2.53 † (2.31–2.78)	5.09 † (4.58–5.66)	6.55 † (5.87–7.29)
Know people positive for COVID-19 (Yes/No *)	1.14 † (1.03–1.26)	0.95 (0.87–1.05)	0.97 (0.88–1.08)	0.86 (0.78–0.95)	0.93 (0.85–1.02)	0.90 (0.82–0.99)	0.88 (0.80–0.97)
Time spent with news (<60 min *) 60–90	1.11 (0.97–1.27)	0.97 (0.85–1.11)	1.01 (0.88–1.17)	0.88 (0.77–1.01)	0.80 † (0.71–0.91)	1.09 (0.96–1.25)	1.08 (0.94–1.24)
90–150	1.33 † (1.15–1.53)	1.09 (0.94–1.25)	1.05 (0.90–1.22)	1.04 (0.90–1.20)	0.74 † (0.65–0.84)	1.48 † (1.28–1.70)	1.42 † (1.23–1.64)
≥150	1.67 † (1.44–1.93)	1.41 † (1.23–1.63)	1.45 † (1.25–1.69)	1.19 † (1.04–1.37)	0.66 † (0.58–0.75)	2.18 † (1.90–2.51)	1.83 † (1.59–2.12)

* Reference category; † $p < 0.001$; ‡ 1 USD = 5.23 BRL.

4. Discussion

This survey evaluated the mental health of Brazilians during the SARS-Cov-2 pandemic and identified characteristics that increased the risk of psychological symptoms. A high prevalence of depression (61.3%), anxiety (44.2%), stress (50.8%), avoidance (59.2%), intrusion (46.8%) and hyperarousal (50.1%) symptoms was observed.

The increase in mental health symptoms in populations during epidemics is not a novelty [8–15], however, the current context deserves attention. In addition to being the largest pandemic in the last 100 years, the eradication of the disease is still a scientific and social challenge, and the effectiveness of control measures (such as hand hygiene, isolation, and quarantine) is thus still unknown,. Thus, the quarantine has been extended, with an unknown end date and the return to normal activities. In addition to the pandemic, the country's economic, political, and social crises related to it contribute to a lack of feeling safe [3–6], creating an environment of multi-faceted vulnerability and unpredictability that affects the general population, especially in those who lack coping skills to manage the conflicts of this scenario.

The lack of feeling safe affected the majority of the study population (84.4%) and significantly increased the risk of developing psychological symptoms. This may be related to both the pandemic itself and the large volume of inaccurate and often conflicting information from the media and the government regarding the coronavirus disease and its control and treatment measures [1,5]. Gao et al. [21] concluded that the amount of false or manipulated information can generate unfounded fear and confuse people. The authors also reported that greater exposure to the news increases the chance of developing symptoms of depression and anxiety, which was also found in the present study. The time spent with the news was a protective factor for the avoidance symptom, indicating that individuals that are more exposed to the news (low avoidance behavior) could be aiming at acquiring the maximum information on the pandemic to gain some control of the situation. However, a false sense of control could aggravate the other psychological symptoms assessed in this study.

Less than one third of individuals reported medical diagnosis related to mental disorders before the pandemic. The prevalence of psychological symptoms among these individuals was extremely high (96.2%) after the beginning of the pandemic. In the total sample, 88.8% of people reported the appearance of one or more psychological symptoms after the beginning of the pandemic. It should be noted that this information was self-reported by the participants. These results are especially important, as they may suggest difficulties in dealing with emotional reactions in the context of the pandemic, whether due to the lack of coping strategies, the unpredictability of the new condition, and/or the feeling of vulnerability. Cullen et al. [35] suggest that psychological intervention measures be provided for the COVID-19-affected communities in primary and emergency healthcare services, especially for people with previous psychological problems.

Actions to raise awareness on mental disorders and help symptom diagnosis are also suggested to reduce psychological distress and prevent new mental health problems [24,35]. In addition, Holmes et al. [2] highlight that individuals with previous symptoms are more vulnerable and have increased risk of physical and psychological effects from the pandemic [35], which was also observed in this study. Moccia et al. [25] point out that people with a depressive or anxious temperament are also more vulnerable. A striking finding in our study was that 85% of those who reported never having received a medical diagnosis related to psychological problems, reported appearance of symptoms during the pandemic, corroborating the findings by Cullen et al. [35] Furthermore, the presence of moderate to severe symptoms of psychological impact (IES-R) can indicate a risk for future development of post-traumatic stress disorder. Therefore, mental health care must be expanded to restrain these symptoms and prevent their aggravation.

In accordance to the literature, psychological symptoms were more common among younger individuals and women [22–29]. The uncertainty of the future, school and university closings and new teaching formats, the breakdown of interpersonal relationships and an immature cognitive and behavioral repertoire to cope with the pandemic demands could explain the greater risk of psychological symptoms in young adults. The results presented by Palgi et al. [26] point out that the feeling of loneliness due to social isolation is greater among young people, which can increase the risk of developing depressive and anxious symptoms. Still, Bruin [27] showed that older individuals report less negative emotions, have better mental health and less responsiveness to daily stressors, which favors a lesser experience of symptoms of depression and anxiety. To explain why stressful factors have a greater impact on women, Almeida and Kessler [36] suggest that women tend to ruminate negative thoughts more, prolonging distress, increasing the effects of stressors on mood, interfering with behaviors, and impeding the development of a strategies to eliminate stressors. Moccia et al. [25] suggest that women's greatest vulnerability to psychological distress is related to genetic, socio-cultural, hormonal, and developmental factors.

The effect of the economic level on psychological symptoms was expected as people in disadvantaged economic and social situations are affected at a much greater extent due to lower access to health care, inability to quarantine without risking losing a job or decreasing income, among several other factors, making this group even more vulnerable.

This study was conducted on a large sample of individuals that covered the entire country and presented valid and reliable findings. However, some limitations should be reported. First, data collection was carried out online, which certainly resulted in more younger individuals and with higher economic level and education being selected. It should be remembered that older people and those with less economic power or education have lower access to or literacy in digital resources. However, this was the feasible strategy for gathering information during the pandemic. Sample selection could also have been biased by the snowball process starting within universities. Despite contacts with NGOs from populations with low income and education levels, the adherence of this group was not representative of the country population, which was confirmed by the absence of a cluster by States in a country with great inequalities among regions. Finally, the cross-sectional study design does not allow causality inference, and therefore, future longitudinal studies should the developed.

Another aspect to be reported is the absence of a national mental health survey that could be used to compare pre, peri and post-pandemic data and/or to monitor the mental health of the Brazilian population. It is expected that the impact generated by the current context of the pandemic may trigger the need to develop this type of tracking in a continuous and rigorous manner, as in the United Kingdom [28].

Despite these limitations, this is the first Brazilian nation-wide study to present quality evidence that deserves a careful look from government officials, managers, and mental healthcare professionals. The development of a national plan is suggested for epidemiological surveillance and minimization of the psychological impacts of the COVID pandemic in the population. As Qiu et al. [24] proposes, a nation-wide program for coordinating psychological first aid [potentially using telemedicine] and establishing a prevention and intervention system could be highly effective. The psychological and psychiatric needs cannot be neglected during any phase of pandemic management, as they play an important role in public policies adherence and dealing with infection threats and possible losses [34]. Moreover, attention to mental care provided during the crisis can help in the reconstruction process of all individuals and provide the skills needed for the post-pandemic world.

5. Conclusions

A high prevalence of mental health symptoms was found in the Brazilian adult population during the SARS-Cov2 pandemic. The impact level of symptoms of depression, anxiety, and stress, and the impact of factors directly related to the current context, emphasizes the importance of mental health care. The probability of having psychological symptoms was affected by several sample characteristics (e.g., sex, age, previous diagnosis of mental health-related disorder, individuals most exposed to pandemic news), which must be considered in the development of support, prevention, and treatment strategies.

Author Contributions: All authors contributed substantially to the work. Conceptualization, J.A.D.B.C., B.G.M. and L.A.C.; Methodology, J.A.D.B.C., B.G.M., L.A.C., J.M., R.A.S. and R.R.; Software, J.A.D.B.C.; Validation, J.A.D.B.C., B.G.M. and L.A.C.; Formal Analysis, J.A.D.B.C. and J.M.; Investigation, J.A.D.B.C., B.G.M., L.A.C., J.M., R.A.S. and R.R.; Resources, J.A.D.B.C.; Data Curation, B.G.M. and L.A.C.; Writing—Original Draft Preparation, J.A.D.B.C. and L.A.C.; Writing—Review & Editing, B.G.M., J.M., R.A.S. and R.R.; Visualization, R.R.; Supervision, J.A.D.B.C. and R.R.; Project Administration, J.A.D.B.C.; Funding Acquisition, J.A.D.B.C. All authors have read and agreed to the published version of the manuscript.

Funding: This research was funded by São Paulo Research Foundation (FAPESP), grant number #2020/08239-6 and in part by the Coordenação de Aperfeiçoamento de Pessoal de Nível Superior-Brasil (CAPES)-Finance Code 001.

Acknowledgments: The authors thank Beatriz Buda Fuller for her assistance in data collection and the people who joined and participated in the project. This study was financed in part by the Coordenação de Aperfeiçoamento de Pessoal de Nível Superior-Brasil (CAPES)-Finance Code 001. We also thank the São Paulo Research Foundation (FAPESP) (grant #2020/08239-6). The authors also thank Calvin Caltvedt for revising the English grammar of the present manuscript.

Conflicts of Interest: The authors declare no conflict of interest.

References

1. Brooks, S.K.; Webster, R.W.; Smith, L.E.; Woodland, L.; Wessely, S.; Greenberg, N.; Rubin, G.J. The psychological impact of quarantine and how to reduce it: Rapid review of the evidence. *Lancet* **2020**, *395*, 912–920. [CrossRef]
2. Holmes, E.A.; O'Connor, R.C.; Perry, V.H.; Tracey, I.; Wessely, S.; Arseneault, L.; Ballard, C.; Christensen, H.; Cohen Silver, R.; Everall, I.; et al. Multidisciplinary research priorities for the COVID-19 pandemic: A call for action for mental health science. *Lancet Psychiatry* **2020**, *7*, 547–560. [CrossRef]
3. Pfefferbaum, B.; North, C.S. Mental Health and the Covid-19 Pandemic. *N. Engl. J. Med.* **2020**, *383*, 510–512. [CrossRef]
4. Rajkumar, R.P. COVID-19 and mental health: A review of the existing literature. *Asian J. Psychatry* **2020**, *52*, 1–4. [CrossRef] [PubMed]
5. Rubin, G.J.; Wessely, S. The psychological effects of quarantining a city. *BMJ* **2020**, *368*, m313. [CrossRef]
6. Usher, K.; Durkin, J.; Bhullar, N. The COVID-19 pandemic and mental health impacts. *Int. J. Ment. Health Nurs.* **2020**, *29*, 315–318. [CrossRef]
7. Wilder-Smith, A.; Freedman, M.D. Isolation, quarantine, social distancing and community containment: Pivotal role for old-style public health measures in the novel coronavirus (2019-nCoV) outbreak. *J. Travel Med.* **2020**, *27*, 1–4. [CrossRef]
8. Bai, Y.; Lin, C.-C.; Lin, C.-Y.; Chen, J.-Y.; Chue, C.-M.P.C. Survey of stress reactions among health care workers involved with the SARS outbreak. *Psychiatr. Serv.* **2004**, *55*, 1055–1057. [CrossRef]
9. Blendon, R.J.; Benson, J.M.; DesRoches, C.M.; Raleigh, E.; Taylor-Clark, K. The public's response to severe acute respiratory syndrome in Toronto and the United States. *Clin. Infect. Dis.* **2004**, *38*, 925–931. [CrossRef]
10. Cava, M.A.; Fay, K.E.; Beanlands, H.J.; McCay, E.A.; Wignall, R. The experience of quarantine for individuals affected by SARS in Toronto. *Public Health Nurs.* **2005**, *22*, 398–406. [CrossRef]
11. Lee, S.; Chan, L.Y.; Chau, A.M.; Kwok, K.P.; Kleinman, A. The experience of SARS-related stigma at Amoy Gardens. *Soc. Sci. Med.* **2005**, *61*, 2038–2046. [CrossRef] [PubMed]
12. Wilken, J.A.; Pordell, P.; Goode, B.; Jarteh, R.; Miller, Z.; Saygar, B.G.; Maximore, L.; Borbor, W.M.; Carmue, M.; Walker, G.W.; et al. Knowledge, attitudes, and practices among members of households actively monitored or quarantined to prevent transmission of Ebola virus disease-Margibi County, Liberia: February–March 2015. *Prehosp. Disaster Med.* **2017**, *32*, 673–678. [CrossRef] [PubMed]
13. Caleo, G.; Duncombe, J.; Jephcott, F.; Lokuge, K.; Mills, C.; Looijen, E.; Theoharaki, F.; Kremer, R.; Kleijer, K.; Squire, J.; et al. The factors affecting household transmission dynamics and community compliance with Ebola control measures: A mixed-methods study in a rural village in Sierra Leone. *BMC Public Health* **2018**, *18*, 248–261. [CrossRef] [PubMed]
14. Wang, Y.; Xu, B.; Zhao, G.; Cao, R.; He, X.; Fu, S. Is quarantine related to immediate negative psychological consequences during the 2009 H1N1 epidemic? *Gen. Hosp. Psychiatry* **2011**, *33*, 75–77. [CrossRef]

15. Braunack-Mayer, A.; Tooher, R.; Collins, J.E.; Street, J.M.; Marshall, H. Understanding the school community's response to school closures during the H1N1 2009 influenza pandemic. *BMC Public Health* **2013**, *13*, 344–359. [CrossRef]
16. Sani, G.; Janiri, D.; Di Nicola, M.; Janiri, L.; Ferretti, S.; Chieffo, D. Mental health during and after the COVID-19 emergency in Italy. *Psychiatry Clin. Neurosci.* **2020**, *74*, 372. [CrossRef]
17. Mao, L.; Jin, H.; Wang, M.; Hu, Y.; Chen, S.; He, Q.; Chang, J.; Hong, C.; Zhou, Y.; Wang, D.; et al. Neurologic Manifestations of Hospitalized Patients With Coronavirus Disease 2019 in Wuhan, China. *JAMA Neurol.* **2020**, *77*, 683–690. [CrossRef]
18. Zheng, F.; Tang, W.; Li, H.; Huang, Y.X.; Xie, Y.L.; Zhou, Z.G. Clinical characteristics of 161 cases of corona virus disease 2019 (COVID-19) in Changsha. *Eur. Rev. Med. Pharmacol. Sci.* **2020**, *24*, 3404–3410.
19. Chen, Q.; Liang, M.; Li, Y.; Guo, J.; Fei, D.; Wang, L.; Sheng, C.; Cai, Y.; Li, X.; Wan, J.; et al. Mental health care for medical staff in China during COVID-19 outbreak. *Lancet Psychiatry* **2020**, *7*, 15–16. [CrossRef]
20. Zhang, W.R.; Wang, K.; Yin, L.; Zhao, W.F.; Xue, Q.; Peng, M.; Min, B.Q.; Tian, Q.; Leng, H.X.; Du, J.L.; et al. Mental Health and Psychosocial Problems of Medical Health Workers during the COVID-19 Epidemic in China. *Psychother. Psychosom.* **2020**, *89*, 242–250. [CrossRef]
21. Gao, J.; Zheng, P.; Jia, Y.; Chen, H.; Mao, Y.; Chen, S.; Wang, Y.; Fu, H.; Dai, J. Mental health problems and social media exposure during COVID-19 outbreak. *PLoS ONE* **2020**, *15*, e0231924. [CrossRef] [PubMed]
22. Wang, C.; Pan, R.; Wan, X.; Tan, Y.; Xu, L.; Ho, C.S.; Ho, R.C. Immediate Psychological Responses and Associated Factors during the Initial Stage of the 2019 Coronavirus Disease (COVID-19) Epidemic among the General Population in China. *Int. J. Environ. Res. Public Health* **2020**, *17*, 1729. [CrossRef]
23. Figueiras, A.; Stults-Kolehmainen, M. The relationship between behavioural and psychosocial factors among brazilians in quarantine due to COVID-19. *Lancet Psychiatry* **2020**. [CrossRef]
24. Qiu, J.; Shen, B.; Zhao, M.; Wang, Z.; Xie, B.; Xu, Y. A nationwide survey of psychological distress among Chinese people in the COVID-19 epidemic: Implications and policy recommendations. *BMJ Gen. Psychiatry* **2020**, *33*, 1–3. [CrossRef]
25. Moccia, L.; Janiri, D.; Pepe, M.; Dattoli, L.; Molinaro, M.; Martin, V.; Chieffo, D.; Janiri, L.; Fiorillo, A.; Sani, G.; et al. Affective treatment, attachment style, and the psychological impact of the COVID-19 outbreak: An early report on the Italian general population. *Brain Behav. Immun.* **2020**, *87*, 75–79. [CrossRef]
26. Palgi, Y.; Shrira, A.; Ring, L.; Bodner, E.; Avidor, S.; Bergman, Y.; Cohen-Fridel, S.; Keisari, S.; Hoffman, Y. The loneliness pandemic: Loneliness anther concomitants of depression, anxiety and their comorbidity during the COVID-19 outbreak. *J. Affect. Disord.* **2020**, *275*, 109–111. [CrossRef]
27. Bruin, W.B. Age Differences in COVID-19 Risk Perceptions and Mental Health: Evidence From a National U.S. Survey Conducted in March 2020. *J. Gerontol. Psychol. Sci.* **2020**, 1–6. [CrossRef]
28. Pierce, M.; Hope, H.; Ford, T.; Hatch, S.; Hotopf, M.; John, A.; Kontopantelis, E.; Webb, R.; Wessely, S.; MacManus, S.; et al. Mental health before and during the COVID-19 pandemic: A longitudinal probability sample survey of the UK population. *Lancet Psychiatry* **2020**, *21*, 1–10.
29. Salari, N.; Hosseinian-Far, A.; Jalali, R.; Vaisi-Raygani, A.; Rasoulpoor, S.; Mohammadi, M.; Rasoulpoor, S.; Khaledi-Paveh, B. Prevalence of stress, anxiety, depression among the general population during the COVID-19 pandemic: A systematic review and meta-analysis. *Glob. Health* **2020**, *16*, 57. [CrossRef] [PubMed]
30. Vignola, R.C.B.; Tucci, A.M. Adaptation and validation of the Depression, Anxiety and Stress Scale (DASS) to Brazilian Portuguese. *J. Affect. Disord.* **2014**, *155*, 104–109. [CrossRef]
31. Martins, B.G.; Silva, W.R.; Maroco, J.; Campos, J.A.D.B. Escala de Depressão, Ansiedade e Estresse: Propriedades psicométricas e prevalência das afetividades. *J. Bras. Psiquiatr.* **2019**, *68*, 32–41. [CrossRef]
32. Caiuby, A.V.S.; Lacerda, S.S.; Quintana, M.I.; Torii, T.S.; Andreoli, S.B. Adaptação transcultural da versão brasileira da Escala do Impacto do Evento—Revisada (IES-R). *Cad. Saúde Pública* **2012**, *28*, 597–603. [CrossRef] [PubMed]
33. Lovibond, S.H.; Lovibond, P.F. Manual for the Depression, Anxiety, Stress Scales. 1995. (update in 26 July 2018). Available online: http://www2.psy.unsw.edu.au/dass/ (accessed on 28 July 2020).
34. Kline, R.B. *Principles and Practice of Structural Equation Modeling*; The Guilford Press: New York, NY, USA, 1998; p. 354.

35. Cullen, W.; Gulati, G.; Kelly, B.D. Mental health in the Covid-19 pandemic. *QJM Int. J. Med.* **2020**, *113*, 311–312. [CrossRef]
36. Almeida, D.M.; Kessler, R.C. Everyday stressors and gender differences in daily distress. *J. Personal. Soc. Psychol.* **1998**, *75*, 670–680. [CrossRef]

Journal of
Clinical Medicine

MDPI

Article

Psychological Impact of COVID-19 Emergency on Health Professionals: Burnout Incidence at the Most Critical Period in Spain

José Ángel Martínez-López [1], Cristina Lázaro-Pérez [2], José Gómez-Galán [3,4,*] and María del Mar Fernández-Martínez [5]

1 Department of Social Work and Social Services, University of Murcia, Avda. Teniente Flomesta, 5-30003 Murcia, Spain; jaml@um.es
2 Department of Sociology, University of Murcia, C/Campus Universitario, 11, 30100 Murcia, Spain; cristina.lazaro2@um.es
3 Department of Education, University of Extremadura, Avda. de Elvas, s/n, 06006 Badajoz, Spain
4 College of Education, Ana G. Méndez University, Cupey Campus, San Juan, PR 00926, USA
5 College of Education Sciences & College of Sociology, Social Work and Public Health, University of Huelva, Campus El Carmen, Avda. de las Fuerzas Armadas, s/n, 21007 Huelva, Spain; mar.fernandez@dstso.uhu.es
* Correspondence: jogomez@uagm.edu

Received: 25 July 2020; Accepted: 18 September 2020; Published: 20 September 2020

Abstract: Background: The health profession is a burnout producer due to the continuous contact with pain and suffering. In addition, excessive workloads can generate stress and psychological distress. Objectives: The aim of this study was to determine the degree of burnout and its main triggers in health professionals in Spain at the most critical period of the COVID-19 emergency. Method: A quantitative research was developed through a simple random sampling in different Spanish hospitals through the period of greatest impact of the pandemic ($N = 157$). Data were collected using a standardized questionnaire from Maslach burnout inventory (MBI) containing 22 items, which measures three subscales: emotional burnout, depersonalization, and self-fulfillment. Results: depersonalization values reached 38.9%. A total of 90.4% of the health professionals considered that psychological care should be provided from the work centers. Furthermore, 43.3% of the health professionals estimated that they might need psychological treatment in the future. Finally, 85.4% stated that the lack of personal protective equipment (PPE) generated an increase in stress and anxiety. Conclusion: This study demonstrates the need to consider specific mental health care services and training in crises to avoid possible psychological disorders. The information obtained is also valuable for the development of future prevention protocols and training of health personnel to face pandemics of these characteristics or emergency scenarios. Having the necessary physical means for their protection, as well to updated regular and accurate information, is essential to avoid feelings of fear and uncertainty. This would promote the health of these professionals.

Keywords: burnout; COVID-19; pandemic; health professionals; stress; anxiety; prevention

1. Introduction

The expansion in March 2020 of the epidemic of the SARS-CoV-2 coronavirus, COVID-19, has meant an unknown scenario for the world's population where panic and fear of contagion has spread rapidly to all continents as a reaction to globalization, taking over almost completely the information transmitted by the media and social networks [1–4]. The disease that began in Wuhan (China) in December 2019, initially associated with pneumonia, quickly became a global epidemic [5]. It became a major global problem, in such a way that on 30 January 2020 the World Health Organization designated the COVID-2019 outbreak as a "public health emergency of international concern" (PHEIC) because of its rapid spread [6].

This pandemic has changed the lives and behaviors of all people (habits, customs, ways of relating, confinement in the digital age, etc.) [7,8] and professionals (health protocols, health alerts, isolation measures, individual and community prevention measures) [9,10]. A single cause has provoked the same collective thinking at a global level and is based on two main lines of action; first, the need to protect ourselves from the virus, and second, to resist the social and economic crisis caused by it.

The actions aimed at surviving the COVID-19 disease also involved managing personal skills and resources to combat the secondary effects that this pandemic may have produced. As many authors have already pointed out, the pandemic has had psychological effects on the general population, but especially on health professionals [11–14]. This group has been exposed for a long period of time to the constant threat of infection with the virus, which is often described as fatal, and which causes a sense of danger and uncertainty in their daily activities among health workers and also in society as a whole [15].

According to the Report on the situation of COVID-19 in health care personnel in Spain, as of 21 May 2020, 40,921 had been infected and 53 deaths had been reported through the SiViES platform of the Centro Nacional de Epidemiología (National Center for Epidemiology) [16]. Considering that the total number of people infected in Spain on that same date was 269,863 [17], the number of health professionals infected exceeds 15%, a sign of the risk to which they have been exposed in their professional work. However, these data should be considered with caution since the number of figures has constantly changed. Updated data from May 29 of the same report shows 40,961 positive cases in health professionals and 52 deaths, fewer than previous counts.

This official report does not include the characteristics related to the professional category of health professionals or other considerations related to professional practice. On 9 May 2020, the Asociación de Médicos Unidos por sus Derechos (Physicians United for their Rights of Association) presented the report "Condiciones de los médicos españoles en la práctica clínica durante la crisis de COVID-19" (conditions of Spanish physicians in clinical practice during the COVID-19 crisis), which included higher figures than those provided by the Ministry, with 48,320 health professionals infected and 76 dead [18]. In addition, this report includes elements that show how health professionals have dealt with the pandemic and under what conditions.

The most relevant data shows that 12% of the physicians had suffered from the disease (data without taking into account those who were asymptomatic); 23% of the physicians suffering from COVID-19 had returned to work without having performed PCR (polymerase chain reaction), that is, without checking through the corresponding diagnostic tests if they were free of the virus or if they had developed antibodies, which would help prevent the virus from spreading in hospitals. Those measures would have help them to prevent the virus from spreading in hospitals; 66.5% had attended patients with COVID-19, 49% considered that they lacked sufficient protective material, highlighting the fact that 1/3 did not have Fpp2 or Fpp3 masks, and one in four physicians had reused their mask for more than a week. Finally, 86.8% of physicians considered that they could have been a vector of the disease because they lacked adequate protective material [18].

This amount of numbers causes uncertainty in the population, especially among health professionals. Altogether, with the lack of personal protective equipment (PPE) and the contradictory information, due to the lack of knowledge of the virus by official sources, are elements that keep the level of professional anxiety very high, and may cause other disorders that would not benefit professional practice at all.

In this scenario, health professionals have carried out a titanic task, with personal unprecedent, work, and social pressure within a context of insufficient PPE to fight this disease. Recent studies [19–22] show how working under pressure from COVID-19 have a significant impact on health professionals, especially those who work in a more precarious context, working long hours, without adequate PPE, etc. In addition, Lai et al. point out that in Wuhan "a considerable proportion of health workers reported experiencing symptoms of depression, anxiety, insomnia and distress, especially women, nurses and frontline health care workers directly involved in the diagnosis, treatment or nursing care of patients with suspected or confirmed COVID-19" [23]. Due to the fact that during the stages prior to the health crisis, in previous studies carried out in Spain, medium-high values of burnout were found [24–28] we asked whether during this phase of increased active cases and overflow of health care facilities caused by the SARS-CoV-2 pandemic, professionals might exhibit evidence of the three components of the Maslach burnout scale [29], emotional exhaustion, depersonalization, and changes in self-fulfilment, as these are the ones that other studies have indicated are most at risk of developing health problems from COVID-19 [23,30]. At the same time, the perception of stress among professionals is closely related to burnout, reporting a higher level of emotional exhaustion and depersonalization [31]. While it is true that burnout is a process that develops over time [32], during the months of March and April the volume, workload and deaths of patients admitted were much higher than in previous months [33], which makes us wonder if this context could have aggravated the situation as occurred in other countries [34,35] in the three subscales of the Maslach burnout inventory.

2. Background

The term burnout was first used in the clinical setting in 1974 by the psychologist Herbert Freudenberger, who carried out a study on the change of attitude of health personnel relating burnout with states of anxiety and depression, considering it "a set of non-specific medical-biological and psychosocial symptoms that develop in work activity as a result of an excessive demand for energy" [36]. From this point, the research stage in Burnout begins [37], characterized by the first clinical analyses of the syndrome and the ratification of its regularity. Later on, Cristina Maslach elaborates a representation of the responses of the workers related to the care environment, when they feel vulnerable due to emotional stress [38]. In 1981, the social psychologist Christina Maslach defined it as "a three-dimensional syndrome characterized by emotional exhaustion, depersonalization and low personal realization that can occur among individuals who work in direct contact with clients and/or patients" [39]. Together with Dr. Jackson, they created one of the most widely used instruments to measure burnout: the Maslach burnout inventory (MBI) by evaluating the three dimensions mentioned.

The most vulnerable professionals to suffer from burnout are those who develop their work in relation to other people such as health and teaching professionals [27,40,41].

Studies on burnout in health professionals have been conducted on numerous occasions relating symptoms of mood disorders, anxiety, and depression as this syndrome consequences [42–44]. Its effects are usually evident within a depressive symptomatology which scope transcends the merely occupational scenario and involves the personal, family, and social sphere [45,46].

Under normal circumstances, the health profession generates work-related stress or burnout for a variety of reasons, including continuous contact with pain and suffering [47,48], as well as monotonous tasks, heavy or excessive workloads, the frequency and amount of time spent with patients, and even work development and management styles [49,50]. On the other hand, there are more personal factors such as one's ability to cope with death and suffering and poor or bad interpersonal relationships, which can also be a cause of stress and psychological distress.

In this sense, and taking into account the clinical point of view, it is considered that work stress, characterized by workload, time pressure, demands, resources or management control, among others, can trigger burnout syndrome (as a state). However, the psychosocial approach considers that it is the work and personal environment that can trigger the appearance of this syndrome (as a process) [51], i.e., it arises as a response to labor stress [52] without there being an exact cause that precipitates it, but the realization of which is not capable of minimizing the dissatisfaction or lack of motivation that is present.

Maslach defined burnout as "a chronic stress produced by contact with clients that leads to emotional exhaustion and alienation from clients in their work" [53]. This definition was widespread during the decades of the late twentieth century [54,55]. Today, however, burnout is defined as a "prolonged response to chronic personal and relational stressors at work, determined from dimensions known as burnout, depersonalization, and professional cynicism and inefficiency" [45].

In the face of a threat such as that posed by COVID-19 disease, as well as other special emergency situations, where rapid action is required and the workload is high, it often happens that the primary reaction is to act, without thinking about the individual's emotional needs. In contrast, we can find protective factors that improve professional practice. In this respect, a recent study by Kisely et al. showed that "clear communication, access to adequate personal protection, adequate rest and both practical and psychological support were associated with a reduction in morbidity" [56].

At the first stage of exposure to the virus, health professionals had to make a great effort, which usually leads to anxiety and consequently the possible intake of anxiolytics, to maintain a constant capacity for work, which could lead to depression on an ongoing basis and after a few months of maintaining this habit, a post-traumatic stress disorder as occurred in other epidemics such as SARS, MERS, influenza A/H1N1 or Ebola [57,58].

At a physical level, burnout syndrome is associated with the appearance of certain disorders that often force the affected person to request sick leave from work [59,60], such as high muscle tension and generalized musculoskeletal pain (fibromyalgia), headaches or backaches, central nervous system dysfunctions, sexual dysfunctions or various cardiovascular and gastrointestinal problems [61].

All these elements guide the need to study the effects that the current pandemic may be having on health professionals from the different subscales of burnout, and thus enable a learning process to prevent possible future situations similar to the COVID-19 pandemic or new waves of this same virus. The World Health Organization [62,63] and many researchers notice the importance of initial and continuing training for health professionals [64–68], especially in the context of emergency situations [69–72].

In this context, training for mental health professionals in these extreme scenarios, which have a huge psychological impact, is essential [73–75]. Most studies focusing on this problem highlight that training and prevention processes can reduce the incidence of burnout syndrome in health professionals [76–84]. It is even argued that a combination of actions (including organizational, support and changes in the work environment) can have an even greater effect [85,86].

However, most of these contributions have focused on the prevention of burnout syndrome in everyday work situations. Although there are studies on professionals working in emergency services [87–92], which would offer similar results, we lack more knowledge when it comes to borderline situations in disasters and catastrophes contexts. These include a global pandemic, a global health emergency that has been unknown for almost a century, when the terrible Spanish flu of 1918–1919 occurred [93]. It is, therefore, necessary, prior to develop programs designed for this purpose, to know the impact on health workers, of a situation of such stress and tension, caused by the COVID-19 epidemic in its most extreme phases.

In this sense, different studies have found that along with service sector workers and teachers, physicians and nurses had high burnout rates [27,94], related to job dissatisfaction, little control over work, lack of recognition, low pay and caring for people in a terminal situation [62,95]. It is, therefore, necessary to establish a description of the state of health professionals, in relation to this important issue, at the most critical moments of the first wave of the pandemic. We are at a critical moment and this data can be very valuable, especially when thinking about the future of health professionals and comparative studies can determine an evolution in this area.

3. Materials and Methods

3.1. Objectives

In the health emergency caused by COVID-19 disease, the occupational stressors and anxiety of health professionals could have been aggravated by the virulence of the pandemic and the shortage of

PPE. In this context, the aim of this research is to find out how the current health crisis has affected health professionals, considering the Maslach and Jackson burnout subscales of the Maslach burnout inventory [55], adapted by Seisdedos [96] and validated by García, Herrero y León [97], during the most critical weeks of the spread of the virus. We decided, therefore, to undertake a study that would describe the situation at that specific moment, in the absence of research at the time, although after this research was carried out, works with similar objectives have been published [98,99] which reinforce the need for knowledge of this problem. In this way, the object of study was centered on the appearance of burnout in health centers in situations of need for an immediate and effective approach, as is the case of the COVID-19 pandemic, where the lives of many patients were in serious danger. This information would be very valuable for the construction of future prevention protocols and training of healthcare personnel in the face of pandemics of these characteristics or borderline scenarios.

3.2. *Study Design and Sample*

The research has been carried out in collaboration with health personnel working in hospital centers in Spain, mainly nurses, physicians, and nursing assistants. The subjects studied were 157. The period in which the questionnaire was administered was between April 6 and 19, in the middle of the confinement stage and where daily deaths and active cases of contagion reached their peak in Spain. Although the sample can be considered small compared to other studies, the need to carry out this research at this historical moment made the benefits greater than the disadvantages. For this reason, it was not possible to carry out research based on a representative sample adjustment in the whole of Spain, but rather an intentional cut-off methodology was followed.

To gain access to health professionals who worked directly with patients affected by COVID-19, representatives of workers, hospital and ICU staff from different Spanish hospitals were contacted directly, who facilitated contact with the workers under study. For this reason, the sample is smaller than what could have been obtained by extending the research to all health professionals. In any case, this methodology made it possible to previously select the subjects who were really working with the disease during this period. Subsequently, an online survey was administered through the application of the University of Murcia (umu.encuestas) to which the participants had access without putting their security at risk, and always guaranteeing their confidentiality and anonymity. Participants must accept the ethical conditions and give their consent before accessing the questionnaire and sending their answers.

In any case, all the requirements of the Ethics Committees that Spanish universities establish for their researchers were followed. Since this is a descriptive study in Spain, the approval of a specific Ethics Committee was not required (unlike studies based on experiments). Despite this, the Codes of Good Practice for Research on Human Beings were followed. Furthermore, it is important to add that the participants gave their informed consent in accordance with the Declaration of Helsinki. The project was registered and signed by the research team with the code number REPRIN-PEM-010.

The research design was a simple random sampling in view of the difficulties aroused from accessing health professionals in such a short period of time-due to the phase of confinement in which the Spanish population found itself after the state of alarm decree—and the need to obtain relevant data on this social phenomenon in such an important historical context.

3.3. *Variables Used*

3.3.1. Dependent Variable

The Maslach burnout inventory (MBI) was used to measure the burnout. This questionnaire was validated by Maslach and Jackson and the final version was published in 1986. A validated and translated version of the original was used, which has already been used in numerous studies in Spain with positive results [60,100–107]. This is a 22-item questionnaire with 7 answer options (Likert scale from 0 to 6) which comprehends the following subscales: emotional exhaustion (EE), understood as the subject's feeling of being emotionally saturated by work; depersonalization (DP), which implies a cold and impersonal response to patients; and personal accomplishment (PA), which encompasses feelings of competence and efficiency at work. With respect to emotional exhaustion, the scores of the different levels are as follows: 0–18 for the low level, 19–26 for the medium level, and 27–54 for the high level. In relation to depersonalization, the low-level ranges from 0–5, the medium level from 6–9, and the high level from 10–30. Finally, regarding personal accomplishment, the scale attributes a low level when values between 0–33 are registered, a medium level when they are between 34–39, and a high level when values between 40–56 are obtained.

In each of the three dimensions, the dependent variable has been established as dichotomous, differentiating between low and medium/high risk. For this purpose, the reference values in each of the subscales were followed to categorize the dependent variable. The medium–high risk in each of the subscales is as follows: emotional exhaustion: 16–54, depersonalization: 6–30 and professional accomplishment: 34–56.

3.3.2. Independent Variables

The following variables were used to predict the burnout: (a) sex (male/female), (b) age (<30 years, 31–40 years, 41–50 years, 51–60 years and >60 years), (c) professional category (nurse, doctor, clinical assistant and others), (d) perception of need for psychological/psychiatric treatment (yes/no), (e) perception about the need to incorporate psychological/psychiatric treatment (yes/no), (f) perception about whether they think they will need psychological/psychiatric treatment in the future (yes/no), (g) if they feel that the lack of PPE may be affecting their level of stress or anxiety (yes/no).

3.4. Statistical Analysis

Firstly, a descriptive analysis of the most representative variables was developed considering sociodemographic aspects and perceptions of stress and anxiety of health professionals. Subsequently, a cross-table analysis was developed with the aim of observing the relationships between the different variables according to their level of significance ($p < 0.005$).

Finally, with the purpose of knowing the probability of the phenomenon of the three subscales of burnout, three logistic regressions were carried out, establishing as a dependent variable in each one of them the risk of suffering a medium-high level of burnout, taking into account the independent variables.

4. Results

The descriptive analysis shows the following results (Table 1). First, with respect to sociodemographic variables, 79% are women and 21% men; the percentage of female participation is higher. This has occurred with other studies with very similar percentages [108–110]. The mean age is 41.8 years. If we make a distribution by age, the sample is widely distributed among all the intervals except among people aged 61 years and older. In terms of professional category, the nurses who accounted for more than 50% of the participants are noteworthy.

As for the MBI scale, the average value is 3.3. If we carry out a more detailed analysis of the MBI scale, we observe that the highest values are concentrated in the depersonalization subscale whose high levels reach 38.9%, almost doubling the values of the EE and PA subscales. Finally, with respect to the data related to subjective issues, the following data were obtained. In the first place, only a small percentage of health professionals consider that they need psychological and psychiatric support, but, nevertheless, 90.4% of the persons surveyed consider that this service should be provided from the work centers in view of the current health crisis.

Related to the above, 43.3% of the persons surveyed considered that they might need psychological or psychiatric treatment in the future. In other words, health professionals do not currently perceive a situation of emotional vulnerability, but they are aware of the intensity of it and the repercussions it may have for them in the future. Finally, when asked how the absence of PPE is affecting their daily work, 85.4% stated that it is generating an increase in their level of stress and anxiety.

Table 1. Descriptive analysis of the variables.

	N	%	Average
Gender			
Woman	124	79.0	
Man	33	21.0	
Age			41.8
<30	35	22.3	
31–40	40	25.5	
41–50	30	19.1	
51–60	36	22.9	
>60	16	10.2	
Job			
Doctor	22	14.0	
Nurse Assistant	29	18.5	
Nurse	80	51.0	
Other	26	16.5	
IMBI Scale Total			
Sub Emotional Exhaustion			
Low	92	58.6	
Medium	33	21.0	
High	32	20.4	
Sub Depersonalization			
Low	50	31.8	
Medium	46	29.3	
High	61	38.9	
Sub Personal Accomplishment			
Low	72	45.9	
Medium	54	34.4	
High	31	19.7	
Need Support P/P			
Yes	42	26.8	
No	112	73.2	
Support Should be Given			
Yes	142	90.4	
No	14	9.6	
He/She'll Need Support P/P			
Yes	68	43.3	
No	87	56.7	
Absence of PPE, Increases Stress/Anxiety			
Yes	134	85.4	
No	20	14.6	

Once the descriptive analysis was done, a cross-table analysis was performed. Before performing this analysis, a classification of burnout risk variables was carried out in each of the subscales of the MBI, differentiating between low/medium risk and medium/high risk.

The results that obtained a Pearson chi-square with a significance level $p < 0.05$ will be presented; that is, those that show a significant relevance and whose association is not determined by chance.

First, it highlights the association between emotional exhaustion and the subjective perception of needing psychological or psychiatric treatment in the future. Regarding this subscale, a significant relationship is also observed between the risk of suffering emotional exhaustion and the professional category. Second, with respect to depersonalization, we observe how the lack of resources of individual protection is associated with this subscale. This result is very interesting given that during the first wave of the pandemic, health professionals had to carry out their work with insufficient resources of individual protection, putting their personal and family health at risk. This fact has important connotations since the lack of individual protection equipment could have caused an increase in the subscale of depersonalization, and with it, cause a detachment of health professionals from their problems, even to blame their patients for the problems caused by the COVID-19 at the professional level. With respect to personal accomplishment, no significant associations were observed. Therefore, the three independent variables that most significantly influence the increase in the level of burnout, taking into account the level of significance of Pearson's chi-square, are: professional category, subjective perception of the need to receive psychological or psychiatric treatment in the future, and the absence of PPE.

Thirdly, we proceeded to use the technique of binary logistic regression to evaluate the effect of sex, age, professional category and subjective perceptions regarding the present and future needs for psychological and psychiatric treatment in health professionals; if this should be provided by hospital centers, as well as if the lack of resources of individual protection is affecting the increase in burnout in health professionals (Table 2). The only subscale that showed an acceptable model was emotional exhaustion.

Table 2. Variables used in binary logistic regression.

1. Gender
Ref. Man
(1) Woman
2. Age
Ref. < 30
(1) 31–40
(2) 41–50
(3) 51–60
(4) >60
3. Job
Ref. Other
(1) Nurse
(2) Doctor
(3) Nurse Assistant
4. Needs Psychological/Psychiatric Support
Ref. No
(1) Yes
5. Psychological/Psychiatric Support Should be Provided at Your Workplace
Ref. No
(1) Yes
6. He/she will Need Psychological/Psychiatric Support
Ref. No
(-1) Yes
7. Increased Stress and Anxiety as a Result of Lack of PPE
Ref. No
(1) Yes

The logistic regression model was statistically significant, X2 = 29.942, $p < 0.0005$. The model explains 24.6% (Nagelkerke's R2) of the variance in the emotional exhaustion subscale and correctly classifies 75.2% of the cases. The Hosmer–Lemeshow test showed that there were no significant differences between the results observed and those predicted in the model with a $p = 0.830$.

From these results, the less significant variables were eliminated through the automatic "forward" or "backward" method. Considering the seven predictor variables, only two were associated with the probability of suffering emotional exhaustion: the professional category and the subjective perception of needing psychological or psychiatric treatment in the future (WNMS). Regarding the professional categories, physicians and nurses have a higher risk of suffering from emotional exhaustion than other professions, including clinical assistants, professionals who in Spain spend the most time with patients performing the most elementary care with basic needs. The results of the logistic regression are shown below (Table 3).

Table 3. Results of logistic regression.

	B	Sig.	Exp(B)	95% C.I. for Exp(B)	
				Lower	Superior
WNMS (1)	−1.412	0.001	0.244	0.109	0.547
Job		0.049			
Nurses	1.330	0.008	3.782	1.419	10.078
Physicians	1.452	0.027	4.270	1.180	15.445
Nurse Assistant	0.926	0.119	2.524	0.787	8.089
Constant	0.650	0.175	1.916		

In the specific case of physicians, the OR was = 4.270, 95%CI (1.180–15.445), $p = 0.027$. Nurses had an OR = 3.782, 95%CI (1.419–10.078), $p = 0.008$. Therefore, physicians and nurses are at risk of suffering from emotional exhaustion. Their risks are 4.27 and 3.78 times greater than other health professionals, respectively. In case of both, physicians and nurses, the contact with patients and the time they spent with them was superior to that of other health professionals, and it was these same professionals, during the time of the greatest number of active cases of COVID-19, who were responsible for trying to restore the health of the patients, at the risk of infecting themselves due to the shortage, in the first few weeks, of personal protective equipment. Likewise, the fact of seeing their patients die every day has been key to the realization that, in the future, when the situation improves, they would need to address this issue in the personal sphere, with professional intervention at the psychological and/or psychiatric level.

Finally, in relation to the subjective perception of needing psychological and psychiatric treatment in the future, the data show OR = 0.244, 95% CI (0.109–0.547), $p = 0.001$. Therefore, and contrary to what might initially be thought, the probability of a person who considers that they may need psychological and psychiatric treatment in the future decreases by 0.24 with respect to those who do not perceive that they consider these treatments necessary. This result suggests that, despite a future perception of the need for psychological treatment, the health demands caused by the COVID-19 pandemic focus their attention on patient care, over and above their own concerns. High-stress situations, in which health personnel do not perceive the need for psychological care, reinforce the fact that they behave homogeneously in the context of this pandemic and that sociodemographic conditions, such as age and sex, are not highlighted. This is essential information that we believe must be considered in any future preventive planning to face these harsh adversities. Prevention is a key factor.

5. Discussion

The results demonstrated us how the burnout syndrome is currently affecting more those aspects related to depersonalization than the rest of the subscales of the MBI. Unlike other studies [15,111–114] it is striking that, during this health crisis, no differences are seen in relation to sex and age as it does on non-exceptional occasions, where it most affects older female health professionals [115].

On the other hand, in relation to the depersonalization scale, we observed a relationship between people who present higher levels in this subscale as a result of the absence of PPE and their subjective perception that it can produce an increase in stress and anxiety levels. Recent studies related to mental health in the face of the COVID-19 pandemic address this phenomenon, demonstrating the fact that health workers face challenges such as the risk of infection, excessive care burden, exposure to family distress and ethical and moral dilemmas [23,57].

This is not a trivial issue, nor is the fact that during the most critical weeks for the health care system, where daily deaths reached almost 1000 people and new infections were counted in the thousands, health care workers lacked PPE, posing a risk to their own health as a group, a point that concurs with the study by Xiang et al. These elements are key to understand that increased anxiety as a result of gaps in pandemic planning and prevention has had an impact on health workers in their personal, family and community spheres, recording burnout values above those found in Spain in previous times [27,115,116]

Moreover, in a remarkable way, in the subscale of emotional exhaustion, we observed from the logistic regression carried out, the higher probability of suffering burnout concentrates in physicians and nurses over other health professionals. The fact that they surpass the clinical assistants, personnel who carry out the most elemental care of the patients, stands out. However, this risk of suffering emotional exhaustion is not the result of the lack of cohesion between the different professional categories, but rather of the lack of foresight from competent professionals regarding the general lack of individual protective equipment among health professionals, especially those who were most exposed to the virus due to increased contact with patients. This can be understood within a context where emotional exhaustion is linked to the capacity to respond to the disease from a more scientific perspective than that of companion and care. In this sense, the work done would be aimed, mainly in certain units such as the intensive care unit, where the demand for beds was higher than the existing capacity, to save the lives of infected patients who, although many could be saved, many others did not. That is to say, the absence of an effective response to COVID-19 disease on the part of these professionals has led to greater emotional exhaustion. Similar results were found in recent studies such as that of Li et al. [117] which indicate that physicians in China experienced an increase in mental health symptoms and fear of violence and a decrease in mood after the outbreak of COVID-19.

On the other hand, a singular fact is taking place in relation to the subjective perception of the need to receive psychological and psychiatric treatment. In this case, the people who have a greater risk of suffering emotional exhaustion are precisely those who, at the time of carrying out the study, consider that they will not need it, a sign of the pressure in which they currently work. This finding is analogous to the results found by Chen et al. [118] who expressed that health professionals were concerned about the insufficiency of PPE and feelings of helplessness when faced with critical patients. Many indicated that they did not need psychological help, but rather more uninterrupted rest and sufficient protective equipment.

It is not difficult to think that this situation will not have repercussions on professionals in the long term, since on many occasions the individual himself is not prepared to face limited situations at the time of greatest tension; often these consequences appear in the future. As Albaladejo and others point out [111], after 10 years from the beginning of a stressful situation, a process of sensitization or de-motivation can occur, losing the vocation that, at the time, made the person choose this profession.

At this point, professional treatment can have significant benefits for the individuals concerned, producing both personal and occupational rewards. In this particular case, characterized by an unprecedented health crisis where there has been a lack of adequate response from health institutions in providing essential PPE to their workers, psychological treatment emerges as a plausible and reasoned need for those health workers who believe they may need this treatment in the future.

In other words, health professionals who do not perceive the need for these treatments, in the face of the adverse health crisis situation, are what may need them most in the future since their emotional exhaustion is increasing without obtaining any compensatory mechanism for the situation of stress and emotional anxiety. Studies such as that previously cited by Chen et al. [106] found similar data; at the first stage of the illness, health professionals were reluctant to participate in the group or individual psychological interventions provided to them for various reasons: becoming infected was not the main concern when they began to work; they were more concerned about the possibility of their relatives worrying about them and about the possibility of bringing the virus home; and finally, the health workers did not know how to act with patients who did not want to be quarantined in the hospital, sometimes because of the panic that ignorance of the disease caused and they did not collaborate with the medical measures.

In this sense, in an emergency context such as the one that occurred during the key months of the COVID-19 outbreak, the measures carried out and the prevention actions at the beginning of the process are more effective. In relation to this issue, Withey [119] considers an emergency situation as a type of stress in which the appearance of several factors lead to the existence of different degrees of fear, anxiety and concern that result in adaptive or non-adaptive efforts; these factors are: the severity of the event, the probability of occurrence and the individual's ability to cope with the crisis and the existing stress. Factors existing during the coronavirus outbreak.

It is also worth asking whether there could be training, both initial and ongoing, for health professionals in dealing with these extreme contingencies, in such a way as to enable them to face these situations with techniques to control their stress, fear and emotions. Academic offerings of specific subjects during the university career or training modules in continuous training processes could be a possibility, but the experiences obtained so far in other scenarios of extreme circumstances do not show that satisfactory results can be guaranteed. As presented by Dreison et al. [76], in a meta-analysis of the effectiveness of interventions against burnout syndrome, the effectiveness is very relative. It is true that training/education appeared in their study as the most effective subtype of organizational intervention, but this was dependent on the context. These authors even recommended that the different interventions carried out be adjusted to the specific needs of the organization and staff, and in long follow-up periods.

However, as we have presented in this study, the situation in which Spanish health professionals have found themselves in this COVID-19 pandemic is what has led to the burnout syndrome having more effect on those aspects related to emotional exhaustion. Further, this has been due, above all, to the fact that they lacked the resources to deal with the virulence of SARS-CoV-2 rather than the lack of prior training or preventive measures in training. The lack of resources of individual protection was one of the highest risks that health professionals have had to face in their professional work, being aware that they were risking their lives and, naturally, those of their loved ones, to whom they could infect. Nevertheless, the work carried out has been admirable, always focusing on the care of patients above their own concerns. In this context, the appearance of the burnout syndrome is evident. If the situation caused by the pandemic has significantly increased the levels of anxiety and stress in the general population, for which interventions are requested [120–122], the experiences of health professionals in Spain, faced in the front line with the most terrible aspects of this disease, and in so many cases without sufficient protection, represent a limited scenario on the psychological level.

Thus, in relation to its meaning, is necessary to emphasize that, unlike the subscales of emotional exhaustion and depersonalization, no significant results were observed in terms of personal accomplishment, neither through the cross tables nor through logistic regression. This is a relevant finding since it can be considered that the previous variables that health professionals highlight as generating stress and anxiety are the lack of PPE and the possible transfer of the virus to relatives and not so much the excessive workload or lack of motivation, which, according to the data, appears intact, despite being in an unprecedented health crisis.

Finally, it should be noted that this research was limited by the accessibility to health professionals at that critical time as a result of the declaration of the state of alarm and the extreme conditions in which they carried out their job. Despite not having developed a stratified research in all the Spain territory, and with a greater sample (the mentioned limitations made it impossible) the results allow access to information of vital importance both for the current management of the health crisis and to design, plan and execute actions to improve the mental health of the health professionals subjected to high levels of anxiety and stress at work. In the context, as we say, of how difficult it has been to carry out the field work, we consider it necessary and essential for all that it could bring us.

Understanding depersonalization as the unemotional and impersonal response to patients, development of negative attitudes and feelings, insensitivity, distancing of patients and colleagues even blaming them for their own frustrations, we find that in this study, the main finding lies in the relationship with the lack of resources of individual protection and the risk of health care workers to be infected and not as a response to fatigue resulting from high workload, time with patients or lack of recognition. In this case, changes in management related to schedules, work shifts, service rotation, training in effective stress management and conflict resolution, tolerance to frustration, as well as the importance of companion and quality of care, would help to minimize this feeling of tiredness and cynicism.

6. Conclusions

This article shows the need to consider mental health care for the health care community, especially those who have been in the front line, working with confirmed and suspected cases of COVID-19, to avoid possible malpractice, but also the development of post-traumatic stress in both health and non-health care extending also to patients who may need it, especially by multidisciplinary teams and in those at risk of suicide.

Up-to-date, regular, and accurate information is essential both, to reduce the high levels of burnout in physicians and nurses and to avoid the feeling of fear and uncertainty that occurred especially in the first weeks of official coexistence with the virus. Both physicians, and nurses have been the health occupations most affected by burnout, precisely those who are most connected in the detection and treatment of the disease. Attention to symptoms such as insomnia, social isolation, information on self-recognition of stress symptoms [123] would have been essential from an institutional intervention. The guidelines adopted and proposed at international level can serve as a guide for possible outbreaks of coronavirus in the healthcare context. It is essential to anticipate what may happen [56,124–126].

Identifying the lack of means of individual protection and the danger of health workers to be infected, with the depersonalization that health workers present, is one of the main contributions of this study since it justifies and relates these reactions of health workers to the work carried out during the COVID-19 pandemic. Therefore, these aspects, which were not avoided and generated a high stress due to the real possibilities of contagion and death, are closely related to the unwanted attitudes inherent to the state of depersonalization of professionals.

This work has some limitations such as reaching a larger sample. However, it must be taken into account that the applied research was carried out in a context of a high level of difficulty in administering the questionnaire to health professionals—submerged in a situation of work stress not known until now—as well as the need to obtain results at the moment of greatest virulence of the COVID-19 disease, it being appropriate not to miss the opportunity to carry out this study at this historical moment. Likewise, and related to the previous limitation, we find the difficulty of carrying out a sample stratification by territories that would have allowed us to analyze the results according to the health policy implemented in each one of them. It would have been convenient to compare the results with other different questionnaires used to measure the existence and level of burnout in health professionals (for example, GAD-7 or PHQ-9), but due to the time pressure and the impossibility of having access to more health professionals due to the conditions they are experiencing, it was not possible. However, there has been a several number of publications on burnout in health professionals in Spain that used the MBI scale which gives consistency and supports the results of this study [127–129].

Author Contributions: Conceptualization, J.Á.M.-L., C.L.-P., J.G.-G.; methodology, J.Á.M.-L., C.L.-P., J.G.G.; validation, J.Á.M.-L., C.L.-P., J.G.-G.; formal analysis, J.Á.M.-L., C.L.-P.; investigation, J.Á.M.-L., C.L.-P., J.G.-G., M.d.M.F.-M.; data curation, J.Á.M.-L., C.L.-P., J.G.-G., M.d.M.F.-M.; writing original draft preparation, J.Á.M.-L., C.L.-P., J.G.-G.; writing, review and editing, J.Á.M.-L., C.L.-P., J.G.-G., M.d.M.F.-M.; supervision, J.Á.M.-L., C.L.-P., J.G.-G., M.d.M.F.-M.; project administration, J.Á.M.-L., C.L.-P., J.G.-G., M.d.M.F.-M. All authors have read and agreed to the published version of the manuscript.

Funding: This research received no external funding.

Acknowledgments: We would like to thank the health staff very much for having given us their valuable time, especially for the very adverse circumstances they were facing, in order to carry out this research.

Conflicts of Interest: The authors declare no conflict of interest.

References

1. Garrett, L. COVID-19: The medium is the message. *Lancet* **2020**, *395*, 942–943. [CrossRef]
2. Vellingiri, B.; Jayaramayya, K.; Iyer, M.; Narayanasamy, A.; Govindasamy, V.; Giridharan, B.; Ganesan, S.; Venugopal, A.; Venkatesan, D.; Ganesan, H.; et al. COVID-19: A promising cure for the global panic. *Sci. Total Environ.* **2020**, *725*, 138277. [CrossRef] [PubMed]
3. Ho, C.S.; Chee, C.Y.; Ho, R.C. Mental health strategies to combat the psychological impact of COVID-19 beyond paranoia and panic. *Ann. Acad. Med. Singap.* **2020**, *49*, 1–3.
4. Lancet, T. COVID-19: Fighting panic with information. *Lancet* **2020**, *395*, 537. [CrossRef]
5. San Martín, M. Coronaviruses and Wuhan pneumonia: COVID-19. *Front. Sci.* **2020**, *7*, 16–22.
6. World Health Organization. *Statement on the Second Meeting of the International Health Regulations (2005). Emergency Committee Regard-ing the Outbreak of Novel Coronavirus (2019-nCoV)*; WHO: Geneva, Switzerland, 2020.
7. Sulkowski, L. Covid-19 pandemic; recession, virtual revolution leading to de-globalization? *J. Intercult. Manag.* **2020**, *12*, 1–11. [CrossRef]
8. Zaki, J. Catastrophe compassion: Understanding and extending prosociality under crisis. *Trends Cogn. Sci.* **2020**. [CrossRef]
9. Vieira, C.M.; Franco, O.H.; Restrepo, C.G.; Abel, T. COVID-19: The forgotten priorities of the pandemic. *Maturitas* **2020**, *136*, 38–41. [CrossRef]
10. Rudnicka, L.; Gupta, M.; Kassir, M.; Jafferany, M.; Lotti, T.; Sadoughifar, R.; Goldust, M. Priorities for global health community in COVID-19 pandemic. *Dermatol. Ther.* **2020**, *33*, e13361. [CrossRef]
11. Qiu, J.; Shen, B.; Zhao, M.; Wang, Z.; Xie, B.; Xu, Y. A nationwide survey of psychological distress among Chinese people in the COVID-19 epidemic: Implications and policy recommendations. *Gen. Psychiatry* **2020**, *33*, e100213. [CrossRef]
12. Bellizzi, S.; Fiamma, M.; Arru, L.; Farina, G.; Manca, A. COVID-19: The daunting experience of health workers in Sardinia, Italy. *Infect. Control Hosp. Epidemiol.* **2020**, 1–2. [CrossRef] [PubMed]
13. Guanche, H. COVID-19. A challenge for healthcare professionals. *MéDicas* **2020**, *19*, e3284.
14. Semple, S.; Cherrie, J. COVID-19: Protecting Worker Health. *Ann. Work Expo. Health* **2020**, *64*, 461–464. [CrossRef] [PubMed]
15. Xiang, Y.; Yang, Y.; Li, W.; Zhang, L.; Zhang, Q. Timely mental health care for the 2019 novel coronavirus. *Lancet Psychiatry* **2020**, *7*, 228–229. [CrossRef]
16. Equipo COVID-19. *Informe Sobre la Situación de COVID-19 en España. Informe COVID-19 nº 32. 21 de mayo de 2020*; Instituto de Salud Carlos III, RENAVE, CNE: Madrid, Spain, 2020.
17. Ministerio de Sanidad. *Situación del COVID-19 en España*; Ministerio de Sanidad: Madrid, Spain, 2020.
18. MUD. *Informe MUD. Condiciones de los Médicos Españoles en la Práctica Clínica Durante la Crisis del COVID-19*; Asociación de Médicos Unidos por tus Derechos: Madrid, Spain, 2020.
19. Aiello, A.; Khayeri, M.Y.; Raja, S.; Peladeau, N.; Romano, D.; Leszcz, M.; Maunder, R.G.; Rose, M.; Adam, M.A.; Pain, C.; et al. Resilience training for hospital workers in anticipation of an influenza pandemic. *J. Contin. Educ. Health Prof.* **2011**, *31*, 15–20. [CrossRef]
20. Liu, Z.; Han, B.; Jiang, R.; Huang, Y.; Ma, C.; Wen, J.; Zhang, T.; Wang, Y.; Chen, H.; Ma, Y. Mental health status of phisicians and nurses during COVID-19 epidemic in China. *Lancet* **2020**. [CrossRef]
21. Maunder, R.G.; Lancee, W.J.; Mae, R.; Vincent, L.; Peladeau, N.; Beduz, M.A.; Hunter, J.J.; Leszcz, M. Computer-assisted resilience training to prepare healthcare workers for pandemic influenza: A randomized trial of the optimal dose of training. *BMC Health Serv. Res.* **2010**, *10*, 72. [CrossRef]
22. Xiao, H.; Zhang, Y.; Kong, D.; Li, S.; Yang, N. The effects of social support on sleep quality of medical staff treating patients with coronavirus disease 2019 (COVID-19) in January and February 2020 in China. *Int. Med. J. Exp. Clin. Res.* **2020**, *26*, e923549.
23. Lai, J.; Ma, S.; Wang, Y.; Cai, Z.; Hu, J.; Wei, N.; Wu, J.; Du, H.; Chen, T.; Li, R.; et al. Factors associated with mental health outcomes among health care workers exposed to coronavirus disease 2019. *JAMA Netw. Open* **2020**, *3*, e203976. [CrossRef]
24. Cumplido, R.; Molina, C. Aproximación al afrontamiento de la muerte en profesionales de cuidados intensivos. *Med. Paliativa* **2011**, *18*, 141–148. [CrossRef]

25. Cañadas, G.; Vargas, C.; San Luis, C.; García, I.; Cañadas, G.R.; De la Fuente, E.I. Risk factors and prevalence of burnout syndrome in the nursing profession. *Int. J. Nurs. Stud.* **2015**, *52*, 240–249. [CrossRef]
26. Navarro, A.; Ayechu, I.; Huarte, P. Prevalencia del síndrome del burnout y factores asociados a dicho síndrome en los profesionales sanitarios de Atención Primaria. *Med. Fam.* **2015**, *41*, 191–198.
27. Falgueras, M.V.; Munoz, C.C.; Pernas, F.O.; Sureda, J.C.; Lopez, M.P.; Miralles, J.D. Burnout y trabajo en equipo en los profesionales de atención primaria. *Atención Primaria* **2015**, *47*, 25–31. [CrossRef] [PubMed]
28. Gómez, J.L.; Monsalve, C.S.; San Luis, C.; Fernández, R.; Aguayo, R.; Cañadas, G.A. Factores de riesgo y niveles de burnout en enfermeras de atención primaria: Una revisión sistemática. *Atención Primaria* **2017**, *49*, 77–85.
29. Joshi, G.; Sharma, G. Burnout: A risk factor amongst mental health professionals during COVID-19. *Asian J. Psychiatry* **2020**, *54*, 102300. [CrossRef] [PubMed]
30. Styra, R.; Hawryluck, L.; Robinson, S.; Kasapinovic, S.; Fones, C.; Gold, W.L. Impact on health care workers employed in high-risk areas during the Toronto SARS outbreak. *J. Psychosom. Res.* **2008**, *64*, 177–183. [CrossRef]
31. Pimble, C. Therapeutic Effectiveness, Stress, and Burnout in Mental Health Professionals. Ph.D. Thesis, Philadelphia College of Osteopathic Medicine, Philadelphia, PA, USA, 2016.
32. Maslach, C. Job burnout new directions in research and intervention. *Curr. Dir. Psychol. Sci.* **2003**, *12*, 189–192. [CrossRef]
33. Blanco-Donoso, L.M.; Moreno-Jiménez, J.; Gálvez-Herrer, M.; Moreno-Jiménez, B.; Garrosa, E. Riesgos psicosociales laborales de los profesionales de la salud ante la crisis producida por el COVID-19: Desde la identificación de estos riesgos hasta la actuación inmediata. *Rev. Int. Av. Estud. Enfermería* **2020**. [CrossRef]
34. Barello, S.; Palamenghi, L.; Graffigna, G. Burnout and somatic symptoms among frontline healthcare professionals at the peak of the Italian COVID-19 pandemic. *Psychiatry Res.* **2020**, *290*, 113129. [CrossRef]
35. Sultana, A.; Sharma, R.; Hossain, M.M.; Bhattacharya, S.; Purohit, N. Burnout among healthcare providers during COVID-19: Challenges and evidence based interventions. *Indian J. Med. Ethics* **2020**. [CrossRef]
36. Maslach, C.; Jackson, S.E.; Leiter, M.P.; Schaufeli, W.B.; Schwab, R.L. *Maslach Burnout Inventory*; Consulting Psychologists Press: Palo Alto, CA, USA, 1986.
37. Maslach, C.; Schaufeli, W.B. Historical and conceptual development of Burnout. In *Professional Burnout: Recent Developments in Theory and Research*; Schaufeli, W.B., Maslach, C., Marek, T., Eds.; Taylor y Francis: Washington, DC, USA, 1993; pp. 1–16.
38. López, A. *El Síndrome de Burnout: Antecedentes y Consecuentes Organizacionales en el Ámbito de la Sanidad Pública Gallega*; EIDO: Vigo, Spain, 2017.
39. Maslach, C.; Jackson, S.E.; Maslach, C.; Jackson, S.E. Maslach Burnout Inventory-Human Services Survey (MBI-HSS). In *Maslach Burnout Inventory Manual*; Maslach, C., Jackson, S.E., Leiter, M.P., Eds.; Consulting Psychologists Press: Palo Alto, CA, USA, 1996; pp. 192–198.
40. Li-Ping, C.; Chung-Yi, L.; Hu, S.C. Job stress and burnout in hospital employees: Comparisons of different medical professions in a regional hospital in Taiwan. *BMJ Open* **2014**, *4*, e004185.
41. Redín, C.I.; Erro-Garcés, A. Stress in teaching professionals across Europe. *Int. J. Educ. Res.* **2020**, *103*, 101623. [CrossRef]
42. Ortega, C.; López, F. El burnout o síndrome de estar quemado en los profesionales sanitarios: Revisión y perspectivas. *Int. J. Clin. Healthy Psichol.* **2004**, *4*, 137–160.
43. Shirom, A.; Melamed, S.; Toker, S.; Berliner, S.; Shapira, I. Burnout and health review: Current knowledge and future research directions. *Int. Rev. Ind. Organ. Psychol.* **2005**, *20*, 269–308.
44. Schonfeld, I.S.; Bianchi, R. Burnout and depression: Two entities or one? *J. Clin. Psychol.* **2016**, *72*, 22–37. [CrossRef] [PubMed]
45. Schaufeli, W.B.; Leiter, M.P.; Maslach, C. Burnout: 35 years of research and practice. *Career Dev. Int.* **2009**, *14*, 204–220. [CrossRef]
46. Maslach, C.; Jackson, S.E.; Leiter, M.P. *Maslach Burnout Inventory Manual*; Mind Garden: Menlo Park, CA, USA, 2010.
47. Simón, M.; Blesa, A.; Calvo, M.; Gómez, C. Estresores laborales y satisfacción en la enfermería de una unidad de críticos. *Enfermería Intensiva* **2005**, *16*, 3–14.
48. Mikolajczak, M.; Gross, J.J.; Stinglhamber, F.; Norberg, A.L.; Roskam, I. Is parental burnout distinct from job burnout and depressive symptomatology? *Clin. Psychol. Sci.* **2020**, 1–50. [CrossRef]

49. Dorevitch, S.; Forst, L. Hazard of emergency physicians. *Am. J. Emerg. Med.* **2000**, *18*, 300–311. [CrossRef]
50. Aguado, J.I.; Bátiz, A.; Quintana, S. El estrés en personal sanitario hospitalario: Estado actual. *Med. Segur. Trab.* **2013**, *59*, 259–275. [CrossRef]
51. Moreno, B.; Oliver, C.; Aragoneses, A. El burnout, una forma específica de estrés laboral. In *Manual de Psicología Clínica Aplicada*; Buela Casal, G., Caballo, V.E., Eds.; Siglo XXI: Madrid, Spain, 1991; pp. 271–284.
52. Grau, A. Cómo prevenir el burnout: Diferentes definiciones e interpretaciones. *Gestión Práctica Riesgos Labor.* **2007**, *43*, 18–27.
53. Maslach, C. Burned out. *Hum. Behav.* **1976**, *5*, 16–22.
54. Maslach, C.; Schaufeli, W.B.; Leiter, M.P. Job burnout. *Annu. Rev. Psychol.* **2001**, *52*, 397–422. [CrossRef]
55. Maslach, C.; Jackson, S. *Maslach Burnout Inventory*; Consulting Psychology Press: Palo Alto, CA, USA, 1981.
56. Kisely, S.; Warren, N.; McMahon, L.; Dalais, C.; Henry, I.; Siskind, D. Occurrence, prevention, and management of the psychological effects of emerging virus outbreaks on healthcare workers: Rapid review and meta-analysis. *BMJ* **2020**, *369*, m1642. [CrossRef] [PubMed]
57. Ibañez-Vizoso, J.E.; Alberdi-Paramo, I.; Díaz-Marsa, M. International Mental Health perspectives on the novel coronavirus SARS-CoV-2 pandemic. *Rev. Psiquiatr. Salud Ment.* **2020**, *13*, 111–113. [CrossRef]
58. Sun, L.; Sun, Z.; Wu, L.; Zhu, Z.; Zhang, F.; Shang, Z.; Jia, Y.; Gu, J.; Zhou, Y.; Wang, Y.; et al. Prevalence and Risk Factors of Acute Posttraumatic Stress Symptoms during the COVID-19 Outbreak in Wuhan, China. *MedRxiv* **2020**. [CrossRef]
59. Tremearne, R.; Calvo, F.; Alonso, J. Síndrome de Burnout en Profesionales Sanitarios. 2005. Available online: https://www.researchgate.net/profile/Fernando_Calvo3/publication/241221960 (accessed on 20 July 2020).
60. Suñer-Soler, R.; Grau-Martín, A.; Flichtentrei, D.; Prats, M.; Braga, F.; Font-Mayolas, S.; Gras, M.E. The consequences of burnout syndrome among healthcare professionals in Spain and Spanish speaking Latin American countries. *Burn. Res.* **2014**, *1*, 82–89. [CrossRef]
61. Mingote Adán, J.C.; Pérez García, S. *Estrés en la Enfermería. El Cuidado del Cuidador*; Ediciones Díaz de Santos: Madrid, Spain, 2003.
62. World Health Organization. *Education and Training of Nurse Teachers and Managers with Special Regard to Primary Health Care: Report of a WHO Expert Committee*; World Health Organization: Geneve, Switzerland, 1984.
63. World Health Organization. *Continuing Education for Health Professionals*; World Health Organization, Genomic Resource Centre: Geneve, Switzerland, 2015.
64. Cook, H.L.; Beery, M.; Sauter, S.V.; DeVellis, R.F. Continuing education for health professionals. *Am. J. Occup. Ther.* **1987**, *41*, 652–657. [CrossRef]
65. Suster, S. On the Importance of Continuing Medical Education. *Arch. Pathol. Lab. Med.* **2019**, *143*, 1442–1443. [CrossRef]
66. Cullen, M.W.; Geske, J.B.; Anavekar, N.S.; McAdams, J.A.; Beliveau, M.E.; Ommen, S.R.; Nishimura, R.A. Reinvigorating Continuing Medical Education: Meeting the Challenges of the Digital Age. *Mayo Clin. Proc.* **2019**, *94*, 2501–2509. [CrossRef]
67. Marinopoulos, S.S.; Dorman, T.; Ratanawongsa, N.; Wilson, L.M.; Ashar, B.H.; Magaziner, J.L.; Miller, R.G.; Thomas, P.A.; Prokopowicz, G.P.; Qayyum, R.; et al. Effectiveness of continuing medical education. *Evid. Rep. Technol. Assess.* **2007**, *149*, 1–69.
68. Bjegovic-Mikanovic, V.; Vukovic, D.; Otok, R.; Czabanowska, K.; Laaser, U. Education and training of public health professionals in the European Region: Variation and convergence. *Int. J. Public Health* **2013**, *58*, 801–810. [CrossRef] [PubMed]
69. Wingate, M.S.; Perry, E.C.; Campbell, P.H.; David, P.; Weist, E.M. Identifying and protecting vulnerable populations in public health emergencies: Addressing gaps in education and training. *Public Health Rep.* **2007**, *122*, 422–426. [CrossRef] [PubMed]

70. Breckjord, E.B.; Stern, S.A.; Shugarman, L.R.; Chandra, A.; Tanielian, T.; Taylor, S.L.; Parker, A.M. Enhancing Emergency Preparedness, Response, and Recovery Management for Vulnerable Populations: Literature Review. 2012. Available online: http://aspe.hhs.gov/daltcp/reports/2008/emergfrA.pdf (accessed on 7 July 2020).
71. Olness, K.; Sinha, M.; Herran, M.; Cheren, M.; Pairojkul, S. Training of health care professionals on the special needs of children in the management of disasters: Experience in Asia, Africa, and Latin America. *Ambul. Pediatrics* **2005**, *5*, 244–248. [CrossRef]
72. Scott, L.A.; Carson, D.S.; Greenwell, I.B. Disaster 101: A novel approach to disaster medicine training for health professionals. *J. Emerg. Med.* **2010**, *39*, 220–226. [CrossRef]
73. Faberow, N.L. (Ed.) *Training Manual for Human Service Workers in Major Disasters*; Diane Publishing: Darby, PA, USA, 1999.
74. Waters, K.A.; Selander, J.; Stuart, G.W. Psychological adaptation of nurses post-disaster. *Issues Ment. Health Nurs.* **1992**, *13*, 177–190. [CrossRef]
75. Antonini, F.C. Psychological training of disaster workers. In *Health and Medical Aspects of Disaster Preparedness*; Duffy, J.C., Ed.; Springer: Boston, MA, USA, 1990; pp. 131–144.
76. Dreison, K.C.; Luther, L.; Bonfils, K.A.; Sliter, M.T.; McGrew, J.H.; Salyers, M.P. Job burnout in mental health providers: A meta-analysis of 35 years of intervention research. *J. Occup. Health Psychol.* **2018**, *23*, 18–30. [CrossRef]
77. Johnson, J.; Hall, L.H.; Berzins, K.; Baker, J.; Melling, K.; Thompson, C. Mental healthcare staff well-being and burnout: A narrative review of trends, causes, implications, and recommendations for future interventions. *Int. J. Ment. Health Nurs.* **2018**, *27*, 20–32. [CrossRef]
78. Salyers, M.P.; Garabrant, J.M.; Luther, L.; Henry, N.; Fukui, S.; Shimp, D.; Wu, W.; Gearhart, T.; Morse, G.A.; York, M.M.; et al. A comparative effectiveness trial to reduce burnout and improve quality of care. *Adm. Policy Ment. Health Ment. Health Serv. Res.* **2019**, *46*, 238–254. [CrossRef]
79. Vargas-Cruz, L.D.; Niño-Cardozo, C.L.; Acosta-Maldonado, J.Y. Estrategias que modulan el síndrome de Burnout en enfermeros (as): Una revisión bibliográfica. *Rev. Cienc. Cuid.* **2017**, *14*, 111–131. [CrossRef]
80. Ruotsalainen, J.; Serra, C.; Marine, A.; Verbeek, J. Systematic review of interventions for reducing occupational stress in health care workers. *Scand. J. Work Environ. Health* **2008**, *34*, 169–178. [CrossRef] [PubMed]
81. Mealer, M.; Conrad, D.; Evans, J.; Jooste, K.; Solyntjes, J.; Rothbaum, B.; Moss, M. Feasibility and acceptability of a resilience training program for intensive care unit nurses. *Am. J. Crit. Care* **2014**, *23*, e97–e105. [CrossRef] [PubMed]
82. Martín-Asuero, A. The mindfulness-based stress reduction program (MBSR) reduces stress-related psychological distress in healthcare professionals. *Span. J. Psychol.* **2010**, *13*, 897–905. [CrossRef] [PubMed]
83. Burton, A.; Burgess, C.; Dean, S.; Koutsopoulou, G.Z.; Hugh-Jones, S. How effective are mindfulness-based interventions for reducing stress among healthcare professionals? A systematic review and meta-analysis. *Stress Health* **2017**, *33*, 3–13. [CrossRef]
84. Lomas, T.; Medina, J.C.; Ivtzan, I.; Rupprecht, S.; Eiroa-Orosa, F.J. A systematic review and meta-analysis of the impact of mindfulness-based interventions on the well-being of healthcare professionals. *Mindfulness* **2019**, *10*, 1193–1216. [CrossRef]
85. Cohen, M.; Gagin, R. Can skill-development training alleviate burnout in hospital social workers? *Soc. Work Health Care* **2005**, *40*, 83–97. [CrossRef]
86. Stanulewicz, N.; Knox, E.; Narayanasamy, M.; Shivji, N.; Khunti, K.; Blake, H. Effectiveness of lifestyle health promotion interventions for nurses: A systematic review. *Int. J. Environ. Res. Public Health* **2020**, *17*, 17. [CrossRef]
87. Howlett, M.; Doody, K.; Murray, J.; LeBlanc-Duchin, D.; Fraser, J.; Atkinson, P.R. Burnout in emergency department healthcare professionals is associated with coping style: A cross-sectional survey. *Emerg. Med. J.* **2015**, *32*, 722–727. [CrossRef]
88. Abraham, L.; Thom, O.; Greenslade, J.H.; Wallis, M.; Johnston, A.N.B.; Carlstrom, E.; Mills, D.; Crilly, J. Morale, stress and coping strategies of staff working in the emergency department: A comparison of two different-sized departments. *Emerg. Med. Australas.* **2018**, *30*, 375–381. [CrossRef]
89. Moukarzel, A.; Michelet, P.; Durand, A.C.; Sebbane, M.; Bourgeois, S.; Markarian, T.; Bompard, C.; Gentile, S. Burnout syndrome among emergency department staff: Prevalence and associated factors. *BioMed Res. Int.* **2019**. [CrossRef]

90. Verougstraete, D.; Hachimi Idrissi, S. The impact of burn-out on emergency physicians and emergency medicine residents: A systematic review. *Acta Clin. Belg.* **2020**, *75*, 57–79. [CrossRef] [PubMed]
91. Brown, J.C. Implementation of Mindfulness with Emergency Nurse Practitioners to Decrease Burnout. Ph.D. Thesis, University of Maryland, Baltimore, MA, USA, 2020.
92. Gaeta, T.J. Need for a holistic approach to reducing burnout and promoting well-being. *J. Am. Coll. Emerg. Physicians Open* **2020**. [CrossRef]
93. Gómez Galán, J. The Black Death and other historical pandemics. *Front. Sci.* **2020**, *7*, 62–75.
94. Bosqued, M. *Quemados: El Síndrome de Burnout, qué es y Cómo Superarlo*; Ed Paidós Ibérica: Barcelona, Spain, 2008.
95. Sobrequés, J.; Cebrià, J.; Segura, J.; Rodríguez, C.; García, M.; Juncosa, S. La satisfacción laboral y el desgaste profesional de los médicos de atención primaria. *Atención Primaria* **2003**, *31*, 227–233.
96. Gil-Monte, P.R. Factorial validity of the Maslach Burnout Inventory (MBI-HSS) among Spanish professionals. *Rev. Saúde Pública* **2005**, *39*, 1–8. [CrossRef]
97. Galán, F.; Sanmartín, A.; Polo, J.; Giner, L. Burnout risk in medical students in Spain using the Maslach Burnout Inventory-Student Survey. *Int. Arch. Occup. Environ. Health* **2011**, *84*, 453–459. [CrossRef]
98. Luceño, L.; Talavera, B.; García, Y.; Martín, J. Symptoms of Posttraumatic Stress, Anxiety, Depression, Levels of Resilience and Burnout in Spanish Health Personnel during the COVID-19 Pandemic. *Int. J. Environ. Res. Public Health* **2020**, *17*, 5514. [CrossRef]
99. González-Sanguino, C.; Ausín, B.; Castellanos, M.A.; Saiz, J.; López-Gómez, A.; Ugidos, C.; Muñoz, M. Mental health consequences during the initial stage of the 2020 Coronavirus pandemic (COVID-19) in Spain. *Brain Behav. Immun.* **2020**, *87*, 172–176. [CrossRef]
100. Suner-Soler, R.; Grau-Martin, A.; Font-Mayolas, S.; Gras, M.E.; Bertran, C.; Sullman, M.J.M. Burnout and quality of life among Spanish healthcare personnel. *J. Psychiatr. Ment. Health Nurs.* **2013**, *20*, 305–313. [CrossRef]
101. Grau, A.; Suñer, R.; García, M.M. Burnout syndrome in health workers and relationship with personal and environmental factors. *Gac. Sanit.* **2005**, *19*, 463–470. [CrossRef]
102. Aguayo, R.; Vargas, C.; Emilia, I.; Lozano, L.M. A meta-analytic reliability generalization study of the Maslach Burnout Inventory. *Int. J. Clin. Health Psychol.* **2011**, *11*, 343–361.
103. Ortega, E.; Ramirez-Baena, L.; la Fuente-Solana, D.; Emilia, I.; Vargas, C.; Gómez-Urquiza, J.L. Gender, marital status, and children as risk factors for burnout in nurses: A meta-analytic study. *Int. J. Environ. Res. Public Health* **2018**, *15*, 2102.
104. González-Rodríguez, R.; López-Castedo, A.; Pastor-Seller, E.; Verde-Diego, C. Burnout syndrome in the Health System: The case of social health workers. *Enfermería Glob.* **2020**, *58*, 152–161.
105. Sanchis, R.; Martínez, M.; García-Aracil, N.; Alcaide, L.; Piquer, T.; Castejón, M.E. Measuring the levels of burnout syndrome and empathy of Spanish emergency medical service professionals. *Australas. Emerg. Care* **2019**, *22*, 193–199. [CrossRef] [PubMed]
106. Gómez, R.; Alonso, M.; Llamazares, M. Factorial validity of the Maslach Burnout Inventory-human services survey (MBI-HSS) in a sample of Spanish social workers. *J. Soc. Serv. Res.* **2019**, *45*, 207–219. [CrossRef]
107. Escudero, A.C.; Segura, A.; Cantero, P.A. Burnout Syndrome in Occupational Therapists in Spain: Prevalence and Risk Factors. *Int. J. Environ. Res. Public Health* **2020**, *17*, 3164. [CrossRef]
108. Moreno, B.; González-Gutiérrez, J.M.; Garrosa, E. Variables sociodemográficas en el proceso de desgaste profesional de enfermería. *Rev. ROL Enfermería* **2002**, *25*, 18–26.
109. Gil-Monte, P.R.; García-Juesas, J.A.; Caro, M. Influencia de la sobrecarga laboral y la autoeficacia sobre el síndrome de quemarse por el trabajo (burnout) en profesionales de enfermería. *Rev. Interam. Psicol.* **2008**, *42*, 113–118.
110. Porras, N. Variables Psicosociológicas y Burnout en Sanitarios. Ph.D. Thesis, University of Salamanca, Salamanca, Spain, 2014.
111. Albaladejo, R.; Villanueva, R.; Ortega, P.; Astasio, P.; Calle, M.; Domínguez, V. Síndrome de burnout en el personal de enfermería de un hospital de Madrid. *Rev. Esp. Salud Pública* **2004**, *78*, 505–516. [CrossRef]
112. LaFaver, K. Age and sex differences in burnout, career satisfaction, and well-being in US neurologists. *Neurology* **2018**. [CrossRef]

113. Wang, C.; Pan, R.; Wan, X.; Tan, Y.; Xu, L.; Ho, C.S.; Ho, R.C. Immediate psychological responses and associated factors during the initial stage of the 2019 coronavirus disease (COVID-19) Epidemic among the general population in China. *Int. J. Environ. Res. Public Health* **2020**, *17*, 1729. [CrossRef] [PubMed]
114. Duan, L.; Zhu, G. Psychological interventions for people affected by the COVID-19 epidemic. *Lancet Psychiatry* **2020**, *7*, 300–302. [CrossRef]
115. Lázaro-Pérez, C. La Conciencia en el Umbral del Tránsito: Experiencias Cercanas a la Muerte. Ph.D. Thesis, University of Murcia, Murcia, Spain, 2016.
116. Jiménez, A.; García, S. Valoración de ansiedad y burnout en los profesionales de enfermería de un servicio de Nefrología. *Enferm. Nefrológicas* **2016**, *19*, 118–124.
117. Li, W.; Frank, E.; Zhao, Z.; Chen, L.; Wang, Z.; Burmeister, M.; Sen, S. Mental Health of Young Physicians in China During the Novel Coronavirus Disease 2019 Outbreak. *JAMA Netw. Open* **2020**, *3*, e2010705. [CrossRef]
118. Chen, Q.; Liang, M.; Li, Y.; Guo, J.; Fei, D.; Wang, L.; He, L.; Sheng, C.; Cai, Y.; Li, X.; et al. Mental health care for medical staff in China during the COVID19 outbreak. *Lancet Psychiatry* **2020**, *7*, e15–e16. [CrossRef]
119. Withey, S.B. Reaction to uncertain threat. In *Man and Society in Disaster*; Baker, G.W., Chapman, D.W., Eds.; Basic Books: New York, NY, USA, 1962.
120. Roy, D.; Tripathy, S.; Kar, S.K.; Sharma, N.; Verma, S.K.; Kaushal, V. Study of knowledge, attitude, anxiety & perceived mental healthcare need in Indian population during COVID-19 pandemic. *Asian J. Psychiatry* **2020**, *51*, 102083. [CrossRef]
121. Gómez Galán, J. Educación frente a la infodemia: Estrategias en el ámbito universitario. In *Innovación Pedagógica Universitaria: Reflexiones y Estrategias*; Reyes-Tejedor, M., Cobos-Sanchiz, D., López-Meneses, E., Eds.; Octaedro: Barcelona, Spain, 2020.
122. Pakpour, A.H.; Griffiths, M.D. The fear of COVID-19 and its role in preventive behaviors. *J. Concurr. Disord.* **2020**. Preprint Version. Available online: http://irep.ntu.ac.uk/id/eprint/39561/ (accessed on 3 August 2020).
123. Center for the Study of Traumatic Stress. Caring for Patient's Mental Well-Being during Coronavirus and other Emerging Infectious Diseases: A Guide for Clinicians. 2020. Available online: https://www.cstsonline.org/assets/media/documents/CSTS_FS_caring_for_patients_mental_wellbeing_during_coronavirus.pdf (accessed on 3 August 2020).
124. Bouillon-Minois, J.B.; Schmidt, J.; Dutheil, F. SARS-CoV-2 pandemic and emergency medicine: The worst is yet to come. *Am. J. Emerg. Med.* **2020**, PMC7286255. [CrossRef]
125. Yang, P.; Wang, X. COVID-19: A new challenge for human beings. *Cell. Mol. Immunol.* **2020**, *17*, 555–557. [CrossRef]
126. Layne, S.P.; Hyman, J.M.; Morens, D.M.; Taubenberger, J.K. New coronavirus outbreak: Framing questions for pandemic prevention. *Sci. Transl. Med.* **2020**, *12*, eabb1469. [CrossRef]
127. Domínguez, J.M.; Herrera, F.; Villaverde, M.C.; Padilla, I.; Martínez, M.L.; Domínguez, J. Síndrome de desgaste profesional en trabajadores de atención a la salud en el área sanitaria de Ceuta. *Atención Primaria* **2012**, *44*, 30–35.
128. Cerrato, P.; Jiménez, M.V.; Marcos, J.; Meneses, M.T. Burnout en enfermería en Ávila. *Rev. Enfermería CyL* **2019**, *11*, 5–10.
129. Fuertes, C.; Aranda, G.; Rezola, N.; Erramuzpe, A.; Palacios, C.; Ibáñez, B. Persistencia a largo plazo de los efectos de un programa de mindfulness y autocompasión en profesionales sanitarios de Atención Primaria. *An. Sist. Sanit. Navar.* **2019**, *42*, 269–280. [PubMed]

Journal of
Clinical Medicine

MDPI

Article

Anxiety in Older Adolescents at the Time of COVID-19

Pietro Smirni [1], Gioacchino Lavanco [2] and Daniela Smirni [2,*]

1 Department of Educational Sciences, University of Catania, 95124 Catania, Italy; pietro.smirni@unict.it
2 Department of Psychology, Educational Science and Human Movement, University of Palermo, viale delle Scienze, Ed.15, 90128 Palermo, Italy; gioacchino.lavanco@unipa.it
* Correspondence: daniela.smirni@unipa.it; Tel.: +39-(0)91-2389-7748

Received: 12 August 2020; Accepted: 21 September 2020; Published: 23 September 2020

Abstract: Corona Virus Disease-19 (COVID-19) is a catastrophic health risk, with psychological, emotional, social, and relational implications. From the early stages of the virus spread, the elderly population was identified as the most vulnerable, and health authorities have rightly focused on this frailer population. Conversely, less attention was given to the emotional and psychological dimensions of children and adolescents. Moreover, even though they were the subjects whose lives and health were at low risk, they, nevertheless, had to face a reality full of anxiety, fears, and uncertainties. The current study investigated the state of anxiety and emotional awareness in a sample of healthy older adolescents, 84 females and 64 males, aged 17 to 19, during the pandemic lockdown, using the Self-Rating Anxiety Scale and the Italian Emotion Awareness Questionnaire. An unexpected anxious phenomenology was found, affecting anxiety and the ideo-affective domain, while somatic symptomatology appeared to be less severe. The highest anxiety symptoms were breathing difficulties. These findings supported the hypothesis that the COVID-19 pandemic may be a risk condition for an increased state of anxiety in older adolescents and suggested the need to provide (1) an effective, empathic communication system with direct participation of older adolescents, (2) a psychological counseling service for the stress management of adolescents.

Keywords: COVID-19 pandemic; virus' transmission; fear of contagion; breathing difficulty; healthy adolescents; emotion awareness; state anxiety

---

1. Introduction

Corona Virus Disease-19 (COVID-19) is a catastrophic health risk, with patients exhibiting symptoms that are often severe, imminent, and/or subtle, leading to very serious psychological, emotional, social, and relational implications for individuals and communities [1–3].

The fear of contagion has become prominent, leading some to believe that the future will be catastrophic and threatening. Fear dominates every other emotion. It is constantly reinforced by media bombardment centered on information about the dead, the number of infections, overcrowded intensive care units, hospitals unable to accommodate the sick, and other news that triggers fears and anxiety. In brief, the news can (oftentimes) spreads discord in society. Widespread panic and hyperarousal symptoms have developed. Individuals must take on a repertoire of somewhat unfamiliar behaviors to protect themselves from the virus and its lethal power. Ritualistic behaviors (with rupophobic and pathophobic imprints) are spreading—useful, perhaps, to contain the virus, but they become distressing signals of alarm and helplessness [2,4,5].

Moreover, the need to reduce the chances of contagion requires social distancing and limiting physical contact. Therefore, relationships between people experience profound changes; for example, direct communication disappears, or, in some cases, people lose the emotional value mediated by non-verbal modalities [2,4,5]. This is especially so since people have been forced to stay home for months. Meetings, places of worship and leisure, production facilities, services, schools, and universities remained closed, forcing students and teachers to experiment with new forms of 'at distance' teaching and learning [6,7].

Worldwide, elderly people were considered most at risk for getting COVID-19, and were more susceptible to fatal complications from the virus. Therefore, international health authorities and governments around the world directed attention and resources towards the health problems of elderly populations. Doctors, health professionals, clinical departments, and hospitals were forced to reduce their institutional interventions to respond, in the first instance, to the COVID emergency, and to treat thousands of elderly people in need of care. Requests have become increasingly demanding and health facilities are increasingly dominated by COVID patients [8].

In this frame, the world of adolescents and their psychological and emotional reactions become less focused, even if fragile individuals (such as adolescents) have high destabilizing and psychological effects. In a developmental stage, in which emotions, cognition, and peer relationships are oriented towards an expanding positive future of expectations and opportunities [9], a sudden, unpredictable, or very serious danger can compromise relationships, sociability, and any immediate and future planning [6].

A growing body of studies has investigated the psychological needs of children and adolescents during epidemics, and reported early data collected in COVID-19–affected areas in China during the outbreak [10]. Although children and adolescents seem to be less vulnerable than older adults to COVID-19, initial reports from Chinese communities reported that children and adolescents have been psychologically and socially affected, and have manifested significant behavioral disturbances [6,10]. The COVID-19 pandemic can worsen existing mental health problems, and lead to more cases among children and adolescents due to the unique combination of the public health crisis, social isolation, and economic recession [7].

In the USA, pre-COVID-19 epidemiological data reported that 35% of adolescents who received mental health services between 2012 and 2015 had turned to school mental health services [11]. Missing school for a prolonged period, therefore, could become an additional risk for the spread of mental disorders in the long-term, especially for more fragile adolescents who exclusively turn to scholastic health services for psychological and behavioral disorders [11].

Similarly, a recent study in the UK proposed a framework for prioritization relevant to psychological, social, and neuroscientific research, for mental health management during the pandemic [12]. The authors prioritize ascertaining and reducing the impact of the effects of school closures for young people seeking assistance [13–15]. Therefore, since adolescents are not indifferent to the dramatic impact of the COVID-19 epidemic, understanding their behaviors and emotions in response to this emergency can certainly be crucial to their psychological well-being, not only in the short-term, but in the long-term.

The literature on emotion regulation and infectious disease epidemics/pandemics highlights the importance of deepening the role of emotion regulation during these troubling times [16]. On the other hand, the impact of pandemics/global health crises, e.g., the Severe Acute Respiratory Syndrome (SARS) outbreak; Hemagglutinin Type 5 and Neuraminidase Type 1 (H5N1- Avian Influenza A) strain; Ebola virus] on the emotional and mental health of individuals has been widely articulated in literature, e.g., [17–19].

The current study aimed to investigate anxiety among a healthy sample of older adolescents, in order to support the need of psychological interventions with adolescents. This developmental stage may be viewed as a significant phase to assess the emotional effects of the pandemic, because it is relatively far off the emotional and behavioral complexity and instability of early adolescence, but not yet emotionally and behaviorally stabilized, as in the young adult stage [9]. The hypothesis of the study was that the COVID-19 pandemic could be a condition that leads to a greater risk of increasing the level of anxiety in healthy older adolescents, compared to the anxiety levels documented by previous literature studies in normal adolescents during non-COVID times.

2. Materials and Methods

2.1. Participants

Participants were recruited via an advertisement sent by email, in which the aims and objectives of the research were explained. Contact details of the participants were provided by school administrators who authorized the data collection.

A sample of 148 Italian students, aged between 17 and 19 (average age 17.9 ± 1.2), 84 females and 64 males, attending the last two years of high school, participated in the study.

Informed consent was obtained from adolescents over the age of 18; parental consent was required for minors to participate in the study. The study respected the anonymity and privacy of each participant, and was conducted in accordance with the Declaration of Helsinki. Moreover, 23 subjects were excluded because their questionnaires were not completed or showed some apparent inconsistencies.

2.2. Measures

To prevent having answers directly related to the anxious reactions to the epidemic, no measures that openly referred to the epidemic were used.

1. To evaluate anxiety, the Zung Self-Rating Anxiety Scale (SAS) was used. It is a standardized self-rating instrument, widely used in research and in clinical practices [20,21]; devised to measure state anxiety (within the previous week) as a clinical entity and an operationally defined disorder (not as a personality trait). It consists of 20 items, rated on a 1–4 Likert type scale. Subjects were asked to rate each item as to how it applied to them within the past week, in the following four quantitative terms: (1) none or a little of the time; (2) some of the time; (3) good part of the time; or (4) most or all of the time, coded respectively as 1, 2, 3, and 4. The total score ranged from 20 (no anxiety at all) to 80 (severe anxiety). Thus, the lower the score, the less anxious the subject, and vice versa.
2. To investigate emotional awareness, the following five subscales of the self-reported Italian Emotion Awareness Questionnaire (EAQ) for children and adolescents [22,23] were used: (1) differentiating emotions, as being aware of one's emotional states and understanding them as distinct states, is composed of seven items, e.g., "it is difficult to know whether I feel sad or angry or something else"; (2) verbal sharing of emotions, as the tendency to share emotional experiences with others, is composed of four items, e.g., "I find it hard to talk to anyone about I feel"; (3) not hiding emotions, as the tendency to refuse to deal with their emotions, is composed of four items, e.g., "when I am angry or upset, I try to hide this"; (4) attending to others' emotions, as the ability to perceive the emotions of others, is composed of five items, e.g., "it is important to know how my friends are feeling"; (5) analyses of one's own emotions, as the ability to detect and recognize one's own feelings, is composed of five items; e.g., "when I am angry or upset, I try to understand why". Participants were asked to rate the degree to which each item was true about them on a 3-point scale (1: Not true; 2: Sometimes true; 3: Often true). Scores ranged from 25 to 75. The higher the score, the better the emotional awareness.

2.3. Methods

Due to mobility restrictions imposed by the Italian government to contain the serious spread of the epidemic, the data were collected online from 15 April to 15 May 2020, a period in which the Italian population was forced to stay home in protective isolation.

Participants were asked to answer two self-rating scales, using their PC or tablet. They were also asked for information about the socio-economic status of their families (parents' occupation and education, geographical origin), and if they, or any of their family members, had been directly infected or exposed to a high risk of contagion.

2.4. Statistical Analysis

Means, standard deviations (SD), and percentages of the responses were computed for each item of the SAS and EAQ questionnaires. For each questionnaire, the items were sorted in descending order of severity.

Following Zung's procedure, an overall SAS index was calculated by dividing the sum of the scores on the 20 items by the maximum score of 80, and multiplying by 100 [20,24]. Similarly, for each item, an SAS index was calculated, considering the maximum score of 4.

The differences between males and females were investigated using the independent t-test.

The Pearson correlation was used to measure the strength of the relationship between SAS and EAQ. A p value < 0.05 was set as an indication of statistical significance for the analyses.

3. Results

None of the participants had been directly affected by COVID or were at high risk of contagion. For demographic conditions, study participants were a homogeneous group. They all had a middle socioeconomic status, and came from three regions of southern Italy (Sicilia, Campania, and Calabria).

Table 1 shows the mean and standard deviation of absolute values out of a maximum score of 4, as well as the SAS index of items of anxiety severity (listed in descending order). The SAS overall mean score was 42.2 ± 4.7 with an SAS index of 52.7. In 12 out of 20 items, the mean agreement score was higher than or equal to 2 (on maximum 4), indicating that, in these items, most participants tended to choose the high anxious agreement responses "good part of the time", coded as 3, or "most or all of the time", coded as 4. The item recording the highest score was item number 13, concerning breathing difficulties ("I can breathe in and out easily"), with a mean of 3.4 ± 0.81 and an SAS index of 85.

Table 1. Self-Rating Anxiety Scale (SAS): mean, standard deviations, and SAS index listed in descending order.

Items	Domain	Mean ± SD	SAS Index
13	breathing	3.4 ± 0.81	85
19	sleep	2.6 ± 1.0	65
1	nervous, anxious	2.5 ± 0.68	62.5
17	hands warm	2.4 ± 1.0	60
3	upset, panicky	2.4 ± 0.78	60
5	fear of future	2.3 ± 0.79	57.5
7	headache	2.3 ± 0.97	57.5
9	calm	2.3 ± 0.78	57.5
16	urinary	2.3 ± 0.83	57.5
8	weak, tired	2.1 ± 0.89	52.5
18	hot face	2.0 ± 0.92	50
10	heartbeat	2.0 ± 0.71	50
2	afraid no reason	1.9 ± 0.80	47.5
20	nightmares	1.9 ± 0.72	47.5
4	falling apart	1.9 ± 0.64	47.5
15	stomach ache	1.8 ± 0.82	45
14	paresthesia	1.8 ± 0.81	45
11	dizzy spells	1.6 ± 0.95	40
6	shake, tremble	1.4 ± 0.78	35
12	fainting spells	1.4 ± 0.63	35
1–20	overall	42.2 ± 4.7	52.7

Similarly, in item 19 of sleep disorder ("I fall asleep easily and get a good night's rest"), the mean was 2.6 ± 0.10. Likewise, for items of anxiety, panic, negative expectations of the future, or somatic signals of anxiety, i.e., item 1, "I feel more nervous and anxious than usual" (mean 2.5 ± 0.68); item 3, "I get upset easily or feel panicky" (mean 2.4 ± 0.78); item 5, "I feel that everything is all right and nothing bad will happen" (mean 2.3 ± 0.79); and item 17 "My hands are usually dry and warm" (mean 2.4 ± 1.0).

On the contrary, the lowest score items referred to somatic disorders, such as item 12, "I have fainting spells or feel like it" (mean 1.4 ± 0.63), where 96% of participants had chosen the lowest scores ("none or a little of the time" coded as 1 or "some of the time" coded as 2), or item 6 "My arms and legs shake and tremble" (mean 1.4 ± 0.78), where participants tended to choose the lowest scores (1 or 2).

Table 2 displays mean values, standard deviations, and the percentage scores in the EAQ and in its individual subscales, in descending order. "Attending to others' emotions", "analyses of own emotions", and "differentiating emotions" were the subscales with the highest scores, indicating high specific emotional abilities. In these subscales, the average agreement score was between two and three, showing that most participants tended to choose between "sometimes true" coded as 2 and "often true", coded as 3.

Table 2. Emotion Awareness Questionnaire (EAQ) and its 5 subscales: means, standard deviations, and percentages listed in descending order.

EAQ Subscale	Mean ± SD	Percentage
4. Attending to others' emotions	13.8 ± 1.9	92.1
5. Analyses of one's own emotions	13.1 ± 2.2	87.3
1. Differentiating emotions	15.2 ± 3.5	72.3
3. Not hiding emotions	8.2 ± 2.1	68.2
2. Verbal sharing of emotions	7.9 ± 2.5	65.7
EAQ total score	58.2 ± 8.2	77.6

Conversely, "verbal sharing of emotions" and "not hiding emotions" subscales reached the lowest scores, indicating a low specific emotional ability. In both scales, the average agreement score was below 2, showing that most participants tended to choose between "not true" coded as 1, or "sometimes true" coded as 2. For example, item 6 of the verbal sharing of emotions subscale: "when I am upset about something, I often keep it to myself" (mean 1.70 ± 0.68); or item 15 of the not hiding emotions' subscale: "when I am upset, I try not to show it" (mean 1.78 ± 0.71).

Furthermore, both SAS and the EAQ scores were examined in relation to sex. Female anxiety total scale scores appeared significantly higher than those of males (43.5 ± 4.6 vs. 39.3 ± 3.7; $t_{146} = 3.06$; $p = 0.003$), but not EAQ scores (57.9 ± 10.4 vs. 58.3 ± 8.3; $t_{146} = 0.15$, $p = 0.88$).

SAS total score and EAQ total score did not correlate and the Pearson correlation index was very close to zero ($r = -0.09$, $p = 0.28$). Correlations between SAS total scores and individual EAQ subscales were similarly low.

4. Discussion

The current study aimed to investigate the state of anxiety and emotional awareness in a sample of healthy older adolescents. It was hypothesized that, because of the effects of the COVID-19 pandemic, the sample would have shown a high level of anxiety. The age group around 18 was chosen to minimize any high anxiety levels or low emotional awareness due to the emotional and affective instability in young adolescence [25–27]. The questionnaires SAS and EAQ were chosen because they did not reference the pandemic.

In the current study, over half of the SAS individual items reached a high anxiety score and, consequently, the SAS total score reached an unusually high anxiety score (SAS index 52.7).

Previous studies, during non-COVID times, found lower total SAS scores, both in large non-clinical samples of college students, in control subjects, and even in several groups of psychiatric patients [20,21,24,28]. For example, normal subjects of Zung's study ($n = 100$) had a mean SAS index significantly lower than all five groups of patients examined (33.8 ± 5.9), while the patient sample

(n = 225) reached mean indices ranging from 45.8 to 58.7. Patients with anxiety disorders showed a mean SAS index significantly higher than those of the other four diagnostic groups (58.7 ± 13.5) [20].

Similarly, in studies comparing normal controls, psychiatric patients, and subjects with anxiety disorders found in healthy groups, SAS indices ranged between 40 and 43 [21,24,28].

Moreover, the Zung rating scale measures state anxiety as a transient expression of a temporary emotional condition, relative to the current period (within the previous week). The state anxiety construct refers to a momentary interruption of an emotional positive continuum expressed in a subjective feeling of tension, worry, restlessness, nervousness, and reactivity, also through the activation of the autonomic nervous system and several physiological activations [29,30]. Conversely, the trait anxiety construct expresses a stable modality of emotional functioning dominated by anxiety, which favors a constant perception of danger and threat, even behind neutral events, or with low anxiety values. Therefore, since the sample was a healthy, non-clinical one, and the SAS measured state and non-trait anxiety, the unusually high anxiety scores observed would not appear to be attributed to the sample's stable emotional functioning, but it is likely due to a temporary condition or feeling of tension and apprehension that favors a leavening of anxious responses.

Analyzing the single items, in the same previous studies, the item of breathing difficulties reached average scores lower than 2, both in normal subjects and in psychiatric patients [21,24,28]. Meanwhile, a study on patients with anxiety disorders [28] documented a score of 3.31 ± 0.99, very close to the score of the current studied adolescents (3.4 ± 0.81). It is interesting to point out that it is widely shared (among public opinion) that breath is a very easy vehicle for virus transmission, and coronavirus mainly affects respiratory functions, while breathing difficulties are among the first manifestations of viral activity in the human body. It is very understandable, therefore, that a high percentage of sample complaints concern not being able to "breathe in and out easily". Moreover, breathing rhythms change in accordance to emotional stress. Anxiety, stress, or panic increase the respiratory rate and the amount of air in the lungs resulting in the feeling of shortness of breath. Chronic respiratory diseases in pediatric age appeared as a significant source of stress, also, for mothers, impacting their personality traits and memory performances [31].

Likewise, items referring to sleep disorder, anxiety, panic, and a negative expectation of the future reached high average scores. Sleep is one of the great anxiety-sensitive functions. Just as the catastrophic expectations of the future, restlessness, and feeling nervous, are symptomatic expressions of anxiety through the motor and neurovegetative pathways.

Coronavirus not only brings death in the short-term, but it also destabilizes behavior patterns in the long-term. The risk and fear of contagion have modified production models, employment policies, social and interpersonal relationships, leisure habits, education, and training systems and every consolidated behavioral repertoire—this is especially so for younger people. Therefore, the overall future becomes nebulous, confused, uncertain, and distressing. An anxious phenomenology develops, affecting anxiety and the ideo-affective dimension, while the somatic symptomatology, such as fainting, tremors, dizziness, and paresthesia, appears to be less severe.

Conversely, on the EAQ, the total emotional awareness score reached quite high levels compared to the maximum score, showing valid emotional abilities in the sample. On the qualitative view, "Attending to others' emotions" and "Analyses of one's own emotions" were the two subscales with the highest scores. The participants considered it important to know, analyze, understand, and care for the emotions of others, as well as their own, both in normal and problematic conditions (i.e., "if a friend is upset"). Contrarily, they self-rated as less willing to verbally share their own emotions with others, and they showed difficulty explaining emotions, i.e., "to talk to anyone about how I feel", believing, for example, that "when I am feeling bad, it is no one else's business". On the one hand, therefore, there was openness and willingness to evaluate and understand the emotions of others and one's own, on the other, less willingness to share one's emotions with others.

In the correlational analysis, anxiety and emotional awareness overall scores appeared as two unrelated variables. Therefore, anxiety observed in the study did not seem associated with emotional awareness and management. Namely, it further confirmed the nature of state anxiety, which occurs temporarily in a particular historical condition, and the hypothesis that the epidemic promotes an increase in anxiety, even in adolescents with good awareness of their own (and others') emotions. These findings supported the hypothesis that the COVID-19 pandemic and its following restrictive measures may be a risk condition for an increased state anxiety level in older adolescents. Widespread anxiety and fear, prolonged isolation in a restricted domestic environment, forced removal from school friends and relatives, the fear of being infected, confused or contradictory information, and the uncertainties of personal and family future likely supported an increase in anxious responses.

Therefore, the group of participants examined, despite showing a good level of emotional awareness at the EAQ, achieved quite high levels of state anxiety in the SAS, which cannot be seen as a stable emotional mode of functioning, but should be associated with the particular anxiety-inducing events during the time of COVID-19. Such data are consistent with similar (recent) studies involving college students in China, indicating that the students were troubled by anxiety concerning COVID-19, for the consequences on their studies [32], future employment [33], and in their interpersonal relationships [34,35].

According to the learned helplessness stress model [36], the COVID-19 pandemic and its following restrictive measures may be viewed as uncontrollable, leading to unpredictable helplessness conditions. Moreover, in line with the cumulative stress hypothesis [37], stressors, such as the physical and psychological problems related to the pandemic and the lockdown, may activate an excessive production of glucocorticoids and a deregulation of cortisol release, increasing, over time, the individual's vulnerability to stress-related pathologies [38,39]. Given its high density of glucocorticoid receptors, the hippocampus appears as a structure particularly involved in stress responses, and in cumulative exposure to high levels of cortisol [40] that could have lasting effects on memory and cognitive processes [39,41–43].

Examining both the EAQ and SAS in relation to sex, female anxiety scale scores appeared significantly higher than those of males, whereas no significant differences were found concerning emotion awareness. It is likely that females feel the distress of the moment with greater anxiety, even though they manifest emotional awareness skills similar to that of boys. This finding was inconsistent with Cao and colleagues [1]—that male and female students in a sample of university students in China experienced similar stresses and negative emotions due to the epidemic.

Concerning psychological community implications, data suggest the need to develop intervention programs focused on the emotional and affective reactions of older adolescents [6,10]. As the pandemic is inevitable, unpredictable, and uncontrollable [44], and as the restrictive measures are the only way to contain the spread of the infection, the golden rule in addressing adolescent anxiety may be to provide 1) an effective, empathic, and reassuring communication system with the direct participation of adolescents, and 2) psychological counseling services for stress management.

In a recent editorial, in order to prevent "the disease of panic", *The Lancet* highlighted that the COVID-19 pandemic cannot be prevented; nevertheless, providing people with accurate information "is the most effective prevention against the disease of panic" [45]. Communication aimed at older adolescents should offer them the possibility of being properly and honestly informed, and of getting out of isolation by sharing with others their fears, anxieties, and irrational beliefs. Such a communication system should not be only factual, but focused on their problems, for example, the management of any physical symptoms potentially related to the infection, the real ways of transmitting the virus, the duration of the restrictive measures, the short-term effects of the pandemic on the school year, lifestyle, leisure activities, interpersonal relationships and the economic conditions of their families, the validity of fake news, and the long-term effects on their futures and their families [46].

Likewise, psychological counseling should provide online services to cope with mental health issues due to anxiety from the pandemic or from intrafamilial interpersonal relations. According to Petersen' suggestion, fear must be handled through "optimistic anxiety"—that is, being anxious enough "to take the advice of the authorities to heart" and optimistic enough to feel that one's actions make a difference [47].

Effective, empathic information, and psychological counseling monitored by experienced adults (directly involving adolescents) can mitigate the anxious reactions of adolescents, and may help them to handle uncertainty and fear contextualizing individual vulnerability.

In conclusion, it is important to underline a limitation of the presented study concerning the sample size. Unfortunately, the unusual condition of forced distancing led us to use a remote data collection method, and to dedicate a large part of the work to build the online task. This has limited us in recruiting a larger sample. The data are descriptive given the sample size, and they must be contextualized to a very specific period and to a unique condition; therefore, they cannot be generalized.

Author Contributions: P.S. and G.L. conceived and designed the experiment; P.S. performed the experiment; P.S. and D.S. analyzed the data; P.S. and G.L. analyzed and supervised the methodology and the form of writing; P.S. and D.S. wrote and revised the manuscript; G.L. acquired the founds; D.S. edited revised versions of the manuscript; P.S., G.L. and D.S. revised and approved the final version of the paper. All authors have read and agreed to the published version of the manuscript.

Funding: This research received no external funding.

Acknowledgments: The authors thank Cristina Leone for her valuable contribution in data collection.

Conflicts of Interest: The authors declare that the research was conducted in the absence of any commercial or financial relationships that could be construed as a potential conflict of interest and in compliance with ethical standards.

References

1. Cao, W.; Fang, Z.; Hou, G.; Han, M.; Xu, X.; Dong, J.; Zheng, J. The psychological impact of the COVID-19 epidemic on college students in China. *Psychiatry Res.* **2020**, *287*, 112934. [CrossRef] [PubMed]
2. Chen, Q.; Liang, M.; Li, Y.; Guo, J.; Fei, D.; Wang, L.; He, L.; Sheng, C.; Cai, Y.; Li, X.; et al. Mental health care for medical staff in China during the COVID-19 outbreak. *Lancet Psychiatry* **2020**, *7*, e15–e16. [CrossRef]
3. Duan, L.; Zhu, G. Psychological interventions for people affected by the COVID-19 epidemic. *Lancet Psychiatry* **2020**, *7*, 300–302. [CrossRef]
4. Yang, Y.; Li, W.; Zhang, Q.; Zhang, L.; Cheung, T.; Xiang, Y.-T. Mental health services for older adults in China during the COVID-19 outbreak. *Lancet Psychiatry* **2020**, *7*, e19. [CrossRef]
5. Li, S.W.; Wang, Y.; Yang, Y.Y.; Lei, X.M.; Yang, Y.F. Analysis of influencing factors of anxiety and emotional disorders in children and adolescents during home isolation during the epidemic of novel coronavirus pneumonia. *Chin. J. Child Health* **2020**, *28*, 1–9.
6. Golberstein, E.; Wen, H.; Miller, B.F. Coronavirus Disease 2019 (COVID-19) and Mental Health for Children and Adolescents. *JAMA Pediatr.* **2020**. [CrossRef]
7. Golberstein, E.; Gonzales, G.; Meara, E. How do economic downturns affect the mental health of children? *Evidence from the National Health Interview Survey. Health Econ.* **2019**, *28*, 955–970.
8. Brooke, J.; Jackson, D. Older people and COVID-19: Isolation, risk and ageism. *J. Clin. Nurs.* **2020**, *29*, 2044–2046. [CrossRef]
9. Smirni, D.; Smirni, P.; Di Martino, G.; Operto, F.F.; Carotenuto, M. Emotional Awareness and Cognitive Performance in Borderline Intellectual Functioning Young Adolescents. *J. Nerv. Ment. Dis.* **2019**, *207*, 365–370.
10. Jiao, W.Y.; Wang, L.N.; Liu, J.; Fang, S.F.; Jiao, F.Y.; Pettoello-Mantovani, M.; Somekh, E. Behavioral and emotional disorders in children during the COVID-19 epidemic. *J. Pediatr.* **2020**, *221*, 264. [CrossRef]
11. Ali, M.M.; West, K.; Teich, J.L.; Lynch, S.; Mutter, R.; Dubenitz, J. Utilization of mental health services in educational setting by adolescents in the United States. *J. Sch. Health* **2019**, *89*, 393–401. [CrossRef] [PubMed]
12. Holmes, E.A.; O'Connor, R.C.; Perry, V.H.; Tracey, I.; Wessely, S.; Arseneault, L.; Ballard, C.; Christensen, H.; Silver, R.C.; Everall, I. Multidisciplinary research priorities for the COVID-19 pandemic: A call for action for mental health science. *Lancet Psychiatry* **2020**, *7*, 547–560. [CrossRef]
13. Collishaw, S. Annual research review: Secular trends in child and adolescent mental health. *J. Child Psychol. Psychiatry* **2015**, *56*, 370–393. [CrossRef] [PubMed]

14. Fazel, M.; Hoagwood, K.; Stephan, S.; Ford, T. Mental health interventions in schools in high-income countries. *Lancet Psychiatry* **2014**, *1*, 377–387. [CrossRef]
15. Schoneveld, E.A.; Lichtwarck-Aschoff, A.; Granic, I. Preventing childhood anxiety disorders: Is an applied game as effective as a cognitive behavioral therapy-based program? *Prev. Sci.* **2018**, *19*, 220–232. [CrossRef]
16. Restubog, S.L.D.; Ocampo, A.C.G.; Wang, L. Taking control amidst the chaos: Emotion regulation during the COVID-19 pandemic. *J. Vocat. Behav.* **2020**, *119*, 103440. [CrossRef]
17. Bults, M.; Beaujean, D.J.M.A.; de Zwart, O.; Kok, G.; van Empelen, P.; van Steenbergen, J.E.; Richardus, J.H.; Voeten, H.A.C.M. Perceived risk, anxiety, and behavioural responses of the general public during the early phase of the Influenza A (H1N1) pandemic in the Netherlands: Results of three consecutive online surveys. *BMC Public Health* **2011**, *11*, 2. [CrossRef]
18. Maunder, R.; Hunter, J.; Vincent, L.; Bennett, J.; Peladeau, N.; Leszcz, M.; Sadavoy, J.; Verhaeghe, L.M.; Steinberg, R.; Mazzulli, T. The immediate psychological and occupational impact of the 2003 SARS outbreak in a teaching hospital. *Cmaj* **2003**, *168*, 1245–1251.
19. Shultz, J.M.; Cooper, J.L.; Baingana, F.; Oquendo, M.A.; Espinel, Z.; Althouse, B.M.; Marcelin, L.H.; Towers, S.; Espinola, M.; McCoy, C.B. The role of fear-related behaviors in the 2013–2016 West Africa Ebola virus disease outbreak. *Curr. Psychiatry Rep.* **2016**, *18*, 104. [CrossRef]
20. Zung, W.W. A Rating Instrument For Anxiety Disorders. *Psychosomatics* **1971**, *12*, 371–379. [CrossRef]
21. Olatunji, B.O.; Deacon, B.J.; Abramowitz, J.S.; Tolin, D.F. Dimensionality of somatic complaints: Factor structure and psychometric properties of the Self-Rating Anxiety Scale. *J. Anxiety Disord.* **2006**, *20*, 543–561. [PubMed]
22. Rieffe, C.; Oosterveld, P.; Miers, A.C.; Terwogt, M.M.; Ly, V. Emotion awareness and internalising symptoms in children and adolescents: The Emotion Awareness Questionnaire revised. *Pers. Individ. Dif.* **2008**, *45*, 756–761.
23. Camodeca, M.; Rieffe, C. Validation of the Italian Emotion Awareness Questionnaire for children and adolescents. *Eur. J. Dev. Psychol.* **2013**, *10*, 402–409.
24. Jegede, R.O. Psychometric attributes of the self-rating anxiety scale. *Psychol. Rep.* **1977**, *40*, 303–306.
25. Giedd, J.N. The teen brain: Insights from neuroimaging. *J. Adolesc. Health* **2008**, *42*, 335–343.
26. Lenroot, R.K.; Giedd, J.N. Brain development in children and adolescents: Insights from anatomical magnetic resonance imaging. *Neurosci. Biobehav. Rev.* **2006**, *30*, 718–729.
27. Spear, L.P. The adolescent brain and age-related behavioral manifestations. *Neurosci. Biobehav. Rev.* **2000**, *24*, 417–463.
28. Lee, J.H. Development of the Korean Form of Zung's Self-Rating Anxiety Scale. *Yeungnam Univ. J. Med.* **1996**, *13*, 279–294.
29. Cattell, R.B.; Scheier, I.H. *The Meaning and Measurement of Neuroticism and Anxiety*; Ronald Press Co.: New York, NY, USA, 1961.
30. Spielberger, C.D.; Gorsuch, R.L.; Lushene, R.E. *State-Trait Anxiety Inventory Manual*; Mind Garden, Inc.: Menlo Park, CA, USA, 1970.
31. Smirni, D.; Carotenuto, M.; Precenzano, F.; Smirni, P.; Operto, F.F.; Marotta, R.; Roccella, M. Memory performances and personality traits in mothers of children with obstructive sleep apnea syndrome. *Psychol. Res. Behav. Manag.* **2019**, *12*, 481–487.
32. Cornine, A. Reducing nursing student anxiety in the clinical setting: An integrative review. *Nurs. Educ. Perspect.* **2020**, *41*, 229–234.
33. Wang, C.; Horby, P.W.; Hayden, F.G.; Gao, G.F. A novel coronavirus outbreak of global health concern. *Lancet* **2020**, *395*, 470–473. [CrossRef]
34. Xiao, C. A novel approach of consultation on 2019 novel coronavirus (COVID-19)-related psychological and mental problems: Structured letter therapy. *Psychiatry Investig.* **2020**, *17*, 175. [CrossRef] [PubMed]
35. Kmietowicz, Z. Covid-19: Highest risk patients are asked to stay at home for 12 weeks. *BMJ* **2020**, *368*, m1170. [CrossRef] [PubMed]
36. Abramson, L.Y.; Seligman, M.E.; Teasdale, J.D. Learned helplessness in humans: Critique and reformulation. *J. Abnorm. Psychol.* **1978**, *87*, 49. [CrossRef]
37. Nederhof, E.; Schmidt, M. V Mismatch or cumulative stress: Toward an integrated hypothesis of programming effects. *Physiol. Behav.* **2012**, *106*, 691–700. [CrossRef]

38. McEwen, B.S. Physiology and neurobiology of stress and adaptation: Central role of the brain. *Physiol. Rev.* **2007**, *87*, 873–904. [CrossRef]
39. Forns, J.; Vegas, O.; Julvez, J.; Garcia-Esteban, R.; Rivera, M.; Lertxundi, N.; Guxens, M.; Fano, E.; Ferrer, M.; Grellier, J. Association between child cortisol levels in saliva and neuropsychological development during the second year of life. *Stress Health* **2014**, *30*, 142–148. [CrossRef]
40. Fuchs, E.; Flügge, G. Chronic social stress: Effects on limbic brain structures. *Physiol. Behav.* **2003**, *79*, 417–427. [CrossRef]
41. Pruessner, J.C.; Baldwin, M.W.; Dedovic, K.; Renwick, R.; Mahani, N.K.; Lord, C.; Meaney, M.; Lupien, S. Self-esteem, locus of control, hippocampal volume, and cortisol regulation in young and old adulthood. *Neuroimage* **2005**, *28*, 815–826. [CrossRef]
42. Lupien, S.J.; Fiocco, A.; Wan, N.; Maheu, F.; Lord, C.; Schramek, T.; Tu, M.T. Stress hormones and human memory function across the lifespan. *Psychoneuroendocrinology* **2005**, *30*, 225–242. [CrossRef]
43. Smirni, D.; Smirni, P.; Di Martino, G.; Cipolotti, L.; Oliveri, M.; Turriziani, P. Standardization and validation of a parallel form of the verbal and non-verbal recognition memory test in an Italian population sample. *Neurol. Sci.* **2018**, *39*, 1391–1399. [CrossRef] [PubMed]
44. Sprang, G.; Silman, M. Posttraumatic stress disorder in parents and youth after health-related disasters. *Disaster Med. Public Health Prep.* **2013**, *7*, 105–110. [CrossRef] [PubMed]
45. The Lancet COVID-19: Fighting panic with information. *Lancet* **2020**, *395*, 537. [CrossRef]
46. Lunn, P.D.; Belton, C.A.; Lavin, C.; McGowan, F.P.; Timmons, S.; Robertson, D.A. Using Behavioral Science to help fight the Coronavirus. *J. Behav. Public Adm.* **2020**, *3*, 15. [CrossRef]
47. Finset, A.; Bosworth, H.; Butow, P.; Gulbrandsen, P.; Hulsman, R.L.; Pieterse, A.H.; Street, R.; Tschoetschel, R.; van Weert, J. Effective health communication—A key factor in fighting the COVID-19 pandemic. *Patient Educ. Couns.* **2020**, *103*, 873. [CrossRef] [PubMed]

Journal of
Clinical Medicine

MDPI

Article

Risk Perception of COVID-19, Meaning-Based Resources and Psychological Well-Being amongst Healthcare Personnel: The Mediating Role of Coping

Dariusz Krok [1] and Beata Zarzycka [2,*]

1 Institute of Psychology, University of Opole, 45-040 Opole, Poland; dkrok@uni.opole.pl
2 Institute of Psychology, John Paul II Catholic University of Lublin, 20-950 Lublin, Poland
* Correspondence: zarzycka@kul.lublin.pl; Tel.: +48-81-4453444

Received: 26 August 2020; Accepted: 5 October 2020; Published: 8 October 2020

Abstract: The well-being of healthcare personnel during the COVID-19 pandemic depends on the ways in which they perceive the threat posed by the virus, personal resources, and coping abilities. The current study aims to examine the mediating role of coping strategies in the relationship between risk perception of COVID-19 and psychological well-being, as well as the relationship between meaning-based resources and psychological well-being amongst healthcare personnel in southern Poland. Two hundred and twenty-six healthcare personnel who worked in hospitals, outpatient clinics, and medical laboratories during the first few months of the coronavirus pandemic (March–May 2020) filled in questionnaires measuring risk perception of COVID-19, meaning-based resources, coping, and psychological well-being. The results demonstrate that risk perception was negatively related to psychological well-being, whereas meaning-based resources were positively associated with well-being. Two coping strategies—problem-focused and meaning-focused coping—mediated the relationship between risk perception and psychological well-being as well as the relationship between meaning-based resources and psychological well-being. This indicates that perception processes and personal factors do not directly influence healthcare personnel's psychological well-being, but rather they do indirectly through coping processes.

Keywords: risk perception of COVID-19; meaning-based resources; psychological well-being; healthcare personnel

1. Introduction

The highly infectious coronavirus SARS-CoV-2 caused an epidemic of acute respiratory syndrome (COVID-19). Between January and April 2020, the epidemic turned into a global pandemic, having spread to most countries around the world [1]. In March 2020, the World Health Organization made the assessment that COVID-19 was as a pandemic. In Poland, the COVID-19 pandemic began on 4 March 2020, and on 5 October 2020 the number of people infected with SARS-CoV-2 had risen to 102,080; of those, 2659 died. The outbreak of the coronavirus disease caused intense stress amongst the public in Poland, and healthcare personnel were one of the most affected groups. Since the outbreak, healthcare personnel have found themselves on the frontline in combating COVID-19, working with an increased workload in terms of working hours and patient numbers and facing the highest risk of infection. Thus, operating under such conditions may have contributed to increased psychological stress, with immediate and perhaps long-term psychological consequences [2].

There have as yet been few studies on the psychological effects of working in a healthcare setting around COVID-19. Research conducted in China showed that after the COVID-19 outbreak, medical staff experienced emotional stress, depression, insomnia, and anxiety [2–4]. Nurses and frontline healthcare workers reported more severe degrees of all measurements of mental health symptoms than other healthcare personnel [3]. Although the psychological effects of outbreaks of COVID-19 disease on healthcare personnel have been demonstrated [2–4], little is known about the combined roles of risk perception and individual resources for well-being, and the mediating effects of coping on their relationships. These factors have also not been studied together in healthcare workers. Thus, it is important that these relationships are examined, because the findings may shed more light on specific factors that contribute significantly to the creation of new intervention programs (e.g., meaning-based approaches that address existential distress and psychological well-being). Healthcare personnel need to protect the well-being of themselves and their colleagues to avoid adverse outcomes for both healthcare workers and patients.

1.1. Risk Perception, Meaning-Based Resources, and Psychological Well-Being

Appraisal-based and resource-based stress theories have been successfully employed in predicting a range of stress outcomes in health contexts [5,6]. Appraisal-based theories, which include the protection motivation theory (PMT), describe how people assess a threat's probability [7], whereas resource-based theories, amongst which the conservation of resources (COR) theory is one of the most prominent, indicate that personal resources enable people to cope effectively with the threat [8].

Protection motivation theory has been successfully applied in the context of health threats to explain the effects of fear on people's reactions and attitudes [7]. It emphasizes the importance of risk perception, which consists of three components: (1) perceived risk of contracting, which is the person's expectation of being exposed to the threat, such as being infected by COVID-19; (2) fear, which plays an indirect role in threat appraisal by affecting the estimation of the danger's severity; and (3) perceived threat, which is the person's estimation of how harmful the consequences of the threat would be to objects they value if the threat were to actually occur (e.g., the judgment that a COVID-19 infection would harm valued things, such as personal health or the health of other people) [9]. Previous studies indicated that perceived risk was negatively related to well-being during the outbreak of severe acute respiratory syndrome (SARS). Research conducted on SARS survivors demonstrated that their subjective interpretation of the infection was related to the level of psychological adjustment measured in terms of emotional distress and perceived health [10]. The few studies carried out so far during the outbreak of COVID-19 amongst the Chinese public revealed that perceived threat was related to a number of undesirable emotional reactions (e.g., an increase in negative emotion) [3] and that self-control moderates the association between perceived threat and mental health problems amongst the Chinese public [11]. Both studies led to the conclusion that the perceived threat of COVID-19 may negatively influence mental health outcomes.

Conservation of resources theory begins with the tenet that individuals strive to obtain, retain, foster, and protect personal resources, defined as "those entities that either are centrally valued in their own right, or act as means to obtain centrally valued ends" [8] (p. 307). The fit of personal resources with external demands determines the direction of stress response and resultant outcomes [5]. Research has demonstrated that resources influence people's abilities to impact their environments successfully, and thus they are typically linked to well-being, positive coping, and global resistance to stress [12]. The studies examining relationships between resources and well-being involve a number of distinctive types of resource [8], among which meaning based resources, e.g., meaning in life (MIL) and existential mattering, are widely studied.

Meaning in life (MIL) has been regarded as a key resource for both coping processes and psychological well-being [13,14]. Meaning in life has been defined as "the extent to which one's life is experienced as making sense, as being directed and motivated by valued goals, and as mattering in the world" [15] (p. 205). Considering the predictive role of MIL on people's psychological health [16–18], examining MIL levels amongst healthcare staff is relevant for many reasons. Meaning in life in healthcare settings plays a vital role in the construction of the individual's identity, and it can provide one of the main sources of inner harmony [19]. In addition, MIL can noticeably influence the ways in which healthcare workers deal with stress and maintain their professional efficiency [20]. Given that the pandemic is considered a prolonged stressful condition, particularly for those who are in the front line in the fight against the virus, the availability of meaning-based resources would help to manage such stress successfully.

Another factor related to meaning-based resources is existential mattering, which has received a considerable deal of empirical attention in recent years [21,22]. This may be described as one's experiences of value, worth, and transcending everyday life conditions, and is regarded as a core dimension of meaning structures in addition to more commonly accepted significance and purpose [23]. Research has demonstrated that mattering is beneficial to developing self-identity, self-concept, sense of belonging, and understanding one's purpose in life [21]. By developing a sense of mattering in their lives, individuals can gain an awareness of being able to make a difference in the world and to lead a valuable life. Mattering was also found to play a crucial role in psychological well-being and health amongst college and university students [24].

The inclusion of meaning-based resources noticeably influenced psychological models of stress and coping due to the internal structures of purpose and value embedded in the resources. They tend to affect the ways in which important events are perceived as well as how these events are managed [20,25]. Being related to different measures of well-being, they are also likely to affect one's coping responses to stressful events (e.g., public health threats or unpredictable infections).

1.2. Coping Strategies as Mediators

Coping is defined as an effort to manage demands that are appraised as exceeding the resources of the person [26]. Two classes of coping are commonly identified: problem-focused and emotion-focused. The former involves efforts to obtain information about what to do as well as how to alter the stressful situation (e.g., information seeking, planning, or taking action). The latter involves efforts to regulate the emotional distress associated with the situation (e.g., seeking emotional support from others or by behavioral disengagement) [27]. More recently, meaning-focused coping—involving changing the appraised meaning of a situation to make it more consistent with individuals' beliefs and goals—was posited [28,29]. Research demonstrated that the three coping strategies often work in tandem; the regulation of anxiety and fear (emotion-focused coping) enables the person to focus on taking a decision (problem-focused coping), or the cognitive restructuring (problem-focused coping) can be guided by underlying values and goals (meaning-focused coping) [29,30]. In addition, different coping strategies appear to be beneficial depending on the particular situation and context, e.g., problem-focused coping was found to be predominantly helpful in high controllability situations, while emotion-focused coping was more effective under low controllability conditions [31].

Previous studies confirmed that coping played a mediating role in relationships between various forms of risk perception and well-being measures. Coping was found to mediate the relationship of ecological risk with depressive symptoms for African Americans [32]. Avoidant coping was a mediator in associations between a form of risk rejection (i.e., evaluative concerns about perfectionism) and distress [33]. In addition, risk perception tended to influence coping strategies in people who had experienced either natural or industrial catastrophe [34]. Environmental risk perception was also confirmed as a predictor of coping behaviors [35].

Coping played an important role in relationships between personal resources and well-being. Coping self-efficacy mediated the associations between self-esteem and optimism and distress experienced in the aftermath of the 1999 earthquake in Turkey [36]. Coping focused on change mediated the relationship between personal resources conceptualized as psychological capital and well-being [37]. Meaning in life was also reported to influence coping behavior after disaster [20] and to be a predictor of the appropriate use of coping and stress management resources at work [19].

These results taken together imply that individuals may use coping in relation to their appraisals of stressful events and personal resources, which will subsequently influence well-being measures [37,38]. There can be also differential predictions for the different strategies as risk perception and personal resources are differently related to the coping strategies. However thus far, no studies have examined the mediating role of coping between risk perception and psychological well-being as well as between meaning-based resources and psychological well-being in the context of the COVID-19 pandemic. A German sample showed that the risk perception of being infected by COVID-19 was higher in women than men and higher in older people than younger people, in conjunction with a more frequent use of problem-focused strategies. The relationship between COVID-19 risk perception and coping strategies was not analyzed [39].

1.3. The Present Study

The present study aims to elucidate the mediating contribution of coping strategies in the association between risk perception of COVID-19 and psychological well-being as well as the association between meaning-based resources and psychological well-being amongst healthcare personnel. Based on the research presented above, three hypotheses were formulated. First, we hypothesized that risk perception of COVID-19 will be negatively and directly associated with psychological well-being, while meaning-based resources will be positively and directly associated with the psychological well-being of healthcare personnel on the frontline in combating COVID-19 (Hypothesis 1). Second, given that the relationship between the individual's appraisal of stressful events and psychological outcomes depends on the way they cope with challenging situations [20,40], we hypothesized that coping strategies will mediate relationships between risk perception of COVID-19 and psychological well-being (Hypothesis 2). Third, given that personal resources play an important role in shaping coping behavior, which consequently determines psychological adjustment [37,38], we hypothesized that coping strategies would mediate the meaning-based resources and psychological well-being link (Hypothesis 3). Table 1 shows the summary of key constructs included in the study.

Table 1. Summary and definitions of the key constructs included in the study.

Construct	Definitions
	Risk perception of COVID-19 (Predictor)
Risk of contracting	Perceived probability of being infected by COVID-19.
Fear	Fear of COVID-19.
Perceived threat	Perceived harmfulness of the consequences of being infected by COVID-19.
	Meaning-based resources (Predictor)
Meaning in life	The extent to which one's life is experienced as making sense, directed and motivated by valued goals.
Mattering	One's experiences of value, worth, and transcending everyday life conditions.
	Coping strategies (Mediators)
Problem focused	Efforts to obtain information about what to do and how to alter the stressful situation.
Emotion focused	Efforts to regulate the emotional distress associated with the situation.
Meaning focused	Changing the appraised meaning of a situation to make it more consistent with individuals' beliefs and goals.
Psychological well-being (Outcome)	Positive psychological functioning and human development.

2. Experimental Section

2.1. Participants and Procedure

In order to generate a representative sample of healthcare workers, quota sampling was used. Quota sampling is a non-probabilistic sampling method in which the population of healthcare workers was divided in equally exclusive subgroups. First, we selected the subgroups of healthcare workers with regard to five criteria: gender, age, types of healthcare professions, years of service, and a level of education. Second, we identified the proportions of these subgroups and then selected subjects from the various subgroups on a basis of these proportions. The aim was to assemble a sample that would have the same proportions of individuals and be representative of the entire population of healthcare workers with respect to the abovementioned characteristics. The final sample consisted of 226 healthcare personnel working in hospitals, outpatient clinics, and medical laboratories in southern Poland during the first few months of the coronavirus pandemic (March–May 2020), and who were consequently exposed to the associated health risks. The group comprised the following professions: doctors ($n = 51$), nurses ($n = 113$), laboratory technicians ($n = 22$), aides and assistants ($n = 29$), and physiotherapists ($n = 11$). Of the participants, 58.8% were female and 41.2% were male. Their average age was 37.36 (SD = 13.59). All were employed either full-time or part-time.

Participants were recruited in hospitals, outpatient clinics, and medical laboratories, with the aim of acquiring a representative sample of healthcare personnel. They were provided with information regarding the purpose and rules of participation and were asked to fill in an online or printed version of the questionnaire. A research assistant was available in case any additional information was requested. The University Ethics Board accepted the research material and procedure.

2.2. Measures

The following scales and questionnaires were used in the study. The summary scores for the study variables were calculated by summing responses to each item.

2.2.1. Risk of Contracting COVID-19

Drawing on the conceptualization of risk perception proposed by Grothmann and Reusswig, who defined it as the extent to which an individual "assesses a threat's probability and damage potential" [9] (p. 104), the risk of contracting COVID-19 scale was developed [41]. The scale comprises 6 items rated from 1 (strongly disagree) to 5 (strongly agree). The sample items are: "Getting infected with coronavirus threatens my health" and "I am worried that I may become infected with coronavirus". A high score reflects a stronger perceived probability of contracting coronavirus. The Cronbach's α reliability for the sample was 0.85.

2.2.2. Fear of COVID-19

The level of fear experienced by individuals in the context of coronavirus was measured with 6 items on a scale ranging from 1 (strongly disagree) to 5 (strongly agree). They represent emotional reactions of anxiety and apprehension caused by the coronavirus pandemic [42]. The sample items are: "I am afraid of serious health complications caused by coronavirus" and "I fear an extended hospital stay in case of being infected by coronavirus". The Cronbach's α reliability for the sample was 0.84.

2.2.3. Perceived Threat of COVID-19

Perceptions of threat severity of coronavirus were evaluated with the perceived threat of COVID-19 scale [41], which includes 6 items rated from 1 (strongly disagree) to 5 (strongly agree). The scale measures perceived threat severity of coronavirus that pertains to the negative personal, societal, and economic consequences people associate with the coronavirus pandemic. The sample items include: "Coronavirus is a serious threat to people" and "The coronavirus pandemic has a damaging impact on the economic situation of our country". The Cronbach's α reliability for the sample was 0.81.

2.2.4. Meaning in Life

Meaning in life was measured with the meaning in life questionnaire [43], which consists of 10 items rated from 1 (strongly disagree) to 7 (strongly agree). The questionnaire includes two dimensions: presence of meaning in life and search for meaning in life. As the aim of our study focuses primarily on the present characteristics of meaning in life experienced by participants, we only used the presence subscale that assesses how much people perceive their lives as meaningful. The Cronbach's α reliability for the sample was 0.83.

2.2.5. Existential Mattering

Existential mattering, which is regarded as the strongest indicator of meaning judgments, was measured with 6 items on a scale ranging from 1 (strongly disagree) to 5 (strongly agree). They assessed existential meaning, which is understood to be the conviction that one's life is significant, important, and valuable in the world [15,23]. The sample items include: "I am sure my life matters" and "I see my life as existentially significant". The Cronbach's α reliability for the sample was 0.80.

2.2.6. Coping

Coping was measured with the coping questionnaire [44], a 37-item instrument that assesses three coping strategies: problem-focused coping, emotion-focused coping, and meaning-focused coping. Participants respond to items on a Likert scale ranging from 1 (not at all) to 5 (very much). The total score was calculated by summing responses to each item. The Cronbach's α reliability for the sample was 0.84 for problem-focused coping, 0.83 for emotion-focused coping, and 0.87 for meaning-focused coping.

2.2.7. Psychological Well-Being

Psychological well-being was measured with the psychological well-being Scale [45] adapted for Polish by Karas and Cieciuch [46]. The short version contains 18 items rated from 1 (strongly disagree) to 6 (strongly agree). The scale comprises six dimensions: self-acceptance, positive relations with others, purpose in life, environmental mastery, personal growth, and autonomy, the score of which gives the total result. Due to the statistical analysis employed in the present study, we only used the total score, which was calculated by summing responses to each item. The Cronbach's α reliability for the sample was 0.84.

2.3. Data Analysis

Pearson's correlations were calculated to examine the relationships among the variables. Then, structural equation modelling (SEM) was used to estimate the statistical models (Amos 21 SPSS, an IBM Company: Chicago, IL, USA) [47]. In accordance with the rules of SEM, we first validated the measurement model by confirmatory factor analyses (CFA) and then we tested the structural relationship between measured variables and latent constructs. The goodness of fit of the model was evaluated by applying different indices: χ^2 statistic, the standardized root-mean-square residual (SRMR), root-mean-square error of approximation (RMSEA), and three modification indices—goodness of fit index (GFI), Tucker Lewis index (TLI), and comparative fit index (CFI). We were removing non-significant parameters and non-significant paths of the original model one at a time in relation to the modification indices to improve the model fit (Table S1, Supplementary Material) [48]. In addition, the modifications were to improve the model fit as long as they were corroborated by the theory. Bootstrapping was used to estimate direct and indirect effects (samples = 5000; 95% bias-corrected confidence intervals; standardized coefficients were presented). This approach enabled us to examine the relationship between risk perception of COVID-19 and psychological well-being as well as the relationship between meaning-based resources and psychological well-being.

3. Results

3.1. Descriptive Statistics and Correlations Amongst Variables

First, the correlations among risk perception of the COVID-19, meaning-based resources, and psychological well-being were tested. They are presented in Table 2.

Table 2. Means, standard deviations, and correlations for risk perception of COVID-19, meaning-based resources, and psychological well-being.

	Variables	M	SD	1.	2.	3.	4.	5.	6.	7.	8.	9.
1.	Risk	4.19	0.63	-								
2.	Fear	3.69	0.87	0.74 ***	-							
3.	Threat	4.44	0.52	0.60 ***	0.57 ***	-						
4.	MIL	5.24	1.18	0.08	0.06	0.11	-					
5.	EM	4.64	0.71	0.02	0.11	0.06	0.39 ***	-				
6.	Problem	3.61	0.57	0.20 **	0.14 **	0.06	0.40 ***	0.49 ***	-			
7.	Emotion	3.40	0.65	0.29 ***	0.36 ***	0.23 ***	0.24 ***	0.37 ***	0.44 ***	-		
8.	Meaning	3.66	0.63	0.21 **	0.22 ***	0.17 ***	0.41 ***	0.62 ***	0.66 ***	0.62 ***	-	
9.	PWB	3.71	0.73	−0.18 **	−0.18 **	−0.16 *	0.51 ***	0.31 ***	0.42 ***	0.20 **	0.29 ***	-

* $p < 0.05$; ** $p < 0.01$; *** $p < 0.001$. Risk—risk of contracting COVID-19; fear—fear of COVID-19; threat—perceived threat of COVID-19; MIL—meaning in life; EM—existential mattering; problem—problem-focused coping; emotion—emotion-focused coping; meaning—meaning-focused coping; PWB—psychological well-being.

Risk of contracting COVID-19 and fear of COVID-19 were positively related to problem-focused coping, emotion-focused coping and meaning-focused coping, and negatively related to psychological well-being. Perceived threat of COVID-19 positively correlated with emotion-focused coping and meaning-focused coping but was negatively associated with psychological well-being. Interestingly, there was no significant correlation between the factors forming risk perception of COVID-19 (risk of contracting, fear, and perceived threat) and meaning-based resources (meaning in life and existential mattering). In contrast, meaning in life and existential mattering were positively related to all coping strategies and psychological well-being. Problem-focused coping, emotion-focused coping, and meaning-focused coping were also positively connected to psychological well-being.

3.2. Direct and Indirect Effects of Risk Perception of COVID-19 and Meaning-Based Resources on Psychological Well-Being: Mediating Effects of Coping

The theoretical model constructed on the basis of previous findings assumed that the relationship of risk perception of COVID-19 and meaning-based resources with psychological well-being could be mediated by coping strategies. To verify these assumptions, structured equation modelling (SEM) analysis and a bootstrapping procedure were applied, as recommended by Preacher and Hayes [47].

3.2.1. Measurement Model

First, the measurement model, including loadings of indicators, was tested in relation to their corresponding latent variables by confirmatory factor analyses (CFA). Two latent factors were specified: (1) risk perception of COVID-19 that represents the individual's negatively-oriented attitude, encompassing risk of contracting, fear, and perceived threat, and (2) meaning-based resources that comprise meaning in life and existential mattering. The CFA results, including two latent factors and five observed variables, confirmed a very satisfactory fit to the data: χ^2 (n = 226) = 7.16, $p < 0.001$; GFI = 0.98; CFI = 0.98; NFI = 0.95; RMSEA = 0.04; SRMR = 0.02. The factor loadings obtained for the latent variables' indicators reached statistical significance ($p < 0.001$) (Table 3).

Table 3. Results of the confirmatory factor analysis: factor loadings (standardized values).

Latent Factors with Indicators	Estimate (Standardised)	SE	*p*
Risk perception of COVID-19			
1. Risk of contracting COVID-19	0.88	0.06	<0.001
2. Fear of COVID-19	0.85	0.06	<0.001
3. Perceived threat of COVID-19	0.71	0.05	<0.001
Meaning-based resources			
1. Meaning in life	0.82	0.06	<0.001
2. Mattering	0.70	0.05	<0.001

3.2.2. Structural Model

Drawing on earlier correlational results, the hypothesized mediation model including direct and indirect paths between two independent variables (risk perception of COVID-19 and meaning-based resources), three mediating variables (coping strategies), and the dependent variable (psychological well-being) was tested (Figure 1). Gender and age were also controlled in our structural analysis. In addition, each mediator was estimated independently, which generated more accurate mediating effects.

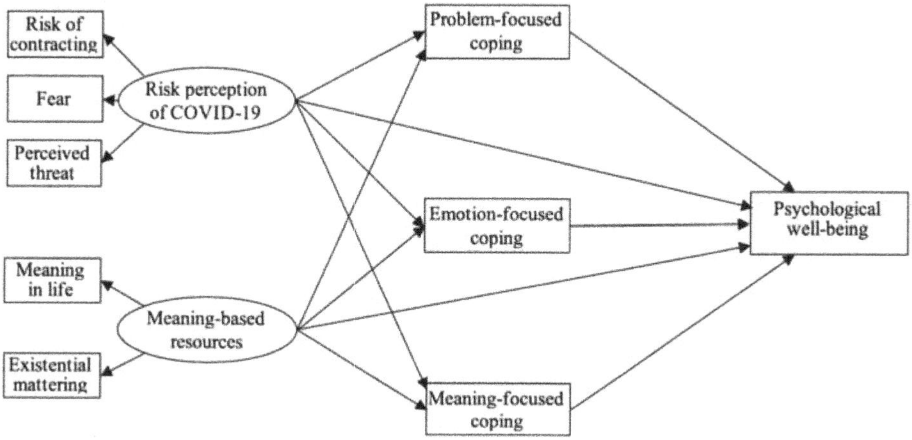

Figure 1. The theoretical model of the relations among risk perception of COVID-19, meaning-based resources, coping, and psychological well-being.

Structured equation modelling analysis revealed that model 1, which included three mediators and direct paths from risk perception of COVID-19 and meaning-based resources to psychological well-being had rather an unsatisfactory fit with the data: χ^2 (20, n = 226) = 59.84, $p < 0.001$; GFI = 0.88; CFI = 0.83; NFI = 0.78; RMSEA = 0.09. Furthermore, some path coefficients were nonsignificant.

The model was thus modified to improve fit in accordance with the modification procedures (the order in which variables and paths were removed is included in a supplement). Emotion-focused coping and nonsignificant paths from risk perception of COVID-19 and meaning-based resources to psychological well-being were deleted. As a consequence, the final model turned out to have significant improvements and a satisfactory fit: χ^2 (15, n = 226) = 38.36, $p < 0.001$; GFI = 0.95; CFI = 0.93; NFI = 0.92; RMSEA = 0.04 (model 2, Figure 2).

The final model contained one statistically significant direct effect ($\beta = -0.43$) from risk perception of COVID-19 to psychological well-being, which indicates that higher risk perception was related to a lower level of psychological well-being. In addition, problem-focused and meaning-focused coping accounted for indirect effects. Risk perception of COVID-19 had indirect relationships with psychological well-being through the two aforementioned coping strategies. The positive directions of those paths suggested that higher risk perception was related to more frequent use of problem- and meaning-focused coping, which again was related to a higher level of psychological well-being. Analogously, there was an indirect relationship between meaning-based resources and psychological well-being through significant positive paths comprising problem-focused coping and meaning-focused coping. More meaning-based resources were associated with more frequent use of problem- and meaning-focused coping, which was then associated with greater psychological well-being.

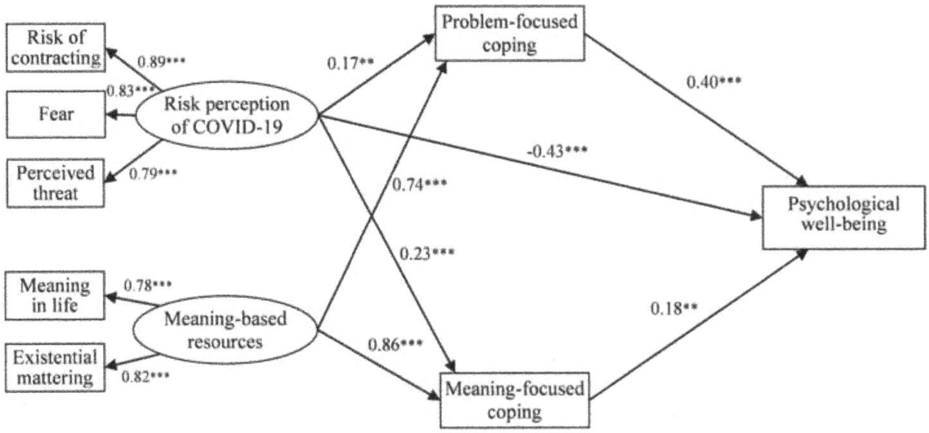

Figure 2. The final mediating model of the relations among risk perception of COVID-19, meaning-based resources, coping, and psychological well-being (standardized coefficients). ** $p < 0.01$; *** $p < 0.001$.

The bootstrapping procedure was applied to examine the mediating effects of problem- and meaning-focused coping on the association between risk perception of COVID-19 and psychological well-being as well as the association between meaning-based resources and psychological well-being (samples = 5000; 95% bias-corrected confidence intervals [47]) (Table 4).

Table 4. Standardized indirect and total effects, standard errors (SE), and 95% confidence intervals (CI).

Model Pathways	Effect	SE	95% CI	
			Lower	Upper
Indirect effects				
Risk perception of COVID-19 → Coping → PWB	0.11 a	0.04	0.04	0.19
Meaning-based resources → Coping → PWB	0.44 a	0.07	0.29	0.56
Total effects				
Risk perception of COVID-19 → PWB	0.31 a	0.07	−0.46	−0.17
Meaning-based resources → PWB	0.44 a	0.07	0.29	0.56

PWB—psychological well-being; a—empirical 95% confidence interval does not overlap with zero.

The results of mediation analysis revealed that problem- and meaning-focused coping mediated the relationship between risk perception of COVID-19 and psychological well-being as well as the relationship between meaning-based resources and psychological well-being. Interestingly, despite conceptual differences between risk perception and meaning-based resources, the mediating effects showed a similar pattern for both paths. Risk perception and meaning-based resources exerted significant indirect effects on the sphere of well-being via problem-focused and meaning-focused coping strategies. The total effects, which denote the sum of the direct and indirect effects, were significant for both paths, which implies therefore that problem-focused coping and meaning-focused coping function in the form of simultaneous mediators.

In addition, we decided to test whether those two indirect effects are significantly different (i.e., whether one or the other of the mediating effects is stronger). The result demonstrates that the mediation for the meaning-based resources–coping–psychological well-being path was significantly stronger than for the risk perception–coping–psychological well-being path (effect = 0.33; SE = 0.06; 95% CI = 0.05 to 0.41).

4. Discussion

The purpose of this study was to examine risk perception of COVID-19 infection and meaning-based resources in relation to coping strategies and psychological well-being amongst healthcare personnel in southern Poland during the COVID-19 outbreak between March and June 2020. We found that risk perception of COVID-19 infection—risk of contracting, fear, and perceived threat of COVID-19—negatively correlated with psychological well-being, whereas meaning-based resources (i.e., MIL and existential mattering) correlated positively with well-being. Moreover, both risk perception of COVID-19 infection and meaning-based resources were related to psychological well-being through the mediating effect of coping strategies.

As was hypothesized, risk perception, which reflects how healthcare personnel assess the probability of COVID-19 infection negatively correlated with psychological well-being. These findings are in line with previous studies that demonstrated perceived risk as a predictor of emotional distress amongst SARS survivors during the SARs epidemic in Hong Kong [10], as well as negative emotions amongst the Chinese population during the COVID-19 pandemic [49]. Our findings complement previous research in two important ways. First, both Cheng et al. [10] and Li et al. [49] studies were carried out amongst the Chinese general population, yet the health workers in Europe are exposed to a greater risk of infection, because of the rapid spread of COVID-19 and the sudden huge influx of patients. Second, SEM analysis revealed that the direct relationship between risk perception and healthcare personnel's well-being remained significant, even after controlling for the mediating effect of coping strategies. This implies the relatively strong character of the relationship between the way in which healthcare personnel interpret risk of contracting, fear, and perceived threat of COVID-19 infection and their psychological well-being.

In contrast, meaning-based resources positively correlated with psychological well-being. Thus, having more meaning-based resources was associated with higher well-being amongst healthcare personnel, which, in turn, can be used to deal with the negative psychological consequences of COVID-19. Healthcare workers who have a strong sense of purpose and value can more efficiently interpret and reorganize daily experiences, identify significant aspects of their life, and constructively pursue their aims. This finding corresponds with previous studies that indicated the predictive role of MIL on people's well-being [16–18] as well as the predictive role of MIL on the construction of individual identity amongst medical staff [19]. However, the direct relationship between meaning-based resources with psychological well-being was not obtained in the SEM analysis, after controlling for coping strategies. Given that SEM is considered to deliver more accurate results than correlations [50], these findings support an indirect rather than a direct relationship between meaning-based resources and well-being amongst healthcare personnel. Therefore, the availability of meaning-based resources can strengthen psychological well-being because they successfully trigger an effective use of coping strategies that can be applied to manage stress during the COVID-19 pandemic. The first hypothesis was only partially confirmed.

The main finding in this study was the mediating role played by coping strategies in the relationships between risk perception of the COVID-19 infection and meaning-based resources with healthcare personnel's psychological well-being. Two coping strategies—problem-focused and meaning-focused—were significant mediators in these relationships. The second and third hypotheses that assumed such relationships were thus confirmed. These results support previous studies that showed how coping strategies played a crucial role when people were facing an adverse situation [34,35,39,40]. They also suggest that perception and resource factors do not operate in "a vacuum" while influencing Polish healthcare personnel's psychological well-being; they are strongly interconnected with coping processes. It highlights the interplay of cognition (risk perception) and motivation (meaning-based resources) in managing stressful events and contributing to successful adaptation to stressors [51]. Problem-focused and meaning-focused coping is thus a dynamic process that varies according to one's cognitive appraisal and personal resources, and, consequently, regulates psychological well-being.

The present study builds on existing findings by revealing the cognitive and motivational mechanisms that underlie the effect of risk perception on psychological well-being in Polish healthcare personnel as they combat COVID-19. The two mediating strategies are predominately based on cognitive (problem-focused coping) and motivational (meaning-focused coping) processes. In contrast, emotional coping proved to be a less significant way of coping with stress during the pandemic. The utility of cognitive coping strategies in dealing with COVID-19 pandemic was confirmed by Gerhold's research [39], which showed that Germans tend to use problem-focused strategies in coping with COVID-19 (e.g., following expert advice and guidelines and thinking carefully about what to do). The current study extends Gerhold's [39] observations, by demonstrating that both problem-focused and meaning-focused coping operate simultaneously as mediators between risk perception and psychological well-being as well as between meaning-based resources and psychological well-being. There is, therefore, a noticeable interplay of cognitive and motivational processes underlying coping mechanisms in dealing with the dangers posed by COVID-19.

These findings suggest that although risk perception of the COVID-19 infection is related to lower psychological well-being, it paradoxically increases coping strategies, particularly problem-focused and meaning-focused coping (i.e., actions that help control the epidemics). In this sense, as noted by Li, Yang, Dou, Wang and colleagues [49], perceived severity can be regarded as a double-edged sword, being both risk and asset, in the encounter of pandemic.

These results can be interpreted within PMT, which posits that people confronted with threats resort to coping strategies that allow them to manage the threat. The decision to employ coping strategies is a consequence of severity, because people must believe that there is some potential harm (e.g., a high probability of infection with COVID-19 for healthcare personnel), and that they are vulnerable to this harm. The perception of threat from COVID-19 enhances the motivation to initiate the coping process [7]. The ability to adopt the recommended coping response may in turn enhance psychological well-being. This is in line with the meta-analysis of PMT findings by Milne et al. [52], which indicated that threat perception made it more likely that people would adopt some coping response because it provided motivational energy.

Our study shows that higher meaning-based resources predicted a more frequent use of problem-focused and meaning-focused coping, which was then related to a higher level of psychological well-being. Thus, personal resources that reflect the individual's convictions about having a significant, meaningful, and valuable life tend to play an important role in shaping coping behavior and, consequently, in predicting the well-being of healthcare personnel. These results can be interpreted within resource-based stress theories, which suggest that individual resources influence people's abilities to manage stress successfully and, consequently, to improve their well-being [12]. Meaning-based resources may be conducive to a constructive use of coping strategies, since a relatively stable pattern of commitment influences the way events are perceived and managed [25]. The predictive role of meaning-based resources in shaping the coping behavior of healthcare personnel is consistent with previous reports regarding the role of meaning in life in strengthening people's coping behavior and influencing their psychological well-being [19,20].

The present study also provides new empirical evidence by demonstrating that risk perception and meaning-based resources can operate together in predicting psychological well-being in healthcare personnel combating COVID-19. Problem-focused and meaning-focused coping mediated both the relationship between risk perception of COVID-19 infection and psychological well-being as well as the relationship between meaning-based resources and psychological well-being. However, the effect test showed that the mediating path for meaning-based resources was significantly stronger than for risk perception. This implies a more important role for coping strategies based on cognitive and motivational processes for healthcare personnel well-being in the case of personal meaning-based resources than the perceived risk of COVID-19 [20,38]. However, the mere availability of meaning-based resources does not contribute automatically to well-being, these resources must rely on coping strategies based on cognitive and motivational processes.

The present study has shortcomings. It should be emphasized that the cross-sectional design limits our ability to make a causal interpretation of the findings. The relationship between risk perception and well-being as well as the relationship between personal resources and well-being can be bilateral; risk perception and personal resources can affect healthcare personnel's well-being, but well-being may also contribute to more positive appraisals and higher meaning-based resources. Second, our explanation of the results of mediation analysis must be treated with caution. The model we tested, (which was confirmed), was based on theories and previous empirical research, but it should also be tested using a longitudinal design. Third, although respondents completed the measures anonymously, response bias could not be controlled, because the study was based on self-report. Therefore, future researchers need to attempt replication of the results with samples where this weakness is minimized.

5. Conclusions

Despite these limitations, the present study demonstrates the value of examining the mediating role of coping in the relationship of risk perception and personal resources with psychological well-being amongst healthcare personnel. Risk perception of COVID-19 infection negatively correlated with psychological well-being, whereas meaning-based resources had a positive correlation with well-being. Both risk perception and meaning-based resources were indirectly related to psychological well-being through the mediating effect of two coping strategies—problem-focused and meaning-focused coping. Higher risk assessment and more meaning-based resources predict more frequent use of problem-focused and meaning-focused coping, which, in turn, is related to a higher level of psychological well-being. The results contribute to a process-oriented approach towards adjustment to adverse situations [20,37,38] amongst healthcare personnel who are often on the frontline in combating COVID-19. They can also provide ideas for the creation of new meaning-based intervention programs that target existential distress and psychological well-being; analogical programs have been found very beneficial in healthcare settings [53,54]. As healthcare workers tend to experience intense stress, fatigue, and anxiety, meaning-based programs can help them find additional sources of meaning in their lives related to e.g., family, goals, values, or personal strengths. It will very likely strengthen the workers' resilience, reduce stress, and increase awareness of professional relationships, which, in turn, will result in higher psychological well-being.

Supplementary Materials: The following are available online at http://www.mdpi.com/2077-0383/9/10/3225/s1. Table S1: The order in which the variables and paths were removed from the initial model on a basis of modification indices.

Author Contributions: Conceptualization, D.K. and B.Z.; methodology, D.K. and B.Z.; formal analysis, B.Z. and D.K.; investigation, D.K.; data curation, D.K.; funding acquisition, B.Z.; writing (original draft preparation), D.K. and B.Z.; writing (review and editing), B.Z. and D.K.; visualization, D.K. All authors have read and agreed to the published version of the manuscript.

Funding: The APC was funded by The John Paul II Catholic University of Lublin.

Acknowledgments: The authors would like to thank healthcare personnel from hospitals, outpatient clinics, and medical laboratories in southern Poland for their contribution to this study.

Conflicts of Interest: The authors declare no conflict of interest.

References

1. Dryhurst, S.; Schneider, C.R.; Kerr, J.; Freeman, A.L.J.; Recchia, G.; van der Bles, A.M.; Spiegelhalter, D.; van der Linden, S. Risk perceptions of COVID-19 around the world. *J. Risk Res.* **2020**. [CrossRef]
2. Cai, H.; Tu, B.; Ma, J.; Chen, L.; Fu, L.; Jiang, Y.; Zhuang, Q. Psychological impacts and coping strategies of front-line medical staff during COVID-19 outbreak in Hunan, China. *Med. Sci. Monit.* **2020**, *26*, e924171-1–e924171-16. [CrossRef] [PubMed]
3. Lai, J.; Ma, S.; Wang, Y.; Cai, Z.; Hu, J.; Wei, N.; Wu, J.; Du, H.; Chen, T.; Li, R.; et al. Factors associated with mental health outcomes among health care workers exposed to coronavirus disease 2019. *JAMA Netw. Open* **2020**, *3*, e203976. [CrossRef] [PubMed]

4. Xiao, H.; Zhang, Y.; Kong, D.; Li, S.; Yang, N. The effects of social support on sleep quality of medical staff treating patients with coronavirus disease 2019 (COVID-19) in January and February 2020 in China. *Med. Sci. Monit. Int. Med. J. Exp. Clin. Res.* **2020**, *26*, e923549-1–e923549-8.
5. Hobfoll, S.E. The influence of culture, community, and the nested-self in the stress process: Advancing conservation of resources theory. *Appl. Psychol.* **2001**, *50*, 337–421. [CrossRef]
6. Szkody, E.; McKinney, C. Appraisal and social support as moderators between stress and physical and psychological quality of life. *Stress Health* **2020**, 1–10. [CrossRef]
7. Floyd, D.L.; Prentice-Dunn, S.; Rogers, R.W. A meta-analysis of research on protection motivation theory. *J. Appl. Soc. Psychol.* **2000**, *30*, 407–429. [CrossRef]
8. Hobfoll, S.E. Social and psychological resources and adaptation. *Rev. Gen. Psychol.* **2002**, *6*, 307–324. [CrossRef]
9. Grothmann, T.; Reusswig, F. People at risk of flooding: Why some residents take precautionary action while others do not. *Nat. Hazards* **2006**, *38*, 101–120. [CrossRef]
10. Cheng, S.K.W.; Chong, G.H.C.; Chang, S.S.Y.; Wong, C.W.; Wong, C.S.Y.; Wong, M.T.P.; Wong, K.C. Adjustment to severe acute respiratory syndrome (SARS): Roles of appraisal and post-traumatic growth. *Psychol. Health* **2006**, *21*, 301–317. [CrossRef]
11. Li, J.B.; Yang, A.; Dou, K.; Cheung, R.Y.M. Self-control moderates the association between perceived severity of coronavirus disease 2019 (COVID-19) and mental health problems among the Chinese public. *Int. J. Environ. Res. Public Health* **2020**, *17*, 4820. [CrossRef] [PubMed]
12. Hobfoll, S.E.; Johnson, R.J.; Ennis, N.; Jackson, A.P. Resource loss, resource gain, and emotional outcomes among inner city women. *J. Pers. Soc. Psychol.* **2003**, *84*, 632–643. [CrossRef] [PubMed]
13. Hooker, S.A.; Masters, K.S.; Park, C.L. A Meaningful life is a healthy life: A conceptual model linking meaning and meaning salience to health. *Rev. Gen. Psychol.* **2018**, *22*, 11–24. [CrossRef]
14. Li, J.-B.; Dou, K.; Liang, Y. The relationship between presence of meaning, search for meaning, and subjective well-being: A three-level meta-analysis based on the meaning in life questionnaire. *J. Happiness Stud.* **2020**. [CrossRef]
15. George, L.S.; Park, C.L. Meaning in life as comprehension, purpose, and mattering: Toward integration and new research questions. *Rev. Gen. Psychol.* **2016**, *20*, 205–220. [CrossRef]
16. Steger, M.F.; Oishi, S.; Kashdan, T.B. Meaning in life across the life span: Levels and correlates of meaning in life from emerging adulthood to older adulthood. *J. Posit. Psychol.* **2009**, *4*, 43–52. [CrossRef]
17. Steger, M.F.; Frazier, P. Meaning in life: One link in the chain from religiousness to well-being. *J. Couns. Psychol.* **2005**, *52*, 574–582. [CrossRef]
18. Zika, S.; Chamberlain, K. On the relation between meaning in life and psychological well-being. *Br. J. Psychol.* **1992**, *83*, 133–145. [CrossRef]
19. Damásio, B.F.; de Melo, R.L.P.; Silva, J.P.d. Sentido de vida, bem-estar psicológico e qualidade de vida em professores escolares. *Paidéia (Ribeirão Preto)* **2013**, *23*, 73–82. [CrossRef]
20. Park, C.L. Meaning making in the context of disasters. *J. Clin. Psychol.* **2016**, *72*, 1234–1246. [CrossRef]
21. Flett, G. *The Psychology of Mattering: Understanding the Human Need to Be Significant*; Academic Press: London, UK, 2018.
22. Prilleltensky, I. Meaning-making, mattering, and thriving in community psychology: From co-optation to amelioration and transformation. *Psychosoc. Interv.* **2014**, *23*, 151–154. [CrossRef]
23. Costin, V.; Vignoles, V.L. Meaning is about mattering: Evaluating coherence, purpose, and existential mattering as precursors of meaning in life judgments. *J. Pers. Soc. Psychol.* **2020**, *118*, 864–884. [CrossRef] [PubMed]
24. Flett, G.L.; Khan, A.; Su, C. Mattering and psychological well-being in college and university students: Review and recommendations for campus-based initiatives. *Int. J. Ment. Health Addict.* **2019**, *17*, 667–680. [CrossRef]
25. Lazarus, R.S.; DeLongis, A. Psychological stress and coping in aging. *Am. Psychol.* **1983**, *38*, 245–254. [CrossRef] [PubMed]
26. Lazarus, R.S.; Folkman, S. *Stress, Appraisal, and Coping*; Springer: New York, NY, USA, 1984; ISBN 978-0-8261-4190-3.
27. Lehavot, K. Coping strategies and health in a national sample of sexual minority women. *Am. J. Orthopsychiatry* **2012**, *82*, 494–504. [CrossRef]

28. Folkman, S.; Moskowitz, J.T. Positive Affect and Meaning-Focused Coping during Significant Psychological Stress. In *The Scope of Social Psychology: Theory and Applications*; Psychology Press: New York, NY, USA, 2007; pp. 193–208. ISBN 978-1-84169-645-4.
29. Riley, K.E.; Park, C.L. Problem-focused vs. meaning-focused coping as mediators of the appraisal-adjustment relationship in chronic stressors. *J. Soc. Clin. Psychol.* **2014**, *33*, 587–611. [CrossRef]
30. Folkman, S. Stress, Coping, and Hope Psychological Aspects of Cancer. In *Psychological Aspects of Cancer*; Carr, B., Steel, J., Eds.; Springer: Boston, MA, USA, 2013; pp. 119–127.
31. Baker, J.P.; Berenbaum, H. Dyadic moderators of the effectiveness of problem-focused and emotional-approach coping interventions. *Cogn. Ther. Res.* **2011**, *35*, 550–559. [CrossRef]
32. Prelow, H.M.; Weaver, S.R.; Swenson, R.R. Competence, self-esteem, and coping efficacy as mediators of ecological risk and depressive symptoms in urban African American and European American youth. *J. Youth Adolesc.* **2006**, *35*, 506–516. [CrossRef]
33. Dunkley, D.M.; Blankstein, K.R.; Halsall, J.; Williams, M.; Winkworth, G. The relation between perfectionism and distress: Hassles, coping, and perceived social support as mediators and moderators. *J. Couns. Psychol.* **2000**, *47*, 437–453. [CrossRef]
34. López-Vázquez, E.; Marván, M.L. Risk perception, stress and coping strategies in two catastrophe risk situations. *Soc. Behav. Pers. Int. J.* **2003**, *31*, 61–70. [CrossRef]
35. de Dominicis, S.; Fornara, F.; Cancellieri, U.G.; Twigger-Ross, C.; Bonaiuto, M. We are at risk, and so what? Place attachment, environmental risk perceptions and preventive coping behaviours. *J. Environ. Psychol.* **2015**, *43*, 66–78. [CrossRef]
36. Sumer, N.; Karanci, A.N.; Berument, S.K.; Gunes, H. Personal resources, coping self-efficacy, and quake exposure as predictors of psychological distress following the 1999 earthquake in Turkey. *J. Trauma. Stress* **2005**, *18*, 331–342. [CrossRef] [PubMed]
37. Rabenu, E.; Yaniv, E.; Elizur, D. The relationship between psychological capital, coping with stress, well-being, and performance. *Curr. Psychol.* **2017**, *36*, 875–887. [CrossRef]
38. Hobfoll, S.E.; Tirone, V.; Holmgreen, L.; Gerhart, J. Conservation of Resources Theory Applied to Major Stress. In *Stress: Concepts, Cognition, Emotion, and Behavior*; Elsevier Academic Press: San Diego, CA, USA, 2016; pp. 65–71. ISBN 978-0-12-800951-2.
39. Gerhold, L. COVID-19: Risk Perception and Coping Strategies. Available online: psyarxiv.com/xmpk4 (accessed on 29 June 2020).
40. Babcicky, P.; Seebauer, S. The two faces of social capital in private flood mitigation: Opposing effects on risk perception, self-efficacy and coping capacity. *J. Risk Res.* **2017**, *20*, 1017–1037. [CrossRef]
41. Krok, D. *The Risk of Contracting COVID-19 and the Perceived Threat of COVID-19 Scales*; Department of Psychology, University of Opole: Opole, Poland, 2020.
42. Dymecka, J. *The Fear of COVID-19 Scale*; Department of Psychology, University of Opole: Opole, Poland, 2020.
43. Steger, M.F.; Frazier, P.; Oishi, S.; Kaler, M. The meaning in life questionnaire: Assessing the presence of and search for meaning in life. *J. Couns. Psychol.* **2006**, *53*, 80–93. [CrossRef]
44. Gruszczynska, E.; Knoll, N. Meaning-focused coping, pain, and affect: A diary study of hospitalized women with rheumatoid arthritis. *Qual. Life Res.* **2015**, *24*, 2873–2883. [CrossRef]
45. Ryff, C.D.; Keyes, C.L.M. The structure of psychological well-being revisited. *J. Pers. Soc. Psychol.* **1995**, *69*, 719. [CrossRef]
46. Karaś, D.; Cieciuch, J. Polish adaptation of Carol Ryff's psychological well-being scales. *Rocz. Psychol.* **2017**, *20*, 837–853. [CrossRef]
47. Preacher, K.J.; Hayes, A.F. Asymptotic and resampling strategies for assessing and comparing indirect effects in multiple mediator models. *Behav. Res. Methods* **2008**, *40*, 879–891. [CrossRef]
48. Kline, R.B. *Principles and Practice of Structural Equation Modeling*, 3rd ed.; The Guilford Press: New York, NY, USA, 2015.
49. Li, J.B.; Yang, A.; Dou, K.; Wang, L.-X.; Zhang, M.-C.; Lin, X. Chinese Public's Knowledge, Perceived Severity, and Perceived Controllability of the COVID-19 and Their Associations with Emotional and Behavioural Reactions, Social Participation, and Precautionary Behaviour: A National Survey. Available online: psyarxiv.com/5tmsh (accessed on 12 June 2020).
50. Iacobucci, D.; Saldanha, N.; Deng, X. A meditation on mediation: Evidence that structural equations models perform better than regressions. *J. Consum. Psychol.* **2007**, *17*, 139–153. [CrossRef]

51. Yih, J.; Kirby, L.D.; Smith, C.A. Profiles of appraisal, motivation, and coping for positive emotions. *Cogn. Emot.* **2020**, *34*, 481–497. [CrossRef] [PubMed]
52. Milne, S.; Sheeran, P.; Orbell, S. Prediction and intervention in health-related behavior: A meta-analytic review of protection motivation theory. *J. Appl. Soc. Psychol.* **2000**, *30*, 106–143. [CrossRef]
53. Applebaum, A.J.; Buda, K.L.; Schofield, E.; Farberov, M.; Teitelbaum, N.D.; Evans, K.; Cowens-Alvarado, R.; Cannady, R.S. Exploring the cancer caregiver's journey through web-based meaning-centered psychotherapy. *Psycho-Oncology* **2017**, *27*, 847–856. [CrossRef] [PubMed]
54. Fillion, L.; Dupuis, R.; Tremblay, I.; Grâce, G.-R.D.; Breitbart, W. Enhancing meaning in palliative care practice: A meaning-centered intervention to promote job satisfaction. *Palliat. Support. Care* **2006**, *4*, 333–344. [CrossRef] [PubMed]

Journal of
Clinical Medicine

MDPI

Article

A Predictive Study of Resilience and Its Relationship with Academic and Work Dimensions during the COVID-19 Pandemic

Silvia San Román-Mata [1], Félix Zurita-Ortega [2], Pilar Puertas-Molero [2], Georgian Badicu [3,*] and Gabriel González-Valero [2]

[1] Nursing Department, University of Granada (Spain), Campus Universitario de Melilla, Calle Santander 1, 52005 Melilla, Spain; silviasanroman@ugr.es

[2] Department of Didactics of Musical, Plastic and Corporal Expression, University of Granada (Spain), Campus de Cartuja, s/n, 18071 Granada, Spain; felixzo@ugr.es (F.Z.-O.); javiconde@correo.ugr.es (P.P.-M.); ggvalero@ugr.es (G.G.-V.)

[3] Department of Physical Education and Special Motricity, Faculty of Physical Education and Mountain Sports, Transilvania University of Brașov, 500068 Brașov, Romania

* Correspondence: georgian.badicu@unitbv.ro; Tel.: +40-769-219-271

Received: 17 August 2020; Accepted: 8 October 2020; Published: 12 October 2020

Abstract: Background: The aim of the present study was to describe the resilience levels in a Spanish population during the Coronavirus (COVID-19) pandemic and to analyze the existing associations between high resilience and socio-demographic, work, and academic parameters. Method: 1176 individuals aged 18–67 years participated in a descriptive cross-sectional study. The participants were administered the 10-item resilience scale developed by Connor-Davidson (CD-RISC-10) and an ad-hoc questionnaire that collected information on socio-demographic, work, and academic variables. Basic descriptive data were used to statistically analyze the data, and a binary logistic regression model was developed incorporating the professional occupation, academic level, whether the respondent worked in emergency services, and whether the respondent had dependents. Results: Slightly more than a quarter of the participants showed low resilience, almost half reported moderate resilience, and slightly more than a quarter had high resilience. Those who were employed were 2.16-times more likely to have high resilience, whilst those with higher education were 1.57-times more likely. Those working in emergency services were 1.66-times more likely, and those with dependents were 1.58-times more likely to have high resilience. Conclusion: In addition to the relationships found, a need to improve the resilience levels in the population was found.

Keywords: resilience; emergency services; COVID-19; adversity; lockdown

1. Introduction

Currently, we find ourselves with a serious public health problem and in a state of global emergency due to the Coronavirus (COVID-19) pandemic [1,2]. This virus first appeared in China at the end of 2019 and in just a few weeks had spread to many other countries around the globe [3,4]. It was responsible for a high number of deaths in the first months after its emergence [5]. Spain was in confinement during the first two weeks of the state of alarm. According to the latest data provided by the Ministry of Health [6], on the 15 March, the number of cases reported nationwide amounted to 7753 (2000 new cases in the last 24 h), representing 16.52 cases per 100,000 inhabitants, including 288 deceased and 382 admitted to the intensive care units.

In this sense, citizens around the globe and those governing them were pushed to take quick and efficient action, complying with the instructions given by the relevant health authorities to slow down this pandemic [7]. The COVID-19 pandemic appears to be a risk factor for psychological illness and sleep disorders, reportedly having a significant impact on these constructs [8,9]. Studies, such as the one carried out by Forte, Favieri, Tambelli, and Casagrande [10] revealed that individuals reported levels of general psychopathological symptoms, anxiety, and post-traumatic stress disorder (PTSD) symptoms that were higher than the cut-off scores.

Resilience capacity, understood as a set of intrinsic factors that characterizes all individuals and is implicated in the process of overcoming adversity [11,12], takes on great importance in relation to the degree of success that can be achieved by health measures. Resilience capacity is also crucial for the promotion of psychological wellbeing in the population [13,14].

Thus, resilience makes up one of the most important dynamic psychological factors with regard to the protection and adaptability of individuals, being malleable to development and improvement through intervention programs [15,16]. In fact, a large amount of scientific literature, currently available within various populations, deals with resilience in general terms, whether this be with children [17,18], adolescents [19], or other populations [20].

In the same way, this skill is currently a hot topic of study in health workers and those working in emergency services because of the arduous work they perform and the stress it entails [21–25]. Studies carried out with patients with different pathologies at different stages of the disease process are also highly relevant, especially those conducted with oncology patients [26–28]. In this way, patients who present lower resilience show greater problems in relation to emotional regulation and, as a consequence, higher levels of stress and anxiety. Such findings were stated by Vaughan et al. [29]

Likewise, research is found that relates resilience with socio-demographic, religious [30], personal, and family factors, in addition to academic performance [31]. It must also be stated that various opinions exist with respect to the resilience capacity and its relationship with gender [32], with studies also emerging within transgender groups [33,34].

Thus, the importance of the resilience capacity to human behavior is clear. As a result of this, confinement and the limitation of movement as a result of the global state of health emergency in which Spain is embroiled, presents a type of adversity to be overcome by the whole population. In this way, there is a need to identify the levels of resilience in the population during this time of crisis. Based on the scarcity of studies tackling the topic of COVID-19 and its relationship with the way in which adversity is tackled and overcome, the present study was proposed with the following objectives: (1) describe the levels of resilience in the Spanish population during the pandemic, and (2) analyze the existing associations between high resilience and socio-demographic, work, and academic parameters.

2. Method

2.1. Participants and Procedure

A total of 1176 individuals from Spain participated in the present descriptive and cross-sectional research study. The participants were aged between 18 and 67 years (M = 35.35 years; SD = 11.900), with 457 (38.9%) being male and 719 (61.1%) being female. The sample was selected through a process of random sampling. In order to be selected, individuals had to be in full possession of their psychological faculties, provide informed consent, be of adult age, not be retired, and not suffer from any type of condition that would impede participation in the research. These requirements made up the inclusion and exclusion criteria. The sample was obtained from all Spanish cities, requesting participation from all those who agreed to do so voluntarily. The study sample was collected in two periods depending on the different states of lockdown. The first period was from 15 to 22 March (n = 727; 61.8%) and the second period was from 23 to 31 March (n = 449; 38.2%).Two questions from the self-reported survey were duplicated to avoid bias in the responses and to check that they were not filled in randomly. We excluded 171 questionnaires after detecting that they had been incorrectly filled out or that the recipients did not meet the inclusion criteria.

The participants were contacted through various calls placed on social networks in diverse social groups so that the sample would be as random as possible. Once contact was made, the potential participants were informed regarding how to fill out the document, informing them that all collected data would be kept totally anonymous and used only for research purposes. The researchers were present in a virtual way during data collection in order to guarantee correct implementation of the process and resolve any doubts. This was achieved by providing a personal Google Meets link associated with the group of researchers, to enable users to connect with the researchers and resolve any questions they might have. The present research received approval from the ethics committee of the University of Granada (641/CEIH/2018).

2.2. Variables and Instruments

The self-registration form (ad-hoc questionnaire), collected data in relation to sex (male or female), age, whether the respondents were responsible for dependents during confinement (older individuals or relatives), whether the respondents knew somebody in their environment who had suffered from or had COVID-19, occupation prior to confinement (student, neither working nor studying, state employee, works with the public, self-employed, or works for a private company), the highest academic level achieved (basic studies, professional training, higher studies (up to baccalaureate), postgraduate studies, or doctorate studies), whether they work in emergency services (categorized as yes or no), and the period of study completion structured according to period 1 (from the 15–22 March) and period 2 (from the 23–31 March).

Resilience test. The Spanish version of the 10-item resilience scale developed by Connor-Davidson (CD-RISC) was used. This comes from the original version of the CD-RISC proposed by Connor and Davidson [35] and adapted into Spanish by Notario-Pacheco et al. [36] and Soler-Sánchez, Meseguer-de Pedro, and García-Izquierdo [37]. The scale is formed by 10 items which request respondents to provide ratings along a Likert type scale thatruns from 0 (totally disagree) to 4 (totally agree). Questions include the example: "I am capable of adapting to changes". Initial studies obtained Cronbach alpha values higher than 0.80, with $\alpha = 0.87$ reported by Soler-Sánchez et al. [37], and $\alpha = 0.85$ reported by Notario-Pacheco et al. [36], whilst the present study obtained a value of $\alpha = 0.89$.

2.3. Data Analysis

For the basic descriptive analysis and cross-tabs, the statistical software package IBM SPSS® was used in version 25.0 for Windows. The normality and homogeneity of the sample was established through the Kolmogorov–Smirnov test.

Following this, binary logistic regression (odds ratio and 95% confidence intervals) was performed. High resilience provided the exposure variable as it was one of the specific objectives being considered. The model examined its association with socio-demographic, work, and academic variables. Likewise, Cox and Snell's R^2 was employed to examine the model fit, whilst the Hosmer–Lemeshow test was used to determine the goodness of fit. Variables were introduced into the model manually if they met the criteria of having shown significant associations in prior bivariate analysis carried out through crosstabs. Variables that did not show significance at this prior stage were excluded from the model ($p \geq 0.05$).

Given that the proposed analysis was binary, participants with low and moderate resilience were categorised into a single "not high resilience" group. Likewise, given the dichotomous nature of analysis, the remaining variables were categorised as follows: Sex (0 = female and 1 = male), professional occupation (0 = employed and 1 = not employed), level of study (0 = without higher education and 1 = higher education), professional occupation related with the emergency services (0 = not emergency services and 1 = emergency services), responsible for dependents (0 = does not have dependents and 1 = has dependents), associated with individuals with COVID-19 (0 = not associated with anybody with COVID-19 and 1 = associated with somebody with COVID-19), and time-period (0 = period from the 15–22 March and 1 = period from the 23–31 March).

3. Results

The 1176 participants of the present study were distributed between both genders, with 61.1% being female and 38.9% being male. Of these, 66.3% stated being responsible for dependents (older adults or children), whilst 33.7% did not. A total of 27.3% were categorized as having high resilience, 46.2% had moderate resilience, and 26.5% had low resilience. With regard to the question asking whether individuals in their immediate environment had contracted COVID-19, 42.7% indicated yes, whilst 57.3% stated that no. In reference to respondents' professional occupation prior to confinement, 34% were public employees, 22.3% were self-employed or lent their services to a private company, 21.8% were students, 18.5% reported studying and working, and 3.4% were neither studying nor working. With regard to their academic level, 50.1% reported their highest level of study being "studies of higher education", 29.3% had postgraduate qualifications, 11.1% had professional training, 6% possessed basic studies, and 3.7% had only third grade studies (Table 1)

Table 1. Descriptive characteristics of the sample.

Sex	Male	38.9% ($n = 457$)	Has dependents	Yes	33.7% ($n = 396$)
	Female	61.1% ($n = 719$)		No	66.3% ($n = 780$)
Resilience	Low	26.5% ($n = 312$)	Close other with corona virus (COVID)-19	Yes	42.7% ($n = 502$)
	Medium	46.2% ($n = 543$)		No	57.3% ($n = 674$)
	High	27.3% ($n = 321$)	Age	M = 35.35; DT = 11.900	
Occupation	Full-time student	21.8% ($n = 256$)	Academic level	Professional training	11.1% ($n = 130$)
	Public employee	34% ($n = 400$)		Doctorate	50.1% ($n = 589$)
	Neither studies nor works	3.5% ($n = 41$)		Postgraduate	29.3% ($n = 344$)
	Studies and works	18.5% ($n = 217$)		Third grade studies	3.7% ($n = 43$)
	Self-employed/works at a private company	22.3% ($n = 262$)		Basic education	6% ($n = 70$)
Works in the Emergency Services	Yes	27.9% ($n = 328$)	Time-point	Period 1	61.8% ($n = 727$)
	No	72.1% ($n = 848$)		Period 2	38.2% ($n = 449$)

Finally, with regard to working in emergency services, 27.9% reported doing so relative to 72.1% who did not. In relation to the time-period as it relates to the state of alarm, 61.8% of the questionnaires were completed during period 1 (from the 15–22 March) and 38.2% during period 2 (from the 23–31 March) (Table 1)

In the relational study of variables relating to the resilience level, statistically significant differences were found (p = 0.015) pertaining to sex. Specifically, low resilience was more common amongst females than males (29.1% relative to 22.5%), with these figures being inverted when high resilience was considered (31.3% for males and 24.9% for females). With regard to being responsible for dependents, differences were shown in the data (p = 0.000), with individuals responsible for dependents showing a greater prevalence of high resilience (35.1%) than those without this responsibility (23.3%).

No association was found (p = 0.248) with regard to whether respondents had individuals in their immediate environment who had contracted COVID-19, whilst participants' occupation prior to confinement did produce statistically significant differences (p = 0.001). Concretely, participants who were working as public employees, were self-employed, or worked for a private company obtained higher values, with 27.5% reporting a high resilience relative to just 16.4% of students who reported the same optimum level.

Regarding the academic levels, statistically significant differences (p = 0.001) emerged. In this case, 33% of respondents with postgraduate or doctorate studies reported high resilience, this being a greater percentage than the 18.6% of individuals with only basic studies who also obtained scores belonging to this category. In relation to whether or not individuals worked in a position related to emergency services, a statically significant association was found (p = 0.002). This was generated because those who did have a relevant profession (32%) presented a higher prevalence of high resilience than those who did not come into contact with emergency services through their work (25.5%). These results were inverted when considering low resilience, with 29.2% of those in contact with emergency services falling into this category, relative to 19.5% of those not in contact. Finally, differences were not detected ($p = 0.243$) with regard to the period of study completion and resilience level. (Table 2)

Table 2. Associations between resilience and all other variables.

Variables		Resilience			
		Low ($n = 312$)	Medium ($n = 543$)	High ($n = 321$)	*Sig*
Sex	Male	22.5% ($n = 103$)	46.4% ($n = 212$)	31.3% ($n = 142$)	0.015 *
	Female	29.1% ($n = 209$)	46.0% ($n = 331$)	24.9% ($n = 179$)	
Has dependents	Yes	22.7% ($n = 90$)	42.2% ($n = 167$)	35.1% ($n = 139$)	0.000 *
	No	28.5% ($n = 222$)	48.2% ($n = 376$)	23.3% ($n = 182$)	
Close others with COVID-19	Yes	24.5% ($n = 123$)	48.8% ($n = 245$)	26.7% ($n = 134$)	0.248
	No	28.0% ($n = 189$)	44.2% ($n = 298$)	27.7% ($n = 187$)	
Occupation	Full-time student	33.6% ($n = 86$)	50% ($n = 128$)	16.4% ($n = 42$)	0.001 *
	Public employee	26.3% ($n = 105$)	46% ($n = 184$)	27.8% ($n = 111$)	
	Neither studies nor works	24.4% ($n = 10$)	53.7% ($n = 22$)	22% ($n = 9$)	
	Studies and works	25.3% ($n = 55$)	41.9% ($n = 91$)	32.7% ($n = 71$)	
	Self-employed/works at a private company	21.4% ($n = 56$)	45% ($n = 118$)	33.6% ($n = 88$)	
Academic level	Professional training	26.2% ($n = 34$)	50.0% ($n = 65$)	23.8% ($n = 31$)	0.001 *
	Doctorate	27.7% ($n = 163$)	48.6% ($n = 286$)	23.8% ($n = 140$)	
	Postgraduate	24.4% ($n = 84$)	41.9% ($n = 144$)	33.7% ($n = 116$)	
	Third grade	27.9% ($n = 12$)	23.3% ($n = 10$)	48.8% ($n = 21$)	
	Basic education	27.1% ($n = 19$)	54.3% ($n = 38$)	18.6% ($n = 13$)	
Works in emergency services	Yes	19.5% ($n = 64$)	48.5% ($n = 159$)	32.0% ($n = 105$)	0.002 *
	No	29.2% ($n = 248$)	45.3% ($n = 384$)	25.5% ($n = 216$)	
Time-point	Period 1	25.0% ($n = 182$)	46.4% ($n = 337$)	28.6% ($n = 208$)	0.243
	Period 2	19.0% ($n = 130$)	45.9% ($n = 206$)	25.2% ($n = 113$)	

Note 1. Statistically significant differences at the level $p < 0.05$ *.

Once the descriptive and relational study was determined, we proceeded to the second study objective, which was to establish a predictive model of high resilience through binary logistic regression. The variables describing close others with COVID-19 and the time-period ($p \geq 0.05$) were excluded. In the first step of analysis, sex did not produce significant outcomes and so it was also excluded from the model. In the second step, good fit was shown through outcomes of the omnibus test ($X^2 = 48.721$; 4df; sig = 0.000), Hosmer–Lemeshow test ($X^2 = 4.095$; 6df; sig = 0.664), Cox and Snell R^2 (0.041), and Nagelkerke statistic (0.059). The model adequately explained 72.7% of cases.

Likewise, as can be seen in the following table, the model identified associations ($p < 0.05$ in the adjusted regression model) between resilience and professional occupation (Exp [B]: 2.160 [1.504–3.101]), academic level (Exp [B]: 1.579 [1.089–2.290]), job related to emergency services (Exp [B]: 1.668 [1.242–2.239]), and responsibility for dependents (Exp [B]: 1.583 [1.194–2.097]) (Table 3).

Table 3. Binary logistic regression model.

	B	Standard Error	Wald	df	Sig.	Exp(B)	95% CI for EXP(B)	
							Lower	Upper
Professional occupation	0.770	0.185	17.415	1	0.000	2.160	1.504	3.101
Academic level	0.457	0.189	5.819	1	0.016	1.579	1.089	2.290
Emergency services	0.511	0.150	11.579	1	0.001	1.668	1.242	2.239
Dependents	0.459	0.144	10.227	1	0.001	1.583	1.194	2.097
Constant	−2.282	0.247	85.259	1	0.000	0.102		

4. Discussion

The present research work was conducted with a sample of 1176 Spanish adults, with 61.1% being represented by females and 38.9% by males. The study sought to determine associative patterns between various aspects associated with resilience, and socio-demographic, work, and academic aspects during the period of confinement caused by the global COVID-19 crisis. In the opinion of the authors of this manuscript, no studies with the characteristics of the present study have been developed to date. Although the results should be considered with caution, positive and predictive relationships of resilience capacity were established with the variables of this study. This study can be used as a starting point for developing resilience-based interventions to help minimize psychological consequences during the COVID-19 pandemic.

First, one of the descriptive results produced in relation to the resilience capacity was that almost half of participants reported values that corresponded to moderate resilience. This finding is similar to that reported by Rodríguez and Ortunio [38], who specified highly similar percentages for this dimension. On the other hand, Szu-Ying et al. [39] stated that slightly more than half of older adults with cardiovascular problems who made up the study sample reported low resilience. This could be due to the fact that they have an illness that causes them stress.

Along similar lines, it is appropriate to highlight that four out of every ten participants in the present study reported having had contact with individuals affected by COVID-19. This could provide an explanation for the medium resilience levels. Fear of the unknown coupled with uncertainty regarding future socio-economics and health can generate mental health problems in the population including the consumption of toxins, somatization, stress, anxiety, and depression that can lead to the risk of suicide [40–42].

When observing scores pertaining to "low resilience", females predominated, whilst males were mostly found in the group of those with "high resilience". This coincides with other studies [12,22,32,38] that allude to both cultural and traditional factors. In this sense, males were traditionally considered responsible for the economic wellbeing of their family. This brought with it skill acquisition and decision making based on the need to take care of their loved ones, leading to rises in resilience.

At the same time, entirely contrasting positions were also found, such as that reported by Laul et al. [43]. These authors showed females to be more resilient, whilst further studies indicated that females were more resilient due to their role as mediator and overseer of the family, with the education and care of members being one of their main functions [44]. Other studies failed to note any sex-based differences, although they did establish resilience-based relationships within health workers [45].

On the other hand, it is interesting to point out the emergence of studies carried out in recent years, especially in transgender groups [33,34]. In the present day, the topic of resilience and gender is somewhat controversial. In this study, sex had to be excluded from the predictive model in the first step of model construction as it was not found to be significantly related.

In relation to professional occupation, the results of the present study indicated that public employees, self-employed workers, and those working at private companies had higher resilience scores. This fact could be explained by the management and planning skills and competencies of individuals at a cognitive, planning, and intellectual level. Individuals draw on these resources to perform tasks, whether this be in the work, social, or academic setting. These resources act as protective factors and help develop resilience [46]. In addition, Zhang et al. [47] added the factor of job commitment as another potentially influential factor.

Thus, at the beginning of this year, a study was conducted in Korea targeting workers that included health workers, in which high levels of work stress, anxiety, and depressive feelings were associated with suicidal ideation, and they found that there was an inverse relationship between resilience and suicidal ideas; that is, high levels of resistance in professionals decreased the incidence of self-injurious thoughts [48].

In fact, Mckinley et al. [45] argued in their study that better scores were obtained by hospital doctors relative to others working in medicine in general. This is likely because dedication and job commitment are greater in hospitals, and this could be considered to be one of the factors related with increased resilience. In the present study, similar figures were found in the proposed regression model, with the likelihood of having high resilience being 2.16-times greater amongst those who were regularly employed.

On the other hand, the scarcity or lack of material necessary to carry out the work with the necessary safety harasses the work environment, favoring the discomfort of the health workers at the mental level. In this sense, the lack of prevention in health supplies was linked to the risk of contagion, user demand, patient morbidity, and the risk of death increasing the burden of stress on health personnel, as well as increasing pressure, concern, and anxiety levels in said personnel [49]. In this line, García-Fernández et al. [50] found, in their research, higher levels of stress and anxiety in health professionals who considered the level of protection in their work environment insufficient or inadequate, while those who had access to adequate protection presented emotional well-being.

At the same time, high resilience scores were uncovered in staff working in the context of emergency services. The ability to overcome adverse situations, adapt to them, and come out stronger the other end, was greater in individuals with stressful occupations as they require emotional management skills to carry out their work [21,22,24,25]. Studies have not only been performed directed towards this population; in fact, research has also been developed at a community level in relation to resilience in hospitals, given the importance of resilience when delivering quality care to service users [23]. In particular, resilience in this setting acts as a protective factor for emergency staff against the potential psychological malaise they might suffer when performing their responsibilities. Thus, our regression model indicated that professionals dedicated to emergency medicine were 1.66-times more likely to have high resilience.

Along similar lines, Zhang et al. [47] outlined the implications of working in different occupational professions as another individual factor. This may influence resilience whilst at the same time improve the quality of work performance, in addition to having a positive association with spiritual health and self-concept [51,52].

All of these observations are also related with the existence of intervention programs designed to improve the resilience levels in nursing staff. An example of such a program is the one developed by Henshall, Davey, and Jackson [53]. This identified the importance of this skill when practicing in the health profession and demonstrated the achievement of better scores following university training [54]. Similarly, in other care settings, such as in social work, resilience is integrated into educational programs, courses, and professional development frameworks. This is due to its importance in carrying out these activities, as has been indicated by Clevelant, Warhurst, and Legood [55].

In this way, academic level is considered to be another factor associated with resilience. Individuals who possess higher education qualifications were shown to be more resilient. This collaborates previously conducted work by Orkaizaguirre-Gómara et al. [31], which found that resilience in university students increased as they progressed through each academic year. Likewise, the results presented by Szu-Ying et al. [39] found higher resilience levels amongst individuals with higher education qualifications. For this reason, this variable was included in the developed regression model, with the outcome confirming that students undertaking higher education were 1.57-times more likely to show high resilience.

Considering the factors we previously mentioned in relation to careers, it is fitting to highlight that individuals with children or dependents were also found to be more resilient than those without. This is illustrated in the regression model via an association between both variables. Thus, it appears that, in some way, the responsibility to care for others leads to development of this skill in such a way that participants with dependents were 1.58-times more likely to present with high resilience.

Finally, with regard to the limitations presented by the present work, there is a scarcity of existing literature conducted on resilience within Spanish populations during the COVID-19 pandemic. Research in other contexts was found in relation to this topic. With regard to the transgender population, no relevant items were included within the gender variable, which could be considered as another study limitation. Another limitation could be the homogeneity of the sample, as it was mostly women who were more willing to answer the survey. Thus, no distinction was made between age groups, this being a possibility for future studies.

Finally, given that Spain found itself in a state of national emergency and health crisis at the time of data collection, it would have been interesting to include the variable of "stress". This would be likely to provide additional information given the large number of studies that have related high resilience with good stress management [56,57] and fewer depressive symptoms [58]. Studies, such as that conducted by Moksnes and Lazarewicz [19], found resilience to play a compensatory role in the relationship between stress and emotional symptoms.

5. Conclusions

In conclusion, individuals who were employed (2.16 times), had higher education (1.57 times), worked in the emergency services setting (1.66 times), and were responsible for dependents (1.58 times) were more likely to report high resilience. In addition to these associations, a clear need was demonstrated to improve resilience levels in general. For this reason, intervention programs must be conducted to develop this capacity from early ages, whilst its dynamic and malleable nature also makes targeting the general population worthwhile. In the same way, future research directives should include additional variables, such as stress, anxiety, and depression.

Uncovering further variables related to the COVID-19 pandemic will also provide priceless information regarding how to manage the stress caused. Similarly, it will be useful to develop psychosocial studies and implement intervention programs that are adapted toward the development of this capacity, whilst also promoting psychological well-being in the population.

Author Contributions: Conceptualization, S.S.R.-M., G.G.-V., and F.Z.-O.; methodology, G.G.-V., F.Z.-O., and S.S.R.-M.; software, G.G.-V. and F.Z.-O.; formal analysis, G.G.-V., F.Z.-O., and P.P.-M.; investigation, G.G.-V., F.Z.-O., S.S.R.-M., and P.P.-M.; data curation, G.G.-V.; writing—original draft preparation, G.G.-V. and S.S.R.-M.; writing—review and editing, S.S.R.-M., G.G.-V., F.Z.-O., P.P.-M., and G.B.; visualization, G.G.-V., G.B., P.P.-M., and F.Z.-O.; supervision, G.G.-V., G.B., S.S.R.-M., and F.Z.-O. All authors have read and agreed to the published version of the manuscript.

Funding: This research received no external funding.

Conflicts of Interest: The authors declare no conflict of interest.

References

1. World Health Organization (WHO). Coronavirus Disease Outbreak (COVID-19): Guidelines for the Public 2020. Available online: http://who.int/es/emergencies/diseases/novel-coronavirus-2019/Advice-for-public (accessed on 12 July 2020).
2. González-Valero, G.; Zurita-Ortega, F.; Lindell-Postigo, D.; Conde-Pipó, J.; Grosz, W.R.; Badicu, G. Analysis of Self-Concept in Adolescents before and during COVID-19 Lockdown: Differences by Gender and Sports Activity. *Sustainability* **2020**, *12*, 7792. [CrossRef]
3. Lee, A. Wuhan novel coronavirus (COVID-19): Why global control is challenging? *Public Health* **2020**, *179*, A1–A2. [CrossRef] [PubMed]
4. Lum, L.H.W.; Tambyah, P.A. Outbreak of COVID-19—An urgent need for good science to silence our fears? *Singap. Med. J.* **2020**, *61*, 55–57. [CrossRef] [PubMed]
5. Gao, P.; Zhang, H.; Wu, Z.; Wang, J. Visualising the expansion and spread of coronavirus disease 2019 by cartograms. *Environ. Plan. A Econ. Space* **2020**, *52*, 698–701. [CrossRef]
6. Ministerio de Sanidad; Departamento de Seguridad Nacional; Gobierno de España. Coronavirus (COVID 19)-15 de marzo 2020. Available online: https://www.mscbs.gob.es (accessed on 22 September 2020).
7. Da Silva, A.A.M. Sobre a possibilidade de interrupção da epidemia pelo coronavírus (COVID-19) com base nas melhores evidências científicas disponíveis. *Rev. Bras. Epidemiol.* **2020**, *23*, e200021. [CrossRef]
8. Casagrande, M.; Favieri, F.; Tambelli, R.; Forte, G. The enemy who sealed the world: Effects quarantine due to the COVID-19 on sleep quality, anxiety, and psychological distress in the Italian population. *Sleep Med.* **2020**, *75*, 12–20. [CrossRef]
9. Favieri, F.; Forte, G.; Tambelli, R.; Casagrande, M. The Italians in the Time of Coronavirus: Psychosocial Aspects of Unexpected COVID-19 Pandemic. *SSRN Electron. J.* **2020**. [CrossRef]

10. Forte, G.; Favieri, F.; Tambelli, R.; Casagrande, M. The Enemy Which Sealed the World: Effects of COVID-19 Diffusion on the Psychological State of the Italian Population. *J. Clin. Med.* **2020**, *9*, 1802. [CrossRef]
11. Eakman, A.M.; Kinney, A.R.; Schierl, M.L.; Henry, K.L. Academic performance in student service members/veterans: Effects of instructor autonomy support, academic self-efficacy and academic problems. *Educ. Psychol.* **2019**, *39*, 1005–1026. [CrossRef]
12. Ramírez-Granizo, I.A.; Sánchez-Zafra, M.; Zurita-Ortega, F.; Puertas-Molero, P.; González-Valero, G.; Ubago-Jiménez, J.L. Multidimensional Self-Concept Depending on Levels of Resilience and the Motivational Climate Directed towards Sport in Schoolchildren. *Int. J. Environ. Res. Public Health* **2020**, *17*, 534. [CrossRef]
13. Asmundson, G.J.; Taylor, S. How health anxiety influences responses to viral outbreaks like COVID-19: What all decision-makers, health authorities, and health care professionals need to know. *J. Anxiety Disord.* **2020**, *71*, 102211. [CrossRef]
14. Birkhead, G.S.; Vermeulen, K. Sustainability of Psychological First Aid Training for the Disaster Response Workforce. *Am. J. Public Health* **2018**, *108*, S381–S382. [CrossRef] [PubMed]
15. Bajaj, B.; Pande, N. Mediating role of resilience in the impact of mindfulness on life satisfaction and affect as indices of subjective well-being. *Pers. Individ. Differ.* **2016**, *93*, 63–67. [CrossRef]
16. Robinson, M.; Hanna, E.; Raine, G.; Robertson, S. Extending the Comfort Zone: Building Resilience in Older People with Long-Term Conditions. *J. Appl. Gerontol.* **2017**, *38*, 825–848. [CrossRef] [PubMed]
17. Jones, L. Adversity and resilience: 10 lessons I have learnt from working with children in humanitarian emergencies. *Arch. Dis. Child.* **2018**, *104*, 833–836. [CrossRef] [PubMed]
18. Román-Mata, S.S.; Puertas-Molero, P.; Ubago-Jiménez, J.L.; González-Valero, G. Benefits of Physical Activity and Its Associations with Resilience, Emotional Intelligence, and Psychological Distress in University Students from Southern Spain. *Int. J. Environ. Res. Public Health* **2020**, *17*, 4474. [CrossRef] [PubMed]
19. Moksnes, U.K.; Lazarewicz, M. The association between stress, resilience, and emotional symptoms in Norwegian adolescents from 13 to 18 years old. *J. Health Psychol.* **2017**, *24*, 1093–1102. [CrossRef]
20. Mata, S.S.R.; Martínez-Martínez, A.; Zurita-Ortega, F.; Cuberos, R.C.; Puertas-Molero, P.; González-Valero, G. Capacidad de resiliencia según tendencia religiosa y género en universitarios. *Rev. Electrón. Investig. Educ.* **2019**, *21*, 1–11. [CrossRef]
21. Arbuzia, M.; Rahnama, M.; Abdollahimohammad, A.; Goli, H.; Akbarizadeh, M.R.; Naderifar, M. The Effect of Resilience Training on Quality of Work Life (QoWL) and Job Stress of Nurses in Emergency Department of Shahid Mohammadi Hospital in Bandar Abbas in 2018. *J. Evol. Med. Dent. Sci.* **2019**, *8*, 3161–3165. [CrossRef]
22. Falavarjani, M.F.; Yeh, C.J. Optimism and distress tolerance in the social adjustment of nurses: Examining resilience as a mediator and gender as a moderator. *J. Res. Nurs.* **2019**, *24*, 500–512. [CrossRef]
23. Ghanaatpisheh, E.; Khankeh, H.; Masoumi, G. Challenges for Hospital Resilience in Emergencies and Disasters: A Qualitative Study in Iran. *J. Clin. Diagn. Res.* **2019**, *13*, 1–8. [CrossRef]
24. Greinacher, A.; Nikendei, A.; Kottke, R.; Wiesbeck, J.; Herzog, W.; Nikendei, C. Secondary Traumatization, Psychological Stress, and Resilience in Psychosocial Emergency Care Personnel. *Int. J. Environ. Res. Public Health* **2019**, *16*, 3213. [CrossRef] [PubMed]
25. Musso, M.W.; Tatum, D.; Hamer, D.; Hammarlund, R.; Son, L.; McMahon, P. The Relationship Between Grit and Resilience in Emergency Medical Service Personnel. *Ochsner. J.* **2019**, *19*, 199–203. [CrossRef]
26. Luo, D.; Eicher, M.; White, K. Individual resilience in adult cancer care: A concept analysis. *Int. J. Nurs. Stud.* **2020**, *102*, 103467. [CrossRef] [PubMed]
27. Saban, K.L.; Tell, D.; Janusek, L. Resilience in African American Women at Risk for Cardiovascular Disease: An Exploratory Study. *J. Hered.* **2018**, *96*, 44–49. [CrossRef]
28. Stegenga, K.; Liu, Q.; Haase, J. Resilience in Pediatric Oncology. *Integr. Pediatr. Oncol.* **2020**, 63–77. [CrossRef]
29. Vaughan, E.; Koczwara, B.; Kemp, E.; Freytag, C.; Tan, W.S.; Beatty, L.J. Exploring emotion regulation as a mediator of the relationship between resilience and distress in cancer. *Psycho-Oncology* **2019**, *28*, 1506–1512. [CrossRef]
30. Crespo, F.J.G.; Alonso, R.F.; Muñiz, J. Resilient and low performer students: Personal and family determinants in European countries. *Psicothema* **2019**, *31*, 363–375.
31. Rn, A.O.; De Miguel, M.S.; Rn, J.O.D.E.; Bs, A.O.D.E. Testing general self-efficacy, perceived competence, resilience, and stress among nursing students: An integrator evaluation. *Nurs. Health Sci.* **2020**, *22*, 529–538. [CrossRef]

32. Zurita-Ortega, F.; Zafra-Santos, E.O.; Valdivia-Moral, P.; Rodríguez-Fernández, S.; Castro-Sánchez, M.; Muros-Molina, J.J. Análisis de la resiliencia, autoconcepto y motivación en judo según el género. *Rev. Psicol. Deporte* **2017**, *21*, 71–82.
33. Akhtar, M.; Bilour, N. State of Mental Health Among Transgender Individuals in Pakistan: Psychological Resilience and Self-esteem. *Community Ment. Health J.* **2019**, *56*, 626–634. [CrossRef] [PubMed]
34. Watson, R.J.; Veale, J.F. Transgender youth are strong: Resilience among gender expansive youth worldwide. *Int. J. Transgend.* **2018**, *19*, 115–118. [CrossRef]
35. Connor, K.M.; Davidson, J.R.T. Development of a new resilience scale: The Connor-Davidson Resilience Scale (CD-RISC). *Depress. Anxiety* **2003**, *18*, 76–82. [CrossRef] [PubMed]
36. Notario-Pacheco, B.; Martínez-Vizcaíno, V.; Serrano-Parra, D.; Bartolomé-Gutiérrez, R.; Campayo, J.G.; Martínez-Vizcaíno, V. Reliability and validity of the Spanish version of the 10-item Connor-Davidson Resilience Scale (10-item CD-RISC) in young adults. *Health Qual. Life Outcomes* **2011**, *9*, 63. [CrossRef] [PubMed]
37. Sánchez, M.I.S.; De Pedro, M.M.; Izquierdo, M.G. Propiedades psicométricas de la versión española de la escala de resiliencia de 10 ítems de Connor-Davidson (CD-RISC 10) en una muestra multiocupacional. *Rev. Latinoam. Psicol.* **2016**, *48*, 159–166. [CrossRef]
38. Rodríguez, A.; Ortunio, M. Resiliencia de trabajadores de la salud de una unidad de cuidados pediátricos. *Rev. Venez. Salud Pública* **2016**, *7*, 27–33.
39. Lee, S.-Y.; Tung, H.-H.; Peng, L.-N.; Chen, L.-K.; Hsu, C.-I.; Huang, Y.-L. Resilience among older cardiovascular disease patients with probable sarcopenia. *Arch. Gerontol. Geriatr.* **2020**, *86*, 103939. [CrossRef]
40. McIntyre, R.S.; Lee, Y. Preventing suicide in the context of the COVID-19 pandemic. *World Psychiatry* **2020**, *19*, 250–251. [CrossRef]
41. Etxebarria, N.O.; Dosil-Santamaria, M.; Picaza-Gorrochategui, M.; Idoiaga-Mondragon, N. Niveles de estrés, ansiedad y depresión en la primera fase del brote del COVID-19 en una muestra recogida en el norte de España. *Cad. Saúde Pública* **2020**, *36*, e00054020. [CrossRef]
42. Bădicu, G.; Grosz, R.W.; Balint, L. Influences of Practicing Leisure Sports Activities on Mental Health in Adult Population. In Proceedings of the European Proceedings of Social & Behavioural Sciences Edu World 2016 7th International Conference, Pitesti, Romania, 4–5 November 2017.
43. Lau, N.; Bradford, M.C.; Steineck, A.; Scott, S.; Bona, K.; Yi-Frazier, J.P.; McCauley, E.; Rosenberg, A.R. Examining key sociodemographic characteristics of adolescents and young adults with cancer: A post hoc analysis of the Promoting Resilience in Stress Management randomized clinical trial. *Palliat. Med.* **2019**, *34*, 336–348. [CrossRef]
44. Stone, A.L.; Nimmons, E.A.; Salcido, R.; Schnarrs, P. "My meemaw is a Cool Ass Person": Family Members as Role Models of Resilience for Sexual and Gender Diverse People of Color. *J. GLBT Fam. Stud.* **2020**, *16*, 241–257. [CrossRef]
45. McKinley, N.; McCain, R.S.; Convie, L.; Clarke, M.; Dempster, M.; Campbell, W.J.; Kirk, S.J. Resilience, burnout and coping mechanisms in UK doctors: A cross-sectional study. *BMJ Open* **2020**, *10*, e031765. [CrossRef] [PubMed]
46. Ortega-González, Z.; Mijares-Llamoza, B. Concepto de resiliencia: Desde la diferenciación de otros constructos, escuelas y enfoques. *Rev. Cient. Electron. Cienc. Hum.* **2018**, *39*, 30–43.
47. Zhang, X.; Bian, L.; Bai, X.; Konng, D.; Liu, L.; Chen, Q.; Li, N. The influence of job satisfaction, resilience and work engagement on turnover intention among villaje doctors in China: A cross-sectional study. *BMC Health Serv. Res.* **2020**, 1–11. [CrossRef]
48. Kim, S.; Kim, H.; Min, K.; Yoo, S.; Shin, Y.; Kim, E.; Jeon, S. Resilence as a protective factor for suicidal ideation among Korean Workers. *Psychiatr. Investig.* **2020**, *17*, 147–156. [CrossRef] [PubMed]
49. Lai, J.; Ma, S.; Wang, Y.; Cai, Z.; Hu, J.; Wei, N.; Wu, J.; Du, H.; Chen, T.; Li, R.; et al. Factors Associated with Mental Health Outcomes Among Health Care Workers Exposed to Coronavirus Disease. *JAMA Netw. Open* **2020**, *3*, e203976. [CrossRef]
50. García-Fernández, L.; Romero-Ferreiro, V.; López-Roldán, P.D.; Padilla, S.; Calero-Sierra, I.; Monzó-García, M.; Pérez-Martín, J.; Rodriguez-Jimenez, R. Mental health impact of COVID-19 pandemic on Spanish healthcare workers. *Psychol. Med.* **2020**, 1–3. [CrossRef]
51. Borji, M.; Memaryan, N.; Khorrami, Z.; Farshadnia, E.; Sadighpour, M. Spiritual Health and Resilience Among University Students: The Mediating Role of Self-Esteem. *Pastor. Psychol.* **2019**, *69*, 1–10. [CrossRef]

52. Zamani Sani, S.H.; Fathirezaie, Z.; Sadeghi-Bazargani, H.; Badicu, G.; Ebrahimi, S.; Grosz, R.W.; Sadeghi Bahmani, D.; Brand, S. Driving Accidents, Driving Violations, Symptoms of Attention-Deficit-Hyperactivity (ADHD) and Attentional Network Tasks. *Int. J. Environ. Res. Public Health* **2020**, *17*, 5238. [CrossRef]
53. Henshall, C.; Davey, Z.; Jackson, D. The implementation and evaluation of a resilience enhancement programme for nurses working in the forensic setting. *Int. J. Ment. Health Nurs.* **2020**, *29*, 508–520. [CrossRef]
54. Babanataj, R.; Mazdarani, S.; Hesamzadeh, A.; Gorji, M.A.H.; Cherati, J.Y. Resilience training: Effects on occupational stress and resilience of critical care nurses. *Int. J. Nurs. Prac.* **2018**, *25*, e12697. [CrossRef]
55. Cleveland, M.; Warhurst, A.; Legood, A. Experiencing Resilience through the Eyes of Early Career Social Workers. *Br. J. Soc. Work* **2019**, *49*, 1434–1451. [CrossRef]
56. Kaiser, T.; Janssen, B.; Schrader, S.; Geerling, G. Depressive symptoms, resilience, and personality traits in dry eye disease. *Arch. Clin. Exp. Ophthalmol.* **2019**, *257*, 591–599. [CrossRef] [PubMed]
57. Yen, J.-Y.; Lin, H.-C.; Chou, W.-P.; Liu, T.-L.; Ko, C.-H. Associations Among Resilience, Stress, Depression, and Internet Gaming Disorder in Young Adults. *Int. J. Environ. Res. Public Health* **2019**, *16*, 3181. [CrossRef]
58. Wang, L.; Xu, B.; Gu, Y.; Zhu, J.; Liang, Y. The mediating and moderating effects of resilience on the relationship between perceived stress and depression in heroin addicts. *J. Community Psychol.* **2018**, *47*, 495–503. [CrossRef] [PubMed]

Journal of
Clinical Medicine

MDPI

Article

Predicting Perceived Stress Related to the Covid-19 Outbreak through Stable Psychological Traits and Machine Learning Models

Luca Flesia [1,†], Merylin Monaro [2,*,†], Cristina Mazza [3], Valentina Fietta [2], Elena Colicino [4], Barbara Segatto [5] and Paolo Roma [3]

1 Associazione Novilunio Onlus, 35020 Ponte San Nicolò (PD), Italy; luca.flesia@ordinepsicologiveneto.it
2 Department of General Psychology, University of Padua, 35131 Padua, Italy; valefietta.vf@gmail.com
3 Department of Human Neuroscience, Sapienza University of Rome, 00185 Rome, Italy; mazzacristina87@gmail.com (C.M.); paolo.roma@uniroma1.it (P.R.)
4 Department of Environmental Medicine and Public Health, Icahn School of Medicine at Mount Sinai, New York, NY 10029, USA; colicinoelena@gmail.com
5 Department of Political Science, Law, and International Studies, University of Padua, 35123 Padua, Italy; barbara.segatto@unipd.it
* Correspondence: merylin.monaro@unipd.it; Tel.: +39-347-107-3377
† These authors contributed equally to this work.

Received: 22 September 2020; Accepted: 14 October 2020; Published: 19 October 2020

Abstract: The global SARS-CoV-2 outbreak and subsequent lockdown had a significant impact on people's daily lives, with strong implications for stress levels due to the threat of contagion and restrictions to freedom. Given the link between high stress levels and adverse physical and mental consequences, the COVID-19 pandemic is certainly a global public health issue. In the present study, we assessed the effect of the pandemic on stress levels in $N = 2053$ Italian adults, and characterized more vulnerable individuals on the basis of sociodemographic features and stable psychological traits. A set of 18 psycho-social variables, generalized regressions, and predictive machine learning approaches were leveraged. We identified higher levels of perceived stress in the study sample relative to Italian normative values. Higher levels of distress were found in women, participants with lower income, and participants living with others. Higher rates of emotional stability and self-control, as well as a positive coping style and internal locus of control, emerged as protective factors. Predictive learning models identified participants with high perceived stress, with a sensitivity greater than 76%. The results suggest a characterization of people who are more vulnerable to experiencing high levels of stress during the COVID-19 pandemic. This characterization may contribute to early and targeted intervention strategies.

Keywords: COVID-19; stress; personality; public health; mental health; coping

1. Introduction

SARS-Cov-2 (severe acute respiratory syndrome coronavirus 2; henceforth referred to as COVID-19) is a strain of coronavirus that can infect humans, attacking the lungs and causing symptoms ranging from those of the common cold to those of severe acute respiratory syndrome (SARS) [1]. While approximately 80% of those who are infected recover with no special treatment (i.e., they are either asymptomatic or suffer from mild pneumonia) [2], recent data have confirmed that older persons (60+ years old) [3] and persons with certain pre-existing medical conditions are more likely to develop serious respiratory distress that can lead to death (3–4% of the population) [4]. COVID-19 spreads very easily between persons and, at the time of writing, no drugs or biologics have proven effective for preventing or treating the virus [5,6].

COVID-19 was first identified in the Chinese region of Wuhan in December 2019 [6]. Between December 2019 and April 2020, the virus spread throughout the world, causing more than 5,000,000 infections and over 300,000 deaths [7]. On 11 March 2020, the World Health Organization (WHO) declared COVID-19 a pandemic [8]. To contain the number of victims and prevent the collapse of the healthcare system, most national governments imposed strict restrictions on residents' freedom, forcing those infected with the virus to self-isolate and requiring all residents (infected or not) to stay at home and move through public areas only for reasons of absolute necessity. Among Western governments, the Italian government was the first to apply such restrictions [9].

1.1. Psychological Impact of the Pandemic

A few weeks after the spread of COVID-19 in China, the first scientific studies investigating the psychological impact of the outbreak highlighted a mild to severe negative psychological impact of the event within a significant proportion of the Chinese population (53.8%); specifically, this impact on mental health was reported to include symptoms of anxiety, depression, and stress [10,11]. More broadly, the literature on the impact of infectious outbreaks on mental health shows that pandemics are extremely stressful events that force people to cope with totally unexpected, ambiguous, and uncertain situations [12]. Specifically, two main aspects of pandemics have been found to affect people's mental state. The first relates to danger (i.e., the fear of contagion), which can increase perceived threat and sometimes lead to panic, behavioral contagion, and an emotional epidemic [13,14]. The second regards the multiple and rapid changes to social, working, and familiar habits, due to self-isolation and social distancing measures [15–19]. The longer the duration of self-isolation, the more people experience frustration and boredom, along with concerns about infection [15].

Well-documented psychological reactions to epidemics include emotional distress, anxiety behaviors, sleeping disorders, fear, anger, depression, health concerns, a sense of powerlessness, and uncertainty [13,16,20–24]. Furthermore, studies examining the long-term consequences of infectious epidemics have shown that some individuals may even develop symptoms of post-traumatic stress disorder (PTSD) [12,25,26]. One review indicated that those who develop PTSD may experience the symptoms for 3 years following the end of the epidemic [15,23].

Stress is defined as an adaptive psycho-physical reaction to a physical, social or psychological stimulus, called a stressor [27]. Stress-related responses may be cognitive, emotional, behavioral, or physiological. Depending on the type, timing, and severity of exposure to a stressor, the resulting stress may become a risk factor for a number of illnesses, including those of a psychiatric or cardiovascular nature [28–32]. An emergency such as the COVID-19 outbreak might rightly be considered a severe stressor, as it is a new and unexpected situation with a potentially serious impact on health (experienced both personally and through loved ones) that also involves social restrictions [13]. Nevertheless, no event, in and of itself, is the precipitating cause of pathology and illness. Rather, it is the perception of stress (i.e., the degree to which one considers the event stressful) that accounts for the varying physical and mental responses to the situation [33]. In this sense, it is important to detect vulnerable persons early, and to promote effective preventive programs in order to treat such persons rapidly and limit negative psychological outcomes. The identification of psycho-social risk and resilience factors for psychological distress during the COVID-19 emergency comprises a significant step in this direction [34].

1.2. Risk and Protective Factors for Psychological Outcomes During the Pandemic

To date, studies on the psychological impact of COVID-19 have mainly focused on the role of sociodemographic variables (e.g., gender, age, education level, and social connections) in moderating reactions to the outbreak [10,11,24,35,36]. The identified sociodemographic risk factors for psychological distress include gender (female), age (18–30 or 60+ years old), student status, education level, perception of the public health system, specific physical symptoms (e.g., coryza, cough, sore throat, headache), and a low reported level of health [10,24,35]. For Chinese students, living in an urban area, having a stable family income, living with parents, and having good social support were also found to protect against anxiety [11].

In addition to investigating sociodemographic factors, many studies have also outlined the role of certain dispositional traits in modulating responses to stressful events. However, these constructs have been poorly investigated in relation to the psychological impact of epidemics and, specifically, COVID-19. More generally, research has shown how individual differences, including dispositional traits, can explain life outcomes [37]. According to the theory of traits (or dispositional theory), individual differences may be explained by certain predispositions (traits), which are expressed in a relatively stable way across situations and time. Traits comprise a person's manner of thinking, feeling, perceiving, and relating to others [37]. Based on these considerations, dispositional traits might play a relevant role in predicting perceived stress in relation to COVID-19.

Coping is one of the most widely studied dispositional traits, and it has been found to be significant in modulating responses to stressful events. Coping is defined as the effort to solve personal and interpersonal problems in an attempt to master, minimize, or tolerate stress and conflict [38]. Distinct coping strategies have been found to be differentially associated with specific emotional responses [39], physiological stress responses [40], and self-efficacy [41,42]. One investigation into the role of coping strategies during a virus outbreak (2009 H1N1 flu pandemic) found coping style to influence the perceived risk of contagion and vaccination intentions among Canadian adults [43]. Another study, based in Singapore, found coping strategies to be associated with post-traumatic outcomes within visitors to community health care services during the national outbreak of SARS [23].

As regards emotional self-regulation and adaptation to the world, self-control may represent a significant protective factor. There is empirical evidence that people with high dispositional self-control have better psychological adjustment and impulse control [44]; this suggests that good self-control may mitigate the influence of a negative environment. Similarly, perceived control over life outcomes has been shown to be positively associated with well-being and health-related quality of life, and negatively associated with emotional distress, in the context of stressful events [45,46]. In this regard, locus of control [47] is a relevant concept, describing the degree to which an individual believes that they have control over the outcome of life events, as opposed to feeling that their life is subject to external forces beyond their control. Finally, among the many individual difference variables that might influence reactions to COVID-19, personality traits merit significant attention. Several studies have highlighted an association between the Big Five personality traits [48] and various health behaviors, such as sedentary behavior [49], sexual health behavior [50], physical activity [51], and alcohol consumption [52].

The first aim of the present study was to investigate the impact of the COVID-19 pandemic and the related government-imposed restrictions on perceived stress in a Western country (i.e., Italy). As reported above, most studies on the psychological impact of COVID-19 have related to the Chinese population. However, countries differ from one another in many important aspects (i.e., social, cultural, political, and economic aspects, to name only a few); consequently, psychological responses may also vary between contexts and communities, revealing unique qualitative and quantitative psychological reactions and psychological needs.

Hypothesis 1 (H1). *Our sample of Italian adults, collected during the COVID-19 outbreak, would show higher levels of perceived stress compared to Italian normative values.*

The second aim of the study was to confirm the role of certain sociodemographic factors in modulating stress responses to the COVID-19 pandemic, as reported in the recent literature.

Hypothesis 2 (H2). *(a) Participants who were female, younger, and students, with a lower level of education and lower income, would report higher levels of stress, and (b) participants who were living with others would report lower levels of psychological distress.*

The third aim of the work was to investigate the association between certain stable psychological traits and psychological distress relating to the current situation. To this end, participants were tested for coping strategies, self-control, locus of control, and select personality traits.

Hypothesis 3 (H3). *(a) Participants with positive coping strategies, higher levels of self-control, an internal locus of control, and higher levels of emotional stability would report lower levels of stress, and (b) participants with negative coping strategies, lower levels of self-control, an external locus of control, and lower levels of emotional stability would report higher levels of stress.*

Finally, with the goal of anticipating persons in need of treatment and improving the targeting and overall effectiveness of preventive programs, we aimed at developing machine learning models to predict individual psychological responses to the COVID-19 pandemic, based on sociodemographic and psychological variables with maximal sensitivity in classifying subjects with high versus low levels of perceived stress.

To summarize, the study was novel in the following two respects: first, it considered the role of not only sociodemographic variables, but also stable psychological traits, as predictors of a stressful reaction to COVID-19; and second, it leveraged machine learning techniques to identify people at the greatest risk of developing severe and negative psychological outcomes due to the pandemic.

2. Materials and Methods

2.1. Measures

To test the abovementioned hypotheses, we implemented a cross-sectional study. Using Google Forms, we designed an ad hoc online questionnaire to collect data on participants' stress reactions to COVID-19, demographical variables, and psychological traits. The questionnaire also assessed the following sociodemographic factors: gender, age, education, number of family members and/or others living in the household, monthly household income, and student status. Subsequently, we administered five standardized questionnaires, as follows:

- The Italian Version of the 10-item Perceived Stress Scale (PSS-10; Cronbach's alpha = 0.74) [53]. The PSS-10 is a frequently used psychological instrument to measure perceived stress [54]. Respondents are asked to answer 10 questions pertaining to the frequency of experiences of stressful situations during the last month on a five-point scale ranging from 0 (never) to 4 (very often) [55,56]. Example items include "In the last month, how often have you been upset because of something that happened unexpectedly?" Higher scores indicate higher levels of perceived stress. Moreover, in the present study, the score corresponding to 1.5 SD above the Italian normative score [53] was used as a cut-off to divide participants into two classes: low perceived stress (males: PSS-10 score <24.35; females: PSS-10 score <24.55) and high perceived stress (males: PSS-10 score ≥24.35; females: PSS score-10 ≥24.55);
- The Italian Shortened Version of the Coping Orientations to the Problems Experienced (COPE-NVI-25; Cronbach's alpha of factors range 0.68–0.95) [57]. The COPE-NVI-25 is a multi-dimensional inventory that assesses individual differences in coping styles. It is comprised of 25 items, which are rated on a 4-point scale ranging from 1 (I usually don't do this at all) to 4 (I usually do this a lot) [58]. The instrument includes five subscales corresponding to five different coping styles: social support, avoidance strategies, positive attitude, problem solving, and turning to religion [59]. An example item is "I admit to myself that I can't deal with it, and quit trying" (avoidance strategies). A higher score on a particular subscale indicates a greater use of that specific coping strategy.
- The Italian translation of the Brief Self-Control Scale (BSCS; Cronbach's alpha = 0.85) [44]. The BSCS measures individual differences in dispositional capacity for self-control. The scale is comprised of 13 items that are rated on a five-point scale ranging from 1 (not at all) to 5 (very much). An example item is "I do certain things that are bad for me, if they are fun." Higher scores on the BSCS

indicate a greater capacity for self-control, and they are also correlated with better psychological adjustment, interpersonal skills, and emotional responses [44];

- The Italian Short Version of the Locus of Control (LOC) Scale [60]. This 20-item questionnaire is used to measure generalized expectancies relating to an internal versus external locus of control, rated via dichotomous options ("Yes" vs. "No"), similar to Rotter's original Internal–External Locus of Control Scale [47]. An example item is "To do well in life, luck is more important than commitment." Respondents with an internal locus of control (i.e., a high score on the internal LOC scale) tend to attribute life outcomes—and general life events—to their own behavior, whereas those with a prevalent external locus of control (i.e., a high score on the external LOC scale) tend to attribute life events to fate, others, or external causes beyond their control [47,61];
- The Italian Version of the 10-item Big Five Inventory (BFI-10; Spearman–Brown coefficients ≥0.50) [62]. The BFI-10 assesses personality traits according to the five-factor approach [63]. It is comprised of 10 items rated on a five-point scale ranging from 1 (strongly disagree) to 5 (strongly agree), measuring five dimensions of personality, which are extraversion, agreeableness, conscientiousness, neuroticism (or, if reversed, emotional stability), and openness [64]. An example item is "I see myself as someone who is outgoing, sociable" (extraversion). The higher the score on a particular subscale, the more that specific dimension represents a characteristic trait of the respondent's personality.

The complete list of 18 variables that were extracted from the responses to the questionnaire is provided in the Supplementary Materials. The present research was designed in accordance with the Declaration of Helsinki and approved by the ethics committee for psychological research at the University of Padova (protocol number 3576, unique code 189B46FE116994F1A8D1077B835D83BB).

2.2. Participants and Procedure

Data were collected during the period of 20–31 March, 2020. Participants were recruited online through an invitation posted on social media (Facebook and WhatsApp). This approach of online recruitment was selected primarily due to the lockdown situation, which prevented us from collecting data in the laboratory. According to the aim of the study, it was necessary for us to capture the psychological state of participants at the time of the pandemic; thus an a posteriori study would not have provided useful and reliable information.

Participants were invited to complete an anonymous online questionnaire to report their personal experiences with the COVID-19 emergency and their mental state. The inclusion criteria were the following: (a) living in Italy at the time of data collection and (b) being aged 18+ years (18 years is the legal age in Italy, defined by the capacity to act and be emancipated). Participation was voluntary. All participants were required to read and provide informed consent before beginning the online questionnaire. They received no compensation for their participation. In total, 2072 volunteers took part in the study. Of these, 19 were excluded on the basis that they responded to the questionnaire twice (we kept only their first response). Thus, the final sample was comprised of 2053 participants, of whom 1555 were female, 480 were male, and 18 were reported as "other." The participants' average age was 35.81 (SD = 13.19; range: 18–83) and their average education level was 15.35 years (SD = 3.43; range: 5–21). A more detailed description of the sample's demographic characteristics is provided in the Supplementary Materials. It has been calculated that a sample size of 2053 is sufficiently large to achieve at least a statistical power $(1-\beta) = 0.90$ in a linear multivariable regression analysis involving 18 predictors, given a significance level $\alpha = 0.05$ and an effect size of 0.356 [65]. Data are provided in the Supplementary Materials.

2.3. Data Analysis Methodology

2.3.1. Statistics

Data analysis was conducted using the JASP software [66]. A single sample t-test (t, two-sided) was performed in relation to the PSS-10 score, in order to determine whether the sample's true mean (μ) was statistically different from that of the known population (m_0). A multivariable regression analysis was run to investigate the relationship between the PSS-10 score and the independent variables that were hypothesized to impact the level of perceived stress. The collinearity assumption was checked prior to running the model, using the tolerance and variance inflation factor (VIF). As a rule of thumb, if VIF >10 and tolerance <0.1, the assumption is greatly violated, whereas if VIF >1 and tolerance <0.2, the model may be biased [67]. The results indicated that the collinearity assumption was not violated by any of the independent variables entered in the regression model. The analysis was performed using the stepwise variable selection method, which identified predictors with a significant ($p < 0.05$) individual association with the outcome (PSS-10 score). The results were reported using unstandardized coefficients, as recommended by Friedrich [68].

2.3.2. Classification Models

Recently, researchers in different scientific fields, including the clinical and social sciences, have emphasized the utility of focusing on prediction, rather than explanation, during data analysis [69–72]. This increased attention to predictive models may be largely attributed to the significant spread of machine learning (ML)—a branch of artificial intelligence that trains algorithms on data samples (i.e., training sets) in order to make predictions on completely new data (i.e., test sets) without being explicitly programmed to do so [73]. As regards psychology, ML techniques have been shown to be particularly useful for predicting human behavior, including high-risk behavior; thus, they may be applied to improve the effectiveness and targeting of preventive programs and interventions [74]. In brief, ML models are capable of predicting the behavior of individual subjects, allowing greater attention to be paid to those considered most critical [69].

In the present study, ML algorithms were trained on psycho-social data to identify subjects who were more likely to present high levels of perceived stress during the COVID-19 emergency, and who were consequently at the greatest risk of developing psychological symptoms, including those of PTSD. For this purpose, participants were split into two classes: high perceived stress and low perceived stress. The high perceived stress class included participants with a PSS-10 score of more than 1.5 *SD* above the Italian population mean (n = 393) for men and women, respectively. Conversely, the low perceived stress class included participants whose PSS-10 did not exceed 1.5 *SD* above the Italian normative value (n = 1642). It should be noted that participants who reported their gender as "other" (n = 18) were excluded from this analysis, as the Italian normative values were available for males and females only [53].

As ML models are built to fit particular data, it is important to test how each model fits new (i.e., unseen) data. For this reason, part of the data (the training set) is generally used to train and validate the model, while another part (the test set) is used to test the model's accuracy on new examples [73,75]. This procedure guarantees the model generalization and increases the replicability of the results [76,77]. In the present study, 20% [73,75] of the participants were randomly chosen and retained as the test set. Accordingly, the training set consisted of 1628 participants (314 with high perceived stress and 1314 with low perceived stress), and the test set consisted of 407 participants (79 with high perceived stress and 328 with low perceived stress).

In the first step, feature selection was performed to remove redundant and irrelevant features and to increase model generalization by reducing overfitting and noise in the data [78]. A good strategy for feature selection is to identify the subset of features that are highly correlated with the class to predict, but not correlated with each other [78]. This procedure was performed in the present study using the correlation-based feature selector (CFS) in the WEKA 3.9 software [79].

The problem of class imbalance was addressed while running the classification algorithms. The ratio between participants with high perceived stress and those with low perceived stress was approximately 1:5. As ML methods work best with balanced datasets, it is necessary to account for any class imbalance, especially when training examples are limited—a condition that is frequently met by datasets in health and clinical psychology [80]. At the same time, it is equally important for ML models to be built on samples that are representative of the population, reflecting real distribution [80].

One strategy to overcome these two limitations consists of altering the relative costs associated with misclassifying the minority and majority classes, in order to compensate for the class imbalance [81]. In the present study, ML algorithms were set in such a way that any algorithmic error made in classifying the minority class (high perceived stress) was weighted four times more than any error in classifying the majority class (low perceived stress). This cost-modifying strategy has been shown to provide better results than other methods in addressing the class imbalance problem [81]. Moreover, it should be noted that, for the goal of the present task, it was more beneficial to minimize false negatives than to minimize false positives (i.e., to have a model with high sensitivity rather than high specificity). In other words, it was more important to identify people who were truly at risk than to avoid misclassifying people who were not truly at risk.

ML models were trained and validated on the training sample (n= 1628) through a 10-fold cross-validation procedure using the WEKA 3.9 software [79]. The different algorithms (i.e., logistic regression [82], support vector machine (SVM) [83], Naïve Bayes [84], random forest [85]) were chosen as representatives of different classification strategies, to ensure that the results would be stable across classifiers and not dependent on specific model assumptions (details on the parameters of the ML classifiers are reported in the Supplementary Materials). K-fold cross-validation is a resampling procedure that seeks to reduce the variance in model performance relative to the performance that may be obtained from a single training set and a single test set. The procedure consists of portioning the sample into k subsets (i.e., folds; in the present study, k = 10), and using k-1 (i.e., 9) subsets to train the model and the remaining subset to validate the model's accuracy. This is repeated k (i.e., 10) times [86]. The final model metrics are obtained by averaging the metrics obtained in all validation subsets. In the present study, the models developed from the 10-fold cross-validation procedure were tested on the test sample (n = 407).

3. Results

The main results of the data analysis are reported in this section. A more complete descriptive analysis of each variable, including the composition of high perceived stress versus low perceived stress samples, is reported in the Supplementary Materials.

3.1. Perceived Stress in Response to the COVID-19 Emergency

The average PSS-10 score of the entire sample was 18.81 (SD = 6.25). Analyzing the responses of males and females separately (note that participants who reported a gender of "other" were excluded from this analysis due to a lack of normative data), males obtained an average score of 16.71 (SD = 6.91) and females obtained an average score of 19.44 (SD = 6.79). To determine whether the sample mean statistically differed from that of the Italian normative population (males: average = 15.2, SD = 6.1; females: average = 16.3, SD = 5.5) [53], a one-sample t-test was run separately for each gender. Statistically significant results emerged for both males ($t_{(479)} = 4.79$, $p < 0.001$, $d = 0.22$, 95% CI for Cohen's d (0.13, 0.31)) and females ($t_{(1554)} = 18.21$, $p < 0.001$, $d = 0.46$, 95% CI for Cohen's d (0.41, 0.510)). The PSS-10 items showing the greatest increase in participants with high perceived stress (1.5 SD above the population mean) were those related to loss of control over one's life (M = 3.09, SD = 0.80) and frequently feeling nervous or stressed (M = 3.51, SD = 0.60) (see Supplementary Materials for an item-by-item analysis).

3.2. The Role of Sociodemographic Variables in Predicting Perceived Stress

A first multiple regression analysis was run, including sociodemographic variables that have been shown to potentially impact the level of perceived stress during a pandemic [10,11,24,35,36]. The PSS-10 score was set as the dependent variable, while gender (male), age, education, monthly income, number of family members, and student status (student) were entered as covariates. The final model accounted for a significant proportion of the variance in the level of perceived stress ($R^2 = 0.103$, adjusted $R^2 = 0.101$, $F\text{-change}_{(1,2029)} = 12.009$, $p < 0.001$). All of the aforementioned variables, with the exception of student status, were found to contribute to the level of perceived stress. Results are reported in Table 1.

Table 1. Multiple Linear Regression Model Predicting the Level of Perceived Stress Based on Sociodemographic Variables.

	ΔR²	Unstandardized Coefficients (B)	S.E.	*t*	*p*	95% CI Lower Bound	95% CI Upper Bound
(Intercept)		25.342	0.987	25.665	$4.845e^{-126}$	23.405	27.278
Age	0.067	−0.121	0.012	−10.506	$3.540e^{-25}$	−0.143	−0.098
Gender (male)	0.024	−2.406	0.345	−6.968	$4.321e^{-12}$	−3.084	−1.729
Education	0.004	−0.081	0.044	−1.842	0.066	−0.168	0.005
Household members	0.003	0.453	0.129	3.500	$4.748e^{-4}$	0.199	0.706
Monthly income	0.005	−0.463	0.134	−3.465	$5.403e^{-4}$	−0.725	−0.201

Note: Root Mean Square Error (RMSE) = 6.56. Analysis of Variance (ANOVA) $F_{(5,2029)} = 46.65$, $p < 0.001$.

3.3. The Role of Stable Psychological Traits in Predicting Perceived Stress

To better understand the role of stable psychological traits in predicting the level of perceived stress (PSS-10 score), a second multiple linear regression was run, adding to the previous model the scores of the five coping styles measured by the COPE-NVI-25 (COPE positive, COPE problem, COPE avoidance, COPE religion and COPE support), the BSCS total score, the internal LOC score, and the scores for the five personality traits measured by the BFI-10 (BFI-10 agreeableness, BFI-10 conscientiousness, BFI-10 emotional stability, BFI-10 extraversion and BFI-10 openness). This second model accounted for a larger proportion of the variance in the level of perceived stress ($R^2 = 0.356$, adjusted $R^2 = 0.352$, $F\text{-change}_{(1,2022)} = 5.908$, $p < 0.05$) compared to the previous model. BFI-10 emotional stability, COPE positive, age, BCSC total score, gender (male), COPE avoidance, internal LOC, number of family members, COPE support, monthly income, and BFI-10 conscientiousness were identified as significant predictors of the level of perceived stress during the COVID-19 epidemic (see Table 2). Education, COPE religion, COPE problem solving, BFI-10 agreeableness, BFI-10 extraversion and BFI-10 openness were excluded.

Table 2. Multiple Linear Regression Model Predicting the Level of Perceived Stress Based on Sociodemographic Variables and Stable Psychological Traits.

	ΔR²	Unstandardized Coefficients (B)	S.E.	*t*	*p*	95% CI Lower Bound	95% CI Upper Bound
(Intercept)	0.000	36.238	1.540	23.531	<0.001	33.218	39.258
BFI-10 emotional stability	0.221	−0.959	0.067	−14.346	<0.001	−1.091	−0.828
COPE positive	0.047	−2.357	0.211	−11.195	<0.001	−2.770	−1.944
Age	0.033	−0.070	0.010	−6.814	<0.001	−0.090	−0.050
BSCS total score	0.018	−0.127	0.019	−6.646	<0.001	−0.165	−0.090
Gender (male)	0.016	−1.883	0.302	−6.228	<0.001	−2.476	−1.290
COPE avoidance	0.007	1.411	0.328	4.307	<0.001	0.768	2.053
Household members	0.003	0.406	0.108	3.751	<0.001	0.194	0.619
BFI-10 conscientiousness	0.003	0.276	0.098	2.809	0.005	0.083	0.469
COPE support	0.002	0.519	0.168	3.087	0.002	0.189	0.849
Monthly income	0.002	−0.283	0.111	−2.543	0.011	−0.502	−0.065
Internal LOC	0.002	−0.145	0.060	−2.431	0.015	−0.262	−0.028

Note: RMSE = 5.57. ANOVA $F_{(12,2022)} = 101.49$, $p < 0.001$. BFI-10 = 10-item Big Five Inventory; COPE = Coping Orientations to the Problems Experienced; BSCS = Brief Self-Control Scale; LOC = Locus of Control.

3.4. Machine Learning Classification Models

Ultimately, the 18 questionnaire variables were considered predictors of perceived stress. The entire list of predictors, along with their descriptions, is provided in the Supplementary Materials. Of these 18 variables, the following 7 were identified as the best set of predictors using correlation-based feature selection: age, monthly income, COPE avoidance, COPE positive, BSCS total score, BFI-10 emotional stability, and BFI-10 agreeableness. Using these predictors, ML algorithms were trained and tested according to the procedure described in the "Data Analysis" section. Classification results for the test set are reported in Table 3, which quantifies predictive performance according to the following metrics: receiver operating characteristic curve (ROC) area, precision, recall and F-measure (F1 score). It is worth noting that the classifiers showed an ROC area ranging from 0.70 to 0.78 in the test set. However, the random forest algorithm highlighted the lower sensitivity (recall) of the high perceived stress class compared to the other classifiers, making it a weaker model for the purposes of prediction.

Table 3. Metrics of the ML Models Tested on the 407 New Participants (Test Set).

Algorithm	ROC Area	Class	Precision	Recall	F-Measure
Logistic	0.782	High perceived stress	0.349	0.759	0.478
		Low perceived stress	0.919	0.659	0.767
SVM	0.697	High perceived stress	0.337	0.747	0.465
		Low perceived stress	0.914	0.646	0.757
Naïve Bayes	0.776	High perceived stress	0.361	0.709	0.479
		Low perceived stress	0.909	0.698	0.790
Random forest	0.776	High perceived stress	0.438	0.532	0.480
		Low perceived stress	0.881	0.835	0.858

Note: ROC = receiver operating characteristic curve; SVM = support vector machine.

4. Discussion and Conclusions

The present study measured the impact of the COVID-19 emergency on perceived levels of stress, taking into account sociodemographic variables and stable psychological traits. The results confirmed that participants perceived the COVID-19 crisis as a stressful experience; in the present sample, the level of perceived stress was higher than that of the general population in a non-emergency condition. Indeed, almost 20% of the sample scored above the results from the normative data on measures of perceived stress. These results are in line with the findings of recent studies on the psychological impact of COVID-19 [10,11,87] and the international literature on epidemic outbreaks [13]. The mean values of the single items of the PSS-10 suggest that, in addition to nervousness and stress, feelings of being unable to control one's personal life accounted for the majority of participants' perceived stress. This suggests that the unpredictability and uncontrollability of the pandemic may play a significant role in determining levels of perceived stress during the crisis. Moreover, it may reflect participants' attitudes toward the significant lifestyle changes demanded of them due to the lockdown and other restrictive measures.

As regards sociodemographic variables, the results suggest that the female gender is associated with higher levels of stress. This is consistent with the literature indicating gender differences in the psychological response to COVID-19 [24,88] and other epidemics [89]; it is also in line with the normative data for the general population. Consistent with other studies (20,30), the present study found an association between higher incomes and lower levels of perceived stress. One explanation for this is that higher incomes might be related to less concern about the economic effects of self-isolation and/or with more comfortable housing solutions (e.g., larger living spaces, access to outdoor spaces (such as gardens), and access to leisure activities). Moreover, people with higher incomes may be more likely to perform work that can easily and fully transition to the online environment, thereby reducing some sources of stress.

In the present sample, older age was found to be associated with lower levels of stress. This finding might appear surprising, since it contradicts both the results of studies on the Chinese population [24,35] and the association between older age and higher COVID-19 mortality. However, the result is in line with recent Italian data [87]. Several studies have indicated age-related differences in coping and locus of control, with older adults presenting greater self-control and emotional self-regulation relative to younger adults [90–92]. Considering the current pandemic, older people may be more used to staying at home, so their daily routines might be less impacted by mandatory self-isolation measures. Data from previous investigations on age differences in stress responses to the SARS epidemic reflect inconsistencies [93,94], but sociopolitical and cultural aspects, such as differences in elder care services and policies, might account for these discrepancies.

The present study did not find education to be a significant predictor of the level of perceived stress. The large percentage of highly educated participants in the sample might partially explain this finding. However, prior research on this subject has generated mixed results—recent studies on the Chinese population [24,35] have found that education does not seem to affect mental health, while data from a Spanish sample [88] and from previous studies on psychological adjustment to SARS [95] have confirmed an association between a higher level of education and better mental health. The present study also found that living alone or with few family members was a protective factor against perceived stress. We might argue that this condition both conveys a sense of protection from contagion and offers continuity with pre-epidemic economic and social conditions. Moreover, when cohabiting with family members, concern for loved ones might contribute to increasing perceived stress.

As regards psychological variables, emotional stability was found to be an important protective factor. According to the five-factors model [63], people with high emotional stability remain calm in response to stressful situations, and view problems in proportion to their importance. As a result, they tend to worry less about problems than do people with low emotional stability [96]. Many studies have found that emotional stability is able to buffer stress responses to adverse events [97,98]. In the present study, conscientiousness and agreeableness were found to predict psychological distress. Generally speaking, individuals who score high on agreeableness tend to dislike conflict and be less suspicious of others; generally, they seek to pacify and mediate. In this sense, agreeable people might be more flexible and accepting when faced with unexpected and undesired situations, such as restrictions and changes to daily routines. Conscientious people are more likely to perceive lower levels of stress (see correlation analysis). According to the literature, they are more aware of their actions and tend to exhibit more goal-oriented behavior. In this sense, in times of self-isolation, conscientious people might have a greater tolerance for frustration and imposition relative to less conscientious people, who might engage in more impulsive behavior [96]. Moreover, previous research has indicated that conscientiousness may influence adaptive behavior, especially in health-related programs [99,100].

The present study found higher levels of dispositional self-control to predict lower levels of psychological distress in response to the COVID-19 emergency. Personal self-control skills may play a role in determining tolerance to restrictions to personal freedom during self-isolation. This result further suggests that self-regulatory processes may have a strong influence on responses to the outbreak. The results regarding dispositional self-control are consistent with those relating to the emotional stability trait of the Big Five model. In fact, these dimensions are often correlated [101], and this specific pattern may indicate the importance of personal skills, such as the ability to remain calm, and maintain emotional balance and a sense of acceptance. In this sense, practices that enhance emotional stability and acceptance, such as mindfulness, could be useful in reducing the stressful impact of the emergency [102,103]. The results concerning coping styles are also in line with this. Besides confirming the protective effect of functional coping styles and the adverse impact of dysfunctional coping styles, the results of the present study suggest that people who use a positive attitude as a coping strategy may be much less likely to experience psychological distress during the present emergency. Such persons may appraise the emergency as a unique opportunity, and feel less need for psychological support. In contrast, the present findings suggest that people who use avoidance strategies may be more likely to experience higher levels of stress during the emergency. These results are consistent with the findings of previous investigations into the relation between coping style and response to an epidemic [23,43,104,105].

The results relating to dispositional locus of control indicate that people with an internal locus of control may be less likely to feel stressed. Again, these results suggest that the more people are inclined to confidently rely on themselves, the better they will cope with uncertainty and change. Several studies have indicated an association between an internal locus of control and self-efficacy and emotional stability [106,107]. Furthermore, previous studies have found a relation between an internal locus of control and the positive appraisal of an emerging infectious disease outbreak [93]. It could be hypothesized that people with an internal locus of control interpret self-isolating as something that they determine and enact for themselves as a protective behavior, rather than something that is imposed on them; this might account for their lower levels of perceived stress.

Overall, the results of the present study identify some population subgroups that may be more vulnerable to experiencing stress during the COVID-19 emergency. Specifically, a set of seven psycho-social variables may identify a high percentage of people experiencing high stress during the COVID-19 pandemic, with sensitivity approaching 0.759 (ROC area of predictive models ranging between 0.70 and 0.78). According to this model, we may develop targeted preventive interventions. Furthermore, self-regulatory skills (including emotional stability, an internal locus of control, and self-control) were shown to be a protective factor, indicating the importance of raising awareness of these skills during the emergency and offering training and education to increase personal abilities in these areas (e.g., mindfulness programs).

The present research aimed at improving our understanding of the possible risk and protective factors for high perceived stress during the COVID-19 outbreak. It is worth noting that all data were collected from an Italian population. Therefore, the findings were inevitably influenced by specific contextual and socio-cultural aspects. Further investigations involving people of different ethnicities and residents of other countries would deepen our understanding of the generalizability of these results, and the effective influence of psychological traits. In this regard, the open access data reported in the Supplementary Materials may contribute to facilitating comparisons between ethnicities, countries, and specific traumatic events.

Some further limitations should be considered when interpreting the findings of this research. First, participants were recruited via an online link posted on social networks. While online recruitment guarantees large samples, it does not guarantee sample representativeness. For this reason, very vulnerable groups, such as homeless or low-income persons, may not be well represented in this study. Similarly, the average age of the sample was young, predominantly female, and largely well educated, as indicative of a sample that is more likely to participate in an online survey. Second, the use of self-report measures did not enable us to verify the reliability of the responses, or to ensure that participants correctly understood the questions. Future research should aim at overcoming these shortcomings.

Finally, future research should also investigate the interplay and mutual interrelationship between protective and risk factors, to improve the targeting and overall effectiveness of preventive programs and interventions. Indeed, the literature suggests that, during a pandemic, it is extremely important for people to sustain their use of psychological services, either online or in the context of social distancing [108,109]. This is particularly essential for those who are more vulnerable to experiencing high levels of stress, and it is important that we ensure that such persons can access timely and high-quality psychological services in order to prevent the development of chronic outcomes, including PTSD.

Supplementary Materials: The following are available online at http://www.mdpi.com/2077-0383/9/10/3350/s1, Table S1: Descriptive statistics, Table S2: Item by item analysis of the PSS-10, Table S3: List of predictors, Table S4: Details on ML classifiers parameters.

Author Contributions: Conceptualization, L.F. and M.M.; methodology, M.M., L.F. and V.F.; formal analysis, M.M., V.F. and E.C.; investigation, M.M., L.F. and V.F.; data curation, M.M. and V.F.; writing—original draft preparation, M.M., L.F. and V.F.; writing—review and editing, M.M., V.F., L.F., C.M., E.C., B.S. and P.R.; supervision, C.M. and P.R.; funding acquisition, P.R. All authors have read and agreed to the published version of the manuscript.

Funding: This research received no external funding.

Conflicts of Interest: The authors declare no conflict of interest.

References

1. Rothan, H.A.; Byrareddy, S.N. The epidemiology and pathogenesis of coronavirus disease (COVID-19) outbreak. *J. Autoimmun.* **2020**, *109*, 102433. [CrossRef] [PubMed]
2. Wu, Z.; McGoogan, J.M. Characteristics of and important lessons from the coronavirus disease 2019 (COVID-19) outbreak in China. *JAMA* **2020**, *323*, 1239. [CrossRef]
3. Kluge, H.H.P.; WHO Regional Office for Europe. Supporting Older People During the COVID-19 Pandemic is Everyone's Business. Available online: https://www.euro.who.int/en/health-topics/health-emergencies/coronavirus-covid-19/news/news/2020/4/supporting-older-people-during-the-covid-19-pandemic-is-everyones-business (accessed on 11 July 2020).
4. Wang, Y.; Wang, Y.; Chen, Y.; Qin, Q. Unique epidemiological and clinical features of the emerging 2019 novel coronavirus pneumonia (COVID-19) implicate special control measures. *J. Med. Virol.* **2020**, *92*, 568–576. [CrossRef]
5. Cunningham, A.C.; Goh, H.P.; Koh, D. Treatment of COVID-19: Old tricks for new challenges. *Crit. Care* **2020**, *24*, 1–2. [CrossRef]
6. Wu, D.; Wu, T.; Liu, Q.; Yang, Z. The SARS-CoV-2 outbreak: What we know. *Int. J. Infect. Dis.* **2020**, *94*, 44–48. [CrossRef] [PubMed]
7. WHO Coronavirus Disease (COVID-19) Dashboard. Available online: https://covid19.who.int (accessed on 11 July 2020).
8. World Health Organization (WHO). WHO Director-General's Opening Remarks at the Mission Briefing on COVID-19. Available online: https://www.who.int/dg/speeches/detail/who-director-general-s-opening-remarks-at-the-mission-briefing-on-covid-19---26-february-2020 (accessed on 11 March 2020).
9. Ren, X. Pandemic and lockdown: A territorial approach to COVID-19 in China, Italy and the United States. *Eurasian Geogr. Econ.* **2020**, 1–12. [CrossRef]
10. Wang, C.; Pan, R.; Wan, X.; Tan, Y.; Xu, L.; Ho, C.S.H.; Ho, R.C.M. Immediate psychological responses and associated factors during the initial stage of the 2019 coronavirus disease (COVID-19) epidemic among the general population in China. *Int. J. Environ. Res. Public Health* **2020**, *17*, 1729. [CrossRef] [PubMed]
11. Cao, W.; Fang, Z.; Hou, G.; Han, M.; Xu, X.; Dong, J.; Zheng, J. The psychological impact of the COVID-19 epidemic on college students in China. *Psychiatry Res.* **2020**, *287*, 112934. [CrossRef]
12. Mak, I.W.C.; Chung, Y.M.G.; Pan, P.C.; Yiu, M.G.C.; Chan, V.L. Long-term psychiatric morbidities among SARS survivors. *Gen. Hosp. Psychiatry* **2009**, *31*, 318–326. [CrossRef]
13. Huremović, D. *Psychiatry of Pandemics: A Mental Health Response to Infection Outbreak*; Springer International Publishing: Cham, Switzerland, 2019.
14. Li, Z.; Ge, J.; Yang, M.; Feng, J.; Qiao, M.; Jiang, R.; Bi, J.; Zhan, G.; Xu, X.; Wang, L.; et al. Vicarious traumatization in the general public, members, and non-members of medical teams aiding in COVID-19 control. *Brain Behav. Immun.* **2020**, *88*, 916–919. [CrossRef]
15. Brooks, S.K.; Webster, R.K.; Smith, E.L.; Woodland, L.; Wessely, S.; Greenberg, N.; Rubin, G.J. The psychological impact of quarantine and how to reduce it: Rapid review of the evidence. *Lancet* **2020**, *395*, 912–920. [CrossRef]
16. Xiang, Y.-T.; Yang, Y.; Li, W.; Zhang, L.; Zhang, Q.; Cheung, T.; Ng, C.H. Timely mental health care for the 2019 novel coronavirus outbreak is urgently needed. *Lancet Psychiatry* **2020**, *7*, 228–229. [CrossRef]
17. Mazza, C.; Ricci, E.; Marchetti, D.; Fontanesi, L.; Di Giandomenico, S.; Verrocchio, M.C.; Roma, P. How personality relates to distress in parents during the COVID-19 lockdown: The mediating role of child's emotional and behavioral difficulties and the moderating effect of living with other people. *Int. J. Environ. Res. Public Health* **2020**, *17*, 6236. [CrossRef]

18. Fontanesi, L.; Marchetti, D.; Mazza, C.; Di Giandomenico, S.; Roma, P.; Verrocchio, M.C. The effect of the COVID-19 lockdown on parents: A call to adopt urgent measures. *Psychol. Trauma Theory Res. Pract. Policy* **2020**, *12*, S79–S81. [CrossRef] [PubMed]
19. Roma, P.; Monaro, M.; Muzi, L.; Colasanti, M.; Ricci, E.; Biondi, S.; Napoli, C.; Ferracuti, S.; Mazza, C. How to Improve Compliance with Protective Health Measures during the COVID-19 Outbreak: Testing a Moderated Mediation Model and Machine Learning Algorithms. *Int. J. Environ. Res. Public Health* **2020**, *17*, 7252. [CrossRef]
20. Cheng, C.; Cheung, M.W.L. Psychological responses to outbreak of severe acute respiratory syndrome: A prospective, multiple time-point study. *J. Pers.* **2005**, *73*, 261–285. [CrossRef]
21. Asmundson, G.J.; Taylor, S. How health anxiety influences responses to viral outbreaks like COVID-19: What all decision-makers, health authorities, and health care professionals need to know. *J. Anxiety Disord.* **2020**, *71*, 102211. [CrossRef] [PubMed]
22. Yu, H.-Y.; Ho, S.C.; So, K.F.E.; Lo, Y.L. The psychological burden experienced by Hong Kong midlife women during the SARS epidemic. *Stress Health* **2005**, *21*, 177–184. [CrossRef]
23. Sim, K.; Chan, Y.H.; Chong, P.N.; Chua, H.C.; Soon, S.W. Psychosocial and coping responses within the community health care setting towards a national outbreak of an infectious disease. *J. Psychosom. Res.* **2010**, *68*, 195–202. [CrossRef]
24. Liu, N.; Zhang, F.; Wei, C.; Jia, Y.; Shang, Z.; Sun, L.; Wu, L.; Sun, Z.; Zhou, Y.; Wang, Y.; et al. Prevalence and predictors of PTSS during COVID-19 outbreak in China hardest-hit areas: Gender differences matter. *Psychiatry Res.* **2020**, *287*, 112921. [CrossRef]
25. Xu, J.; Zheng, Y.; Wang, M.; Zhao, J.; Zhan, Q.; Fu, M.; Wang, Q.; Xiao, J.; Cheng, Y. Predictors of symptoms of posttraumatic stress in Chinese university students during the 2009 H1N1 influenza pandemic. *Med. Sci. Monit.* **2011**, *17*, PH60–PH64. [CrossRef] [PubMed]
26. Di Crosta, A.; Palumbo, R.; Marchetti, D.; Ceccato, I.; La Malva, P.; Maiella, R.; Cipi, M.; Roma, P.; Mammarella, N.; Verrocchio, M.C.; et al. Individual differences, economic stability, and fear of contagion as risk factors for PTSD symptoms in the COVID-19 emergency. *Front. Psychol.* **2020**, *11*. [CrossRef] [PubMed]
27. McEwen, B.S. Neurobiological and systemic effects of chronic stress. *Chronic Stress* **2017**, *1*, 247054701769232. [CrossRef]
28. Toussaint, L.; Shields, G.S.; Dorn, G.; Slavich, G.M. Effects of lifetime stress exposure on mental and physical health in young adulthood: How stress degrades and forgiveness protects health. *J. Health Psychol.* **2014**, *21*, 1004–1014. [CrossRef] [PubMed]
29. Yang, L.; Zhao, Y.; Wang, Y.; Liu, L.; Zhang, X.; Li, B.; Cui, R. The effects of psychological stress on depression. *Curr. Neuropharmacol.* **2015**, *13*, 494–504. [CrossRef]
30. Mayer, S.E.; Lopez-Duran, N.L.; Sen, S.; Abelson, J.L. Chronic stress, hair cortisol and depression: A prospective and longitudinal study of medical internship. *Psychoneuroendocrinology* **2018**, *92*, 57–65. [CrossRef]
31. Schultebraucks, K.; Rombold-Bruehl, F.; Wingenfeld, K.; Hellmann-Regen, J.; Otte, C.; Roepke, S. Heightened biological stress response during exposure to a trauma film predicts an increase in intrusive memories. *J. Abnorm. Psychol.* **2019**, *128*, 645–657. [CrossRef]
32. Colodro-Conde, L.; Couvy-Duchesne, B.; Zhu, G.; Coventry, W.L.; Byrne, E.M.; Gordon, S.; Wright, M.J.; Montgomery, G.W.; Madden, P.A.F.; Ripke, S.; et al. A direct test of the diathesis–stress model for depression. *Mol. Psychiatry* **2017**, *23*, 1590–1596. [CrossRef]
33. Lazarus, R.S. Psychological stress and coping in adaptation and illness. *Int. J. Psychiatry Med.* **1974**, *5*, 321–333. [CrossRef]
34. Zhang, J.; Wu, W.; Zhao, X.; Zhang, W. Recommended psychological crisis intervention response to the 2019 novel coronavirus pneumonia outbreak in China: A model of West China Hospital. *Precis. Clin. Med.* **2020**, *3*, 3–8. [CrossRef]
35. Qiu, J.; Shen, B.; Zhao, M.; Wang, Z.; Xie, B.; Xu, Y. A nationwide survey of psychological distress among Chinese people in the COVID-19 epidemic: Implications and policy recommendations. *Gen. Psychiatry* **2020**, *33*, e100213. [CrossRef] [PubMed]
36. Li, S.; Wang, Y.; Xue, J.; Zhao, N.; Zhu, T. The impact of COVID-19 epidemic declaration on psychological consequences: A study on active weibo users. *Int. J. Environ. Res. Public Health* **2020**, *17*, 2032. [CrossRef] [PubMed]

37. Roberts, B.W.; Kuncel, N.R.; Shiner, R.; Caspi, A.; Goldberg, L.R. The Power of Personality: The comparative validity of personality traits, socioeconomic status, and cognitive ability for predicting important life outcomes. *Perspect. Psychol. Sci.* **2007**, *2*, 313–345. [CrossRef]
38. Folkman, S.; Lazarus, R.S. An analysis of coping in a middle-aged community sample. *J. Health Soc. Behav.* **1980**, *21*, 219. [CrossRef]
39. Folkman, S.; Lazarus, R.S. Coping as a mediator of emotion. *J. Pers. Soc. Psychol.* **1988**, *54*, 466–475. [CrossRef] [PubMed]
40. Connor-Smith, J.K.; Compas, B.E. Coping as a moderator of relations between reactivity to interpersonal stress, health status, and internalizing problems. *Cogn. Ther. Res.* **2004**, *28*, 347–368. [CrossRef]
41. Bandura, A. Human agency in social cognitive theory. *Am. Psychol.* **1989**, *44*, 1175. [CrossRef] [PubMed]
42. Bandura, A. *Self-Efficacy: The Exercise of Control*; Freeman: New York, NY, USA, 1997.
43. Taha, S.A.; Matheson, K.; Anisman, H. The 2009 H1N1 influenza pandemic: The role of threat, coping, and media trust on vaccination intentions in Canada. *J. Health Commun.* **2013**, *18*, 278–290. [CrossRef]
44. Tangney, J.P.; Baumeister, R.F.; Boone, A.L. High self-control predicts good adjustment, less pathology, better grades, and interpersonal success. *J. Pers.* **2004**, *72*, 271–324. [CrossRef]
45. Smith, N.B.; Sippel, L.M.; Presseau, C.; Rozek, D.; Mota, N.; Gordon, C.; Horvath, M.; Harpaz-Rotem, I. Locus of control in US combat veterans: Unique associations with posttraumatic stress disorder 5-factor model symptom clusters. *Psychiatry Res.* **2018**, *268*, 152–156. [CrossRef]
46. Rizza, F.; Gison, A.; Bonassi, S.; Dall'Armi, V.; Tonto, F.; Giaquinto, S. 'Locus of control', health-related quality of life, emotional distress and disability in Parkinson's disease. *J. Health Psychol.* **2015**, *22*, 844–852. [CrossRef] [PubMed]
47. Rotter, J.B. Generalized expectancies for internal versus external control of reinforcement. *Psychol. Monogr. Gen. Appl.* **1966**, *80*, 1–28. [CrossRef]
48. McCrae, R.R.; Costa, P.T. *Personality in Adulthood*; The Guilford Press: New York, NY, USA, 1990.
49. Allen, M.S.; Walter, E.E.; McDermott, M.S. Personality and sedentary behavior: A systematic review and meta-analysis. *Health Psychol.* **2017**, *36*, 255–263. [CrossRef] [PubMed]
50. Allen, M.S.; Walter, E.E. Linking big five personality traits to sexuality and sexual health: A meta-analytic review. *Psychol. Bull.* **2018**, *144*, 1081–1110. [CrossRef]
51. Wilson, K.E.; Dishman, R.K. Personality and physical activity: A systematic review and meta-analysis. *Pers. Individ. Differ.* **2015**, *72*, 230–242. [CrossRef]
52. Malouff, J.M.; Thorsteinsson, E.B.; Rooke, S.E.; Schutte, N.S. Alcohol involvement and the five-factor model of personality: A meta-analysis. *J. Drug Educ.* **2007**, *37*, 277–294. [CrossRef]
53. Mondo, M.; Sechi, C.; Cabras, C. Psychometric evaluation of three versions of the Italian Perceived Stress Scale. *Curr. Psychol.* **2019**, 1–9. [CrossRef]
54. Maroufizadeh, S.; Foroudifard, F.; Navid, B.; Ezabadi, Z.; Sobati, B.; Omani-Samani, R. The Perceived Stress Scale (PSS-10) in women experiencing infertility: A reliability and validity study. *Middle East Fertil. Soc. J.* **2018**, *23*, 456–459. [CrossRef]
55. Cohen, S.; Kamarck, T.; Mermelstein, R. A global measure of perceived stress. *J. Health Soc. Behav.* **1983**, *24*, 385. [CrossRef]
56. Cohen, S.; Hoberman, H.M. Positive events and social supports as buffers of life change Stress1. *J. Appl. Soc. Psychol.* **1983**, *13*, 99–125. [CrossRef]
57. Caricati, L.; Foà, C.; Fruggeri, L.; Tonarelli, A. COPE-NVI-25: Validazione italiana della versione ridotta della Coping orientation to the problems experienced (COPE-NVI). *Psicol. Salut.* **2015**, *2*, 123–140. [CrossRef]
58. Carver, C.S.; Scheier, M.F.; Weintraub, J.K. Assessing coping strategies: A theoretically based approach. *J. Pers. Soc. Psychol.* **1989**, *56*, 267–283. [CrossRef]
59. Sica, C.; Magni, C.; Ghisi, M.; Altoè, G.; Sighinolfi, C.; Chiri, L.R.; Franceschini, S. Coping orientation to problems experienced-nuova versione italiana (COPE-NVI): Uno strumento per la misura degli stili di coping. *Psicoter. Cogn. Comport.* **2008**, *14*, 27–53.
60. Meazzini, P. *Vivere Con il Sole in Tasca: Cos' è la Psicologia Positiva E Cosa Può Fare per Noi*; FrancoAngeli: Milan, Italy, 2017.
61. Nigro, G. Contributo alla taratura italiana della scala di controllo interno-esterno (I-E) di Rotter. *Boll. Psicol. Appl.* **1983**, *168*, 29–41.

62. Guido, G.; Peluso, A.M.; Capestro, M.; Miglietta, M. An Italian version of the 10-item Big Five Inventory: An application to hedonic and utilitarian shopping values. *Pers. Individ. Differ.* **2015**, *76*, 135–140. [CrossRef]
63. McCrae, R.R.; Costa, P. The stability of personality: Observations and evaluations. *Curr. Dir. Psychol. Sci.* **1994**, *3*, 173–175. [CrossRef]
64. Rammstedt, B.; John, O.P. Measuring personality in one minute or less: A 10-item short version of the Big Five Inventory in English and German. *J. Res. Pers.* **2007**, *41*, 203–212. [CrossRef]
65. Faul, F.; Erdfelder, E.; Lang, A.-G.; Buchner, A. G*Power 3: A flexible statistical power analysis program for the social, behavioral, and biomedical sciences. *Behav. Res. Methods* **2007**, *39*, 175–191. [CrossRef]
66. JASP, Version0.14. Available online: https://jasp-stats.org/2020/10/14/introducing-jasp-0-14/ (accessed on 14 October 2020).
67. Goss-Sampson, M.A. Statistical Analysis in JASP: A Guide for Students. Available online: https://static.jasp-stats.org/Statistical%20Analysis%20in%20JASP%20-%20A%20Students%20Guide%20v2.pdf (accessed on 1 October 2018).
68. Friedrich, R.J. In defense of multiplicative terms in multiple regression equations. *Am. J. Polit. Sci.* **1982**, *26*, 797. [CrossRef]
69. Yarkoni, T.; Westfall, J. Choosing prediction over explanation in psychology: Lessons from machine learning. *Perspect. Psychol. Sci.* **2017**, *12*, 1100–1122. [CrossRef]
70. Mazza, C.; Orrù, G.; Burla, F.; Monaro, M.; Ferracuti, S.; Colasanti, M.; Roma, P. Indicators to distinguish symptom accentuators from symptom producers in individuals with a diagnosed adjustment disorder: A pilot study on inconsistency subtypes using SIMS and MMPI-2-RF. *PLoS ONE* **2019**, *14*, e0227113. [CrossRef] [PubMed]
71. Mazza, C.; Monaro, M.; Orrù, G.; Burla, F.; Colasanti, M.; Ferracuti, S.; Roma, P. Introducing machine learning to detect personality faking-good in a male sample: A new model based on minnesota multiphasic personality inventory-2 restructured form scales and reaction times. *Front. Psychiatry* **2019**, *10*. [CrossRef] [PubMed]
72. Orrù, G.; Mazza, C.; Monaro, M.; Ferracuti, S.; Sartori, G.; Roma, P. The development of a short version of the SIMS using machine learning to detect feigning in forensic assessment. *Psychol. Injury Law* **2020**. [CrossRef]
73. Orrù, G.; Monaro, M.; Conversano, C.; Gemignani, A.; Sartori, G. machine learning in psychometrics and psychological research. *Front. Psychol.* **2020**, *10*. [CrossRef] [PubMed]
74. Dwyer, D.B.; Efallkai, P.; Koutsouleris, N. Machine learning approaches for clinical psychology and psychiatry. *Annu. Rev. Clin. Psychol.* **2018**, *14*, 91–118. [CrossRef]
75. Nelles, O. Nonlinear system identification. In *From Classical Approaches to Neural Networks and Fuzzy Models*; Springer: Berlin/Heidelberg, Germany, 2001.
76. Cumming, G. Replication and p intervals: P values predict the future only vaguely, but confidence intervals do much better. *Perspect. Psychol. Sci.* **2008**, *3*, 286–300. [CrossRef] [PubMed]
77. Dwork, C.; Feldman, V.; Hardt, M.; Pitassi, T.; Reingold, O.; Roth, A. The reusable holdout: Preserving validity in adaptive data analysis. *Science* **2015**, *349*, 636–638. [CrossRef] [PubMed]
78. Hall, M.A. Correlation-Based Feature Selection for Machine Learning. Ph.D. Thesis, University of Waikato, Hamilton, New Zealand, 1999.
79. Hall, M.; Frank, E.; Holmes, G.; Pfahringer, B.; Reutemann, P.; Witten, I.H. The WEKA data mining software. *ACM SIGKDD Explor. Newsl.* **2009**, *11*, 10–18. [CrossRef]
80. Japkowicz, N. (Ed.) The class imbalance problem: Significance and strategies. In Proceedings of the International Conference on Artificial Intelligence (ICAI), Las Vegas, NV, USA, 28 June–1 July 2000; pp. 111–117.
81. Japkowicz, N.; Stephen, S. The class imbalance problem: A systematic study1. *Intell. Data Anal.* **2002**, *6*, 429–449. [CrossRef]
82. Le Cessie, S.; Van Houwelingen, J.C. Ridge estimators in logistic regression. *J. R. Stat. Soc. Ser. C Appl. Stat.* **1992**, *41*, 191. [CrossRef]
83. Keerthi, S.S.; Shevade, S.K.; Bhattacharyya, C.; Murthy, K.R.K. Improvements to Platt's SMO algorithm for SVM classifier design. *Neural Comput.* **2001**, *13*, 637–649. [CrossRef]
84. John, G.H.; Langley, P. Estimating continuous distributions in Bayesian classifiers. In Proceedings of the 11th Conference on Uncertainty in Artificial Intelligence, Montreal, QC, Canada, 18–20 August 1995; pp. 338–345.
85. Breiman, L. Random forest. *Mach. Learn.* **2001**, *45*, 5–32. [CrossRef]

86. Kohavi, R. A study of cross-validation and bootstrap for accuracy estimation and model selection. In Proceedings of the 14th International Joint Conference on Artificial Intelligence, Morgan Kaufmann, San Mateo, CA, USA, August 1995; pp. 1137–1143.
87. Mazza, C.; Ricci, E.; Biondi, S.; Colasanti, M.; Ferracuti, S.; Napoli, C.; Roma, P. A nationwide survey of psychological distress among Italian people during the COVID-19 pandemic: Immediate psychological responses and associated factors. *Int. J. Environ. Res. Public Health* **2020**, *17*, 3165. [CrossRef] [PubMed]
88. Losada-Baltar, A.; Jiménez-Gonzalo, L.; Gallego-Alberto, L.; Pedroso-Chaparro, M.D.S.; Fernandes-Pires, J.; Márquez-González, M. "We Are Staying at Home." Association of self-perceptions of aging, personal and family resources, and loneliness with psychological distress during the lock-down period of COVID-19. *J. Gerontol. Ser. B* **2020**. [CrossRef]
89. Chew, Q.H.; Wei, K.C.; Vasoo, S.; Chua, H.C.; Sim, K. Narrative synthesis of psychological and coping responses towards emerging infectious disease outbreaks in the general population: Practical considerations for the COVID-19 pandemic. *Singap. Med. J.* **2020**, *61*, 350–356. [CrossRef]
90. Labouvie-Vief, G. Dynamic integration: Affect, cognition, and the self in adulthood. *Curr. Dir. Psychol. Sci.* **2003**, *12*, 201–206. [CrossRef]
91. Cummings, E.M.; Greene, A.L.; Karraker, K.H. *Life-Span Developmental Psychology: Perspectives on Stress and Coping*; Lawrence Erlbaum Associates, Inc.: Hillsdale, NJ, USA, 1991.
92. Carstensen, L.L. Social and emotional patterns in adulthood: Support for socioemotional selectivity theory. *Psychol. Aging* **1992**, *7*, 331. [CrossRef]
93. Peng, E.Y.-C.; Lee, M.-B.; Tsai, S.-T.; Yang, C.-C.; Morisky, D.E.; Tsai, L.-T.; Weng, Y.-L.; Lyu, S.-Y. Population-based post-crisis psychological distress: An example from the SARS outbreak in Taiwan. *J. Formos. Med Assoc.* **2010**, *109*, 524–532. [CrossRef]
94. Main, A.; Zhou, Q.; Ma, Y.; Luecken, L.J.; Liu, X. Relations of SARS-related stressors and coping to Chinese college students' psychological adjustment during the 2003 Beijing SARS epidemic. *J. Couns. Psychol.* **2011**, *58*, 410–423. [CrossRef]
95. Mak, W.W.; Law, R.W.; Woo, J.; Cheung, F.M.; Lee, D. Social support and psychological adjustment to SARS: The mediating role of self-care self-efficacy. *Psychol. Health* **2009**, *24*, 161–174. [CrossRef]
96. Caprara, G.V.; Barbaranelli, C.; Borgogni, L.; Perugini, M. The "big five questionnaire": A new questionnaire to assess the five factor model. *Pers. Individ. Differ.* **1993**, *15*, 281–288. [CrossRef]
97. Rodríguez-Ramos, Á.; Moriana, J.A.; García-Torres, F.; Ruiz-Rubio, M. Emotional stability is associated with the MAOA promoter uVNTR polymorphism in women. *Brain Behav.* **2019**, *9*, e01376. [CrossRef]
98. Cohrdes, C.; Mauz, E. Self-Efficacy and emotional stability buffer negative effects of adverse childhood experiences on young adult health-related quality of life. *J. Adolesc. Health* **2020**, *67*, 93–100. [CrossRef] [PubMed]
99. Sanatkar, S.; Baldwin, P.; Clarke, J.; Fletcher, S.; Gunn, J.; Wilhelm, K.; Campbell, L.; Zwar, N.; Harris, M.; Lapsley, H.; et al. The influence of personality on trajectories of distress, health and functioning in mild-to-moderately depressed adults with type 2 diabetes. *Psychol. Health Med.* **2019**, *25*, 296–308. [CrossRef]
100. Fisher, L.; Hessler, D.; Masharani, U.; Strycker, L. Impact of baseline patient characteristics on interventions to reduce diabetes distress: The role of personal conscientiousness and diabetes self-efficacy. *Diabet. Med.* **2014**, *31*, 739–746. [CrossRef] [PubMed]
101. Digman, J.M. Higher-order factors of the Big Five. *J. Pers. Soc. Psychol.* **1997**, *73*, 1246. [CrossRef]
102. Alexander, M. Let's conquer COVID-19 and sustain our abilities. *Spinal Cord Ser. Cases* **2020**, *6*, 19. [CrossRef]
103. Pascoe, M.C.; Thompson, D.R.; Jenkins, Z.M.; Ski, C.F. Mindfulness mediates the physiological markers of stress: Systematic review and meta-analysis. *J. Psychiatr. Res.* **2017**, *95*, 156–178. [CrossRef] [PubMed]
104. Phua, D.H.; Tang, H.K.; Tham, K.Y. Coping responses of emergency physicians and nurses to the 2003 severe acute respiratory syndrome outbreak. *Acad. Emerg. Med.* **2005**, *12*, 322–328. [CrossRef]
105. Teasdale, E.; Yardley, L.; Schlotz, W.; Michie, S. The importance of coping appraisal in behavioural responses to pandemic flu. *Br. J. Health Psychol.* **2011**, *17*, 44–59. [CrossRef]
106. Judge, T.A.; Bono, J.E. Relationship of core self-evaluations traits—self-esteem, generalized self-efficacy, locus of control, and emotional stability—with job satisfaction and job performance: A meta-analysis. *J. Appl. Psychol.* **2001**, *86*, 80–92. [CrossRef] [PubMed]
107. Ajzen, I. Perceived behavioral control, self-efficacy, locus of control, and the theory of planned behavior 1. *J. Appl. Soc. Psychol.* **2002**, *32*, 665–683. [CrossRef]

108. Duan, L.; Zhu, G. Psychological interventions for people affected by the COVID-19 epidemic. *Lancet Psychiatry* **2020**, *7*, 300–302. [CrossRef]
109. Zhou, X.; Snoswell, C.L.; Harding, L.E.; Bambling, M.; Edirippulige, S.; Bai, X.; Smith, A.C. The role of telehealth in reducing the mental health burden from COVID-19. *Telemed. e-Health* **2020**, *26*, 377–379. [CrossRef] [PubMed]

Publisher's Note: MDPI stays neutral with regard to jurisdictional claims in published maps and institutional affiliations.

Journal of
Clinical Medicine

MDPI

Article

Increased Psychological Distress during COVID-19 and Quarantine in Ireland: A National Survey

Tom Burke [1,*], Anna Berry [1,2], Laura K. Taylor [1,3], Owen Stafford [1], Eddie Murphy [1,2], Mark Shevlin [4], Louise McHugh [1] and Alan Carr [1]

1 School of Psychology, University College Dublin, D04 F6X4 Dublin, Ireland; annanibheara@gmail.com (A.B.); laura.taylor@ucd.ie (L.K.T.); stafford.owen@yahoo.co.uk (O.S.); eddie.murphy2@hse.ie (E.M.); louise.mchugh@ucd.ie (L.M.); alan.carr@ucd.ie (A.C.)

2 Health Service Executive, CHO 8 (Laois/Offaly), R34 YFW6 Laois, Ireland

3 School of Psychology, Queen's University Belfast, Belfast BT7 1NN, UK

4 Department of Psychology, University of Ulster (Psychology), Coleraine BT52 1SA, UK; m.shevlin@ulster.ac.uk

* Correspondence: tom.m.burke@ucd.ie

Received: 31 August 2020; Accepted: 23 October 2020; Published: 28 October 2020

Abstract: Background: The emergence of the coronavirus pneumonia (COVID-19) resulted in a global pandemic. The psychological impact of an epidemic is multifaceted and acute, with long-term consequences. Methods: A cross-sectional online survey-based design was employed, assessing the psychological impact of COVID-19 on members of the Irish public during the quarantine period of COVID-19 in Ireland. Participants were invited to complete the Depression, Anxiety, and Stress Scale-21 (DASS-21) retrospectively (prior to quarantine) and during the quarantine period, as well as measures of illness perceptions, well-being, and a bespoke measure (the Effects of COVID Questionnaire, ECQ), which assessed perceptions of COVID-related stresses associated with personal concerns, caring for children, caring for aging parents, as well as gratitude. Results: A total of $n = 1620$ entered the survey platform, with a total of $n = 847$ surveys completed by members of the Irish public. Entry into COVID-19 quarantine was associated with significant increases in clinically significant symptoms of depression, stress, and anxiety. The ECQ reliably assessed a range of COVID-19-related stresses and had large and significant correlations with the DASS-21. Conclusions: The COVID-19 quarantine was associated with stresses and significant increases in symptoms of depression, anxiety, and stress in a national Irish cohort. The public require increased access to mental health services to meet this increase in COVID-19-related psychological distress.

Keywords: psychological distress; public; quarantine; COVID-19; mental health; Ireland

---

1. Introduction

December 2019 saw the emergence of a novel severe acute respiratory syndrome, coronavirus pneumonia (COVID-19) outbreak, which subsequently became a global pandemic [1]. COVID-19 elicits challenging psychological and psychiatric responses due to its sudden and unpredictable nature, creating a sense of uncertainty and vulnerability, while challenging individuals' sense of personal and societal safety [2]. This may be amplified by the treatment-resistant nature of COVID-19 to common medications and the delay in contraction to symptom onset [3]. Patients, health professionals, and the general public face increasing psychological demands and pressure which may in itself lead to challenges with anxiety, fear, depression, and sleep difficulties, all of which need to be considered and targeted in the overall deployment of the disease control measures [4].

COVID-19 is associated with a significant mental health burden both in the acute phase and the long-term from people who are exposed to the virus and those not directly exposed. Anxiety, depression, cognitive impairment, delirium, psychosis, irritability, insomnia, and post-traumatic stress disorder are prevalent following COVID-19 infection [5–8]. One-third of the first 153 COVID-19 cases in the UK were diagnosed with new-onset mental health problems including psychosis (43%), cognitive decline (26%), and affective disorder (17%) [9]. Further to the psychological response to COVID-19, in a recent COVID-19 study using a national cross-sectional survey based design in Italy [10], it was found that previous history of trauma and medical problems, or having an acquaintance infected was associated with higher levels of depression and anxiety.

With a view to reduce infection and control the outbreak of a virus, many countries undertake stepped measures such as social distancing, the reduction and cancellation of large public gatherings, self-isolation recommendations, quarantine in a dedicated facility, and mass public quarantine (Public Health England, 2020). While quarantine can be necessary during major infectious disease outbreaks from a population-health perspective, a recent systematic review suggests that quarantine itself is often associated with negative psychological and physical effects [1,11]. For some, the psychological impact of being in a pandemic is wide-ranging [11], significant, and long-lasting [12,13], requiring effective and accessible psychological support be put in place as early as possible.

In recent years, much of the research into the psychological sequalae following public quarantine has resulted from similar epidemics (e.g., Severe Acute Respiratory Syndrome (SARS) circa. 2003; Equine influenza circa. 2008; and Swine Flu circa. 2009 [H1N1 Influenza]). Research suggests that quarantine may result in a higher prevalence of symptoms of psychological distress [14], emotional disturbance [15], depression [16], stress [17], low mood with irritability and insomnia [18], post-traumatic stress symptoms [19], anger [20], and emotional exhaustion [21]. Low mood (73% of 903) and irritability (57% of 903) are among the most prevalent symptoms of psychological distress reported [18]. People quarantined because of being in close contact with those who potentially had SARS [19] reported various negative responses during the quarantine period: over 20% (230 of 1057) reported fear, 18% (187) reported nervousness, 18% (186) reported sadness, and 10% (101) reported guilt. However, not all studies have found evidence of psychological distress following quarantine. For example, [22] compared undergraduates who had been quarantined with those not quarantined immediately after the quarantine period and found no significant difference between the groups in terms of post-traumatic stress symptoms or general mental health problems. Recently, the typical responses to COVID-19 have been reported as panic, fear to go out, excessive disinfection, disappointment, fear, irritability, aggressive behavior, and extreme optimism or pessimism [23].

Mental health risks associated with COVID-19 have yet to be systematically studied; however, the emerging literature on COVID-19 as well as previous studies on infectious disease outbreaks provide insights into probable risk factors and correlates of mental health challenges and chronic psychological distress [24]. There is also emerging evidence that specific members of society, e.g., parents, may be experiencing additional psychological distress due to increased and unstable financial demands, school closures, and suspended recreational outlets, which would have support personal and familial coping [25,26]. A better classification and quantification of mental health and psychological needs following COVID-19 will allow for the appropriate consideration of therapeutic frameworks, service-based funding considerations, intervention integration through non-routine modalities, and to consider service models and accessibility for those vulnerable and in need [27].

The primary aim of the study was to investigate the mental health and well-being of adults in Ireland during the quarantine period of the COVID-19 crisis and examine the reliability and validity of a new instrument for assessing stresses and things for which people felt grateful that were specifically related to the COVID-19 crisis (the Effects of COVID-19 Questionnaire [ECQ, Berry and Carr, 2020]). For the purpose of this study, the quarantine period is defined as the period of time in which the initial national lockdown occurred in Ireland. The following specific questions were addressed:

- Were mean levels and rates of depression, anxiety, and stress significantly higher during the quarantine period?

- Did mean levels and rates of depression, anxiety, and stress differentially increase significantly for those caring for children or older aging parents during the quarantine period?
- What were the rates of stresses and things that people felt grateful for that were specifically related to the COVID-19 crisis (as assessed the ECQ)?
- What were the psychometric properties of the ECQ?
- Were the COVID-19-related stresses and gratitude assessed by the ECQ correlated with indices of mental health and well-being?

2. Materials and Methodology

2.1. Participants

A cross-sectional survey-based design was employed to recruit a public sample through the use of media outlets, social media, and professional networking websites in Ireland, during the period of mass public quarantine (effective 27 March 2020 to 8 June 2020, as per Irish government authorization). A total of $n = 1620$ entered the survey platform, with a total of $n = 847$ completing each of the survey questionnaires fully. The response sample was predominantly female, and the age range was reflected between 18 and 76 years of age. Further details on the participant results are below. Inclusion criteria were being over the age of 18; living in Ireland at the time of quarantine; and participants were required to read an information sheet and provide consent before proceeding to the questionnaire. Participants were excluded if they did not meet the inclusion criteria.

2.2. Materials

All information provided was self-reported and completed online through the use of *Qualtrics* (SPA, London, England). Demographic information regarding gender, age, marital status, household and family composition, and years of education were collected. The following scales were used: the Depression, Anxiety, and Stress Scale (DASS-21) [28], the Warwick–Edinburgh Mental Well-Being Scale (WEMWBS) [29], the Brief Illness Perception Questionnaire (BIPQ) [30], and the ECQ (Berry and Carr 2020).

The DASS-21, which yields scores for depression, anxiety, and stress, was the primary measure for this study. Each scale contains 7 items. The Depression scale assesses dysphoria, hopelessness, devaluation of life, self-deprecation, lack of interest/involvement, anhedonia, and inertia. The Anxiety scale assesses autonomic arousal, skeletal muscle effects, situational anxiety, and subjective experience of anxious affect. The stress scale is sensitive to levels of chronic non-specific arousal. It assesses difficulty relaxing, nervous arousal, and being easily upset/agitated, irritable/over-reactive, and impatient. Scores for depression, anxiety and stress are calculated by summing the scores for the relevant items per scale; then, the DASS-21 subscale total is multiplied by 2 to give the final score for categorization into Normal, Mild, Moderate, Severe, or Extremely Severe. The reliability of the DASS-21 was considered acceptable [31] and has "good" Cronbach's alpha values of 0.81 and 0.89 for the depression and anxiety subscales, respectively. The alpha value for the stress subscale was observed at 0.78, which is considered "fair" [31].

The WEMWBS is a 14-item measure that focuses on the positive aspects of mental health and well-being including optimism, autonomy, agency, curiosity, clarity of thought, positive relationships, positive affect confidence, and having energy to spare [29]. High scores indicate greater well-being. The reliability of the WEMWBS is noted to be "good" within a student sample, with an observed Cronbach's alpha of 0.89 [31].

The BIPQ assesses the cognitive and emotional representations of illness. For this survey, we included the "Cognitive Perceptions" subscale adapted for COVID-19, which asks about the effect of COVID-19 on life (item 1); perceived duration of COVID-19 (item 2); control over COVID-19 (item 3); beliefs about the effectiveness of treatment for COVID-19 (item 4); and experience of COVID-19 symptoms (item 5). We further employed a single item to capture understanding of COVID-19 (item

7); items 1–5 are summed to give a total score for the "Cognitive Perceptions" scale. High BIPQ scores reflect negative perceptions of COVID-19. The reliability of the BIPQ has been shown to have a "good" Cronbach's alpha value of 0.85 [31].

The ECQ is a bespoke 34-item tool that measures perceptions of COVID-related stresses as well as gratitude arising from the COVID-19 crisis, as developed by the second and senior author following a review of the literature and discussions as part of a doctoral thesis (Supplementary Table S1). Items 1–25 are about COVID-19-related stresses. Items 26–34 are about things participants felt grateful for arising from the COVID-19 crisis. For COVID-19-related stresses, participants were asked, "In the past month, how much stress have you experienced as a result of the following things?" For COVID-19-related gratitude, participants were asked, "In the past month, how much has your experience of the COVID-19 crisis led you to feel grateful for the following things?" For all items, there are 5 response options: none, a little, some, quite a lot, and a great deal. The ECQ contains four a priori scales: Personal Stress (items 1–13), Parenting Stress (items 14–21), Older Aging Parent Stress (items 22–25) and Gratitude (items 26–34). Items in the Personal Stress scale cover financial hardship, difficulty getting supplies, loss of social contact, loss of routine, family conflict, conflicting media information about COVID-19, witnessing or worrying about COVID-19-related illness, hospitalization, death, and long-term effects for oneself and one's family. Items in the Parenting Stress scale (which are only relevant to respondents with children) cover school closure, preventing children having social contact with extended family and friends, helping children observe social distancing, handwashing, cough etiquette, and worrying about their health due to the presence an underlying condition that makes them vulnerable to COVID-19-related adverse outcomes. Items in the Older Aging Parent Stress scale (which are only relevant to respondents with aging parents) cover worrying about the impact of COVID-19 on older aging parents, especially loneliness, difficulty getting supplies, risk of illness, and risk of not receiving adequate medical care. Items in the Gratitude scale cover things that the COVID-19 crisis has made one feel grateful for including personal and family health, relationships, employment, social, sports and cultural events, community, schools, children's friendships, children's involvement in activities, and aging parents' health and safety. The ECQ is included in the supplemental materials.

2.3. Procedure

This study was approved by the host institution's research ethics committee (HS-E-20-66-Burke). Study information was disseminated through the use of a national online media outlet, informing readers of the nature of the study and inviting interested participants to take part. Social media, and other online platforms were also engaged to support recruitment. Then, interested participants followed a link to access the study information sheet, consent, and questions via *Qualtrics*. Once participant screening questions were completed, i.e., confirmation of being in Ireland during the national quarantine period, and inclusion criteria were confirmed, consent was obtained, and participants provided demographic information. Following this, participants were requested to complete the outcome measures. Participants were invited to complete the survey during the quarantine period and also to consider retrospectively their well-being, distress, and mood prior to the quarantine period. Participants were informed of that a participation raffle would take place, and they could opt in to be entered into the draw to win one of 3 €50 vouchers. Participants were made aware that they may withdraw from the study at any time during data collection by simply exiting the browser window.

2.4. Statistical Analysis and ECQ Validation

For continuous variables, comparisons were undertaken using MANOVA, ANOVA, and t-tests. For categorical variables, chi-square tests were used for comparisons. Bonferroni corrections were used where multiple comparisons were made. Pearson product moment correlation coefficients were used to determine associations between variables. Internal consistency reliability of ECQ scales was assessed with Cronbach's alpha. Exploratory factor analysis was used to assess the factor structure of the ECQ. K-means clustering was used as a non-hierarchical method to quantify the responses on the

ECQ subscales, with an a priori cluster set to 5, to create a categorical stratification of the DASS-21 (Normal, Mild, Moderate, Severe, Extremely Severe). IBM Statistical Software Package for the Social Sciences (SPSS) 26.0 (IBM, Armonk, NY, USA) was used for analyses.

3. Results

A total of $n = 1620$ entered the survey platform, with a total of $n = 847$ surveys completed. There were no significant differences on age or gender in those who completed the survey completely and those who did not, who had entered demographic details prior to exiting. The median time taken to complete the survey was 14.93 min for those who completed the survey fully. As reported in Table 1, participants were mostly female (83%), and age ranged from 18 to 76 years. The household income, education status, and relationship status can be seen in Table 1, as well as a full demographic breakdown for participants who were: (1) people who had older aging parents (OAPs; $n = 433$); (2) parents of children under 18 years of age (Parents; $n = 269$, of whom, $n = 33$ had a child but did not have older aging parents); and (3) participants who had neither children nor an older aging parent (Neither; $n = 145$) at the time of completing the survey. Within each cohort, >50% of the respondents continued to work during the COVID-19 pandemic. Supplementary Table S2 shows the outcome data under the same stratification.

Table 1. Demographics of the total group stratified by group membership.

			Total Cohort ($n = 847$)	**Parent to a Child ($n = 269$) ***	**Older Aging Parent ($n = 433$)**	**Neither ($n = 145$)**
Gender	Female	%	83.6	83	84.8	80
Age	(Range:18–76)	M ± SD	36.07 ± 10.29	41.07 ± 6.95	33.26 ± 8.61	35.19 ± 15.49
Household income	0–24	%	9	6	9.7	13.1
	25–49		26	16.4	28.9	35.2
	50–74		24.4	24.9	25.6	20.0
	75–99		19.1	23.8	17.1	16.6
	100–149		15.1	18.6	13.9	12.4
	≥150 k		6	10.4	4.4	2.8
Education	≤School	%	22.5	23.2	16.7	24.8
	Degree		38.7	34.9	41.9	36.6
	Masters		32.5	27.9	35	33.8
	Doctorate		5.28	5.6	5.3	4.1
	Post-doc		0.8	0.4	1.2	0.7
Relationship Status	Single	%	7.6	3	8.3	13.1
	Engaged		10.5	5.6	11.8	14.5
	Married		43	76.2	27.7	22.8
	Committed		38.9	3.8	50.1	48.3
Currently Working?	Yes	%	64.4	64.3	68.6	51.7

Note: "Neither" refers to neither a child nor an older aging parent; * Of which, $n = 33$ only have a child as illustrated in Figure 1.

3.1. Did Mean Levels of Depression Anxiety and Stress Increase Significantly during the Quarantine Period?

Mean DASS-21 depression, anxiety, and stress scores for the whole sample are given in the first panel of results in Table 2. When comparing the pre-quarantine outcomes to those reported during the quarantine period, there was a significant increase in mean levels of depression (pre-quarantine $M = 7.46$, quarantine $M = 10.54$, $t = 10.50$, $p < 0.001$), anxiety (pre-quarantine $M = 5.39$, quarantine $M = 6.02$, $t = 3.39$, $p = 0.001$), and stress (pre-quarantine $M = 11.99$, quarantine $M = 12.86$, $t = 2.82$, $p = 0.005$). See Figure 1 for illustration.

Table 2. DASS-21 depression, anxiety, and stress mean scores before and during quarantine.

Variable		Total Sample	Parent to a Child	Older Aging Parent	Neither
n		847	269	433	145
Depression	Pre-Q	7.46 ± 7.78	6.59 ± 6.81	8.12 ± 8.04	7.09 ± 8.54
	Q	10.54 ± 9.46	9.14 ± 8.74	11.41 ± 7.12	10.51 ± 9.89
Anxiety	Pre-Q	5.39 ± 5.87	4.71 ±5.71	5.82 ± 5.88	5.34 ± 6.04
	Q	6.02 ± 6.86	5.29 ± 6.67	6.63 ± 7.12	5.56 ± 6.26
Stress	Pre-Q	11.99 ± 7.74	11.41 ± 7.40	12.46 ± 8.00	11.62 ± 7.49
	Q	12.86 ± 9.09	11.73 ± 8.63	13.45 ± 9.24	13.20 ± 9.33

Note: DASS-21 = Depression, Anxiety, and Stress Scale. Pre-Q = Pre-quarantine. Q = During Quarantine. Standard deviations are given after ±. For each variable, means with different superscripts differ significantly at $p < 0.01$.

3.2. Did Mean Levels of Depression Anxiety and Stress Differentially Increase Significantly for those Caring for Children or Older Aging Parents during the Quarantine Period?

Mean DASS-21 depression, anxiety, and stress scores for parents caring for children, adults caring for older aging parents, and those caring for neither type of dependant are given in the last three panels of results in Table 2. A Groups × Time MANOVA, with three groups (parent to a child, older aging parent, and neither) and two time periods (pre-quarantine and quarantine) yielded a significant Groups × Time interaction ($p = 0.006$). Post-hoc analyses show that increases in depression, anxiety, and stress from pre-quarantine to quarantine were significantly associated with having older aging parents. Post-hoc analyses with Bonferroni adjustment showed participants with older aging parents were found to have significantly elevated Anxiety pre-quarantine ($p = 0.024$) and significantly elevated Anxiety ($p = 0.038$) and Depression ($p = 0.002$) during the quarantine period, with the largest difference relative to parents with children.

3.3. Did Rates of Depression, Anxiety, and Stress Increase Significantly during the Quarantine Period?

Rates of mild, moderate, severe, and very severe symptoms on DASS-21 scales for the whole sample are given in the first panel of results in Table 3. When cases in mild, moderate, severe, and very severe categories were combined and compared to those in the normal category, there were increases in rates of symptoms on all three DASS-21 scales from pre-quarantine to the quarantine period. The rate of depression increased from 30 to 46.3% (X^2 (1, n = 847) = 67.92, $p < 0.0001$). The rate of anxiety increased from 30.7 to 32.5% (X^2 (1, n = 847) = 121.71, $p < 0.0001$). The rate of stress increased from 27.7 to 34% (X^2 (2, n = 847) = 4.99, $p = 0.025$).

3.4. Did Rates of Depression, Anxiety, and Stress Differentially Increase Significantly for those Caring for Children or Older Aging Parents during the Quarantine Period?

Rates of mild, moderate, severe, and very severe symptoms on DASS-21 scales for parents caring for children, adults caring for older aging parents, and those caring for neither type of dependant are given in the last three panels of results in Table 3. To determine if there was an association between being a parent to a child, caring for an older aging parent, or having neither sort of dependent, on the one hand and symptom rates before and during quarantine on the other, 3 × 2, Group x Time, chi square tests were conducted on frequencies of symptoms outside the normal range in the three groups on both occasions.

There were significant Group × Time associations for both depression and anxiety from pre-quarantine to the quarantine period for parents caring for children, adults caring for older aging parents, and those caring for neither type of dependant ($p < 0.001$, respectively) but not specifically for stress. As reported through a detailed breakdown of the percentage of caseness and severity in Table 3, this reflects an increased severity of symptoms over time as a result of entering the quarantine period.

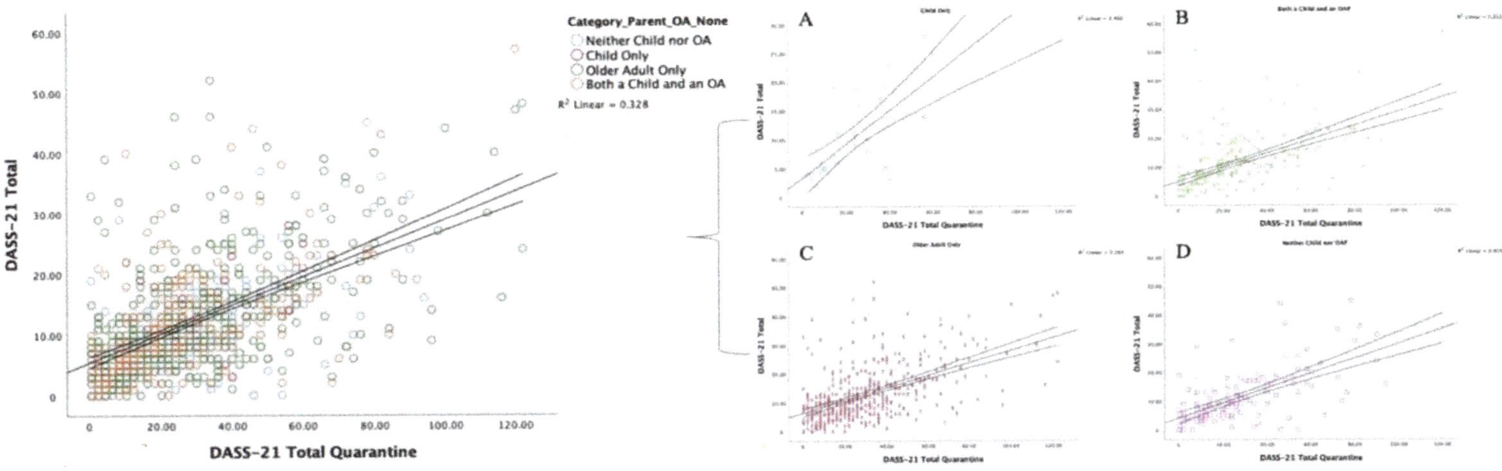

Figure 1. Outcomes for the summed score of the Depression, Anxiety, and Stress subscales (DASS-21) prior to, and during, the quarantine. Group stratification is illustrated as: Left: Total cohort with color demarcation; (**A**) parents with a child only i.e., no older aging parents [$R^2 = 0.490$]; (**B**) both a child and an older aging parent [$R^2 = 0.352$]; (**C**) older aging parents only [$R^2 = 0.283$]; (**D**) neither a child nor an older aging parent [$R^2 = 0.403$].

Table 3. A summary of the total percentage of the cohort who score within the cut-off categories of the DASS-21 for Stress, Anxiety, and Depression, stratified by group membership.

			Total Cohort (n = 847)				Parents of Children (n = 269) *				Older Aging Parents (n = 433)				Neither Children nor Older Aging Parent (n = 145)			
Variable	DASS-21 Classification	Range	Before [1] (%)	Mean ± SD [2]	During [3] (%)	Mean ± SD [2]	Before (%)	Mean ± SD	During (%)	Mean ± SD	Before (%)	Mean ± SD	During (%)	Mean ± SD	Before (%)	Mean ±SD	During (%)	Mean ± SD
Stress	Normal	0–14	72.3	8.22 ± 4.21	66	7.62 ± 4.69	76.4	8.24 ± 4.34	71.3	7.32 ± 4.77	69.7	8.27 ± 4.15	64	7.93 ± 4.60	72.9	4.01 ± 2.09	62.3	3.63 ± 2.38
	Mild	15–18	11.5	16.92 ± 1.01	12.3	16.90 ± 1.01	9.7	17.04 ± 1.01	9.8	16.56 ± 0.916	12.6	16.90 ± 1.00	13.4	16.98 ± 1.00	11.8	8.41 ± 0.507	13.8	8.57 ± 0.507
	Moderate	19–25	10.1	21.78 ± 1.53	10.8	22.04 ± 1.58	9.3	21.50 ± 1.21	9.4	22.08 ± 1.50	10.4	21.86 ± 1.69	10.9	22.00 ± 1.59	10.4	11.00 ± 0.755	13	11.05 ± 0.872
	Severe	26–33	4	28.36 ± 1.96	7.7	28.38 ± 2.04	3.5	28.88 ± 1.45	7.9	28.10 ± 2.10	4.5	28.10 ± 2.05	8	28.42 ± 2.16	3.5	14.20 ± 1.30	6.5	14.44 ± 0.726
	Extremely Severe	≥34	2.1	36.94 ± 3.17	3.1	37.68 ± 3.24	1.2	39.55 ± 3.05	1.6	37.00 ± 3.82	2.8	36.33 ± 3.28	3.6	38.00 ± 3.09	1.4	18.50 ± 0.707	4.3	17.66 ± 1.03
Anxiety	Normal	0–7	69.3	2.22 ± 2.16	67.5	2.26 ± 2.17	73.8	1.95 ± 2.19	72.8	1.97 ± 2.16	66.4	2.14 ± 2.12	63.9	2.53 ± 2.17	70	2.04 ± 2.16	68.3	2.06 ± 2.13
	Mild	8–9	8.9	8.00 ± 0.00	8.2	8.00 ± 0.00	7.4	8.00 ± 0.00	7	8.00 ± 0.00	10.9	8.00 ± 0.00	9.2	8.00 ± 0.00	5.7	8.00 ± 0.00	7.2	8.00 ± 0.00
	Moderate	10–14	14.8	11.45 ± 1.61	14.8	11.53 ± 1.54	13.3	11.52 ± 1.63	11.7	11.66 ± 1.39	15.4	11.47 ± 1.63	16.2	11.37 ± 1.56	15.7	11.27 ± 1.57	16.5	11.82 ± 1.69
	Severe	15–19	2.6	16.38 ± 0.80	3.7	17.20 ± 0.99	2.3	16.00 ± 0.00	1.9	17.60 ± 0.894	2.4	16.60 ± 0.996	4.6	17.15 ± 1.01	3.6	16.40 ± 0.894	4.3	17.00 ± 1.09
	Extremely Severe	≥20	4.4	23.27 ± 3.82	5.8	25.82 ± 5.48	3.1	24.75 ± 4.65	6.6	24.11 ± 4.27	5	23.14 ± 3.26	6.1	27.20 ± 5.85	5	22.00 ± 4.47	3.6	24.80 ± 6.41
Depression	Normal	0–9	70	3.36 ± 2.66	53.7	3.64 ± 2.75	74	3.28 ± 2.65	60.5	3.41 ± 2.77	66.1	3.52 ± 2.65	49.4	3.89 ± 2.70	74.5	3.10 ± 2.70	54	3.46 ± 2.85
	Mild	10–13	11.5	10.88 ± 0.99	15.1	11.20 ± 0.982	9.5	11.04 ± 1.01	12.6	11.06 ± 1.01	13.2	10.75 ± 0.977	15.8	11.23 ± 0.980	9.9	11.14 ± 1.02	17.3	11.33 ± 0.963
	Moderate	14–20	11.7	16.43 ± 2.29	17.1	16.43 ± 2.19	12.6	16.24 ± 2.22	15.4	16.30 ± 2.22	12	16.31 ± 2.37	19.5	16.55 ± 2.15	9.2	17.38 ± 2.06	12.9	16.22 ± 2.36
	Severe	21–27	3.5	24.06 ± 1.64	7.0	23.78 ± 1.60	2.3	23.33 ± 1.63	5.5	23.14 ± 1.51	4.9	24.19 ± 1.66	7.1	23.93 ± 1.64	1.4	25.00 ± 1.41	9.4	24.15 ± 1.51
	Extremely Severe	≥28	3.3	33.40 ± 4.76	7.2	33.72 ± 4.99	1.5	34.50 ± 5.74	5.9	31.86 ± 4.03	3.8	32.62 ± 4.36	8.3	33.94 ± 5.24	5	34.57 ± 5.50	6.5	36.00 ± 4.79

Note: [1] "Before" refers to the time period before the government-enforced quarantine restrictions; [2] The mean and standard deviation of the group performance within the DASS-21 Classification, stratified into Stress, Anxiety, and Depression subscales; [3] "During" refers to the time period during the quarantine. * Of which, n = 33 only have a child, as illustrated in Figure 1.

3.5. What Were the Rates of COVID-19-Related Stresses and Feelings of Gratitude?

Rates of COVID-19-related stresses and feelings of gratitude based on responses to ECQ items are given in Table 4. For each item, percentages are given for those who answered "quite a lot" or "a great deal". Percentages are based on the number of participants for whom the items were relevant. Items 1–13 and 26–30 were relevant to all 847 participants. Items 14–21 and 31–33 were relevant to 268 parents of children. Items 22–25 and 34 were relevant to 433 people with older, aging parents.

Table 4. COVID-19-related sources of stress and feelings of gratitude.

Item No.	COVID-19-Related Personal Stress for all Participants (n = 847)	%
	In the past month, how much stress have you experienced as a result of the following things?	"Quite a lot" or "A great deal"
3	Not being able to meet with your extended family and friends	69.9
13	Worrying about the effects COVID-19 on you or your family, now or in the future	47.5
5	Loss of your own or your family's daily routine (such as sleeping patterns; meal times; work, school and recreation schedules)	39.9
9	Worrying that you may become infected with COVID-19 and then infect other people	35.8
10	You, or members of your family being hospitalized for COVID-19 illness	26.4
11	Death of a family member or very close friend as a result of COVID-19	23.3
12	Witnessing others in your community suffering because of COVID-19	20.3
7	Getting a lot of conflicting information and misinformation online and in the media about COVID-19	17.9
8	You or members of your family becoming ill with COVID-19	16.3
1	Financial hardship for you or your family arising from the COVID-19 crisis due to job loss or loss of earnings	15.7
2	Having difficulty getting supplies when you need them, including face masks, hand sanitizers, medicines, food, drinks, or other essentials	12.6
6	Family conflict arising from the COVID-19 crisis due to arguing or fighting with other family members more than usual because you are spending more time together at home	9
4	Not being able to go to your church or place of religious worship	4.9
	COVID-19-related stresses for parents to a child (n = 268)	
16	Helping your child keep a safe distance from members of your extended family or preventing them from visiting with the extended family (for example grandparents)	11.9
14	Your child's school closing	9.9
17	Helping your child avoid crowded places and activities that they like, such as going to sports or musical events, scouts or guides, clubs, the playground, or to church	8.5
15	Helping your child keep a safe distance from their friends or preventing them from mixing with their friends	8.1
18	Helping your child to not shake hands, hug, or touch other people	5.2
19	Helping your child to wash or sanitize their hands regularly	4.8
21	Being worried that your child will catch COVID-19 because they have an underlying medical condition such as cancer or asthma, which makes them vulnerable to severe illness if they become infected	3.8
20	Helping your child remember to cough or sneeze into their elbow	2.8

Table 4. *Cont.*

Item No.	COVID-19-Related Personal Stress for all Participants (n = 847)	%
	In the past month, how much stress have you experienced as a result of the following things?	"Quite a lot" or "A great deal"
	COVID-19-related stresses for people with older, aging parents (n = 433)	
24	Worrying that your aging parents will become infected with COVID-19	44.7
25	Worrying that your aging parents will not receive adequate medical care if they become infected with COVID-19	36.9
22	Worrying that your aging parents will become lonely during the COVID-19 crisis	34.1
23	Worrying that your aging parents will not get supplies during the COVID-19 crisis	15.6
	COVID-19-related feelings gratitude	
	In the past month, how much has your experience of the COVID 19 crisis led you to feel grateful for the following things?	
26	Your health and the health of your family (n = 847)	85.4
27	Your relationships with your extended family and friends (n = 847)	81.7
34	Your aging parents' health and safety (n = 433)	67.9
28	Your job (n = 847)	61.9
29	Attending social, sports, and cultural events (n = 847)	59.7
30	Your community (n = 847)	45.6
32	Your child's relationships with their friends (n = 268)	21.7
31	Your child's regular attendance at school (n = 268)	20.7
33	Your child's involvement in activities such as sports, music, scouts, guides, clubs, etc. (n = 268)	15.9

From Table 4, it may be seen that for COVID-19-related personal stresses relevant to all participants, the top three were (1) not being able to meet with extended family and friends (Item 3: 69.9%); (2) worrying about the effects of COVID-19 on themselves or their family, now or in the future (Item 13: 47.5%); (3) loss of their own or family routine i.e., sleeping patterns, meal times, and/or work/school/recreational schedules (Item 5: 39.9%).

The top three COVID-19-related stresses for parents of children were (1) helping to keep their child a safe distance from extended family, and preventing them from visiting extended family i.e., grandparents (Item 16: 11.9%); (2) their child's school closing (Item 14: 9.9%); and helping their child avoid crowded places and activities they like (Item 17: 8.5%).

The top three COVID-19-related stresses for people with older, aging parents were (1) worrying that their aging parents would become infected with COVID-19 (Item 24: 44.7%); (2) worrying that aging parents will not receive adequate medical care if they become infected with COVID-19 (Item 25: 36.9%); and worrying that their aging parents will become lonely during the COVID-19 crisis (Item 22: 34.1%).

The top three COVID-19-related feelings of gratitude were personal and familial health (Item 26: 85.4%), relationships with extended family and friends (Item 27: 81.7%), and their job (Item 28: 61.9%). Participants with aging parents were most grateful for their aging parents' health and safety (Item 34; 67.9%). Participants with children were most grateful for their child's relationships with their friends (Item 32: 21.7%).

3.6. What Were the Psychometric Properties of the ECQ?

Each a priori ECQ scale had satisfactory internal consistency reliability: Personal Stress, items 1–13, alpha = 0.79; Parenting Stress, items 14–21, alpha = 0.90; Older Parent Stress, items 22–25 alpha = 0.80; and Gratitude, items 26–34, alpha = 0.72.

An exploratory factor analysis of ECQ items yielded factors that corresponded to a priori subscales with one exception. Items in the Personal Stress subscale loaded on two separate factors that assessed "Routines and Resources" (items 2, 3, 5, 6, 7, and 13; alpha = 0.61) and "Worry and Well-being" (items 8–12; alpha = 0.87). Since the alpha value for the 13-item Personal Distress scale was satisfactory (0.79), this scale rather than the two subfactors was used in the main analysis.

A five-band severity classification was devised based on the categorization of the DASS-21, which the ECQ was compared to. Within the ECQ subscales, the following ranges were derived through k-means clustering for Personal Distress: Normal 0–12; Mild 13–2; Moderate 20–26; Severe 27–33; Extremely Severe >34; Older Aging Parents: Normal 0–4; Mild 5–2; Moderate 8–11; Severe 12–15; Extremely Severe >16; Parents to children: Normal 0–8; Mild 9–2; Moderate 16–21; Severe 22–29; Extremely Severe >30.

3.7. Were the COVID-19 Related Stresses and Gratitude Assessed by the ECQ Correlated with Indices of Mental Health and Well-Being?

Table 5 shows correlations between the ECQ and other scales. The ECQ Personal Stress, Parenting Stress, and Older Parent Stress scales had significant ($p < 0.001$) correlations with DASS-21 Depression, Anxiety, and Stress scales completed to reflect distress during quarantine, the WEMWBS well-being scale, and the BIPQ Perception of COVID-19 and Emotional Impact of COVID-19 scales. All correlations were in the expected direction. High levels of COVID-19-related stresses assessed with the ECQ were associated with greater depression, anxiety, and stress assessed with the DASS-21; lower levels of well-being assessed with the WEMWBS; and greater negative perceptions of and emotional reactions to COVID-19 assessed with the BIPQ. The ECQ Gratitude scale had non-significant correlations with the DASS-21 Depression, Anxiety and Stress Scale when stratified by group. The ECQ Gratitude scale correlated positively and significantly with the WEMWBS for people with older aging parents and individuals with neither older aging parents nor children. There was a positive, non-significant correlation for parents of children. There were also positive and significant correlations between the ECQ Gratitude measure and the BIPQ Perception of COVID-19 for all group stratifications. The Emotional Impact of COVID-19, as measured by the BIPQ, correlated positively and significantly with the ECQ Gratitude scale for parents and people with older parents. The BIPQ Knowledge about COVID-19 had a significant correlation with the ECQ Gratitude scale for parents of children. Supplementary Tables S3 and S4 report the correlation coefficients across all measures, stratified by group.

Table 5. Correlations between ECQ scales and DASS, WEMWBS, and BIPQ scales.

	ECQ Scales					
Scale	Personal Stress	Parenting Stress	Older Parent Stress	Gratitude Scale		
				Personal	Parents	Older Parent
n	847	269	433	145	269	433
Quarantine DASS-21 Depression	0.39 **	0.45 **	0.24 **	0.01	−0.007	0.002
Quarantine DASS-21 Anxiety	0.46 **	0.46 **	0.32 **	0.03	0.089	0.06
Quarantine DASS-21 Stress	0.48 **	0.52 **	0.36 **	0.04	0.104	0.07
WEMWBS Well-being	−0.34 **	−0.42 **	−0.23 **	0.107 **	0.054	0.085 *

Table 5. *Cont.*

Scale	ECQ Scales					
	Personal Stress	Parenting Stress	Older Parent Stress	Gratitude Scale		
				Personal	Parents	Older Parent
n	847	269	433	145	269	433
BIPQ Perception of COVID-19	0.30 **	0.21 **	0.22 **	0.183 *	0.150 *	0.240 **
BIPQ Emotional impact of COVID-19	0.53 **	0.35 **	0.41 **	0.05	0.192 **	0.178 **
BIPQ Knowledge about COVID-19	0.01	−0.02	0.03	0.031	0.161 **	0.082

Note: ECQ = Effects of COVID-19 Questionnaire. DASS-21 = Depression, Anxiety, and Stress Scale. WEMWBS = Warwick–Edinburgh Mental Well-Being Scale. BIPQ = Brief Illness Perception Questionnaire. * $p < 0.05$. ** $p < 0.001$.

4. Discussion

This study utilized a cross-sectional online survey-based approach to investigate stress, anxiety, depression, and psychological well-being with members of the Irish public recruited through national media and social media outlets. We investigated changes in psychological distress during the COVID-19 pandemic comparing psychological outcomes before and during the quarantine period in Ireland with a sample of individuals ranging age from 18 to 76 years. Participants were asked to retrospectively comment on their "before lockdown" experience of mood and well-being. We addressed a series of five research questions. With regard to the first question concerning mean levels and rates of depression, anxiety, and stress, we found that both mean levels of all three variables and clinical levels of symptoms increased significantly during the quarantine period. The greatest increase in case severity occurred for depression. This is in line with current research specific to the COVID-19 pandemic [10]. With regard to the second question concerning mean reports of depression, anxiety, and stress in subgroups of the sample, we found that increases in depression, anxiety and stress from pre-quarantine to quarantine were not significantly affected by having responsibility for caring for a child or older, aging parents. With regard to the third question concerning rates of stresses and things for which people felt grateful that were specifically related to the COVID-19 crisis, the most frequently identified stressors by the whole sample related to social isolation, personal and familial well-being, and loss of routines such as sleeping patterns and recreational schedules. For those caring for children, the most frequently identified stressors related to keeping their child safe, keeping their child away from crowded areas, and their child's school closing, which was in line with expected outcomes [25]. For those with older, aging parents, the most frequently identified stress was them contracting COVID-19. There was also concern over the availability of medical treatment for their parent should they need it, followed by stress that their older aging parent may become lonely during the pandemic. The most frequently identified thing that people indicated the COVID-19 crisis made them grateful for was their own personal and familial health, close relationships, and their current employment.

The fourth question concerned the psychometric properties of the ECQ. We found that the four a priori subscales had acceptable levels of internal consistency reliability, and that the structure of the ECQ was partially supported by factor analytic results. We also created severity classification bands for the ECQ based on the DASS-21, which has been used to identify high levels of psychological distress during the COVID-19 pandemic through a national survey in Italy [10]. The final question concerned the association between COVID-19-related stresses and gratitude assessed by the ECQ and indices of mental health and well-being. We found that three of the four ECQ scales had significant correlations in expected directions with depression, anxiety, stress, and each correlated as expected with mental health well-being and perceptions of COVID-19.

A limitation of the current study is the profiling of parents, children, and older aging parents. While our public sample allows for stratification into these groups to better understand relative distress, our questionnaire was not designed to specifically investigate specific additional stressors, i.e., parents who may be managing behaviors that challenge during the quarantine period, or caregiving demands for older aging parents. It is well reported in the literature that externalizing behavior in children is among the most prevalent causes of parental stress across a number of clinical morbidities [32], and quarantine, social isolation, school closure, and reduced access to routine coping strategies may result in greater parental stress. However, such a conclusion cannot be drawn from this study [25,26]. A further limitation is the lack of male participants (16.4%), which future research could aim to recruit specifically, as this may implicate the generalizability of the findings. Lastly, the cross-sectional nature of the study, which included a retrospective component, may be subject to memory bias, and thusly participants may have reported lower scores on measures of distress prior to quarantine. Future research could prospectively conduct serial assessments. Our study is in line with the existing literature on psychological outcomes in response to both COVID-19 and what we know of the psychological impact of quarantine [11,23,27,33].

5. Conclusions

The Irish general public requires increased access to mental health services to meet the increase in COVID-19-related psychological problems identified in this study. In particular, access to evidence-based psychological interventions are needed that support the development and maintenance of coping mechanisms, in order to improve mental health and psychological well-being. Specifically, this research highlights the need to support people and their families across the lifespan (18–76 years) within our healthcare systems, with both traditional and non-traditional intervention strategies, ensuring accessibility is considered. This research suggests that features of depression have significantly increased as a result of the COVID-19 pandemic, which are further perpetuated by the quarantine and imposed restriction, albeit necessary steps for infection control.

Supplementary Materials: The following are available online at http://www.mdpi.com/2077-0383/9/11/3481/s1, Table S1: Effects of COVID-19 questionnaire (ECQ); Table S2: Mean and standard deviation of the psychological outcome measures for the total cohort, and the stratified group membership; Table S3: Correlations for the psychological outcome variables for the total group and the stratification of those who had neither a child nor an older aging parent; Table S4: Correlations for the psychological outcome variables stratified by those who were parents of children, as well as participants with older aging parents.

Author Contributions: Conceptualization, T.B., A.B., L.K.T., E.M., L.M. and A.C; Methodology, T.B., A.B., L.K.T., E.M., L.M. and A.C.; formal analysis, T.B., L.K.T., O.S., M.S. and A.C.; Writing—original draft preparation, T.B.; Writing—review and editing, T.B., A.C., L.M., O.S., L.K.T., A.B., E.M. and M.S.; Visualization, T.B.; Supervision, T.B. and A.C.; Funding acquisition, T.B. and A.C. All authors have read and agreed to the published version of the manuscript.

Funding: This research received no external funding.

Acknowledgments: The authors would like to thank the participants of this survey, who took part amid the global COVID-19 pandemic and local national quarantine.

Conflicts of Interest: The authors declare no conflict of interest.

References

1. Wang, C.; Horby, P.W.; Hayden, F.G.; Gao, G.F. A novel coronavirus outbreak of global health concern. *Lancet* **2020**, *395*, 470–473. [CrossRef]
2. Marazziti, D. The COVID-19 outbreak: The latest challenge to psychological and psychiatric intervention. *Clin. Neuropsychiatry* **2020**, *17*, 39–40.
3. Cheng, Z.J.; Shan, J. 2019 Novel coronavirus: Where we are and what we know. *Infection* **2020**, *48*, 155–163. [CrossRef] [PubMed]
4. Li, W.; Yang, Y.; Liu, Z.H.; Zhao, Y.J.; Zhang, Q.; Zhang, L.; Cheung, T.; Xiang, Y.T. Progression of Mental Health Services during the COVID-19 Outbreak in China. *Int. J. Biol. Sci.* **2020**. [CrossRef]
5. Kotfis, K.; Williams Roberson, S.; Wilson, J.E.; Dabrowski, W.; Pun, B.T.; Ely, E.W. COVID-19: ICU delirium management during SARS-CoV-2 pandemic. *Crit. Care* **2020**. [CrossRef] [PubMed]

6. Zambrelli, E.; Canevini, M.; Gambini, O.; D'Agostino, A. Delirium and sleep disturbances in COVID–19: A possible role for melatonin in hospitalized patients? *Sleep Med.* **2020**, *77*, 111. [CrossRef] [PubMed]
7. Romano, M. Between intensive care and palliative care at the time of CoViD-19. *Recenti Prog. Med.* **2020**. [CrossRef]
8. Salins, N.; Mani, R.K.; Gursahani, R.; Simha, N.; Bhatnagar, S. Symptom Management and Supportive Care of Serious COVID-19 Patients and their Families in India. *Indian J. Crit. Care Med.* **2020**, *24*, 435.
9. Varatharaj, A.; Thomas, N.; Ellul, M.; Davies, N.W.S.; Pollak, T.; Tenorio, E.L.; Sultan, M.; Easton, A.; Breen, G.; Zandi, M. UK-Wide Surveillance of Neurological and Neuropsychiatric Complications of COVID-19: The First 153 Patients. *Lancet Psychiatry* **2020**, in press. [CrossRef]
10. Mazza, C.; Ricci, E.; Biondi, S.; Colasanti, M.; Ferracuti, S.; Napoli, C.; Roma, P. A nationwide survey of psychological distress among italian people during the covid-19 pandemic: Immediate psychological responses and associated factors. *Int. J. Environ. Res. Public Health* **2020**, *17*, 3165. [CrossRef]
11. Brooks, S.K.; Webster, R.K.; Smith, L.E.; Woodland, L.; Wessely, S.; Greenberg, N.; Rubin, G.J. The psychological impact of quarantine and how to reduce it: Rapid review of the evidence. *Lancet* **2020**, *395*, 912–920. [CrossRef]
12. Jeong, H.; Yim, H.W.; Song, Y.J.; Ki, M.; Min, J.A.; Cho, J.; Chae, J.H. Mental health status of people isolated due to Middle East Respiratory Syndrome. *Epidemiol. Health* **2016**. [CrossRef] [PubMed]
13. Liu, X.; Kakade, M.; Fuller, C.J.; Fan, B.; Fang, Y.; Kong, J.; Guan, Z.; Wu, P. Depression after exposure to stressful events: Lessons learned from the severe acute respiratory syndrome epidemic. *Compr. Psychiatry* **2012**. [CrossRef] [PubMed]
14. Mihashi, M.; Otsubo, Y.; Yinjuan, X.; Nagatomi, K.; Hoshiko, M.; Ishitake, T. Predictive Factors of Psychological Disorder Development During Recovery Following SARS Outbreak. *Health Psychol.* **2009**. [CrossRef] [PubMed]
15. Yoon, M.K.; Kim, S.Y.; Ko, H.S.; Lee, M.S. System effectiveness of detection, brief intervention and refer to treatment for the people with post-traumatic emotional distress by MERS: A case report of community-based proactive intervention in South Korea. *Int. J. Ment. Health Syst.* **2016**. [CrossRef]
16. Hawryluck, L.; Gold, W.L.; Robinson, S.; Pogorski, S.; Galea, S.; Styra, R. SARS control and psychological effects of quarantine, Toronto, Canada. *Emerg. Infect. Dis.* **2004**. [CrossRef]
17. DiGiovanni, C.; Conley, J.; Chiu, D.; Zaborski, J. Factors influencing compliance with quarantine in Toronto during the 2003 SARS outbreak. *Biosecur. Bioterror.* **2004**. [CrossRef]
18. Lee, S.; Chan, L.Y.Y.; Chau, A.M.Y.; Kwok, K.P.S.; Kleinman, A. The experience of SARS-related stigma at Amoy Gardens. *Soc. Sci. Med.* **2005**. [CrossRef]
19. Reynolds, D.L.; Garay, J.R.; Deamond, S.L.; Moran, M.K.; Gold, W.; Styra, R. Understanding, compliance and psychological impact of the SARS quarantine experience. *Epidemiol. Infect.* **2008**. [CrossRef]
20. Marjanovic, Z.; Greenglass, E.R.; Coffey, S. The relevance of psychosocial variables and working conditions in predicting nurses' coping strategies during the SARS crisis: An online questionnaire survey. *Int. J. Nurs. Stud.* **2007**. [CrossRef]
21. Maunder, R.; Hunter, J.; Vincent, L.; Bennett, J.; Peladeau, N.; Leszcz, M.; Sadavoy, J.; Verhaeghe, L.M.; Steinberg, R.; Mazzulli, T. The immediate psychological and occupational impact of the 2003 SARS outbreak in a teaching hospital. *CMAJ* **2003**, *168*, 1245–1251. [PubMed]
22. Wang, Y.; Xu, B.; Zhao, G.; Cao, R.; He, X.; Fu, S. Is quarantine related to immediate negative psychological consequences during the 2009 H1N1 epidemic? *Gen. Hosp. Psychiatry* **2011**. [CrossRef] [PubMed]
23. Dong, L.; Bouey, J. Early Release-Public Mental Health Crisis during COVID-19 Pandemic, China. *EID J.* **2020**, *26*. [CrossRef]
24. Boyraz, G.; Legros, D.N. Coronavirus Disease (COVID-19) and Traumatic Stress: Probable Risk Factors and Correlates of Posttraumatic Stress Disorder. *J. Loss Trauma* **2020**. [CrossRef]
25. Fontanesi, L.; Marchetti, D.; Mazza, C.; Di Giandomenico, S.D.; Roma, P.; Verrocchio, M.C. The Effect of the COVID-19 Lockdown on Parents: A Call to Adopt Urgent Measures. *Psychol. Trauma Theory Res. Pract. Policy* **2020**. [CrossRef]
26. Mazza, C.; Ricci, E.; Marchetti, D.; Fontanesi, L.; Di Giandomenico, S.; Verrocchio, M.C.; Roma, P. How personality relates to distress in parents during the COVID-19 lockdown: The mediating role of child's emotional and behavioral difficulties and the moderating effect of living with other people. *Int. J. Environ. Res. Public Health* **2020**, *17*, 6236. [CrossRef]

27. Vostanis, P.; Bell, C.A. Counselling and psychotherapy post-COVID-19. *Couns. Psychother. Res.* **2020**, *20*, 389–393. [CrossRef]
28. Lovibond, S.H.; Lovibond, P.F. *Manual for the Depression Anxiety Stress Scales*; Psychology Foundation: Sydney, Australia, 1995; ISBN 7334-1423-0.
29. Tennant, R.; Hiller, L.; Fishwick, R.; Platt, S.; Joseph, S.; Weich, S.; Parkinson, J.; Secker, J.; Stewart-Brown, S. The Warwick-Dinburgh mental well-being scale (WEMWBS): Development and UK validation. *Health Qual. Life Outcomes* **2007**. [CrossRef]
30. Broadbent, E.; Petrie, K.J.; Main, J.; Weinman, J. The Brief Illness Perception Questionnaire. *J. Psychosom. Res.* **2006**. [CrossRef]
31. Cicchetti, D.V. Guidelines, Criteria, and Rules of Thumb for Evaluating Normed and Standardized Assessment Instruments in Psychology. *Psychol. Assess* **1994**. [CrossRef]
32. Barroso, N.E.; Mendez, L.; Graziano, P.A.; Bagner, D.M. Parenting Stress through the Lens of Different Clinical Groups: A Systematic Review & Meta-Analysis. *J. Abnorm. Child Psychol.* **2018**, *46*, 449–461. [PubMed]
33. Liang, L.; Ren, H.; Cao, R.; Hu, Y.; Qin, Z.; Li, C.; Mei, S. The Effect of COVID-19 on Youth Mental Health. *Psychiatr. Q.* **2020**. [CrossRef]

Journal of
Clinical Medicine

MDPI

Article

Does Physical Activity Matter for the Mental Health of University Students during the COVID-19 Pandemic?

Aleksandra M. Rogowska [1,*], Iuliia Pavlova [2], Cezary Kuśnierz [3], Dominika Ochnik [4], Ivanna Bodnar [2] and Petro Petrytsa [5]

1 Institute of Psychology, University of Opole, 45-052 Opole, Poland
2 Theory and Methods of Physical Culture Department, Lviv State University of Physical Culture, 79007 Lviv, Ukraine; pavlova.j.o@gmail.com (I.P.); ivannabodnar@ukr.net (I.B.)
3 Faculty of Physical Education and Physiotherapy, Opole University of Technology, 45-378 Opole, Poland; c.kusnierz@po.edu.pl
4 Faculty of Medicine, University of Technology, 40-555 Katowice, Poland; dominika.ochnik@gwsh.pl
5 Department of Physical Education, Ternopil Volodymyr Hnatiuk National Pedagogical University, 46027 Ternopil, Ukraine; petrytsa@tnpu.edu.ua
* Correspondence: arogowska@uni.opole.pl

Received: 29 September 2020; Accepted: 22 October 2020; Published: 29 October 2020

Abstract: Research indicates that university and college students are at higher risk of experiencing mental health problems than other populations. This study aims to examine the relationship between Physical Activity (PA) and the mental health of Ukrainian university students during the Corona Virus Disease 2019 (COVID-19) pandemic lockdown. The conventional sample consisted of 1512 students from 11 Ukrainian universities, with a mean age of 20 years (M = 20.06, SD = 3.05) and 69% of whom were female. The cross-sectional online survey was disseminated through the most popular social media channels in Ukraine (i.e., Facebook, Viber, Telegram) and included the Generalized Anxiety Disorder (GAD-7) scale to measure anxiety and the Patient Health Questionnaire (PHQ-9) to assess depression. Data were collected from 14 May to 4 June 2020 during the COVID-19 pandemic outbreak in Ukraine. Among university students, 43% were engaged in PA $\geq$ 150 min weekly, 24% met the criteria of GAD, and 32% met the criteria of depression. More students were involved in PA before the COVID-19 outbreak than during the national lockdown. Students with anxiety and depression were almost two times less likely to engage in PA than their counterparts without mental health disorders. The inactive group had higher scores of anxiety and depression than the physically active group. The relationship of PA with anxiety and depression was statistically significant but weak during the COVID-19 pandemic.

Keywords: anxiety; depression; PHQ-9; GAD-7; physical activity (PA); undergraduates; university students

1. Introduction

1.1. *Coronavirus Disease in Ukraine*

This study examines the mental health of Ukrainian university students during the first two months of the Corona Virus Disease 2019 (COVID-19) outbreak. On 3 March 2020, Ukraine announced the first confirmed case of the coronavirus disease. On 30 April 2020, approximately 10,860 cases of COVID-19 were recorded. Merely one month later (on 31 May 2020), the number of cases was confirmed as 24,012. The Cabinet of Ministers of Ukraine adopted a resolution on preventing the spread of the coronavirus COVID-19 in Ukraine on 11 March 2020. Following the resolution, quarantine was enforced in the territory of Ukraine from 12 March 2020. Students were prohibited from attending or visiting any type of educational establishment and mass events were canceled and banned. On the same day, the Ministry of Education and Science published a letter stating the need to comply with the rules of the quarantine. As a consequence, kindergartens, schools, colleges, and universities were closed, and e-learning using remote technologies was implemented. Lockdown was introduced in all regions of Ukraine. State borders were closed, and a minimum period was granted for the return of citizens who were abroad at that time. On 16 March, Ukraine closed international air, rail, and bus services. On 18 March, domestic rail, air, and bus services were suspended. In addition, intercity and interregional passenger traffic, pedestrian traffic, and the use of public transport were also significantly restricted. Social distancing and the wearing of face masks were introduced as obligatory requirements.

According to government decrees in early April, it was forbidden to visit parks, squares, recreation areas, coastal areas, sports areas, and children's playgrounds. Moving in groups of more than two people was also banned. Citizens were not allowed to stay outside their homes or be on the streets without documents. The police and the military were involved in monitoring the self-isolation regime. The penalty for the violation of quarantine conditions was a fine or imprisonment. A five-step program for quarantine alleviation was implemented after 22 May 2020, dependent on the epidemiological situation in each region. In June 2020, educational institutions' work was only carried out remotely. Social distancing and the wearing of facemasks were still required.

1.2. Mental Health during the COVID-19 Pandemic

Although a lockdown increases the chance of effectively dealing with COVID-19, it also contributes to a decrease in people's well-being [1–4], invoking several adverse emotional reactions such as anger, fear, confusion, irritability, frustration, elevated stress, insomnia, and nervousness [1,4,5]. Thousands of people have lost their work and socio-economic status during the COVID-19 pandemic. Numerous studies have reported an increase in anxiety and depression among people around the world [5–18]. A review study indicated that, up to the time of its publishing, the prevalence of anxiety and depression ranged between 16–28% of the Chinese population during the COVID-19 pandemic [13]. Furthermore, it was found that women were at higher risk of coronavirus-related mental health disorders than men [16,19–23]. Research also indicated that younger adults were at higher risk of anxiety, depression, and alcohol use than adults with an average age and above [6,9,10,19,22,23].

A growing body of literature has recently focused on examining mental health among undergraduates [18,20,21,24–29]. Those studies suggest that university and college students experience higher rates of anxiety than it has been reported in other population groups [18,20,21,24,28]. However, a disparity in the prevalence of mental health disorders was also noted between particular studies, dependent on cross-cultural differences and the measurement methods used to assess anxiety and depression. When a seven-item General Anxiety Disorder (GAD-7) scale was used, Cao et al. [24] found that approximately 30% of Chinese students (n = 7143) reported symptoms of mild (21.3%), moderate (2.7%), and severe (0.9%) anxiety during the COVID-19 pandemic. In research by Feng et al. [25], anxiety was reported for 32% (in the GAD-7) of Chinese students, and depression was found in 28%, using a nine-item Patient Health Questionnaire (PHQ-9). The prevalence of general anxiety disorder (using GAD-7) among Polish university students (n = 914) was 67%, including 32% with mild, 21% with moderate, and 14% with severe symptoms. Among nursing students, the prevalence of moderate and severe anxiety (using the GAD-7) was 42.8% and 13.1%, respectively, during the third week of the national lockdown in Israel [28]. Sallam et al. [21] found a mean anxiety score of 8.4 (assessed using GAD-7), with statistically significant higher scores among males (M = 7.7) compared to females (M = 8.6).

It is important to note that the high risk of anxiety and depression disorders was noted among university and college students before the pandemic started, and this trend has been observed in research for years. A review of previous studies conducted before the COVID-19 pandemic showed that depression was present on average in 30.6% of undergraduates [30,31], with significantly higher rates among women. Studies revealed that anxiety has been diagnosed in 12–43% of college and university students [31–33]. Thus, there is a need to develop and integrate various prevention and intervention programs at university campuses to cope with stress, anxiety, and depression. One of the ways to reduce the levels of anxiety and depression is engagement in healthy behavior, such as physical activity (PA).

1.3. Physical Activity and Health

The beneficial effect of PA on mental health is well-documented in many studies e.g., [34–40]. Regular exercise improves sleep, mood, endurance, and cardiovascular fitness; reduces cholesterol, body weight, tiredness; and helps boost stress relief, energy, and interest in sex. Therefore, exercise is recommended as a prescription for patients with various conditions including respiratory system diseases [41]. Recent research found that enhanced aerobic capacity could improve immune functions, decrease COVID-19 severity, and may help prevent infection [42].

Although home-based physical training was recommended during the COVID-19 lockdown [43–45], some research suggested that the intensity of PA decreased among people in Asia, America, Africa, and Europe [23,34,46,47]. On the other hand, a general increase in PA was observed in Belgium [48] and Canada [49] during the coronavirus outbreak. This inconsistency regarding the changes in the intensity of PA during the pandemic should be monitored, particularly in the groups of the population at higher risk of mental health disorders such as university and college students.

Here, we examine the relationship between PA and both anxiety and depression in a large sample of university students in Ukraine during the national lockdown. Previous research conducted prior to the COVID-19 pandemic indicates that 58% of college students met the WHO physical activity guidelines (i.e., ≥150 min per week of PA) in Canada [50]. Furthermore, Ghrouz et al. [51] showed that Indian college students with moderate and high PA levels (49% of the total sample) reported significantly lower anxiety and depression scores than their counterparts with a low PA level. To the best of our knowledge, only one study has explored the PA level and mental health of college students during the COVID-19 pandemic so far [18]. That study indicated that approximately 56% of Chinese students were engaged in moderate and high levels of PA during the coronavirus outbreak [18]. It was also shown that PA alleviated negative emotions and depression.

The following research questions were posed in the present study: (1) What is the prevalence of anxiety and depression disorders during the coronavirus pandemic in a sample of university students in Ukraine? (2) How many Ukrainian undergraduates meet the PA level consistent with the WHO recommendation (≥150 min per week) during the COVID-19 lockdown? (3) Has the level of PA changed from before the pandemic? (4) What is the association between PA, anxiety, and depression in the study sample? Due to differences between the sexes found in previous studies on PA, anxiety, and depression during the COVID-19 pandemic, sex will be controlled in this study as a covariate.

We formulated the following hypotheses:

1. Based on previous research, we expected approximately one-third of university students to have suffered from various forms of depression and anxiety, experiencing moderate to severe symptoms [6,9,10,13,16–18,20,21,25,52].
2. We expected approximately half of the university students to meet the recommended criteria of sufficient PA level (≥150 min per week) during the COVID-19 pandemic, as previously suggested [18].
3. We expected that the level of PA would have changed during the COVID-19 pandemic compared to the typical PA level before the coronavirus outbreak [23,34,46–49].
4. We expected physically active university students to demonstrate lower scores in anxiety and depression than their inactive counterparts [18,51]. The appropriate level of PA (≥150 min/week) can predict levels of anxiety and depression.

2. Materials and Methods

2.1. Participants

The sample consisted of 1512 students whose age ranged between 18–51 (M = 20.06, SD = 3.05), most of whom were female (n = 1038, 68.65%). The target population was comprised of undergraduates from 18 Ukrainian universities located in 11 cities: Kyiv (National Aviation University, National University of Food Technologies), Kharkiv (Yaroslav Mudryi National University, Kharkiv National Kotlyarevsky University of Arts), Lviv (Lviv Polytechnic National University, Ivan Franko National University of Lviv, Lviv State University of Physical Culture named after Ivan Boberskyj), Drohobych (Drohobych Ivan Franko State Pedagogical University), Ternopil (Ternopil Volodymyr Hnatiuk National Pedagogical University), Lutsk (Lesya Ukrainka Eastern European National University, Lutsk National Technical University), Mykolaiv (Petro Mohyla Black Sea National University, Mykolaiv V.O.Sukhomlynskyi National University), Poltava (National University "Yuri Kondratyuk Poltava Polytechnic"), Cherkasy (Bohdan Khmelnytsky Cherkasy National University), Chernivtsi (Yuriy Fedkovych Chernivtsi National University), and Ivano-Frankivsk (Vasyl Stefanyk Precarpathian National University). Territorially, the study covered 10 of the 27 Ukrainian regions. Students represented various university majors at various levels of higher education. Table 1 outlines the demographic characteristics of the sample (age, gender, faculty, and level, year, and type of study).

Table 1. Demographic characteristics of the study sample.

Demographic Variables	n	%
Sex		
Female	1038	68.65
Male	474	31.35
Place of Residence		
Village	494	32.67
Small town	535	35.38
Big city	434	28.70
Urban agglomeration	49	3.24
Level of Study		
Bachelor	1374	90.87
Master	127	8.40
Doctoral	11	0.73
Branches of Study Science		
Social Science	531	35.12
Formal Science	109	7.21
Natural Science	141	9.32
Health Science	731	48.35
Year of Study		
First	610	40.34
Second	346	22.88
Third	243	16.07
Fourth	222	14.68
Fifth	91	6.02
Type of Study		
Stationary	1417	93.72
Extramural	95	6.28

The total number of students in Ukraine is about 1.5 million people. According to state statistics in Ukraine [53], the largest group consists of state institutions of higher education (universities, academies, institutes, colleges, technical schools, colleges), amounting to 456 institutions (381 when excluding separate units); there are 191 private institutions 191 (140 when excluding separate units). The number of institutions of the highest level of accreditation (universities, institutes, academies) was 282, with 78 private institutions at this level. Of the total number of students, 400,000 are in extramural study and 106,000 are in private higher education institutions. Approximately 90% of students in universities, institutes, and academies are aged 17–24 years.

There are more females in higher education. This trend at universities has been stable over the past ten years [53]. With regard to study majors, constant changes began in higher education from 2015. The available statistics [53,54] offer only a partial understanding of the structure of student distribution by field of study. The majority of students choose social sciences (38.3%); natural sciences (6.4%); engineering, architecture, and construction (19–21%); education and pedagogy (8%); service industries (6.9%); and health and social security (8%).

In the present survey, we tried to avoid questions concerning ethnicity (Ukrainian, Russian) due to the military actions in eastern Ukraine provoked and initiated by the Russian Federation. The questionnaire was written in Ukrainian and was intended only for local students who spoke Ukrainian at the native speakers' level. According to national statistics [55], 96.2% of young people aged 18–29 consider themselves ethnic Ukrainians, 2.8% Russians, and 0.7% of other nationalities. For 2019, the number of international students did not exceed 5%. Among students of other nationalities (foreign students) studying in Ukraine are citizens from India (n = 14,958), Morocco (n = 7390), Azerbaijan (n = 6228), Turkmenistan (n = 5033), Nigeria (n = 3552), Egypt (n = 3412), Turkey (n = 3254), China (n = 2721), Israel (n = 2460), and Georgia (n = 2397) [53]. Most international students traditionally choose Ukrainian medical colleges and universities, but we did not collect data from students in this type of higher education.

2.2. Measures

2.2.1. Exposure to COVID-19

Exposure to COVID-19 was assessed based on eight questions about the consequences of the coronavirus: (1) Have you experienced symptoms that could indicate coronavirus infection? (2) Have you been tested for coronavirus? (3) Were you hospitalized by coronavirus? (4) Did you have to be in strict quarantine for at least 14 days, that is, in isolation from loved ones because of the coronavirus infection? (5) Has anyone in your family or friend group been infected with coronavirus? (6) Have any of your relatives died of coronavirus? (7) Have you or a loved one lost their job because of coronavirus? (8) Are you currently experiencing a worsening of your functioning or economic status due to the effects of the coronavirus pandemic? Individuals answered each of these questions with 1 = Yes and 0 = No.

2.2.2. Perceived Impact of Coronavirus

The perceived impact of COVID-19 on the student's life was measured using five statements. Participants used a 5-item Likert scale (from 1 = Strongly disagree, to 5 = Definitely agree) to express how much they were afraid that the current situation associated with the coronavirus pandemic (COVID-19) may negatively affect their life in each of the following five areas: (1) Completing the semester and graduation; (2) finding a job and professional development; (3) financial situation (e.g., subsistence during studies); (4) relationships with loved ones and family; (5) relations with colleagues and friends. Next, the scores obtained from the five items were summarized to give a total score of perceived coronavirus impact (PCI). Higher scores indicated greater coronavirus-related concerns. The internal reliability of the scale was acceptable with Cronbach's $\alpha = 0.65$.

2.2.3. Physical Activity

Physical activity during the coronavirus-related lockdown was assessed using the following question: "How many days a week did you exercise physically or pursue sports activities at home or away from home, at the university, in clubs or at the gym, in the last month?". Participants answered this question on an eight-point scale (from 0 = Not one day to 7 = Seven days a week). Next, the students answered the open question "how many minutes a day (on average) did you practice?", writing an average number of minutes of PA per day. The next question was as follows: "How many days a week did you do physical exercise or sports activities at home or away from home, at the university, in clubs or at the gym, within a month before the general coronavirus quarantine?", with the same scales used as in the answers for the previous questions. The number of days was multiplied by the number of minutes per day to calculate the PA level the previous week. Those students who performed 150 min weekly or more were included in the Active (A) group, whereas the Inactive (I) sample comprised those individuals who devoted less than 150 min per week to PA, according to the WHO recommendation [45].

2.2.4. Anxiety

A seven-item generalized anxiety disorder (GAD-7) is a self-reported measure designed to screen for symptoms following the Diagnostic and Statistical Manual of Mental Disorders (DSM-IV) criteria [56]. People rated, on a 4-point Likert scale (0 = Not at all, 1 = Several days, 2 = More than half the days, and 3 = Nearly every day), how often they experienced anxiety symptoms in the past 2 weeks. The GAD-7 scores ranged between 0–4, indicating no or minimal anxiety, between 5–9 mild, between 10–14 moderate, and between 15–21 severe GAD [57]. Scores above 10 points indicated an anxiety disorder. In this study, the Cronbach's α for the GAD-7 was 0.90.

2.2.5. Depression

A patient health questionnaire (PHQ-9) was used to measure symptoms of depression among university students. PHQ-9 consisted of nine items, corresponding to the DSM-IV diagnostic criteria [58,59]. Participants answered questions about how often over the past two weeks they had been bothered by nine depression symptoms, using a Likert-like response scale ranging from 0 = Not at all, to 3 = Nearly every day. The PHQ-9 scores may be interpreted as normal between 0–4, mild major depressive disorder between 5–9, moderate between 10–14, moderately severe between 15–19, and severe between 20–27 [58]. At a score of 10 or above, it is recommended to screen for a major depressive disorder [58,60,61]. In this study, the Cronbach's α for the PHQ-9 was 0.85.

2.2.6. Demographics

The survey also included eight questions related to demographic variables. The questions referred to age, gender, place of residence (village, small town, big city, and urban agglomeration), field of study, study major, level of study (i.e., first degree, secondary studies, uniform five-year studies, doctoral studies), year of the study (ranging 1–5), and mode (i.e., stationary or extramural). Table 2 presents the frequency of the given response category in the study sample.

Table 2. Coronavirus-related variables.

Variable	*n*	%
Physical Activity ≥150 min Weekly		
Before Coronavirus Pandemic	703	46.49
During Coronavirus Pandemic	653	43.19
Exposure To COVID-19		
Symptoms of Coronavirus Infection	111	7.34
Testing for Coronavirus	34	2.25
Hospitalization Because of Coronavirus	8	0.53
Strict Quarantine For At Least 14 Days	122	8.07
Coronavirus Infection Among Close Relatives	83	5.49
Death of Coronavirus Among Close Relatives	7	0.46
Unemployment Because Of The Coronavirus	602	39.81
Worse Functioning or Lower Economic Status	1063	70.30

Table 2. *Cont.*

Variable	*n*	%
Anxiety (GAD-7)		
Normal (0–4)	618	40.87
Mild (5–9)	534	35.32
Moderate (10–14)	243	16.07
Severe (15–21)	117	7.74
Depression (PHQ-9)		
Normal (0–4)	476	31.48
Mild (5–9)	557	36.84
Moderate (10–14)	290	19.18
Moderately severe (15–19)	127	8.40
Severe (20–27)	62	4.10
Neither Depression nor Anxiety Diagnosis (Scores ≤ 10)	958	63.36
Anxiety Only Diagnosis (GAD-7 ≥ 10)	75	4.96
Depression Only Diagnosis (PHQ-9 ≥ 10)	194	12.83
Dual Anxiety and Depression Diagnosis (Scores ≥ 10)	285	18.85

2.3. Procedure

A cross-sectional study was performed using a self-reported Google Forms survey. This study was part of an international research project preregistered in the Open Science Framework (OSF) [62]. Researchers collaborated with students' trade unions and student government organizations to disseminate an invitation to participate in the study among the students of target universities. The invitation was distributed by Facebook groups, Viber groups, and Telegram channels. The data were collected from 14 May to 4 June 2020 and 99% of the responses were dated between 14 May and 1 June. The first website of the Google Forms survey consisted of information about the study and an informed consent form. All students were informed about the purpose of the study and participation was voluntary. They were also assured about the anonymity and confidentiality of the survey and that they may refuse to participate in the study at any time. Initially, 1542 students visited the website with the survey. However, 30 undergraduates did not agree to participate in the study. Ultimately, 1512 respondents gave their informed consent and completed the questionnaire (98.1% response rate). This study was approved by the Institutional Research Board (IRB) of the Lviv State University of Physical Culture (No. 4/2020.04.01) and was conducted according to the principles of the Declaration of Helsinki.

Statistical Analysis

Descriptive statistics, such as the mean (*M*), standard deviation (SD), range, standard error (SE), and 95% confidential intervals (CI) with lower limit (LL) and upper limit (UL) calculated for the total sample. Pearson's χ^2 test of independence was performed to find an association between physical activity (PA) before and during the coronavirus pandemic. A two-way ANOVA was performed to examine sex and PA differences (considered as dichotomous discrete variables) in anxiety (continuous variable). The effect size was measured by partial eta-squared ($\eta_p{}^2$), which describes the ratio of variance explained in the dependent variable by a predictor in the ANOVA model. The Tukey's honest significant difference test (HSD) was performed to examine post hoc differences between mean scores. The associations between mental health and PA were examined using binominal logistic regression analysis. The relationships between anxiety, COVID-19 impact, physical activity, and sex were examined using Pearson's correlation analysis. Finally, multiple linear regression analysis was conducted to find the moderation effect of physical activity and sex on the relationship between COVID-19 impact and anxiety. All analyses were performed using Statistica 13.3. (Statsoft Polska Sp. z o.o., Kraków, Poland)

3. Results

3.1. Prevalence of Anxiety and Depression among Undergraduates during the COVID-19 Pandemic

Anxiety criteria (GAD-7 $\geq$ 10) were met by 360 undergraduates (24%), while depression (PHQ-9 $\geq$ 10) was found in 479 university students (32%). Overall, people with clinically significant depression and/or anxiety totaled 554 (37%), whereas 958 (63%) of people did not display significant symptoms of mental disorder. In the study sample, individuals meeting exclusively anxiety criteria numbered 75 (5%), those exclusively with depression criteria numbered 194 (13%), and those with dual depression and anxiety symptoms totaled 285 undergraduates (19%). The contingency table showed that the difference between people with singular and dual symptoms was statistically significant, χ^2 (1) = 492.28, $p < 0.001$, $\phi = 0.57$. Descriptive statistics for anxiety and the impact of COVID-19 on students' well-being are shown in Table 3.

Table 3. Descriptive statistics.

Variable	Range	M	SD	95% CI LL	95% CI UL
Anxiety	0–21	6.43	4.94	6.19	6.68
Depression	0–27	7.79	5.48	7.51	8.06
Perceived Impact of Coronavirus on Life	5–25	15.86	4.17	15.65	16.07
Completing the Semester and Graduation	1–5	3.36	1.26	3.30	3.42
Finding A Job and Professional Development	1–5	3.67	1.20	3.61	3.73
Financial Situation	1–5	3.82	1.18	3.76	3.88
Relationships with Loved Ones, Family	1–5	2.44	1.43	2.37	2.51
Relations with Colleagues, Friends	1–5	2.57	1.36	2.50	2.64

3.2. Prevalence of PA before and during the COVID-19 Pandemic

Tables 1 and 2 demonstrate the number and proportion of individuals exposed to the coronavirus disease and engaged in PA at a sufficient level ($\geq$150 min/week, according to the WHO recommendations) before and during the national coronavirus quarantine. As shown in Table 2, most students reported being inactive both before and during the COVID-19 quarantine. During the COVID-19 outbreak, 43% of university students were engaged in PA at the desired level. In comparison, 46% of students reported being active before lockdown. A Pearson's χ^2 test of independence indicated that the differences between active and inactive participants significantly changed over time; χ^2 (1) = 254.93, $p < 0.001$, $\phi = 0.41$. The same status of PA before and during the coronavirus pandemic was reported by 457 active individuals (30.22%) and 613 (40.54%) inactive individuals. People active before the quarantine but becoming inactive during the COVID-19 pandemic numbered 246 (16.27%). Conversely, those inactive before the pandemic outbreak but becoming active during the coronavirus lockdown totaled 196 (12.96%). It suggests that students with a reduced level of PA during the COVID-19 pandemic outnumbered those becoming more active.

3.3. Differences in Anxiety and Depression between Physically Active and Inactive University Students

Results of the binominal logistic regression suggest that, during the COVID-19 pandemic, university students that met the clinical criteria for depression (the PHQ-9 scores $\geq$ 10) were 1.6 times less likely to engage in PA ($\geq$150 min PA weekly) than those without clinically significant depression χ^2 (1) = 19.04, OR = 1.64, 95% CI (1.31, 2.05), B = 0.49, SE B = 0.11, t(1510) = 4.32, $p < 0.001$, Wald χ^2 = 18.67. Undergraduates that met the clinical criteria for anxiety (the GAD-7 scores $\geq$ 10) were 1.7 times less likely to exercise than their counterparts without clinically significant anxiety disorders, χ^2(1) = 17.98, OR = 1.69, 95% CI (1.32, 2.17), B = 0.53, SE B = 0.13, t(1510) = 4.18, $p < 0.001$, Wald χ^2 = 17.47. Undergraduates with the dual clinical criteria of depression and anxiety (scores in the PHQ-9 $\geq$ 10 and GAD-7 $\geq$ 10) were 1.9 times less likely to be physically active than people without clinically significant mental health symptoms, χ^2 (1) = 22.84, OR = 1.95, 95% CI (1.47, 2.58), B = 0.67, SE B = 0.14, t(1241) = 4.68, $p < 0.001$, Wald $\chi^2 = 21.89$.

Table 4 and Figure 1 demonstrate some results of the two-way ANOVA test with anxiety as the dependent variable and sex (female, male) and PA groups (inactive, active) as the independent variables. A significant effect was found for sex and PA separately (Table 4). The Tukey HSD post hoc test showed that females scored significantly higher in anxiety than males and physically inactive female students (those who were engaged in PA less than 150 min weekly during the coronavirus pandemic). Levels of anxiety were similar in physically active and inactive female students. Physically active and inactive male university students did not differ in their anxiety levels. The effect of interaction between gender and PA was also not statistically significant.

Table 4. Means, standard deviations, and two-way ANOVA statistics for anxiety.

Variable	Female		Male		ANOVA			
	M	SD	M	SD	Effect	F (1, 1508)	p	$\eta_p{}^2$
PA Groups					S	41.27	<0.001	0.03
Inactive	6.58	4.98	4.87	4.52	PA	5.88	0.015	0.00
Active	7.29	4.96	5.49	4.67	S × PA	0.03	0.861	0.00

n = 1512. ANOVA = analysis of variance; S = sex, PA = physical activity.

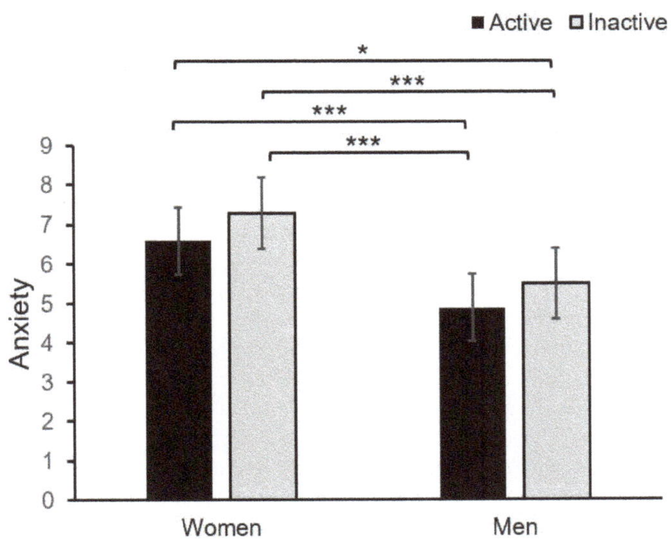

Figure 1. Mean anxiety scores for groups of undergraduates differing in sex (women, men) and engagement in physical activity (active, inactive). Error bars show standard errors. * $p < 0.05$, *** $p < 0.001$.

A two-way ANOVA was conducted for depression as a dependent variable and sex (female, male) and PA groups (inactive, active) as independent variables (see Table 5 and Figure 2 for more details). Both sex and PA were statistically significant factors for depression but without an interaction effect. The Tukey HSD post hoc test showed that physically active women differ significantly in depression to inactive female students, as well as active and inactive males. Significant differences were also found between inactive women and active men.

Table 5. Means, standard deviations, and two-way ANOVA statistics for depression.

Variable	Female		Male		ANOVA			
	M	SD	M	SD	Effect	F (1, 1508)	p	η_p^2
PA groups					S	44.59	<0.001	0.03
Active	7.82	5.30	5.88	5.09	PA	10.33	0.001	0.01
Inactive	8.87	5.62	6.78	5.06	S × PA	0.06	0.812	0.00

n = 1512. ANOVA = analysis of variance; S = sex, PA = physical activity.

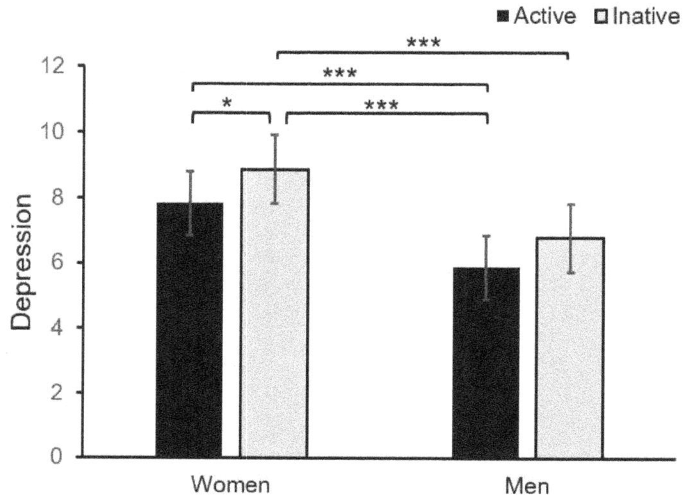

Figure 2. Mean depression scores for groups of undergraduates differing in sex (women, men) and engagement in physical activity (active, inactive). Error bars show standard errors. * $p < 0.05$, *** $p < 0.001$.

3.4. Predictors of Anxiety and Depression

Correlation analysis showed that anxiety was positively associated with exposure to COVID-19 (r = 0.25, $p < 0.001$) and the perceived coronavirus impact (PCI) on students' well-being (r = 0.16, $p < 0.001$). Hierarchical multiple linear regression was conducted separately for anxiety and depression as an explanatory variable and sex, exposure to COVID-19, the impact of COVID-19 on well-being, and physical activity (PA) as predictor variables. Both regression models were tested in a preliminary analysis to ensure that they met the assumptions of residual normality, linearity, homoscedasticity, and non-collinearity (using VIF < 10). All criteria were met. As presented in Table 6, all variables were found to be significant predictors of anxiety. Sex alone explained about 3% of anxiety variability, F(1, 1510) = 48.41, $p < 0.001$. The negative correlation found between sex and anxiety indicated that females (coded as "0") presented higher anxiety levels than males (coded as "1"). When exposure to COVID-19 was included in the regression in the second step, the model explained 9% of anxiety variability, F(2, 1509) = 73.23, $p < 0.001$. The change in variance explained was 6%, F(1, 1509) = 95.04, $p < 0.001$. The third model of regression included the impact of COVID-19 on students' well-being. The variability explained significantly increased to 13% (F(3, 1508) = 74.50, $p < 0.001$), with 4% of change in variance explained (F(1, 1508) = 70.30, $p < 0.001$). The fourth step of regression analysis included PA, which significantly changed the variance explained to 14% (F(4, 1507) = 61.92, $p < 0.001$). The variability explained changed significantly by about 1% (F(1, 1507) = 21.21, $p < 0.001$). The negative association between PA and anxiety indicates that those university students who spent less than 150 min doing PA every week during the COVID-19 pandemic experienced higher levels of anxiety than their counterparts who engaged in more than 150 min PA per week.

Table 6. Hierarchical regression results for anxiety.

Variable	95% CI for *B*						
	B	LL	UL	SE B	β	R^2	ΔR^2
Step 1						0.03 ***	0.03 ***
Constant	8.47 ***	8.15	8.80	0.17			
Sex	−2.17 ***	−2.78	−1.61	0.30	−0.19 ***		
Step 2						0.09 ***	0.06 ***
Constant	6.75 ***	6.26	7.24	0.25			
Sex	−2.11 ***	−2.68	−1.54	0.29	−0.18 ***		
Exposure to COVID–19	1.26 ***	0.99	1.53	0.14	0.23 ***		
Step 3						0.13 ***	0.04 ***
Constant	2.92 ***	1.88	3.95	0.53			
Sex	−2.21 ***	−2.77	−1.65	0.29	−0.19 ***		
Exposure to COVID–19	0.99 ***	0.72	1.27	0.14	0.18 ***		
Impact of COVID–19 (PCI)	0.27 ***	0.20	0.33	0.03	0.20 ***		
Step 4						0.14 ***	0.01 ***
Constant	4.42 ***	3.31	5.53	0.57			
Sex	−2.08 ***	−2.63	−1.53	0.28	−0.18 ***		
Exposure to COVID–19	0.99 ***	0.72	1.26	0.14	0.18 ***		
Impact of COVID–19 (PCI)	0.27 ***	0.21	0.34	0.03	0.21 ***		
Physical activity (PA)	−0.46 ***	−0.60	−0.33	0.07	−0.16 ***		

*** $p < 0.001$.

Depression was found to be positively associated with exposure to COVID-19 (r = 0.23, $p < 0.001$) and PCI (r = 0.23, $p < 0.001$). Hierarchical multiple regression analysis showed that all variables included in the model were significant predictors of depression (Table 7). Similar to the previous analysis, sex explained about 3% of depression variability (F(1, 1510) = 54.01, $p < 0.001$), with higher depression among female students than male. In the second step, gender and exposure to COVID-19 explained for 8% of anxiety variability, F(2, 1509) = 70.46, $p < 0.001$. The change in variance explained equaled 5%, F(1, 1509) = 83.95, $p < 0.001$. When PCI was included in the third regression model, the percentage of variability explained significantly increased to 12% (F(3, 1508) = 71.29, $p < 0.001$), with 4% of change in variance explained (F(1, 1508) = 66.81, $p < 0.001$). The fourth model of regression included PA, which significantly changed the variance explained to 15% (F(4, 1507) = 66.64, $p < 0.001$). The variability explained changed significantly by about 3% (F(1, 1507) = 46.26, $p < 0.001$). In comparison with the hierarchical regression model for anxiety, PA seems more important for depression than for anxiety.

Table 7. Hierarchical regression results for depression.

Variable	95% CI for B						
	B	LL	UL	SE B	β	R^2	ΔR^2
Step 1						0.03 ***	0.03 ***
Constant	8.47 ***	8.14	8.80	0.17			
Gender	−2.20 ***	−2.78	−1.61	0.30	−0.19 ***		
Step 2						0.08 ***	0.05 ***
Constant	6.75 ***	6.27	7.24	0.25			
Gender	−2.11 ***	−2.68	−1.54	0.29	−0.18 ***		
Exposure to COVID–19	1.26 ***	0.99	1.53	0.14	0.23 ***		
Step 3						0.12 ***	0.04 ***
Constant	2.92 ***	1.88	3.95	0.53			
Gender	−2.21 ***	−2.77	−1.65	0.29	−0.19 ***		
Exposure to COVID–19	0.99 ***	0.72	1.27	0.14	0.18 ***		
Impact of COVID–19 (PCI)	0.27 ***	0.20	0.33	0.03	0.20 ***		
Step 4						0.15 ***	0.03 ***
Constant	4.42 ***	3.31	5.53	0.57			
Gender	−2.08 ***	−2.63	−1.53	0.28	−0.18 ***		
Exposure to COVID–19	0.99 ***	0.72	1.26	0.14	0.18 ***		
Impact of COVID–19 (PCI)	0.27 ***	0.21	0.34	0.03	0.21 ***		
Physical activity (PA)	−0.46 ***	−0.60	−0.33	0.07	−0.16 ***		

*** $p < 0.001$.

4. Discussion

4.1. Mental Health in Ukrainian University Students

This study aimed to examine PA's relationship with the mental health of university students during the COVID-19 pandemic. Results suggest that 37% of the study sample suffered from moderate to severe anxiety and/or depression. Symptoms of depression were significantly more frequently found than symptoms of anxiety. In addition, more people had dual clinically significant mental disorders (anxiety and depression simultaneously) than those who met the singular criteria of the PHQ-9 and GAD-7. Approximately one-quarter of students may suffer from general anxiety disorders, while nearly one-third may be affected by depression. Furthermore, almost one-fifth of university students manifested symptoms of anxiety and depression concurrently. This means that the vast majority of individuals with anxiety symptoms experienced the comorbidity of depression.

The hypothesis that approximately one-third of the university student population suffered from various forms of depression and anxiety (from moderate to severe symptoms) was confirmed in this research regarding depression, but anxiety levels were lower than expected. The present result is consistent with the study of Feng et al. [25] but differs from certain previous studies performed in the student population during the COVID-19 pandemic [18,20,21,28]. The prevalence of depression in the present study sample was 32%. In comparison, between 23% [18] and 32% [25] of depression was reported among college and university students in China. General anxiety disorder was found in approximately 24% of Ukrainian university students, as compared to 4% [24], 28% [25] and 45% [18] among Chinese college students, 35% of Polish university students [20], and 56% in nursing students from Israel [28]. The mean anxiety score was 6.43 in the present sample of Ukrainian university students, while Jordanian students reported a mean anxiety score of 8.4 [21]. Anxiety in the present study was lower than in most previous studies reported for both students and general populations.

A review indicated that the prevalence of anxiety and depression ranged between 16–28% of the Chinese population during the COVID-19 pandemic at the time of publishing [13]. However, differences between particular studies can be seen in mental health symptoms during the COVID-19 pandemic. More specifically, moderate to severe anxiety was noted in 29%, whereas moderate to severe depression was reported in 16% of the population living in China during the COVID-19 pandemic outbreak [16,17]. Among Chinese people younger than 35, 38% reported general anxiety disorder (GAD), and 22% reported depression symptoms [9,10]. Ahmed et al. [6] found 19% of people suffered from anxiety and 27% suffered from symptoms of depression ranging from moderate to severe among 1074 Chinese people living in Hubei province. The prevalence of depression, anxiety, and comorbidity of depression and anxiety was 48.3%, 22.6%, and 19.4%, respectively, among people from Wuhan province in China [52]. Approximately 23% of individuals from Cyprus reported moderate to severe anxiety symptoms, and 9% reported moderate to severe depression symptoms [22].

The differences between particular studies may be determined, besides cross-cultural differences, by the various methods used to measure anxiety and depression, the distinct quality of the study, and the various cut-off criteria for diagnosing anxiety and depression. A recent meta-analysis indicated that the prevalence of depression assessed using the PHQ-9 scores ≥10 are often overestimated when compared to a diagnosis of major depression on the base of Structured Clinical Interview for Diagnostic and Statistical Manual of Mental Disorders (SCID) [63]. On the other hand, the PHQ is a self-reported screening questionnaire used to detect a risk of depression by an average non-clinician person, so overestimating seems to be a desired feature in this case. Another systematic review and meta-analysis [64] showed that PHQ-9 has acceptable diagnostic properties for major depressive disorders (with cut-off points between 8–11), and diagnostic accuracy was reasonably consistent despite the clinical heterogeneity of the included studies. Most likely, certain anxiety and depression measures present better sensitivity, specificity, and reliability than others. A previous meta-analysis showed a wide range of differences in the global prevalence of anxiety among medical students, which may also be related to cross-cultural differences [65]. Moreover, research was conducted at different stages of the COVID-19 outbreak. Many countries in the world introduced several coronavirus-related restrictions in traveling; shopping; access to education, medical and social services; outdoor physical activity; gatherings; and meetings with friends and family. However, these restrictions were changed systematically within each country. As a consequence, a reliable comparison of mental health during the COVID-19 pandemic may be very difficult to achieve.

Consistent with most of the previous research, the analysis of variance showed that female Ukrainian university students score higher than men in anxiety and depression [16,18–23]. However, it is essential to note that these differences are rather weak, since the effect size was very small ($\eta_p^2 = 0.03$), and sex was not found to be a predictor for both anxiety and depression. Previous research indicated that the fear of the COVID-19 disease was positively related to a younger age, being female, and those more likely to keep smoking and drinking alcohol among medical students in Vietnam [26]. Among Jordanian university students, higher anxiety was reported in females, individuals with the lowest monthly income, those with less coronavirus knowledge, and those who believed the disease was part of a conspiracy [21].

The present results do not differ substantially from previous research conducted before the coronavirus pandemic outbreak [30–33]. It is confirmed that university and college students experience consistently higher rates of mental health disorders than other populations, which may be slightly elevated by the COVID-19 pandemic and lockdown restrictions. The findings from the regression analysis suggest that exposure to COVID-19 and individual differences in the perception of the coronavirus impact (PCI) showed significant but weak associations with anxiety and depression, so other factors may be more important in explaining mental health among Ukrainian university students.

However, the COVID-19 pandemic has given rise to many new concerns among the academic population. Besides the usual restrictions, university students have to contend with virtual learning during the COVID-19 pandemic. Online learning was not available to many students due to the lack of computers or internet access. During the pandemic, neither the students nor the teachers had been trained in the use of large-scale web-based teaching platforms and technology. Teachers were not familiar with the new online learning methodology. They had to change learning plans to adapt to the unique situation rapidly. Thus, the virtual classes were stressful for both teachers and students [18,66–69].

Furthermore, most of the students lost their part-time jobs which supported them while studying and offered them financial independence [70]. Adults who lived in dormitories had to return to their family homes and be dependent on their parents. During the first months of the outbreak of the pandemic, a prevalence of uncertainty regarding the near future, examinations, completing classes and finishing studies, the financial situation, and housing and social situation was evident [69]. Cao et al. [24] showed that economic factors affected daily life during the COVID-19 pandemic and that delays in academic activities were positively related to anxiety symptoms among Chinese college students. Furthermore, Qiu et al. [19] suggested that young adults tend to obtain a large amount of information from social media, which may elevate stress. Overall, the SARS-CoV-2 was perceived as a moderately dangerous disease by most students [21].

4.2. Relationship between PA and Mental Health

The present study suggests that 43% of university students were physically active during the coronavirus lockdown, according to the WHO recommendation (≥150 min/week of PA) [45]. A previous study found that 56% of Chinese college students were physically active at moderate or vigorous levels during the national quarantine [18]. The results suggest that the sample of Ukrainian students may be less involved in PA than the group of Chinese undergraduates. However, the previous research [18] used different measurement methods (i.e., a seven-item International Physical Activity Questionnaire—IPAQ) to assess weekly PA during the last two weeks according to three categories: light, moderate, and vigorous. Thus, the previous and present studies are not fully comparable.

Furthermore, the number of active students decreased significantly in comparison to the situation before the COVID-19 outbreak in Ukraine, which is consistent with some previous studies [23,34,46,47]. Stanton et al. [23] showed that negative physical activity changes are associated with increased depression, anxiety, and stress symptoms. Research indicates that exercise withdrawal may consistently result in an increase in depressive symptoms and anxiety [71].

Consistent with other research [18,51], this study indicates that there is a significant and inverse relationship between PA and anxiety and depression during the COVID-19 pandemic. A longitudinal survey showed that PA directly alleviated general negative emotions in college students during the peak time of the COVID-19 outbreak in China [18]. The volume of moderate-to-vigorous leisure-time PA (MVPA) was also positively associated with mental health and negatively related to the symptoms of anxiety and depression among post-secondary students aged between 16–24 years [72]. Furthermore, increasing PA during the COVID-19 lockdown was related to lower anxiety and improved well-being among individuals who were inactive before the pandemic [49].

Ukrainian undergraduates with anxiety and depression symptoms are between 1.6 and 1.9 times less likely to be physically active than their counterparts without mental health problems. This result is consistent with the previous population study of DeMello et al. [73], which showed that individuals who do not engage in PA are two times more likely to exhibit symptoms of depression and anxiety compared with those who regularly pursue PA. Furthermore, the highest association with PA was found in this study for participants with a dual anxiety and depression diagnosis. Forte et al. [74] also found that severe depression was most common among adolescents with comorbid anxiety and low PA levels.

The anti-depressive and anxiolytic effects of physical activity on clinical and non-clinical populations were evidenced in a great number of studies e.g., [70,71,75,76]. A systematic review and meta-analysis showed that PA reduces depression by a medium effect and anxiety by a small effect, in non-clinical populations [77,78]. Previous meta-analyses found a moderate-to-strong negative relationship between PA and depression and inconsistent association of PA with anxiety (ranged between not statistically significant effect to a moderate beneficial effect of PA on anxiety) in clinical populations. Previous findings suggest that high PA significantly reduced the prevalence of depressive problems, but not anxiety disorders, among Chinese first-year college students [25]. In contrast, this study found a statistically significant but rather weak association of PA with anxiety and depression. The hierarchical regression model with PA, sex, exposure to COVID-19, and PCI as predictors explained only 14% of anxiety and 15% of depression variability. PA can solely explain 1% of anxiety variability and 3% of depression variability, as shown in the hierarchical regression model in the fourth step of the analysis. Thus, more research is necessary to explain the specific relationship between these variables.

4.3. Limitations of the Study

There are certain limitations to this study. First, the online recruitment method has several limitations. As the research was performed during the lockdown related to the COVID-19 pandemic, all students used remote web-based technologies to learn in virtual educational platforms. An online survey was the only way to perform research on student well-being during the general quarantine. However, the invitation was distributed via Facebook groups, Viber groups, and Telegram channels, so students who do not use these websites could not respond. The online survey results may not be consistent with "paper and pencil" questionnaires. Although the study sample was substantial, there were more female respondents. This proportion is consistent with sex prevalence in typical universities (although technical universities comprise more males). Further research may include a more balanced proportion of the sexes in the study sample. As this research was performed in universities exclusively, the results of this study may not be generalized into more technically focused types of universities. Moreover, this study's results cannot be generalized into other adult populations, since participants in this study were exclusively university students. Some demographic variables, such as ethnicity, income, employment, marital status, or household members, were not included in the questionnaire. Thus, we do not know if these variables would be more useful as covariates in analyzing the relationship between PA and mental disorder. Further research should include more demographic variables related to the mental health of university students. We used a simple, dichotomous division of people into active and inactive groups according to the WHO recommendation of PA level over the past week. However, other survey questions concerning more details of the level of PA (mild, moderate, vigorous) or time of each of the types could be used in future research. Finally, due to the cross-sectional character of research, the results of the regression analysis should be treated with caution.

5. Conclusions

This study confirmed that a significant proportion of Ukrainian students experience high levels of anxiety and depression. Both anxiety and depression are, to some extent, related to gender and PA, but the relationship is rather weak though statistically significant. PA seems a relatively inexpensive and effective way to cope with the effects of the COVID-19 pandemic. Thus, the present research results may be used in the prevention and treatment of coronavirus-related mental health burdens on university campuses. Mailey et al. [79] recommended an internet-delivered physical activity intervention, which should be implemented with psychological counseling for college students suffering from anxiety and depression. Clemente-Suárez [80] suggests that the combination of psychological therapy with aerobic physical activity and nutritional recommendations can decrease anxiety and depression symptoms in just six sessions. WHO recommends a minimum of 150 min of physical activity weekly [45]. According to a recent study [18], just 108 min of mild PA, 80 min of moderate PA, or 45 min of vigorous PA per day is enough to prevent mental health disorders and maintain well-being during the COVID-19 pandemic, and this is a recommended intervention in university student populations. We propose the introduction of online PA training on e-learning platforms (e.g., Moodle, MS Teams, Zoom), conducted by a professional sports coach in the field of aerobic and anaerobic exercises varying in intensity level (light, moderate, and vigorous), to be chosen by students depending on their movement abilities and interests. Exercises should last a minimum of one hour and should be proposed online twice a day (morning and evening) each day.

We believe that this PA training can be useful for all students in preventing mental health disorders. For university students with severe symptoms of anxiety and depression, supportive interventions can include physical exercises performed in conjunction with individual psychological online therapy.

Author Contributions: Conceptualization, A.M.R., I.P., C.K. and D.O.; methodology, A.M.R. and D.O., software, A.M.R.; validation, A.M.R., I.P., C.K., D.O., I.B. and P.P.; formal analysis, A.M.R.; investigation, I.P., I.B. and P.P.; resources, A.M.R., I.P., C.K., D.O., I.B. and P.P.; data curation, A.M.R., I.P., I.B. and P.P.; writing—original draft preparation, A.M.R., I.P., C.K., D.O., I.B. and P.P.; writing—review and editing, A.M.R., I.P., C.K., D.O., I.B. and P.P.; visualization, A.M.R.; supervision, C.K.; project administration, I.P.; funding acquisition, C.K. All authors have read and agreed to the published version of the manuscript.

Funding: The APC was funded by the Opole University of Technology.

Conflicts of Interest: The authors declare no conflict of interest. The APC funders had no role in the design of the study; in the collection, analyses, or interpretation of data; in the writing of the manuscript, or in the decision to publish the results.

References

1. Brooks, S.K.; Webster, R.K.; Smith, L.E.; Woodland, L.; Wessely, S.; Greenberg, N.; Rubin, G.J. The psychological impact of quarantine and how to reduce it: A rapid review of the evidence. *Lancet* **2020**, *395*, 912–920. [CrossRef]
2. Chaturvedi, S.K. COVID-19, coronavirus, and mental health rehabilitation at times of crisis. *J. Psychosoc. Rehabil. Ment. Health* **2020**, *7*, 1–2. [CrossRef]
3. Ding, Y.; Xu, J.; Huang, S.; Li, P.; Lu, C.; Xie, S. Risk perception and depression in public health crises: Evidence from the COVID-19 crisis in China. *Int. J. Environ. Res. Public Health* **2020**, *17*, 5728. [CrossRef] [PubMed]
4. Li, J.B.; Yang, A.; Dou, K.; Cheung, R.Y.M. Self-Control Moderates the Association between Perceived Severity of Coronavirus Disease 2019 (COVID-19) and Mental Health Problems among the Chinese Public. *Int. J. Environ. Res. Public Health* **2020**, *17*, 4820. [CrossRef] [PubMed]
5. Ahorsu, D.K.; Lin, C.Y.; Imani, V.; Saffari, M.; Griffiths, M.D.; Pakpour, A.H. The Fear of COVID-19 Scale: Development and Initial Validation. *Int. J. Ment. Health Addict.* **2020**, 1–9. [CrossRef] [PubMed]
6. Ahmed, Z.; Ahmed, O.; Aibao, Z.; Hanbin, S.; Siyu, L.; Ahmad, A. Epidemic of COVID-19 in china and associated psychological problems. *Asian J. Psychiatr.* **2020**, *51*, 102092. [CrossRef] [PubMed]
7. Choi, E.P.H.; Hui, B.P.H.; Wan, E.Y.F. Depression and anxiety in Hong Kong during COVID-19. *Int. J. Environ. Res. Public Health* **2020**, *17*, 3740. [CrossRef] [PubMed]
8. Hao, F.; Tan, W.; Jiang, L.; Zhang, L.; Zhao, X.; Zou, Y.; Hu, Y.; Luo, X.; Jiang, X.; McIntyre, R.S.; et al. Do psychiatric patients experience more psychiatric symptoms during COVID-19 pandemic and lockdown? A case-control study with service and research implications for immunopsychiatry. *Brain Behav. Immun.* **2020**, *87*, 100–106. [CrossRef]
9. Huang, Y.; Zhao, N. Chinese mental health burden during the COVID-19 pandemic. *Asian J. Psychiatr.* **2020**, *51*, 102052. [CrossRef]
10. Huang, Y.; Zhao, N. Generalized anxiety disorder, depressive symptoms and sleep quality during COVID-19 outbreak in China: A web-based cross-sectional survey. *Psychiatry Res.* **2020**, *288*, 112954. [CrossRef]
11. Kim, Y.-J.; Cho, J.-H.; Kim, E.-S. Differences in sense of belonging, pride, and mental health in the Daegu Metropolitan Region due to COVID-19: Comparison between the presence and absence of National Disaster Relief Fund. *Int. J. Environ. Res. Public Health* **2020**, *17*, 4910. [CrossRef]
12. Liang, L.; Ren, H.; Cao, R.; Hu, Y.; Qin, Z.; Li, C.; Mei, S. The Effect of COVID-19 on Youth Mental Health. *Psychiatr Q.* **2020**, *91*, 841–852. [CrossRef]
13. Rajkumar, R.P. Covid-19 and mental health: A review of the existing literature. *Asian J. Psychiatr.* **2020**, *52*, 102066. [CrossRef] [PubMed]
14. Ran, L.; Wang, W.; Ai, M.; Kong, Y.; Chen, J.; Kuang, J. Psychological resilience, depression, anxiety, and somatization symptoms in response to COVID-19: A study of the general population in China at the peak of its epidemic. *Soc. Sci. Med.* **2020**, *262*, 113261. [CrossRef] [PubMed]
15. Shi, L.; Lu, Z.A.; Que, J.Y.; Huang, X.L.; Liu, L.; Ran, M.S.; Gong, Y.M.; Yuan, K.; Yan, W.; Sun, Y.K.; et al. Prevalence of and Risk Factors Associated with Mental Health Symptoms among the General Population in China during the Coronavirus Disease 2019 Pandemic. *JAMA Netw. Open* **2020**, *3*, e2014053. [CrossRef]

16. Wang, C.; Pan, R.; Wan, X.; Tan, Y.; Xu, L.; Ho, C.S.; Ho, R.C. Immediate Psychological Responses and Associated Factors during the Initial Stage of the 2019 Coronavirus Disease (COVID-19) Epidemic among the General Population in China. *Int. J. Environ. Res. Public Health* **2020**, *17*, 1729. [CrossRef]
17. Wang, C.; Pan, R.; Wan, X.; Tan, Y.; Xu, L.; McIntyre, R.S.; Choo, F.N.; Tran, B.; Ho, R.; Sharma, V.K.; et al. A longitudinal study on the mental health of general population during the COVID-19 epidemic in China. *Brain Behav. Immun.* **2020**, *87*, 40–48. [CrossRef]
18. Zhang, Y.; Zhang, H.; Ma, X.; Di, Q. Mental health problems during the COVID-19 pandemics and the mitigation effects of exercise: A longitudinal study of college students in China. *Int. J. Environ. Res. Public Health* **2020**, *17*, 3722. [CrossRef]
19. Qiu, J.; Shen, B.; Zhao, M.; Wang, Z.; Xie, B.; Xu, Y. A nationwide survey of psychological distress among Chinese people in the COVID-19 epidemic: Implications and policy recommendations. *Gen. Psychiatr.* **2020**, *33*, e100213. [CrossRef] [PubMed]
20. Rogowska, A.; Kuśnierz, C.; Bokszczanin, A. Examining anxiety, life satisfaction, general health, stress and coping styles during COVID-19 pandemic in Polish sample of university students. *Psychol. Res. Behav. Manag.* **2020**, *13*, 797–811. [CrossRef]
21. Sallam, M.; Dababseh, D.; Yaseen, A.; Al-Haidar, A.; Ababneh, N.A.; Bakri, F.G.; Mahafzah, A. Conspiracy Beliefs Are Associated with Lower Knowledge and Higher Anxiety Levels Regarding COVID-19 among Students at the University of Jordan. *Int. J. Environ. Res. Public Health* **2020**, *17*, 4915. [CrossRef]
22. Solomou, I.; Constantinidou, F. Prevalence and predictors of anxiety and depression symptoms during the COVID-19 pandemic and compliance with precautionary measures: Age and sex matter. *Int. J. Environ. Res. Public Health* **2020**, *17*, 4924. [CrossRef] [PubMed]
23. Stanton, R.; To, Q.G.; Khalesi, S.; Williams, S.L.; Alley, S.J.; Thwaite, T.L.; Fenning, A.S.; Vandelanotte, C. Depression, anxiety and stress during COVID-19: Associations with changes in physical activity, sleep, tobacco and alcohol use in Australian adults. *Int. J. Environ. Res. Public Health* **2020**, *17*, 4065. [CrossRef]
24. Cao, W.; Fang, Z.; Hou, G.; Han, M.; Xu, X.; Dong, J.; Zheng, J. The psychological impact of the COVID-19 epidemic on college students in China. *Psychiatry Res.* **2020**, *287*, 112934. [CrossRef] [PubMed]
25. Feng, Y.; Zong, M.; Yang, Z.; Gu, W.; Dong, D.; Qiao, Z. When altruists cannot help: The influence of altruism on the mental health of university students during the COVID-19 pandemic. *Global. Health* **2020**, *16*, 61. [CrossRef]
26. Nguyen, H.T.; Do, B.N.; Pham, K.M.; Kim, G.B.; Dam, H.T.B.; Nguyen, T.T.; Nguyen, T.T.P.; Nguyen, Y.H.; Sørensen, K.; Pleasant, A.; et al. Fear of COVID-19 Scale—Associations of its scores with health literacy and health-related behaviors among medical students. *Int. J. Environ. Res. Public Health* **2020**, *17*, 4164. [CrossRef] [PubMed]
27. Ryu, S.; Ali, S.T.; Lim, J.-S.; Chun, B.C. Estimation of the excess COVID-19 cases in Seoul, South Korea by the students arriving from China. *Int. J. Environ. Res. Public Health* **2020**, *17*, 3113. [CrossRef]
28. Savitsky, B.; Findling, Y.; Ereli, A.; Hendel, T. Anxiety and coping strategies among nursing students during the covid-19 pandemic. *Nurse Educ. Pract.* **2020**, *46*, 102809. [CrossRef]
29. Taghrir, M.H.; Borazjani, R.; Shiraly, R. COVID-19 and Iranian medical students: A survey on their related-knowledge, preventive behaviors and risk perception. *Arch. Iran. Med.* **2020**, *23*, 249–254. [CrossRef]
30. Ibrahim, A.K.; Kelly, S.J.; Adams, C.E.; Glazebrook, C. A systematic review of studies of depression prevalence in university students. *J. Psychiatr. Res.* **2013**, *47*, 391–400. [CrossRef]
31. Zeng, Y.; Wang, G.; Xie, C.; Hu, X.; Reinhardt, J.D. Prevalence and correlates of depression, anxiety and symptoms of stress in vocational college nursing students from Sichuan, China: A cross-sectional study. *Psychol. Health Med.* **2019**, *24*, 798–811. [CrossRef] [PubMed]
32. Liu, X.; Ping, S.; Gao, W. Changes in undergraduate students' psychological well-being as they experience university life. *Int. J. Environ. Res. Public Health* **2019**, *16*, 2864. [CrossRef] [PubMed]
33. Pedrelli, P.; Nyer, M.; Yeung, A.; Zulauf, C.; Wilens, T. College students: Mental health problems and treatment considerations. *Acad. Psychiatry* **2015**, *39*, 503–511. [CrossRef]
34. Wang, X.; Lei, S.M.; Le, S.; Yang, Y.; Zhang, B.; Yao, W.; Gao, Z.; Cheng, S. Bidirectional Influence of the COVID-19 Pandemic Lockdowns on Health Behaviors and Quality of Life among Chinese Adults. *Int. J. Environ. Res. Public Health* **2020**, *17*, 5575. [CrossRef] [PubMed]
35. Fibbins, H.; Ward, P.B.; Watkins, A.; Curtis, J.; Rosenbaum, S. Improving the health of mental health staff through exercise interventions: A systematic review. *J. Ment. Health* **2018**, *27*, 184–191. [CrossRef] [PubMed]
36. Guszkowska, M. Effects of exercise on anxiety, depression and mood. *Psychiatr. Pol.* **2004**, *38*, 611–620.

37. Heijnen, S.; Hommel, B.; Kibele, A.; Colzato, L.S. Neuromodulation of Aerobic Exercise—A Review. *Front. Psychol.* **2016**, *6*, 1890. [CrossRef]
38. Paluska, S.A.; Schwenk, T.L. Physical activity and mental health: Current concepts. *Sports Med.* **2000**, *29*, 167–180. [CrossRef]
39. Sharma, A.; Madaan, V.; Petty, F.D. Exercise for mental health. *Prim. Care Companion J. Clin. Psychiatry* **2005**, *8*, 106. [CrossRef]
40. Warburton, D.E.; Nicol, C.W.; Bredin, S.S. Health benefits of physical activity: The evidence. *CMAJ* **2006**, *174*, 801–809. [CrossRef]
41. Luan, X.; Tian, X.; Zhang, H.; Huang, R.; Li, N.; Chen, P.; Wang, R. Exercise as a prescription for patients with various diseases. *J. Sport Health Sci.* **2019**, *8*, 422–441. [CrossRef]
42. Mohamed, A.; Alawna, M. Role of increasing the aerobic capacity on improving the function of immune and respiratory systems in patients with coronavirus (COVID-19): A review. *Diabetes Metab. Syndr.* **2020**, *14*, 489–496. [CrossRef] [PubMed]
43. Chen, P.; Mao, L.; Nassis, G.P.; Harmer, P.; Ainsworth, B.E.; Li, F. Coronavirus disease (COVID-19): The need to maintain regular physical activity while taking precautions. *J. Sport Health Sci.* **2020**, *9*, 103–104. [CrossRef]
44. Hammami, A.; Harrabi, B.; Mohr, M.; Krustrup, P. Physical activity and coronavirus disease 2019 (COVID-19): Specific recommendations for home-based physical training. *Manag. Sport Leis.* **2020**, 1–6. [CrossRef]
45. WHO. Be Active during COVID-19. Available online: https://www.who.int/emergencies/diseases/novel-coronavirus-2019/question-and-answers-hub/q-a-detail/be-active-during-covid-19 (accessed on 5 June 2020).
46. Ammar, A.; Brach, M.; Trabelsi, K.; Chtourou, H.; Boukhris, O.; Masmoudi, L.; Bouaziz, B.; Bentlage, E.; How, D.; Ahmed, M.; et al. Effects of COVID-19 Home Confinement on Eating Behaviour and Physical Activity: Results of the ECLB-COVID19 International Online Survey. *Nutrients* **2020**, *12*, 1583. [CrossRef]
47. López-Bueno, R.; Calatayud, J.; Andersen, L.L.; Balsalobre-Fernández, C.; Casaña, J.; Casajús, J.A.; Smith, L.; López-Sánchez, G.F. Immediate Impact of the COVID-19 Confinement on Physical Activity Levels in Spanish Adults. *Sustainability* **2020**, *12*, 5708. [CrossRef]
48. Constandt, B.; Thibaut, E.; De Bosscher, V.; Scheerder, J.; Ricour, M.; Willem, A. Exercising in Times of Lockdown: An Analysis of the Impact of COVID-19 on Levels and Patterns of Exercise among Adults in Belgium. *Int. J. Environ. Res. Public Health* **2020**, *17*, 4144. [CrossRef] [PubMed]
49. Lesser, I.A.; Nienhuis, C.P. The Impact of COVID-19 on Physical Activity Behavior and Well-Being of Canadians. *Int. J. Environ. Res. Public Health* **2020**, *17*, 3899. [CrossRef] [PubMed]
50. Li, Y.C.; Chirico, D.; Graham, J.D.; Kwan, M.; Cairney, J. Motor Coordination and Moderate-to-Vigorous Physical Activity in Emerging Adults: Mediating Effect of Physical Self-Concept. *Int. J. Environ. Res. Public Health* **2020**, *17*, 3748. [CrossRef] [PubMed]
51. Ghrouz, A.K.; Noohu, M.M.; Dilshad Manzar, M.; Warren Spence, D.; BaHammam, A.S.; Pandi-Perumal, S.R. Physical activity and sleep quality in relation to mental health among college students. *Sleep Breath.* **2019**, *23*, 627–634. [CrossRef] [PubMed]
52. Gao, J.; Zheng, P.; Jia, Y.; Chen, H.; Mao, Y.; Chen, S.; Wang, Y.; Fu, H.; Dai, J. Mental health problems and social media exposure during COVID-19 outbreak. *PLoS ONE* **2020**, *15*, e0231924. [CrossRef]
53. Kvit, S.; Yeremenko, O.; Stukalo, N.; Butenko, A.; Nazarov, A.; Artyuxov, A.; Vynnyczkyj, M.; Shypilov, L.; Ksheveczkyj, V.; Tereshhuk, V. *Annual Report of the National Agency for Quality Assurance in Higher Education for 2019*; National Agency for Quality Assurance in Higher Education: Kyiv, Ukraine, 2020. Available online: https://naqa.gov.ua/wp-content/uploads/2020/02/%D0%97%D0%B2%D1%96%D1%82-2020.pdf (accessed on 19 October 2020).
54. Finikov, T.V.; Sharov, O.I. *Monitoring the Integration of the Ukrainian Higher Education System into the European Higher Education Area and Research: Monitoring Study: Analytical Report*; Edupolicy: Kyiv, Ukraine, 2014; Available online: http://www.edupolicy.org.ua/_dx/assets/images/Analit2ua_web.pdf (accessed on 19 October 2020).
55. Ruzumkov Center. *Basic Principles and Ways of Formation of Common Identity of Citizens of Ukraine*; Information and Analytical Materials for the Round Table on April 12 2017; Ruzumkov Center: Kyiv, Ukraine, 2017; Available online: https://razumkov.org.ua/images/Material_Conference/2017_04_12_ident/2017-Identi-3.pdf (accessed on 19 October 2020).
56. Spitzer, R.L.; Kroenke, K.; Williams, J.B.W.; Löwe, B. A brief measure for assessing generalized anxiety disorder. *Arch. Intern. Med.* **2006**, *166*, 1092–1097. [CrossRef] [PubMed]

57. Löwe, B.; Decker, O.; Müller, S.; Brähler, E.; Schellberg, D.; Herzog, W.; Herzberg, P.Y. Validation and standardization of the Generalized Anxiety Disorder Screener (GAD-7) in the general population. *Med. Care* **2008**, *46*, 266–274. [CrossRef]
58. Kroenke, K.; Spitzer, R.L.; Williams, J.B. The PHQ-9: Validity of a brief depression severity measure. *J. Gen. Intern. Med.* **2001**, *16*, 606–613. [CrossRef] [PubMed]
59. Löwe, B.; Kroenke, K.; Herzog, W.; Gräfe, K. Measuring depression outcome with a brief self-report instrument: Sensitivity to change of the Patient Health Questionnaire (PHQ-9). *J. Affect. Disord.* **2004**, *81*, 61–66. [CrossRef]
60. Kocalevent, R.-D.; Hinz, A.; Brähler, E. Standardization of the depression screener Patient Health Questionnaire (PHQ-9) in the general population. *Gen. Hosp. Psychiatry* **2013**, *35*, 551–555. [CrossRef]
61. Manea, L.; Gilbody, S.; McMillan, D. A diagnostic meta-analysis of the Patient Health Questionnaire-9 (PHQ-9) algorithm scoring method as a screen for depression. *Gen. Hosp. Psychiatry* **2015**, *37*, 67–75. [CrossRef]
62. Rogowska, A.M.; Kuśnierz, C.; Ochnik, D.; Schütz, A.; Kafetsios, K.; Slan, I.; Pavlova, I.; Benatov, J.; Arzenšek, A.; Jakubiak, M.; et al. *Wellbeing of Undergraduates during the COVID-19 Pandemic*; International Study; OSF: Charlottesville, VA, USA, 2020. [CrossRef]
63. Levis, B.; Benedetti, A.; Ioannidis, J.; Sun, Y.; Negeri, Z.; He, C.; Wu, Y.; Krishnan, A.; Bhandari, P.M.; Neupane, D.; et al. Patient Health Questionnaire-9 scores do not accurately estimate depression prevalence: Individual participant data meta-analysis. *J. Clin. Epidemiol.* **2020**, *122*, 115–128.e1. [CrossRef]
64. Manea, L.; Gilbody, S.; McMillan, D. Optimal cut-off score for diagnosing depression with the Patient Health Questionnaire (PHQ-9): A meta-analysis. *CMAJ* **2012**, *184*, 191–196. [CrossRef]
65. Quek, T.T.; Tam, W.W.; Tran, B.X.; Zhang, M.; Zhang, Z.; Ho, C.S.; Ho, R.C. The Global Prevalence of Anxiety among Medical Students: A Meta-Analysis. *Int. J. Environ. Res. Public Health* **2019**, *16*, 2735. [CrossRef]
66. Daniel, S.J. Education and the COVID-19 pandemic. *Prospects* **2020**. [CrossRef]
67. García-González, M.A.; Torrano, F.; García-González, G. Analysis of stress factors for female professors at online universities. *Int. J. Environ. Res. Public Health* **2020**, *17*, 2958. [CrossRef] [PubMed]
68. Olmos-Gómez, M.C. Sex and Careers of University Students in Educational Practices as Factors of Individual Differences in Learning Environment and Psychological Factors during COVID-19. *Int. J. Environ. Res. Public Health* **2020**, *17*, 5036. [CrossRef]
69. Zhang, X. Thoughts on large-scale long-distance web-based teaching in colleges and universities under novel Coronavirus pneumonia epidemic: A case of Chengdu University. In Proceedings of the 4th International Conference on Culture, Education and Economic Development of Modern Society (ICCESE 2020), Moscow, Russia, 13–14 March 2020; pp. 1222–1225. [CrossRef]
70. Gautam, R.; Sharma, M. 2019-nCoV pandemic: A disruptive and stressful atmosphere for Indian academic fraternity. *Brain Behav. Immun.* **2020**, *88*, 948–949. [CrossRef] [PubMed]
71. Weinstein, A.A.; Koehmstedt, C.; Kop, W.J. Mental health consequences of exercise withdrawal: A systematic review. *Gen. Hosp. Psychiatry* **2017**, *49*, 11–18. [CrossRef]
72. Doré, I.; O'Loughlin, J.L.; Beauchamp, G.; Martineau, M.; Fournier, L. Volume and social context of physical activity in association with mental health, anxiety and depression among youth. *Prev. Med.* **2016**, *91*, 344–350. [CrossRef]
73. DeMello, M.T.; Lemo, V.A.; Antunes, H.K.M.; Bittencourt, L.; Santos-Silva, R.; Tufik, S. Relationship between physical activity and depression and anxiety symptoms: A population study. *J. Affect. Disord.* **2013**, *149*, 241–246. [CrossRef] [PubMed]
74. Forte, C.; McDowell, C.; MacDonncha, C.; Herring, M.P. Depressive symptoms differ across Physical Activity Status based on comorbid anxiety and depression status among adolescents. *Ment. Health Phys. Act.* **2020**, *19*, 100338. [CrossRef]
75. Hallgren, M.; Kandola, A.; Stubbs, B.; Nguyen, T.-T.-D.; Wallin, P.; Andersson, G.; Ekblom-Bak, E. Associations of exercise frequency and cardiorespiratory fitness with symptoms of depression and anxiety—A cross-sectional study of 36,595 adults. *Ment. Health Phys. Act.* **2020**, *19*, 100351. [CrossRef]
76. Ströhle, A. Physical activity, exercise, depression and anxiety disorders. *J. Neural. Trans.* **2009**, *116*, 777–784. [CrossRef]
77. Rebar, A.L.; Stanton, R.; Geard, D.; Short, C.; Duncan, M.J.; Vandelanotte, C. A meta-meta-analysis of the effect of physical activity on depression and anxiety in non-clinical adult populations. *Health Psychol. Rev.* **2015**, *9*, 366–378. [CrossRef] [PubMed]

78. Siefken, K.; Junge, A.; Laemmle, L. How does sport affect mental health? An investigation into the relationship of leisure-time physical activity with depression and anxiety. *Hum. Mov.* **2019**, *20*, 62–74. [CrossRef]
79. Mailey, E.L.; Wójcicki, T.R.; Motl, R.W.; Hu, L.; Strauser, D.R.; Collins, K.D.; McAuley, E. Internet-delivered physical activity intervention for college students with mental health disorders: A randomized pilot trial. *Psychol. Health Med.* **2010**, *15*, 646–659. [CrossRef] [PubMed]
80. Clemente-Suárez, V.J. Multidisciplinary intervention in the treatment of mixed anxiety and depression disorder. *Physiol. Behav.* **2020**, 112858. [CrossRef]

Publisher's Note: MDPI stays neutral with regard to jurisdictional claims in published maps and institutional affiliations.

Journal of
Clinical Medicine

MDPI

Article

Impact of COVID-19 Lockdown Measures on Spanish People with Chronic Pain: An Online Study Survey

Rubén Nieto [1,*,†], Rebeca Pardo [2,3,†], Beatriz Sora [4,5], Albert Feliu-Soler [6,7,‡] and Juan V. Luciano [6,‡]

1 eHealth Lab Research Group, Faculty of Health Sciences, Universitat Oberta de Catalunya, 08018 Barcelona, Spain
2 Centro de Psicología Aplicada, Universidad Autónoma de Madrid, 28049 Madrid, Spain; rebeca.pardocebrian@gmail.com
3 Facultad de Ciencias Biológicas, Universidad Europea de Madrid, 28670 Villaviciosa de Odón, Spain
4 eHealth Lab Research Group, Faculty of Psychology and Education, Universitat Oberta de Catalunya, 08018 Barcelona, Spain; beatriz.sora@urv.cat
5 Faculty of Educational Sciencies and Psychology, Psychology Department, Universitat Rovira i Virgili, 43007 Tarragona, Spain
6 Parc Sanitari Sant Joan de Déu, 08830 Sant Boi de Llobregat, Spain; albert.feliu@uab.cat (A.F.-S.); jvluciano@pssjd.org (J.V.L.)
7 Faculty of Psychology, Universitat Autònoma de Barcelona, 08193 Barcelona, Spain
* Correspondence: rnietol@uoc.edu; Tel.: +34-933-263-538
† Both authors contributed equally and should be considered as co-first authors.
‡ These authors share senior authorship.

Received: 17 October 2020; Accepted: 2 November 2020; Published: 5 November 2020

Abstract: The corona virus disease 2019 (COVID-19) pandemic is one of the most important healthcare and societal challenges to have emerged in the last century. It may have effects on both physical and psychosocial health, but studies considering the impact on vulnerable populations, such as people with chronic pain, are needed. In this cross-sectional study, an online survey of relevant chronic pain domains, coping strategies, triggers and potential related variables was answered by 502 Spanish individuals with chronic pain. Participants were mainly women (88%) with longstanding chronic pain and moderate to high pain intensity and disability. The perception of pain aggravation and the most pain-related outcomes were observed. Contextual variables such as job insecurity, worries about the future, people cohabiting, being close to someone who had passed away, or being potentially infected with COVID-19 were related to worse outcomes. More than half the participants altered their pain management style (e.g., increased medication intake) and several changes occurred with respect to pain triggers (cognitions, feelings of insecurity and loneliness, and sleeping problems were more frequently reported as triggers during lockdown). Our preliminary results highlight the negative effects of lockdown on patients with chronic pain as well as the need to make available cost-effective and remotely accessible healthcare resources for counteracting them.

Keywords: COVID-19; chronic pain; lockdown; triggers; coping; well-being

1. Introduction

The corona virus disease 2019 (COVID-19) pandemic is one of the most important worldwide healthcare and societal challenges to have emerged in the last century, and it has had dramatic consequences on the population. Providing exact data on the number of infected people and mortality rates is complicated since the health crisis is not yet under control and the death toll is growing daily. For example, in mid-July 2020, there were more than 13,000,000 cases and 574,464 deaths reported to the World Health Organization [1].

Available data on the effects of the crisis and lockdown measures on people's quality of life and wellbeing remain scant. Wang et al. [2] conducted a study in mainland China in the initial phase of the pandemic and found that 53.8% of the people surveyed ($n = 1200$) reported a moderate to severe psychological impact. There are also reports suggesting an increase in anxiety, depression and stress [3], as well as a rise in suicide rates [4]. Prior pandemics and lockdowns also provide insight into how much of an impact a situation like this can have in these areas. For example, Hawryluck et al. [5] found a high prevalence of depression and post-traumatic stress related to the quarantine brought on by severe acute respiratory syndrome (SARS). The European Foundation for the Improvement of Living and Working Conditions [6] conducted an online survey exploring the effects of COVID-19 in different regards. Although final results have yet to be published, in their preliminary April 2020 report they observed an overall decrease in people's reported well-being (lowered life satisfaction, happiness, optimism and mental well-being).

Apart from its detrimental impact on health, the pandemic is jeopardizing the worldwide economy, too. For example, there has been an increase in the worldwide unemployment rate [7]. In the United States, it was estimated that 20 million jobs were lost in April [8]. In a preliminary report by the Eurofound [6], 5% of respondents reported losing their jobs permanently and 23%, temporarily. Moreover, 38% of people reported that their financial situation was worse than before the pandemic. In turn, unemployment and job uncertainty have negative effects on individuals' and communities' psychological and social well-being [9].

Besides these few studies, there is little research on how people living through the COVID-19 crisis or those having been infected with the disease perceive and experience the situation [10]. Of particular interest for exploration are the views and experiences of people with chronic pain, as COVID-19 can have a greater impact on them [11], as well as on individuals with physical disabilities in general [3]. This is because, among other factors, chronic pain is more frequent in older people and is strongly related to disability, and access to pain management facilities has been disrupted as a consequence of lockdown, to prevent the risk of spreading the COVID-19 disease [11,12]. Chronic pain management difficulties can increase pain, pain-related disability and psychological issues such as depression [13]. In this regard, international panels of experts have recently highlighted the importance of ensuring continued pain treatment, and promote telemedicine from a biopsychosocial approach [14].

It is also important to highlight that some of the reported consequences of the pandemic and resulting lockdown can be triggers of pain. We are referring to factors such as stress. As previously stated, available data suggest that stress increases as a consequence of the pandemic and lockdown. The link between stress and chronic pain has been widely studied in recent decades. For example, we already know that exposure to certain stressful situations increases the risk of developing chronic pain [15]. General anxiety levels and general stress have also been related in general with a poorer adjustment to chronic pain [16,17]. Social isolation, which might have increased for some people as a consequence of lockdown, has a well-known impact on pain [18–20]. Similarly, lack of exercise or lack of activity in general can worsen functioning in people with pain [21]. Likewise, sleep problems have also been described during lockdown, and have been related to higher levels of intolerance to uncertainty, concern about COVID-19, loneliness, and severe depressive symptoms [22]. The relationship between sleep disturbances and pain is bidirectional (as is the relationship between stress and pain), so that pain disturbs sleep quality and lack of sleep further exacerbates pain [23,24].

As far as we know, there are no data available at this moment regarding the impact of the COVID-19 pandemic and home lockdown measures on people with chronic pain. Therefore, we conducted a preliminary exploratory study to address this important issue. Our intention was to provide a general perspective, basically descriptive, from a cross-sectional online data survey, contextualized in one of the most affected countries worldwide: Spain. Specifically, we wanted to know how people with chronic pain felt in relation to different important domains, to analyze changes in their general health, and to explore changes in the coping strategies they have used and in their pain itself.

2. Methods

A cross-sectional online survey methodology was used. The Universitat Oberta de Catalunya's Ethics Board evaluated and approved the study protocol on 22 April 2020.

2.1. Procedure

An online survey was created and implemented with the widely used online software Qualtrics (Qualtrics LLC, Provo, UT, USA). The survey was developed by the research group taking into account previous relevant literature about chronic pain prevalence and impact, available measures, and core outcome domains for chronic pain [25]. An important point was to make it as brief as possible to increase the response rate.

Once the research group reached a consensus regarding the survey content, it was sent to a panel of experts for review. At this stage, the questionnaire was fully reviewed by a methodologist with experience in health promotion, a researcher with experience in e-health and survey design, a psychologist with experience in health promotion research, a psychologist with experience in chronic pain management and research, and two psychologists with experience in clinical and health psychology research. Two people with chronic pain were also asked to answer the survey. If considered appropriate, their comments were included and the final survey was ready for dissemination. The online survey included a consent to participate in the study as well as statements on data protection laws. Below we describe the battery of variables gathered by this online survey.

The survey was open from 27 April to 25 May 2020. Spain was in a state of emergency from 13 March to 21 June, with restrictions placed on people's movement. During this period, the Spanish population was required to stay at home, although different steps were taken until the country reached the so-called "new normality". In this vein, for example, from 4 May people were allowed to exercise outside and walk with children, and from 11 to 25 May restaurants opened with some restrictions and only in some places. Therefore, there was high variability depending, basically, on the region where people resided and their work situation. In any case, all Spanish people had restrictions and their movement was limited during the emergency period. To make a clear point of reference for respondents, we asked them about the period since the lockdown started, which was the same for the whole country (14 March). No compensation was given for completing the survey and the average estimated time for completion was approximately 15 to 20 min.

2.2. Participants

Potential participants were contacted through the researchers' social media, massive electronic mailing, and by emailing the survey through a long list of patient and regional chronic pain associations and social media channels. The final sample consisted of 502 people. Inclusion criteria were: (1) adults (aged 18 or older); (2) Spanish residents; (3) persistent or chronic pain (>3 months) reported, with at least two pain episodes per week; and (4) completion of at least 80% of the online survey.

2.3. Measures

2.3.1. Sociodemographic Variables and Contextual Variables

We gathered sociodemographic data on age (in ranges of 10 years) and sex. We used multiple choice questions for civil status and education. We included other sociodemographic contextual variables in the survey that we hypothesized could affect the home lockdown situation: number of people living in the home, people in a situation of dependence living in the home, and number of people under 18 or above 65 years old living in the home. We also collected self-reported data about their personal COVID-19 infection status (positive, negative, unknown, COVID-like symptoms), infected people close to them and people close to them that had died due to COVID-19.

Job insecurity, or concern about the possibility of job loss, was measured through a 4-item scale developed by de Witte [26]. An example item is: "Chances are I will soon lose my job."

Participants give their responses on a 5-point Likert scale ranging from 1 (strongly disagree) to 5 (strongly agree). Cronbach's alpha for this measure in our sample was 0.91. Worries about the future were measured through the 9-item scale developed by Höge et al. [27]. This measure was composed of three dimensions: labor, material and social worries. Labor worries reflected concerns about not maintaining their work conditions in the future and interference in their professional career (e.g., "I am worried about my future job conditions."). Material worries addressed worries about reduced income in the future and having fewer possibilities to satisfy material needs and wishes (e.g., "I am worried about a future decline in my income."). Social worries reflected worries about not maintaining and nurturing satisfactory family lives, partnerships, friendships, and other social contacts (e.g., "I am worried about not being able to have a happy family life or partnership in the future."). Responses ranged from 1 (strongly disagree) to 5 (strongly agree). Cronbach's alphas in our sample were 0.87 for labor worries, 0.87 for material worries and 0.77 for social worries.

2.3.2. Description of Participants' Pain Characteristics

We asked subjects to indicate how many months had passed since the onset of their chronic/persistent pain and what type of chronic pain they had, using a multiple-choice question as per the proposal by Treede et al. [28] for the classification of chronic pain for the ICD-11 diagnosis system. Therefore, the following entities were included: chronic primary pain, chronic cancer pain, chronic postsurgical and post-traumatic pain, chronic neuropathic pain, chronic headache and orofacial pain, chronic visceral pain and chronic musculoskeletal pain. A figure of the human body was used for gathering information about pain location and also for the location of the most bothersome pain problem. Pain frequency was measured by asking subjects about their usual frequency of pain through a multiple-choice question based on the work by Breivik et al. [29].

Besides these previous questions, we used the Spanish version of the Chronic Pain Grade Questionnaire [30], an 8-item measure widely used in epidemiological studies. It typically comprises a first item asking for pain frequency during the last six months and seven additional items in a 11-point Likert scale (from 0 = "no pain" to 10 = "the worst pain imaginable") asking for patient's status during the last three months. These items allow the calculation of (a) the characteristic pain intensity index (CPGQ-P; including items of worst and mean pain intensity during the last three months and current pain intensity; 0–30 range score); and (b) a disability score (CPGQ-D; with items of mean of interference in performing daily tasks, activities of daily life, work, and social occupations; 0–40 range score). The time frame of the questionnaire was slightly adapted in our study, since subjects were asked to rate their situation since the beginning of the home lockdown situation. According to Ferrer-Peña et al. [30], the Spanish version of the CPGQ shows adequate internal consistency ($\alpha = 0.87$).

2.3.3. Changes in Pain and Pain-Related Outcomes Associated with Lockdown

Taking the IMMPACT (Initiative on Methods, Measurement, and Pain Assessment in Clinical Trials) assessment domains [25] and the CPGQ as references, we designed a short questionnaire to assess the perceived changes in respondents' situation since the beginning of home lockdown in comparison to their situation pre-lockdown. We asked them to rate their status on a scale from −10 (it has decreased extremely) to 10 (it has increased extremely), with 0 meaning no changes, for the following variables: pain intensity, frequency of pain episodes, pain interference in everyday activities, pain interference on work capacity (including homework), pain interference on hobbies, pain interference on social and familiar activities, distress caused by pain, support received from others when they were in pain, effects of pain on sleep and on physical activity.

2.3.4. Changes in Functional Domains

The Patient Global Impression of Change (PGIC) and the Pain-Specific Impression of Change (PSIC) instruments [31] were used as self-reporting measures of perception of global change and change in specific domains. These measures are frequently used as indicators of patient-meaningful change in interventions for chronic pain and are scored on a 7-point Likert scale (from 1 = "much better" to 7 = "much worse"). Regarding specific domains evaluated in the PSIC, perceived changes in physical and social functioning, work-related activities, mood, and pain intensity were collected. In total, the six items from the two questionnaires were administered and adapted for asking about changes since the beginning of lockdown.

2.3.5. Pain-Related Coping Strategies and Triggers

We asked participants with a single yes/no question if they had changed their pain coping strategies during lockdown. If they responded affirmatively, they were asked to inform if they had incorporated or stopped using the following strategies (they also had the option of choosing that they had neither incorporated nor stopped using them): increase of pain-related medication intake, stretching, physical exercise, resting, social support seeking, online health information seeking, and drinking.

Finally, we included a list of perceived pain triggers, and participants were asked to report whether each one had prompted pain episodes (Yes/No/Not sure) before and during lockdown. Perceived triggers included: stress, familiar or social conflicts, inadequate diet, uncertainty or worries about the future, sleep problems, feelings of insecurity, negative thoughts, feelings of sadness, feelings of loneliness, work-related factors, sedentarism, weather changes and fear of being infected with coronavirus.

2.4. *Data Analysis*

We computed descriptive statistics for each of the variables measured. We also tested if reported changes in pain and pain consequences were related to sociodemographic variables and lockdown background variables. We used Pearson correlations for continuous variables (e.g., relationship between CPGQ-P scores and changes in usual pain intensity) and a *t*-test for dichotomic variables (e.g., for testing differences between those participants who are and are not living with someone in dependence regarding changes in frequency of pain episodes). The same procedure was carried out to test the relationships with the changes in global domains assessed by the PSIC and the PGIC.

Apart from descriptive statistics, we tested triggers using McNemar's test if there were significant differences between the percentage of people who informed of each specific variable as a trigger before and during the lockdown period. All the tests used were bilateral and the significance level was set at $\alpha < 0.05$. All analyses were performed using IBM SPSS statistical software version 20.0 (IBM, Armonk, NY, USA).

3. Results

3.1. *Sociodemographic, Contextual Variables and Job Perceptions*

A total of 998 people visited our online survey, confirmed that they fulfilled the inclusion criteria, and agreed to participate, but 232 did not answer a single question. Of the remaining 766 subjects, 663 confirmed their residence in Spain with a multiple choice question. Of those, 536 were confirmed to meet the pain-related inclusion criteria through a question designed for this purpose. In the end, a total of 502 subjects completed at least 80% of the survey (most of them, 94.2%, completed the entire survey) and comprised the final sample. Most respondents were women (88%), between 30 and 59 years old (80.7%). Most were married (66.9%) and had reached secondary education or higher (87.8%). Socio-demographic data are displayed in Table 1.

Table 1. Sociodemographic and pain characteristics of the study sample.

Variable	%
Age ranges	
18–29	7%
30–39	21.90%
40–49	31.30%
50–59	27.50%
60–69	10.40%
70–79	1.60%
80–89	0.40%
Marital status	
Married/Living with a partner	66.90%
Separated/Divorced	10.20%
Single	20.50%
Widowed	2.40%
Education level	
No studies	0.20%
Primary school	12%
Secondary school	40.40%
University	26.90%
Postgraduate studies	20.50%
Employment status	
Temporary employment	8.90%
Permanent employment	44.30%
Self-employed	7.80%
Unemployed but searching for a job	7.80%
Unemployed and not searching for a job	8%
Student	2.70%
Retired	7.60%
Others	12.90%
Type of pain *	
Primary pain	53.20%
Musculoskeletal pain	52.20%
Headache and orofacial pain	26.70%
Other	26.30%
Neuropathic pain	19.50%
Visceral pain	12.50%
Postsurgical/posttraumatic pain	10.40%
Cancer pain	1.60%
Most bothersome pain location	
Low back	18.10%
Abdomen	18.10%
Neck	17.30%
Buttocks	13.10%
Legs	10.40%
Head	7.80%
Upper back	4.80%
Shoulder	3%
Hands	2.40%
Arms	2.40%
Feet	2%
Chest	0.60%
Pain frequency	
Always	39.60%
Daily	36.10%
Several times per week	17.50%

Table 1. *Cont.*

Variable	%
Once per week **	1%
Several times per month	5%
Once per month	0.60%
Less than once per month	0.20%

* These were multiple choice questions; ** Inclusion criteria for the study were having chronic pain with a duration of at least three months and at least two episodes per week. All respondents indicated meeting these criteria, but some of them, in the question related to frequency, indicated a range lower than two times per week. We understand that they were probably undergoing a period of less frequency.

Regarding contextual variables, 10.2% of the participants defined themselves as individuals in a situation of dependence, and 8% stated they were living together with someone in a status of dependence during lockdown. A total of 70.5% were not cohabitating with people under 18 during the lockdown. Of those cohabitating with children or adolescents, most were living with one or two (20.3% and 8.6%, respectively). The mean number of people living at home during the lockdown was 2.60 (standard deviation (SD): 1.06; range 1–7).

Finally, in relation to labor concerns (considering only those subjects of the sample who were working; n = 274), means were as follows: 2.60 (SD: 1.21) for job insecurity, 3.63 (SD: 1.21) for labor worries, 3.61 (SD: 1.15) for economic worries, and 3.02 (SD: 1.24) for personal worries.

In relation to COVID-19 infection, 1.6% of the sample had been infected, and 30.5% stated that they were not sure if they had been infected. A further 24.1% reported having someone close to them being infected and 16.9% reported that they were not sure if someone close to them had been infected by COVID-19. Finally, 13.5% reported having someone close to them die due to COVID-19.

3.2. Participant's Pain Characteristics

Most of the participants (87.6%) reported pain in more than one pain location (mean pain locations: 5.01; SD: 3.18), with the abdomen, lower back and neck being the most frequently reported locations. The majority of the sample reported pain with a frequency of several times per week or more (93.2%). Mean pain duration was around seven years (79.33 months; SD = 90.73). See Table 1 for more details about specific diagnoses selected, most bothersome pain locations and pain frequency.

Mean for characteristic pain intensity since the beginning of lockdown assessed with CPGQ was 68.1 (SD = 17.62); for the disability score, the mean was 60 (SD = 25.43).

3.3. Changes in Pain and Pain-Related Outcomes Associated with Lockdown

Mean scores of all the scales are presented in Table 2, which also displays the frequency of participants who obtained a score less than 0 (indicating an improvement), a score of 0 (no change) or a score greater than 0 (indicating a worsening). As can be seen, most of the participants experienced worsening or no changes in pain and pain-related outcomes. Domains with more people reporting a worsening (and with higher mean scores), around 80%, were distress, sleep and interference of pain in physical activities. On the other hand, the area with a higher proportion of people reporting no changes or even an improvement was "support received from others".

Correlations between each domain (changes in pain and pain-related outcomes) with CPGQ scores, age, duration of pain, labor perceptions and number of people living at home are also displayed in Table 2. There were significant positive correlations between CPGQ-P and CPGQ-D and each pain-related outcome. Pain duration was negatively and significantly correlated with changes in perceived social support (greater duration was related with greater diminution in the support received). Job perceptions were positively and significantly related with all domains except for support received. Age was not correlated with any of the domains. Number of people cohabiting was significantly related to greater distress caused by pain, greater effects on sleep, and increase in perceived social support, although the correlations were of small magnitude.

Regarding the *t*-tests, cohabitating with someone in a situation of dependence, gender and having someone close to you infected by coronavirus did not have a significant impact on any of the domains. Those who indicated having had someone close to them die due to COVID-19 reported a significantly greater effect of pain on physical activity (mean of 6.1 and 4.95, respectively; $t = 2.07$; $p = 0.04$). Those who were not sure of being infected by COVID-19 had significantly greater trouble sleeping than those who claimed not to have been infected (mean of 5.39 and 4.43, respectively; $t = -2.26$; $p = 0.02$). We could not compare those who reported being infected with those who did not or those who were unsure due to sample size limitations (only 8 participants confirmed that they had been infected).

3.4. Changes in Functional Domains

Descriptive statistics for the PSIC domains and global changes in the PGIC are presented in Table 3. Scores for the 6 items were significantly and positively correlated with the CPGQ-P, CPGQ-D, and with labor perceptions (the exception being the correlation between material worries and social activities). As can be seen in Table 3, the lowest correlations were between the CPGQ scores and changes in social activities, and the highest, between CPGQ scores and global well-being. In relation to labor perceptions, the highest correlations were with emotional state. Pain duration was not related to any of the 6 items. Number of people cohabiting was only significantly related with emotional state. Age was significantly related to small positive correlations with changes in physical capacity and labor and social activities.

Those living with someone in a situation of dependence had significantly worse outcomes in general health since the lockdown (mean of 5.41 and 4.95, respectively; $t = -2.13$; $p = 0.03$), physical capacity (mean of 5.54 and 5.12, respectively; $t = -1.97$; $p < 0.05$), and social activities (mean of 5.56 and 5.15, respectively; $t = -2.01$; $p < 0.05$). Those who were not sure of COVID-19 infection had worse outcomes compared to those who claimed not to be infected regarding changes in global well-being (mean of 5.17 and 4.91, respectively; $t = -2.06$; $p = 0.04$) and in changes in emotional state since the lockdown (mean of 5.58 and 4.16, respectively; $t = -3.36$; $p = 0.001$). Having someone close to them infected with COVID-19 or dying because of it and gender did not have a significant impact on any of the assessed domains.

Table 2. Perceived changes in pain and pain-related outcomes, and correlations between study variables.

Descriptives			Correlations with Pain Characteristics		Correlations with Sociodemographic and Contextual Variables						
VARIABLE	Mean (SD)	Proportion (%) of Improvement, no Change and Worsening	CPGQ-P	CPGQ-D	Age	Pain Duration	Job Insecurity	Labor Worries	Material Worries	Social Worries	Number People Cohabitating
Usual pain intensity	3.4 (3.89)	9.3–19.9–70.8	0.43 *	0.40 *	0.04	0.04	0.16 ***	0.26 *	0.22 *	0.20 **	0.04
Frequency of pain episodes	3.55 (4)	8.7–19.7–71.6	0.42 *	0.41 *	0.05	0.01	0.13 ***	0.23 *	0.18 ***	0.21 **	0.007
Pain interference in everyday activities	3.47 (4.1)	8.5–22–69.5	0.48 *	0.50 *	0.07	0.002	0.18 ***	0.35 *	0.26 *	0.29 *	0.01
Pain interference on work capacity	3.76 (4.14)	7.1–20.1–72.8	0.48 *	0.53 *	0.07	−0.02	0.19 ***	0.34 *	0.26 *	0.28 *	0.04
Pain interference on leisure, social and familiar activities	3.41 (4.22)	8.1–22.8–69.1	0.48 *	0.54 *	0.04	−0.01	0.19 **	0.38 *	0.28 *	0.32 *	0.07
Distress caused by pain	5 (4.45)	6.7–13.2–80.1	0.43 *	0.45 *	−0.02	−0.04	0.15 ***	0.34 *	0.28 *	0.28 *	0.11 ***
Support received from others	2.56 (5.14)	55.7–29.5–14.8	0.15 **	0.16 *	0.05	−0.11 ***	0.03	0.04	0.08	0.03	0.13 ***
Effects on sleep	4.69 (4.37)	6.5–14.4–79.1	0.38 *	0.36 *	−0.06	0.03	0.19 ***	0.30 *	0.25 *	0.23 *	0.09 ***
Effects on physical activity	5.11 (4.26)	5.5–14.6–79.9	0.41 *	0.47 *	−0.02	−0.001	0.10	0.33 *	0.26 *	0.23 *	0.04

Note: * $p < 0.0001$; ** $p < 0.001$; *** $p < 0.05$; CPGQ-P = Characteristic Pain Intensity Index; CPGQ-D = Disability Score.

Table 3. Descriptives in Pain-Specific Impression of Change (PSIC) domains and global changes (Patient Global Impression of Change (PGIC)) and correlations between study measures.

Descriptives		Correlations with Pain Characteristics		Correlations with Sociodemographic and Contextual Variables						
VARIABLE	Mean (SD)	CPGQ-P	CPGQ-D	Age	Pain Duration	Job Insecurity	Labor Worries	Material Worries	Social Worries	Number People Cohabitating
Global well-being	4.99 (1.29)	0.43 *	0.4 *	0.05	0.004	0.18 **	0.29 *	0.22 **	0.22 *	0.06
Activity/physical capacity	5.16 (1.27)	0.27 *	0.30 *	0.09 ***	0.04	0.15 ***	0.26 *	0.19 **	0.24 *	−0.02
Social activities	5.18 (1.24)	0.14 **	0.19 *	0.11 ***	0.02	0.15 ***	0.18 **	0.08	0.21 **	0.02
Laboral activities	5 (1.25)	0.31 *	0.38 *	0.09 ***	−0.01	0.17 **	0.22 *	0.20 **	0.18 **	0.09
Emotional state	5.29 (1.32)	0.41 *	0.38 *	−0.007	−0.02	0.26 *	0.31 *	0.27 *	0.29 *	0.11 ***
Pain	5.14 (1.29)	0.47 *	0.42 *	0.05	0.06	0.15 ***	0.25 *	0.23 *	0.25 *	0.04

Note: * $p < 0.0001$; ** $p < 0.005$; *** $p < 0.05$; CPGQ-P = Characteristic Pain Intensity Index; CPGQ-D = Disability Score.

3.5. Changes in Pain-Coping Strategies

More than half the sample reported having experienced changes in their way of coping with pain (54.5%). Table 4 displays the proportion of these people who incorporated, refrained from using, or neither incorporated nor dismissed each of the proposed coping strategies. As can be seen in Table 4, a substantial proportion of the participants incorporated new coping strategies during lockdown, with resting (54.5%), stretching (48.2%) and increase in medication intake (46.7%) being the most usually incorporated.

Table 4. Changes in coping strategies during lockdown.

Coping Strategy	Incorporated (%)	Dismissed (%)	Neither Incorporated nor Dismissed (%)
Resting	54.5	7.5	38.0
Stretching	48.2	9.0	42.7
Increase in medication intake	46.7	3.1	50.2
Exercising	32.1	28.6	39.3
Using internet resources	33.6	6.3	60.2
Social support	26.8	12.8	60.3
Alcohol consumption	7.8	11.4	80.8

3.6. Changes in Perceived Pain Triggers

Frequency of perceived pain triggers before and during lockdown can be seen in Table 5. Stress was the trigger most frequently reported before lockdown, followed by weather changes and sleep problems. During lockdown, there was a significant increase in the proportion of participants who thought that the following variables triggered pain: worries about the future, sleep problems, feelings of insecurity, negative thoughts, sadness, loneliness, sedentarism, and fear of suffering from COVID−19. In contrast, the proportion of participants indicating that stress triggered pain was reduced during lockdown significantly.

Table 5. Changes in perceived pain triggers before and during lockdown.

	Before			During			
Trigger	Yes (%)	No (%)	Not Sure (%)	Yes (%)	No (%)	Not Sure (%)	McNemar's Test p Value
Stress	83.5	8.2	8.2	76.3	13.5	10.1	<0.0001
Weather changes	67.7	21.1	11.2	68.5	20.7	10.8	0.62
Sleep problems	66.0	26.6	7.4	79.1	15.9	5.1	<0.0001
Working issues	60.3	30.0	9.7	57.5	33.8	8.7	0.18
Worries about the future	59.8	27.3	12.9	71.2	17.1	11.6	<0.0001
Familiar or social conflicts	58.8	30	11.2	60.7	30.0	9.3	0.36
Sedentarism	57.9	31.3	10.8	75.5	16.7	7.8	<0.0001
Sadness	55.0	33.0	12.1	68.1	21.1	10.8	<0.0001
Negative thoughts	49.5	35.7	14.8	61.5	26.0	12.5	<0.0001
Feelings of insecurity	48.2	37.4	14.4	62.6	25.2	12.3	<0.0001
Diet	40.2	36.4	23.5	43.6	33.8	22.6	0.06
Loneliness	37.2	50.1	12.7	45.2	42.3	12.5	<0.0001
Fear of suffering from COVID-19	20.3	67.9	11.8	39.1	48.2	12.7	<0.0001

Note: respondents who said "No" or "Not Sure" were grouped together to perform McNemar's test.

4. Discussion

Our study sample was predominantly made up of women (88%) who typically suffered pain in more than one location and had longstanding problems. These characteristics are similar to those found in epidemiological studies. However, although a higher percentage of women is usual, it is not usually as high as it is in our study. For example, the proportion of women in one recent epidemiological study in Italy was 67% [32]. Our major proportion of women may be due to the fact that we sent information about our study to pain associations and groups via social media in which women tend to participate more frequently [33]. Available literature also confirms that women are more likely to participate in online surveys [34].

Characteristic pain intensity and disability scores from the beginning of lockdown assessed with the CPGQ were in the upper range (mean of 68.1 and 60, respectively). Although comparison between studies is quite complicated, our data suggest worse scores on both scales than those reported in other studies using the same questionnaire and reporting scores for the two scales [35]. Changes in pain and pain-related outcomes since the beginning of lockdown were correlated with pain intensity and disability scores and confirmed a worsening in all assessed domains (except for support received from others, which increased). There was an increase in pain intensity, frequency of pain episodes, pain interference (in everyday activities, work capacity, and leisure activities), distress caused by pain, and effects of pain on sleep and on physical activity. Higher mean scores (suggesting greater worsening) were found for distress, quality of sleep and physical activity. Similar results were found for PSIC domains and global changes. Specifically, when respondents were asked about changes (not necessarily related to pain) mean scores showed a worsening in physical activity, social activities, labor activities, emotional state and global well-being (mean scores were quite similar, around 5, for all the scales). These data highlight the importance of paying attention to people with chronic pain during health crises, since their pain problem and general health can worsen, as has been pointed out by experts [13]. Moreover contextual variables such as job insecurity, worries about the future, and number of people cohabiting are related with changes in pain and pain-related outcomes, and with global changes. Having someone close to you died because of COVID-19 and not being sure whether you were infected with the virus were also related with worse outcomes. Along the same lines, a recent study on the general population reported that a greater psychological effect was related to those with self-reported symptoms of COVID-19, with changes in employment activity [36] and with those cohabiting with two to four people (vs. those living alone or cohabiting with one person). In any case, here we consider longitudinal studies essential for studying causal relationships, building sound statistical models and truly understanding the experience of those people suffering from chronic pain. However, these preliminary data suggest the importance of taking into account the context in which people with chronic pain are involved during crises such as that caused by COVID-19.

More than half the participants reported changes in their way of managing their pain as a consequence of the pandemic. Of those, more than half reported having incorporated resting and around half informed of having increased their intake of medication. Resting can be a dangerous coping strategy if used permanently, as it can increase disability [37]. Medication intake is also something to take into account, requiring future research to explore whether people with chronic pain increase intake with or without a professional prescription. This is because medication patterns (particularly with prescription drugs such as opioids) require strict supervision by health professionals, and overdose of non-prescription analgesics represents a non-negligible risk [38]. In contrast, a good point is that nearly half the participants reported having started to use stretching to cope with pain, and nearly one third started using exercise (although almost another one third stopped exercising to cope with pain, probably due to the impossibility of doing so from home). Literature widely supports the benefit of stretching and exercising for managing pain [39], and the mass media and relevant stakeholders (e.g., patients' associations and health-related websites) likely helped during this period since the idea of being active at home was widespread. For example, the Spanish Society for Pain's website [40] encouraged people with chronic pain to stay active and exercise. It is also noteworthy that more than one third of the participants reported starting to use Internet resources to cope with pain. This is congruent with the fact that information and communication technologies (ICT) have great potential for facilitating access to pain management interventions [41], especially taking into account the difficulties in accessing pain management facilities as a consequence of the pandemic [11]. Considering the current health situation, it is probably an area in which society should invest more resources. It would also be interesting to work on the creation of online community networks, since people going through catastrophes need to feel they belong to a community [42].

An important contribution made by our work is the study of participants' perceived triggers. This is because few studies have asked people with pain which factors they consider to trigger their pain [43–46]. It is interesting to explore whether people's perceptions coincide with scientific literature and if these perceptions change as a consequence of the pandemic. Along these lines, stress was the most recognized factor as a trigger in our study prior to lockdown. As commented in the introduction, there is a lot of evidence of its role in pain literature [16,17]. However, it is curious that during the lockdown a slightly lower (yet significant) proportion of the participants chose stress as a pain trigger. This is probably because other triggers gained representativeness during the pandemic. Along these lines, there was a significant increase in people who stated that triggers related to cognitions (i.e., worries about the future, fear of being infected by COVID-19, and negative thoughts) triggered pain during the lockdown. The proportion of people who stated that sadness and loneliness triggered pain also increased significantly. Cognitions and emotions are constantly interacting with each other and with pain, and their role is widely recognized and supported in scientific literature [18–20,47]. The situation of uncertainty and emergency likely magnified all these factors. Finally, also in relation with available literature [23,24] sleeping problems were also widely recognized as triggers and their role increased during lockdown (being the most frequently mentioned by participants as a trigger).

The main implications of our results can be found in Table 6.

Table 6. Main implications of the results.

- Lockdown seems to be related to a worsening in pain, pain-related domains and global changes.
- Management of pain was negatively affected during the lockdown for many people who tended to use resting and increased medication consumption; however, as a positive effect, some people started stretching and exercising for pain.
- Worries about the future, sleep problems, feelings of insecurity, negative thoughts, sadness, loneliness, sedentarism, and fear of suffering from COVID-19 gained representativeness as triggers during the lockdown.
- Particular attention should be given to those with chronic pain problems in emergency healthcare situations; and eHealth probably has the power to maintain care for vulnerable populations, such as people with chronic pain during global healthcare emergencies.

Besides these important implications, we have to acknowledge some limitations of our work. First, although online assessment has proven to generate reliable data [48], it has inherent limitations, such as self-selection bias and sample representativeness [49]. For instance, there are difficult-to-reach people characterized by digital illiteracy. Second, we did not use a stratified random sampling technique, which may have an impact on the generalizability of our findings. Third, as commented, the design was not longitudinal, which prevents it from exploring causal models. Fourth, a more in-depth assessment (e.g., including interviews with people in pain) would have been very useful to obtain a more global picture. However, despite these limitations, our results are important, as they show a clear impact on pain and general well-being and highlight some factors (and triggers) that can be helpful for creating prevention programs or guidelines for health professionals. Firstly, among the measures to be implemented, it may be useful to consider those that have been indicated for the general population. These include the use of psychological first aid, after evaluating critical needs, and intervening early on stress [50]. E-health has emerged as a clear need and should be implemented for general health and pain interventions while lockdown and social distancing measures are in place [11,51]. Lastly, and more specifically, in future lockdown situations it would probably be useful to help people with chronic pain to curb uncertainty, provide online support communities, manage loneliness, and take care of sleeping habits.

Author Contributions: All the authors contributed (R.N., R.P., B.S., A.F.-S., J.V.L.) to the conceptualization, manuscript preparation and conducting the research (design of the survey and dissemination of the study).

Analyses were led by B.S., and writing the first draft was led by R.N. and R.P. All authors have read and agreed to the published version of the manuscript.

Funding: J.V.L. has a "Miguel Servet" research contract from the Instituto de Salud Carlos III (ISCIII; CPII19/00003). This specific project did not receive external funding.

Acknowledgments: We greatly appreciated the participation of all the people with chronic pain and patients' associations, groups and professionals who help with the dissemination of the study.

Conflicts of Interest: The authors declare no conflict of interest.

References

1. World Health Organization. WHO Coronavirus Disease (COVID-19) Dashboard. Available online: https://covid19.who.int (accessed on 17 October 2020).
2. Wang, C.; Pan, R.; Wan, X.; Tan, Y.; Xu, L.; Ho, C.S.; Ho, R.C. Immediate Psychological Responses and Associated Factors during the Initial Stage of the 2019 Coronavirus Disease (COVID-19) Epidemic among the General Population in China. *Int. J. Environ. Res. Public Health* **2020**, *17*, 1729. [CrossRef] [PubMed]
3. Huarcaya, J. Consideraciones sobre la salud mental en la pandemia de Covid-19. *Rev. Peru. Med. Exp. Salud Pública* **2020**, *37*, 327–334. (In Spanish) [CrossRef]
4. Gunnell, D.; Appleby, L.; Arensman, E.; Hawton, K.; John, A.; Kapur, N.; Khan, M.; O'Connor, R.C.; Pirkis, J.; Caine, E.D.; et al. Suicide risk and prevention during the COVID-19 pandemic. *Lancet Psychiatry* **2020**, *7*, 468–471. [CrossRef]
5. Hawryluck, L.; Gold, W.L.; Robinson, S.; Pogorski, S.; Galea, S.; Styra, R. SARS Control and Psychological Effects of Quarantine, Toronto, Canada. *Emerg. Infect. Dis.* **2004**, *10*, 1206–1212. [CrossRef] [PubMed]
6. Eurofound. Living, Working and COVID-19 First Findings—April 2020. Available online: https://www.eurofound.europa.eu/publications/report/2020/living-working-and-covid-19-first-findings-april-2020 (accessed on 17 October 2020).
7. International Labor Organization. Almost 25 Million Jobs Could Be Lost Worldwide as a Result of COVID-19, Says ILO. Available online: https://www.ilo.org/global/about-the-ilo/newsroom/news/WCMS_738742/lang--en/index.htm (accessed on 17 October 2020).
8. Coibion, O.; Gorodnichenko, Y.; Weber, M. Labor Markets during the COVID-19 Crisis: A Preliminary View. *SSRN Electron. J.* **2020**. [CrossRef]
9. Meltzer, H.; Bebbington, P.; Brugha, T.; Jenkins, R.; McManus, S.; Stansfeld, S. Job insecurity, socio-economic circumstances and depression. *Psychol. Med.* **2009**, *40*, 1401–1407. [CrossRef] [PubMed]
10. Romeyke, T.; Noehammer, E.; Stummer, H. COVID-19 Case Report: An 84-Year-Old Man with Exacerbation of Multiple Comorbidities Due to COVID-19 Managed by a Multidisciplinary Team Using Patient-Reported Outcomes. *Am. J. Case Rep.* **2020**, *21*, e926694-1. [CrossRef] [PubMed]
11. Eccleston, C.; Blyth, F.M.; Dear, B.F.; Fisher, E.A.; Keefe, F.J.; Lynch, M.E.; Palermo, T.M.; Reid, M.C.; Williams, A.C.D.C. Managing patients with chronic pain during the COVID-19 outbreak. *Pain* **2020**, *161*, 889–893. [CrossRef]
12. Murray, C.J.; Atkinson, C.; Bhalla, K.; Birbeck, G.; Burstein, R.; Chou, D.; Murray, U.S. The State of US Health, 1990-2016: Burden of Diseases, Injuries, and Risk Factors among US States. *JAMA* **2013**, *310*, 591–608. [CrossRef]
13. El-Tallawy, S.N.; Nalamasu, R.; Pergolizzi, J.V.; Gharibo, C. Pain Management during the COVID-19 Pandemic. *Pain Ther.* **2020**, 1–14. [CrossRef]
14. Shanthanna, H.; Strand, N.H.; Provenzano, D.A.; Lobo, C.A.; Eldabe, S.; Bhatia, A.; Wegener, J.; Curtis, K.; Cohen, S.P.; Narouze, S. Caring for patients with pain during the COVID-19 pandemic: Consensus recommendations from an international expert panel. *Anaesthesia* **2020**, *75*, 935–944. [CrossRef]
15. Burke, N.N.; Finn, D.P.; McGuire, B.E.; Roche, M. Psychological stress in early life as a predisposing factor for the development of chronic pain: Clinical and preclinical evidence and neurobiological mechanisms. *J. Neurosci. Res.* **2016**, *95*, 1257–1270. [CrossRef] [PubMed]
16. Crettaz, B.; Marziniak, M.; Willeke, P.; Young, P.; Hellhammer, D.; Stumpf, A.; Burgmer, M. Stress-Induced Allodynia—Evidence of Increased Pain Sensitivity in Healthy Humans and Patients with Chronic Pain after Experimentally Induced Psychosocial Stress. *PLoS ONE* **2013**, *8*, e69460. [CrossRef]

17. Ortego, G.; Villafañe, J.H.; Doménech-García, V.; Berjano, P.; Bertozzi, L.; Herrero, P. Is there a relationship between psychological stress or anxiety and chronic nonspecific neck-arm pain in adults? A systematic review and meta-analysis. *J. Psychosom. Res.* **2016**, *90*, 70–81. [CrossRef] [PubMed]
18. Aremka, L.M.; Andridge, R.R.; Fagundes, C.P.; Alfano, C.M.; Povoski, S.P.; Lipari, A.M.; Agnese, D.M.; Arnold, M.W.; Farrar, W.B.; Yee, L.D.; et al. Pain, depression, and fatigue: Loneliness as a longitudinal risk factor. *Health Psychol.* **2014**, *33*, 948–957. [CrossRef]
19. Smith, T.O. "On their own": Social isolation, loneliness and chronic musculoskeletal pain in older adults. *Qual. Ageing Older Adults* **2017**, *18*, 87–92. [CrossRef]
20. Smith, T.O.; Dainty, J.R.; Williamson, E.; Martin, K.R. Association between musculoskeletal pain with social isolation and loneliness: Analysis of the English Longitudinal Study of Ageing. *Br. J. Pain* **2018**, *13*, 82–90. [CrossRef] [PubMed]
21. Booth, J.; Moseley, G.L.; Schiltenwolf, M.; Cashin, A.; Davies, M.; Hübscher, M. Exercise for chronic musculoskeletal pain: A biopsychosocial approach. *Musculoskelet. Care* **2017**, *15*, 413–421. [CrossRef]
22. Voitsidis, P.; Gliatas, I.; Bairachtari, V.; Papadopoulou, K.; Papageorgiou, G.; Parlapani, E.; Syngelakis, M.; Holeva, V.; Diakogiannis, I. Insomnia during the COVID-19 pandemic in a Greek population. *Psychiatry Res.* **2020**, *289*, 113076. [CrossRef]
23. Mills, S.E.; Nicolson, K.P.; Smith, B.H. Chronic pain: A review of its epidemiology and associated factors in population-based studies. *Br. J. Anaesth.* **2019**, *123*, e273–e283. [CrossRef]
24. Smith, M.T.; A Haythornthwaite, J.A. How do sleep disturbance and chronic pain inter-relate? Insights from the longitudinal and cognitive-behavioral clinical trials literature. *Sleep Med. Rev.* **2004**, *8*, 119–132. [CrossRef]
25. Turk, D.C.; Dworkin, R.H.; Allen, R.R.; Bellamy, N.; Brandenburg, N.; Carr, D.B.; Cleeland, C.; Dionne, R.; Farrar, J.T.; Galer, B.S.; et al. Core outcome domains for chronic pain clinical trials: IMMPACT recommendations. *Pain* **2003**, *106*, 337–345. [CrossRef]
26. De Witte, H. *Langdurig Werkozen: Tussen Optimisten en Teruggetrokkenen*; Hoger Instituut van de Arbeid: Leuven, The Netherdlands, 1992. (In Dutch)
27. Höge, T.; Sora, B.; Weber, W.G.; Peiró, J.M.; Caballer, A. Job insecurity, worries about the future, and somatic complaints in two economic and cultural contexts: A study in Spain and Austria. *Int. J. Stress Manag.* **2015**, *22*, 223–242. [CrossRef]
28. Treede, R.-D.; Rief, W.; Barke, A.; Aziz, Q.; Bennett, M.I.; Benoliel, R.; Cohen, M.; Evers, S.; Finnerup, N.B.; First, M.B.; et al. A classification of chronic pain for ICD-11. *Pain* **2015**, *156*, 1003–1007. [CrossRef]
29. Breivik, H.; Collett, B.; Ventafridda, V.; Cohen, R.; Gallacher, D. Survey of chronic pain in Europe: Prevalence, impact on daily life, and treatment. *Eur. J. Pain* **2006**, *10*, 287–333. [CrossRef]
30. Ferrer-Peña, R.; Gil Martinez, A.; Pardo-Montero, J.; Jiménez-Penick, V.; Gallego-Izquierdo, T.; La Touche, R. Adaptación y validación de la Escala de gradación del dolor crónico al español. *Reumatol. Clín.* **2016**, *12*, 130–138. (In Spanish) [CrossRef]
31. Scott, W.; McCracken, L.M. Patients' Impression of Change Following Treatment for Chronic Pain: Global, Specific, a Single Dimension, or Many? *J. Pain* **2015**, *16*, 518–526. [CrossRef] [PubMed]
32. Latina, R.; De Marinis, M.G.; Giordano, F.; Osborn, J.F.; Giannarelli, D.; Di Biagio, E.; Varrassi, G.; Sansoni, J.; Bertini, L.; Baglio, G.; et al. Epidemiology of Chronic Pain in the Latium Region, Italy: A Cross-Sectional Study on the Clinical Characteristics of Patients Attending Pain Clinics. *Pain Manag. Nurs.* **2019**, *20*, 373–381. [CrossRef]
33. Chen, G.M. Why do women bloggers use social media? Recreation and information motivations outweigh engagement motivations. *New Media Soc.* **2013**, *17*, 24–40. [CrossRef]
34. Blasius, J.; Brandt, M. Representativeness in Online Surveys through Stratified Samples. *Bull. Sociol. Methodol.* **2010**, *107*, 5–21. [CrossRef]
35. Salaffi, F.; Stancati, A.; Grassi, W. Reliability and validity of the Italian version of the Chronic Pain Grade questionnaire in patients with musculoskeletal disorders. *Clin. Rheumatol.* **2006**, *25*, 619–631. [CrossRef] [PubMed]
36. Odriozola-González, P.; Planchuelo-Gómez, Á.; Irurtia, M.J.; De Luis-García, R. Psychological effects of the COVID-19 outbreak and lockdown among students and workers of a Spanish university. *Psychiatry Res.* **2020**, *290*, 113108. [CrossRef]

37. Foster, N.E.; Anema, J.R.; Cherkin, D.; Chou, R.; Cohen, S.P.; Gross, D.P.; Ferreira, P.; Fritz, J.M.; Koes, B.; Peul, W.; et al. Prevention and treatment of low back pain: Evidence, challenges, and promising directions. *Lancet* **2018**, *391*, 2368–2383. [CrossRef]
38. Wolf, M.S.; King, J.; Jacobson, K.; Di Francesco, L.; Bailey, S.C.; Mullen, R.; McCarthy, D.; Serper, M.; Davis, T.C.; Parker, R.M. Risk of Unintentional Overdose with Non-Prescription Acetaminophen Products. *J. Gen. Intern. Med.* **2012**, *27*, 1587–1593. [CrossRef]
39. Kroll, H.R. Exercise Therapy for Chronic Pain. *Phys. Med. Rehabil. Clin. N. Am.* **2015**, *26*, 263–281. [CrossRef]
40. Sociedad Española del Dolor. Información y Recomendaciones de la SED para Pacientes con Dolor Crónico ante la Pandemia por Covid-19. Available online: https://www.sedolor.es/infirmacion-y-recomendaciones-de-la-sed-para-pacientes-con-dolor-cronico-ante-la-pandemia-por-covid-19/ (accessed on 23 October 2020). (In Spanish)
41. Nieto, R. Secondary prevention of chronic pain: Can internet help? *Pain Manag.* **2014**, *4*, 285–291. [CrossRef]
42. Reissman, D.B.; Watson, P.J.; Klomp, R.W.; Tanielian, T.L.; Prior, S.A. Pandemic Influenza Preparedness: Adaptive Responses to an Evolving Challenge. *J. Homel. Secur. Emerg. Manag.* **2006**, *3*. [CrossRef]
43. Crowe, M.; Whitehead, L.; Gagan, M.J.; Baxter, G.D.; Panckhurst, A. Self-management and chronic low back pain: A qualitative study. *J. Adv. Nurs.* **2010**, *66*, 1478–1486. [CrossRef]
44. Kawi, J. Chronic low back pain patients' perceptions on self-management, self-management support, and functional ability. *Pain Manag. Nurs.* **2014**, *15*, 258–264. [CrossRef] [PubMed]
45. Roth-Isigkeit, A. Pain among Children and Adolescents: Restrictions in Daily Living and Triggering Factors. *Pediatrics* **2005**, *115*, e152–e162. [CrossRef]
46. Setchell, J.; Costa, N.; Ferreira, M.; Hodges, P.W. What decreases low back pain? A qualitative study of patient perspectives. *Scand. J. Pain* **2019**, *19*, 597–603. [CrossRef]
47. Martinez-Calderon, J.; Jensen, M.P.; Morales-Asencio, J.M.; Luque-Suarez, A. Pain Catastrophizing and Function In Individuals with Chronic Musculoskeletal Pain. *Clin. J. Pain* **2019**, *35*, 279–293. [CrossRef]
48. Gwaltney, C.J.; Shields, A.L.; Shiffman, S. Equivalence of Electronic and Paper-and-Pencil Administration of Patient-Reported Outcome Measures: A Meta-Analytic Review. *Value Health* **2008**, *11*, 322–333. [CrossRef]
49. Wright, K.B. Researching Internet-Based Populations: Advantages and Disadvantages of Online Survey Research, Online Questionnaire Authoring Software Packages, and Web Survey Services. *J. Comput. Commun.* **2006**, *10*, 1034. [CrossRef]
50. Ramírez-Ortiz, J.; Castro-Quintero, D.; Lerma-Córdoba, C.; Yela-Ceballos, F.; Escobar-Córdoba, F. Consecuencias de la Pandemia COVID-19 en la Salud Mental Asociadas al Aislamiento Social. 2020, 5. Scientific Electronic Library Online. Available online: https://preprints.scielo.org/index.php/scielo/preprint/view/303 (accessed on 3 November 2020).
51. Tull, M.T.; Edmonds, K.A.; Scamaldo, K.M.; Richmond, J.R.; Rose, J.P.; Gratz, K.L. Psychological Outcomes Associated with Stay-at-Home Orders and the Perceived Impact of COVID-19 on Daily Life. *Psychiatry Res.* **2020**, *289*, 113098. [CrossRef] [PubMed]

Journal of
Clinical Medicine

MDPI

Article

Relationship of Forced Social Distancing and Home Confinement Derived from the COVID-19 Pandemic with the Occupational Balance of the Spanish Population

Jerónimo J. González-Bernal [1], Mirian Santamaría-Peláez [1,*], Josefa González-Santos [1,*], Paula Rodríguez-Fernández [1], Benito León del Barco [2] and Raúl Soto-Cámara [1]

[1] Department of Health Sciences, University of Burgos, 09001 Burgos, Spain; jejavier@ubu.es (J.J.G.-B.); prf0011@alu.ubu.es (P.R.-F.); rscamara@ubu.es (R.S.-C.)

[2] Department of Psychology, Faculty of Teacher Training College, University of Extremadura, 10071 Caceres, Spain; bleon@unex.es

* Correspondence: mspelaez@ubu.es (M.S.-P.); mjgonzalez@ubu.es (J.G.-S.)

Received: 4 October 2020; Accepted: 6 November 2020; Published: 9 November 2020

Abstract: Abrupt interruption in the performance of everyday occupations as a consequence of forced social distancing and home confinement, coupled with a lack of regulatory capacities and skills, can trigger harmful effects on people's health and well-being. This study aimed to determine the factors related to the occupational balance in the Spanish population during home confinement as a consequence of the coronavirus disease 19 (COVID-19) pandemic. A total of 3261 subjects completed an online survey, which was disseminated through the mainstream social media platforms in Spain and included the Occupational Balance Questionnaire (OBQ), sociodemographic variables, and factors related to COVID-19 infection. The mean age of the participants (81.69% women) was 40.53 years (SD ± 14.05). Sociodemographic variables were related to a greater occupational balance, and the multivariate analysis showed that age ($\beta = 0.071$; $p = 0.001$), the perception of having received enough information ($\beta = 0.071$; $p \leq 0.001$), not telecommuting ($\beta = -0.047$; $p = 0.022$), and not being infected by COVID-19 ($\beta = 0.055$; $p = 0.007$) contributed to a better occupational balance. There were profiles of people less likely to suffer disturbances in occupational balance during home confinement, but more studies are needed to help understand and analyze the effects of the COVID-19 pandemic on people's occupational and mental health.

Keywords: occupational balance; pandemic; COVID-19; social distancing; home confinement

1. Introduction

Occupational balance is defined as the state in which there is a positive evaluation between the number of occupations and their variations [1]. Traditionally, and from an intrapersonal perspective, occupational balance has been described as a satisfactory pattern that the subject presents when carrying out their occupations [2–4]. Occupations are defined as all types of life activities in which people, groups, or populations participate, including activities of daily living, instrumental activities of daily living, rest and sleep, education, work, play, leisure, and socializing [5]. In this sense, the actions cited by Meyer [5]—work, play, rest, and sleep—should always be taken into account when considering what each person needs to achieve balance, even in difficult situations.

In order to maintain an occupational balance over time, there must be harmony and variation in occupations, capacity and resources to be able to manage them, and congruence between occupational commitment, values, and personal meaning [6]. However, despite the fact that an adequate occupational balance has been positively related to the health and well-being [7,8] of a person, recent research has highlighted the importance of the interpersonal perspective, which involves having to satisfy needs, such as family, or to avoid harming others [9–11].

Factors such as quality and satisfaction with life [7] and subjective health [12] can affect the achievement of this balance by hindering access to necessary resources. In this situation, states of underemployment or overoccupation may occur as a consequence of a deficient or exaggerated processing of occupational and environmental stimuli, of few or too many occupational opportunities, or of understimulating, overstimulating, or inappropriate environments [7]. It is therefore a dynamic process in which occupations, roles, personal factors, and external factors vary throughout the lifecycle, with the existence of a certain degree of disturbances in occupational balance being normal, as long as it is not too intense and durable over time and the person has the necessary capacities and resources to adapt and regain balance by readjusting their occupations [13].

A lack of regulatory capacities and abilities can be detrimental to a person's health and lead to illness. Responses to the understimulating occupations or excess occupations, such as boredom or exhaustion, respectively, are the most frequent forms of stress when occupational balance is disturbed. These forms of stress are associated with a poor state of health and can lead to more severe medical conditions [14]. Based on all of the above, this disturbance is defined as any perception of decompensation in daily occupations, which translates into personal dissatisfaction and difficulty in adapting to particular circumstances [15]. It can be caused by both positive and negative situations [16]. In the former, it is the person himself who has chosen the disturbances directly, such as going to university or starting a new job. In the latter, the disturbances are not voluntarily chosen by the person, such as being unemployed, contracting a disease, or experiencing a global pandemic.

In the general population, the measures adopted by the Health Authorities to contain the spread of the coronavirus disease (COVID-19) outbreak, mainly focused on forced social distancing and home confinement, have produced negative psycho-emotional effects due to the loss of leisure and work, alterations in lifestyles, and the generation of stress [17]. The abrupt interruption in the performance of daily occupations has favored the adoption of health risk behaviors, such as physical inactivity, sedentary lifestyles, and excessive alcohol consumption [18], producing high levels of anxiety and depression [19–21]. All of this suggests that the lack of occupational balance translates into a general shortage of regulatory skills and capacities, with negative effects on health, which can lead to serious illnesses [22–25]. The feelings of loss of control and loneliness, caused by confinement and social distancing, have increased the incidence of daytime stress, altered sleep patterns [21,26–28], and increased irritability [21], as well as the almost-complete loss of structured occupations (school, work, and training) in young adults, one of the groups most affected by the effects of this situation [29,30]. In addition, adverse situations may encourage new lifestyle demands to exceed the individual's capacities to face them, negatively affecting their health status [14].

The analysis of the impact of confinement on occupational balance is key to provide meaningful data that allow an approach to the situation focused on reducing or eliminating changes in behaviors and lifestyles produced by the pandemic, increasing quality of life, and reducing its effects on psycho-emotional health. We hypothesized that there was a relationship between sociodemographic and COVID-19-related factors and occupational balance in the Spanish population during the forced social distancing. Therefore, the objective of this study was to determine the factors related to occupational balance in the Spanish population during the confinement that occurred as a consequence of the COVID-19 outbreak.

2. Materials and Methods

2.1. Study Design—Participants

A cross-sectional study was designed. The study population consisted of people aged 18 years or above, who resided in Spain during the forced home confinement phase confinement that occurred as a consequence of the COVID-19 outbreak, and who had the necessary means and resources to access the study survey.

2.2. Procedure—Data Collection

The participants were selected by a non-probabilistic convenience sampling based on the voluntary character of the study. The data was obtained using an online survey through Google Forms, and the link was broadcasted through mainstream social media platforms, such as Facebook, Instagram, Twitter, and WhatsApp. This procedure represented the best data collection strategy in the phase of forced social distancing, allowing us to reach the largest number of people. The survey was available from 16 March to 10 May 2020, the time interval between the first working day of forced home confinement and the first working day on which the forced home confinement rules were relaxed. In the first part of the survey, a brief presentation informed the participants about the aims of the study, requesting their anonymous and voluntary participation. Participants could withdraw from the study at any time, without providing any justification, and the data were not saved. To guarantee anonymity, no personal data which could allow the identification of participants were collected. The completed return of the survey implied the electronic informed consent of the person to participate in the study. Only the questionnaire data that had a complete set of answers were considered. The required time to answer the survey was approximately 15–20 min.

The study received a favorable report from the Bioethics Committee of the Burgos University (Reference IR 14/2020) and was conducted in accordance with the ethical principles of the Declaration of Helsinki.

2.3. Main Outcomes—Instruments

Occupational balance was evaluated by the Occupational Balance Questionnaire (OBQ), designed by Wagman and Håkansson in 2014 [31] and validated for the Spanish population by Peral Gómez in 2017 [32]. This self-administered questionnaire includes 13 items and explores the balance between the different types of activities, their significance, time spent on each activity, and perceived satisfaction. Each item must be answered using a six-point Likert scale, according to the degree of agreement with the content of the sentence, where 0 corresponds to "completely disagree" and 5 to "totally agree." The total score can range from 0 to 65, with higher scores indicating greater occupational balance [31]. Participants had to answer this questionnaire twice. In the first questionnaire, their responses had to refer to the week before the forced home confinement, while in the second one, responses referred to the time of the survey completion. The variation in occupational balance was the main outcome of the study, which was assessed by calculating the differential scores between each questionnaire.

Other variables were collected through an ad hoc questionnaire, previously piloted in a sample of 15 people, who were not part of the subsequent analysis. These variables were classified as sociodemographic (age, sex, marital status, employment status, educational level, home size and number of stays, number of people who make up the family nucleus, possibility of private access to the outside, setting), or COVID-19-related aspects (days of confinement at the time of completing the questionnaire, employment status, telecommuting, suffering or having suffered from COVID-19, experiencing required home isolation, perception of the information received).

2.4. Statistical Analysis

Descriptive analyses were conducted to describe sociodemographic characteristics, COVID-19-related aspects, and occupational balance. The categorical variables were expressed as absolute frequencies and percentages, while the continuous variables were expressed in terms of mean and standard deviation (SD). The compliance of the normality criteria of the quantitative variables was assessed by the Kolmogorov–Smirnov test. In cases where the normal distribution could not be assumed, the contributions made by Blanca et al. [33] were considered. To evaluate the association between the variation in the occupational balance and the categorical variables, the analysis of variance (ANOVA) and the post-hoc less significant differences (LSD) test were used. The effect size differences were calculated using partial eta squared (η^2 p) or Hedge's g and interpreted according to the following criteria: If $0 \leq \eta^2$ p or $g < 0.01$, there is no effect; if $0.01 \leq \eta^2$ p or g < 0.06, the effect is minimal; if $0.06 \leq \eta^2$ p or g < 0.14, the effect is moderate; and if η^2 p or g ≥ 0.14, the effect is strong. The relationship between the differential score obtained in the OBQ and the quantitative variables was analyzed using the Pearson correlation. A forward stepwise multiple lineal regression analysis, adjusted by sex and age, was performed to identify possible independent predictive factors, related to COVID-19 infection, for a higher occupational balance. In this model, variables with a p-value < 0.05 in the univariate analysis were included. Statistical analysis was performed with SPSS version 25 software (IBM-Inc, Chicago, IL, USA). For the analysis of statistical significance, a value of $p < 0.05$ was established.

3. Results

The study sample comprised 3261 subjects, with a majority of women over men (81.69% versus 18.31%). The age of the participants ranged from 18 to 93, with a mean of 40.53 years (SD ± 14.05). Of the 2412 participants who were previously working or studying, 66.92% (n = 1614) continued working or telecommute during the home confinement phase. At the time of completing the survey, 3.25% of participants reported that they had suffered or were currently suffering from COVID-19 infection. The perception of having received insufficient information about the infection by COVID-19 was generalized, with 2043 persons reporting it. The time elapsed between the beginning of home confinement and the filling of the questionnaire ranged between 4 and 57 days. The mean differential score obtained in the OBQ was (−10.45) (SD ± 18.25).

When comparing the differential scores of the occupational balance with the sociodemographic variables, marital status, educational level, employment status, private access to the outside, and housing size were related to disturbances in occupational balance (Table 1). Widowers were the group with the lowest occupational balance during home confinement when compared with married ($p < 0.001$) and single ($p = 0.003$) people. In terms of employment status, subjects with active employment status presented a greater occupational balance than students ($p < 0.001$), unemployed people ($p = 0.001$), and retired people ($p < 0.001$). Likewise, a higher occupational balance was observed in the students in relation to the unemployed ($p = 0.05$). A greater trend toward occupational balance was observed with higher levels of education and larger housing sizes. Private access to the outside showed a strong effect size on the differential scores of the occupational balance ($p = 0.001$; η^2 $p = 0.212$), whereas the effect size of the employment status was minimal ($p < 0.001$; g = 0.14).

Likewise, the differential scores of occupational balance were weakly and positively correlated with age ($p = 0.048$) and the number of children under 18 years old at home ($p = 0.003$), and were weakly and negatively with the number of days in confinement ($p < 0.001$), with a greater mismatch over the days. At home, the number of people living together ($p = 0.252$), the number of dependents ($p = 0.061$), and the number of rooms ($p = 0.232$) did not show a significant relationship with the differential scores of occupational balance produced by confinement (Table 2).

The comparison of the differential scores of occupational balance according to the COVID-19-related variables showed a lower occupational balance in people who were not telecommuting previously ($p = 0.033$; g = 0.087), people who were infected by the virus ($p = 0.004$; g = 0.470) or isolated ($p = 0.048$; g = 0.165) at the time of filling in the form, and people who perceived the information received regarding the pandemic as insufficient ($p < 0.001$; g = 0.191) (Table 3). All of these factors showed a strong effect size on the differential scores of occupational balances except telecommuting, for which it was moderate.

Table 1. Comparison of differential scores in the OBQ according to sociodemographic variables.

	n (%)	Differential Score in OBQ		p-Value	Effect Size
		Mean	SD		
Sex					
Female	2664 (81.69)	(−10.30)	18.72	0.332	0.044 *
Male	597 (18.31)	(−11.10)	15.95		
Marital status					
Single/Separated—Divorced	1154 (35.39)	(−10.98)	18.93	0.002	0.004 **
Married—Living with a partner	2040 (62.56)	(−9.92)	17.80		
Widower	67 (20.55)	(−17.25)	18.35		
Educational level					
Primary studies	269 (8.25)	(−11.71)	19.61	<0.001	0.008 **
Secondary studies	367 (11.25)	(−13.43)	20.12		
Vocational training studies	547 (16.77)	(−11.00)	17.69		
University studies	1480 (45.38)	(−10.36)	17.98		
Post-university studies	586 (17.97)	(−7.88)	17.07		
No formal studies	12 (0.37)	(−0.75)	21.72		
Employment status					
Active	1891(57.99)	(−8.63)	17.96	<0.001	0.014 **
Unemployed—Home chores	606 (18.58)	(−11.96)	18.59		
Student	521 (15.98)	(−14.09)	19.21		
Retired	243 (7.45)	(−12.66)	15.61		
Residence area					
Urban	2271 (69.64)	(−10.69)	18.08	0.241	0.044 **
Rural	990 (30.36)	(−9.88)	18.61		
Private access to the outside					
Yes	2045 (62.71)	(−9.00)	17.88	0.001	0.212 *
No	1216 (37.29)	(−12.87)	18.60		
Housing size					
<30 m^2	36 (1.10)	(−16.41)	21.12	0.003	0.005 **
30–60 m^2	450 (13.80)	(−12.02)	19.39		
60–90 m^2	1294 (39.68)	(−11.06)	18.49		
90–120 m^2	997 (30.57)	(−9.68)	17.40		
>120 m^2	504 (15.45)	(−8.51)	17.72		

n: Number of patients; OBQ: Occupational Balance Questionnaire; SD: Standard deviation; Effect size: * Hedge's' g, ** Partial eta squared (n^2 p).

Table 2. Correlation between differential OBQ scores and sociodemographic variables.

	Mean	SD	r Pearson with Differential Score in OBQ	p-Value
Age	40.53	14.05	0.035	0.048
Days of home confinement	22.69	13.29	(−0.101)	<0.001
Number of people at home	2.96	1.23	(−0.020)	0.252
Number of children under 18 years at home	0.49	0.87	0.052	0.003
Number of dependents at home	0.18	0.51	(−0.033)	0.061
Number of rooms at home	5.27	2.17	0.021	0.232

OBQ: Occupational Balance Questionnaire; SD: Standard deviation.

Multivariate analysis showed that the major contributors to higher occupational balance during the confinement phase were age, the perception of having received enough information, not telecommuting, and not being infected by the COVID-19 at the time of filling out the form (Table 4). Other factors included in the regression model were not significantly associated with occupational balance.

Table 3. Comparison of differential scores in the OBQ according to COVID-19-related variables.

	n (%)	Differential Score in OBQ		*p*-Value	Effect Size
		Mean	SD		
Employment status due to COVID-19					
Stopped working—No telecommuting	798 (33.08)	(−9.70)	20.21	0.228	0.011
Working—Telecommuting	1614 (66.92)	(−9.91)	17.39		
Telecommuting					
Yes	1105 (45.81)	(−8.97)	17.67	0.033	0.087
No	1307 (54.19)	(−10.57)	18.91		
Currently infected by COVID-19					
Yes	38 (1.17)	(−18.89)	19.71	0.004	0.470
No	3223 (98.83)	(−10.34)	18.21		
Infected by COVID-19					
Yes	68 (2.09)	(−11.83)	20.99	0.402	0.078
No	3193 (97.91)	(−10.41)	18.18		
Isolation					
Yes	150 (4.60)	(−13.32)	18.69	0.048	0.165
No	3111 (95.40)	(−10.31)	18.21		
Perception of the information received					
Enough	1218 (37.35)	(−8.27)	16.36	<0.001	0.191
Insufficient	2043 (62.65)	(−11.74)	19.17		

n: Number of patients; OBQ: Occupational Balance Questionnaire; SD: Standard deviation; Effect size: Hedge´s; COVID-19: Coronavirus disease.

Table 4. Multiple linear regression analysis of independent predictive factors related to COVID-19 infection for a higher occupational balance.

Independent Predictive Factors	Standard Error	β	t	*p*-Value
Age	0.03	0.071	3.75	0.001
Perception of received enough information	0.78	0.071	3.34	<0.001
Being not currently infected by COVID-19	3.30	0.055	2.71	0.007
Telecommuting	0.76	0.047	−2.29	0.022

COVID-19: Coronavirus disease.

4. Discussion

The measures adopted to contain the spread of the COVID-19 outbreak, based on forced social distancing and home confinement, were not significantly related to occupational balance in the Spanish population. A low educational level, being unemployed, being a widower or not having a partner, living in small house without private access to the outside, having a fewer number of children under 18 years old at home, being isolated, and spending a greater number of days in home confinement were related to a lower occupational balance. Regarding the variables related to COVID-19 infection, being older, the perception of having received enough information during the pandemic, not telecommuting, and not being infected at the time of filling out the form were independent predictive factors of a higher occupational balance.

People are born with an innate occupational nature, which drives them to occupy themselves and build their occupational identity. However, heterogeneity in what each person considers important makes it difficult to determine who is most vulnerable to suffering disturbances in occupational balance [34].

Despite being one of the first studies to describe the factors related to the occupational balance during home confinement, some research has already explored the differences between sociodemographic groups. Matuska et al. [13] observed that the profile of the people with a higher occupational balance was those 61 years or older, who had earned a master´s degree, and who had children under their care. Similar results were found in this study.

People with active employment, including those who went to the workplace in person and those who telecommuted from home, did not suffer a revealing disturbance in occupational balance compared to those who were unemployed, retired, or students. This result is consistent with previous research, in which financial security, provided by having a job, was a determining factor in achieving balance with occupations and with life [34,35].

The study by Wagman et al. [34], whose objective was to explore the factors that people consider to be more or less relevant to occupational balance, showed the importance of social relationships. A systematic review by Kamalakannan and Chakraborty [36] highlighted the limited attention paid to occupations during the COVID-19 outbreak compared to previous pandemics. In addition, these authors observed that people whose most significant occupations were related to social and leisure activities were most affected by home confinement. In this study, despite the lack of evidence of a significant relationship between the number of people living at home and occupational balance, widowers showed lower occupational balance than single people and people who lived with a partner, as well as those who were isolated in a single room at some point in home confinement. These findings reiterate the importance of social relationships in achieving occupational balance, highlighting the interpersonal perspective mentioned above [11].

There is a trend for a worse occupational balance as the days of home confinement progress, probably due to increased levels of stress, anxiety and depression [23]. Occupational balance is significantly and positively correlated with physical and mental health [6,22,34,37] and predicts the perceived stress by the general population [13], with a higher incidence in so-called risk groups [38].

In a recent study carried out in the Spanish population, it was shown that certain sociodemographic characteristics, such as being female, having minor children, and having a low educational level, increased the perception of threat of COVID-19 infection, facilitating the appearance of symptoms of anxiety or stress [38]. The results of another study, whose objective was to analyze the relation between the psychological impact of the pandemic and the national confinement experienced in Spain, concluded that excessive exposure to the mass media, living with individuals with chronical illness, and living with children under 12 years old increased fears of COVID-19 infection and its emotional consequences. However, an older age, a higher income level, working outside the home, having a private garden at home, and having positive affection have been considered protective factors [39]. The abovementioned results partially coincide with those obtained in this study, since factors such as age, the perception of having received enough information, working outside the home, and not being infected by COVID-19 at the time of filling out the form contributed to a better occupational balance during home confinement.

This study gives a picture of the occupational balance of the Spanish population during the COVID-19 pandemic. However, the study findings must be considered within the context of their limitations. Despite the large sample size, it was not possible to overcome the limitation of a cross-sectional study, and we were unable to determine a causal relationship between the variables. The use of an online survey presented a selection bias in participant recruitment, which was expressed by some characteristics of the sample, such as the high number of females. Measuring occupational balance on a single occasion, but referring to two different moments in time, may have influenced the responses given by the participants. However, using this data collection strategy made it possible to determine the occupational balance of the participants prior to the forced social distancing phase to avoid the participants´ loss during the follow-up period. The use of a convenience sampling may have induced the collection of responses primarily from people who felt strongly about the considered issue. Also, the lack of studies on this topic made it difficult to contrast the results obtained. These limitations can reduce the generalizability of the findings and may have influenced the results of the study. The strengths of this study include the collection of data on a large sample of Spanish adults and the analysis of a wide set of variables, including novel data such as length of confinement, telecommuting, and private access to the outside.

This type of research can promote social and health initiatives for the prevention and treatment of the possible effects of the pandemic and home confinement on the most vulnerable population, for example, by providing psychological and social support, promoting access to resources that reduce social isolation, or proposing measures to stop COVID-19 that take into account the needs of the population which affect their life balance.

Future studies are recommended to help understand and analyze the effects of the COVID-19 pandemic on people's occupational and mental health.

5. Conclusions

The disturbances in occupational balance, caused by the home confinement derived from the COVID-19 pandemic, increased as the days progressed. Sociodemographic variables, such as marital status, educational level, employment situation, private access to the outside, and the size of the house, significantly affected the occupational balance. Specifically, married people, with an active work, a higher educational level, large houses, and with private access to the outside reported a better occupational balance during home confinement. Regarding the variables related to COVID-19, the main contributors to a greater occupational balance were age, the perception of having received enough information, working outside the home, and not currently being infected.

Author Contributions: Conceptualization, J.J.G.-B. and M.S.-P.; methodology, J.J.G.-B., M.S.-P., J.G.-S. and R.S.-C.; software, J.J.G.-B., P.R.-F. and R.S.-C.; validation, M.S.-P. and B.L.d.B.; formal analysis, J.J.G.-B., P.R.-F. and R.S.-C.; investigation, J.J.G.-B., M.S.-P., J.G.-S., P.R.-F. and R.S.-C.; data curation, J.J.G.-B., M.S.-P., J.G.-S. and R.S.-C.; writing—original draft preparation, P.R.-F. and B.L.d.B.; writing—review and editing, J.J.G-B, J.G.-S. and R.S.-C.; visualization, J.J.G.-B., M.S.-P., J.G.-S., P.R.-F., B.L.d.B. and R.S.-C.; supervision, J.J.G.-B. and M.S.-P.; project administration, J.J.G.-B. and M.S.-P. All authors have read and agreed to the published version of the manuscript.

Funding: This research received no external funding.

Conflicts of Interest: The authors declare no conflict of interest.

References

1. Wagman, P.; Håkansson, C.; Björklund, A. Occupational balance as used in occupational therapy: A concept analysis. *Scand. J. Occup. Ther.* **2012**, *19*, 322–327. [CrossRef] [PubMed]
2. Edgelow, M.; Krupa, T. Randomized controlled pilot study of an occupational time-use intervention for people with serious mental illness. *Am. J. Occup. Ther.* **2011**, *65*, 267–276. [CrossRef] [PubMed]
3. Eklund, M.; Leufstadius, C.; Bejerholm, U. Time use among people with psychiatric disabilities: Implications for practice. *Psychiatr. Rehabil. J.* **2009**, *32*, 177–191. [CrossRef] [PubMed]
4. Hultqvist, J.; Lund, K.; Argentzell, E.; Eklund, M. Predictors of clinically important improvements in occupational and quality of life outcomes among mental health service users after completion and follow-up of a lifestyle intervention: Multiple regression modelling based on longitudinal data. *BMC Psychol.* **2019**, *7*, 83. [CrossRef]
5. Meyer, A. The philosophy of occupation therapy. Reprinted from the Archives of Occupational Therapy, Volume 1, pp. 1–10, 1922. *Am. J. Occup Ther.* **1977**, *31*, 639–642. [PubMed]
6. Eklund, M.; Orban, K.; Argentzell, E.; Bejerholm, U.; Tjörnstrand, C.; Erlandsson, L.K.; Håkansson, C. The linkage between patterns of daily occupations and occupational balance: Applications within occupational science and occupational therapy practice. *Scand. J. Occup. Ther.* **2017**, *24*, 41–56. [CrossRef] [PubMed]
7. Bejerholm, U. Occupational balance in people with Schizophrenia. *Occup. Ther. Ment. Health* **2010**, *26*, 1–17. [CrossRef]
8. Forhan, M.; Backman, C. Exploring Occupational Balance in Adults with Rheumatoid Arthritis. *OTJR Occup. Particip. Health* **2010**, *30*, 133–141. [CrossRef]

9. Wada, M.; Backman, C.L.; Forwell, S.J. Men's discursive constructions of balance in everyday life. *Community Work Fam.* **2015**, *18*, 117–133. [CrossRef]
10. Wada, M.; Backman, C.L.; Forwell, S.J.; Roth, W.M.; Ponzetti, J.J. Balance in everyday life: Dual-income parents' collective and individual conceptions. *J. Occup. Sci.* **2014**, *21*, 259–276. [CrossRef]
11. Wagman, P.; Håkansson, C. Occupational balance from the interpersonal perspective: A scoping review. *J. Occup. Sci.* **2019**, *26*, 537–545. [CrossRef]
12. Wagman, P.; Håkansson, C. Exploring occupational balance in adults in Sweden. *Scand. J. Occup. Ther.* **2014**, *21*, 415–420. [CrossRef]
13. Matuska, K.; Bass, J.; Schmitt, J.S. Life balance and perceived stress: Predictors and demographic profile. *OTJR Occup. Particip. Health* **2013**, *33*, 146–158. [CrossRef] [PubMed]
14. Wilcock, A.A.; Chelin, M.; Hall, M.; Hamley, N.; Morrison, B.; Scrivener, L.; Towsend, M.; Treen, K. The relationship between occupational balance and health: A pilot study. *Occup. Ther. Int.* **1997**, *4*, 17–30. [CrossRef]
15. Guest, D.E. Perspectives on the study of work-life balance. *Soc. Sci. Inf.* **2002**, *41*, 255–279. [CrossRef]
16. Clark, S.C. Work Cultures and Work/Family Balance. *J. Vocat. Behav.* **2001**, *58*, 348–365. [CrossRef]
17. Hossain, M.M.; Sultana, A.; Purohit, N. Mental Health Outcomes of Quarantine and Isolation for Infection Prevention: A Systematic Umbrella Review of the Global Evidence. *SSRN Electron. J.* **2020**, *42*, 11. [CrossRef]
18. Wang, C.; Pan, R.; Wan, X.; Tan, Y.; Xu, L.; Ho, C.S.; Ho, R.C. Immediate Psychological Responses and Associated Factors during the Initial Stage of the 2019 Coronavirus Disease (COVID-19) Epidemic among the General Population in China. *Int. J. Environ. Res. Public Health* **2020**, *17*, 1729. [CrossRef]
19. Fleming, K.M.; Campbell, M.; Herring, M.P. Acute effects of Pilates on mood states among young adult males. *Complement. Ther. Med.* **2020**, *49*, 102313. [CrossRef]
20. Lin, C.Y.; Park, J.H.; Hsueh, M.C.; Sun, W.J.; Liao, Y. Prevalence of Total Physical Activity, Muscle-Strengthening Activities, and Excessive TV Viewing among Older Adults; and Their Association with Sociodemographic Factors. *Int. J. Environ. Res. Public Health* **2018**, *15*, 2499. [CrossRef]
21. Jiao, W.Y.; Wang, L.N.; Liu, J.; Fang, S.F.; Jiao, F.Y.; Pettoello-Mantovani, M.; Somekh, E. Behavioral and Emotional Disorders in Children during the COVID-19 Epidemic. *J. Pediatr.* **2020**, *221*, 266. [CrossRef] [PubMed]
22. Ammar, A.; Trabelsi, K.; Brach, M.; Chtourou, H.; Boukhris, O.; Masmoudi, L.; Bouazizet, B.; Bentlage, E.; How, D.; Ahmed, M.; et al. Effects of home confinement on mental health and lifestyle behaviours during the COVID-19 outbreak: Insight from the «ECLB-COVID19» multi countries survey. *Biol. Sport* **2020**, *38*, 9–21. [CrossRef]
23. López-Bueno, R.; Calatayud, J.; Casaña, J.; Casajús, J.A.; Smith, L.; Tully, M.A.; Andersen, L.L.; López-Sánchez, G. COVID-19 Confinement and Health Risk Behaviors in Spain. *Front. Psychol.* **2020**, *11*, 1426. [CrossRef] [PubMed]
24. Ashworth, N.L.; Chad, K.E.; Harrison, E.L.; Reeder, B.A.; Marshall, S.C. Home versus center based physical activity programs in older adults. *Cochrane Database Syst. Rev.* **2005**, *1*, CD004017. [CrossRef] [PubMed]
25. Nollet, M.; Wisden, W.; Franks, N.P. Sleep deprivation and stress: A reciprocal relationship. *Interface Focus* **2020**, *10*, 20190092. [CrossRef]
26. Shuja, K.H.; Aqeel, M.; Jaffar, A.; Ahmed, A. Covid-19 pandemic and impending global mental health implications. *Psychiatr. Danub.* **2020**, *32*, 32–35. [CrossRef]
27. Rubin, G.J.; Wessely, S. The psychological effects of quarantining a city. *BMJ* **2020**, *368*, m313. [CrossRef]
28. Usher, K.; Durkin, J.; Bhullar, N. The COVID-19 pandemic and mental health impacts. *Int. J. Ment. Health Nurs.* **2020**, *29*, 315–318. [CrossRef]
29. Power, E.; Hughes, S.; Cotter, D.; Cannon, M. Youth Mental Health in the time of COVID-19. *Ir. J. Psychol. Med.* **2020**, 1–5. [CrossRef]
30. Matthews, T.; Danese, A.; Caspi, A.; Fisher, H.L.; Goldman-Mellor, S.; Kepa, A.; Moffitt, T.E.; Odgers, C.L.; Arseneault, L. Lonely young adults in modern Britain: Findings from an epidemiological cohort study. *Psychol. Med.* **2019**, *49*, 268–277. [CrossRef] [PubMed]
31. Wagman, P.; Håkansson, C. Introducing the Occupational Balance Questionnaire (OBQ). *Scand. J. Occup. Ther.* **2014**, *21*, 227–231. [CrossRef]
32. Peral Gómez, P. Equilibrio ocupacional en Estudiantes de Terapia Ocupacional. Ph.D. Thesis, Universidad Miguel Hernández, Alicante, Spain, 2017.

33. Blanca, M.J.; Alarcón, R.; Arnau, J.; Bono, R.; Bendayan, R. Non-normal data: Is ANOVA still a valid option? *Psicothema* **2017**, *29*, 552–557. [CrossRef]
34. Wagman, P.; Håkansson, C.; Jacobsson, C.; Falkmer, T.; Björklund, A. What is considered important for life balance? Similarities and differences among some working adults. *Scand. J. Occup. Ther.* **2012**, *19*, 377–384. [CrossRef] [PubMed]
35. Wagman, P.; Hakansson, C.; Matuska, K.M.; Björklun, A.; Falkmer, T. Validating the model of lifestyle balance on a working Swedish population. *J. Occup. Sci.* **2012**, *19*, 106–114. [CrossRef]
36. Kamalakannan, S.; Chakraborty, S. Occupational therapy: The key to unlocking locked-up occupations during the COVID-19 pandemic. *Wellcome Open Res.* **2020**, *5*, 153. [CrossRef]
37. Diez García, C.; López Expósito, C.; Palatucci García, A.; Sesé Sanz, E.; Tapiador Velasco, N. Crisis económica y disfunción ocupacional: Efectos y propuestas de cambio en contexto de crisis. *TOG* **2014**, *11*, 12.
38. Molero Jurado, M.M.; Herrera-Peco, I.; Pérez-Fuentes, M.C.; Gázquez Linares, J.J. Analysis of the threat perceived by the COVID-19 in the Spanish population. *Aten. Primaria* **2020**, *52*, 515–516. [CrossRef]
39. Sandin, B.; García-Escalera, J.; Valiennte, R.; Chorot, P. Impacto psicológico de la pandemia de COVID-19: Efectos negativos y positivos en población española asociados al periodo de confinamiento nacional. *Rev. Psicopatol. Psicol. Clin.* **2020**, *25*, 1–22. [CrossRef]

Journal of
Clinical Medicine

MDPI

Article

Mental Health, Sense of Coherence, and Interpersonal Violence during the COVID-19 Pandemic Lockdown in Germany

Stefanie Jung [1], Jonas Kneer [1] and Tillmann H. C. Krüger [1,2,*]

[1] Department of Psychiatry, Social Psychiatry and Psychotherapy, Division of Clinical Psychology and Sexual Medicine, Hannover Medical School, Carl-Neuberg-Str. 1, 30625 Hannover, Germany; jung.stefanie@mh-hannover.de (S.J.); kneer.jonas@mh-hannover.de (J.K.)

[2] Center for Systems Neuroscience, Bünteweg 2, 30559 Hannover, Germany

* Correspondence: krueger.tillmann@mh-hannover.de; Tel.: +49-511-532-2407

Received: 27 October 2020; Accepted: 16 November 2020; Published: 18 November 2020

Abstract: Preliminary data indicates that the Coronavirus SARS-CoV-2 disease (COVID-19) pandemic may have a substantial impact on mental health and well-being. We assessed mental health in response to the lockdown in Germany between 1 April 2020 and 15 April 2020 using a cross-sectional online survey (n = 3545) with a mixed-methods approach. We found increased levels of psychosocial distress (Patient Health Questionnaire (PHQ) stress module), anxiety, depressive symptoms (PHQ-4), irritability, and a decrease in overall well-being (WHO-Five Well-Being Index (WHO-5)), sense of coherence (Short Form of the Sense of Coherence Scale (SOC-L9)), sexual contentment, and sleep quality. The four-week-prevalence of interpersonal violence was yet at 5% and included verbal, physical, and sexual violence. Participants reported finding comfort in family, friends, conversation, exercise, and activity. Findings are also in line with research showing that women seem to have more trouble coping with the pandemic and lockdown measures. Our observations demonstrate that the COVID-19 pandemic and related measures lead to a mental health burden even in a highly developed Western country and should, therefore, be taken seriously. The findings for interpersonal violence are alarming. Thus, we should sharpen our focus on the matter and activate and enhance supporting systems to help protect those affected.

Keywords: COVID-19; coronavirus; lockdown; mental health; depression; interpersonal violence; sense of coherence

1. Introduction

The novel, highly contagious corona virus SARS-CoV-2 is currently spreading all over the world. First cases of Coronavirus SARS-CoV-2 disease (COVID-19) were reported in Wuhan, China, in early December 2019. Symptoms mainly include respiratory distress, fever, coughing, and fatigue. As of 13 November 2020, 53,126,651 cases of COVID-19 and 1,312,170 COVID-19 related deaths have been confirmed worldwide (for Germany: 771,976 cases of COVID-19 and 12,270 COVID-19-related deaths) (John Hopkins University) [1]. The diseases' course has, thus, proven to be potentially fatal. In order to flatten the curve, measures like social distancing, wearing of a protective mask, enhanced hygiene concepts, and temporary lockdown have been taken in most countries worldwide. The current focus on COVID-19 infections, however, might distract attention from mental health issues related to the outbreak and the measures taken in order to prevent further spreading [2]. In fact, besides its impact on physical health for those infected, the pandemic and the measures taken seem to have a substantial impact on mental health and well-being. Preliminary data from China indicated increased levels of psychological distress, anxiety, depressive symptoms, and insomnia [3,4]. Another Chinese survey found that more than half of the general population rated the outbreak's psychological impact as moderate or severe [5].

Studies related to mental health during the COVID-19 pandemic are still scarce, but more results indicate that anxiety and depression increase with an overall decrease in psychological well-being [6]. Increasing feelings of isolation, fear, worry, and sadness may cause depression and abuse of alcohol, drugs, and prescription medication and may also lead to violence toward the self or others [7]. Some authors even go so far as to describe the current situation as a public mental health crisis [8], the next mental health pandemic [9], or a mental health emergency [10]. Factors associated with a current decrease in mental health include female gender, lower socioeconomic status, lower education, and poor sleep quality [6]. Pandemic-related symptoms of depression and post-traumatic stress disorder (PTSD) have also been found to be linked to female gender and lower socioeconomic status [11].

In March 2020, the German government agreed upon a substantial catalogue of lockdown measures including contact bans that came into effect on 22 March 2020. Such measures were unprecedented for the majority of people and may affect their lives tremendously. As for now, few studies from Europe have been published [6] and yet it seems of vital importance to surveil the psychosocial consequences of the current pandemic. Here, we present data that was taken during the height of lockdown measures in Germany from 1 April 2020 to 15 April 2020.

For one, we assume an increase in depression, anxiety, impaired sleep, and domestic violence as well as changes in alcohol and food consumption. Measures taken against the spreading of the coronavirus included a strict social distancing protocol that also meant a nationwide lockdown with people being advised to stay at home and to only leave the house for essential activities such as work, shopping for essential goods, and care of pets. These measures lead to an involuntary decrease in social contact. Lack of contact with other humans can cause feelings of loneliness, which may lead to depression [12], negative self-esteem, anxiety, feeling unsafe [13], and impaired sleep [14,15]. Moreover, perceived loneliness impairs the capacity to self-regulate [16], which could lead to dysfunctional behavioral changes such as an increase in alcohol or food consumption [17,18]. In addition, when combined with confined domestic circumstances, a decrease in self-regulation could lead to an increase in domestic violence. Second, we assume that the sense of coherence decreased, leaving the German population vulnerable to stress. Sense of coherence is a theoretical concept that offers a framework for overall coping in life. It combines three key aspects: comprehensibility, manageability, and meaningfulness [19]. Whether we understand the things happening to us, whether we believe that we have the necessary resources and skills to manage, and whether things in life are worthwhile and have a purpose, greatly defines how we cope with and how we perceive stressful events. We believe that the pandemic and the measures taken against it constitute such a stressful event. At the beginning of the pandemic, there was little understanding concerning why and how the virus spread or which measures were useful. The uncertainty and the lockdown may have increased feelings of powerlessness and, thus, reduced feelings of manageability.

The current survey was developed in order to systematically assess mental health in response to the pandemic and the measures taken in order to contain it. We sought out to replicate and expand findings from China for the German population and to explore perceived risks and remedies in order to derive much-needed implications for politics and healthcare.

2. Experimental Section

The development of the current study started as the COVID-19 pandemic gathered speed and an implementation of lockdown measures in Germany was starting to become conceivable. Since the population was advised to stay at home, we agreed upon conducting an online survey. We put together a test battery including quantitative as well as qualitative measurements. Apart from demographics, quantitative instruments included the Patient Health Questionnaire-4 (PHQ-4), the Patient Health Questionnaire stress module (PHQ stress module), the WHO-5 Well-being Index (WHO-5), and the

Sense of Coherence Scale–short form Leipzig (SOC-L9). Moreover, using comparative questions on 3-point and 5-point Likert scales, we asked participants to indicate changes to pre-lockdown times (workplace changes, feelings of aggression, sleep quality, quality and quantity of nutritional intake, quality and quantity of sexual activity, availability of time, and experience of violence). We constructed the comparative questions using a multi-step procedure. After reviewing current research from China that already pointed toward the psychosocial areas that might be affected by the pandemic and the measures taken, we brought together the first set of items. Initial items were subsequently revised by experts and members of our department until we reached agreement upon the additional items concerning changes to pre-lockdown times. Additionally, we included a multiple selection question concerning how participants spend their time and two open-ended questions concerning what helped participants during this time and which opportunities they expected to stem from the COVID-19 pandemic and the measures taken against it.

2.1. Patient Health Questionnaire-4 (PHQ-4)

The PHQ-4 briefly measures anxiety and depression. It consists of the first two items of the Generalized Anxiety Disorder-7 scale (GAD-7) and the Patient Health Questionnaire-8 (PHQ-8) and shows good reliability [20].

2.2. Patient Health Questionnaire Stress Module (PHQ Stress Module)

The PHQ stress module is a 15-item questionnaire measuring psychosocial risk factors that contribute to the development of psychiatric disease. It consists of the PHQ items 12a–12j and shows good reliability [21].

2.3. WHO-5 Well-Being Index (WHO-5)

The WHO-5 is a five-item scale measuring current mental well-being while referencing the previous two weeks. It shows high clinometric validity [22].

2.4. Sense of Coherence Scale—Short Form Leipzig (SOC-L9)

The SOC-L9 is a nine-item short form scale derived from the original 29-item questionnaire. It measures sense of coherence, which is a construct referring to a person's attitude or confidence that intrapsychic and environmental events are predictable and manageable. Sense of coherence is believed to be a protective factor for mental health. The scale shows good reliability and validity [23].

Access to the online survey was spread and made available through social media (Instagram, Facebook), mailing lists, the Hannover Medical Schools' website, and TV as well as radio appearances by T.H.C. Krüger. Participants from 18 years up were invited to participate. Deliberately, there were no further inclusion and exclusion criteria as we sought out to reach as many citizens as possible.

2.5. Statistical Analysis

Data was analyzed using SPSS Statistics 26 (IBM® Corporation, Amonk, NY, USA) and tested for normal distribution and non-violence of assumptions, which were applicable prior to further analysis. We mainly report means and standard deviations, group comparisons (using t-tests and Mann-Whitney-U-tests with Bonferroni-Holm adjustment), and frequencies (in percent).

2.6. Analysis of Qualitative Data

Our qualitative data analysis was guided by qualitative content analysis [24]. After sifting through raw data in order to get an overview, filler words like and, the, in … were excluded from further analysis. After data cleansing, we applied the summary method that aims at reducing the material in a way in which essential content is retained. Using abstraction, we build a corpus that represents the raw material and clustered keywords into contextual theme blocks. Our coding was inductive.

Thus, categories were derived from raw data. Since the sample size for men is rather small and the gender differences we found showed only small effect sizes, we will report qualitative data for women and men as one sample.

The survey was approved by the local ethics committee at Hannover Medical School, Germany (Nr. 9002_BO_K_2020). Data was collected during the height of lockdown measures in Germany from 1 April 2020 to 15 April 2020. Participants were informed about the survey content and consented by starting the questionnaire.

3. Results

Demographics. A total of 3545 volunteers took part in this cross-sectional survey. Mean age was M = 40.36 years, standard deviation (SD) = 11.70, n = 2946 (83.1%) female, n = 539 (15.2%) male, n = 60 (1.7%) diverse or missing), mean educational years 15.87 (SD = 4.19), 30.6% held a university degree, 9.9% were unemployed, and 23.9% reported living alone. Acute or chronic disease was reported by 36.7% (physical) and 24.7% (mental) of subjects. Mean duration for completion of the survey was at M = 1134.53 seconds (18.9 min) (SD = 575.35 seconds, 9.6 min). Due to the imbalanced gender distribution, we will report further results separately for women and men.

Depression, Anxiety, and Distress. Depression and anxiety as assessed by PHQ-4 was at M = 3.91 (SD = 3.05) for women and at M = 3.21 (SD = 2.86) for men. Reference samples show mean scores of M = 1.71 (SD = 2.19) for women and M = 1.31 (SD = 1.88) for men [25]. Thus, PHQ-4 scores were significantly higher in our sample for both genders (($t(4254) = -23.66$, $p < 0.001$) for women and ($t(1700) = -16.28$, $p < 0.001$) for men with Bonferroni-Holm-adjustment). Psychosocial distress as measured with the PHQ stress module was at M = 6.40 (SD = 3.88) for women and at M = 6.19 (SD = 4.00) for men, implying mild psychosocial distress (range 5–9) for both genders. The mean well-being score (WHO-5) was at M = 51.44 (SD = 23.88) for women and at M = 47.52 (SD = 22.52) for men (range 0–100). Healthy individuals usually score at M = 75.00 and subjects with major depression usually score at M = 37.50 (WHO, 1998) [26]. Brähler et al. [27] reported the following values for the psychometric validation and standardization of the WHO-5 German version: M = 72.6, SD = 4.90 for men and M = 68.28, SD = 4.98 for women. See Figures 1 and 2. Bonferroni-Holm-adjusted calculation of gender differences revealed higher scores for depression and anxiety ($t(3459) = 4.93$, $p < 0.001$), but also a higher well-being score (($t(3451) = 3.52$, $p < 0.001$)) in women. Effect sizes reported as Cohen's d, however, demonstrate small effects with $d = 0.24$ for depression and anxiety and $d = 0.17$ for well-being.

Sense of Coherence and Coping. Sense of coherence as measured with SOC-L9 was at M = 41.77 (SD = 10.07) for women and at M = 44.11 (SD = 9.71) for men. Reference samples show mean scores of M = 46.70 (SD = 9.00) for women and M = 48.50 (SD = 8.80) for men [28]. Thus, SOC-L9 scores were significantly lower in our sample for both genders ($t(3756) = 14.17$, $p < 0.001$), for women ($t(1372) = 8.56$, $p < 0.001$), and for men with Bonferroni-Holm-adjustment). The majority of subjects (58.1% women, 70.3% men) indicated very good or fairly subjective coping with the pandemic and the corresponding measures, while 28.7% women and 18.2% men indicated poor or very poor subjective coping. Bonferroni-Holm-adjusted calculation of gender differences revealed poorer subjective coping (U = 678156, $p < 0.001$) and lower sense of coherence ($t(3125) = -4.75$, $p < 0.001$) in women. Effect sizes reported as Cohen's d and Pearson's r, however, demonstrate small effects with $d = 0.24$ for sense of coherence and $r = 0.1$ for coping.

Sleeping, Eating, and Sexual Activity. Using comparative questions, 46.5% of all women and 39.5% of all men indicated worsened sleep compared to pre-pandemic times. Bonferroni-Holm-adjusted calculation of gender differences revealed poorer sleep quality in women (U = 740746, $p < 0.05$), even though the effect size shows a small effect ($r = 0.05$). Of all women, 29.2% reported eating less healthy, compared to 18.9% reporting eating healthier. Moreover, 38.1% reported eating more, compared to 16.2% reporting eating less. Of all men, 23.6% reported eating less healthy, compared to 18% reporting eating healthier. Moreover, 26.3% reported eating more, compared to 14.5% reporting eating less. Regarding sexual activity, 20.5% of all women reported having less sexual intercourse, compared to 7.5% reporting having more sexual intercourse. Of all men, 20.4% reported having less sexual intercourse, compared to 7.4% reporting having more sexual intercourse. Furthermore, 21.6% of all women reported decreased sexual contentment, compared to 4.6% reporting increased sexual contentment. Of all men, 29.5% reported decreased sexual contentment, compared to 4.1% reporting increased sexual contentment.

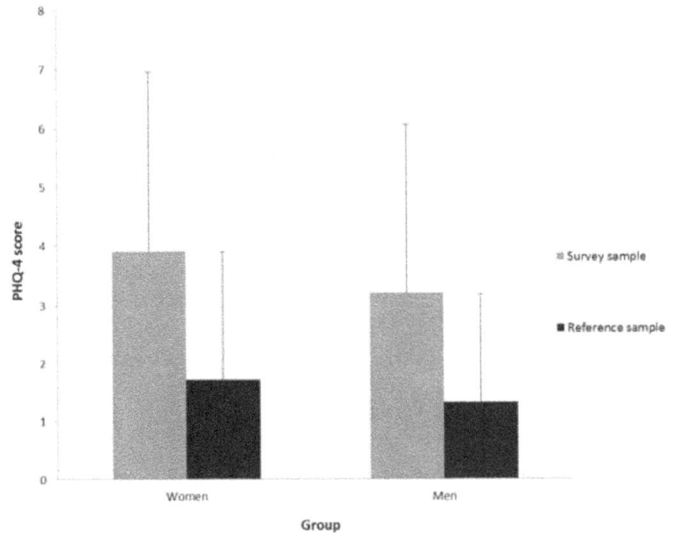

Figure 1. Anxiety and Depression (Patient Health Questionnaire (PHQ-4)): Means and standard deviation of PHQ-4 score for depression and anxiety for women and men in the reference and survey sample.

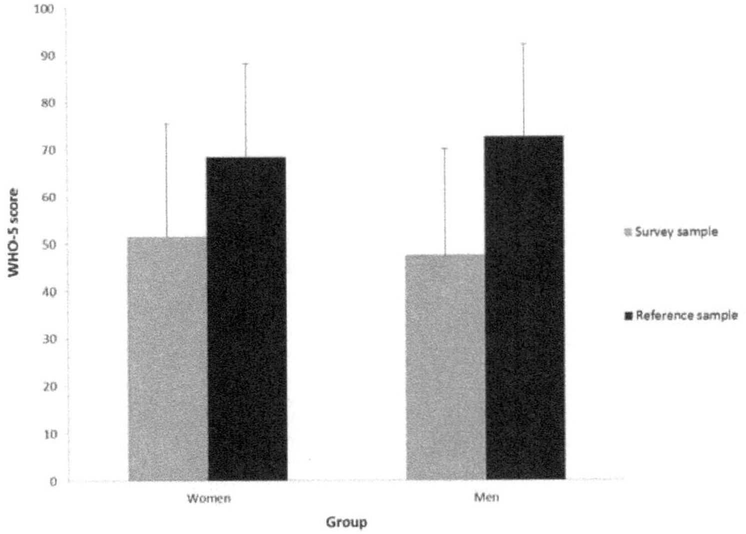

Figure 2. Well-being (WHO-Five Well-Being Index (WHO-5)): Means and standard deviation of WHO-5 well-being score for women and men in reference and survey sample.

3.1. Anger and Violence

3.1.1. Women

A total of 22.8% of all women reported being slightly more easily angry/aggressive, compared to 6.7% reporting feeling slightly less easily angry/aggressive. Furthermore, 7.5% of all women reported experiencing way more anger and aggression, compared to 6.3% experiencing way less. Of those women, who experienced way more anger and aggression, 66.2% directed their anger and aggression at others, while 33.8% directed it at themselves.

3.1.2. Men

Additionally, 20.2% of all men reported being slightly more easily angry/aggressive, compared to 7.6% reporting feeling slightly less easily angry/aggressive. In addition, 2.6% of all men reported experiencing way more anger and aggression, compared to 4.8% experiencing way less. Of those men, who experienced way more anger and aggression, 71.9% directed their anger and aggression at others, while 28.1% directed it at themselves.

Most importantly, 5% of all participants (5.1% of all women and 4.1% of all men) reported experiencing interpersonal violence (IPV) on a verbal (98% of all women and 100% of all men who experienced IPV), physical (38.4% of all women and 63.6% of all men who experienced IPV), or a sexual (26.5% of all women and 50% of all men who experienced IPV) level. In case of verbal violence, 76.8% of all women and 78.2% of all men reported experiencing more verbal violence lately. Regarding physical violence, 14.5% of all women and 21.4% of all men reported experiencing increased levels and, in case of sexual violence, 2.6% of all women but none of the men reported experiencing increased sexual violence lately. Of note, Bonferroni-Holm-adjusted calculation of gender differences revealed more experience of physical violence in men (U = 1206, $p < 0.05$), even though the effect size demonstrates a small effect with $r = 0.18$.

Pastime. While women reported to mostly spend their time doing household chores (65.2%), cooking (54%), and watching movies/TV (50.1%), men reported to mostly spend their time watching movies/TV (51.9%), working (47.3%), and doing household chores (46.6%) (also see Table 1).

Table 1. Pastime.

Women		Men	
Activity	%	Activity	%
1. Household Chores	65.2	1. Watching Movies/TV	51.9
2. Cooking	54.0	2. Work	47.3
3. Watching Movies/TV	50.1	3. Household Chores	46.6
4. Taking A Walk	45.0	4. Spending Time with Family/Partner	
5. Spending Time with Family/Partner	43.8	5. Reading/Watching News	41.9
6. Work	42.3	6. Playing on the Computer/Console/Smartphone	38.0
7. Cleaning	39.9	7. Taking a Walk	36.7
8. Reading/Watching News	37.6	8. Distraction Using Media	35.8
9. Write Text Messages/Chat with Friends/Family	37.1	9. Cooking	35.3
10. Chat with Friends/Family Via Telephone/Video	34.9	10. Listening to Music	28.8

Notes. $n = 3545$, $n = 2946$ female, $n = 539$ male.

Pre-existing mental and physical health conditions. The results show that 24.7% of participants reported pre-existing mental health issues. In order to analyze the impact on our outcome measures, we compared participants with and without mental disease. Bonferroni-Holm-adjusted calculation of differences revealed more anxiety and depression (PHQ-4) in participants with pre-existing mental conditions (U = 548645, $p < 0.001$) with a small to medium effect with $r = 0.39$. Moreover, Bonferroni-Holm-adjusted calculation of differences revealed lower well-being (WHO-5) in participants with pre-existing mental conditions (U = 582613, $p < 0.001$) with a small to medium effect with $r = 0.37$. Furthermore, Bonferroni-Holm-adjusted calculation of differences revealed a lower sense of coherence (SOC-L9) in participants with pre-existing mental conditions (U = 378028, $p < 0.001$) with a small to medium effect with $r = 0.44$. Additionally, Bonferroni-Holm-adjusted calculation of differences revealed worse coping in participants with pre-existing mental conditions (U = 830145, $p < 0.001$), even though the effect size demonstrates a small effect with $r = 0.23$. Lastly, Bonferroni-Holm-adjusted calculation of differences revealed more stress (PHQ stress module) in participants with pre-existing mental conditions (U = 933171, $p < 0.05$), even though the effect size demonstrates a very small effect with $r = 0.04$ (also see Tables 2–4). Pre-existing physical health conditions were reported by 36.7% of participants. Although we found statistically significant differences for outcome measures between participants with and without pre-existing physical health conditions, the effect sizes indicate negligible effects (see Tables S1–S3).

Table 2. Mann-Whitney-U-tests for group differences between participants with (WMHC) and without (WOMHC) pre-existing mental health conditions.

Variable	*z*-Value	*p*-Value	*r*-Value	Mean Rank $_{WMHC}$ [a]	Mean Rank $_{WOMHC}$ [b]
PHQ-4	−23.22	<0.001	0.39	2438.65	1526.21
WHO-5	−21.61	<0.001	0.37	2389.74	1536.61
SOC-L9	−24.88	<0.001	0.44	875.40	1813.63
Coping	−13.46	<0.001	0.23	2140.43	1638.00
PHQ stress	−2.57	0.035	0.04	1703.36	1605.70

Notes. [a] = with mental health condition, $n = 877$, [b] = without mental health condition, $n = 2651$. PHQ-4 = Patient Health Questionnaire-4, WHO-5 = WHO-5 Well-being Index, SOC-L9 = Sense of Coherence Scale–short form Leipzig, PHQ stress module = Patient Health Questionnaire stress module.

Table 3. Means and standard deviations for PHQ-4, WHO-5, SOC-L9, and PHQ stress module for participants with (WMHC) and without (WOMHC) pre-existing mental health conditions.

Variable	M_{WMHC} [a]	SD_{WMHC} [a]	M_{WOMHC} [b]	SD_{WOMHC} [b]
PHQ-4	6.02	3.34	3.06	2.53
PHQ Stress	6.67	3.95	6.26	3.87
WHO-5	16.50	5.43	11.43	5.55
SOC-L9	33.98	9.69	44.79	8.67

Notes. [a] = with mental health condition, $n = 877$ [b] = without mental health condition, $n = 2651$. PHQ-4 = Patient Health Questionnaire-4, PHQ stress module = Patient Health Questionnaire stress module, WHO-5 = WHO-5 Well-being Index, SOC-L9 = Sense of Coherence Scale–short form Leipzig.

Table 4. Answers for item Coping (in percentage) for participants with (WMHC) and without (WOMHC) pre-existing mental health conditions.

How Well Are You Coping?	Percentage $\%_{WMHC}$ [a]	Percentage $\%_{WOMHC}$ [b]
Very good	8.1	16.2
Good	34.3	49.8
Neither nor	13.9	12.6
Not very good	33.8	18.5
Not good at all	9.9	2.9

Notes. [a] = with mental health condition, $n = 877$ [b] = without mental health condition, $n = 2651$.

3.2. Qualitative Data

What does help you during the COVID-19 pandemic? With 35.3%, participants mainly reported finding comfort in their families (including partner and children). Talking to others (18.3%), friends (17.3%), exercise (15.5%), and staying active/occupied and distracted (14.9%) were also perceived as helpful (also see Table 5).

Table 5. What does help you during the COVID-19 * pandemic?

Theme	*n*	%
Family/Partner/Children	1036	35.3
Conversation/Communication	538	18.3
Friends	507	17.3
Exercise	456	15.5
Distraction/Activity/Occupation	437	14.9
Contact	179	6.1
Having More Time	167	5.7
Garden/Nature	143	4.9
Pets	133	4.5
Fine Weather	109	3.7
Nothing	98	3.3

Notes. We will report data up to 3%. $n = 3545$ with $n = 606$ not stated, percentage related to remaining $n = 2939$.
* Coronavirus SARS-CoV-2 disease.

Opportunities stemming from the COVID-19 pandemic. The biggest perceived opportunity stemming from the current pandemic seems to be appreciation/thankfulness (19.6%). Moreover, participants believed that environmental and climate protection (16.1%) as well as reevaluation and rethinking current values (15.1%) and solidarity/willingness to help (11.4%) might be positive outcomes. Beyond, participants named health care system (9.2%), society/community (7.8%), and together (7.4%) as opportunities stemming from the ongoing pandemic (see Table 6).

Table 6. Opportunities stemming from the COVID-19 * pandemic.

Theme	*n*	%
Appreciation/Thankfulness	553	19.6
Environmental Protection/Climate Protection	453	16.1
Reevaluation/Rethinking/Consciousness	425	15.1
Solidarity/Willingness to help	322	11.4
Healthcare System/Care-Giver	260	9.2
Society/Community	219	7.8
Together	209	7.4
Slow Movement	163	5.8
Home Office	137	4.9
Family	114	4.0
Digitalization	109	3.9

Notes. We will report data up to 3%. $n = 3545$ with $n = 723$ not stated, percentage related to remaining $n = 2822$.
* Coronavirus SARS-CoV-2 disease.

4. Discussion

This is one of the first and largest surveys on mental health during the current COVID-19 pandemic in a European society. Although the cohort reflects a relatively well educated and financially secure sample, we found evidence for a substantial mental burden with increased levels of psychosocial distress, irritability (anger/aggression), anxiety, and depressive symptoms. Moreover, participants reported overall lower well-being, lower sense of coherence, decreased sexual contentment, less healthy diet, and almost half of the sample indicated worsened sleep. Our results further indicate that participants with pre-existing mental conditions show more depression and anxiety, less well-being, less sense of coherence, and worse coping skills in terms of the pandemic and the measures taken. Most importantly and also most concerning is the finding of a one-month prevalence of 5% IPV, which is already close to one-year prevalence rates [29] and for which there were indices that this has currently increased. Both women and men experienced more anger and aggression. Both predominantly directed their anger at others rather than themselves.

While we do not present an analysis of risk factors, in line with current research [6], we found that women showed higher levels of anxiety and depression and worse coping, even though small effect sizes restrict these findings. One explanation, however, might be that women seem to lapse into traditional roles. While women report to predominantly spend their time with household chores and cooking, men mainly reported watching movies/TV and going to work. It seems conceivable that an imbalanced distribution of child care and household responsibilities led to fear of or actual work place changes for women, which might, in turn, have further increased women's burden.

Besides the negative impact the current COVID-19 pandemic seems to have on our world population, participants also reported opportunities and pointed out what seemed helpful and beneficial. Almost one-fifth of the sample noted that the current pandemic offers the opportunity to be thankful for and appreciate what we have with 15% assuming that a process of reevaluation might take place. As many as 16% believe that the situation might lead to a sharpened view for environmental and climate issues. More than one-third found comfort in their families, children, and life partners. Almost one-fifth experienced talking to others and friends as beneficial. Exercise and staying active also seemed to help people coping with the COVID-19 pandemic.

The current study offers several strengths and limitations. While some authors argue that sample sizes between $n = 1000$ and $n = 3000$ are usually sufficient enough to make assertions for the general population [30], despite the large sample size, norm deviations for various demographics lead to limitations concerning representativeness. First, in our data set, we found a large gender imbalance. The German population consists of 50.66% women and 49.34% men [31]. Yet, in our study, we found 83.1% females and 15.2% males. However, the phenomenon of gender imbalance in online surveys with women representing the majority is established, as women are more likely to participate in online surveys [32]. Moreover, gender imbalance has been observed in other recent COVID-19 online surveys. Di Renzo et al. [33] reported 80% female respondents and Hsing-Ying Ho et al. [34] reported 66% female respondents. Further potential explanations might be the following: (1) women are more likely to use social media [35] (2) with women staying more at home during the lockdown than men, they had the occasion to participate in surveys, (3) the title of the survey included the term "mental health," which may have spoken more to women than to men, and (4) women are impacted by affective disorders twice as much as men, so they may have had a higher incentive to participate. Second, our sample was well educated. While 17.6% of the German population hold a university degree [36], in our sample we found 30.6% with a Bachelor's degree, a Master's degree or diploma. The unemployment rate in our sample was higher than in the German population (9.9% in our sample and 6.2% in the German population [37]). Mean age (40.36 years in our sample and 44.5 years in the German population [38]) and household status (23.9% reported living alone in our sample vs. 21.13% single households in Germany [39]), however, did not seem to differ widely. Taken together, the demographic deviations from the norm restrict representativeness. Moreover, we did not investigate depression and anxiety rates before the pandemic. Thus, we can only draw a comparison between current pandemic values and reference values. We did, however, check for pre-existing mental and physical illness. Concerning pre-existing mental conditions, the occurrence corresponds to point prevalence in Germany [40]. Thus, a resulting bias cannot be expected. Further on, we did not explore the extent to which women were involved in child care during the lockdown, which included closing of day care and schools. Beyond that, we did not control for social desirability effects. These aspects should be taken into account for future studies. Yet, using a mixed-methods approach, we present comprehensive European data that gives a valuable insight into potential challenges and protective factors for mental health during the height of lockdown measures in Germany.

5. Conclusions

Although there is reason to expect that mental health will increase with the successful containment of the COVID-19 pandemic [41], the spreading course of the coronavirus seems to be coming and going in waves. The populations' mental health can, thus, be assumed to be equally dynamic. The latest numbers from the U.S., for example, demonstrate that, related to the pandemic, 40% of respondents showed signs of anxiety, depression, or increased use of substances with 25% even reporting symptoms of trauma-related and stressor-related disorders [42]. By now, COVID-19 case numbers worldwide have gone up again and measures are being intensified globally. Therefore, it is of vital importance to continuously monitor the mental health of the general public during this pandemic and its aftermath to identify associated protective factors and to carefully screen for IPV and its risk factors such as stress, sleep problems, and anger [43].

Supplementary Materials: The following are available online at http://www.mdpi.com/2077-0383/9/11/3708/s1, Table S1: Mann-Whitney-U-tests for group differences between participants with and without pre-existing physical health conditions, Table S2: Means and standard deviations for PHQ-4, WHO-5, SOC-L9 and PHQ stress module for participants with and without pre-existing physical health conditions., Table S3: Answers for item "coping" (percentage) for participants with and without pre-existing physical health conditions.

Author Contributions: Conceptualization, S.J., J.K. and T.H.C.K.; methodology, S.J., J.K. and T.H.C.K.; validation, S.J., J.K. and T.H.C.K.; formal analysis, S.J. and J.K.; investigation, S.J.; resources, S.J. and T.H.C.K.; data curation, S.J. and J.K.; writing—original draft preparation, S.J.; writing—review and editing, S.J., J.K. and T.H.C.K.; visualization, S.J. and J.K.; supervision, T.H.C.K.; project administration, S.J. and T.H.C.K. All authors have contributed to the scientific work and have read and agreed to the published version of the manuscript.

Funding: This research received no external funding.

Conflicts of Interest: The authors declare no conflict of interest.

References

1. Johns Hopkins University. Johns Hopkins Coronavirus Resource Center. JHU. Available online: https://coronavirus.jhu.edu/map.html (accessed on 13 November 2020).
2. Torales, J.; O'Higgins, M.; Castaldelli-Maia, J.M.; Ventriglio, A. The outbreak of COVID-19 coronavirus and its impact on mental health. *Int. J. Soc. Psychiatry* **2020**, *66*, 317–320. [CrossRef] [PubMed]
3. Lai, J.; Ma, S.; Wang, Y.; Cai, Z.; Hu, J.; Wei, N.; Wu, J.; Du, H.; Chen, T.; Li, R.; et al. Factors associated with mental health outcomes among health care workers exposed to coronavirus disease 2019. *JAMA Netw. Open* **2020**, *3*, e203976. [CrossRef] [PubMed]
4. Huang, Y.; Zhao, N. Generalized anxiety disorder, depressive symptoms and sleep quality during COVID-19 outbreak in China: A web-based cross-sectional survey. *Psychiatry Res.* **2020**, *288*, 112954. [CrossRef] [PubMed]
5. Wang, C.; Pan, R.; Wan, X.; Tan, Y.; Xu, L.; Ho, C.S.H.; Ho, R.C.M. Immediate psychological responses and associated factors during the initial stage of the 2019 coronavirus disease (COVID-19) epidemic among the general population in China. *Int. J. Environ. Res. Public. Health* **2020**, *17*, 1729. [CrossRef] [PubMed]
6. Vindegaard, N.; Benros, M.E. COVID-19 pandemic and mental health consequences: Systematic review of the current evidence. *Brain Behav. Immun.* **2020**. [CrossRef]
7. Lieberman, J.A.; Olfson, M. Meeting the mental health challenge of the COVID-19 pandemic. Psychiatric Times. Available online: https://www.psychiatrictimes.com/view/meeting-mental-health-challenge-covid-19-pandemic (accessed on 12 August 2020).
8. Dong, L.; Bouey, J. Public mental health crisis during COVID-19 pandemic, China. *Emerg. Infect Dis.* **2020**, *26*, 3201. [CrossRef]
9. Parrish, E. The next pandemic: COVID-19 mental health pandemic. *Perspect. Psychiatr. Care* **2020**, *56*, 485. [CrossRef] [PubMed]
10. Kelly, B.D. Coronavirus disease: Challenges for psychiatry. *Br. J. Psychiatry.* **2020**, *217*, 352–353. [CrossRef]
11. Mowbray, H. In Beijing, coronavirus 2019-nCoV has created a siege mentality. *BMJ* **2020**. [CrossRef]
12. Cacioppo, J.T.; Hughes, M.E.; Waite, L.J.; Hawkley, L.C.; Thisted, R.A. Loneliness as a specific risk factor for depressive symptoms: Cross-sectional and longitudinal analyses. *Psychol. Aging* **2006**, *21*, 140–151. [CrossRef]
13. Cacioppo, J.T.; Hawkley, L.C.; Ernst, J.M.; Burleson, M.; Berntson, G.G.; Nouriani, B.; Spiegel, D. Loneliness within a nomological net: An evolutionary perspective. *J. Res. Pers.* **2006**, *40*, 1054–1085. [CrossRef]
14. Cacioppo, J.T.; Hawkley, L.C.; Crawford, L.E.; Ernst, J.M.; Burleson, M.H.; Kowalewski, R.B.; Malarkey, W.B.; Van Cauter, E.; Berntson, G.G. Loneliness and health: Potential mechanisms. *Psychosom. Med.* **2002**, *64*, 407–417. [CrossRef] [PubMed]

15. Mahon, N.E. Loneliness and sleep during adolescence. *Percept. Mot. Ski.* **1994**, *78*, 227–231. [CrossRef] [PubMed]
16. Hawkley, L.C.; Cacioppo, J.T. Loneliness matters: A theoretical and empirical review of consequences and mechanisms. *Ann. Behav. Med.* **2010**, *40*, 218–227. [CrossRef] [PubMed]
17. Lauder, W.; Mummery, K.; Jones, M.; Caperchione, C. A comparison of health behaviours in lonely and non-lonely populations. *Psychol. Health Med.* **2006**, *11*, 233–245. [CrossRef] [PubMed]
18. Akerlind, I.; Hornquist, J.O. Loneliness and alcohol abuse: A review of evidences of an interplay. *Soc. Sci. Med.* **1992**, *34*, 405–414. [CrossRef]
19. Antonovsky, A. *Unraveling the Mystery of Health—How People Manage Stress and Stay Well*; Jossey-Bass Publishers: San Francisco, CA, USA, 1987.
20. Kroenke, K.; Spitzer, R.L.; Williams, J.B.W.; Löwe, B. An ultra-brief screening scale for anxiety and depression: The PHQ–4. *Psychosomatics* **2009**, *50*, 613–621.
21. Gräfe, K.; Zipfel, S.; Herzog, W.; Löwe, B. Screening psychischer störungen mit dem "Gesundheitsfragebogen für Patienten (PHQ-D)". *Diagnostica* **2004**, *50*, 171–181. [CrossRef]
22. Topp, C.W.; Østergaard, S.D.; Søndergaard, S.; Bech, P. The WHO-5 well-being index: A systematic review of the literature. *Psychother. Psychosom.* **2015**, *84*, 167–176. [CrossRef]
23. Lin, M.; Bieda, A.; Margraf, J. Short form of the sense of coherence scale (SOC-L9) in the US, Germany, and Russia: Psychometric properties and cross-cultural measurement invariance test. *Eur. J. Psychol. Assess.* **2019**. [CrossRef]
24. Mayring, P. *Qualitative Inhaltsanalyse. Grundlagen und Techniken*, 11th ed.; Beltz: Weinheim, Germany, 2010.
25. Kroenke, K.; Spitzer, R.L.; Williams, J.B.; Monahan, P.O.; Lowe, B. Anxiety disorders in primary care: Prevalence, impairment, comorbidity, and detection. *Ann. Intern. Med.* **2007**, *146*, 317–325. [CrossRef] [PubMed]
26. *Wellbeing Measures in Primary Health Care/the Depcare Project*; Report on a WHO Meeting: Stockholm, Swedish, 1998.
27. Brähler, E.; Mühlan, H.; Albani, C.; Schmidt, S. Teststatistische prüfung und normierung der deutschen versionen des eurohis-qol lebensqualität-index und des WHO-5 wohlbefindens-index. *Diagnostica* **2007**, *53*, 83–96. [CrossRef]
28. Singer, S.; Brähler, E. *Die "Sense of Coherence Scale"*; Vandenhoeck & Ruprecht: Göttingen, Germany, 2007.
29. Makaroun, L.K.; Brignone, E.; Rosland, A.M.; Dichter, M.E. Association of health conditions and health service utilization with intimate partner violence identified via routine screening among middle-aged and older women. *JAMA Netw. Open* **2020**, *3*, e203138. [CrossRef] [PubMed]
30. Schnell, R.; Hill, P.B.; Esser, E. *Methoden der Empirischen Sozialforschung*, 2nd ed.; Oldenbourg: München, Germany, 1989.
31. Statistisches Bundesamt. Available online: https://www.destatis.de/DE/Themen/Gesellschaft-Umwelt/Bevoelkerung/Bevoelkerungsstand/_inhalt.html;jsessionid=DE922D7E04B48DCE2930CF8398773356.internet8742 (accessed on 20 October 2020).
32. Moore, D.L.; Tarnai, J. Survey nonresponse. In *Evaluating Nonresponse Error in Mail Surveys*; Groves, R.M., Dillman, D.A., Eltinge, J.L., Little, R.J.A., Eds.; John Wiley & Sons, Inc.: New York, NY, USA, 2002; pp. 197–211.
33. Di Renzo, L.; Gualtieri, P.; Cinelli, G.; Bigioni, G.; Soldati, L.; Attinà, A.; Bianco, F.F.; Caparello, G.; Camodeca, V.; Carrano, E.; et al. Psychological aspects and eating habits during covid-19 home confinement: Results of EHLC-COVID-19 Italian online survey. *Nutrients* **2020**, *12*, 2152. [CrossRef] [PubMed]
34. Ho, H.-Y.; Chen, Y.-L.; Yen, C.-F. Different impacts of COVID-19-related information sources on public worry: An online survey through social media. *Internet Interv.* **2020**, *22*, 100350. [CrossRef]
35. Perrin, A. "Social Networking Usage: 2005–2015" Pew Research Center. Available online: http://www.pewinternet.org/2015/10/08/2015/Social-Networking-Usage-2005-2015/ (accessed on 15 February 2016).
36. Statistisches Bundesamt. Available online: https://www.destatis.de/DE/Themen/Gesellschaft-Umwelt/Bildung-Forschung-Kultur/Bildungsstand/_inhalt.html (accessed on 20 October 2020).
37. Arbeitsagentur. Available online: https://www.arbeitsagentur.de/news/arbeitsmarkt-2020 (accessed on 20 October 2020).
38. Statistisches Bundesamt. Available online: https://de.statista.com/statistik/daten/studie/723069/umfrage/durchschnittsalter-der-bevoelkerung-in-deutschland-nach-staatsangehoerigkeit/ (accessed on 20 October 2020).

39. Statistisches Bundesamt. Available online: https://de.statista.com/statistik/daten/studie/156951/umfrage/anzahl-der-einpersonenhaushalte-in-deutschland-seit-1991/ (accessed on 20 October 2020).
40. DGPPN. Basisdaten Psychische Erkrankungen. Available online: https://www.dgppn.de/_Resources/Persistent/a2e357dac62be19b5050a1d89ffd8603cfdb8ef9/20201008_Factsheet.pdf (accessed on 27 October 2020).
41. Sønderskov, K.M.; Dinesen, P.T.; Santini, Z.I.; Østergaard, S.D. Increased psychological well-being after the apex of the COVID-19 pandemic. *Acta Neuropsychiatr.* **2020**. [CrossRef]
42. Czeisler, M.É.; Lane, R.I.; Petrosky, E.; Wiley, J.F.; Christensen, A.; Njai, R.; Weaver, M.D.; Robbins, R.; Facer-Childs, E.R.; Barger, L.K.; et al. Mental health, substance use, and suicidal ideation during the COVID-19 pandemic — United States, June 24–30, 2020. *MMWR. Morb. Mortal. Wkly. Rep.* **2020**, *69*, 1049–1057. [CrossRef]
43. DeWolfe, D.J. *Training Manual for Mental Health and Human Service Workers in Major Disasters*, 2nd ed.; Federal Emergency Management Agency: Washington, DC, USA, 2000.

Publisher's Note: MDPI stays neutral with regard to jurisdictional claims in published maps and institutional affiliations.

Journal of
Clinical Medicine

MDPI

Article

Psychological and Emotional Impact of Patients Living in Psychiatric Treatment Communities during Covid-19 Lockdown in Italy

Jessica Burrai [1,2,*], Paolo Roma [3], Benedetta Barchielli [1], Silvia Biondi [3], Pierluigi Cordellieri [2], Angelo Fraschetti [2], Alessia Pizzimenti [4], Cristina Mazza [5], Stefano Ferracuti [3] and Anna Maria Giannini [2]

1 Department of Dynamic and Clinical Psychology, Sapienza University of Rome, Via Degli Apuli 1, 00185 Rome, Italy; benedetta.barchielli@gmail.com

2 Department of Psychology, Sapienza University of Rome, Via dei Marsi 78, 00185 Rome, Italy; pierluigi.cordellieri@uniroma1.it (P.C.); angelo.fraschetti@uniroma1.it (A.F.); annamaria.giannini@uniroma1.it (A.M.G.)

3 Department of Human Neuroscience, Sapienza University of Rome, Viale dell'Università 30, 00185 Rome, Italy; paolo.roma@uniroma1.it (P.R.); silviabiondi14@gmail.com (S.B.); stefano.ferracuti@uniroma1.it (S.F.)

4 SRTR Villa Costanza, gruppo Sage, Via Belmonte 74, 00079 Rome, Italy; info@alessiapizzimenti.it

5 Department of Neuroscience, Imaging and Clinical Sciences, G. d'Annunzio University of Chieti-Pescara, Via dei Vestini 33, 66100 Chieti-Pescara, Italy; cristina.mazza@uniroma1.it

* Correspondence: jessica.burrai@uniroma1.it

Received: 28 October 2020; Accepted: 21 November 2020; Published: 23 November 2020

Abstract: Most studies on well-being during the COVID-19 pandemic have focused on the mental health of the general population; far less attention has been given to more specific populations, such as patients with mental illness. Indeed, it is important to examine the psychiatric population, given its vulnerability. The present study aimed at assessing the psychological and emotional impact of isolation on patients in Residential Rehabilitation Communities, compared to healthy controls. A questionnaire was administered cross-sectionally on an online survey platform and both psychiatric patients and healthy controls accessed via a designed link. The results showed significant differences between psychiatric patients and controls on Anxiety, Stress, Worry, and Risk Perception variables. Psychiatric patients scored lower on Stress compared to healthy controls and higher on Anxiety, Perceived Risk of getting infected with COVID-19 and Worry about the emergency situation. The results showed that, during the Italian lockdown, psychiatric patients living in residential communities received unbroken support from peers and mental health professionals, maintained their usual medication treatment, and were informed of COVID-19 consequences. This finding provides insight into the differences between residential and healthy populations and highlights the importance of continuous support for psychiatric patients, especially during stressful situations such as a pandemic.

Keywords: Covid-19; psychiatric patients; stress; anxiety; depression; coping; worry; risk perception; mental illness

1. Introduction

Over the past century, there have been several pandemics, with many devastating consequences. In a pandemic situation, when there is no pre-existing immunity to pandemic pathogens, no effective pharmacological treatment, and no vaccine, individuals' only preventive health measure is to practice good hygiene (e.g., wash hands) and social distancing [1]. Thus, in the wake of the global spread of SARS-CoV-2 and its associated disease (COVID-19), governments have implemented significant containment measures, including quarantines and lockdowns and the closure of schools, offices, and non-essential shops [2].

Research on individual and community responses to restrictive measures in the context of previous infectious disease outbreaks (e.g., Severity Acute Respiratory Syndrome [SARS]; H1N1; Ebola; Middle East Respiratory Syndrome [MERS]; equine influenza) have studied the psychological effects of isolation, social distancing, and lack of physical contact. The findings have demonstrated a significant psychological impact on individual well-being, characterized by higher levels of Anxiety, Depression, and Stress [3–8]. Recent studies conducted during the COVID-19 pandemic have shown similar consequences of the lockdown on psychophysical wellness in the general population [9–15].

Most studies on well-being during the COVID-19 pandemic have focused on the mental health of the general population; far less attention has been given to more specific populations, such as patients with mental illness [16]. In this context, it is important for researchers to examine the psychiatric population, given its vulnerability. It has already been shown that both older adults and those who are immunocompromised (including psychiatric patients) are at greater risk for developing complications when infected with COVID-19 (e.g., comorbidity with other medical disorders, see, e.g., [17]).

In addition, the co-occurrence of mental illness and substance use disorders [18] as risk factor for COVID-19 infection, and risk adverse outcomes related to cardiovascular, pulmonary and metabolic disease associated to an extent with chronic use of alcohol and other drugs need to be taken into account [19].

Moreover, social isolation is part of the symptomatology of many psychiatric disorders. For this reason, at first it could be assumed that lockdown policies could reduce the stress related to compliance with social norms; on the other hand, it should be considered that the long-term outcomes could be an increase of rumination and decompensation due to a possible exacerbation of loneliness and despair relating to social isolation [20].

Furthermore, the psychiatric population may increase their suffering in reaction to forced isolation and compromise their ability to adequately understand the emergency and implement appropriate containment behaviors.

Very few studies have addressed the effects of comprehensive restrictive public health measures on psychiatric patients. To the best of our knowledge, during the SARS epidemic, only one study [21] investigated the effect of the epidemic on the clinical state of psychiatric inpatients with schizophrenia, finding them to present lower levels of Anxiety, Depression, and Fear compared to a control group of health staff. The authors explained these findings as indicative of the in-patients' greater denial of the importance and personal relevance of the epidemic.

With respect to the COVID-19 pandemic, contrasting results have emerged, showing a higher sensitivity in psychiatric patients due to pandemic-related Stress [22]. Hao et al. [22] studied the psychological impact of the pandemic on psychiatric patients and healthy controls during the peak of viral spread in China. The psychiatric patients (who had been diagnosed with Major Depressive Disorder, Generalized Anxiety Disorder, Panic Disorder, and/or mixed Anxiety and Depressive Disorder) showed significantly higher levels of Post-Traumatic Stress Disorder (PTSD), Depression, Anxiety, Stress, and insomnia, compared to the healthy controls. More specifically, 31.6% of the psychiatric sample fulfilled the diagnostic criteria for PTSD, while 23.6% showed moderate to severe anxiety symptoms and 22.4% showed moderate to severe depressive symptoms. Finally, more than 25.0% of the psychiatric patients suffered from moderately severe to severe insomnia [22]. The authors suggested that the worse outcomes shown by their psychiatric patient group may have been caused by their lack of access to mental health services during the emergency.

During the COVID-19 pandemic, people with mental illness were also shown to demonstrate stronger emotional responses compared to the general population, as a result of their higher susceptibility to Stress [16]. Psychiatric patients were also found to experience higher levels of Distress, which could play a mediating role in elevating levels of Anxiety [23].

All of the abovementioned studies were conducted online, using samples of in-patients at hospitals and psychiatric units. To the best of knowledge, no prior study has assessed psychiatric patients in a rehabilitation community. In such communities, psychiatric patients have adjusted to conditions of less personal autonomy and community engagement; they no longer attend school and/or internships and they do not leave the facility to visit family and friends. Thus, the typical residential conditions are similar to a quarantine or lockdown situation.

The present study aimed at assessing the psychological and emotional impact of isolation on patients in these psychiatric communities, compared to healthy controls. In more detail, we wondered whether there might be significant differences between psychiatric patients and healthy controls during the COVID-19 lockdown in relation to Coping Style, Risk Perception, and Worry, as well as levels of Depression, Anxiety, and Stress. Furthermore, we sought to identify potential risk and protective factors for psychological distress, taking into account sociodemographic variables (i.e., age, gender, education), Worry, Risk Perception, and—particularly—the presence or absence of a psychiatric diagnosis.

2. Experimental Section

2.1. Participants

A questionnaire was administered cross-sectionally on an online survey platform, which participants (both psychiatric patients and healthy controls) accessed via a designed link. The respondents were 82 Italian psychiatric patients, living in two rehabilitation communities in the Lazio region during the COVID-19 lockdown, and 106 healthy control subjects, recruited online and randomly chosen from a larger sample on the basis of mean age. The two communities are accredited by the National Health Service and provide healthcare assistance through qualified personnel 24 h per day. Various professional figures work closely with psychiatric patients within the community: psychiatrists, educators, psychologists, nurses and social assistants. During the lockdown, all the professionals continued to work in the community guaranteeing psychiatric patients' continuity of care and treatment. In both communities, an attempt was made to maintain a link with the patients' affections and families through remote communication systems, strengthening the Internet connection and helping psychiatric patients with video calls. Several meetings have been held within the community between the mentioned professionals in order to organize specific therapy groups for the psychiatric patients. Positive reinforcement techniques were used to encourage participation in therapy groups to prepare the patients to face social isolation and emotional flattening.

The psychiatric patients were aged 18 years or older and had been diagnosed with at least one psychotic disorder; healthy controls were aged 18 years or older and had no psychiatric diagnosis. All participants voluntarily responded to the anonymous survey and indicated their informed consent. The procedures were clearly explained, and participants could interrupt or quit the survey at any point without providing explanation. As regards the questionnaire administered to psychiatric patients, the first items were intended for the community administrators who helped patients respond to the measure. The remaining items were administered for patient self-report.

Five psychiatric patients and six healthy controls were excluded from the analysis because they did not complete the entire survey. The final sample consisted of 177 participants. The psychiatric patient sample comprised 77 participants: 51 males (M_{years} = 47.29; SD = 13.26) and 26 females (M_{years} = 45.27; SD = 12.03), aged 22–73 years, with a mean age of 46.61 (SD = 12.81). Most psychiatric patients did not have children and were either retired or recipients of state support. The healthy control sample comprised 100 participants: 50 males (M_{years} = 48.38; SD = 12.79) and 50 females (M_{years} = 44.42; SD = 9.81), aged 20–69 years, with a mean age of 46.40 (SD = 11.52). No significant difference was found between groups in age [F (1,176) = 0.013, p = 0.909], while significant differences were found in gender [χ^2 (1) = 4.679, p = 0.031] and education [F (1,176) = 14.796, $p \leq 0.001$] (see Table 1).

Table 1. Descriptive statistics of the study sample.

		Psychiatric Patients	Healthy Controls
Characteristic	Group	*N* (%) = 77	*N* (%) = 100
Age	*M* (*SD*)	46.61 (12.81)	46.40 (11.52)
	Min–Max	22–73	20–69
Gender	Female	26 (33.8%)	50 (50%)
	Male	51 (66.2%)	50 (50%)
Education	Primary school diploma	6 (7.8%)	4 (4%)
	Middle school diploma	37 (48.1%)	28 (28%)
	High school diploma	28 (36.4%)	47 (47%)
	Graduate	5 (6.5%)	21 (21%)
	Unknown	1 (1.3%)	0 (0%)

Data were collected between April and May 2020, before the end of the lockdown period in Italy. Expedited ethics approval was obtained from the Institutional Board of the Department of Human Neuroscience, Faculty of Medicine and Dentistry, "Sapienza" University of Rome (IRB-2020-6), in conformity with the principles of the Declaration of Helsinki.

Descriptive statistics are reported in Table 1.

Most psychiatric patients (93.5%) received training and education on COVID-19 and its transmission by the referred community, hence we assessed patients' knowledge about the COVID-19 pandemic using three items (i.e., "How did you become aware of the spread of COVID-19?"; "What is COVID-19?"; "Did you participate in community training sessions on this health emergency?"). Each of these items enabled more than one response option to be indicated. Furthermore, the first two items were also administered by the healthy control group, in order to assess where they had retrieved information about the virus and their awareness about it. Possible responses to the first item differed between groups, since the psychiatric patients were living in the rehabilitation communities and had contact with the operators. Table 2 reports the response frequency of these items.

Table 2. Descriptive statistics of the sample, in regard to knowledge about COVID-19.

Questions	Options	Psychiatric Patients *N* (%)	Healthy Controls *N* (%)
Information about COVID-19 retrieved from	Media	60	82
	Social networks	13	37
	Family	9	18
	Community operators *	37	-
	Community hosts *	7	-
	Organized communication from community staff *	25	-
	Other	4	2
What is COVID-19	Seasonal flu	2	5
	Respiratory syndrome	39	42
	Respiratory insufficiency	35	38
	High temperature	18	15
	Fake news	0	2
	Terrorist attack	2	0
	Other	9	3
Participation in formative meetings about COVID-19 *	Yes	72 (93.5%)	-
	No	5 (6.5%)	-

Note. * indicates responses/questions administered only to the psychiatric patients.

2.2. Materials

The Depression, Anxiety and Stress Scale–21 items (DASS-21) [24] was used to assess participants' mental health. The DASS-21 is a set of three self-report scales designed to measure the emotional states of Depression, Anxiety, and Stress. All subscales are rated on a 4-point Likert scale ranging from 0 (never) to 3 (almost always). In our sample, Cronbach's alphas were 0.82, 0.83, and 0.87 for the Depression, Anxiety, and Stress Subscales, respectively.

The Brief Resilient Coping Scale (BRCS) [25] is a four-item questionnaire designed to capture highly adaptive Stress coping tendencies. It is rated on a 5-point Likert scale ranging from 1 (does not describe me at all) to 5 (describes me very well). Total scores range from 4–20, with scores of 4–13 indicating low resilient coping, scores of 14–16 indicating medium resilient coping, and scores of 17–20 indicating high resilient coping. In the present sample, the BRCS showed a Cronbach's alpha of 0.64.

Risk Perception was assessed through two variables, perceived severity and perceived likelihood, using items adapted from Cho and Lee [26] and Liao et al. [27]. Perceived severity was measured through four items (e.g., "If I got COVID-19, it would be severe") and perceived likelihood was measured through two items ("How likely is it that you will get COVID-19 in this period?"). Twelve questions were assessed on a 5-point Likert scale ranging from 1 (not likely at all) to 5 (certain). In the present sample, the items showed good reliability, with Cronbach's alpha of 0.72.

Worry was assessed using six items (e.g., "In the past week, you have been worried about contracting the COVID-19") designed to measure Worry about the present emergency situation, risk of contracting COVID-19, and perspectives on the future. Items were assessed on a 5-point Likert scale ranging from 1 (hardly) to 5 (extremely). The items showed good reliability, with Cronbach's alpha of 0.63.

2.3. Statistical Analysis

Descriptive statistics of both the psychiatric patient and the healthy control groups were collected in order to summarize the variables. Analysis of variance (ANOVA) tests were run to identify differences between groups in their scores for Risk Perception, the BRCS, Worry, and DASS-21 Depression, Anxiety, and Stress. Two multiple linear regressions were performed using the enter and stepwise methods, respectively, to compute associations between sociodemographic variables (i.e., age, gender, education), the presence/absence of diagnosis, Risk Perception, and Worry (used as independent variables); and DASS-21 Anxiety and Stress (used as dependent variables). DASS-21 Depression was excluded because no differences were found between groups. All statistical analyses were conducted using the software package SPSS, version 25.

3. Results

3.1. Between Groups Comparison (ANOVAs)

As reported in Table 3, psychiatric patients demonstrated lower scores on DASS-21 Anxiety, BRCS, Risk Perception, and Worry. In more detail, ANOVAs showed a significant difference between groups on DASS-21 Anxiety and Stress, Risk Perception, and Worry. In particular, psychiatric patients scored lower on Stress and higher on Anxiety, Perceived Risk of getting infected with COVID-19 and Worry about the emergency situation, compared to healthy controls.

Table 3. Between groups comparison (ANOVAs).

	Psychiatric Patients N = 77	Healthy Controls N = 100	F	p	parη2
DASS-21 Depression	4.58 (4.10)	5.77 (5.53)	2.488	0.116	0.014
DASS-21 Anxiety	**4.04 (4.39)**	**2.66 (3.98)**	**4.776**	**0.030**	**0.027**
DASS-21 Stress	**5.94 (4.83)**	**7.92 (5.53)**	**6.252**	**0.013**	**0.034**
BRCS	14.58 (3.03)	15.13 (2.84)	1.513	0.220	0.009
Risk Perception	**41.96 (7.77)**	**18.50 (2.87)**	**772.276**	**<0.001**	**0.817**
Worry	**15.80 (3.79)**	**8.88 (2.05)**	**207.898**	**<0.001**	**0.543**

Note. BRCS: Brief Resilient Coping Scale. Emboldened results were found to be significant, with $p < 0.05$.

No significant differences were found between groups on DASS-21 Depression and the BRCS.

3.2. Multiple Linear Regression

The final multiple linear regression model accounted for a significant portion of the variance in DASS-21 Anxiety [R2 = 0.27 (Adj R2 = 0.25), F-change = 8.997, p = 0.003]. Lower age, together with a psychiatric diagnosis and higher scores on the Worry measure, were found to be significant predictors of DASS-21 Anxiety. Risk Perception (B = 0.052, p = 0.764) was excluded (see Table 4).

Table 4. Multiple linear regression of DASS-21 Anxiety.

	Unstandardized Coefficients B	Std. Error	Standardized Coefficient B	t	p
(Constant)	−1.559	2.407		−0.648	0.518
Age	**−0.047**	**0.023**	**−0.133**	**−1.985**	**0.049**
Gender	−0.993	0.579	−0.117	−1.716	0.088
Education	−0.281	0.362	−0.055	−0.776	0.439
Diagnosis, ref. no	**2.549**	**0.850**	**0.300**	**2.999**	**0.003**
Worry	**0.609**	**0.098**	**0.627**	**6.215**	**<0.001**

Note. Emboldened results were found to be significant, with $p < 0.05$.

The final multiple linear regression model accounted for a significant portion of the variance in DASS-21 Stress [$R^2 = 0.28$ ($Adj\ R^2 = 0.26$), F-change = 30.920, $p \leq 0.001$]. Lower age, a psychiatric diagnosis, and higher scores on the Worry measure were found to be significant predictors of DASS-21 Depression. Risk Perception (B = 0.118, p = 0.492) was excluded (see Table 5).

Table 5. Multiple linear regression of DASS-21 Stress.

	Unstandardized Coefficients B	Std. Error	Standardized Coefficient B	t	p
(Constant)	2.520	3.009		0.837	0.404
Age	**−0.098**	**0.029**	**−0.222**	**−3.345**	**0.001**
Gender	−1.252	0.723	−0.117	−1.731	0.085
Education	−0.490	0.453	−0.076	−1.083	0.280
Diagnosis, ref. no	**6.413**	**1.062**	**0.599**	**6.037**	**<0.001**
Worry	**0.681**	**0.123**	**0.556**	**5.561**	**<0.001**

Note. Emboldened results were found to be significant, with $p < 0.05$.

Since no differences were found between groups on the DASS-21 Depression subscale, it was excluded, and the regression analysis was not carried out for this specific variable.

4. Discussion

The present study evaluated the impact of the COVID-19 pandemic on Risk Perception, Worry, Depression, Anxiety, Stress, and Coping Strategies among Italian psychiatric patients living in a rehabilitation community, compared to healthy controls. The results showed significant differences between psychiatric patients and controls on Anxiety, Stress, Worry, and Risk Perception variables. Concerning the DASS-21, psychiatric patients scored lower on all three subscales than the comparative clinical sample studied by Bottesi et al. [24], who registered mean scores of 5.5 (SD = 4.6), 7.7 (SD = 5.6), and 8.9 (SD = 4.2) for the Depression, Anxiety, and Stress subscales, respectively. Although psychiatric patients in the current study generated lower DASS-21 scores, all scores were within a normal range, according to Lovibond and Lovibond's [28] version of the scale. In contrast, other studies of both non-residential psychiatric patients and the general population have identified higher DASS-21 scores during the COVID-19 lockdown [11,22].

The lower scores registered in the present study could be explained by the residential care condition of our study sample. As reported by Tansella [29], it is possible to hypothesize that residents of psychiatric rehabilitation communities, unlike psychiatric inpatients in a hospital setting, experience greater support from mental health workers and peers, present higher perceived security, and, above all, enjoy minimal coercion and maximal freedom. Moreover, unlike the population of non-residential psychiatric patients who were forced to reduce their access to psychiatric care and pharmacological and psychological support during the lockdown [30], the residential psychiatric patients in our sample were able to maintain their typical levels of care and support. This could explain their DASS-21 scores in the normal range.

Residence in a psychiatric rehabilitation community during lockdown may have been an important factor in limiting psychiatric patients' increase in depressive, anxious, and stressful symptoms. However, psychiatric patients did still show higher levels of Anxiety relative to healthy controls. While this significant difference might be explained by the impact of COVID-19 on psychopathology and mental health [31], it could also be related to psychiatric pathology. In fact, there is a higher prevalence of Anxiety disorders in people diagnosed with schizophrenia or other spectrum psychotic disorders, with 6.3% of this population presenting at least one lifetime Anxiety disorder [32–34].

In the present study, psychiatric patients presented with lower Stress compared to controls. This result could relate to their pre-existing adaptation to conditions of restricted personal freedom (i.e., limits imposed by the psychiatric community), in contrast to healthy controls, who were not accustomed to the limitations of freedom required by the lockdown. Considering that the lockdown implied separation from loved ones, loss of freedom, and boredom, higher Stress levels would be expected, as supported by research on the impact of quarantine on the general population [35].

In addition, psychiatric patients obtained a medium score on the BRCS, demonstrating a medium level of resilience [25]. Resilience and gratitude are considered protective mechanisms in conditions of trauma [36], and the resilience exhibited by the present psychiatry patients may have made them less vulnerable to COVID-19 stressors.

Furthermore, psychiatric patients scored higher than healthy controls on the Perceived Risk of getting infected with COVID-19. They received training and education on COVID-19 and its transmission by their rehabilitation community, and this might explain their higher perception of risk relative to healthy controls, as measured by the relevant survey items (e.g., "If I got COVID-19, it would be severe").

Moreover, psychiatric patients showed higher levels of Worry than the control group, particularly with respect to worries about their health and contraction of the virus [37]. Overall, the presence of a psychiatric diagnosis and higher scores on the Worry measure were found to be significant predictors of DASS-21 Anxiety and Stress. As testified by the cognitive behavioral model [38], Worry may produce negative interpretations of information. For example, Internet search results (e.g., graphic images of the surge of contagion, alarmism, fake news, conspiracy theories) could exacerbate fear, Stress, and Anxiety and, in some people, manifest nightmares and intrusive thoughts concerning COVID-19 [39].

It is worth noting that the present sample mainly consisted of younger adults (psychiatric patients: $M = 46.61$, $SD = 12.81$; healthy controls: $M = 46.40$, $SD = 11.52$). Previous studies on the COVID-19 epidemic have found a different age and gender association with Perceived Risk and Worry, with older adults demonstrating a higher risk perception and younger adults demonstrating greater Worry [40]. In the present study, both psychiatric patients and healthy controls scored higher on Worry than Risk Perception. Our results also found an association between having a psychiatric disorder and increased Anxiety and Stress.

To the best of our knowledge, the present study was the first to provide data on a population of psychiatric patients who, during the lockdown in Italy, lived within a psychiatric community that provided continuous support and care. However, the study has some limitations. First, we were limited in our ability to draw comparisons between psychiatric patients and healthy controls, due to significant differences in gender and educational level. Previous studies have investigated the impact of education level on individual responses to COVID-19, showing that, in healthy controls, a lower level of education is correlated with a lower awareness of COVID-19; this may be due to limited access to health information, reduced access to health care, and increased financial burden [41]. Furthermore, this study was conducted in only two communities in the Lazio region and may not reflect trends observed in similar contexts. The present study also used an observational design; therefore, no assumptions of causation can be made, as baseline evaluations for the psychological variables investigated were not available. Despite these limitations, this is, to the best of our knowledge, the first study to have examined the psychological impact of the threat of COVID-19 on psychiatric patients living in rehabilitation communities during the lockdown.

5. Conclusions

While quarantine and lockdown measures have been successful in limiting the spread of COVID-19, they have also resulted in isolation and loneliness, which might trigger or aggravate pre-existing mental illnesses [42]. However, despite their pervasive and long-lasting psychological impact, such measures still remain the best available containment strategy, and may be considered the lesser of two evils.

The present findings paint a general picture of the psychological impact of COVID-19 on the psychiatric residential population, in comparison with the general population, and provide a baseline for future research on the impact of COVID-19 on individuals and specific populations.

The results showed that, during the lockdown in Italy, psychiatric patients living in residential communities received unbroken support from peers and mental health professionals, maintained their usual medication treatment, and were informed of the possible consequences of COVID-19 and which strategies to implement to protect against contagion. Consequently, they had significantly lower levels of Stress than the non-residential psychiatric population. This finding provides insight into the differences between residential and non-residential psychiatric populations and highlights the importance of continuous support for psychiatric patients, especially during stressful situations such as a pandemic.

Author Contributions: Substantial contribution to conception and design: J.B., P.R., B.B., P.C. and A.M.G. Acquisition of data: A.P. Analysis and interpretation of data: P.R., S.B. and A.F. Drafting the manuscript: J.B., P.R., B.B., S.B. Revising the manuscript critically for important intellectual content: S.F., C.M. and A.M.G. All authors have read and agreed to the published version of the manuscript.

Funding: This research received no external funding.

Acknowledgments: The data of this study were collected thanks to participation of the Manager and Staff of SRTR Villa Costanza, Gruppo Sage.

Conflicts of Interest: The authors declare no conflict of interest.

References

1. Taylor, S. *The Psychology of Pandemics: Preparing for the Next Global Outbreak of Infectious Disease*; Cambridge Scholars Publishing: Newcastle upon Tyne, UK, 2019.
2. Hsiang, S.; Allen, D.; Annan-Phan, S.; Bell, K.; Bolliger, I.; Chomgh, T.; Wu, T. The effect of large-scale anti-contagion policies on the COVID-19 pandemic. *Nature* **2020**, *584*, 262–267. [CrossRef] [PubMed]
3. Roma, P.; Monaro, M.; Muzi, L.; Colasanti, M.; Ricci, E.; Biondi, S.; Napoli, C.; Ferracuti, S.; Mazza, C. How to Improve Compliance with Protective Health Measures during the COVID-19 Outbreak: Testing a Moderated Mediation Model and Machine Learning Algorithms. *Int. J. Environ. Res. Public Health.* **2020**, *17*, 7252. [CrossRef] [PubMed]
4. Flesia, L.; Monaro, M.; Mazza, C.; Fietta, V.; Colicino, E.; Segatto, B.; Roma, P. Predicting Perceived Stress Related to the Covid-19 Outbreak through Stable Psychological Traits and Machine Learning Models. *J. Clin. Med.* **2020**, *9*, 3350. [CrossRef] [PubMed]
5. Di Crosta, A.; Palumbo, R.; Marchetti, D.; Ceccato, I.; La Malva, P.; Maiella, R.; Cipi, M.; Roma, P.; Mammarella, N.; Verrocchio, M.C.; et al. Individual Differences, Economic Stability, and Fear of Contagion as Risk Factors for PTSD Symptoms in the COVID-19 Emergency. *Front. Psychol.* **2020**, *567367*. [CrossRef]
6. Hawryluck, L.; Gold, W.L.; Robinson, S.; Pogorski, S.; Galea, S.; Styra, R. SARS control and psychological effects of quarantine, Toronto, Canada. *Emerg. Infect. Dis.* **2004**, *10*, 1206–1212. [CrossRef] [PubMed]

7. Jeong, H.; Yim, H.W.; Song, Y.J.; Ki, M.; Min, J.A.; Cho, J.; Chae, J.H. Mental health status of people isolated due to Middle East Respiratory Syndrome. *Epidemiol. Health* **2016**, *38*. [CrossRef] [PubMed]
8. Main, A.; Zhou, Q.; Ma, Y.; Luecken, L.J.; Liu, X. Relations of SARS-related stressors and coping to Chinese college students' psychological adjustment during the 2003 Beijing SARS epidemic. *J. Couns Psychol.* **2011**, *3*, 410–423. [CrossRef]
9. Fontanesi, L.; Marchetti, D.; Mazza, C.; Di Giandomenico, S.; Roma, P.; Verrocchio, M.C. The effect of the COVID-19 lockdown on parents: A call to adopt urgent measures. *Psychol. Trauma* **2020**. [CrossRef]
10. Marchetti, D.; Fontanesi, L.; Mazza, C.; Di Giandomenico, S.; Roma, P.; Verrocchio, M.C. Parenting-related exhaustion during the italian COVID-19 lockdown. *J. Pediatric Psychol.* **2020**, *45*. [CrossRef]
11. Mazza, C.; Ricci, E.; Biondi, S.; Colasanti, M.; Ferracuti, S.; Napoli, C.; Roma, P. A Nationwide Survey of Psychological Distress among Italian People during the COVID-19 Pandemic: Immediate Psychological Responses and Associated Factors. *Int. J. Environ. Res. Public Health* **2020**, *17*, 3165. [CrossRef]
12. Roma, P.; Monaro, M.; Colasanti, M.; Ricci, E.; Biondi, S.; Di Domenico, A.; Verrocchio, M.C.; Napoli, C.; Ferracuti, S.; Mazza, C. A 2-Month Follow-Up Study of Psychological Distress among Italian People during the COVID-19 Lockdown. *Int. J. Environ. Res. Public Health.* **2020**, *17*, 81. [CrossRef] [PubMed]
13. Mazza, C.; Ricci, E.; Marchetti, D.; Fontanesi, L.; Di Giandomenico, S.; Verrocchio, M.C.; Roma, P. How Personality Relates to Distress in Parents during the Covid-19 Lockdown: The Mediating Role of Child's Emotional and Behavioral Difficulties and the Moderating Effect of Living with Other People. *Int. J. Environ. Res. Public Health* **2020**, *17*, 6236. [CrossRef] [PubMed]
14. Marchitelli, S.; Mazza, C.; Lenzi, A.; Ricci, E.; Gnessi, L.; Roma, P. Weight Gain in a Sample of Patients Affected by Overweight/Obesity with and without a Psychiatric Diagnosis during the Covid-19 Lockdown. *Nutrients* **2020**, *12*, 3525. [CrossRef] [PubMed]
15. Qiu, J.; Shen, B.; Zhao, M.; Wang, Z.; Xie, B.; Xu, Y. A nationwide survey of psychological distress among Chinese people in the COVID-19 epidemic: Implication and policy recommendations. *Gen. Psychiatry* **2020**, *33*, e100213. [CrossRef] [PubMed]
16. Yao, H.; Chen, J.H.; Xu, Y.F. Patients with mental health disorders in the COVID-19 epidemic. *Lancet Psychiatry* **2020**, *7*, e21. [CrossRef]
17. Kuzman, M.R.; Curkovic, M.; Wasserman, D. Principles of mental health care during the COVID-19 pandemic. *Eur. Psychiatry* **2020**, *63*, 1–11. [CrossRef]
18. Brems, C.; Johnson, M.E.; Wells, R.S.; Burns, R.; Kletti, N. Rates and sequelae of the coexistence of substance use and other psychiatric disorders. *Int. J. Circumpolar Health* **2002**, *61*, 224–244. [CrossRef]
19. Zhou, F.; Yu, T.; Du, R.; Fan, G.; Liu, Y.; Liu, Z. Clinical course and risk factors for mortality of adult inpatients with COVID-19 in Wuhan, China: A retrospective cohort study. *Lancet* **2020**, *395*, 1054–1062. [CrossRef]
20. Moesmann Madsen, M.; Dines, D.; Hieronymus, F. Optimizing psychiatric care during the COVID-19 pandemic. *Acta Psychiatr. Scand.* **2020**. [CrossRef]
21. Iancu, I.; Strous, R.; Poreh, A.; Kotler, M.; Chelben, Y. Psychiatric inpatients' reactions to the SARS epidemic: An Israeli survey. *Isr. J. Psychiatry Relat. Sci.* **2005**, *42*, 258.
22. Hao, F.; Tan, W.; Jiang, L.; Zhang, L.; Zhao, X.; Zou, Y.; Tam, W. Do psychiatric patients experience more psychiatric symptoms during COVID-19 pandemic and lockdown? A case-control study with service and research implications for immunopsychiatry. *Brain Behav. Immun.* **2020**, *87*, 100–106. [CrossRef] [PubMed]
23. Iasevoli, F.; Fornaro, M.; D'Urso, G.; Galletta, D.; Casella, C.; Paternoster, M.; de Bartolomeis, A. The COVID-19 in Psychiatry Study Group. Psychological distress in patients with serious mental illness during the COVID-19 outbreak and one-month mass quarantine in Italy. *Psychol. Med.* **2020**, 1–3. [CrossRef] [PubMed]
24. Bottesi, G.; Ghisi, M.; Altoè, G.; Conforti, E.; Melli, G.; Sica, C. The Italian version of the Depression Anxiety Stress Scales-21: Factor structure and psychometric properties on community and clinical samples. *Compr. Psychiatry* **2015**, *60*, 170–181. [CrossRef] [PubMed]
25. Sinclair, V.G.; Wallston, K.A. The development and psychometric evaluation of the Brief Resilient Coping Scale. *Assessment* **2004**, *11*, 94–101. [CrossRef] [PubMed]
26. Cho, H.; Lee, J.S. The influence of self-efficacy, subjective norms, and risk perception on behavioral intentions related to the H1N1 flu pandemic: A comparison between Korea and the US. *Asian J. Soc. Psychol.* **2015**, *18*, 311–324. [CrossRef]

27. Liao, Q.; Cowling, B.J.; Lam, W.W.; Ng, D.M.; Fielding, R. Anxiety worry and cognitive risk estimate in relation to protective behaviors during the 2009 influenza A/H1N1 pandemic in Hong Kong: Ten cross-sectional surveys. *BMC Infect. Dis.* **2014**, *14*, 169. [CrossRef] [PubMed]
28. Lovibond, S.H.; Lovibond, P.F. *Manual for the Depression Anxiety Stress Scales*, 2nd ed.; Psychology Foundation of Australia: Sydney, NSW, Australia, 1995.
29. Tansella, M. Alternatives to standard acute in-patient care for people with mental disorders: From systematic description to evaluative research. *Br. J. Psychiatry* **2010**, *197*, s1–s3. [CrossRef]
30. Vinkers, C.H.; van Amelsvoort, T.; Bisson, J.I.; Branchi, I.; Cryan, J.F.; Domschke, K.; van der Wee, N. Stress resilience during the coronavirus pandemic. *Eur. Neuropsychopharmacol.* **2020**, *35*, 12–16. [CrossRef]
31. Muruganandam, P.; Neelamegam, S.; Menon, V.; Alexander, J.; Chaturvedi, S.K. COVID-19 and Severe Mental Illness: Impact on patients and its relation with their awareness about COVID-19. *Psychiatry Res.* **2020**, *291*, 113265. [CrossRef]
32. Achim, A.M.; Maziade, M.; Raymond, E.; Olivier, D.; Merette, C.; Roy, M.A. How prevalent are anxiety disorders in schizophrenia? A meta-analysis and critical review on a significant association. *Schizophr. Bull.* **2011**, *37*, 811–821. [CrossRef]
33. Somers, J.M.; Goldner, E.M.; Waraich, P.; Hsu, L. Prevalence and incidence studies of anxiety disorders: A systematic review of the literature. *Can. J. Psychiatry* **2006**, *51*, 100–113. [CrossRef] [PubMed]
34. Roy, M.A.; Mérette, C.; Maziade, M. Subtyping schizophrenia according to outcome or severity: A search for homogeneous subgroups. A review of the literature. *Schizophr. Bull.* **2001**, *27*, 115–137. [CrossRef] [PubMed]
35. Brooks, S.K.; Webster, R.K.; Smith, L.E.; Woodland, L.; Wessely, S.; Greenberg, N.; Rubin, G.J. The psychological impact of quarantine and how to reduce it: Rapid review of the evidence. *Lancet* **2020**, *395*, 912–920. [CrossRef]
36. Vieselmeyer, J.; Holguin, J.; Mezulis, A. The role of resilience and gratitude in posttraumatic stress and growth following a campus shooting. *Psychol. Trauma* **2017**, *9*, 62–69. [CrossRef]
37. Colizzi, M.; Bortoletto, R.; Silvestri, M.; Mondini, F.; Puttini, E.; Cainelli, C.; Zoccante, L. Medically unexplained symptoms in the times of Covid-19 pandemic: A case-report. *Brain Behav. Immun.* **2020**, *5*, 100073. [CrossRef]
38. Taylor, S.; Asmundson, G.J.G. *Treating Health Anxiety: A Cognitive-Behavioral Approach*; Guilford: New York, NY, USA, 2004.
39. Taylor, S.; Landry, C.A.; Paluszek, M.M.; Fergus, T.A.; McKay, D.; Asmundson, G.J.G. COVID stress syndrome: Concept, structure, and correlates. *Depress. Anxiety* **2020**, *37*. [CrossRef]
40. Barber, S.J.; Kim, H. COVID-19 Worries and Behavior Changes in Older and Younger Men and Women. *J. Gerontol. Ser. B* **2020**. [CrossRef]
41. Wolf, L.J.; Haddock, G.; Manstead, A.S.; Maio, G.R. The importance of (shared) human values for containing the COVID-19 pandemic. *Br. J. Soc. Psychol.* **2020**, *59*, 618–627. [CrossRef]
42. Vahia, I.V.; Blazer, D.G.; Smith, G.S.; Karp, J.F.; Steffens, D.C.; Forester, B.P.; Reynolds, C.F. COVID-19, mental health and aging: A need for new knowledge to bridge science and service. *Am. J. Geriatr. Psychiatry* **2020**, *28*, 695–697. [CrossRef]

Journal of
Clinical Medicine

MDPI

Article

Effects of Spirituality, Knowledge, Attitudes, and Practices toward Anxiety Regarding COVID-19 among the General Population in INDONESIA: A Cross-Sectional Study

Yohanes Andy Rias [1,2], Yafi Sabila Rosyad [3], Roselyn Chipojola [1], Bayu Satria Wiratama [4], Cikra Ikhda Safitri [5], Shuen Fu Weng [6,7], Chyn Yng Yang [8,9] and Hsiu Ting Tsai [1,9,*]

1 School of Nursing, College of Nursing, Taipei Medical University, Taipei 11031, Taiwan; yohanes.andi@iik.ac.id (Y.A.R.); rosechipojola@gmail.com (R.C.)
2 Faculty of Health and Medicine, College of Nursing, Institut Ilmu Kesehatan Bhakti Wiyata, Kediri 64114, Indonesia
3 Faculty of Health and Medicine, College of Nursing, Sekolah Tinggi Ilmu Kesehatan Yogyakarta, Yogyakarta 55281, Indonesia; rosyad2yafi@gmail.com
4 Department of Epidemiology and Biostatistics, Faculty of Medicine Public Health and Nursing, Universitas Gadjah Mada, Yogyakarta 55281, Indonesia; bayu.satria@ugm.ac.id
5 Department of Pharmacology, College of Pharmacology, Akademi Farmasi Mitra Sehat Mandiri Sidoarjo, Sidoarjo 61262, Indonesia; cikraikhda@gmail.com
6 Division of Endocrinology and Metabolism, Department of Internal Medicine, Taipei Medical University Hospital, Taipei 11031, Taiwan; sfweng@ntu.edu.tw
7 Division of Endocrinology and Metabolism, Department of Internal Medicine, School of Medicine, College of Medicine, Taipei Medical University, Taipei 11031, Taiwan
8 Integrated Medical Examination Center, Taipei Medical University Hospital, Taipei 11031, Taiwan; caring@h.tmu.edu.tw
9 Post-Baccalaureate Program in Nursing, College of Nursing, Taipei Medical University, Taipei 11031, Taiwan
* Correspondence: hsiuting@tmu.edu.tw; Tel.: +886-2-2736-1661 (ext. 6330)

Received: 4 November 2020; Accepted: 23 November 2020; Published: 24 November 2020

Abstract: Background: Currently, the determinants of anxiety and its related factors in the general population affected by COVID-19 are poorly understood. We examined the effects of spirituality, knowledge, attitudes, and practices (KAP) on anxiety regarding COVID-19. Methods: Online cross-sectional data (n = 1082) covered 17 provinces. The assessment included the Daily Spiritual Experiences Scale, the Depression, Anxiety, and Stress Scale, and the KAP-COVID-19 questionnaire. Results: Multiple linear regression revealed that individuals who had low levels of spirituality had increased anxiety compared to those with higher levels of spirituality. Individuals had correct knowledge of early symptoms and supportive treatment (K3), and that individuals with chronic diseases and those who were obese or elderly were more likely to be severe cases (K4). However, participants who chose incorrect concerns about there being no need for children and young adults to take measures to prevent COVID-19 (K9) had significantly lower anxiety compared to those who responded with the correct choice. Participants who disagreed about whether society would win the battle against COVID-19 (A1) and successfully control it (A2) were associated with higher anxiety. Those with the practice of attending crowded places (P1) had significantly higher anxiety. Conclusions: Spirituality, knowledge, attitudes, and practice were significantly correlated with anxiety regarding COVID-19 in the general population.

Keywords: anxiety; attitudes; COVID-19; knowledge; practices; spirituality; Indonesia

1. Introduction

The novel coronavirus disease 2019 (COVID-19) is a group of complex respiratory syndromes caused by a beta-coronavirus called severe acute respiratory syndrome coronavirus 2 (SARS-CoV-2) [1]. COVID-19 is currently fostering a rapidly growing global health disaster [2]. As of 26 October 2020, the World Health Organization (WHO) has estimated that the prevalence of people infected with COVID-19 globally had reached 42,966,344 [3]. In particular, this threat has emerged in Indonesia, where COVID-19 prevalence is estimated to be around 394,454 with a mortality rate of 3.4% [4]. Currently, the struggle against COVID-19 is still ongoing in Indonesia [5]. The rising menace of the pandemic has led to a global climate of mental health concerns due to social distancing, travel restrictions, and rumors spreading misinformation [6–8]. Unfortunately, mental health problems may trigger a series of physiological events and reduce immunity, and good mental health is vital in curbing infectious transmission [9–11].

A recent study in China revealed that vicarious traumatization scores of the general population were significantly more likely to be higher than those of front-line medical professionals [12]. Consequently, these situations urgently need guidelines and/or public health authorities to promote crisis management and safeguard the mental health of the population [13,14]. More than 80% of the general population is aware that mental health concerns need to be addressed [15]. Approximately 8.1%, 16.5%, and 28.8%, of the general Chinese population, respectively have stress, depression, and anxiety symptoms due to the COVID-19 pandemic [6]. Another study from Turkey observed that 115 (45.1%) people were experiencing feelings of anxiety [16]. Moreover, an extensive study determined that 2053 (19.1%) people of an Iranian population exhibited severe symptoms of anxiety, 2291 (21.3%) of them had moderate symptoms, and 1128 (10.5%) had mild symptoms [17]. When anxiety levels increase, individuals may become vague and irrational when reacting to the COVID-19 pandemic [6,18–20]. In contrast, individuals with a low level of anxiety are associated with a highly relaxed manner, which consequently improves self-control and encourages adherence to personal protective health practices [19]. However, no epidemiological research has investigated the correlation between anxiety and the COVID-19 pandemic in Indonesia. Thus, a study of the threat of anxiety in Indonesia should immediately be conducted.

Knowledge, attitudes, and practices (KAP) towards COVID-19 play major roles in assessing the willingness of a community to adopt behavioral change initiatives during the pandemic [21,22]. KAP empirical studies can reveal fundamental information to determine the types of intervention which can effectively curb an infectious disease. Consequently, improving KAP is a potentially valuable strategy for better insight into addressing misconceptions [22–24]. Moreover, good levels of knowledge were positively associated with optimistic attitudes and appropriate practices [21,25]. Meanwhile, lessons learned from the 2003 SARS outbreak showed that knowledge and practice towards infectious diseases were significantly related to a low level of anxiety [26], which might further complicate efforts to prevent the spread of a disease. However, levels of anxiety in India and China were high, even though the general population of India [15] and China [11] had a reasonably good level of knowledge and attitudes. Moreover, KAP and their associations with amelioration of anxiety have not been clarified in Indonesia. As Indonesia is currently experiencing difficult impacts due to the COVID-19 pandemic [5], relationships between KAP and the level of anxiety need to be clarified.

Spirituality as a complementary treatment in health care is a key factor in reducing psychological outcomes, especially anxiety [27,28]. Generally speaking, spirituality and religiosity are often used interchangeably in studies [27–30]. Spirituality can contribute to reduce anxiety and support health protection by the power of faith [29,30]. Indonesia is unique because most of the population has a higher level of positive spirituality related to health conditions [31,32]. Improving the level of spirituality is potentially a valuable strategy to restrain mental illness [32], psychological impacts, post-traumatic stress disorder, and anxiety [33]. However, personal spirituality may become the source of host resistance and/or resilience [34]. Therefore, a reasonably high level of spirituality may be associated with reduced or increased anxiety. However, such relationships require clarification, especially in Indonesia.

Previous studies have showed that COVID-19 causes psychological problems [6,8,11,14,15]. Thus, survey findings are of great practical significance to all levels of government for the provision of KAP and spirituality to reduce high levels of anxiety. Therefore, this study assessed the prevalence of anxiety and identified positively and negatively associated factors contributing to anxiety in Indonesia as a unique part of the world.

2. Methods

2.1. Study Design and Population

Primary data were collected using a community-based cross-sectional study design to select members of the general population in 17 provinces from western, central, and eastern regions of Indonesia. Convenience sampling was carried out by distributing an online survey through a Google Form link via WhatsApp, Instagram, Facebook, and Twitter, which are the most popular and accessible social media platforms in Indonesia. While Instagram and Twitter are more popular among the younger generation, Facebook is generally preferred by older Indonesians. We utilized different approaches to targeting as many respondents as possible from across the region during the 7 April–30 May 2020 data collection period. This involves relying on researchers' technical and personal networks and engaging with and sharing the survey through social media influencers and community lenders. The inclusion criteria to fill in the Google form were: Indonesian civilian, adult aged 17~65 years, able to speak Bahasa Indonesia, and willing to fill out the informed consent form. We reached 1114 participants through the Google form. We excluded 32 participants because they had duplicate responses when filling out the survey. The final sample size was 1082 participants.

2.2. Procedures

On the first page of the online questionnaire, participants were given an explanation as to the purpose of the survey, the objectives, and that they were agreeing to voluntary participation and consent by completing the questionnaire. In addition, they participated by completing the questionnaire, and in a thank you note at the end, participants were encouraged to invite new respondents from their contact list. Ethical clearance was reviewed and approved by the Institutional Review Board of Institut Ilmu Kesehatan Strada Indonesia (IRB-1911/KEPK/IV/2020). All responses were anonymous and provided with informed consent. There was no monetary compensation for completing the questionnaire.

2.3. Measurements

Participants were asked to complete the online sociodemographic questionnaire consisting of information on age, gender, ethnicity, region, marital status, religion, educational level, and health. In terms of participants' living conditions, extended family included grandparent(s), parent(s) and child(ren) of three or more generations; nuclear family included conventional family of parent(s) and child(ren); and alone defined a Single person household. The physiological impact of anxiety against COVID-19 was assessed using the Depression, Anxiety, and Stress Scale (DASS-21). According to previous studies, a major physiological problem was anxiety, compared to depression and stress [6,16]. Anxiety was assessed by seven items [35]. A higher score indicates a higher level of anxiety. Response options were "never", "sometimes", "frequently", and "every time", with respective scores of 0, 1, 2, and 3. Cronbach's α value for the Indonesian version was 0.85 [36].

Participants' knowledge, attitudes, and practices (KAP) towards COVID-19 were assessed using a KAP questionnaire developed by Zhong et al. (2020) and included statements about clinical presentations, transmission routes, and the prevention and control of COVID-19 (a 12-item scale). The response options were "true", "false", and "do not know"; a correct answer was given a score of 1 and an incorrect or "do not know" response was given a score of 0. The total possible knowledge score (K1~K12) ranged from 0–12; a higher score indicates better knowledge of COVID-19. Cronbach's α value for the KAP-COVID-19 study was 0.71, indicating good internal consistency [21]. Items of attitude in this study were measured by two questions (A1 and A2), including agreement about ultimate control of the disease with three response options, namely agree = 0, disagree, and unknown = 1, and confidence of winning the battle against COVID-19 (agree = 0 and disagree = 1). Moreover, the assessment of participants' practices consisted of two behavioral questions (P1 and P2), including going to crowded places (yes = 1; no = 0), and wearing a mask when leaving home these days (yes = 0; no = 1). The KAP-COVID-19 questionnaire was developed in China and is available in English. A back-translation method was used to translate the items from English into Bahasa Indonesia and to ensure linguistic and conceptual equivalence using an item discriminant analysis with a p value of <0.001.

The Daily Spiritual Experiences Scale (DSES) contains 16 questions, each of which has a 6-point Likert scale ranging from 1 (never or seldom) to 6 (every time). The scale measures ordinary experiences encountered in daily life related to feelings of transcendence [37]. The Indonesian version of the 16-item DSES questionnaire had good internal consistency with Cronbach's alpha of 0.86 [38]. The more points an individual has, the greater their experience of spirituality.

2.4. Statistical Analysis

Descriptive statistics were used to evaluate sociodemographic characteristics, knowledge, attitudes, and practices, additional health information, and spiritual variables between groups, and results are presented as frequencies (n) and percentages (%). The percentage of responses was determined according to the total respondents per response for the total question. Continuous variables are presented as the mean and standard deviation (SD) and were evaluated using an independent t-test or one-way ANOVA. Absolute values for skewness and kurtosis were used to assess normality of the data; skewness value of 1.779 and kurtosis value of 3.716 indicated a normal distribution [39]. Multicollinearity was calculated using a variance inflation factor (VIF) of <10 [40]. This analysis had a maximum VIF of 2.51, suggesting that the results had low multicollinearity effects. The adjusted beta-coefficients with 95% confidence intervals (CIs) were obtained by performing a multiple linear regression for anxiety related to exposures of interest (spirituality, knowledge, attitudes, and practices) after adjusting for potential confounding variables, including gender, age, ethnicity, region, marital status, religion, educational level, whether the participant was living with family or alone, and the source of health information (family members, professional health education, or online and offline media). SPSS Version 25.0 (Chicago, IL, USA) was used for all statistical analyses, and a p value of <0.05 indicated statistically significant.

3. Results

Table 1 shows participants' demographic characteristics. Overall, totals for female participants and non-Javanese participants were 62.1% and 61.7%, respectively; 67.3% of participants had a higher educational level. Most participants were aged 25~39 years (43.9%), were single (51.4%), were Moslem (64.7%), and were from the western part of Indonesia (76.2%). Except for marital status and professional health education information, there were significantly different levels of anxiety in all sociodemographic variables (all $p < 0.05$; Table 1).

Table 1. Comparisons of participants' sociodemographic characteristics and anxiety towards the corona virus disease 2019 (COVID-19) pandemic in an Indonesian population (n = 1082).

Variables	Total Participants	Anxiety	
	n (%)	Mean (SD)	p-Value [a]
Age (years)			
17~24	376 (34.8)	5.13 (5.07)	0.005 [b]
25~39	475 (43.9)	4.07 (4.37)	
>40	231 (21.3)	4.14 (5.84)	
Gender			
Male	410 (37.9)	5.11 (5.72)	0.001
Female	672 (62.1)	4.05 (4.43)	
Ethnicity			
Javanese	414 (38.3)	3.68 (4.01)	<0.001
Non-Javanese	668 (61.7)	4.93 (5.44)	
Region			
Western part of Indonesia	824 (76.2)	3.58 (3.90)	<0.00 [b]
Central part of Indonesia	148 (13.7)	7.77 (7.21)	
Eastern part of Indonesia	110 (10.2)	6.55 (5.97)	
Marital status			
Married	526 (48.6)	4.24 (5.22)	0.174
Single	556 (51.4)	4.65 (4.74)	
Religion			
Moslem	700 (64.7)	5.70 (6.15)	<0.001
Non-Moslem	382 (35.3)	3.77 (4.05)	
Education			
ISCED ≥ 3	728 (67.3)	3.54 (4.06)	<0.001
ISCED < 3	354 (32.7)	6.32 (6.07)	
Participants live			
With an extended family	247 (22.8)	5.34 (5.87)	0.006 [b]
With a nuclear family	811 (75.0)	4.19 (4.66)	
Alone	24 (2.2)	4.08 (4.66)	
Sources of information: Online media			
Yes	329 (30.4)	5.16 (5.51)	0.002
No	753 (69.6)	4.14 (4.70)	
Sources of information: Offline media			
Yes	56 (5.2)	6.61 (5.98)	0.001
No	1026 (94.8)	4.33 (4.89)	
Sources of information: Family members			
Yes	116 (10.7)	5.90 (5.24)	0.001
No	966 (89.3)	4.28 (4.92)	
Sources of information: Professional health			
Yes	119 (11.0)	4.08 (5.26)	0.394
No	963 (89.0)	4.50 (4.94)	

Note: ISCED, International Standard Classification of Education; SD, standard deviation. Data were presented as mean ± SD, frequency and percentage, and p-values were calculated using [a] independent sample t-test, [b] one-way ANOVA. A p-value of <0.05 indicates statistical significance.

The determinants, including KAP and spirituality, of anxiety are presented in Table 2. Interestingly, there were no significant differences between anxiety scores in terms of the following two determinants of KAP: main clinical symptoms of COVID-19 (K1); and residents wearing medical masks to prevent spread of the infection (K8). Levels of anxiety were significantly higher in participants who justified the response (chose 'correct') for the following information: unlike the common cold, a stuffy nose, runny nose, and sneezing are less common in persons infected with the COVID-19 virus (K2). Moreover, participants had significantly lower anxiety scores who justified the response (chose 'correct') for the following information: currently there is no effective treatment for COVID-19, but early symptomatic and supportive treatment can help most patients recover from the infection (K3); not all persons with COVID-19 will develop severe cases; only those who are elderly, obese, and have chronic illnesses are more likely to be severe cases (K4); the COVID-19 virus can spread via respiratory droplets from infected people (K7); avoiding going to crowded places can prevent the spread of infection (K10); the isolation and treatment of infected people are effective ways to reduce the spread of the virus (K11); and people who have contact with someone infected with the COVID-19 virus should be immediately isolated in a proper place (K12). However, levels of anxiety were significantly lower in participants who justified the response (chose 'incorrect') for the information that eating or having contact with wild animals would result in being infected with the COVID-19 virus (K5); persons with COVID-19 cannot spread the virus to others when a fever does not appear (K6); and it is not necessary for children and young adults to take measures to prevent the COVID-19 virus infection (K9). Also, there was a significant association between the total knowledge score of knowledge and level of anxiety due to COVID-19. However, there was not a significant association after adjusting for other covariates. The mean and standard deviation (SD) for anxiety were significantly higher (all p values of <0.001) in participants who disagreed that Indonesians will be successful in controlling (A1) and winning the battle against COVID-19 (A2). In analyzing participants' personal practices, those who reported going to crowded places (P1) and not wearing a mask when outside the home (P2) were significantly correlated with high anxiety scores (both $p < 0.001$). A significantly higher score of anxiety was found in participants with a lower level of spirituality ($p < 0.001$; Table 2).

The adjusted beta-coefficients and 95% CIs of KAP and spirituality for anxiety are presented in Table 3. Three items of knowledge (K3, K4, and K9) were the strongest predictors of the anxiety score, but other items of knowledge (K2, K5, K6, and K7) were not significantly predictors of anxiety score after adjustment for covariates. Participants who justified (chose 'correct') that early symptomatic and supportive treatment can help most patients recover from the COVID-19 infection (K3) and people with chronic diseases, who are obese, and who are elderly are more likely to have a possibility of being a severe case (K4) had a significantly lower anxiety score compared to those who responded with 'incorrect' after adjusting for covariates. Individuals who justified (chose 'incorrect') concerns about the necessity for children and young adults to take measures to prevent the COVID-19 virus infection (K9) had a significantly lower anxiety score compared to those who responded with 'correct' after adjusting for covariates. The adjusted beta-coefficients and 95% CIs of the three items of knowledge that predicted the anxiety score were −0.74 (95% CI = −1.47~−0.02), −0.73 (95% CI = −1.43~−0.03), and −0.96 (95% CI = −1.82~−0.09), respectively. Participants who disagreed with the statement that Indonesia could successfully control COVID-19 (A1) and had confidence that Indonesia could win the battle against COVID-19 (A2) had significantly higher anxiety scores ($\beta = 3.23$, 95% CI = 2.19~4.26; and $\beta = 2.34$, 95% CI = 1.29~3.40, respectively) after adjusting for confounders. Participants with the practice of going to crowded places (P1) had a significantly higher anxiety score ($\beta = 1.23$, 95% CI = 0.62~1.83) after controlling for confounding factors. However, there was no significant correlation between the practice of wearing a mask (P2) when leaving the house after controlling for confounding variables. Further analyses revealed that having low spirituality was significantly correlated with a higher anxiety score with an adjusted β of 1.23 (95% CI = 0.65~1.81) among the Indonesian population (Table 3).

Table 2. Comparisons of participant's knowledge, attitudes, practices, and spirituality with their anxiety scores towards the COVID-19 pandemic among an Indonesian population (n = 1082).

Variables	Total Participants	Anxiety	
	n (%)	Mean (SD)	p-Value [a]
Knowledge (K) Main clinical symptoms of COVID-19 are a fever, fatigue, dry cough, and myalgia/muscle pain. (K1)			
Incorrect	124 (11.5)	4.52 (4.73)	0.877
Correct	958 (88.5)	4.44 (5.02)	
Unlike the common cold, a stuffy nose, runny nose, and sneezing are less common in persons infected with the COVID-19 virus. (K2)			
Incorrect	325 (30.0)	3.87 (4.09)	0.011
Correct	757 (70.0)	4.70 (5.30)	
Currently, there is no effective treatment for COVID-19, but early symptomatic and supportive treatment can help most patients recover from the infection. (K3)			
Incorrect	189 (17.5)	6.82 (6.74)	<0.001
Correct	893 (82.5)	3.95 (4.36)	
Not all persons with COVID-19 will develop severe disease. Only those who are elderly, obese, and have chronic illnesses are more likely to be severe cases. (K4)			
Incorrect	191 (17.7)	6.04 (6.50)	<0.001
Correct	891 (82.3)	4.11 (4.52)	
Eating or having contact with wild animals could result in being infected with the COVID-19 virus. (K5)			
Correct	662 (61.2)	5.10 (5.42)	<0.001
Incorrect	420 (38.8)	3.42 (3.98)	
Persons with COVID-19 cannot spread the virus to others when a fever does not appear. (K6)			
Correct	281 (26.0)	5.81 (5.75)	<0.001
Incorrect	801 (74.0)	3.98 (4.59)	
The COVID-19 virus spreads via respiratory droplets of infected people. (K7)			
Incorrect	72 (6.7)	6.72 (6.12)	<0.001
Correct	1010 (93.3)	4.29 (4.85)	
Residents can wear medical masks to prevent COVID-19 virus infection. (K8)			
Incorrect	308 (28.5)	4.13 (4.41)	0.181
Correct	774 (71.5)	4.58 (5.18)	
Isolation and treatment of people infected with COVID-19 virus are effective ways to reduce the virus spread. (K11)			
Incorrect	164 (15.2)	7.42 (6.69)	<0.001
Correct	918 (84.8)	3.92 (4.41)	
People who have had contact with someone infected with the COVID-19 virus should immediately be isolated in a proper place. In general, the observation period is 14 days. (K12)			
Incorrect	52 (4.8)	7.43 (6.28)	<0.001
Correct	1030 (95.2)	4.30 (4.86)	

Table 2. *Cont.*

Variables	Total Participants	Anxiety	
	n (%)	Mean (SD)	*p*-Value [a]
Total score of knowledge			
High (score ≥10) Low (score <9)	34 (3.1) 1048 (96.9)	9.12 (7.12) 4.30 (4.82)	<0.001
Attitudes (A) Do you agree that COVID-19 will be successfully controlled? (A1)			
Agree Disagree	39 (3.6) 1043 (96.4)	9.90 (7.05) 4.25 (4.77)	<0.001
Do you have any confidence that Indonesia can win the battle against the COVID-19 virus? (A2)			
Agree Disagree	680 (62.8) 402 (37.2)	3.72 (4.72) 5.70 (5.90)	<0.001
Practices (P) Recently, have you gone to a crowded place? (P1)			
No Yes	969 (89.6) 113 (10.4)	3.77 (4.21) 10.31 (6.85)	<0.001
Recently, have you worn a mask when leaving home? (P2)			
Yes No	976 (90.2) 106 (9.8)	3.84 (4.29) 10.06 (7.03)	<0.001
Spirituality			
High (score ≥ 72) Low (score < 72)	786 (72.6) 296 (27.4)	3.65 (3.94) 6.57 (6.58)	<0.001

Note: A, attitude; K, knowledge; P, practices; SD, standard deviation. [a] Data were presented as mean ± SD, frequency and percentage, and *p*-values were calculated using independent sample *t*-test, A *p*-value of <0.05 indicates statistical significance.

Table 3. Adjusted beta-coefficients and 95% confidence intervals (CIs) of knowledge, attitudes, and practices, and anxiety towards the COVID-19 pandemic among the Indonesian population ($n = 1082$).

Variables	Anxiety	
	Unadjusted β-Coef. (95% CI)	Adjusted β-Coef. (95% CI)
Currently, there is no effective treatment for COVID-2019, but early symptomatic and supportive treatment can help most patients recover from the infection. (K3)		
Incorrect Correct	Ref. −2.86 (−3.63~−2.10) **	Ref. −0.74 (−1.47~−0.02) *
Not all persons with COVID-2019 will develop to severe cases. Only those who are elderly, are obese, and have chronic illnesses are more likely to be severe cases. (K4)		
Incorrect Correct	Ref. −1.93 (−2.70~−1.16) **	Ref. −0.73 (−1.43~−0.03) *

Table 3. *Cont.*

Variables	Anxiety	
	Unadjusted β-Coef. (95% CI)	Adjusted β-Coef. (95% CI)
It is not necessary for children and young adults to take measures to prevent COVID-19 virus infection. (K9)		
Correct	Ref.	Ref.
Incorrect	−3.49 (−4.30~−2.69) **	−0.96 (−1.82~−0.09) *
Do you agree that COVID-19 will be successfully controlled? (A1)		
Agree	Ref.	Ref.
Disagree	6.55 (5.66~7.44) **	3.23 (2.19~4.26) **
Do you have any confidence that Indonesia can win the battle against the COVID-19 virus? (A2)		
Agree	Ref.	Ref.
Disagree	6.21 (5.29~7.14) **	2.34 (1.29~3.40) **
Recently, have you gone to a crowded place? (P1)		
No	Ref.	Ref.
Yes	2.91 (2.27~3.58) **	1.23 (0.62~1.83) **
Recently, have you worn a mask when leaving home? (P2)		
Yes	Ref.	Ref.
No	3.84 (2.85~4.82) **	0.66 (−0.27~1.59)
Spirituality		
High (score ≥ 72)	Ref.	Ref.
Low (score < 72)	3.08 (2.51~3.65) **	1.23 (0.65~1.81) **

Note: Adjusted beta-coefficients (coef.) and 95% confidence intervals (CIs) were estimated using a multiple linear regression after adjusting for age, gender, ethnicity, region, marital status, religion, educational level, the source of health information, and whether the participants are living with an extended or nuclear family, or alone. * $p < 0.05$; ** $p < 0.001$.

4. Discussion

This is the first community-based cross-sectional research study with a large sample to determine associations of KAP and spirituality with anxiety among a population during the COVID-19 pandemic in Indonesia. Anxiety symptoms are more likely to occur in the population than in medical professionals and those who have been spending much energy, time, and money on the pandemic [12]. Our findings support an accurate understanding of the source literature related to anxiety among the Indonesian population. In particular, this study revealed that participants who had knowledge and confidence of winning the battle against the disease, agreed with the possibility that the COVID-19 pandemic could be successfully controlled, did not go to crowded places, and had higher spirituality were statistically associated with decreased anxiety in the population. Interestingly, an unexpected result demonstrated that the practice of wearing a mask when leaving home was not significantly correlated with anxiety after adjusting for covariates.

Previous studies revealed that knowledge of the availability and effectiveness of medicines for COVID-19 was negatively correlated with higher anxiety [8]. In a study by Wang et al. [8], children, young adults, those with obesity, those with chronic diseases, and the elderly were also correlated with anxiety. Notably, these findings are in line with the current study: identifying knowledge related to the absence of an effective treatment for COVID-19 and that early symptomatic and supportive treatment will help most patients recover from the infection is positively correlated with a lower level of anxiety.

Thus, participants' knowledge needs to be assessed, especially for children, young adults, those who are obese, those with chronic diseases, and the elderly among the general population, as related to anxiety. A similar study which evaluated knowledge found that most participants had inadequate knowledge and experienced anxiety [41,42]. Good knowledge may help individuals recognize aspects of their emotional experience and learn how to apply emotional regulation and adaptive strategies, particularly for anxiety [43]. Several other studies of hypochondriasis and anxiety disorder suggested that the development and maintenance of health anxiety were subject to selective attention to internal or external health risks [44,45], which may help provide deeper insights into poor knowledge of the disease, and consequently would allow improved psychological regulation control strategies. Our results were inconsistent with other studies, in which no significant correlation between a higher level of knowledge and a low anxiety level was found [11,46,47]. These inconsistent findings might be explained by the fact that participants who seek health information to improve their knowledge of risk factors may play a dominant role, rather than misconceptions about COVID-19 due to rumors, false propaganda, and inaccurate information [46]. These conditions may provoke anxiety, such as panic buying among people during the early phase of the COVID-19 pandemic. Therefore, the specifics of each knowledge question [6,8] or specific psychological knowledge [48] concerning anxiety about COVID-19 need to be re-evaluated during and after the pandemic in terms of psychological problems, including individuals who experienced anxiety during this pandemic period. Consequently, health authorities and health professionals should provide accurate health information through psychological counselling services for stress management, primarily based on evidence regarding knowledge in the general population, to avoid adverse anxiety responses.

In general, having a positive attitude was the most important predictor for a lower level of anxiety [11]. Specifically, our data suggested that individuals with a negative attitude towards confidence that COVID-19 would be successfully controlled, and that Indonesia would win the battle against the disease were independently correlated with higher levels of anxiety. Similar to this study, people who thought that they were unlikely to survive COVID-19 had a 3.9% higher anxiety score [6]. Attitudes agreeing that COVID-19 will be successfully controlled and the battle against it will be won were also effectively correlated with adherence, which further attenuated physiological problems [49,50]. Moreover, several studies revealed that the disadvantages of poor attitudes, such as a high perception of susceptibility and severity, may contribute to higher anxiety problems among the population [11,51,52]. In reality, acute respiratory syndrome resulting from COVID-19 can consequently increase the neutrophil-to-lymphocyte ratio (NLR) in the respiratory tract [53]. Importantly, it was reported that individuals with a more pessimistic attitude regarding their illness were correlated with elevated NLR levels, which might cause more severe symptoms, such as high levels of anxiety [54], leading to a poor quality of life [55]. Therefore, researchers have suggested that those with a positive attitude exhibited declines in inflammation biomarkers, such as NLR [54]. This might subsequently contribute to decreased mental health symptoms, including anxiety [54]. As the pandemic advances and mitigation strategies progress, understanding attitudes is critical among the general population. Importantly, a good attitude is also a key factor in commitment to prevention, as well as decreasing anxiety during this epidemic.

Other evidence of lessons learned from COVID-19 concerns the effects of infectious diseases; this pandemic has altered precautionary practice patterns, which negatively influence anxiety regarding infection among the population [8]. Correspondingly, this study also revealed that the practice of wearing a proper mask when leaving home during the pandemic was not significantly correlated with anxiety. However, avoiding crowded places was significantly correlated with reduced anxiety, and is one of the most important things an individual can do to protect themselves from this infectious pandemic disease. This result is similar to that of a recent review explaining that negative psychological effects during pandemic situations are associated with adverse effects, such as anger, confusion, and stress [56]. In particular, a cross-sectional study of 4700 people in Istanbul, Turkey suggested that the practice of avoiding crowded places had a 0.12-fold lower protective factor against fatigue;

however, no significant correlation between wearing a mask to prevent COVID-19 was suggested after adjusting for covariates [57]. Unexpectedly, an inquiry found that wearing masks was not correlated with a low level of anxiety. These inconsistent results might be explained by two possible behaviors among the Indonesian population. First, wearing a mask in public is not a habit among the Indonesian population. The lack of availability of masks indicated that many people could not get them. This was a global problem [58,59]. Second, the Ministry of Health of Indonesia announced that only those with COVID-19 symptoms or relevant diseases should wear medical masks. Uncertainty possibly occurred, created by different recommendations of the Ministry of Health of Indonesia and the Ministry of Health of other countries, such as China, Malaysia, and Vietnam [8,22]. Thus, this issue contributed to various responses when wearing a mask in public areas. In reality, the target of uncovering practices is to modify innate and maladaptive responses, such as fear and anxiety. Anxiety, fear, anger, and a lack of immunity increases pro-inflammatory cytokines and psycho-neuro-immunity against COVID-19. These conditions might provide insights into the pathway that affects how anxiety can increase proinflammatory cytokines [10,60], which further attenuates behaviors or practices [60]. Consequently, health providers or stakeholders should make clear rules related to the use of masks, the time in which to wear them, and the type of mask, in order to ameliorate panic, fear, and confusion, especially for individuals with no access to masks. Strong public support for these practices indicates an opportunity to normalize healthy behaviors and encourage continued use of these and other personal protective behaviors to reduce anxiety as well as mitigate further COVID-19 spread as jurisdictions reopen.

Interestingly, the existence of concerns raised by the COVID-19 pandemic suggests the seriousness of spirituality [30,61]. This finding is in line with a study that explored potential factors affecting anxiety in Spain, in which the authors found that participants with a high score for spirituality had a 0.320-fold lower level of anxiety [33]. Current studies also found that spirituality was correlated with anxiety [62,63]. Spirituality is, indeed, generally helpful for people dealing with major life stressors, as positive psychological concepts including an individual's core values, deep connections, orientation, and beliefs relate to physical and mental health [64,65]. Additionally, Indonesia has a diverse society with diverse spiritual practices. This unique condition embodies a holistic care approach that recognizes diverse bio-psycho-social-spiritual needs. Therefore, health professionals should develop regulations to achieve holistic mental health services in Indonesia [66]. Conceivably, anxiety is induced by immune system activation and is associated with proinflammatory cytokines, such as interleukin (IL)-6. Increased IL-6 is considered to be correlated with cortisol and could be a risk factor for psychological problems, such as depression and anxiety. Religious psychological concepts also indicate that spirituality mediates the indirect influence of anxiety on IL-6 [64]. The increase in COVID-19-related anxiety cases in Indonesia requires further advocacy of holistic mental health services with spirituality prevention or growth, in which spirituality is recommended among people with anxiety.

When considering anxiety related to the COVID-19 pandemic, providing people with accurate information is the most reasonable prevention against the anxiety. Governments must ascertain the proper propagation of COVID-19 related information. In this pandemic situation, when considering mental health issues due to anxiety, online consultation services might also be more useful in constructing mental health interventions. Finally, these findings and periodic assessments of public KAP, anxiety and spirituality can also advise future planning if subsequent outbreak waves occur, to prevent the dissemination of a new pandemic.

Our study has several strengths. To the best of our knowledge, this is the first paper to estimate associations of spirituality, knowledge, attitude, and practices and their effects on anxiety among the general population in Indonesia. These variables are potentially valuable and might contribute to the recognition and encouragement of strategies for ameliorating anxiety, targeted on encouraging spirituality and KAP. Moreover, a large-scale multisite and cluster-randomized study would provide more-comprehensive evidence regarding individual effects of both KAP and spirituality and other determinants on anxiety in the population that could guide future research implemented in community or clinical settings.

Along with its strengths, this study also had some limitations. We found that the self-reported score of anxiety by participants might not always be aligned with objective measurements by psychological health professionals. Nonetheless, anxiety, based on personal feelings, is a primary factor during COVID-19 when ensuring the availability of essential preventive and curative healthcare programs [6]. The online assessment approach had a selection bias problem because the Google form was only circulated through social media platforms (WhatsApp, Facebook, Instagram, and Twitter). As a result, there is a possibility that members of the general population without social media may not have been able to access this form. Another limitation is related to the KAP instrument, especially that, regarding attitudes and practices, only two simple questions were used in this study. However, the instrument was adapted from a survey that had been previously tested and used in China [21], Malaysia [22], Jordan, Saudi Arabia, and Kuwait [24]. A further limitation is the lack of participants from the central and easters region, participants living alone, and other sources of information, which future studies could aim to recruit specifically, as this may implicate the generalizability of the findings. However, we adjusted for a considerable number of potential confounding factors by performing a multiple linear regression, thus minimizing the effect of an unequal distribution

5. Conclusions

In summary, the present study presents a thorough analysis of Indonesian population's knowledge, attitudes, and practices regarding anxiety towards the COVID-19 pandemic. These findings indicate crucial roles for health professional educators and practitioners in recognizing and implementing therapeutic approaches, such as improving knowledge, attitudes, and practices to ameliorate anxiety. Hence, it is important to actively monitor the general population's distress during this pandemic and its aftermath, to detect related protective factors and test for mental health issues, in order to improve policies. Our findings also highlight ensuring the continuity of spirituality during the pandemic.

Author Contributions: Conceptualization, Y.A.R., Y.S.R., R.C. and H.T.T.; methodology, Y.A.R., B.S.W., S.F.W. and H.T.T.; data curation, Y.A.R., Y.S.R., R.C., B.S.W., C.I.S., S.F.W., C.Y.Y. and H.T.T.; formal analysis, Y.A.R. and B.S.W.; validation, S.F.W., C.Y.Y. and H.T.T.; writing—original draft preparation, Y.A.R., C.I.S. and R.C.; writing—review and editing, Y.A.R., Y.S.R., R.C., B.S.W., C.I.S., S.F.W., C.Y.Y. and H.T.T.; visualization, Y.A.R., S.F.W., C.Y.Y. and H.T.T.; supervision, S.F.W., C.Y.Y. and H.T.T.; project administration, Y.A.R. and Y.S.R.; funding acquisition, S.F.W., C.Y.Y. and H.T.T. All authors have read and agreed to the published version of the manuscript.

Funding: This research was funded by Grants Ministry of Science and Technology, Taiwan (MOST), grant number 106-2314-B-038-013-MY3 and 109-2314-B-038-110-MY3 and The APC was funded by Taipei Medical University, Taiwan.

Acknowledgments: We would like to thank the Ethics Committee of Institut Ilmu Kesehatan Strada Indonesia, the Ministry of Science and Technology, Taiwan, Taipei Medical University, the study participants, and the data collection team members.

Conflicts of Interest: The authors declare no conflict of interest. The funders had no role in the design of the study; in the collection, analyses, or interpretation of data; in the writing of the manuscript, or in the decision to publish the results.

References

1. Huang, C.; Wang, Y.; Li, X.; Ren, L.; Zhao, J.; Hu, Y.; Zhang, L.; Fan, G.; Xu, J.; Gu, X. Clinical features of patients infected with 2019 novel coronavirus in Wuhan, China. *Lancet* **2020**, *395*, 497–506. [CrossRef]
2. Sohrabi, C.; Alsafi, Z.; O'Neill, N.; Khan, M.; Kerwan, A.; Al-Jabir, A.; Iosifidis, C.; Agha, R. World Health Organization declares global emergency: A review of the 2019 novel coronavirus (COVID-19). *Int. J. Surg.* **2020**, *76*, 71–76. [CrossRef] [PubMed]
3. World Health Organization. WHO Coronavirus Disease (COVID-19) Dashboard. Available online: https://covid19.who.int/ (accessed on 29 September 2020).

4. Gugus Tugas Percepatan Penanganan COVID-19. Infografis COVID-19. Available online: https://covid19.go.id/peta-sebaran (accessed on 27 October 2020).
5. Setiati, S.; Azwar, M.K. COVID-19 and Indonesia. *Acta Med. Indones.* **2020**, *52*, 84. [PubMed]
6. Wang, C.; Pan, R.; Wan, X.; Tan, Y.; Xu, L.; McIntyre, R.S.; Choo, F.N.; Tran, B.; Ho, R.; Sharma, V.K.; et al. A longitudinal study on the mental health of general population during the COVID-19 epidemic in China. *Brain Behav. Immun.* **2020**, *87*, 40–48. [CrossRef] [PubMed]
7. World Health Organization. *Mental Health and Psychosocial Considerations during the COVID-19 Outbreak, 18 March 2020*; World Health Organization: Geneva, Switzerland, 2020; Available online: https://www.who.int/docs/default-source/coronaviruse/mental-health-considerations.pdf (accessed on 28 April 2020).
8. Wang, C.; Pan, R.; Wan, X.; Tan, Y.; Xu, L.; Ho, C.S.H.; Ho, R.C.M. Immediate Psychological Responses and Associated Factors during the Initial Stage of the 2019 Coronavirus Disease (COVID-19) Epidemic among the General Population in China. *Int. J. Environ. Res. Public Health* **2020**, *17*, 1729. [CrossRef]
9. Marsland, A.L.; Walsh, C.; Lockwood, K.; John-Henderson, N.A. The effects of acute psychological stress on circulating and stimulated inflammatory markers: A systematic review and meta-analysis. *Brain Behav. Immun.* **2017**, *64*, 208–219. [CrossRef]
10. Kim, S.-W.; Su, K.-P. Using psychoneuroimmunity against COVID-19. *Brain Behav. Immun.* **2020**, *87*, 4–5. [CrossRef]
11. Lin, Y.; Hu, Z.; Alias, H.; Wong, L.P. Knowledge, Attitudes, Impact, and Anxiety Regarding COVID-19 Infection Among the Public in China. *Front. Public Health* **2020**, *8*, 236. [CrossRef]
12. Li, Z.; Ge, J.; Yang, M.; Feng, J.; Qiao, M.; Jiang, R.; Bi, J.; Zhan, G.; Xu, X.; Wang, L.; et al. Vicarious traumatization in the general public, members, and non-members of medical teams aiding in COVID-19 control. *Brain Behav. Immun.* **2020**, *88*, 916–919. [CrossRef]
13. Rubin, E.J.; Baden, L.R.; Morrissey, S.; Campion, E.W. Medical Journals and the 2019-nCoV Outbreak. *N. Engl. J. Med.* **2020**, *382*, 866. [CrossRef]
14. Vindegaard, N.; Benros, M.E. COVID-19 pandemic and mental health consequences: Systematic review of the current evidence. *Brain Behav. Immun.* **2020**, *89*, 531–542. [CrossRef] [PubMed]
15. Roy, D.; Tripathy, S.; Kar, S.K.; Sharma, N.; Verma, S.K.; Kaushal, V. Study of knowledge, attitude, anxiety & perceived mental healthcare need in Indian population during COVID-19 pandemic. *Asian J. Psychiatry* **2020**, *51*, 102083. [CrossRef]
16. Özdin, S.; Özdin Şükriye, B. Levels and predictors of anxiety, depression and health anxiety during COVID-19 pandemic in Turkish society: The importance of gender. *Int. J. Soc. Psychiatry* **2020**, *66*, 504–511. [CrossRef] [PubMed]
17. Moghanibashi-Mansourieh, A. Assessing the anxiety level of Iranian general population during COVID-19 outbreak. *Asian J. Psychiatry* **2020**, *51*, 102076. [CrossRef]
18. Qiu, J.; Shen, B.; Zhao, M.; Wang, Z.; Xie, B.; Xu, Y. A nationwide survey of psychological distress among Chinese people in the COVID-19 epidemic: Implications and policy recommendations. *Gen. Psychiatry* **2020**, *33*, e100213. [CrossRef]
19. Asmundson, G.J.G.; Taylor, S. How health anxiety influences responses to viral outbreaks like COVID-19: What all decision-makers, health authorities, and health care professionals need to know. *J. Anxiety Disord.* **2020**, *71*, 102211. [CrossRef]
20. Stein, M.B. COVID-19 and Anxiety and Depression in 2020. *Depress. Anxiety* **2020**, *37*, 302. [CrossRef]
21. Zhong, B.-L.; Luo, W.; Li, H.-M.; Zhang, Q.-Q.; Liu, X.-G.; Li, W.-T.; Li, Y. Knowledge, attitudes, and practices towards COVID-19 among Chinese residents during the rapid rise period of the COVID-19 outbreak: A quick online cross-sectional survey. *Int. J. Biol. Sci.* **2020**, *16*, 1745. [CrossRef]
22. Azlan, A.A.; Hamzah, M.R.; Tham, J.S.; Ayub, S.H.; Mohamad, E. Public knowledge, attitudes and practices towards COVID-19: A cross-sectional study in Malaysia. *PLoS ONE* **2020**, *15*, e0233668. [CrossRef]
23. Honarvar, B.; Lankarani, K.B.; Kharmandar, A.; Shaygani, F.; Zahedroozgar, M.; Haghighi, M.R.R.; Ghahramani, S.; Honarvar, H.; Daryabadi, M.M.; Salavati, Z.; et al. Knowledge, attitudes, risk perceptions, and practices of adults toward COVID-19: A population and field-based study from Iran. *Int. J. Public Health* **2020**, *65*, 731–739. [CrossRef]
24. Naser, A.Y.; Dahmash, E.Z.; Alwafi, H.; Alsairafi, Z.; Al Rajeh, A.M.; Alhartani, Y.J.; Turkistani, F.M.; Alyami, H.S. Knowledge and practices towards COVID-19 during its outbreak: A multinational cross-sectional study. *medRxiv* **2020**. [CrossRef]

25. Geldsetzer, P. Knowledge and Perceptions of COVID-19 Among the General Public in the United States and the United Kingdom: A Cross-sectional Online Survey. *Ann. Intern. Med.* **2020**, *173*, 157–160. [CrossRef]
26. Chan, S.S.; So, W.K.; Wong, D.C.; Lee, A.C.; Tiwari, A. Improving older adults' knowledge and practice of preventive measures through a telephone health education during the SARS epidemic in Hong Kong: A pilot study. *Int. J. Nurs. Stud.* **2007**, *44*, 1120–1127. [CrossRef] [PubMed]
27. Hai, A.H.; Franklin, C.; Park, S.; DiNitto, D.M.; Aurelio, N. The efficacy of spiritual/religious interventions for substance use problems: A systematic review and meta-analysis of randomized controlled trials. *Drug Alcohol Depend.* **2019**, *202*, 134–148. [CrossRef]
28. Gonçalves, J.P.B.; Lucchetti, G.; Menezes, P.R.; Vallada, H. Religious and spiritual interventions in mental health care: A systematic review and meta-analysis of randomized controlled clinical trials. *Psychol. Med.* **2015**, *45*, 2937–2949. [CrossRef] [PubMed]
29. Koenig, H.G. Ways of Protecting Religious Older Adults from the Consequences of COVID-19. *Am. J. Geriatr. Psychiatry* **2020**, *28*, 776–779. [CrossRef] [PubMed]
30. Koenig, H.G. Maintaining Health and Well-Being by Putting Faith into Action During the COVID-19 Pandemic. *J. Relig. Health* **2020**, *59*, 2205–2214. [CrossRef] [PubMed]
31. Rochmawati, E.; Wiechula, R.; Cameron, K. Centrality of spirituality/religion in the culture of palliative care service in Indonesia: An ethnographic study. *Nurs. Health Sci.* **2018**, *20*, 231–237. [CrossRef]
32. Suryani, L.K.; Lesmana, C.B.J.; Tiliopoulos, N. Treating the untreated: Applying a community-based, culturally sensitive psychiatric intervention to confined and physically restrained mentally ill individuals in Bali, Indonesia. *Eur. Arch. Psychiatry Clin. Neurosci.* **2011**, *261*, 140. [CrossRef]
33. González-Sanguino, C.; Ausín, B.; Castellanos, M.; Ángel Saiz, J.; López-Gómez, A.; Ugidos, C.; Muñoz, M. Mental health consequences during the initial stage of the 2020 Coronavirus pandemic (COVID-19) in Spain. *Brain Behav. Immun.* **2020**, *87*, 172–176. [CrossRef]
34. Levin, J. The Faith Community and the SARS-CoV-2 Outbreak: Part of the Problem or Part of the Solution? *J. Relig. Health* **2020**, 1–14. [CrossRef] [PubMed]
35. Lovibond, P.; Lovibond, S. The structure of negative emotional states: Comparison of the Depression Anxiety Stress Scales (DASS) with the Beck Depression and Anxiety Inventories. *Behav. Res. Ther.* **1995**, *33*, 335–343. [CrossRef]
36. Oei, T.P.S.; Sawang, S.; Goh, Y.W.; Mukhtar, F. Using the Depression Anxiety Stress Scale 21 (DASS-21) across cultures. *Int. J. Psychol.* **2013**, *48*, 1018–1029. [CrossRef] [PubMed]
37. Underwood, L.G.; Teresi, J.A. The daily spiritual experience scale: Development, theoretical description, reliability, exploratory factor analysis, and preliminary construct validity using health-related data. *Ann. Behav. Med.* **2002**, *24*, 22–33. [CrossRef] [PubMed]
38. Fath, N.M.D.E. Hubungan Antara Spiritualitas dengan Penerimaan Orang tua pada Orang tua yang Memiliki Anak Autis. Universitas Negeri Makasar. 2015. Available online: http://eprints.unm.ac.id/5117/ (accessed on 23 November 2020).
39. Kim, H.-Y. Statistical notes for clinical researchers: Assessing normal distribution (2) using skewness and kurtosis. *Restor. Dent. Endod.* **2013**, *38*, 52–54. [CrossRef]
40. García, C.; García, J.; Martín, M.L.; Salmerón, R. Collinearity: Revisiting the variance inflation factor in ridge regression. *J. Appl. Stat.* **2015**, *42*, 648–661. [CrossRef]
41. Rakhmanov, O.; Dane, S. Knowledge and anxiety levels of African university students against COVID-19 during the pandemic outbreak by an online survey. *Int. Dent. J.* **2020**, *8*, 53–56.
42. Nemati, M.; Ebrahimi, B.; Nemati, F. Assessment of Iranian Nurses' Knowledge and Anxiety toward COVID-19 During the Current Outbreak in Iran. *Arch. Clin. Infect. Dis.* **2020**, *15*, 15. [CrossRef]
43. Leonidou, C.; Panayiotou, G. Maintaining Mechanisms of Health Anxiety: Current State of Knowledge. In *Somatoform and Other Psychosomatic Disorders*; Springer: Berlin/Heidelberg, Germany, 2018; pp. 1–21.
44. Olatunji, B.O.; Deacon, B.J.; Abramowitz, J.S. Is hypochondriasis an anxiety disorder? *Br. J. Psychiatry* **2009**, *194*, 481–482. [CrossRef]
45. Scarella, T.M.; Laferton, J.A.C.; Ahern, D.K.; Fallon, B.A.; Barsky, A.J. The Relationship of Hypochondriasis to Anxiety, Depressive, and Somatoform Disorders. *J. Psychosom. Res.* **2016**, *57*, 200–207. [CrossRef]

46. Lei, L.; Huang, X.; Zhang, S.; Yang, J.; Yang, L.; Xu, M. Comparison of Prevalence and Associated Factors of Anxiety and Depression Among People Affected by versus People Unaffected by Quarantine During the COVID-19 Epidemic in Southwestern China. *Med. Sci. Monit.* **2020**, *26*, e924609-1. [CrossRef] [PubMed]
47. Huang, Y.; Zhao, N. Generalized anxiety disorder, depressive symptoms and sleep quality during COVID-19 outbreak in China: A web-based cross-sectional survey. *Psychiatry Res.* **2020**, *288*, 112954. [CrossRef] [PubMed]
48. Wang, Z.-H.; Yang, H.-L.; Yang, Y.-Q.; Liu, D.; Li, Z.-H.; Zhang, X.-R.; Zhang, Y.-J.; Shen, D.; Chen, P.-L.; Song, W.-Q.; et al. Prevalence of anxiety and depression symptom, and the demands for psychological knowledge and interventions in college students during COVID-19 epidemic: A large cross-sectional study. *J. Affect. Disord.* **2020**, *275*, 188–193. [CrossRef] [PubMed]
49. Gara, K.H.; Kartheek, A.S.V.; Vanamali, D.R. Knowledge, attitude and practices towards COVID-19 among Indian residents during the pandemic: A cross-sectional online survey. *J. Dr. NTR Univ. Health Sci.* **2020**, *9*, 107. [CrossRef]
50. Kontoangelos, K.; Economou, M.; Papageorgiou, C. Mental Health Effects of COVID-19 Pandemia: A Review of Clinical and Psychological Traits. *Psychiatry Investig.* **2020**, *17*, 491. [CrossRef]
51. Leung, G.M.; Ho, L.-M.; Chan, S.K.K.; Ho, S.-Y.; Bacon-Shone, J.; Choy, R.Y.L.; Hedley, A.J.; Lam, T.-H.; Fielding, R. Longitudinal Assessment of Community Psychobehavioral Responses During and After the 2003 Outbreak of Severe Acute Respiratory Syndrome in Hong Kong. *Clin. Infect. Dis.* **2005**, *40*, 1713–1720. [CrossRef]
52. Rubin, G.J.; Amlôt, R.; Page, L.; Wessely, S. Public perceptions, anxiety, and behaviour change in relation to the swine flu outbreak: Cross sectional telephone survey. *BMJ* **2009**, *339*, b2651. [CrossRef]
53. Lagunas-Rangel, F.A. Neutrophil-to-lymphocyte ratio and lymphocyte-to-C-reactive protein ratio in patients with severe coronavirus disease 2019 (COVID-19): A meta-analysis. *J. Med Virol.* **2020**, *92*, 1733–1734. [CrossRef] [PubMed]
54. Hu, Y.; Chen, Y.; Zheng, Y.; You, C.; Tan, J.; Hu, L.; Zhang, Z.; Ding, L. Factors related to mental health of inpatients with COVID-19 in Wuhan, China. *Brain Behav. Immun.* **2020**, *89*, 587–593. [CrossRef] [PubMed]
55. Rias, Y.A.; Kurniasari, M.D.; Traynor, V.; Niu, S.-F.; Wiratama, B.S.; Chang, C.W.; Tsai, H.T. Synergistic Effect of Low Neutrophil–Lymphocyte Ratio With Physical Activity on Quality of Life in Type 2 Diabetes Mellitus: A Community-Based Study. *Biol. Res. Nurs.* **2020**, *22*, 378–387. [CrossRef] [PubMed]
56. Brooks, S.K.; Webster, R.K.; Smith, L.E.; Woodland, L.; Wessely, S.; Greenberg, N.; Rubin, G.J. The psychological impact of quarantine and how to reduce it: Rapid review of the evidence. *Lancet* **2020**, *395*, 912–920. [CrossRef]
57. Morgul, E.; Bener, A.; Atak, M.; Akyel, S.; Aktaş, S.; Bhugra, D.; Ventriglio, A.; Jordan, T.R. COVID-19 pandemic and psychological fatigue in Turkey. *Int. J. Soc. Psychiatry* **2020**. [CrossRef] [PubMed]
58. Djalante, R.; Lassa, J.; Setiamarga, D.; Sudjatma, A.; Indrawan, M.; Haryanto, B.; Mahfud, C.; Sinapoy, M.S.; Djalante, S.; Rafliana, I.; et al. Review and analysis of current responses to COVID-19 in Indonesia: Period of January to March 2020. *Prog. Disaster Sci.* **2020**, *6*, 100091. [CrossRef]
59. Ricca, M. Don't Uncover that Face! Covid-19 Masks and the Niqab: Ironic Transfigurations of the ECtHR's Intercultural Blindness. *Int. J. Semiot. Law-Rev. Int. Sémiotique Jurid.* **2020**, 1–25. [CrossRef] [PubMed]
60. Miller, A.H. Mechanisms of cytokine-induced behavioral changes: Psychoneuroimmunology at the translational interface. *Brain Behav. Immun.* **2009**, *23*, 149–158. [CrossRef]
61. Peteet, J.R. COVID-19 Anxiety. *J. Relig. Health* **2020**, *5*, 2203–2204. [CrossRef] [PubMed]
62. Saiz, J.; Pung, M.A.; Wilson, K.L.; Pruitt, C.; Rutledge, T.; Redwine, L.; Taub, P.R.; Greenberg, B.; Mills, P.J. Is Belonging to a Religious Organization Enough? Differences in Religious Affiliation versus Self-Ratings of Spirituality on Behavioral and Psychological Variables in Individuals with Heart Failure. *Healthcare* **2020**, *8*, 129. [CrossRef]
63. Alshraifeen, A.; Alnuaimi, K.; Al-Rawashdeh, S.; Ashour, A.; Al-Ghabeesh, S.; Al-Smadi, A. Spirituality, Anxiety and Depression Among People Receiving Hemodialysis Treatment in Jordan: A Cross-Sectional Study. *J. Relig. Health* **2020**, 1–16. [CrossRef]
64. Ai, A.L.; Pargament, K.I.; Appel, H.B.; Kronfol, Z. Depression following open-heart surgery: A path model involving interleukin-6, spiritual struggle, and hope under preoperative distress. *J. Clin. Psychol.* **2010**, *66*, 1057–1075. [CrossRef]

65. Seybold, K.S. Physiological Mechanisms Involved in Religiosity/Spirituality and Health. *J. Behav. Med.* **2007**, *30*, 303–309. [CrossRef]
66. Liem, A. "Doing My Profession is also Part of Worship": How Clinical Psychologists Address Aspects of Spirituality and Religion in Indonesia. *J. Relig. Health* **2019**, *59*, 1434–1457. [CrossRef] [PubMed]

Publisher's Note: MDPI stays neutral with regard to jurisdictional claims in published maps and institutional affiliations.

Journal of
Clinical Medicine

MDPI

Article

Forced Cohabitation during Coronavirus Lockdown in Italy: A Study on Coping, Stress and Emotions among Different Family Patterns

Emanuela Mari [1,*,†], Angelo Fraschetti [1,†], Giulia Lausi [1], Alessandra Pizzo [1], Michela Baldi [1], Elena Paoli [2], Anna Maria Giannini [1] and Francesco Avallone [3]

1 Department of Psychology, Sapienza University of Rome, 00185 Rome, Italy; angelo.fraschetti@uniroma1.it (A.F.); giulia.lausi@uniroma1.it (G.L.); ale.18.pizzo@gmail.com (A.P.); michela.baldi@uniroma1.it (M.B.); annamaria.giannini@uniroma1.it (A.M.G.)

2 Department of Dynamic and Clinical Psychology, Sapienza University of Rome, 00185 Rome, Italy; elena.paoli@uniroma1.it

3 Department of Legal and Economic Sciences, Unitelma Sapienza University of Rome, Viale Regina Elena 295, 00161 Rome, Italy; segretariogenerale@fondbg.it

* Correspondence: e.mari@uniroma1.it; Tel.: +39-06-49917534

† These authors contributed equally to this work.

Received: 10 October 2020; Accepted: 30 November 2020; Published: 1 December 2020

Abstract: Background: At the beginning of 2020, a pandemic caused by a new strain of coronavirus occurred. On March 9th, the Italian population was forced to lockdown to prevent the spread of this new virus. This event forced families and cohabitants to spend their entire days and weeks in the same physical space, interacting with partners and children with a very different degree of intimacy than in the earlier situation. The present study investigated the effects of being forced to live together on different family patterns, on various dimensions such as stress, coping strategies, time perception and quality evaluation of cohabitation. Method: A total sample consisting of 1750 individuals was recruited through a random sample of probability across the Italian country. Due to the lockdown condition, an online questionnaire was set up; several validated scales were chosen, and some open-ended items were included for the thoughts of the participants. Results: The results showed statistically significant differences between the three family patterns examined. Conclusion: During the forced period of living together, a positive effect could be inferred as given by the presence of children and the collaborative coping strategies that have been adopted; the results have been discussed according to the literature on the topic.

Keywords: quality of life; COVID-19; stress disorder; living together; emotional bond; coronavirus disease

1. Introduction

When talking about cohabitation, we refer to the process of sharing an experience, and to "living with" in a common and defined time and space. It can be described as a process that allows individuals, organizations and communities to manage meaningful and stable relationships in a physical and symbolic space [1,2]. Living together can be described according to three levels of relationship: social, organizational and emotional. When we talk about the social level, the relationships of cohabitation refer to the context of civic society, the interactions in the community and, in a broader sense, in the global social context. Studies on social coexistence are various and mainly concern the debate and encounter between different ethnic groups, cultures, religions and political orientations [3–5], the effects of immigration and social integration processes [6], conflicts related to tolerance, discrimination or crime [7,8], and the construction of a multi-ethnic and multicultural citizenship [9,10]. At the organizational level, the relationships of cohabitation concern those within the workplace; in this case, individuals do not normally choose each other, and the choice of professional environment is also subject to constraints. The organizational context, on the other hand, is a place wherein many individuals spend a large part of their lives, build relationships and set up shared ways of being together, investing energy, emotions and hopes. The studies that have dealt with areas and dimensions related to organizational cohabitation refer, in particular, to cultures and organizational climate [11–13], organizational citizenship [14,15], and organizational well-being and health [16–18]. Thirdly, on an emotional level, cohabitation relationships concern those within the family of origin, between parents and children or between relatives within an extended family, or relationships as a couple within marriage or outside of marriage, where the members of the couple share a common project and imagine a future together. Studies on emotional cohabitation address the issue of family relationships between parents and children and between siblings [19,20], the reasons for the success or failure of couples' relationships [21,22], and living together in peer groups [23]. Other studies have investigated emotional cohabitation in particular situations, such as the complexity faced by families in managing new lifestyles and relationships [24], cohabitation in a family with a seriously ill child [25], and changes in cohabitation following catastrophic events [26].

At the beginning of 2020 an unexpected event occurred: a pandemic caused by a new strain of coronavirus—never previously identified in humans—which took the name SARS-CoV-2 (Severe Acute Respiratory Syndrome–Coronavirus–2) according to the indications of the International Committee on Taxonomy of Viruses (ICTV), which deals with the designation and naming of viruses. Italy, for some weeks, has been the second country in terms of number of infections after China. On 24 February, the first decrees of restrictions and social distancing for schools and shops in two northern regions were approved, restrictions that were extended to the whole nation on March 9 by the Ministry of Health.

This pandemic has deeply altered the rhythms and styles of the emotional, as well as working and social, coexistence of millions of individuals following the measures adopted by the Italian Government to deal with the epidemiological emergency (Decree-Law no. 19 of 25 March 2020; Decree-Law no. 33 of 16 May 2020). Strong restrictions were imposed on the free circulation of individuals, and they were forbidden to leave their place of residence except for proven reasons. This has kept some individuals from reaching their homes and their families; it has interrupted, for a large majority of citizens, sociality and organizational coexistence by forcing smart-working. It has forced families and cohabitants to spend their entire days and weeks in the same physical space, interacting with partners and children with a very different degree of intimacy than in the earlier situation.

The issue of the opportunities and difficulties of living together, already well known in the life experience of all individuals, has acquired new attention in terms of investigating its possible effects on the level of affective coexistence that more than two months of confinement have entailed.

The aim of the research is to investigate, through an online questionnaire, the effects of cohabitation caused by COVID-19 lockdown on different types of living together (partner, partner and children, relatives), on various dimensions such as stress, coping strategies, time perception and quality evaluation of cohabitation.

2. Method

2.1. Procedure

Data were collected from 1 April 2020 to 30 April 2020. Participants completed a secure online survey, optimized for its use on computers, tablets, and mobile devices. The Qualtrics Survey Platform was used to widely distribute the questionnaire throughout Italy. A non-probabilistic and convenience sampling technique was used, in order to successfully attract as many voluntary participants as possible, motivated by interest and curiosity about the research topic.

The questionnaire was distributed through different channels, such as the authors' official working platforms, by word of mouth and through social networks. After reading the informed consent, each respondent was able to voluntarily decide to join the research and start answering the digital survey. Maximum confidentiality in the handling and analysis of the responses was guaranteed.

2.2. Participants

In total, 1750 participants joined the research; 72.7% were female (N = 1273), and the age ranged from 18 to 85 years (M = 36.81; SD = 13.56).

In total, 24.7% of the sample was from the north of Italy, 57.1% from Central Italy and 18.2% were from the south; 47.3% of the sample was single, 44.1% married, 4.7% in a civil union, 1.6% separated, 1.7% divorced and 0.6% widowed (shown in Table 1).

Table 1. Demographic characteristics of the sample classified by living together patterns.

		Partner	Partners with Children	Relatives
Gender	Male	119	154	204
	Female	362	466	445
Geographic Area	North Italy	167	173	92
	Central Italy	245	321	434
	South Italy	69	126	123
Marital Status	Single	195	52	581
	Married	217	511	44
	Civil Union	48	29	6
	Legal Separation	7	13	8
	Divorced	13	10	6
	Widow	1	5	4
Total		481	620	649

Regarding the educational degree, 10.1% of the sample had a middle school diploma, 6.1% a professional diploma, 28.8% a high school diploma, 16.1% has a bachelor's degree, 23.8% a master's degree, and 14.3% had a post-graduate degree, while 0.8% had a different degree.

In total, 25.7% of the sample were students, 12.1% were unemployed, 58.7% were workers and 3.5% were retired.

2.3. Materials

For the purpose of the present study, an online questionnaire consisting of different sections was developed. First, a short summary of demographic data (i.e., age, gender, living conditions), then, the questionnaire included the following measures.

2.3.1. Attitudes and Moods about the New Coronavirus

This scale was developed by the authors in order to investigate the attitudes and moods of respondents about the new coronavirus through items such as, for example, "The Coronavirus is a mysterious and highly lethal virus capable of decimating the world's population" or "The mass media have generated an exaggerated alarm about the real dangers of the Coronavirus". The 8 items on the scale were evaluated on a 5-point Likert scale, from "Completely disagree" (1) to "Completely agree" (5).

2.3.2. Perceived Stress Scale (PSS)

This scale is widely used to measure stress perception [27]; it aims to understand how participants perceive their lives as unpredictable, uncontrollable and overloaded, and includes questions about their levels of experienced stress. The 10 items of the PSS ask about feelings and thoughts over the past month; respondents are asked how often they feel in a particular way and all responses are on a five-point answer scale from "never" (0) to "very often" (4).

2.3.3. Semantic Differential

The authors developed a semantic differential (a five points scale) to measure attitudes to forced cohabitation during lockdown. It consists of 13 pairs of bipolar nouns, on which respondents had to subjectively place themselves (i.e., "Calm—Excitement" or "Fun—Boredom").

2.3.4. Cohabitation Scales

The authors elaborated a sequence of scales for the evaluation of the cohabitation construct with respect to the different housing contexts (positive and negative relationship scale). In particular, three different types of scales were developed to measure cohabitation habits in cases where the respondent lived with their partner, their partner and their children or family members/relatives. For two of the cohabitation scales, 10 items were developed, while the scale on cohabitation with children included 12 items; all were evaluated on a 5-point Likert scale from "Never" (1) to "Very often" (5).

2.3.5. Coping Orientation to Problem Experienced—New Italian Version (COPE-NVI)

This scale evaluates coping styles and asks participants to evaluate the frequency with which they perform specific coping strategies in difficult or stressful situations [28]. The instructions ask participants not to refer to a specific episode, but rather to think about how they usually behave in stressful situations.

In this study only 8 out of the original 25 items were selected; the response alternatives of the chosen items were on a five-point scale ranging from "Never" (0) to "Very often" (4).

2.3.6. Stanford Time Perspective Inventory (STPI—Short Form)

This instrument provides a simple way to measure multiple temporal perspectives of individuals, and is built on a theoretical basis that examines the emotional, social, cognitive and motivational processes that are supposed to contribute to, and are in turn influenced by, the functioning of the temporal perspective [29]. Based on the specific purpose of this study, a selection of the original 22-item scale was made, whereby only 9 items were used, and all the answers were on five-point response scales ranging from "Never" (0) to "Very often" (4).

2.3.7. Future Forecasts

Finally, the authors developed a scale in relation to the future forecasts expressed by respondents. Thirteen items were elaborated (for example, "Overall health management will improve"), with a 5-point Likert scale response from "Completely unlikely" (0) to "Very likely" (4).

2.3.8. Social Lockdown Perception

A single item was formulated to investigate thoughts and moods related to the lockdown; participants were asked to answer the question "Try to define in a few words this period of relational and social life restrictions".

2.4. Data Analysis

Participants were divided into three groups and were compared across some different scales, such as stress, coping strategies, time perception and quality evaluation of cohabitation. After performing basic descriptive analyses, a content analysis for Social Perception was performed. Then, differences between groups were examined using the analysis of variance (One-way ANOVA), and statistical significance in post-hoc analysis was determined using Bonferroni correction. Statistical significance was defined as $p < 0.05$. The IBM SPSS software version 25 was used for statistical analysis.

3. Results

3.1. Demographic Statistics

As far as concerns the current working condition, 6.3% of the participants were entrepreneurs or managers, 18.7% were qualified professionals (e.g., lawyer, psychologist, accountant), 12.2% were managers or officials, 20.9% were executives, 6.0% were manual workers, 0.3% worked in agriculture, 4% were law enforcement officers, 6.4% were doctors, 12.6% were teachers, and 12.5% were employed in a different profession from those listed above.

The sample consisted of three different family configurations: 27.5% of the participants lived with the partner, 35.4% with their partner and children, while 37.1% lived with their parents or family members, and 48.1% of participants had a pet.

Finally, regarding housing conditions, 5.4% lived in a house of less than 50 sqm, 44.3% in a house between 51 and 90 sqm, and finally 50.3% in a house over 91 sqm. A second question investigated concerned the presence of outdoor spaces in the house. In this case, 40.9% had at least one balcony, 44.1% had a private terrace or garden and 10.1% had a communal terrace or garden, and 4.9% had no outdoor spaces.

3.2. Social Lockdown Perception

Regarding Social lockdown perception, participants were asked to freely define through a maximum of three words (not sentences) the lockdown period. It was not required to enter words with a specific positive or negative value.

A total of 7209 terms was recorded and then they were grouped through a double-blind procedure into 1045 clusters (terms such as prepositions, articles, and adverbs were removed); in order to minimize the possible experimenter inferences, no changes were made to the different words. Therefore, no adjectives were changed into nouns and vice versa, but only words with the same semantic root and different desinence (e.g., masculine/feminine, singular/plural) were grouped together.

Frequencies analysis results are shown in Figure 1. The 10 most used words were, in descending order: "stressful", with 227 instances (31.5%) followed by "thinking", with 185 instances (25.6%); "sad", with 177 instances (24.5%); "boredom", with 172 instances (23. 8%); "necessary" with 131 instances (18.2%); "missing" with 123 instances (17.6%); "family" with 119 instances (16.5%); "restrictive" with 115 instances (15.9%); "difficult" with 111 instances (15.4%) and "anxiety" with 19 instances (15.1%).

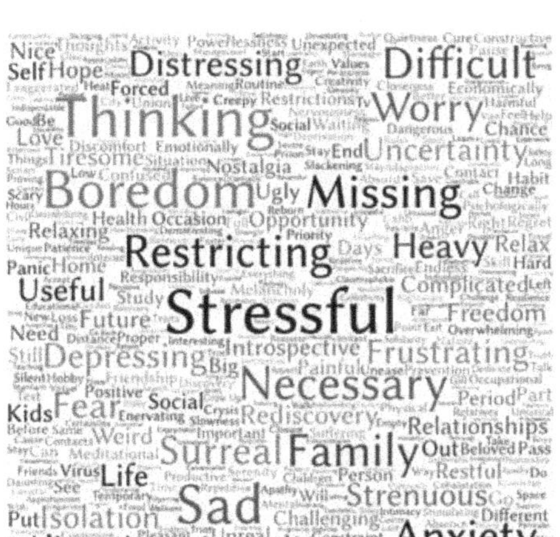

Figure 1. Visual representation of the words related to lockdown social perception.

It is important to underline that, while the most frequent words have a negative or neutral meaning, the first words with a full positive connotation appeared after position 23, and are: "useful" (0.8%), "rediscovered" (0.7%), "freedom" (0.7%) and "hope" (0.5%).

3.3. Semantic Differential

Through a semantic differential, attitudes and emotions with regard to forced cohabitation during lockdown were queried. The 13 pairs of bipolar nouns were analyzed using a one-way ANOVA in order to identify any differences between the three groups (Figure 2) through post-hoc comparison. Lower mean values are closer to positive nouns, while higher mean values are oriented towards the negative nouns.

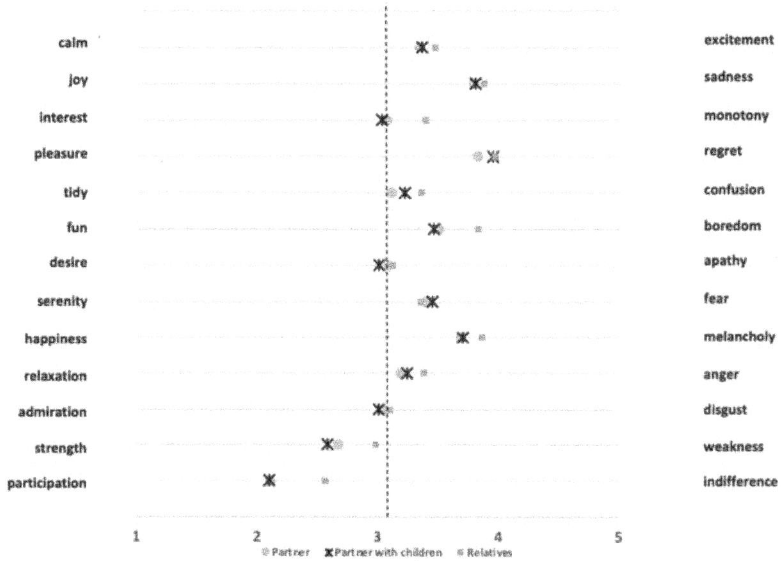

Figure 2. Graphic representation of the semantic differential concerning emotions, group comparison.

Statistically significant differences have been found, through post-hoc comparisons, between individuals in the three groups. More in detail, in Interest–Monotony, $F_{(2, 1747)} = 14.94$, $p < 0.001$ between individuals living with relatives (M = 3.39, SD = 1.27) and individuals living with the partner (M = 3.07, SD = 1.26), and between individuals living with relatives and individuals living with partners and children M = 3.03, SD = 1.29. In Pleasure–Regret $F_{(2, 1747)} = 3.73$, $p < 0.05$ between the relatives group (M = 3.97, SD = 0.92) and partner group (M = 3.82, SD = 1.00). In Tidy–Confusion $F_{(2, 1747)} = 6.38$, $p < 0.001$ between individuals living with relatives (M = 3.36, SD = 1.18) and individuals living with the partner (M = 3.11, SD = 1.19). In Fun–Boredom $F_{(2, 1747)} = 27.12$, $p < 0.001$ between the relatives group (M = 3.83, SD = 0.94) and partner group (M = 3.50, SD = 0.96), and between relatives and partners with children M = 3.46, SD = 1.02. In Happiness–Melancholy $F_{(2, 1747)} = 6.09$, $p < 0.01$ between individuals living with relatives (M = 3.86, SD = 0.92) and individuals living with the partner (M = 3.69, SD = 0.94), and between individuals living with relatives and individuals living with partners and children M = 3.70, SD = 0.98. In Relaxation–Anger $F_{(2, 1747)} = 5.18$, $p < 0.01$ between relatives the group (M = 3.38, SD = 1.07) and partner group (M = 3.19, SD = 1.08), and between the relatives and partners with children groups M = 3.24, SD = 1.06. In Strength–Weakness $F_{(2, 1747)} = 20.82$, $p < 0.001$ between individuals living with relatives (M = 2.98, SD = 1.17) and individuals living with the partner (M = 2.67, SD = 1.09), and between individuals living with relatives and individuals living with partners and children M = 2.58, SD = 1.15. In Participation–Indifference $F_{(2, 1747)} = 38.50$, $p < 0.001$

between the relatives group (M = 2.56, SD = 1.13) and partner group (M = 2.11, SD = 1.01), and between the relatives and partner with children groups M = 2.10, SD = 1.02. In each case, the individuals living with the partner reported positive pole-oriented scores for the adjective couple.

As far as comparisons between individuals living with the partner and individuals living with partners and children are concerned, no statistically significant differences have been identified.

3.4. Attitudes and Moods about The New Coronavirus

Regarding the "Attitudes and moods about the new Coronavirus" scale, there are some interesting results. In particular, with respect to the item "The Coronavirus is a mysterious and highly deadly virus capable of decimating the world's population", 7.2% declared to "Completely disagree", 18.3% to "Quite disagree", 17.4% to "Neither agree nor disagree", 37.4% declared to "Quite agree" and 19.7% to "Completely agree". Additionally, the item "The authorities were right in closing bars, restaurants, shops, etc. and inviting the population to stay at home" had some interesting answers, with 70.8% declaring to "Completely agree" and 22.7% to "Quite agree", while the remaining 6.5% is distributed between "Completely disagree" (1%), "Quite disagree" (2%) and "Neither disagree nor agree" (3.5%). Finally, as regards the item "The Italian population behaved responsibly respecting the limitations imposed by the authorities", the respondents were grouped as follows: 6% "Completely disagree", 26.5% "Quite disagree", 17.7% "Neither disagree nor agree", 44.3% "Quite agree" and only 5.5% "Completely agree", showing a general confidence in the population, but also a certain degree of criticism towards some behaviors.

3.5. Future Forecasts Scale

Regarding the "Future forecasts" scale, the results show some interesting outcomes. For example, the items related to a "hope" dimension show the general confidence of the population in the possibility that things will improve. The item "Overall health management will improve" reported a 45.5% response of "Probable". To the item "Overall school management will improve", 33.9% said that it would be "Probable", and with respect to the item "Individuals will learn to manage their health better" 38.8% considered it "Probable". Other interesting items are those related to the "political" dimension (to the item "It will be discovered that the policy of closing cities has been wrong", 35.1% answered with "Very unlikely" and 39% with "Unlikely") and to the "corruption" dimension (in particular, the item "Corruption in Italy will decrease" shows that 51.5% believe that this will be "Very unlikely"). Important too are the forecasts made by respondents regarding the items "Separations between spouses will increase" (to which 47.8% responded with "Probable") and "Domestic violence will increase" (46.2% believe that this will be "Probable").

3.6. Cohabitation Scales: Positive Relationship

A one-way ANOVA was conducted to compare the three groups regarding "Positive Relationship Cohabitation Scales" (shown in Table 2), and statistically significant results emerged on "We had a good level of confidence and complicity", in which the partner group differed both from partner and children and relatives ($F_{(2, 1747)} = 58.49$, $p < 0.001$); however, post-hoc comparisons using Bonferroni correction revealed a statistically significant difference between the groups partner (M = 4.11, SD = 0.86), partner and children (M = 3.77, SD = 1.00) and relatives (M = 3.48, SD = 1.03). For the item "In some moments of discomfort, I could rely on her/him/them", the partner group differed both from partners and children, and relatives ($F_{(2, 1747)} = 58.61$, $p < 0.001$), and in post-hoc comparisons there was a statistically significant difference between partner (M = 4.16, SD = 1.02), partner and children (M = 3.84, SD = 1.16) and relatives (M = 3.42, SD = 1.27).

Table 2. Positive relationship cohabitation scale: "In the last month, with the partner I live with … ", group comparison. Note: PwC = partners with children; R = relatives; P = partner.

		ANOVA								
		Sum of Squares	df	Mean Square	F	Sig.	Multiple Comparison	Mean Difference	Sig.	η^2
I freely faced every thought or emotion	Between Groups	177.098	2	88.549	94.666	0.000	P vs. R	0.713	0.000	0.10
	Within Groups	1634.116	1747	0.935			PwC vs. R	0.606	0.000	
	Total	1811.214	1749							
We had a good level of confidence and complicity	Between Groups	111.657	2	55.828	58.486	0.000	P vs. PwC	0.342	0.000	0.06
	Within Groups	1667.614	1747	0.955			P vs. R	0.635	0.000	
	Total	1779.271	1749				PwC vs. R	0.293	0.000	
We have divided up the household management tasks equally	Between Groups	92.066	2	46.033	36.949	0.000	P vs. R	0.541	0.000	0.04
	Within Groups	2176.506	1747	1.246			PwC vs. R	0.397	0.000	
	Total	2268.571	1749							
In some moments of discomfort, I could rely on him/her/them	Between Groups	159.002	2	79.501	58.613	0.000	P vs. PwC	0.326	0.000	0.06
	Within Groups	2369.569	1747	1.356			P vs. R	0.748	0.000	
	Total	2528.571	1749				PwC vs. R	0.423	0.000	
Together we faced the difficulties	Between Groups	142.670	2	71.335	62.978	0.000	P vs. PwC	0.188	0.011	0.07
	Within Groups	1978.815	1747	1.133			P vs. R	0.677	0.000	
	Total	2121.486	1749				PwC vs. R	0.489	0.000	
We have been able to listen to each other and respect our differences of opinion	Between Groups	137.417	2	68.709	64.896	0.000	P vs. PwC	0.263	0.000	0.07
	Within Groups	1849.651	1747	1.059			P vs. R	0.687	0.000	
	Total	1987.068	1749				PwC vs. R	0.424	0.000	
We had pleasant intimate interactions	Between Groups	72.364	2	36.182	26.253	0.000	P vs. PwC	0.490	0.000	0.03
	Within Groups	2407.750	1747	1.378			PwC vs. R	−0.349	0.000	
	Total	2480.115	1749							
We shared responsibility	Between Groups	165.387	2	82.693	85.301	0.000	P vs. R	0.661	0.000	0.09
	Within Groups	1693.5858	1747	0.969			PwC vs. R	0.615	0.000	
	Total	1858.972	1749							
We have been patient enough to tolerate some annoying character from each other	Between Groups	103.454	2	51.727	58.807	0.000	P vs. PwC	0.216	0.000	0.06
	Within Groups	1536.654	1747	0.880			P vs. R	0.593	0.000	
	Total	1640.108	1749				PwC vs. R	0.377	0.000	
We agreed to make the sacrifices and renunciations that the new situation has entailed	Between Groups	74.531	2	37.265	49.036	0.000	P vs. R	0.436	0.000	0.05
	Within Groups	1327.661	1747	0.760			PwC vs. R	0.420	0.000	
	Total	1402.192	1749							

There were statistically significant differences between three groups ($F_{(2, 1747)} = 64.90$, $p < 0.001$) on the item "We have been able to listen to each other and respect our differences of opinion", wherein the partner group (M = 4.00, SD = 0.92) differed from partner and children (M = 3.74, SD = 0.98) and relatives (M = 3.31, SD = 1.15). Ultimately, statistically significant results emerged for "We have been patient enough to tolerate some annoying character from each other", in which the partner group differed both from partners and children and relatives ($F_{(2, 1747)} = 58.81$, $p < 0.001$); however, post-hoc comparisons using Bonferroni correction revealed a statistically significant difference between partner (M = 3.96, SD = 0.83), partner and children (M = 3.75, SD = 0.89) and relatives (M = 3.37, SD = 1.05).

3.7. Cohabitation Scales: Negative Relationship

A one-way ANOVA was conducted to compare the three groups regarding "negative relationship cohabitation scales" (shown in Table 3), and statistically significant results emerged on "We have had verbal arguments and disagreements" in which the relatives group differed both from the partners and children and the partner group ($F_{(2, 1747)} = 15.34$, $p < 0.001$); however, post-hoc comparisons using Bonferroni correction revealed a statistically significant difference between relatives (M = 2.75, SD = 0.89), partners and children (M = 2.61, SD = 0.83) and partner (M = 2.47, SD = 0.83).

Statistically significant results emerged on "Mutual trust has been compromised", in which the relatives group differed both from partners and children and partner ($F_{(2, 1747)} = 16.88$, $p < 0.001$); however, post-hoc comparisons using Bonferroni correction revealed a statistically significant difference between relatives (M = 1.83, SD = 1.00), partners and children (M = 1.66, SD = 0.96) and partner (M = 1.50, SD = 0.83).

Lastly, for the item "Our differing views were unbearable", the relatives group differed both from partners and children and partner ($F_{(2, 1747)} = 20.91$, $p < 0.001$), and in post-hoc comparisons there was a statistically significant difference between relatives (M = 2.15, SD = 1.11), partners and children (M = 1.93, SD = 1.06) and partner (M = 1.75, SD = 0.96).

3.8. Stanford Time Perspective Inventory

A one-way ANOVA was conducted to compare the three groups regarding "Stanford Time Perspective Inventory" (shown in Table 4), and statistically significant results emerged on the item "I believe that my future is beautiful and well planned," in which the partners and children group differed both from the partner group and the relatives group ($F_{(2, 1747)} = 29.98$, $p < 0.001$); however, post-hoc comparisons using Bonferroni correction revealed a statistically significant difference between partners and children (M = 2.17, SD = 0.91), partner (M = 1.99, SD = 1.00) and relatives (M = 1.73, SD = 1.10).

Table 3. Negative relationship cohabitation scale: "In the last month, with the partner I live with … ", group comparison. Note: PwC = partners with children; R = relatives; P = partner.

		ANOVA								
		Sum of Squares	df	Mean Square	F	Sig.	Multiple Comparison	Mean Difference	Sig.	η^2
We have had verbal arguments and disagreements	Between Groups	22.207	2	11.103	15.339	0.000	P vs. PwC	−0.138	0.023	0.02
	Within Groups	1264.633	1747	0.724			P vs. R	−0.282	0.000	
	Total	1286.839	1749				PwC vs. R	−0.144	0.008	
There have been barriers and obstacles between us	Between Groups	24.987	2	12.494	12.815	0.000	P vs. PwC	−0.252	0.000	0.01
	Within Groups	1703.150	1747	0.975			P vs. R	−0.280	0.000	
	Total	1728.138	1749							
Matters of power and responsibility have emerged	Between Groups	34.871	2	17.436	16.709	0.000	P vs. R	−0.342	0.000	0.02
	Within Groups	1823.001	1747	1.044			PwC vs. R	−0.224	0.000	
	Total	1857.872	1749							
Mutual trust has been compromised	Between Groups	30.048	2	15.024	16.878	0.000	P vs. PwC	−0.155	0.021	0.02
	Within Groups	1555.111	1747	0.890			P vs. R	−0.327	0.000	
	Total	1585.159	1749				PwC vs. R	−0.172	0.003	
Distance and indifference have increased	Between Groups	15.371	2	7.686	7.019	0.001	P vs. PwC	−0.230	0.001	0.01
	Within Groups	1912.821	1747	1.095			P vs. R	−0.180	0.013	
	Total	1928.192	1749							
Our differing views were unbearable	Between Groups	46.288	2	23.144	20.906	0.000	P vs. PwC	−0.181	0.014	0.02
	Within Groups	1933.992	1747	1.107			P vs. R	−0.405	0.000	
	Total	1980.279	1749				PwC vs. R	−0.224	0.000	
Intimacy interactions have been unsatisfactory	Between Groups	30.945	2	15.473	9.295	0.000	P vs. PwC	−0.189	0.049	0.01
	Within Groups	2908.166	1747	1.665			PwC vs. R	0.311	0.000	
	Total	2939.111	1749							
Certain annoying traits about the other have turned out to be intolerable	Between Groups	76.290	2	38.145	32.879	0.000	P vs. R	−0.497	0.000	0.04
	Within Groups	2026.808	1747	1.160			PwC vs. R	−0.354	0.000	
	Total	2103.098	1749							
Violent verbal contrasts have come between us	Between Groups	38.473	2	19.237	22.587	0.000	P vs. R	−0.349	0.000	0.03
	Within Groups	1487.840	1747	0.852			PwC vs. R	−0.259	0.000	
	Total	1526.314	1749							
Verbal violence almost turned into physical violence	Between Groups	6.140	2	18.018	19.605	0.000	P vs. R	−0.136	0.000	0.01
	Within Groups	486.146	1747	0.278			PwC vs. R	−0.109	0.000	
	Total	492.286	1749							

Table 4. Time perspective inventory, group comparison. Note: PwC = partners with children; R = relatives; P = partner.

	ANOVA									
		Sum of Squares	df	Mean Square	F	Sig.	Multiple Comparison	Mean Difference	Sig.	η^2
When I want to achieve something, I set goals and consider specific means for reaching those goals.	Between Groups	0.775	2	0.387	0.668	0.513				0.00
	Within Groups	989.811	1707	0.580						
	Total	990.585	1709							
I try to live my life as fully as possible one day at a time.	Between Groups	2.343	2	1.171	1.047	0.351				0.00
	Within Groups	1907.196	1705	1.119						
	Total	1909.539	1707							
If things do not get done on time, I do not worry about it.	Between Groups	19.246	2	9.623	8.431	0.000	PwC vs. P	−0.190	0.013	0.01
	Within Groups	1944.956	1704	1.141			PwC vs. R	0.239	0.000	
	Total	1964.202	1706							
I believe that my future is beautiful and well planned.	Between Groups	60.793	2	30.396	29.984	0.000	P vs. PwC	−0.176	0.014	0.03
	Within Groups	1727.458	1704	1.014			P vs. R	0.263	0.000	
	Total	1788.251	1706				PwC vs. R	0.439	0.000	
It does not make sense to worry about the future since there is nothing to do about it anyway.	Between Groups	3.637	2	1.819	1.769	0.171				0.00
	Within Groups	1751.182	1703	1.028						
	Total	1754.819	1705							
I feel that it's more important to enjoy what you're doing than to get work done on time.	Between Groups	0.144	2	0.072	0.063	0.939				0.00
	Within Groups	1933.559	1700	1.137						
	Total	1933.703	1702							
It gives me pleasure to think about my past.	Between Groups	2.432	2	1.216	1.201	0.301				0.00
	Within Groups	1721.072	1700	1.012						
	Total	1723.503	1702							
I do things impulsively and I take decisions at the moment.	Between Groups	7.627	2	3.813	4.292	0.014	P vs. PwC	−0.161	0.018	0.01
	Within Groups	1510.427	1700	0.888						
	Total	1518.054	1702							
I take risks to put excitement in my life.	Between Groups	16.834	2	8.417	10.055	0.000	P vs. R	−0.246	0.000	0.01
	Within Groups	1423.099	1700	0.837			PwC vs. R	−0.140	0.021	
	Total	1439.933	1702							

3.9. Perceived Stress and Coping Orientation to Emotions and Problems

A one-way ANOVA was conducted to compare the three groups regarding PSS (shown in Table 5). The results show statistically significant differences, especially between relatives and the two other groups, partners with children and partners, both with respect to negative items (for example, "In the last month, how often have you felt nervous and «stressed»" ($F_{(2, 1747)} = 16.22$, $p < 0.001$, with relatives M = 2.41, SD = 0.99; partners with children M = 2.17, SD = 0.90; partners M = 2.12, SD = 0.91)) and positive items (for example, "In the last month, how often have you felt that you were on top of things" ($F_{(2, 1747)} = 18.06$, $p < 0.001$, with relatives M = 1.82, SD = 0.79; partners with children M = 2.20, SD = 0.82; partners M = 2.13, SD = 0.82)). The results highlight that there is greater perceived stress in relatives in comparison to partners with children and partners, which report lower average scores for all items on the scale. In addition, the three groups were compared with respect to the positive ($F_{(2, 1747)} = 47.64$, $p < 0.001$) and negative ($F_{(2, 1747)} = 16.13$, $p < 0.001$) sub-dimensions of the PSS, and post-hoc comparisons using Bonferroni correction showed statistically significant differences in the PSS-negative dimension between partners and children (M = 10.69, SD = 3.95), partners (M = 10.79, SD = 4.24) and relatives (M = 11.9, SD = 4.27). Statistically significant differences were also found in the PSS-positive dimension between partners and children (M = 10.35, SD = 2.28), partners (M = 10.25, SD = 2.41) and relatives (M = 9.11, SD = 2.74). The results therefore show that relatives, compared to partners with children and partners, generally have more negative perceived stress and less positive perceived stress.

A one-way ANOVA was also conducted to compare the three groups regarding "Coping Orientation to Problem Experienced" (shown in Table 6). Once again, relatives showed more general statistically significant differences from partners with children and partners (e.g., "I think about how I might best handle the problem", $F_{(2, 1747)} = 16.93$, $p < 0.001$ with relatives M = 2.99, SD = 0.87; partners with children M = 3.24, SD = 0.77; partners M = 3.18, SD = 0.75). Moreover, the three groups were compared with respect to the emotion ($F_{(2, 1747)} = 8{,}45$, $p < 0.001$) and problem ($F_{(2, 1747)} = 7{,}79$, $p < 0.001$) sub-dimensions of the COPE, and post-hoc comparisons using Bonferroni correction outlined statistically significant differences in the COPE–emotion dimension between partners and children (M = 8.24, SD = 2.46), partners (M = 7.62, SD = 2.49) and relatives (M = 7.65, SD = 2.64). Statistically significant differences were also found in the COPE–problem dimension between partners and children (M = 10.84, SD = 2.23), partners (M = 10.56, SD = 2.29) and relatives (M = 10.32, SD = 2.49). The results show, once again, that relatives, compared to partners with children and partners, report lower average scores when compared to problem-focused coping strategies, while partners with children report higher average scores with respect to emotion-focused coping strategies.

Table 5. Perceived stress, group comparison. Note: PwC = partners with children; R = relatives; P = partner.

		ANOVA								
		Sum of Squares	df	Mean Square	F	Sig.	Multiple Comparison	Mean Difference	Sig.	η^2
In the last month, how often have you been upset because of something that happened unexpectedly	Between Groups	0.831	2	0.416	0.477	0.621				0.00
	Within Groups	1522.404	1747	0.871						
	Total	1523.235	1749							
In the last month, how often have you felt that you were unable to control the important things in your life	Between Groups	6.118	2	3.059	3.068	0.047	PwC vs. R	−0.138	0.042	0.00
	Within Groups	1742.093	1747	0.997						
	Total	1748.211	1749							
In the last month, how often have you felt nervous and "stressed"	Between Groups	28.411	2	26.499	16.226	0.000	P vs. R	−0.289	0.000	0.02
	Within Groups	1529.452	1747	0.652			PwC vs. R	−0.239	0.000	
	Total	1557.863	1749							
In the last month, how often have you felt confident about your ability to handle your personal problems	Between Groups	44.996	2	22.498	33.849	0.000	P vs. R	0.291	0.000	0.04
	Within Groups	1161.143	1747	0.665			PwC vs. R	0.356	0.000	
	Total	1206.139	1749							
In the last month, how often have you felt that things were going your way	Between Groups	52.999	2	26.499	40.668	0.000	P vs. R	0.316	0.000	0.04
	Within Groups	1138.359	1747	0.652			PwC vs. R	0.387	0.000	
	Total	1191.358	1749							
In the last month, how often have you found that you could not cope with all the things that you had to do	Between Groups	16.111	2	8.056	9.678	0.000	P vs. R	−0.202	0.001	0.01
	Within Groups	1454.141	1747	0.832			PwC vs. R	−0.196	0.000	
	Total	1470.252	1749							
In the last month, how often have you been able to control irritations in your life	Between Groups	28.914	2	14.457	21.929	0.000	P vs. R	0.287	0.000	0.02
	Within Groups	1151.706	1747	0.659			PwC vs. R	0.247	0.000	
	Total	1180.619	1749							
In the last month, how often have you felt that you were on top of things	Between Groups	26.361	2	13.181	18.064	0.000	P vs. R	0.247	0.000	0.02
	Within Groups	1274.738	1747	0.730			PwC vs. R	0.259	0.000	
	Total	1301.099	1749							
In the last month, how often have you been angered because of things that were outside of your control	Between Groups	29.780	2	14.890	16.832	0.000	P vs. R	−0.231	0.000	0.02
	Within Groups	1545.398	1747	0.885			PwC vs. R	−0.292	0.000	
	Total	1575.178	1749							
In the last month, how often have you felt difficulties were piling up so high that you could not overcome them	Between Groups	36.036	2	18.018	19.605	0.000	P vs. R	−0.286	0.000	0.02
	Within Groups	1605.561	1747	0.919			PwC vs. R	−0.305	0.000	
	Total	1641.598	1749							

Table 6. Coping orientation to emotions and problems, group comparison. Note: PwC = partners with children; R = relatives; P = partner.

		ANOVA								
		Sum of Squares	**df**	**Mean Square**	**F**	**Sig.**	**Multiple Comparison**	**Mean Difference**	**Sig.**	η^2
I have been saying to myself "this is not real"	Between Groups	16.422	2	3.059	3.068	0.003	P vs. PwC	−0.243	0.002	0.01
	Within Groups	2383.272	1740	0.997			P vs. R	−0.173	0.042	
	Total	2399.694	1742							
I concentrate my efforts on doing something about it	Between Groups	49.483	2	24.741	42.896	0.000	P vs. PwC	−0.181	0.000	0.05
	Within Groups	1002.997	1739	0.577			P vs. R	0.214	0.000	
	Total	1052.480	1741				PwC vs. R	0.395	0.000	
I look for something good in what is happening	Between Groups	22.145	2	11.072	12.241	0.000	P vs. R	0.165	0.012	0.01
	Within Groups	1572.997	1739	0.905			PwC vs. R	0.262	0.000	
	Total	1595.142	1741							
I think about how I might best handle the problem	Between Groups	21.750	2	10.875	16.931	0.000	P vs. R	0.194	0.000	0.02
	Within Groups	1116.930	1739	0.642			PwC vs. R	0.251	0.000	
	Total	1138.680	1741							
I try to get emotional support from friends or relatives	Between Groups	36.615	2	18.307	14.712	0.000	P vs. R	−0.226	0.002	0.02
	Within Groups	2163.952	1739	1.244			PwC vs. R	−0.334	0.000	
	Total	2200.567	1741							
I think hard about what steps to take	Between Groups	3.709	2	1.855	2.046	0.130				0.00
	Within Groups	1576.186	1739	0.906						
	Total	1579.895	1741							
I pray more than usual	Between Groups	59.639	2	29.819	20.129	0.000	P vs. PwC	−0.372	0.000	0.02
	Within Groups	2573.232	1737	1.481			PwC vs. R	0.398	0.000	
	Total	2632.871	1739							
I try to get advice from someone about what to do	Between Groups	18.012	2	9.006	9.696	0.000	P vs. R	−0.184	0.005	0.01
	Within Groups	1613.319	1737	0.929			PwC vs. R	−0.226	0.000	
	Total	1631.330	1739							

4. Discussions

The results of this research allow different considerations on the influence that interpersonal relationships have on the quality of living together, in particular on the emotional level. Several studies report the importance of the type of relationship in living together [19,21]; in this study, we aimed to investigate the possible effect of the relationship as a mediator on stress, future perspectives and coping strategies during the COVID-19 lockdown in Italy.

PSS results showed that perceived stress is greater in the relatives group. In particular, negative perceived stress showed higher scores in the relatives group, instead of the partner and partners with children groups, while positive perceived stress showed higher scores in the partners with children and partner groups compared to the relatives one. Furthermore, an important fact arises from the comparison between the three groups: in general, partners with children showed statistically higher scores in COPE-NVI. In particular, the results showed that the partners with children group engaged coping strategies related to emotions and problem solving more frequently than other groups, suggesting that children could play a moderating role in the implementation of stress coping strategies. Similar results emerged from the STPI; in fact, as far as concerns the future perspective, the group partners with children showed higher values than the other two groups, showing a greater tendency towards planning for future events. These results can be explained through the positive dyadic coping and collaborative coping constructs; these coping constructs consider stress management as a collective and not individualistic process—the subject does not manage stress in a void but within an interpersonal context [30]. Giving support to the partner in stressful situations would increase the quality of the conjugal relationship, but also the physical and psychological well-being of the family members, both in cases of daily stress and in extraordinary stressful events [31–33]. In highly stressful situations, significant others, especially the partner, are a great support source, but so too are active participants in family management and the influence of the management process itself [34,35], and activate shared coping strategies [34].

Moreover, according to Berg and colleagues [36], there is a positive association between dyadic coping and partner well-being. More specifically, when partners reported more collaborative coping, they reported more positive emotions. This result seems to be in line with the present study result; in fact, from the data that emerged from the semantic differential on the perceived emotions during lockdown, it could be noted that positive emotions are more likely to be experienced by individuals who live with their partner, and with partners and children.

From the data analysis, an interesting finding seems to emerge from the comparison between the future forecasts scale and the positive and negative relationships scales. According to participants' future forecasts, as a result of the COVID-19 emergency an increase in spousal separations is likely to occur, as well as in domestic violence. However, according to the positive and negative relationships data, the results seem to be in contrast with the future forecasts scale. In fact, while in future forecasts negative aspects at a relational level (i.e., separations) emerge, on the other side, items from the positive relationships scale, referring to complicity, trust, listening and respect, show above-average scores, both in the general sample and especially in those who reported living with the partner only, and with partners and children. The same thing happens, on the contrary, with the negative relationships scale (e.g., indifference, arguments, differences of opinion, but also verbal and physical violence), on which scores were quite low, in contrast with the risk perception of increasing separations and domestic violence. This apparent contradiction between the data could be explained through fundamental attribution error [37], which is the tendency to underestimate the role of situational determinants and overestimate the degree to which social actions and outcomes reflect the dispositions of relevant actors.

Finally, from the qualitative analysis, a prevalence of negative words and ideas emerges, referring to the experience during lockdown and forced cohabitation caused by the Ministerial Decrees (Decree-Law no. 19 of 25 March 2020; Decree-Law no. 33 of 16 May 2020). Since responses were not sentences and only three words were asked for, it was not necessarily possible to assign a meaning (e.g., positive, negative or neutral) to the terms, but these analysis results allowed a broader interpretation of the emerging data; however, it could be noteworthy that the first word with a fully positive meaning (i.e., "useful") appeared in the twenty-third position, while the previous words all had a negative (i.e., "stressful") or neutral (i.e., "thinking") meaning. From what emerges, most people have reported to experience the lockdown as a difficult period, reporting heavy and meaningful words, often related to strong psychological distress conditions (i.e., alienating, depressing, anxiety, crisis).

Overall, it can be hypothesized that during the COVID-19 lockdown, interpersonal relationships with people living together had an important impact on psychological well-being. An emotional bond seems to be an important mediator in the management of stress and negative emotions; moreover, the COVID-19 outbreak has generated a unique situation with specific characteristics related to stress, coping strategies and living together, creating a new multifaceted form of cohabitation, highlighting the need to create and validate instruments which can be used in unexpected events. New studies could investigate the effects of forms of cohabitation without emotional bonds (e.g., roommates), also by using these ad hoc instruments, in order to validate them for use among the scientific community.

This study may give rise to a consideration for future research considering the possible mediating effect of the caregiver role. In fact, the partners with children group suggested the possible positive effect on stress and coping strategies of being a caregiver; however, those living with relatives could equally be caregivers for both children and elderly or disabled relatives. Therefore, it could be investigated if it is the caregiver role that act as a mediator in the experience of positive emotions—for example, differentiating within the relatives group between those who take care of a cohabitant relative and those who do not—or if it is the presence of children which activates positive emotions.

These results may have important practical and clinical implications—emotional cohabitation plays a key role in stress and coping management, proving to be a good basis for possible counseling interventions, but also for the development of awareness and preventions projects related to COVID-19's psychological consequences that are also linked to educational programs on living together and emotional relationships. Since lockdown has led to intense stress, fatigue and anxiety [38,39], this kind of study may help identify potential action fields and protocols in order to reduce stress and increase awareness of cohabitant relationships, which will result, in turn, in greater psychological well-being.

Author Contributions: Conceptualization, E.M., A.F., G.L., A.P., M.B., E.P., A.M.G. and F.A.; data curation, E.M., A.F., G.L. and A.P.; formal analysis, E.M., A.F. and G.L.; investigation, E.M. and A.F.; methodology, E.M., A.F., G.L. and F.A.; project administration, A.M.G. and F.A.; resources, E.M. and A.F.; software, E.M., A.F. and M.B.; supervision, A.M.G. and F.A.; validation, E.M., A.F., A.P., M.B., E.P. and A.M.G.; visualization, G.L., A.P., M.B., E.P., A.M.G. and F.A.; writing—original draft, E.M., A.F., G.L. and A.P.; writing—review and editing, E.M., A.F., G.L., A.P., M.B., E.P., A.M.G. and F.A. All authors have read and agreed to the published version of the manuscript.

Funding: This research received no external funding.

Conflicts of Interest: The authors declare no conflict of interest.

References

1. Avallone, F. *Psicologia del Lavoro e Delle Organizzazioni: Costruire e Gestire Relazioni nei Contesti Professionali e Sociali*; Carocci, Ed: Roma, Italia, 2011.
2. Avallone, F.; Farnese, M.L.; Pepe, S.; Paplomatas, A. Il processo di convivenza. Indagine esplorativa delle dimensioni della convivenza affettiva, organizzativa, sociale. *Rass. Psicol.* **2007**, *1*, 9–33.
3. Besozzi, E. L'incontro tra culture e la possibile convivenza. *Studi Sociol.* **2001**, *39*, 65–81.
4. Cesari, J. *When Islam and Democracy Meet: Muslims in Europe and in the United States*; Palgrave Macmillan: New York, NY, USA, 2004. [CrossRef]
5. De Rudder, V. Interethnic Relationships in Cohabitation. *Crit. Sociol.* **1989**, *89*, 39–60.
6. Katz, R. Effects of migration, ethnicity, and religiosity on cohabitation. *J. Comp. Fam. Stud.* **2001**, *32*, 587–599. [CrossRef]
7. Atrey, S. *Intersectional Discrimination*; Oxford University Press: Oxford, MS, USA, 2019.
8. Collier, P. *Breaking the Conflict Trap: Civil War and Development Policy*; World Bank Publications: Washington, DC, USA, 2003.

9. Cohen, A. The relationship between multiple commitments and organizational citizenship behavior in Arab and Jewish culture. *J. Vocat. Behav.* **2006**, *69*, 105–118. [CrossRef]
10. Uberoi, V.; Modood, T. Inclusive Britishness: A multiculturalist advance. *Political Stud.* **2013**, *61*, 23–41. [CrossRef]
11. Alvesson, M. *Understanding Organizational Culture*; Sage: London, UK, 2012. [CrossRef]
12. Schein, E.H. *Organizational Culture and Leadership (Jossey-Bass Business & Management Series)*; Jossey Bass Incorporated: San Francisco, CA, USA, 2004.
13. Schneider, B.; Barbera, K.M. *Introduction: The Oxford Handbook of Organizational Climate and Culture*; Oxford University Press: New York, NY, USA, 2014. [CrossRef]
14. Bateman, T.S.; Organ, D.W. Job satisfaction and the good soldier: The relationship between affect and employee "citizenship". *Acad. Manag. J.* **1983**, *26*, 587–595. [CrossRef]
15. Podsakoff, P.M.; MacKenzie, S.B.; Podsakoff, N.P. Organizational citizenship behavior: Introduction and overview of the handbook. In *The Oxford Handbook of Organizational Citizenship Behavior*; Oxford University Press: New York, NY, USA, 2018; pp. 1–6. [CrossRef]
16. Avallone, F.; Paplomatas, A. *Salute Organizzativa: Psicologia del Benessere nei Contesti Lavorativi*; Raffaello Cortina: Milano, Italia, 2005.
17. Bennet, J.B.; Cook, R.F.; Pelletier, K.R. *Toward an Integrated Framework for Comprehensive Organizational Wellness: Concepts, Practices, and Research in Workplace Health Promotion*; American Psychological Association: Washington, DC, USA, 2003. [CrossRef]
18. Cartwright, S.; Cooper, C.L. (Eds.) The Psychological Impact of Merger. In *Managerial, Occupational and Organizational Stress Research*; Routledge: London, UK, 2018.
19. Baril, M.E.; Crouter, A.C.; McHale, S.M. Processes linking adolescent well-being, marital love, and coparenting. *J. Fam. Psychol.* **2007**, *21*, 645. [CrossRef]
20. Fine, M.A.; Fincham, F.D. (Eds.) *Handbook of Family Theories: A Content-Based Approach*; Routledge: London, UK, 2013.
21. Markman, H.J.; Hahlweg, K. The prediction and prevention of marital distress: An international perspective. *Clin. Psychol. Rev.* **1993**, *13*, 29–43. [CrossRef]
22. Kurdek, L.A. The link between facets of neuroticism and dimensions of relationship commitment: Evidence from gay, lesbian, and heterosexual couples. *J. Fam. Psychol.* **1997**, *11*, 503. [CrossRef]
23. Schneider, B.H.; Fonzi, A.; Tomada, G.; Tani, F. A cross-national comparison of children's behavior with their friends in situations of potential conflict. *J. Cross-Cult. Psychol.* **2000**, *31*, 259–266. [CrossRef]
24. Arcidacono, C.; Procentese, F. (Eds.) *Madri e Padri tra Famiglia e Lavoro. Teoria e Prassi Delle Politiche di Conciliazione Nella Provincia di NAPOLI*; Filema: Napoli, Italia, 2008; pp. 57–128.
25. Vermaes, I.P.; van Susante, A.M.; van Bakel, H.J. Psychological functioning of siblings in families of children with chronic health conditions: A meta-analysis. *J. Pediatr. Psychol.* **2012**, *37*, 166–184. [CrossRef] [PubMed]
26. Lowe, S.R.; Rhodes, J.E.; Scoglio, A.A. Changes in marital and partner relationships in the aftermath of Hurricane Katrina: An analysis with low-income women. *Psychol. Women Q.* **2012**, *36*, 286–300. [CrossRef] [PubMed]
27. Cohen, S.; Kamarck, T.; Mermelstein, R. A global measure of perceived stress. *J. Health Soc. Behav.* **1983**, 24. [CrossRef]
28. Sica, C.; Magni, C.; Ghisi, M.; Altoè, G.; Sighinolfi, C.; Chiri, L.R.; Franceschini, S. Coping Orientation to Problems Experienced-Nuova Versione Italiana (COPE-NVI): Uno strumento per la misura degli stili di coping. *Psicoter. Cogn. Comport.* **2008**, *14*, 27.
29. D'Alessio, M.; Guarino, A.; De Pascalis, V.; Zimbardo, P.G. Testing Zimbardo's Stanford time perspective inventory (STPI)-short form. *Time Soc.* **2003**, *12*, 333–347. [CrossRef]
30. Donato, S. Il coping diadico, ovvero far fronte allo stress insieme: Una rassegna della letteratura. *G. Ital. Psicol.* **2014**, *41*, 473–504. [CrossRef]
31. Bodenmann, G.; Atkins, D.C.; Schär, M.; Poffet, V. The association between daily stress and sexual activity. *J. Fam. Psychol.* **2010**, *24*, 271. [CrossRef]
32. Papp, L.M.; Witt, N.L. Romantic partners' individual coping strategies and dyadic coping: Implications for relationship functioning. *J. Fam. Psychol.* **2010**, *24*, 551. [CrossRef]
33. Sullivan, K.T.; Pasch, L.A.; Johnson, M.D.; Bradbury, T.N. Social support, problem solving, and the longitudinal course of newlywed marriage. *J. Personal. Soc. Psychol.* **2010**, *98*, 631. [CrossRef]

34. Revenson, T.A.; Kayser, K.E.; Bodenmann, G.E. *Couples Coping with Stress: Emerging Perspectives on Dyadic Coping*; American Psychological Association: Washington, DC, USA, 2005.
35. Rohrbaugh, M.J.; Mehl, M.R.; Shoham, V.; Reilly, E.S.; Ewy, G.A. Prognostic significance of spouse we talk in couples coping with heart failure. *J. Consult. Clin. Psychol.* **2008**, *76*, 781. [CrossRef] [PubMed]
36. Berg, C.A.; Wiebe, D.J.; Butner, J.; Bloor, L.; Bradstreet, C.; Upchurch, R.; Hayes, J.; Stephenson, R.; Nail, L.; Patton, G. Collaborative coping and daily mood in couples dealing with prostate cancer. *Psychol. Aging* **2008**, *23*, 505. [CrossRef] [PubMed]
37. Ross, L.D.; Amabile, T.M.; Steinmetz, J.L. Social roles, social control, and biases in social-perception processes. *J. Personal. Soc. Psychol.* **1977**, *35*, 485. [CrossRef]
38. Xiong, J.; Lipsitz, O.; Nasri, F.; Lui, L.; Gill, H.; Phan, L.; Chen-Li, D.; Iacobucci, M.; Ho, R.; Majeed, A.; et al. Impact of COVID-19 pandemic on mental health in the general population: A systematic review. *J. Affect. Disord.* **2020**, *277*, 55–64. [CrossRef]
39. Pieh, C.; Budimir, S.; Probst, T. The effect of age, gender, income, work, and physical activity on mental health during coronavirus disease (COVID-19) lockdown in Austria. *J. Psychosomatic Res.* **2020**, *136*, 110186. [CrossRef]

Publisher's Note: MDPI stays neutral with regard to jurisdictional claims in published maps and institutional affiliations.

Journal of
Clinical Medicine

MDPI

Article

The Italian COVID-19 Psychological Research Consortium (IT C19PRC): General Overview and Replication of the UK Study

Giovanni Bruno [1], Anna Panzeri [1], Umberto Granziol [1], Fabio Alivernini [2], Andrea Chirico [2], Federica Galli [2], Fabio Lucidi [2], Andrea Spoto [1] and Marco Bertamini [1,3,*]

1 Department of General Psychology, University of Padua, 35122 Padova, Italy; giovanni.bruno.4@phd.unipd.it (G.B.); anna.panzeri@phd.unipd.it (A.P.); umberto.granziol@unipd.it (U.G.); andrea.spoto@unipd.it (A.S.); giulio.vidotto@unipd.it (G.V.)
2 Department of Developmental and Social Psychology, University of Rome, 00185 Roma, Italy; fabio.alivernini@gmail.com (F.A.); andrea.chirico@uniroma1.it (A.C.); federica.galli@uniroma1.it (F.G.); fabio.lucidi@uniroma1.it (F.L.)
3 Department of Psychological Sciences, University of Liverpool, Liverpool L69 3BX, UK
* Correspondence: m.bertamini@liv.ac.uk

Abstract: The COVID-19 pandemic represents a major stressor for the psychological health of people worldwide. In the UK, the COVID19-Psychological Research Consortium Study (C19PRC) launched to evaluate the psychological impact of COVID-19 in the general population and its implications. The project was then extended to Italy and several other countries. This article provides an overview of the Italian C19PRC study and its replication of two specific findings from the UK C19PRC. In the first part, the relationship between anxiety and somatic symptomatology is examined. In the second part, we analyze the association between several factors and psychological health outcomes: depression/anxiety, traumatic stress, COVID-19 anxiety. In line with the study conducted in the UK, an online survey was administered to the adult Italian general population. The sample included 1038 respondents (age, mean = 49.94, SD = 16.14, 51.15% females) taken from four regions: Lombardia, Veneto, Lazio, and Campania. The relationship between predictors and outcomes was evaluated by means of logistic regression models. Somatic indices showed a positive association with anxiety, worse somatic symptoms were associated with mourning a loss of a beloved one due to COVID-19 and with precarious health conditions. Females showed a higher incidence of psychological issues. No differences in anxiety, depression, and traumatic stress were found across regions but the Campania region showed the most severe somatic symptomatology. In the second analysis, the factors associated with more severe psychological outcomes (i.e., anxiety and/or depression, traumatic stress, and COVID-19 related anxiety) were younger age, the presence of minors in the household, traumatic stressors, and precarious health conditions. No differences across regions emerged. The Italian results correspond to the UK findings for anxiety, depression, and traumatic stress. Both in the UK and Italy, the factors associated with worse psychological health were gender (female), younger age, having children, pre-existing health issues (both for oneself or someone close), and the moderate/high perceived risk of contracting COVID-19 within one month. In Italy, unlike the UK, lower household income and having (had) COVID-19 were not associated with poorer mental health. The psychological impact of COVID-19 can last for months; future research should explore all aspects of the psychological burden of COVID-19 in order to implement psychological interventions and promote psychological health.

Keywords: COVID-19; psychological health; general population; somatic symptoms; anxiety; depression

Citation: Bruno, G.; Panzeri, A.; Granziol, U.; Alivernini, F.; Chirico, A.; Galli, F.; Lucidi, F.; Spoto, A.; Vidotto, G.; Bertamini, M. The Italian COVID-19 Psychological Research Consortium (IT C19PRC): General Overview and Replication of the UK Study. *J. Clin. Med.* **2021**, *10*, 52. https://doi.org/10.3390/jcm10010052

Received: 30 November 2020
Accepted: 22 December 2020
Published: 25 December 2020

1. Introduction

Coronavirus-19 (COVID-19) is a virus first identified in 2019 that has led to an ongoing health emergency worldwide, with high infection rates and mortality [1]. The World

Health Organization recognized the outbreak as a Public Health Emergency of International Concern in January 2020, and as a pandemic in March 2020. Infection can cause systemic organ disease and some categories of people are more at risk in developing severe health consequences, such as those over 70 years old, pregnant women, and those who have pre-existing health conditions (e.g., cardiovascular disease) [2]. However, everyone can be infected and the long-term health consequences—also in its milder presentations—are still not fully understood.

Given the high transmissibility of COVID-19, to contain contagion many countries have adopted restrictive measures such as lockdown, quarantine, social distancing, and limits to movements and travel. These measures have serious economic as well as social implications. Therefore, these aspects of the pandemic extend beyond the health domain. The lives of millions of people have been affected, potentially increasing anxiety, loneliness, and distress. Some of these behavioral responses have been noted and commented in the media. Moreover, the measures have produced various responses, ranging from resistance, stockpiling of food supplies, denial, and beliefs in conspiracy theories. Some behavioral changes have the potential to affect the course of the pandemic itself [3].

The impact of the pandemic can be analyzed from social, psychological, and economic perspectives. Some authors have claimed that we are in the presence of a mental health emergency [4]. Over time fear, anxiety, worry, and depression have grown among people [5]. According to some, the psychological impact of COVID-19 may be greater than the threat represented by the physical disease itself, especially for vulnerable individuals [6]. A growing number of studies have highlighted psychological symptoms and issues in the clinical and general population [7–9].

A focus on the clinical population and on specific risk categories (e.g., young adults, pregnant women, health professionals, caregivers, the elderly) is useful to highlight the needs of these groups [10–12]. However, at the same time, it is important to direct attention to the general population to identify psychological and behavioral patterns.

Several studies have been conducted during the acute phase when contagions reached their peak. The effect of stressors and the psychological symptoms may persist or evolve over periods or months [13]. This is the case when people experience fear (for self and for significant others), stigmatization, and severe psychological symptoms [14].

Italy was one of the first countries to face the COVID-19 emergency and in an especially intense manner. In China, the city of Wuhan was put under quarantine on the 9th of January 2020. Already on/by the 21st of February 16 cases were confirmed in Lombardia and two in Veneto (two Italian regions in the North). Cases grew quickly leading to shortfalls of hospital beds, especially in intensive care units (ICU). The impact on the individual, social, and economic life in Italy was significant. In Italy, as in other countries, the pandemic did not affect all regions equally. Thus, national statistics can be misleading. An analysis by region is important for at least two reasons: first, the north of Italy is divided in eight regions but there are large differences in the impact even between these. Second, in Italy the national health service has a regional structure, and different measures were taken by different regions, (e.g., different testing effort, quarantine policy, individual mobilities, the progression of social distancing, and local capacity of medical infrastructure) [15]. Third, the timeline of the virus varied by region. Lombardia was the first region to be affected and remained also the region with most cases over time. This is a wealthy region with high population density and its capital Milan is the second largest city in Italy.

In March 2020, a longitudinal, multi-country project was launched by the COVID-19 Psychological Research Consortium (C19PRC) in the UK and then enlarged to other countries [16]. The present study represents the opening article of the Italian C19PRC project. Data was collected in Italy from 13 to 28 July 2020, after the contagion peak (end of March) and after the end of the strict national lockdown (18 May). Many commercial and social activities had restarted, and people were allowed to move beyond their own towns. In mid-July, the number of contagions had a stable and decreasing trend, but there were still preventive measures in place (e.g., social distancing, hygiene practices, masks).

There was an awareness in the population that a second wave of contagions was possible in all regions.

This study focused on four Italian regions selected because of their geographical location, from the north (Lombardia, Veneto), center (Lazio), and south (Campania), and because of their infection rate when the survey was launched–at the beginning of July 2020–from higher (Lombardia = 95,118 cases, Veneto = 19,432) to medium-lower (Lazio = 8389, Campania = 4788) [17]. Indeed, when data was collected, from 13 to 18 July, in Italy a total of 243,230 cases of COVID-19 had been registered, with 35,042 deaths. The regions that registered the highest number of contagions were Lombardia and Veneto, while in the center and south the outbreak was more contained.

According to the Italian Ministry of Health, the health services and policies are the same in the Italian regions, but some independent regional choices are allowed. In the North, Lombardia ran fewer tests than Veneto and Emilia Romagna. These regions adopted proactive testing modalities and treatment strategies, testing a large number of people and treating positive patients with mild symptoms at home. Therefore, we chose to compare Lombardia and Veneto. Veneto is geographically next to Lombardia, they both have a mix of large cities and small towns and, with respect to population, Lombardia is the largest (10 million) and Veneto is the 5th largest region in Italy (nearly 5 million). The other two regions also include some large cities (Rome in Lazio and Naples in Campania) and are relatively large (5.8 million each). From 17 May 2020 the government passed responsibility to single regions under the overall supervision of the Ministry of Health [18]; different measures in different regions were motivated by the underlying infections and death trends.

Data from a substantial sample of the general population are useful to plan effective interventions. A range of variables have to be assessed due to the complexity of the psychological, social, and cultural context of the pandemic. Some of them are: demographics; socioeconomic status; political opinions; belongingness in the community; public health knowledge; news broadcasting; risk perceptions; hygienic and preventive practices; decision making (e.g., whether to vaccinate or not). Among the psychological ones, post-traumatic stress, loneliness, anxiety, and depression should be assessed as well as self-esteem, personality, and resilience.

Aims

This Italian C19PRC study uses data collected on a range of demographic, social, and psychological variables from a sample of the general population in Italy. The aim is to describe the effects of the pandemic in adults. Here we provide an overview of the project, and an initial analysis, while additional detailed analyses will require further work. In particular in this paper we focus on anxiety, depression, and stress related to COVID-19 and on the comparison with the same measurements from the first wave of the UK C19PRC study [19,20]. Moreover, comparisons across four Italian regions—selected according to geographic location and infection rate—are provided.

2. Methodological Section

2.1. Study Plan

The original complete survey from the UK is described by McBride and colleagues [16]. Our goal was to maintain the Consortium aims and measures, applying them to the Italian population. Part of this data will be used to conduct further in-depth studies focusing on specific topics described in detail in following papers. In line with the UK survey, the Italian C19PRC study relied on an online survey provided by Qualtrics. R software was used for all analyses [21]. The survey was administered in four Italian regions—Campania, Lazio, Lombardia and Veneto. Ethical approval for this study was provided by the Ethical Committee for Psychological Research of the University of Padua (protocol: 3818).

2.2. Participants

The inclusion criteria were living in Italy and at least 18 years old. Participants were excluded if survey completion time was below 11 minutes and 11 seconds or above three days. All participants were informed about the study's aims, their rights, and privacy policies. All of them provided informed consent before completing the survey of the study, conducted according to Ethical Principles and Code of Conduct of the Italian Association of Psychology.

Adult participants (n = 1038) were recruited by the survey company Qualtrics from an online research panel using stratified quota sampling to guarantee that the sample characteristics of gender, age, household income, and region (Campania, Lazio, Lombardia, and Veneto) matched the Italian population. After the completion of the survey online (median time of completion = 41 min), each participant was reimbursed by Qualtrics.

The mean age of the total sample was 49.94 years (median = 51, SD = 16.14, range = 18–87), and 51.15% were female (n = 531). Participants were recruited from the four selected regions based on their population size: Campania (n = 227), Lazio (n = 234), Lombardia (n = 391), Veneto (n = 186). Most of the participants were Italian (96.61%, n = 1003) and with Caucasian ethnicity (74.66%, n = 775). A minority had only elementary or some secondary education (8.28%, n = 86), nearly half had completed high school (48.74%, n = 506) with a further 42.97% having attained a higher level of education. Less than half were in full employment (44.41%, n = 461), with 24.18% retired (n = 251). Married participants comprised 57.99% (n = 602) whereas never married participants comprised 26.59% of the sample (n = 276).

Only 14 participants tested positive for COVID-19 (1.35%). Two and a half percent of the sample confirmed the presence of coronavirus cases among individuals living in the same house, and 17.82% among friends or relatives. Finally, 10.50% of the participants mourning a loss due to confirmed cases of COVID-19. Further information about demographics is available in the Supplementary Materials (S1, Tables S1–S20 and https://osf.io/nx2zd/).

2.3. Measures

In line with the aim of the original C19PRC-UK study, the measures remained the same in order to allow cross-cultural comparison. Below, the measures that are relevant for the present analysis are described. Items were translated into Italian. The full list is available as Supplementary Material (Supplementary File S1 and https://osf.io/nx2zd/).

Sociodemographic variables: we collected the same information as the original C19PRC-UK study [16]: location, presence of adults or minors in the house, income, and previous health issues. We integrated these with further information (region, mourning for COVID-19 human losses, perceived risk to contract COVID-19).

The Patient Health Questionnaire-15 (PHQ-15) [22] is a 15-item self-report measure based on a 3-point Likert scale. It asks about the presence of somatic symptoms in the last 14 days. In this study, we use both the total scores and the four subscales pain symptoms (0–6), gastrointestinal symptoms (0–8), cardiopulmonary symptoms (0–8), and fatigue symptoms (0–4). As in previous works [16–23] and for the same reasons, item 4 and item 13 were excluded, lowering the maximum score to 26.

The Patient Health Questionnaire-9 (PHQ-9) [24] was used to measure nine symptoms of depression, asking participants how often they have been bothered by each symptom over the last 14 rated on a four-point Likert scale. The maximum score is 27, which is indicative of a high level of depression. A cut-off score of 10 was used, corresponding to moderate levels of depression [25].

The Generalized Anxiety Disorder 7-item Scale (GAD-7) [26] is a seven-item self-report measure based on a four-point Likert scale. It asks participants about anxiety symptoms in the last 14 days. The maximum score is 21, which is indicative of high levels of generalized anxiety. A cut-off of 10 was used, corresponding to a moderately severe level of anxiety [27].

The International Trauma Questionnaire (ITQ) [28] is a nine-item self-report measure based on a 5-point Likert scale. Consistently with ICD-11 [29], it asks participants about particular events or behaviors in the last 30 days, across the three symptom clusters of re-experiencing, avoidance, and sense of threat (two items each). Another three items measure functional impairment caused by these symptoms. The maximum score is 24, and a score of $\geq$2 (*Moderately*) is considered endorsement of that symptom. A PTSD diagnosis requires the endorsement of the three clusters and at least one indicator of functional impairment [30,31].

COVID-19-related anxiety was measured through a single item, 'How anxious are you about the coronavirus COVID-19 pandemic?', rated on a continuous scale from 0 to 100. Higher values correspond to higher COVID-19 related anxiety.

2.4. Analytic Methods

In Section 3.1, scores of the COVID-19 anxiety variable were categorized into quintiles, and the quintiles were dummy-coded with the lowest one used as the reference category [20] Regression models were used to estimate the relationship between the COVID-19 anxiety quintiles and the PHQ-15 subscales (pain, gastrointestinal, cardiopulmonary, and fatigue). Model 1 included the four dummy-coded COVID-19 anxiety variables as predictors of the four PHQ-15 subscales. The regression coefficient for each dummy-coded variable is interpreted as the mean difference between each quintile and the lowest one. Model 1 was also run separately with the total PHQ-15 summed scale score replacing the subscales. In Model 2 the covariates (age, gender, income, pre-existing health problems, and GAD) were included as predictors, with the addition of Italian region mourning for COVID-19 losses factors.

In Section 3.2, measures of depression (PHQ-9), generalized anxiety (GAD-7), trauma symptoms relating to the pandemic (ITQ) and COVID-19 anxiety were considered as dependent variables for three binary logistic regression models [19]. The predictor variables were age, gender, living location, living alone, presence of children in the household, income, pre-existing health conditions in self and someone close, and perceived risk of infection over the next month. Italian region and mourning for COVID-19 losses factors were included.

3. Results

3.1. Somatic Symptoms

Correlations for all the variables included in Models 1 and 2 are shown in Table 1. The PHQ-15 subscales and the total score were positively and significantly correlated with COVID-19 anxiety, as well as with GAD-7 total score. These correlations are in line with results from the first wave of the UK study [20]. Figure 1 shows the relationship between COVID-19 anxiety and somatic symptoms.

Table 1. Correlation table for all the variables included in Model 1.

	Age	Gender	Income	C-19 Human Losses	P.H.I.	C-19 Anxiety	PHQ-15 (Pain)	PHQ-15 (Gastro)	PHQ-15 (Cardio)	PHQ-15 (Fatigue)	PHQ-15 (Total)
Gender	0.19 ***										
Income	0.00	0.12 ***									
C-19 Human Losses	−0.12 ***	−0.09 **	−0.04								
P.H.I.	0.21 ***	0.09 **	−0.07 *	−0.05							
GAD-7 (Total)	−0.23 ****	−0.13 ****	−0.02	−0.28 ***	0.06						
C-19 Anxiety	−0.06	−0.14 ****	−0.05	0.31 ****	0.01	0.23 ****					
PHQ-15 (Pain)	0.07 *	−0.09 **	−0.08 *	0.15 ****	0.19 ****	0.25 ****	0.10 **				
PHQ-15 (Gastro)	−0.23 ****	−0.15 ****	0.00	0.25 ****	0.10 **	0.35 ****	0.10 **	0.46 ****			
PHQ-15 (Cardio)	−0.09 **	−0.13 ****	0.00	0.29 ****	0.19 ****	0.40 ****	0.12 ***	0.43 ****	0.59 ****		
PHQ-15 (Fatigue)	−0.07 *	−0.13 ****	−0.04	0.18 ****	0.18 ****	0.31 ****	0.13 ***	0.5***	0.56 ****	0.51 ****	
PHQ-15 (Total)	−0.08 *	−0.15 ****	−0.04	0.24 ****	0.20 ****	0.36 ****	0.12 ***	0.75 ****	0.82 ****	0.71 ****	0.81 ****

Note. * $p < 0.05$; ** $p < 0.01$; *** $p < 0.001$; **** $p < 0.0001$ (adjusted controlling the false discovery rate [32]). Abbreviations: C-19: COVID-19; P.H.I.: Previous Health Issues; GAD-7: Generalized Anxiety Disorder 7-item; PGQ-15: Patient Health Questionnaire-15.

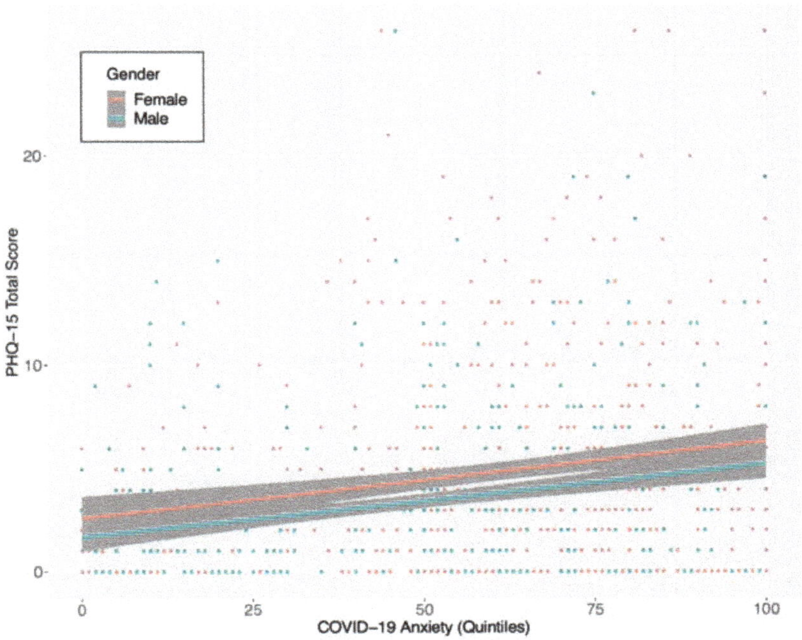

Figure 1. Relationship of COVID-19 anxiety on somatic symptoms (Model 2).

Table 2 shows the estimates from the regression models. In Model 1, considering COVID-19 first quintile as no-anxiety, we can observe significant differences between the baseline and the other quantiles both in PHQ-15 subscales and in its total score. In the sample, the aggravation of the somatic symptoms between quintiles seems to be characterized by a more linear increase than in the UK data, with a similar wider effect over the 5th quintile.

In Model 2, the control variables were taken into account. The effect of COVID-19 anxiety on somatic symptoms was weaker but similar to Model 1, especially referred to the total scale score. The presence of pre-existing health problems and high scores on GAD-7 significantly worsen specific and general somatic symptoms, confirming UK's findings. Mourning for COVID-19 losses also has a detrimental effect on psychological health. No effect of household income was found. In terms of regions, Campania showed higher scores of somatic symptoms than the other regions. Campania scores were high in the PHQ-15 pain subscale and in the gastrointestinal subscale, but also overall.

Table 2. Regression coefficients from models predicting PHQ-15 scale and subscale scores.

	Pain	Gastro	Cardio	Fatigue	Total Score
Model 1					
COVID-19 anxiety					
Quintile 1	-	-	-	-	-
Quintile 2	0.18	0.61 **	0.33 *	0.23 *	1.36 **
Quintile 3	0.26 *	0.91 ***	0.55 ***	0.30 **	2.03 ***
Quintile 4	0.26 *	0.89 ***	0.53 ***	0.47 ***	2.15 ***
Quintile 5	0.56 ***	1.20 ***	0.90 ***	0.72 ***	3.40 ***
R^2	0.02 ***	0.04 ***	0.03 ***	0.04 ***	0.05 ***
Model 2					
COVID-19 anxiety					
Quintile 1	-	-	-	-	-
Quintile 2	0.13	0.42 *	0.22	0.14	0.92 *
Quintile 3	0.12	0.46 *	0.26	0.10	0.95 *
Quintile 4	0.08	0.37	0.19	0.23	0.87
Quintile 5	0.25 *	0.38	0.32	0.32 *	1.27 *
Control variables					
Age	0.006 **	−0.01 ***	0.00	0.00	−0.02
Gender (Male)	−0.18 *	−0.30 *	−0.24 *	−0.20 *	−0.93 **
Income (Max)	−0.12	0.08	0.10	0.00	0.04
Health Problem (Yes)	0.52 ***	0.63 ***	0.60 ***	0.50 ***	2.27 ***
GAD-7 $\geq$ 10	0.75 ***	1.82 ***	1.48 ***	0.87 ***	4.93 ***
Region					
Lazio	−0.19	−0.17	−0.12	−0.14	−0.63
Lombardia	−0.21 *	−0.15	−0.09	−0.19	−0.64
Veneto	−0.26 *	−0.38	−0.19	−0.18	−1.03 *
Human Losses due to COVID-19					
Yes	0.30 *	0.71 ***	0.37 *	0.41 ***	1.80 ***
Not sure	0.43 *	0.34	0.09	0.34*	1.21
R^2	0.14 ***	0.24 ***	0.22 ***	0.18 ***	0.27 ***

Note. * $p < 0.05$; ** $p < 0.01$; *** $p < 0.001$ (adjusted controlling the false discovery rate [32]).

3.2. Anxiety, Depression, and Traumatic Stress

We focused on anxiety, depression, traumatic stress and COVID-19 related anxiety, following Shevlin et al. (2020). In order to be consistent with the original study, traumatic stress and COVID-19 related anxiety where treated independently, whereas a new variable was computed to describe participants with anxiety, depression, or both. Sample size, percentages and adjusted odds ratio are summarized in Tables 3–5.

Table 3. Multiple logistic regression results predicting anxiety or depression.

	n	Anxiety/Depression (*n*%)	Adjusted OR (95% CI)
Age			
	1038	271 (26.10%)	0.962 (0.951–0.973) ***
Gender			
Female	531	165 (31.07%)	-
Male	507	106 (20.90%)	0.728 (0.406–1.048)
Living Location			
Rural	49	11 (22.45%)	-
Town	297	57 (19.19%)	0.960 (0.162–1.815)
Suburb	123	41 (33.33%)	1.648 (0.796–2.551)
City	569	162 (28.47%)	1.365 (0.592–2.200)
Lone Adult			
No	899	238 (26.47%)	-
Yes	139	33 (23.74%)	1.258 (0.759–1.744)
Children			
No	680	131 (19.26%)	-
Yes	358	140 (39.10%)	1.552 (1.203–1.902) **
Income			
−15.000 €/yr	218	66 (30.27%)	-
−28.000 €/yr	214	50 (23.36%)	0.709 (0.224–1.189)
−55.000 €/yr	212	50 (23.59%)	0.880 (0.380–1.377)
−75.000 €/yr	211	67 (31.75%)	1.039 (0.543–1.534)
+75.000 €/yr	183	38 (20.54%)	0.559 (0.009–1.100)
Pre-Existing Health Condition, Self			
No	869	222 (25.54%)	-
Yes	169	49 (29.00%)	1.356 (0.911–1.813)
Pre-Existing Health Condition, Relatives			
No	811	192 (23.67%)	-
Yes	227	79 (34.80%)	1.526 (1.145–1.906) **
Human Losses due to COVID-19			
No	888	217 (24.43%)	-
Yes	109	38 (34.86%)	1.519 (1.017–2.012) *
Not Sure	41	16 (39.02%)	2.027 (1.267–2.771) **
Region			
Campania	227	65 (28.63%)	-
Lazio	234	61 (26.06%)	0.972 (0.504–1.440)
Lombardia	391	94 (24.04%)	0.728 (0.292–1.165)
Veneto	186	51 (27.42%)	0.912 (0.407–1.414)
Personal Risk at 1 Month			
Low	269	33 (12.26%)	-
Moderate—Low	252	46 (18.25%)	1.435 (0.924–1.955)
Moderate—High	261	75 (28.73%)	1.930 (1.453–2.423) ***
High	256	117 (45.70%)	2.565 (2.104–3.047) ***

Note. * $p < 0.05$; ** $p < 0.01$; *** $p < 0.001$ (adjusted controlling the false discovery rate [32]).

Table 4. Multiple logistic regression results predicting COVID-19-related anxiety.

	n	C-19 Related Anxiety (*n*%)	Adjusted OR (95% CI)
Age			
	1038	190 (26.10%)	1.001 (0.989–1.014)
Gender			
Female	531	126 (23.73%)	-
Male	507	64 (12.62%)	0.336 (−0.028–693) ***
Living Location			
Rural	49	5 (10.20%)	-
Town	297	62 (20.87%)	2.111 (1.147–3.265) *
Suburb	123	26 (21.14%)	1.648 (0.796–2.551)
City	569	97 (17.04%)	2.035 (0.994–3.238)
Lone Adult			
No	899	170 (18.90%)	-
Yes	139	20 (14.38%)	0.629 (0.051–1.168)
Children			
No	680	112 (16.47%)	-
Yes	358	78 (21.79%)	1.001 (1.595–1.402)
Income			
−15.000 €/yr	218	51 (23.39%)	-
−28.000 €/yr	214	42 (19.62%)	0.721 (0.214–1.223)
−55.000 €/yr	212	28 (13.20%)	0.219 (−0.353–0.775)
−75.000 €/yr	211	33 (15.64%)	0.389 (−0.171–0.937)
+75.000 €/yr	183	36 (19.67%)	0.949 (0.386–1.507)
Pre-Existing Health Condition, Self			
No	869	157 (18.06%)	-
Yes	169	33 (19.52%)	1.015 (0.510–1.501)
Pre-Existing Health Condition, Relatives			
No	811	136 (16.77%)	-
Yes	227	54 (23.7%)	1.325 (0.904–1.738)
Human Losses due to COVID-19			
No	888	159 (17.90%)	-
Yes	109	23 (21.1%)	1.099 (0.541–1.628)
Not Sure	41	8 (19.51%)	1.283 (0.355–2.108)
Region			
Campania	227	49 (21.58%)	-
Lazio	234	42 (17.95%)	0.913 (0.402–1.421)
Lombardia	391	64 (16.37%)	0.719 (0.250–1.190)
Veneto	186	35 (18.81%)	0.935 (0.390–1.473)
Personal Risk at 1 Month			
Low	269	17 (6.32%)	-
Moderate–Low	252	33 (13.09%)	1.747 (1.134–2.392) *
Moderate–High	261	43 (16.47%)	1.956 (1.366–2.585) **
High	256	97 (37.89%)	3.196 (2.647–3.798) ***

Note. * $p < 0.05$; ** $p < 0.01$; *** $p < 0.001$ (adjusted controlling the false discovery rate [32]).

Table 5. Multiple logistic regression results predicting traumatic stress.

	n	Traumatic Stress (n%)	Adjusted OR (95% CI)
Age	1038	269 (25.91%)	0.968 (0.957–0.979) ***
Gender			
Female	531	157 (29.56%)	-
Male	507	112 (22.09%)	0.850 (0.532–1.168)
Living Location			
Rural	49	13 (26.53%)	-
Town	297	59 (19.86%)	0.670 (−0.092–1.475)
Suburb	123	33 (26.83%)	0.940 (0.109–1.803)
City	569	164 (28.82%)	1.049 (0.312–1.832)
Lone Adult			
No	899	236 (26.25%)	-
Yes	139	33 (23.74%)	1.243 (0.749–1.722)
Children			
No	680	134 (19.70%)	-
Yes	358	135 (37.70%)	1.520 (1.169–1.87) **
Income			
−15.000 €/yr	218	60 (27.52%)	-
−28.000 €/yr	214	52 (24.30%)	0.906 (0.425–1.386)
−55.000 €/yr	212	58 (27.36%)	1.259 (0.771–1.749)
−75.000 €/yr	211	63 (29.85%)	1.099 (0.600–1.597)
+75.000 €/yr	183	36 (19.67%)	0.657 (0.102–1.203)
Pre-Existing Health Condition, Self			
No	869	216 (24.85%)	-
Yes	169	53 (31.36%)	1.587 (1.148–2.023) **
Pre-Existing Health Condition, Relatives			
No	811	197 (24.29%)	-
Yes	227	72 (31.71%)	1.219 (0.836–1.597)
Human Losses due to COVID-19			
No	888	219 (24.66%)	-
Yes	109	33 (30.27%)	1.207 (0.696–1.702)
Not Sure	41	17 (41.46%)	2.130 (1.386–2.886) **
Region			
Campania	227	70 (30.83%)	-
Lazio	234	57 (24.36%)	0.686 (0.223–1.146)
Lombardia	391	92 (23.53%)	0.519 (0.092–946) *
Veneto	186	50 (26.88%)	0.663 (0.168–1.154)
Personal Risk at 1 Month			
Low	269	29 (10.78%)	-
Moderate–Low	252	51 (20.24%)	1.782 (1.272–2.307) **
Moderate–High	261	69 (26.43%)	2.008 (1.519–2.518) ***
High	256	120 (46.87%)	2.815 (2.345–3.310) ***

Note. * $p < 0.05$; ** $p < 0.01$; *** $p < 0.001$ (adjusted controlling the false discovery rate [32]).

The rate of anxiety (GAD-7) in the overall sample was 21.59% (95% CI: 15.93%–20.72%), with no differences between regions ($\chi^2_{(3)} = 4.07$, $p = 0.25$) and with more women above the anxiety cut-off (11.75%, men: 6.45%; $\chi^2_{(1)} = 15.94$, $p < 0.001$). Depression (PHQ-9), with a rate of 21.4% (95% CI: 18.95%–24.03%), showed no differences between regions ($\chi^2_{(3)} = 0.29$, $p = 0.96$) but was significantly higher among women (12.52%), compared to men (8.86%; $\chi^2_{(1)} = 5.82$, $p = 0.016$).

The rate of anxiety and/or depression was 26.11 (95% CI: 23.48%–28.91%). No significant differences between regions were detected ($\chi^2_{(3)} = 1.78$ $p = 0.61$), whereas the gender difference was confirmed (women: 15.90%, men: 10.21%; $\chi^2_{(1)} = 13.37$, $p < 0.001$).

Using the ITQ scale, 25.92% of the sample was above the traumatic stress cut-off score (95% CI: 23.34%–28.77%). No difference was found between regions ($\chi^2_{(3)} = 4.30$, $p = 0.23$), while the gender effect was again significant (women: 15.11%, men: 10.88%; $\chi^2_{(1)} = 7.16$, $p = 0.007$). Finally, COVID-19 related anxiety was 18.30% overall (95% CI: 16.02%–20.82%). Regions showed a similar rate ($\chi^2_{(3)} = 2.66$, $p = 0.44$) whereas a gender difference was found (women: 12.14%, men: 6.17%; $\chi^2_{(1)} = 20–65$, $p < 0.001$).

We considered anxiety and/or depression, traumatic stress, and COVID-19-related Anxiety as dependent variables in three separate multiple logistic regressions (respectively, Tables 3–5). Figure 2 shows the plot of the odds ratio for the model of traumatic stress.

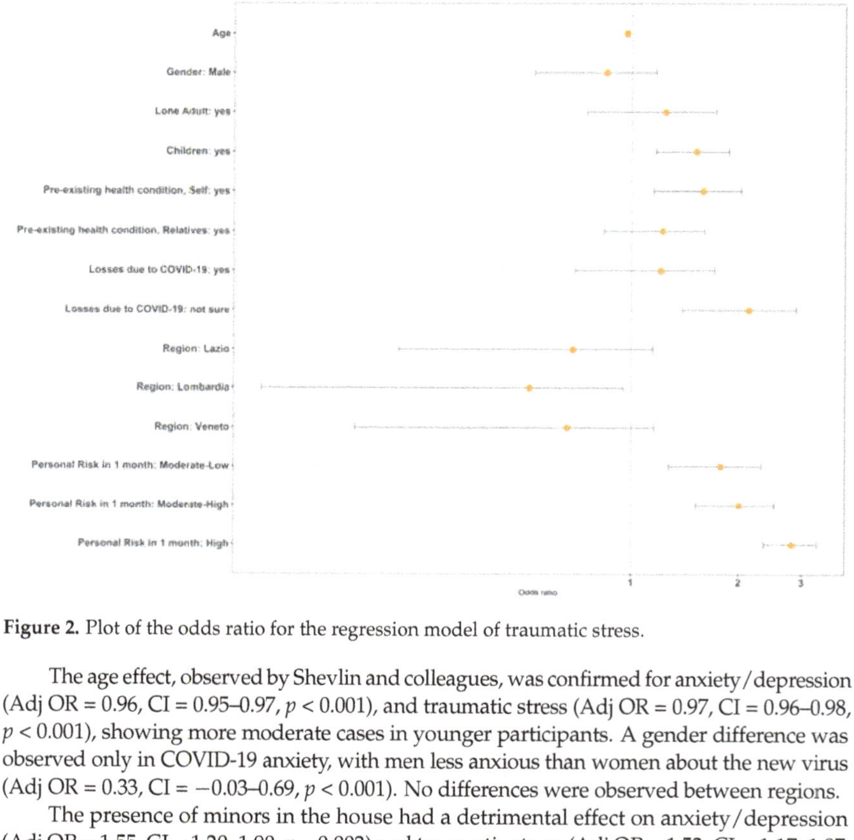

Figure 2. Plot of the odds ratio for the regression model of traumatic stress.

The age effect, observed by Shevlin and colleagues, was confirmed for anxiety/depression (Adj OR = 0.96, CI = 0.95–0.97, $p < 0.001$), and traumatic stress (Adj OR = 0.97, CI = 0.96–0.98, $p < 0.001$), showing more moderate cases in younger participants. A gender difference was observed only in COVID-19 anxiety, with men less anxious than women about the new virus (Adj OR = 0.33, CI = −0.03–0.69, $p < 0.001$). No differences were observed between regions.

The presence of minors in the house had a detrimental effect on anxiety/depression (Adj OR = 1.55, CI = 1.20–1.90, $p = 0.002$) and traumatic stress (Adj OR = 1.52, CI = 1.17–1.87, $p = 0.004$), as did the presence of pre-existing health conditions in others (anxiety/depression; Adj OR = 1.53, CI = 1.14–1.91, p = 0.006) and themselves (traumatic stress; Adj OR = 1.59, CI = 1.15–2.02; $p = 0.008$).

Interestingly, an increase in perceived risk to contract COVID-19 in the following four weeks had an effect on depression/anxiety (LR $\chi^2_{(3)} = 54.24$, $p < 0.001$), traumatic stress (LR $\chi^2_{(3)} = 66.14$, $p < 0.001$), and COVID-19 anxiety (LR $\chi^2_{(3)} = 84.74$, $p < 0.001$), mostly in the third and fourth quartile.

4. Discussion

This report provides an overview of the Italian C19CRP study to investigate the psycho-social impact of the COVID-19 pandemic in the adult population. We aimed at replicating the analyses of the first two UK studies [19,20]. First, we focused on replicating the analyses by Shevlin et al. [20] about the somatic symptomatology and their relationship with anxiety. All the psychosomatic subscales showed positive correlations both with COVID-19 anxiety and general anxiety (GAD-7) (Table 1). In our regression analysis, higher COVID-19 anxiety was associated with more severe somatic symptomatology (Model 1, Table 2). Compared to the UK, in Italy the somatic symptoms showed a more linear relation between COVID-19 related anxiety and the somatic subscales and total score.

In Model 2, the individuals with higher COVID-19 anxiety displayed more severe somatic symptoms. When considering covariates, gender, health problems, GAD-7 $\geq$ 10, and human losses due to COVID-19 had a significant effect on somatic symptomatology. No consistent effect of region or household income were observed, with the exception of higher levels of somatic symptoms registered in the Campania region followed by the Veneto region.

In a second part of the analysis, we replicated the approach by Shevlin et al. [19]. We conducted three logistic regressions with different outcomes: presence of moderate anxiety/depression; presence of moderate traumatic stress symptoms; presence of high COVID-19-related anxiety.

When the outcome variable was the presence of moderate symptoms of anxiety and/or depression (Table 3), the factors associated with moderate symptoms of anxiety and/or depression were younger age, having children, having pre-existing precarious health conditions, mourning for COVID-19 losses, and perceiving a moderate to high risk of contracting the COVID-19 virus within one month. Regarding the regions, no significant results emerged.

If COVID-19 related anxiety is used as outcome (Table 4), being male had a protective effect, whilst living in a town and perceiving a low-moderate to high risk of getting COVID-19 within one month were associated with higher COVID-19 related anxiety.

When considering as dependent variable the presence of traumatic stress symptoms above the clinical cut-off (Table 5), younger age, having children, having pre-existing precarious health conditions, thinking about having lost someone due to COVID-19, and perceiving a low-moderate/high risk of contracting COVID-19 within one month were associated with more severe traumatic stress symptoms. Regarding, regional differences, living in Lombardia compared to Campania was associated with lower traumatic stress symptoms.

Across these models, an increase in the perceived risk to contract COVID-19 in the following month was associated with depression/anxiety, traumatic stress, and COVID-19 anxiety.

Summarizing, these results are in line with those of the UK study about anxiety, depression, and traumatic stress [19]. The UK and Italian data identify factors associated with worst psychological health: being a woman, younger age, having children, pre-existing health issues of self or someone close, and the moderate to high perceived risk of contracting COVID-19 within one month. Unlike Italy, in the UK lower household incomes and having (had) the COVID-19 were associated with worst psychological health outcomes.

Despite the similar variables used in Italy and in UK, the comparison has to take into account the differences in data collection in regard to the evolution of the epidemic. The first wave in the UK was launched at the beginning of the lockdown while the Italian first wave took place two months after the end of the first lockdown, thus focusing on the adaptation to life with COVID-19. The literature shows that psychological distress symptoms can last for years [13,33–35] and data from Italy confirms that the levels of psychological distress are still considerable two months after the end of the lockdown. Moreover, the literature about other infectious respiratory diseases (IRDs) (e.g., H1N1, MERS, SARS) shows that it is important to monitor psychological health also after the peak [34–36].

Regarding the differences among Italian regions, results suggest that in July 2020 the Campania and Lazio regions suffered a strong psychological impact of the COVID-19 pandemic. In particular in Campania somatic symptoms were more severe, compared to Lombardia and Veneto (Model 2). COVID-19-related anxiety was higher in Campania than in Lombardia (Table 3). This is counterintuitive given that Lombardia had been affected earlier and to a larger extent. There were no significant regional differences between regions in term of anxiety/depression and traumatic stress. As for COVID-19 related anxiety, this result appears counterintuitive, because on the basis of the differences in infection rate and media coverage one may have expected Lombardia to have higher scores than other regions.

There are a few factors that may have affected these results. As always, findings should be contextualized with respect to the time and circumstances of data collection. Lombardia and Veneto experienced COVID-19 issues for a longer period and had more contagions than Lazio and Campania. Resilience may have increased over time [37]. Another possible explanation concerns the role of media in transmission of threatening information, when the data was gathered people in areas with higher infection rates (e.g., north vs. south; Italy vs. UK) already received more threatening information, thus increasing their risk perception but also their strength. A second factor is that in July 2020 attention was focused on the central and southern regions because of seasonal tourism. This may be related to the higher anxiety and somatic issues in the Campania region at this point in time. Finally, as discussed in the introduction, one reason both Lombardia and Veneto were included in our study is because they are geographically contiguous but had been differentially affected by the pandemic. If differences reflect geography rather than extent of the health emergency, these may also relate to differences in attitudes or approach to the survey in different regions. Further investigations are necessary to clarify similarities and differences between regions.

These findings from the Italian general population suggest that two months after the end of lockdown the psychological distress was still present, and it was high for certain categories of the population, such as women, the younger, and those with children. Our results are in line with the current literature about the impact of COVID-19 in Italy [10,38–40] and worldwide [41] both in clinical and general population as well. To date, most of studies focused on the negative consequences of COVID-19. An Italian study in general population showed the COVID-19 massive effects with rates of psychological issues ranging around 41.8% for high distress, 32.1% for high anxiety, and 7.6% for PTSD symptomatology linked to the virus [38]. Other Italian studies focused on the mental health of specific categories, as parents [40] at higher risk of experiencing distress and young adults [39] who showed an increase in internalizing and externalizing problems, anxiety, depression, somatic complaints, and aggressive and rule-breaking behaviors.

The anxiety related to COVID-19 was associated with somatic symptomatology beyond general anxiety, thus suggesting that COVID-related issues (e.g., degree and type of exposure to COVID-19) deserve clinical consideration. Moreover, results highlighted the socio-demographic risk-factors associated with more severe psychological outcomes. These indicators are useful to identify at-risk groups in the population which may need targeted psychological interventions. Noteworthy, the perceived risk of contracting COVID-19 was considerable in the population. This may influence a number of outcomes ranging from psychological issues, hygiene practices, precautionary behavior, attitudes toward vaccine, trust in institutions, and beliefs in conspiracy theories. Future studies will focus on the role of other aspects that are relevant for adaptation to living with the COVID-19 in the Italian context.

The limitations of this study should be acknowledged. An online administration methodology was used, this may bias the results because there may be differences between the paper-pen administration and the online version. Self-report measures were used, with potential well-known biases related to social desirability and misleading answers. When the study was launched in UK, a broad number of measurement tools were used, including already validated measures and tools developed ad hoc in order to reflect the current psychological issues related to the COVID-19 emergency. Given that the same measures were administered in Italy, socio-cultural differences suggest caution in interpretation and in the direct comparison [20].

An observational cross-sectional study design was used, whilst a longitudinal design would be desirable to monitor the evolution of the COVID-19 impact. Future waves of the survey would provide valuable information. Our analyses can only show association and not causation. Finally, despite the well-balanced sample, a larger sample would better capture and represent minorities.

The Italian C19PRC can contribute to ongoing research on health issues such as: the factors hindering resilience, the relationship between conspiracy theories and denial, the link between trust in Institutions and compliance, the burden and clinical characteristics of psychological issues, and the psychological heath of specific subgroups at higher risk for adverse psychophysical outcomes. Moreover, comparing results in a broader international framework allows cross-cultural comparisons. In addition to Italy and the UK, the international consortium now includes the Republic of Ireland (from March 2020), Spain (from April 2020), the United Arab Emirates (from April 2020), and Saudi Arabia (from May 2020).

Regarding the strengths of this research, respondents were recruited by using an online research panel with stratified quota sampling to ensure that the sample would meet the characteristics of sex, age, household income of the Italian population. Moreover, the C19PRC Study was designed drawing from studies that investigated previous IRDs epidemics and their psychosocial impact (e.g., H1N1, MERS, SARS). To do so, several factors were assessed to capture the complexity of the phenomenon from an ecological perspective, taking into account the demographic, social, political, economic, and psychological influences. The findings of this project may be useful to understand and manage the psycho-social implications of the COVID-19 pandemic.

5. Conclusions

The social and psychological impact of the COVID-19 pandemic is believed to be severe and long-lasting. Behavioral changes and psychological impact need to be studied over time and across countries. Therefore, the Italy COVID-19 study was modelled on the UK COVID-19 study. This paper is only a first summary of the Italian data. Analyzing and combining large datasets will allow a better understanding of the phenomena and in turn the development of measure to safeguard the psychological health of individuals.

Supplementary Materials: The following are available online at https://www.mdpi.com/2077-0383/10/1/52/s1, Table S1: Age; Table S2: Ethnicity (frequencies); Table S3: Level of education (frequencies); Table S4: Occupation (frequencies); Table S5: Income (frequencies); Table S6: Financial concern (1–10); Table S7: Religious belief (frequencies); Table S8: Marital status (frequencies); Table S9: Individual and family health issues (frequencies); Table S10: COVID-19-related anxiety (0–100); Table S11: Perceived personal risk in the next 30 days (0–100); Table S12: COVID-19 total participants tested and confirmed cases (participants, relatives, friends); Table S13: Patient health questionnaire (PHQ-15, range: 0–30); Table S14: PHQ-15, pain symptoms (range 0–6); Table S15: Gastrointestinal symptoms (range 0–8); Table S16: PHQ-15, cardiopulmonary symptoms (range 0–8); Table S17: PHQ-15, fatigue symptoms (range 0–4); Table S18: Patient Health Questionnaire-9 (PHQ-9, range 0–27); Table S19: *International Trauma Questionnaire* (ITQ, range 0–36); Table S20: Generalized Anxiety Disorder 7-item Scale (GAD-7, range 0–21).

Author Contributions: Study conceptualization: M.B. and the C19PRC-UK; survey translation and adaptation to Italian: all the authors; survey construction: G.B.; data collection: provided by Qualtrics via University of Roma and University of Padua; data cleaning: G.B.; data analysis: G.B. and U.G.; funding acquisition: G.V., F.L.; writing original draft: A.P. and G.B. (methods and results sections); writing—review and editing: M.B., G.V.; supervision: M.B., G.V., A.S. All authors have read and agreed to the published version of the manuscript.

Funding: This research was funded by the University "La Sapienza" of Roma and the Department of General Psychology of the University of Padua.

Institutional Review Board Statement: The study was conducted according to the guidelines of the Declaration of Helsinki, and approved by the Ethics Committee of the University of Padua (Area 17, protocol code 3818, date of approval 03/11/2020).

Informed Consent Statement: Informed consent was obtained from all subjects involved in the study.

Data Availability Statement: Data is contained within the article or supplementary material. The data presented in this study are available in [Supplementary material S1 and Tables S1–S20].

Acknowledgments: The present work was carried out within the scope of the research program "Dipartimenti di Eccellenza" from MIUR to the Department of General Psychology, University of Padua.

Conflicts of Interest: The authors declare no conflict of interest.

References

1. Baud, D.; Qi, X.; Nielsen-Saines, K.; Musso, D.; Pomar, L.; Favre, G. Real estimates of mortality following COVID-19 infection. *Lancet Infect. Dis.* **2020**, *20*, 773. [CrossRef]
2. Zaim, S.; Chong, J.H.; Sankaranarayanan, V.; Harky, A. COVID-19 and Multiorgan Response. *Curr. Probl. Cardiol.* **2020**, *45*, 100618. [CrossRef] [PubMed]
3. Funk, S.; Salathé, M.; Jansen, V.A.A. Modelling the influence of human behaviour on the spread of infectious diseases: A review. *J. R. Soc. Interface* **2010**, *7*, 1247–1256. [CrossRef] [PubMed]
4. Wind, T.R.; Rijkeboer, M.; Andersson, G.; Riper, H. The COVID-19 pandemic: The 'black swan' for mental health care and a turning point for e-health. *Internet Interv.* **2020**, *20*, 100317. [CrossRef]
5. Forte, G.; Favieri, F.; Tambelli, R.; Casagrande, M. The Enemy Which Sealed the World: Effects of COVID-19 Diffusion on the Psychological State of the Italian Population. *J. Clin. Med.* **2020**, *9*, 1802. [CrossRef]
6. Torales, J.; O'Higgins, M.; Castaldelli-Maia, J.M.; Ventriglio, A. The outbreak of COVID-19 coronavirus and its impact on global mental health. *Int. J. Soc. Psychiatry* **2020**, *66*, 317–320. [CrossRef]
7. Cellini, N.; Canale, N.; Mioni, G.; Costa, S. Changes in sleep pattern, sense of time and digital media use during COVID-19 lockdown in Italy. *J. Sleep Res.* **2020**, *29*, e13074. [CrossRef]
8. Cerami, C.; Santi, G.C.; Galandra, C.; Dodich, A.; Cappa, S.F.; Vecchi, T.; Crespi, C. COVID-19 Outbreak in Italy: Are We Ready for the Psychosocial and Economic Crisis? Baseline Findings from the Longitudinal PsyCovid Study. *SSRN Electron. J.* **2020**. [CrossRef]
9. Rossi, A.; Panzeri, A.; Pietrabissa, G.; Manzoni, G.M.; Castelnuovo, G.; Mannarini, S. The Anxiety-Buffer Hypothesis in the Time of COVID-19: When Self-Esteem Protects from the Impact of Lone-liness and Fear on Anxiety and Depression. *Front. Psychol.* **2020**, *11*, 2177. [CrossRef]
10. Rossi, R.; Socci, V.; Pacitti, F.; Di Lorenzo, G.; Di Marco, A.; Siracusano, A.; Rossi, A. Mental Health Outcomes Among Frontline and Second-Line Health Care Workers During the Coronavirus Disease 2019 (COVID-19) Pandemic in Italy. *JAMA Netw. Open* **2020**, *3*, e2010185. [CrossRef]
11. Yang, Y.; Li, W.; Zhang, Q.; Zhang, L.; Cheung, T.; Xiang, Y.-T. Mental health services for older adults in China during the COVID-19 outbreak. *Lancet Psychiatry* **2020**, *7*, e19. [CrossRef]
12. Yao, H.; Chen, J.-H.; Xu, Y.-F. Patients with mental health disorders in the COVID-19 epidemic. *Lancet Psychiatry* **2020**, *7*, e21. [CrossRef]
13. Kang, L.; Wang, G.; Liu, Z. Targeted long-term mental health services in Wuhan dealing with COVID-19. *Eur. Arch. Psychiatry Clin. Neurosci.* **2020**, 1–3. [CrossRef]
14. Gardner, P.J.; Moallef, P. Psychological impact on SARS survivors: Critical review of the English language literature. *Can. Psychol. Can.* **2015**, *56*, 123–135. [CrossRef]
15. Gatto, M.; Bertuzzo, E.; Mari, L.; Miccoli, S.; Carraro, L.; Casagrandi, R.; Rinaldo, A. Spread and dynamics of the COVID-19 epidemic in Italy: Effects of emergency containment measures. *Proc. Natl. Acad. Sci. USA* **2020**, *117*, 10484–10491. [CrossRef] [PubMed]
16. McBride, O.; Murphy, J.; Shevlin, M.; Gibson-Miller, J.; Hartman, T.K.; Hyland, P.; Levita, L.; Mason, L.; Martinez, A.P.; McKay, R.; et al. Monitoring the psychological, social, and economic impact of the COVID-19 pandemic in the population: Context, design and conduct of the longitudinal COVID-19 psychological research consortium (C19PRC) study. *Int. J. Methods Psychiatr. Res.* **2020**, e1861. [CrossRef] [PubMed]
17. Ministero della Salute, Istituto Superiore della Sanità. Report Monitoraggio Settimanale Covid-19: "Lieve Aumento dei Casi. Rispettare Misure di Precauzione". Available online: http://www.salute.gov.it/portale/nuovocoronavirus/dettaglioNotizieNuovoCoronavirus.jsp?menu=notizie&p=dalministero&id=4971 (accessed on 15 November 2020).
18. Berardi, C.; Antonini, M.; Genie, M.G.; Cotugno, G.; Lanteri, A.; Melia, A.; Paolucci, F. The COVID-19 pandemic in Italy: Policy and technology impact on health and non-health outcomes. *Health Policy Technol.* **2020**, *9*, 454–487. [CrossRef]
19. Shevlin, M.; McBride, O.; Murphy, J.; Miller, J.G.; Hartman, T.K.; Levita, L.; Mason, L.; Martinez, A.P.; McKay, R.; Stocks, T.V.A.; et al. Anxiety, depression, traumatic stress and COVID-19-related anxiety in the UK general population during the COVID-19 pandemic. *BJPsych Open* **2020**, *6*. [CrossRef]
20. Shevlin, M.; Nolan, E.; Owczarek, M.; McBride, O.; Murphy, J.; Gibson Miller, J.; Hartman, T.K.; Levita, L.; Mason, L.; Martinez, A.P.; et al. COVID-19-related anxiety predicts somatic symptoms in the UK population. *Br. J. Health Psychol.* **2020**, *25*, 875–882. [CrossRef]
21. R Core Team. *R: A Language and Environment for Statistical Computing*; R Foundation for Statistical Computing: Vienna, Austria, 2018.
22. Kroenke, K.; Spitzer, R.L.; Williams, J.B.W. The PHQ-15: Validity of a New Measure for Evaluating the Severity of Somatic Symptoms. *Psychosom. Med.* **2002**, *64*, 258–266. [CrossRef]

23. Cano-García, F.J.; Muñoz-Navarro, R.; Abad, A.S.; Moretti, L.S.; Medrano, L.A.; Ruiz-Rodríguez, P.; González-Blanch, C.; Moriana, J.A.; Cano-Vindel, A. Latent structure and factor invariance of somatic symptoms in the patient health questionnaire (PHQ-15). *J. Affect. Disord.* **2020**, *261*, 21–29. [CrossRef] [PubMed]
24. Kroenke, K.; Spitzer, R.L.; Williams, J.B.W. The Patient Health Questionnaire (PHQ-9)—Overview. *J. Gen. Intern. Med.* **2001**, *16*, 606–616. [CrossRef] [PubMed]
25. Manea, L.; Gilbody, S.; McMillan, D. Optimal cut-off score for diagnosing depression with the Patient Health Questionnaire (PHQ-9): A meta-analysis. *Can. Med Assoc. J.* **2011**, *184*, E191–E196. [CrossRef] [PubMed]
26. Spitzer, R.L.; Kroenke, K.; Williams, J.B.W.; Löwe, B. A Brief Measure for Assessing Generalized Anxiety Disorder: The GAD-7. *Arch. Intern. Med.* **2006**, *166*, 1092. [CrossRef]
27. Hinz, A.; Klein, A.M.; Brähler, E.; Glaesmer, H.; Luck, T.; Riedel-Heller, S.G.; Wirkner, K.; Hilbert, A. Psychometric evaluation of the Generalized Anxiety Disorder Screener GAD-7, based on a large German general population sample. *J. Affect. Disord.* **2017**, *210*, 338–344. [CrossRef]
28. Cloitre, M.; Shevlin, M.; Brewin, C.R.; Bisson, J.I.; Roberts, N.P.; Maercker, A.; Karatzias, T.; Hyland, P. The International Trauma Questionnaire: Development of a self-report measure of ICD-11 PTSD and com-plex PTSD. *Acta Psychiatr. Scand.* **2018**, *138*, 536–546. [CrossRef]
29. World Health Organization. International Classification of Diseases for Mortality and Morbidity Statistics (11th Revision, 2018). Available online: https://icd.who.int/browse11/l-m/en (accessed on 15 November 2020).
30. Ben-Ezra, M.; Karatzias, T.; Hyland, P.; Brewin, C.R.; Cloitre, M.; Bisson, J.I.; Roberts, N.P.; Lueger-Schuster, B.; Shevlin, M. Posttraumatic stress disorder (PTSD) and complex PTSD (CPTSD) as per ICD-11 proposals: A population study in Israel. *Depress. Anxiety* **2018**, *35*, 264–274. [CrossRef]
31. Cloitre, M.; Hyland, P.; Bisson, J.I.; Brewin, C.R.; Roberts, N.P.; Karatzias, T.; Shevlin, M. ICD-11 Posttraumatic Stress Disorder and Complex Posttraumatic Stress Disorder in the United States: A Population-Based Study. *J. Trauma. Stress* **2019**, *32*, 833–842. [CrossRef]
32. Benjamini, Y.; Hochberg, Y. Controlling the false discovery rate: A practical and powerful approach to multiple testing. *J. R. Stat. Soc. Ser. B Stat. Methodol.* **1995**, *57*, 289–300. [CrossRef]
33. Bonanno, G.A.; Ho, S.M.Y.; Chan, J.C.K.; Kwong, R.S.Y.; Cheung, C.K.Y.; Wong, C.P.Y.; Wong, V.C.W. Psychological resilience and dysfunction among hospitalized survivors of the SARS epidemic in Hong Kong: A latent class approach. *Health Psychol.* **2008**, *27*, 659–667. [CrossRef]
34. Chen, J.; Wu, J.; Hao, S.; Yang, M.; Lu, X.; Chen, X.; Li, L. Long term outcomes in survivors of epidemic Influenza A (H7N9) virus infection. *Sci. Rep.* **2017**, *7*, 1–8. [CrossRef] [PubMed]
35. Lee, A.M.; Wong, J.G.W.S.; McAlonan, G.M.; Cheung, V.; Cheung, C.; Sham, P.C.; Chu, C.-M.; Wong, P.-C.; Tsang, K.W.T.; Chua, S.E. Stress and Psychological Distress among SARS Survivors 1 Year after the Outbreak. *Can. J. Psychiatry* **2007**, *52*, 233–240. [CrossRef] [PubMed]
36. Esterwood, E.; Saeed, S.A. Past Epidemics, Natural Disasters, COVID19, and Mental Health: Learning from History as we Deal with the Present and Prepare for the Future. *Psychiatr. Q.* **2020**, *91*, 1121–1133. [CrossRef] [PubMed]
37. Seery, M.D.; Holman, E.A.; Silver, R.C. Whatever does not kill us: Cumulative lifetime adversity, vulnerability, and resilience. *J. Pers. Soc. Psychol.* **2010**, *99*, 1025–1041. [CrossRef]
38. Casagrande, M.; Favieri, F.; Tambelli, R.; Forte, G. The enemy who sealed the world: Effects quarantine due to the COVID-19 on sleep quality, anxiety, and psychological distress in the Italian population. *Sleep Med.* **2020**, *75*, 12–20. [CrossRef]
39. Parola, A.; Rossi, A.; Tessitore, F.; Troisi, G.; Mannarini, S. Mental Health through the COVID-19 Quarantine: A Growth Curve Analysis on Italian Young Adults. *Front. Psychol.* **2020**, *11*, 567484. [CrossRef]
40. Spinelli, M.; Lionetti, F.; Pastore, M.; Fasolo, M. Parents and Children Facing the COVID-19 Outbreak in Italy. *SSRN Electron. J.* **2020**. [CrossRef]
41. Xiong, J.; Lipsitz, O.; Nasri, F.; Lui, L.M.W.; Gill, H.; Phan, L.; Chen-Li, D.; Iacobucci, M.; Ho, R.; Majeed, A.; et al. Impact of COVID-19 pandemic on mental health in the general population: A systematic review. *J. Affect. Disord.* **2020**, *277*, 55–64. [CrossRef]

Journal of
Clinical Medicine

MDPI

Article

The Impact of COVID-19 Pandemic and Lockdown Measures on Quality of Life among Italian General Population

Maria Stella Epifanio [1], Federica Andrei [2], Giacomo Mancini [3,*], Francesca Agostini [2], Marco Andrea Piombo [2], Vittoria Spicuzza [1], Martina Riolo [1], Gioacchino Lavanco [1], Elena Trombini [2] and Sabina La Grutta [1]

[1] Department of Psychology, Educational Science and Human Movement, University of Palermo, 90128 Palermo, Italy; mariastella.epifanio@unipa.it (M.S.E.); vittoriaspicuzza@hotmail.it (V.S.); martina.riolo93@gmail.com (M.R.); gioacchino.lavanco@unipa.it (G.L.); sabina.lagrutta@unipa.it (S.L.G.)
[2] Department of Psychology "Renzo Canestrari", Alma Mater Studiorum, University of Bologna, 40127 Bologna, Italy; federica.andrei2@unibo.it (F.A.); f.agostini@unibo.it (F.A.); marcoandrea.piombo2@unibo.it (M.A.P.); elena.trombini@unibo.it (E.T.)
[3] Department of Education Studies "Giovanni Maria Bertin", Alma Mater Studiorum, University of Bologna, 40126 Bologna, Italy
* Correspondence: giacomo.mancini7@unibo.it; Tel.: +39-051-2091490

Abstract: The COVID-19 pandemic that has hit the world in the year 2020 has put a strain on our ability to cope with events and revolutionized our daily habits. On 9 March, Italy was forced to lockdown to prevent the spread of the infection, with measures including the mandatory closure of schools and nonessential activities, travel restrictions, and the obligation to spend entire weeks in the same physical space. The aim of this study was to assess the impact of the COVID-19 pandemic and lockdown measures on quality of life (QoL) in a large Italian sample, in order to investigate possible differences in QoL levels related to both demographic and pandemic-specific variables. A total of 2251 Italian adults (1665 women, mainly young and middle adults) were recruited via a snowball sampling strategy. Participants were requested to answer to an online survey, which included demographic and COVID-related information items, and the World Health Organization Quality of Life BREF questionnaire (WHOQOL-BREF). The results showed statistically significant differences in QoL depending on a number of variables, including sex, area of residence in Italy, and being diagnosed with a medical/psychiatric condition. To our knowledge, this is the first study to assess QoL during COVID-19 pandemic in Italy, therefore the present findings can offer guidelines regarding which social groups are more vulnerable of a decline in QoL and would benefit of psychological interventions.

Keywords: COVID-19; Quality of Life; pandemic; lockdown; gender differences; WHOQOL-BREF; health; health psychology; general population; Italy

Citation: Epifanio, M.S.; Andrei, F.; Mancini, G.; Agostini, F.; Piombo, M.A.; Spicuzza, V.; Riolo, M.; Lavanco, G.; Trombini, E.; La Grutta, S. The Impact of COVID-19 Pandemic and Lockdown Measures on Quality of Life among Italian General Population. *J. Clin. Med.* **2021**, *10*, 289. https://doi.org/10.3390/jcm10020289

Received: 24 December 2020
Accepted: 11 January 2021
Published: 14 January 2021

1. Introduction

During pandemics, the population's psychological responses to infection play an important role in both the spreading and containment of the disease, influencing the extent to which psychological distress and social disorder occur [1]. This may be partly explained by those emotional states that frequently mark pandemics, such as uncertainty, confusion, and sense of urgency [2]. In the early stages of a pandemic, feelings of uncertainty prevail, due to the fear of becoming infected and not having the right information about the best methods of prevention and management [3–5]. Furthermore, pandemics are associated with various psychosocial stressors, including health threats to oneself and loved ones; significant changes in daily routine, such as restriction in the physical activity behavior (PA) [6–8]; separation from family and friends; shortages of food and medicine; wage loss; social isolation due to quarantine or other social distancing measures; and school closures [9]. Serious economic difficulties can also occur if a family's primary wage earner is unable to work due to illness [1].

For these reasons, the effects of the current COVID-19 pandemic would be more pronounced, more widespread, and longer-lasting than the purely somatic effects of infection, with serious impairment on peoples' actual and perceived quality of life (QoL). The COVID-19 pandemic that has hit the world in the last 12 months has indeed put a strain on our ability to cope with events and revolutionized our daily habits. In Italy, a state of emergency was declared by the Italian government on 31 January 2020 [10], when two Chinese tourists in Rome tested positive for the SARS-CoV-2. The first case in Italy was recorded in February 2020, and the epidemic rapidly spread, reaching 220 infections on 24 February [11]. The government responded by implementing prevention measures and infection control on 11 March, when the number of infections reached 12,462 and the total deaths were 827. Despite the fact that the infection spread differently between the northern and southern regions of Italy, the increasingly restrictive containment measures led to a total lockdown throughout the country (11 March–3 May 2020). Lockdown measures included the mandatory closure of schools and nonessential commercial activities and industries, in addition to travel restrictions both inside and outside the country. After 3 May, the number of infections dropped below 1221 new cases and many restrictions were gradually eased [12]. On 3 June, freedom of movement across regions and European countries was restored and other nonessential activities reopened.

Most of the early studies on the psychological impact of COVID-19, published at the beginning of the pandemic, have compared the current situation with the SARS epidemic in 2003 [13–16]. These studies highlighted the risk for people with suspected or certain infections to experience uncontrolled fear over a long period, not only in relation to the disease but also to the condition of quarantine. During the previous SARS epidemic, a peak of incidence of many psychiatric disorders, such as depression, anxiety, panic attacks, psychomotorial agitation, and suicide, had been reported. Kwek and colleagues [17] brought out the long-term consequences of the pandemic on health and claimed that SARS impaired significantly both QoL and mental functioning at three months from the acute episode. A small number of additional studies conducted during a previous pandemic also showed the consequences of the pandemic on psychological well-being of infected people, highlighting various factors associated with greater psychological distress, including sociodemographic variables, such as being a woman and middle aged adult or having a lower level of education [3,5]. Moreover, the majority of the studies recently reviewed by Brooks and co-workers [18] reported on the negative psychological effects of quarantine, including symptoms of post-traumatic stress, confusion, and anger. Examples of relevant stressors were a long quarantine period, fear of infection, frustration, boredom, inadequate supplies of personal security systems, inadequate information, financial losses, and social stigma.

This evidence has been further supported by an increasing number of publications on mental health demonstrating higher levels of psychological distress among the population during COVID-19 pandemic [19–22]. For instance, a large Italian study by Rossi and colleagues [19] showed an increase in anxiety and depressive symptoms for people who had lived four weeks of lockdown, and found 37% of the sample with post-traumatic stress symptoms, whereby female gender and younger age were risk factors for worse mental health.

However, while the attention on the consequences of COVID-19 over mental health has been increasing, there is a limited number of international studies on its effects over QoL. Among already published studies, Pieh and co-workers [23] found an average psychological score of the World Health Organization Quality of Life BREF (WHOQOL-BREF) questionnaire significantly lower compared to a study published in 2015 [24]; the study also reported lower scores for younger adults, women, individuals without work, and those with low income. Horesh, Kapel Lev-Ari, and Hasson-Ohayon [25] also reported higher stress levels and lower QoL for women, younger participants, and for people with pre-existing chronic illness. However, to our knowledge, there have been no studies investigating QoL in Italian populations during the COVID-19 pandemic [23,25–28].

In addition to sociodemographic variables, it has been suggested that other factors might influence QoL during pandemics, such as the difficulty in accessing healthcare services [26,27] and social isolation [29]. Van Ballegooijen and colleagues [27] described considerable levels of stress, a lower QoL, and concerns about access to healthcare during the first eight weeks of the COVID-19 lockdown in the Netherlands and Belgium. With respect to the difficulty in accessing healthcare, a Chinese study showed that the relevant index of QoL decreased with increasing age, due to the presence of chronic diseases in this segment of the population [26]. Regarding social isolation, a British study reported lower levels of wellbeing and QoL for people who felt more isolated than usual during lockdown, whereas the level of perceived social support showed significant positive correlations with QoL [29]. Another study from a Chinese sample showed relatively lower levels of physical and psychological domains of QoL but, interestingly, not in the social and environmental domains [28].

These studies highlight that the pandemic situation, including the measures put in place to contain it, involves various aspects of life and health. Monitoring the state of health requires the measurement of indicators capable of grasping the many subjective and functional dimensions of well-being and QoL. Particularly, the assessment of QoL is increasingly often considered as an integral part of any intervention that aims to promote health and wellness. QoL is actually viewed as an overall and multidimensional indicator of general wellbeing. Indeed, the WHO defines QoL as "an individual's perception of their position in life in the context of the culture and value systems in which they live, and in relation to their goals, expectations, standards and concern" (p. 1405) [30]. In measuring QoL, the WHOQOL group takes the subjective dimension strongly into account [31]. The ability to feel a certain well-being, regardless of living conditions, is a subjective variable directly related to other dimensions: genetic variables, personality, and life events. It is a set of factors dynamically interacting with each other in a different way through the life span and across different cultures. QoL is not a simple and linear entity, it is indeed a complex, multidimensional construct that, according to the WHO, includes six domains: physical, psychological, social, level of independence, environment, and spirituality/religions/personal beliefs.

The present study aimed to explore the impact that both the COVID-19 emergency and the resulting restrictive measures had on the perception of QoL among Italian general adult population. Additionally, this study aimed to investigate possible differences in QoL depending on sociodemographic variables, such as sex, age, marital status, occupational status, level of education, and area of residence in Italy, as well as specific factors related to the COVID-19 outbreak (e.g., changes in employment status and location, family members or friends infected with Sars-Cov-2, adherence to control and precautions measures, household size during COVID-19 outbreak). Particular reference will be given to the physical, psychological, social, and environmental domains of QoL as measured by the WHOQOL-BREF.

2. Materials and Methods

2.1. Procedure

An online cross-sectional survey was performed with Qualtrics® (Qualtrics, Provo, UT, USA) Survey Platform. Such a data collection strategy was chosen as it allowed us to reach as many voluntary participants as possible in a phase of forced social distancing. The survey started after 7 weeks of quarantine in Italy (25 April 2020) and was performed for about 6 weeks, until the end of lockdown measures (2 June 2020). This measurement point was selected because significant changes in individuals' QoL need some time to be perceived by the person. Moreover, this timeframe potentially allowed the population to adjust to the new situation. The sample was recruited via a snowball sampling strategy. A link to Qualtrics questionnaires were sent via e-mail, social networks (Facebook and WhatsApp), and official working platforms (website of the University of Palermo, Italy). The link was shared with personal contacts of the research group members, who in turn passed the survey to their friends and acquaintances. A brief presentation informed the participants about the aims of the study and electronic informed consent, assuring maximum confidentiality in the handling and analysis of the responses, was requested from each participant before starting the investigation. The survey took approximately 30 min to complete. Participation was voluntary and free of charge. To guarantee anonymity, no personal data, which could allow the identification of participants, were collected. Participants could withdraw from the study at any time without providing any justification, and the data were not saved. Only the questionnaire data with a complete set of answers by respondents were considered. The study was conducted in accordance with the Declaration of Helsinki and was approved by the Bioethics Committee of the University of Palermo (n. 4/2020).

2.2. Participants

Italian individuals over 18 years of age who were living in Italy at the time of quarantine were eligible for participation to data collection. The recruited sample size through the online survey included 2332 Italian adults, with an attrition rate of approximately 20%. Of 2332 who completed the survey 71 respondents were excluded because of missing demographic data, while a further 10 participants were excluded as they were residents outside Italy at the time of data collection. Our final sample comprised 2251 respondents. Demographic characteristics of the study sample are presented in Table 1.

Table 1. Frequencies (%) of the main demographic characteristics for men, women, and global sample.

Sample Characteristics	Men (n = 586)	Women (n = 1665)	Total (n = 2251)	p Value
Age range (years)				0.022
18–34	247 (42.2)	691 (41.6)	938 (41.7)	
35–64	290 (49.5)	885 (53.1)	1175 (52.2)	
≥65	49 (8.3)	89 (5.3)	138 (6.1)	
Area of residence in Italy				0.087
North	244 (41.6)	686 (41.2)	930 (41.3)	
Center	19 (3.3)	92 (5.5)	111 (4.9)	
South	323 (55.1)	887 (53.3)	1210 (53.8)	
Level of education [a]				0.001
Secondary school	37 (6.3)	57 (3.4)	94 (4.2)	
High school	249 (42.5)	578 (34.7)	827 (36.7)	
University	211 (36.0)	722 (43.4)	933 (41.4)	
Post-graduate	72 (12.3)	247 (14.8)	319 (14.2)	
Marital status				0.573
Single	269 (45.9)	783 (47.2)	1052 (46.7)	
Married	259 (44.2)	721 (32.0)	980 (43.5)	
Divorced/separated	49 (8.4)	127 (7.7)	176 (7.9)	
Widowed	9 (1.5)	34 (2.1)	43 (1.9)	
Employment status				0.000
Student	114 (19.4)	341 (20.5)	455 (20.2)	
Employed	389 (66.4)	1013 (60.8)	1402 (62.3)	
Unemployed	38 (6.5)	216 (13.0)	254 (11.3)	
Retired	45 (7.7)	95 (5.7)	140 (6.2)	
Currently diagnosed with psychiatric condition				0.012
Yes	23 (3.9)	113 (6.8)	136 (6.1)	
No	563 (96.1)	1552 (93.2)	2115 (93.9)	
Currently diagnosed with medical condition				0.239
Yes	112 (19.1)	282 (16.9)	394 (17.5)	
No	474 (80.9)	1383 (83.1)	1857 (82.5)	

[a] Global sample size for this variable was 2173, as 61 women and 17 men did not report data on their education level.

2.3. Measures

2.3.1. Demographic and COVID-Related Information Questionnaire

An ad hoc questionnaire was created to collect demographic data (such as sex, age, marital status, education level, occupational status, region of residence in Italy, and presence of medical and psychiatric diagnosis) and COVID-related information (i.e., changes in employment status and location, number of people residing with the respondent during quarantine, adherence to control measures, knowing someone who tested positive for COVID-19).

2.3.2. World Health Organization Quality of Life BREF Assessment Instrument (WHOQOL-BREF)

The Italian version of the WHOQOL-BREF was used to assess QoL [32,33]. The WHOQOL-BREF is a short version of the WHOQOL-100, developed by the WHO for use in situations in which time is restricted and respondent burden must be minimized, such as in epidemiological surveys. It is a 26 items self-rating questionnaire, and a person-centered instrument, giving scores to overall QoL and its four dimensions: physical health (e.g., sleep quality, energy and tiredness), psychological health (e.g., positive emotion, self-esteem, personal beliefs), social relationships (e.g., social support and sexual activity), and environment (e.g., climate, transportation, and healthcare assistance). Items ask respondents to rate their QoL during the last two weeks and each of them are rated on a 5-point Likert scale. Similarly to the Italian validation study and to the original version of the questionnaire [29,30], internal consistencies for the WHOQOL-BREF were satisfactory, with Cronbach's alpha values ranging from 0.57 for social relationships and 0.79 for physical health. Reliability for the global score of the WHOQOL-BREF was good (Cronbach's alpha = 0.88).

2.4. Statistical Analyses

Descriptive statistics and frequency analysis were used to investigate demographic characteristics and COVID-related information. Comparisons on these variables by sex (men vs. women) and age range (young, middle, and older adults) were performed using Pearson's χ^2 test and Student's t test for independent samples for nominal and continuous demographic variables, respectively.

Analysis of variance (ANOVA) was used to analyze the difference in respondents' levels of QoL at the global score of the WHOQOL-BREF, while multivariate analysis of variance (MANOVA) was employed to analyze the differences in levels of QoL at domain scores of the WHOQOL-BREF. Statistical analyses were performed using SPSS (version 25) for Windows [34]. In all statistical tests, a p value of less than 0.05 was considered significant.

3. Results

3.1. Demographic Characteristics

As Table 1 shows, the final sample comprised 2251 participants (74% females) collected mainly from the north (41.3%) and south (53.8%) regions of Italy. Respondents were mostly young (age 18–34) and middle (age 35–64) aged adults (41.7% and 52.2% of the entire sample, respectively), while the group of older adults (age 65 and older) was smaller (6.1% of the total sample). Most of them had a university degree (41.2%) or a high school diploma (36.7%), were employed (62.3%), and either single (46.7%) or married (43.5%). With respect to university students (20.2% of the sample), they were enrolled in either social sciences and humanities (53.2%), biotechnical sciences (29.3%), and medical (14.2%) study programs, while a few students did not report their major (3.3%).

With regards to comparisons between men and women in demographic variables, we found statistically significant sex differences in employment status ($\chi^2 = 21.25$, $p < 0.001$), level of education ($\chi^2 = 23.34$, $p = 0.001$), and age range ($\chi^2 = 7.59$, $p = 0.022$). Particularly, women were less often employed than men, so much so that 80% of the unemployed respondents were women, although with higher levels of education (see Table 1). In fact, women reported more often than men to have a university degree (43.4% vs. 36.0% for women and men, respectively) or a postgraduate title (such as PhD; 14.8% vs. 12.3% for women and men, respectively). Moreover, with regards to age distribution, female respondents were mainly from the group of middle adults, while fewer of them fell into the older adults group compared to men.

Table 1 reports that 136 respondents (6.1%) had a psychiatric diagnosis at the time of data collection, with the highest prevalence in women compared to men ($\chi^2 = 6.25$, $p = 0.012$). Within this group, 47.1% individuals have been diagnosed with anxiety disorders, 41.2% with mood disorders, while the remaining 11.7% with other conditions (e.g., eating and personality disorders).

Yet, 394 participants (17.5%) reported to be in treatment for a medical condition, mainly for circulatory system diseases (24.1%), such as hypertension and heart failure, and endocrine system diseases (19%), such as diabetes and hypothyroidism. No significant differences in the distribution between men and women were detected ($\chi^2 = 1.38$, $p = 0.239$).

3.2. COVID-Related Information

Table 2 shows the results obtained from epidemic-related information. Most participants had their job/study activity moved at home (50.9%), didn't have any family members or friends diagnosed with COVID-19 (93.6%), were always adherent to control and precautions measures against COVID-19 (62.9%), and had a household size of mainly three to four persons (55.3%).

Concerning sex differences among these variables, we found a significantly different distribution of answers between men and women in the adherence to control and precautions measures against COVID-19 ($\chi^2 = 10.28$, $p = 0.006$). Particularly, most women (64.4%) reported to be more inclined to always adhere to control and precautions measures against COVID-19, rather than often or not that much, compared to men (58.8%). We did not find any significant sex difference with regards to the distribution of changes in job/study activity ($\chi^2 = 5.12$, $p = 0.163$), presence of family members or friends infected by COVID-19 ($\chi^2 = 1.25$, $p = 0.263$), and household size during the outbreak of the disease ($\chi^2 = 6.28$, $p = 0.099$).

With respect to age range differences, we found a significantly different distribution of answers in the variables changes in job/study activity ($\chi^2 = 74.92$, $p < 0.001$) and household size during the outbreak of the disease ($\chi^2 = 80.45$, $p < 0.001$). Particularly, young (50.4%) and middle (53.9%) adults reported to have mainly their job activity moved at home, as well as a household size of three to four persons during lockdown (58.7% and 55.0% for young and middle adults, respectively), compared to older adults who reported no changes in job or job moved at home to the same extent (29% for both), and a house composition of mainly two persons (44.2%). No significant age differences in the adherence to control and precautions measures against COVID-19 ($\chi^2 = 1.57$, $p = 0.815$), nor in the presence of family members or friends infected by COVID-19 ($\chi^2 = 3.62$, $p = 0.163$), were detected.

3.3. Quality of Life during the Outbreak of COVID-19

Table 3 presents means and standard deviations for WHOQOL-BREF global and domain scores. The overall average score at the WHOQOL-BREF for our sample was 54.48 ($SD = 7.77$). Analyses performed on the single items, showed that the item with the lowest scores was 14 (about the use of spare time), given that 932 (41.4%) participants reported to have little or no time for leisure at the time of data collection; said item refers to the domain environment of the WHOQOL-BREF. Regarding the other three domains of the WHOQOL, items with lowest scores were: item 15 for the physical domain, as 1019 (45.3%) participants reported little or no possibility to do physical activity; item 5 for the psychological domain, with 712 (31.6%) respondents reporting that they were not enjoying their lives at the time of data collection; and item 21 for social relationships, as 843 (37.4%) respondents reported that they were little or not at all satisfied with their sexual life.

Table 2. Frequencies (%) of COVID-related information for men, women, and global sample by age range.

	Men				Women				Global Sample			
Sample Characteristics	**Young Adults (*n* = 247)**	**Middle Adults (*n* = 290)**	**Older Adults (*n* = 49)**	**Total (*n* = 586)**	**Young Adults (*n* = 691)**	**Middle Adults (*n* = 885)**	**Older Adults (*n* = 89)**	**Total (*n* = 1665)**	**Young Adults (*n* = 938)**	**Middle Adults (*n* = 1175)**	**Older Adults (*n* = 138)**	**Total (*n* = 2251)**
Changes in employment status and location												
No changes	62 (25.1)	62 (21.4)	15 (30.6)	139 (23.7)	166 (24.0)	165 (18.6)	25 (28.1)	356 (21.3)	228 (24.3)	227 (19.3)	40 (29.0)	495 (22.0)
Job/study activity moved at home	118 (47.8)	154 (53.1)	16 (32.6)	288 (49.1)	355 (51.4)	478 (54.0)	24 (27.0)	857 (51.5)	473 (50.4)	632 (53.8)	40 (29.0)	1145 (50.9)
Job/study activity suspended	44 (17.8)	51 (17.6)	7 (14.3)	102 (17.4)	110 (15.9)	132 (14.9)	9 (10.1)	251 (15.1)	154 (16.4)	183 (15.6)	16 (11.6)	353 (15.7)
Unemployed prior to COVID-19	23 (9.3)	23 (7.9)	11 (22.5)	57 (9.8)	60 (8.7)	110 (12.5)	31 (34.8)	201 (12.1)	83 (8.9)	133 (11.3)	42 (30.4)	258 (11.4)
Family member or friend infected with Sars-Cov-2												
Yes	13 (5.3)	20 (6.9)	0 (0)	33 (5.6)	44 (6.4)	67 (7.6)	5 (5.6)	116 (7.0)	57 (6.1)	87 (7.4)	5 (3.6)	145 (6.4)
No	234 (94.7)	270 (93.1)	49 (100)	553 (94.4)	647 (93.6)	818 (92.4)	84 (94.4)	1549 (93.0)	881 (93.9)	1088 (92.6)	133 (96.4)	2106 (93.6)
Adherence to the precautions and control measures												
Always	140 (56.7)	170 (58.6)	31 (63.3)	341 (58.2)	445 (64.4)	570 (64.4)	57 (64.1)	1072 (64.4)	585 (62.4)	740 (63.0)	88 (63.8)	1413 (62.9)
Often	94 (38.1)	100 (34.5)	15 (30.6)	209 (35.7)	193 (27.9)	260 (29.4)	23 (25.8)	476 (28.6)	287 (30.6)	360 (30.6)	38 (27.5)	685 (30.2)
Not that much	13 (5.2)	20 (6.9)	3 (6.1)	36 (6.1)	53 (7.7)	55 (6.2)	9 (10.1)	117 (7.0)	66 (7.0)	75 (6.4)	12 (8.7)	153 (6.9)
Household size during COVID-19 outbreak												
1 person	25 (10.0)	42 (14.5)	7 (14.3)	74 (12.6)	38 (5.5)	95 (10.7)	19 (21.3)	152 (9.1)	63 (6.7)	137 (11.7)	26 (18.8)	226 (10.0)
2 persons	52 (21.1)	69 (23.8)	22 (44.9)	143 (24.4)	152 (22.0)	228 (25.8)	39 (43.8)	419 (25.2)	204 (21.8)	297 (25.3)	61 (44.2)	562 (25.0)
3–4 persons	137 (55.5)	155 (53.4)	18 (36.7)	310 (52.9)	414 (60.0)	492 (55.6)	28 (31.5)	934 (56.1)	551 (58.7)	647 (55.0)	46 (33.3)	1244 (55.3)
5 persons or more	33 (13.4)	24 (8.3)	2 (4.1)	59 (10.1)	87 (12.5)	70 (7.9)	3 (3.4)	160 (9.6)	120 (12.8)	94 (8.0)	5 (3.7)	219 (9.7)

3.3.1. Differences in Sex and Age Range

Results of ANOVA analyses showed that WHOQOL global scores differed between male and female participants (F (1, 2250) = 9.34, p = 0.002), with women reaching lower scores compared to men. No significant differences were found for age range (F (2, 2250) = 1.91, p = 0.148). About the factor scores of the WHOQOL, two separate MANOVAs were run by taking into account sex and age range as the only between-subject factor. The model where sex was considered showed a significant main effect for this variable (F (1, 2250) = 13.51, p < 0.001); between-subject tests showed significant differences between men and women in the areas of physical (F (1, 2250) = 17.58, p < 0.001), psychological (F (1, 2250) = 25.85, p < 0.001), and environmental (F (1, 2250) = 7.00, p = 0.008) domains. As can be seen in Table 3, women reported overall worse psychological, physical, and environmental QoL during the pandemic compared to men.

Age range also resulted in a significant between-subject factor for the detection of differences across WHOQOL-BREF domains (F (1, 2250) = 11.93, p < 0.001). About this, results showed significant differences among groups in the psychological (F (2, 2251) = 11.69, p < 0.001) and environmental (F (2, 2251) = 11.96, p < 0.001) domains. Particularly, young adults reported the lowest levels of psychological QoL, which were significantly lower compared to both middle (p < 0.001) and older (p = 0.019) adults, as attested by Bonferroni's post hoc comparisons. As shown by Table 3, middle adults had the lowest scores at the environment domain compared to both young (p < 0.001) and older (p = 0.005) adults. No significant differences emerged in both physical (F (2, 2251) = 0.39, p = 0.675) and social relationship (F (2, 2251) = 1.82, p = 0.161) domains.

3.3.2. Differences in Demographic and COVID-Related Variables

The effects of 10 further relevant variables (i.e., area of residence in Italy, level of education, marital status, employment status, currently diagnosed with psychiatric condition, currently diagnosed with medical condition, changes in employment status and location, family member or friend infected with Sars-Cov-2, adherence to the precautions and control measures, household size during COVID outbreak) were tested over WHOQOL global and domain scores. In light of the results on sex and age range, sex was controlled in all additional ANOVAs, while both sex and age in all MANOVA models. Table 4 presents means, standard deviations and statistics of ANOVA and MANOVA analyses. Overall, no interaction term was significant, therefore statistics were not reported within the Table. As reported by Table 4, results show that seven out of ten variables significantly differed in WHOQOL global score (global level of QoL), while five other WHOQOL factor scores did not (physical, psychological, environmental health, and social relationships; p < 0.05). Overall, three variables, namely marital status, family member or friend infected with Sars-Cov-2, and household size during COVID outbreak, had no significant effect over both global and factor scores of the WHOQOL (ps = n.s.).

Regarding WHOQOL global score, results from Table 4 show that individuals with the poorest QoL during the outbreak of the disease (as their global score of the WHOQOL was significantly lower compared to the other groups) had the following characteristics: lived in the South of Italy, had lower education levels (secondary or high school diploma), were unemployed or university students, had been diagnosed with psychiatric and medical syndromes, had their job activity suspended, and did not comply with the restriction measures to contrast COVID-19 pandemic.

Table 3. Means ± standard deviations of quality of life indicators for all respondents during the outbreak of COVID-19 (N = 2251) by sex and age range.

	Young Adults			Middle Adults			Older Adults			Global Sample		
Variables	**Women (*n* = 691)**	**Men (*n* = 247)**	**Total (*N* = 938)**	**Women (*n* = 885)**	**Men (*n* = 290)**	**Total (*N* = 1175)**	**Women (*n* = 89)**	**Men (*n* = 49)**	**Total (*N* = 138)**	**Women (*n* = 1665)**	**Men (*n* = 586)**	**Total (*n* = 2251)**
WHOQOL												
Total score	54.11 ± 8.01	54.97 ± 8.05	54.34 ± 8.03	54.07 ± 7.56	55.59 ± 7.69	54.44 ± 7.61	54.18 ± 7.74	55.32 ± 7.80	54.48 ± 7.77	54.18 ± 7.75	55.32 ± 7.80	54.48 ± 7.77
Physical health	14.11 ± 2.38	14.55 ± 2.29	14.23 ± 2.36	14.02 ± 2.23	14.54 ± 2.24	14.15 ± 2.24	14.24 ± 2.40	14.32 ± 2.04	14.27 ± 2.27	14.07 ± 2.30	14.53 ± 2.25	14.19 ± 2.29
Psycho-logical health	12.82 ± 2.66	13.36 ± 2.54	12.97 ± 2.66	13.30 ± 2.31	13.98 ± 2.38	13.46 ± 2.34	13.39 ± 2.16	13.93 ± 2.32	13.26 ± 2.49	13.11 ± 2.46	13.71 ± 2.50	13.26 ± 2.49
Environ-mental health	13.56 ± 2.11	13.92 ± 2.16	13.65 ± 2.13	13.18 ± 2.27	13.43 ± 2.15	13.24 ± 2.24	13.96 ± 1.99	13.68 ± 1.91	13.86 ± 1.96	13.38 ± 2.20	13.66 ± 2.14	13.45 ± 2.19
Social relations	13.61 ± 3.15	13.13 ± 3.18	13.49 ± 3.16	13.57 ± 2.88	13.65 ± 2.85	13.59 ± 2.88	14.23 ± 2.50	13.58 ± 2.33	14.00 ± 2.45	13.63 ± 2.98	13.42 ± 2.96	13.57 ± 2.98

Table 4. Means ± standard deviations and statistics of ANOVA and MANOVA analyses pertaining respondents' quality of life during the outbreak of COVID-19 (*n* = 2251).

	WHOQOL						
	Total Score		**Physical Health**	**Psychological Health**	**Environmental Health**	**Social Relations**	
Variables		***F*, *p* Value**					***F*, *p* Value**
Area of residence in Italy		3.86, 0.021					3.34, 0.001
North	55.11 ± 7.28		14.32 ± 2.19	13.45 ± 2.38	13.75 ± 2.08	13.59 ± 2.80	
Center	55.08 ± 7.96		14.26 ± 2.33	13.48 ± 2.36	13.61 ± 2.11	13.73 ± 3.23	
South	53.94 ± 8.09		14.08 ± 2.36	13.10 ± 2.57	13.21 ± 2.25	13.55 ± 3.08	
Level of education [a]		4.56, 0.003					3.84, 0.003
Secondary school	54.35 ± 9.13		14.26 ± 2.65	13.51 ± 2.81	12.63 ± 2.29	13.94 ± 3.28	
High school	53.71 ± 8.12		14.05 ± 2.41	12.98 ± 2.55	13.16 ± 2.19	13.51 ± 3.06	
University	54.54 ± 7.50		14.22 ± 2.18	13.32 ± 2.43	13.43 ± 2.05	13.57 ± 2.90	
Post-graduate	55.56 ± 7.25		14.37 ± 2.26	13.67 ± 2.35	13.83 ± 2.02	13.67 ± 2.89	

Table 4. *Cont.*

	WHOQOL						
	Total Score		**Physical Health**	**Psychological Health**	**Environmental Health**	**Social Relations**	
Variables		***F*, *p* Value**					***F*, *p* Value**
Marital status		0.235, 0.872					1.38, 0.169
Single	54.42 ± 7.81		14.28 ± 2.30	13.08 ± 2.58	13.64 ± 2.08	13.40 ± 3.05	
Married	54.55 ± 7.80		14.09 ± 2.29	13.40 ± 2.38	13.28 ± 2.56	13.77 ± 2.92	
Divorced/separated	54.22 ± 7.34		14.08 ± 2.24	13.45 ± 2.38	13.22 ± 2.24	13.46 ± 2.82	
Widowed	55.51 ± 8.44		14.51 ± 2.31	13.78 ± 2.56	13.57 ± 2.54	13.64 ± 2.72	
Employment status		4.54, 0.004					1.32, 0.198
Student	53.62 ± 7.91		14.02 ± 2.31	12.71 ± 2.67	13.65 ± 2.07	13.25 ± 3.11	
Employed	55.03 ± 7.53		14.31 ± 2.26	13.53 ± 2.37	13.46 ± 2.20	13.72 ± 2.88	
Unemployed	52.75 ± 8.76		13.79 ± 2.44	12.74 ± 2.71	12.91 ± 2.30	13.32 ± 3.34	
Retired	54.87 ± 7.18		14.19 ± 2.23	13.26 ± 2.49	13.71 ± 2.07	13.63 ± 2.71	
Currently diagnosed with psychiatric condition		6.38, 0.012					2.02, 0.089
Yes	52.33 ± 8.66		13.59 ± 2.74	12.42 ± 2.79	13.48 ± 2.36	12.84 ± 3.17	
No	54.62 ± 7.70		14.23 ± 2.26	13.32 ± 2.46	13.45 ± 2.18	13.62 ± 2.96	
Currently diagnosed with medical condition		4.15, 0.042					2.46, 0.043
Yes	53.54 ± 7.94		13.66 ± 2.52	13.12 ± 2.52	13.21 ± 2.23	13.56 ± 2.79	
No	54.67 ± 7.74		14.30 ± 2.23	13.29 ± 2.48	13.51 ± 2.18	13.57 ± 3.02	
Changes in employment status and location		5.78, 0.001					1.94, 0.025
No changes	55.37 ± 7.83		14.41 ± 2.32	13.52 ± 2.55	13.59 ± 2.21	13.85 ± 2.86	
Job/study activity moved at home	54.64 ± 7.22		14.25 ± 2.15	13.32 ± 2.36	13.59 ± 2.10	13.48 ± 2.88	
Job/study activity suspended	53.88 ± 8.52		14.08 ± 2.47	13.06 ± 2.62	13.15 ± 2.31	13.59 ± 3.24	
Unemployed prior to COVID-19	52.87 ± 8.65		13.66 ± 2.52	12.80 ± 2.64	12.97 ± 2.27	13.44 ± 3.22	
Family member or friend infected with Sars-Cov-2		0.164, 0.686					0.96, 0.430
Yes	54.33 ± 7.48		14.12 ± 2.31	13.14 ± 2.39	13.50 ± 1.92	13.56 ± 2.95	
No	54.49 ± 7.80		14.19 ± 2.29	13.27 ± 2.49	13.45 ± 2.21	13.57 ± 2.98	
Adherence to the precautions and control measures		7.26, 0.001					2.03, 0.039
Always	54.88 ± 7.96		14.21 ± 2.35	13.37 ± 2.53	13.59 ± 2.14	13.71 ± 3.00	
Often	54.18 ± 7.41		14.24 ± 2.18	13.22 ± 2.41	13.37 ± 2.15	13.34 ± 2.97	
Not that much	52.05 ± 7.16		13.73 ± 2.24	12.47 ± 2.27	12.53 ±2.52	13.32 ± 2.70	

Table 4. *Cont.*

	WHOQOL						
	Total Score		Physical Health	Psychological Health	Environmental Health	Social Relations	
Variables		F, p Value					F, p Value
Household size during COVID outbreak		1.92, 0.125					0.91, 0.531
1 person	55.43 ± 7.06		13.46 ± 2.10	13.63 ± 2.43	13.80 ± 2.10	13.53 ± 2.59	
2 persons	54.76 ± 7.95		14.19 ± 2.36	13.32 ± 2.43	13.42 ± 2.29	13.82 ± 2.95	
3–4 persons	54.33 ± 7.80		14.17 ± 2.28	13.20 ± 2.51	13.42 ± 2.17	13.53 ± 3.04	
5 persons or more	53.62 ± 7.81		13.97 ± 2.36	13.07 ± 2.55	13.34 ± 2.12	13.24 ± 3.04	

[a] Global sample size for this variable was 2173, as 61 women and 17 men did not report data on their education level.

With respect to the factor scores of the WHOQOL, significant effects were found for the following variables: area of residence in Italy, level of education, having a diagnosis of a medical condition, changes in employment status and location, and for adherence to precaution measures. None of such effects pertained the dimension of the WHOQOL assessing social relationships (all *p*s = n.s.). When area of residence in Italy was considered, between-subject tests revealed that only the differences pertaining the dimension of environmental health were significant (F (2, 2250) = 11.16, $p < 0.001$), with respondents living in the south reporting overall worse conditions of their environment, which were significantly different compared to respondents from the north of Italy ($p < 0.001$).

Between-subject tests for level of education showed that environmental (F (3, 2145) = 5.43, $p = 0.001$) and psychological health (F (3, 2145) = 3.45, $p = 0.016$) were significantly different across groups. Particularly, Bonferroni post hoc tests showed that individuals with a high school diploma had significantly lower levels of psychological health compared to respondents who had either a university degree ($p = 0.028$) or a postgraduate title ($p < 0.001$). Yet, individuals with a postgraduate title reported the highest scores for environmental health, which were significantly different to that of individuals with a secondary ($p < 0.001$) or high school ($p < 0.001$) diploma, as well as with a university degree ($p = 0.040$).

With respect to medical conditions, between-subject tests showed that physical (F (3, 2145) = 8.91, $p = 0.003$), psychological (F (3, 2145) = 4.03, $p = 0.045$), and environment (F (3, 2145) = 4.90, $p = 0.027$) domains of QoL were significantly lower for those respondents reporting a diagnosis of a medical condition.

Between-subject tests relevant to changes in employment status and location showed significant differences across groups in both physical (F (3, 2250) = 5.97, $p < 0.001$) and psychological domains (F (3, 2250) = 4.21, $p = 0.006$). Specifically, respondents who were unemployed prior to the COVID-19 outbreak reported worse levels of both physical and psychological health, which were significantly lower compared to individuals who had their job/study activity with no changes ($p < 0.001$ for both physical and psychological domains) or moved to home ($p = 0.001$ and $p = 0.012$ for physical and psychological domains, respectively).

With respect to the variable adherence to control measures, between-subject tests showed that the domain environment (F (3, 2145) = 6.15, $p = 0.002$) was significantly different across groups, with individuals who reported lower levels of adherence to control measures having the poorest QoL pertaining to environment, compared to respondents who reported either always or often (both *p*s < 0.001).

4. Discussion

The study aimed to assess the impact of the COVID-19 pandemic and lockdown measures on QoL in a large Italian sample. The main objective was to investigate possible differences in QoL levels related to both demographic and pandemic-specific factors, with particular attention to physical, psychological, social, and environmental dimensions of QoL. Our results show a number of significant differences in QoL levels related to several relevant variables.

Although the WHOQOL does not have cut-off scores allowing a precise definition of QoL as "poor" or "good", and despite the absence of recent data available on Italian QoL assessed with the WHOQOL, already existing literature can be taken into account to make some general considerations. Our results showed that, during the lockdown period, the mean of both the global and dimensions scores of the WHOQOL were lower compared to those obtained by both the Italian validation study of the questionnaire [33] and an international study comparing the main psychometric properties of WHOQOL-BREF among 23 countries [31]. Along this line, it is interesting to note that our results showed a poorer QoL for our sample compared to the data reported by another Italian study, in which the goal was to estimate QoL changes over an 18-month period in an adult population sample after the L'Aquila 2009 earthquake [35]. These results emphasize that the current situation due to the pandemic emergency and the lockdown measures had a severe impact on the QoL of the Italian general population, as confirmed by ISTAT (The Italian National Institute of Statistics) report [36]. It was, and still is, an actual collective trauma. In fact, although only 7.4% of the respondents reported to have a friend or relatives hit by COVID-19, we did not find significant differences in QoL compared to participants who had no friends or relatives infected by the virus. People's lives during lockdown were affected by an abrupt and sudden change in their habits, a sense of precariousness, the indefiniteness of the future, and a strong worry for their health. All these factors may have affected general QoL levels.

Looking into this even further, we found that the items that overall had the lowest scores were: "To what extent do you have the opportunity for leisure activities?" (item 14—environment dimension), "How well are you able to get around?" (item 15—physical domain), "How much do you enjoy life?" (item 5—psychological domain), and "How satisfied are you with your sex life?" (item 21—social domain). Through these items, it is possible to grasp the considerable impact that the lockdown measures have had on the dimensions of life satisfaction and pleasure, favoring an impairment of the ability to enjoy life. Particular attention should be given to the psychological domain, which seems to indicate a relapse to depressive nuances related to the loss of pleasure for one's life. Furthermore, it might be that the shelter-in-place order could have led to restrictions in physical activity behavior [6], with a possible significant negative impact on psychological well-being and QoL. In fact, recent literature suggests that daily physical activity helped to offset the psychological burden and negative emotions caused by COVID-19 pandemic [6–8]. A possible explanation is that regular exercise is linked to change in hypothalamic–pituitary–adrenal (HPA) axis, with reduced adrenal, autonomic, and psychological responses to a psychosocial stressor [37].

With respect to the influence of demographics on QoL, results showed significant differences between men and women. In line with the literature on QoL, women reported overall worse psychological, physical, and environmental QoL during the pandemic compared to men [31,33]. For instance, Girgus and Yang [38] showed that women's increased psychological vulnerability might be due to a higher tendency to ruminate and to use internal attribution for negative events. Pineles, Hall, and Rasmusson reported more cognitive symptoms of PTSD, such as self-blame, in women compared to men [39]. It is important to notice that in our sample, 80% of unemployed respondents were women, although with higher levels of education than men. Yet, within the 6.1% of respondents that had a psychiatric diagnosis, the highest prevalence was represented by women. With this regard, epidemiological data have shown that in Italy, despite a higher longevity, women get more illnesses and tend to have a lower quality of physical and psychological health than men [40,41]. According to Bekker [42], gender differences in health-related phenomena can be explained through a holistic approach, in which the relationships between biological sex, gender, and health are various, diverse, operative at many levels, and complex. In fact, this relationship can be moderated by daily life or social circumstances, person-related characteristics, and healthcare factors [42]. With respect to daily life and social circumstances, we can assume that, as a consequence of school closures, during the COVID-19 lockdown Italian women experienced a greater overload in care and work, favoring an organizational family shock [35,43].

With regards to age range differences, young adults (18-34) reported the lowest levels of psychological health, which were significantly lower compared to both middle and older adults. Middle adults had the lowest levels of environment dimension compared to both young and older adults. No significant differences emerged for both physical and social domains. Compared to other age groups and in the context of the pandemic, younger adults represent the most psychologically fragile subjects. Additionally, their age is characterized by important transformations (starting university, graduation, first access to work, precarious work condition, unemployment, sentimental projects), which during the pandemic situation might have exposed them to higher risks for their psychological wellbeing. Students, unemployed young people, or young people in the process of building a family or achieving working objectives have suddenly seen a threat to their projects and prospects for the future (finding a job, getting married). Young adults have certainly experienced more negative emotions and loss of self-confidence, with a possible impact on reasoning ability, learning, memory, and concentration, for example for university performances. In fact, emotional skills are crucial to cognitive processes as they affect cognitive styles, use of learning strategies [44], and, consequently, performance [45].

Other studies conducted during lockdown [19,23,25] showed a lower QoL and high levels of stress, anxiety, and depression in younger adults. Pieh and colleagues [23] reported a clear age-related effect in all tested mental health scales, in which the younger adult groups showed the worst scores, in contrast to a previous study before COVID-19. The authors hypothesized various explanations for these findings, such as more uncertain conditions and financial difficulties that occurred in COVID-19 lockdown. According to Horesh and co-workers [25], instead, older age seemed to act as a protective factor for psychological health and this could be attributed to their richer life experience [46] and a possible reduced fear of illness and death, despite the fact that the elderly are constantly being identified as a high-risk population [26,47–49]. Middle adults showed less impact on mental health but greatest dissatisfaction with the availability of financial resources, accessibility and quality of health and social care [26,27], the domestic environment conditions, access to information and sense of safety for their own health regarding to the physical environment, and to the possibility to access to means of transport in safety, compared to younger and older ones.

During lockdown, about 50% of young people and 53% of middle adults underwent changes in work conditions (moved home). This can also explain the dissatisfaction about housing conditions, in which simultaneously parents and children shared the same spaces to carry out their activities, with a probable lack of personal space, but about 18% of middle adults and about 14% of older had to stop their work activities, and this could have led to dissatisfaction with their own financial resources, with these not being considered adequate to meet their needs. In addition, in the first weeks after the declaration of emergency state, mass media were overwhelmed by information, which was not always accurate given the little knowledge on the contagion and the care of COVID-19. People probably felt a sense of uncertainty, confusion, and serious threat for their own physical safety. High intolerance of uncertainty has been found to exacerbate the relation between daily stressors and increased anxiety [50] and, not unexpectedly, increased intolerance of uncertainty as well as the desire to reduce uncertainty was found to predict increased information seeking and monitoring of a situation [51]. Therefore, obtaining information that only provides uncertain estimates related to viral threats may serve to increase perceptions of uncertainty and thus increase anxiety [5].

Our results also showed that individuals who were living in the south of Italy at the moment of the lockdown, had lower education levels (secondary or high school diploma), were unemployed or university students, were diagnosed with psychiatric and medical syndromes, had their job activity suspended, and did not comply with the control measures to contrast COVID-19 pandemic had the poorest QoL during the outbreak of the disease. It is interesting to point out that southern Italy, during the first period of lockdown, was less affected by the epidemic, yet the population showed lower levels of satisfaction with their general state of life. On the one hand, this can be related with structural differences that have always recorded lower QoL levels in the south than in the regions of northern Italy [52], especially with regard to the environment dimension (availability of financial resources, access to healthcare services, housing conditions, quality of public transport). Starting from these structural differences between the north and south of Italy, it is possible to assume that the population of southern Italy has perceived greater concern and distrust in the ability to cope with the pandemic. To support this, Rossi and colleagues [19] showed higher odds of several psychological outcomes, such as anxiety, depression, perceived stress, and insomnia in people who lived in southern Italy.

In regards to the relationship between low education level and low scores in the quality of life measure, it appears that the most compromised dimensions were psychological health and the interaction with the environment. Skevington [53] reported worse QoL levels in people without education, especially in some areas of QoL (lack of positive feelings; inadequate financial resources; little information and skills; few opportunities of recreation and leisure; weak spiritual, religious, and personal beliefs). Vice versa, most highly educated respondents reported a more positive environmental QoL, in terms of financial resources and physical environment, e.g., pollution and access to information and skills [53,54]. It is conceivable that, during lockdown, a lower educational level probably impaired more well-being because it hindered access to nonalienated paid work and economic resources, and may have reduced the sense of control over one's life, as well as the access to stable social relationships, especially marriage. Then, a lower educational level could increase emotional distress (including depression, anxiety, and anger), physical distress (including aches and pains and malaise), and levels of dissatisfaction.

As to work conditions, individuals who were unemployed prior to the COVID-19 outbreak reported overall worse levels of both physical and psychological QoL, which were significantly lower compared to individuals who had maintained their job/study activity with no changes nor moved to home. These findings are supported by previous studies highlighting a relationship between unemployment and poorer health-related QoL, explained by the economic and social consequences of unemployment [55,56]. Work has a central part in most individuals' lives. It meets the requirements of both material needs (income security and social protection) and social needs (self-esteem and identity, social interaction, time structure, and feeling of purpose and participation in society) [57], and these requirements are further compromised by limitations about job search activities during lockdown [36].

With reference to persons suffering from medical diseases, they reported lower scores in the physical and psychological domains, but also in the interaction with the environment, probably due to the difficulties of access to healthcare services (e.g., concern about cancelled/postponed care). During the pandemic, Italian hospitals were converted into COVID hospitals, and entire wards and surgeries were closed, making it difficult to access for all those with chronic or acute non-COVID-19 medical conditions. Furthermore, as assumed by Van Ballegoijen and co-workers [27], patients could have been anxious to visit their physician due to fear of infection or to avoid further burdening the healthcare system. This could lead to secondary healthcare problems, such as delay in diagnosis of critical medical conditions and exacerbation of existing health conditions. Horesh and colleagues [25] hypothesized that having a pre-existing medical condition is associated to distress, because COVID-19 is more dangerous for those with existing illness and, for that reason, these patients may have felt more vulnerable.

Most of our participants said they adhered to the government-enacted measures much or very much, and there was a significant difference between women and men in favor of the former. These data are in line with the study of Carlucci, D'Ambrosio, and Balsamo [58], where it was assumed that the increased adherence of women to containment measures can explain sex differences in mortality and vulnerability [59,60] to the COVID-19 disease. In this case, women's adherence has been a protective factor. As suggested by findings from previous studies regarding age and gender patterns of risk-taking behaviors [61,62], men would be more likely to engage in risk taking behaviors.

Finally, the present results have also highlighted that people who felt a greater dissatisfaction in all areas of QoL, especially the environment dimension, had a lower adherence to containment measures. After all, QoL is given by the interaction between environmental and personal factors, and it is possible that people who have perceived higher dissatisfaction with the availability of financial resources, physical safety, and accessibility and quality of health and social assistance may have had a more passive attitude linked to the sense of helplessness, concerning the real possibility that their personal contribution could contain the spread of contagion. Moreover, feelings of helplessness and passivity in dealing with the threat may result from high perception of risk that can promote the adoption of strategies to minimize infection [63].

5. Conclusions

There are limited international studies that have investigated how severe the impact of COVID-19 pandemic is on QoL and to our knowledge there have been no studies on the Italian population [23,25–28]. We believe that the assessment of QoL represents an important indicator of global health, which allows us to grasp the state of health of a population in a multidimensional way, especially in this particular moment in which all the dimensions of life have been disrupted.

Our study highlights significant differences in QoL and its dimensions (physical, psychological, environmental, and social) depending on a number of variables, including sex, age, status of employment, area of residence in Italy, and being diagnosed with a medical/psychiatric condition during the COVID-19 pandemic and lockdown. Strengths of the present study include the focus on a large Italian representative sample, which could be reached in a relatively short time period since the pandemic situation developed rapidly, and the use of an internationally validated questionnaire. Of course, the present study has some shortcomings, such as gender imbalance, cross-sectional data collection, the lack of information on the population of the central regions of Italy, and no exclusion criteria except minors under the age of 18 and those not living in Italy during COVID-19 lockdown.

We are aware that we have analyzed only some of multiple aspects that influence QoL and many others should be tested and considered in further research, such as the role of physical activity on psychological well-being. However, based on our findings, attention should be given to people showing a combination of risk factors, including younger age, female gender, unemployed status, having a pre-existing illness, and living in the south of Italy, thereby assisting them in coping with the pandemic, especially now that the continued exposure to the epidemic and to the necessary measures to contain it, above all in Italy, could lead to further impairment of the people's quality of life.

We believe that subjective well-being measures are needed to assess a society's population and it is important to add them to the health and economic indicators that are now favored by policymakers. Such measures include QoL, which may be conceptualized as a multidimensional construct that is influenced by personal and objective factors, as well as by their interactions. The subjective evaluation that people make about their living conditions, their expectations, and their beliefs, could also play a very important role for the adherence to both contagion containment measures and vaccination.

Actually, health authorities have devoted relatively little attention to the identification and management of psychological and social factors likely to significantly influence a person's QoL. Our results can offer guidelines regarding which social groups may be at a high risk of decreasing QoL, revealing areas of vulnerability during a pandemic. This line of research is particularly important for the management of public health interventions, especially in regards to the need for an optimal allocation of resources. Findings suggest the following recommendations for future interventions: (1) more attention needs to be paid to vulnerable groups such as the young, women, unemployed, and people living in the south of Italy, implementing psychological interventions for vulnerable individuals who cope with the long-term consequences of this pandemic; (2) accessibility to medical resources and the public health service systems should be further strengthened and improved; (3) comprehensive crisis prevention and psychological intervention are needed to reduce distress and prevent further impairment of QoL.

Author Contributions: Conceptualization, M.S.E. and S.L.G.; methodology, F.A. (Federica Andrei); software, M.S.E. and F.A. (Federica Andrei); validation, E.T. and S.L.G.; formal analysis, F.A. (Federica Andrei); investigation, M.S.E. and G.M.; data curation, F.A. (Federica Andrei) and M.R.; writing—original draft preparation, M.S.E., F.A. (Federica Andrei) and V.S.; writing—review and editing, G.M. and F.A. (Francesca Agostini); visualization, M.A.P., V.S., and M.R.; supervision, S.L.G. and E.T.; project administration, G.L. All authors have read and agreed to the published version of the manuscript.

Funding: This research received no external funding.

Institutional Review Board Statement: The study was conducted according to the guidelines of the Declaration of Helsinki, and in agreement with the ethical norms laid down by the Italian National Psychological Association.

Informed Consent Statement: Informed consent was obtained from all subjects involved in the study.

Data Availability Statement: Data available on request due to restrictions (privacy).

Acknowledgments: With grateful thanks to Marianna Franco, Simona Piraino, and Sofia Scordato to help us to data collection.

Conflicts of Interest: The authors declare no conflict of interest.

References

1. Taylor, S. *The Psychology of Pandemics: Preparing for the Next Global Outbreak of Infectious Disease*; Cambridge Scholars Publishing: Newcastle upon Tyne, UK, 2019.
2. World Health Organization. *WHO Checklist for Influenza Pandemic Preparedness Planning*; No. WHO/CDS/CSR/GIP/2005.4; World Health Organization: Geneva, Switzerland, 2005.
3. Taylor, M.R.; Agho, K.E.; Stevens, G.J.; Raphael, B. Factors influencing psychological distress during a disease epidemic: Data from Australia's first outbreak of equine influenza. *BMC Public Health* **2008**, *8*, 347. [CrossRef] [PubMed]
4. Kanadiya, M.K.; Sallar, A.M. Preventive behaviors, beliefs, and anxieties in relation to the swine flu outbreak among college students aged 18–24 years. *J. Public Health* **2011**, *19*, 139–145. [CrossRef] [PubMed]
5. Taha, S.; Matheson, K.; Cronin, T.; Anisman, H. Intolerance of uncertainty, appraisals, coping, and anxiety: The case of the 2009 H 1 N 1 pandemic. *Br. J. Health Psychol.* **2014**, *19*, 592–605. [CrossRef] [PubMed]
6. Carriedo, A.; Cecchini, J.A.; Fernandez-Rio, J.; Méndez-Giménez, A. COVID-19, Psychological Well-being and Physical Activity Levels in Older Adults during the Nationwide Lockdown in Spain. *Am. J. Geriatr. Psychiatry* **2020**. [CrossRef] [PubMed]
7. Zhang, Y.; Zhang, H.; Ma, X.; Di, Q. Mental Health Problems during the COVID-19 Pandemics and the Mitigation E ects of Exercise: A Longitudinal Study of College Students in China. *Int. J. Environ. Res. Public Health* **2020**, *17*, 3722. [CrossRef]
8. Maugeri, G.; Castrogiovanni, P.; Battaglia, G.; Pippi, R.; D'Agata, V.; Palma, A.; Di Rosa, M.; Musumeci, G. The impact of physical activity on psychological health during Covid-19 pandemic in Italy. *Heliyon* **2020**, *6*, e043152. [CrossRef] [PubMed]
9. Shultz, J.M.; Espinel, Z.; Flynn, B.W.; Hoffmann, Y.; Cohen, R.E. *DEEP PREP: All-Hazards Disaster Behavioral Health Training*; DEEP Centre: Miami, FL, USA, 2008.
10. Available online: http://www.governo.it/it/articolo/comunicato-stampa-del-consiglio-dei-ministri-n-27/13937 (accessed on 7 September 2020).
11. Available online: https://opendatadpc.maps.arcgis.com/apps/opsdashboard/index.html#/b0c68bce2cce478eaac82fe38d4138b1 (accessed on 7 September 2020).
12. Available online: http://www.governo.it/node/14613 (accessed on 9 October 2020).
13. Qiu, J.; Shen, B.; Zhao, M.; Wang, Z.; Xie, B.; Xu, Y. A nationwide survey of psychological distress among Chinese people in the COVID-19 epidemic: Implications and policy recommendations. *Gen. Psychiatry* **2020**, *33*. [CrossRef]
14. Wang, C.; Pan, R.; Wan, X.; Tan, Y.; Xu, L.; McIntyre, R.S.; Ho, C. A longitudinal study on the mental health of general population during the COVID-19 epidemic in China. *Brain Behav. Immun.* **2020**. [CrossRef]
15. Jin, Z.; Zhao, K.; Xia, Y.; Chen, R.; Yu, H.; Tamutana, T.T. Psychological responses to the Coronavirus Disease (COVID-19) outbreak. *China* **2020**, *14*, 1.
16. Xiang, Y.T.; Yang, Y.; Li, W.; Zhang, L.; Zhang, Q.; Cheung, T.; Ng, C.H. Timely mental health care for the 2019 novel coronavirus outbreak is urgently needed. *Lancet Psychiatry* **2020**, *7*, 228–229. [CrossRef]
17. Kwek, S.K.; Chew, W.M.; Ong, K.C.; Ng, A.W.K.; Lee, L.S.U.; Kaw, G.; Leow, M.K.S. Quality of life and psychological status in survivors of severe acute respiratory syndrome at 3 months post discharge. *J. Psychosom. Res.* **2006**, *60*, 513–519. [CrossRef] [PubMed]
18. Brooks, S.K.; Webster, R.K.; Smith, L.E.; Woodland, L.; Wessely, S.; Greenberg, N.; Rubin, G.J. The psychological impact of quarantine and how to reduce it: Rapid review of the evidence. *Lancet* **2020**. [CrossRef]
19. Rossi, R.; Socci, V.; Talevi, D.; Mensi, S.; Niolu, C.; Pacitti, F.; Di Lorenzo, G. COVID-19 pandemic and lockdown measures impact on mental health among the general population in Italy. *Front. Psychiatry* **2020**, *11*, 790. [CrossRef] [PubMed]

20. Cao, W.; Fang, Z.; Hou, G.; Han, M.; Xu, X.; Dong, J.; Zheng, J. The psychological impact of the COVID-19 epidemic on college students in China. *Psychiatry Res.* **2020**, 112934. [CrossRef] [PubMed]
21. Marroquín, B.; Vine, V.; Morgan, R. Mental health during the COVID-19 pandemic: Effects of stay-at-home policies, social distancing behavior, and social resources. *Psychiatry Res.* **2020**, *293*, 113419. [CrossRef] [PubMed]
22. Zhang, Y.; Ma, Z.F. Impact of the COVID-19 pandemic on mental health and quality of life among local residents in Liaoning Province, China: A cross-sectional study. *Int. J. Environ. Res. Public Health* **2020**, *17*, 2381. [CrossRef]
23. Pieh, C.; Budimir, S.; Probst, T. The effect of age, gender, income, work, and physical activity on mental health during coronavirus disease (COVID-19) lockdown in Austria. *J. Psychosom. Res.* **2020**, *136*, 110186. [CrossRef]
24. Austria, S.; Klimont, J. Österreichische Gesundheitsbefragung. In *Hauptergebnisse des Austrian Health Interview Survey (ATHIS) und Methodische Dokumentation*; Im Auftrag des Bundesministerium für Gesundheit und der Bundesgesundheitsagentur: Wienna, Austria, 2015.
25. Horesh, D.; Kapel Lev-Ari, R.; Hasson-Ohayon, I. Risk factors for psychological distress during the COVID-19 pandemic in Israel: Loneliness, age, gender, and health status play an important role. *Br. J. Health Psychol.* **2020**, *25*, 925–933. [CrossRef]
26. Ping, W.; Zheng, J.; Niu, X.; Guo, C.; Zhang, J.; Yang, H.; Shi, Y. Evaluation of health-related quality of life using EQ-5D in China during the COVID-19 pandemic. *PLoS ONE* **2020**, *15*, e0234850. [CrossRef]
27. Van Ballegooijen, H.; Goossens, L.; Bruin, R.H.; Michels, R.; Krol, M. Concerns, quality of life, access to care and productivity of the general population during the first 8 weeks of the coronavirus lockdown in Belgium and the Netherlands. *medRxiv* **2020**. [CrossRef]
28. Wang, X.; Lei, S.M.; Le, S.; Yang, Y.; Zhang, B.; Yao, W.; Cheng, S. Bidirectional influence of the COVID-19 pandemic lockdowns on health behaviors and quality of life among Chinese adults. *Int. J. Environ. Res. Public Health* **2020**, *17*, 5575. [CrossRef] [PubMed]
29. White, R.G.; Van Der Boor, C. Impact of the COVID-19 pandemic and initial period of lockdown on the mental health and well-being of adults in the UK. *BJPsych Open* **2020**, *6*. [CrossRef]
30. WHOQOL Group. The World Health Organization quality of life assessment (WHOQOL): Position paper from the World Health Organization. *Soc. Sci. Med.* **1995**, *41*, 1403–1409. [CrossRef]
31. Skevington, S.M.; Lotfy, M.; O'Connell, K.A. The World Health Organization's WHOQOL-BREF quality of life assessment: Psychometric properties and results of the international field trial. A report from the WHOQOL group. *Qual. Life Res.* **2004**, *13*, 299–310. [CrossRef] [PubMed]
32. Group, T.W. The World Health Organization quality of life assessment (WHOQOL): Development and general psychometric properties. *Soc. Sci. Med.* **1998**, *46*, 1569–1585. [CrossRef]
33. De Girolamo, G.; Rucci, P.; Scocco, P.; Becchi, A.; Coppa, F.; D'Addario, A.; Marson, C. Quality of life assessment: Validation of the Italian version of the WHOQOL-Brief. *Epidemiol. Psychiatr. Sci.* **2000**, *9*, 45–55. [CrossRef]
34. IBM Corp. *Released 2017*; IBM SPSS Statistics for Windows, Version 25.0; IBM Corp.: Armonk, NY, USA, 2017.
35. Valenti, M.; Masedu, F.; Mazza, M.; Tiberti, S.; Di Giovanni, C.; Calvarese, A.; Sconci, V. A longitudinal study of quality of life of earthquake survivors in L'Aquila, Italy. *BMC Public Health* **2013**, *13*, 1143. [CrossRef]
36. Available online: https://www.istat.it/storage/rapporto-annuale/2020/Rapportoannuale2020.pdf (accessed on 15 October 2020).
37. Rimmele, U.; Seilerb, R.; Martic, B.; Wirtzd, P.H.; Ehlertd, U.; Heinrichs, M. The level of physical activity affects adrenal andcardiovascular reactivity to psychosocial stress. *Psychoneuroendocrinology* **2009**, *34*, 190–198. [CrossRef]
38. Girgus, J.S.; Yang, K. Gender and depression. *Curr. Opin. Psychol.* **2015**, *4*, 53–60. [CrossRef]
39. Pineles, S.L.; Hall, K.A.A.; Rasmusson, A.M. Gender and PTSD: Different pathways to a similar phenotype. *Curr. Opin. Psychol.* **2017**, *14*, 44–48. [CrossRef]
40. ISTAT. La Soddisfazione dei Cittadini per le Condizioni di vita 2011. Available online: https://www.istat.it/it/archivio/44575 (accessed on 15 October 2020).
41. Rollero, C. Salute in una prospettiva di genere. In *Salute e Qualità di vita Nella Società del Benessere*; De Piccoli, N., Ed.; Prospettive interdisciplinari, Carocci Editore: Roma, Italy, 2014.
42. Bekker, M.H.J. Investigating gender within health research is more than sex disaggregation of data: A Multi-Facet Gender and Health Model. *Psychol. Health Med.* **2003**, *8*, 231–243. [CrossRef]
43. Power, K. The COVID-19 pandemic has increased the care burden of women and families. *Sustain. Sci. Pract. Policy* **2020**, *16*, 67–73. [CrossRef]
44. Vega-Hernández, M.C.; Patino-Alonso, M.C.; Cabello, R.; Galindo-Villardón, M.P.; Fernández-Berrocal, P. Perceived emotional intelligence and learning strategies in Spanish university students: A new perspective from a canonical non-symmetrical correspondence analysis. *Front. Psychol.* **2017**, *8*, 1888. [CrossRef] [PubMed]
45. Perera, H.N. The role of trait emotional intelligence in academic performance: Theoretical overview and empirical update. *J. Psychol.* **2016**, *150*, 229–251. [CrossRef] [PubMed]
46. Ardelt, M.; Landes, S.D.; Gerlach, K.R.; Fox, L.P. Rediscovering internal strenghts of the aged: The beneficial impact of wisdom, mastery, purpose in life, and spirituality on aging well. In *Positive Psychology: Advances in Understanding Adult Motivation*; Sinnot, J.D., Ed.; Springer Science+Business Media: New York, NY, USA, 2013; pp. 97–119.
47. Burström, K.; Johannesson, M.; Diderichsen, F. Swedish population health-related quality of life results using the EQ-5D. *Qual. Life Res.* **2001**, *10*, 621–635. [CrossRef] [PubMed]
48. Johnson, J.A.; Coons, S.J. Comparison of the EQ-5D and SF-12 in an adult US sample. *Qual. Life Res.* **1998**, *7*, 155–166. [CrossRef]

49. Fortner, B.V.; Neimeyer, R.A.; Rybarczyk, B. Correlates of death anxiety in older adults: A comprehensive review. *Death Attitudes Older Adult Theor. Concepts Appl.* **2000**, 95–108. [CrossRef]
50. Chen, C.Y.; Hong, R.Y. Intolerance of uncertainty moderates the relation between negative life events and anxiety. *Personal. Individ. Differ.* **2010**, *49*, 49–53. [CrossRef]
51. Rosen, N.O.; Knäuper, B.; Sammut, J. Do individual differences in intolerance of uncertainty affect health monitoring? *Psychol. Health* **2007**, *22*, 413–430. [CrossRef]
52. Available online: https://www.istat.it/storage/rapporto-annuale/2019/Rapportoannuale2019.pdf (accessed on 15 October 2020).
53. Skevington, S.M. Qualities of life, educational level and human development: An international investigation of health. *Soc. Psychiatry Psychiatr. Epidemiol.* **2010**, *45*, 999–1009. [CrossRef]
54. Ross, C.E.; Van Willigen, M. Education and the subjective quality of life. *J. Health Soc. Behav.* **1997**, 275–297. [CrossRef]
55. Norström, F.; Waenerlund, A.K.; Lindholm, L.; Nygren, R.; Sahlén, K.G.; Brydsten, A. Does unemployment contribute to poorer health-related quality of life among Swedish adults? *BMC Public Health* **2019**, *19*, 457. [CrossRef] [PubMed]
56. McKee-Ryan, F.; Song, Z.; Wanberg, C.R.; Kinicki, A.J. Psychological and physical well-being during unemployment: A meta-analytic study. *J. Appl. Psychol.* **2005**, *90*, 53. [CrossRef] [PubMed]
57. Brydsten, A.; Hammarström, A.; Strandh, M.; Johansson, K. Youth unemployment and functional somatic symptoms in adulthood: Results from the Northern Swedish cohort. *Eur. J. Public Health* **2015**, *25*, 796–800. [CrossRef]
58. Carlucci, L.; D'Ambrosio, I.; Balsamo, M. Demographic and attitudinal factors of adherence to quarantine guidelines during COVID-19: The Italian Model. *Front. Psychol.* **2020**, *11*, 2702. [CrossRef]
59. Chen, N.; Zhou, M.; Dong, X.; Qu, J.; Gong, F.; Han, Y.; Yu, T. Epidemiological and clinical characteristics of 99 cases of 2019 novel coronavirus pneumonia in Wuhan, China: A descriptive study. *Lancet* **2020**, *395*, 507–513. [CrossRef]
60. Wenham, C.; Smith, J.; Morgan, R. COVID-19: The gendered impacts of the outbreak. *Lancet* **2020**, *395*, 846–848. [CrossRef]
61. Pawlowski, B.; Atwal, R.; Dunbar, R.I.M. Sex differences in everyday risk-taking behavior in humans. *Evol. Psychol.* **2008**, *6*. [CrossRef]
62. Cobey, K.D.; Laan, F.; Stulp, G.; Buunk, A.P.; Pollet, T.V. Sex differences in risk taking behavior among Dutch cyclists. *Evol. Psychol.* **2013**, *11*. [CrossRef]
63. Leppin, A.; Aro, A.R. Risk perceptions related to SARS and Avian influenza: Theoretical foundations of current empirical research. *Int. J. Behav. Med.* **2009**, *16*, 7–29. [CrossRef]

Journal of
Clinical Medicine

MDPI

Article

Predictors of Threat from COVID-19: A Cross-Sectional Study in the Spanish Population

María del Carmen Pérez-Fuentes [1,*], Iván Herrera-Peco [2,3,*], María del Mar Molero Jurado [1,*], Nieves Fátima Oropesa [1] and José Jesús Gázquez Linares [4,*]

1 Department of Psychology, Faculty of Psychology, University of Almería, 04120 Almería, Spain; foropesa@ual.es
2 Nursing Department, Faculty of Health Sciences, Alfonso X El Sabio University, 28691 Madrid, Spain
3 Alfonso X El Sabio Foundation, 28691 Madrid, Spain
4 Department of Psychology, Universidad Autónoma de Chile, Providencia 7500000, Chile
* Correspondence: mpf421@ual.es (M.d.C.P.-F.); iherrpec@uax.es (I.H.-P.); mmj130@ual.es (M.d.M.M.J.); jlinares@ual.es (J.J.G.L.)

Abstract: One of the first measures for fighting the worldwide spread of the COVID-19 pandemic is social isolation or quarantine. The perceived threat from COVID-19 in this situation, maintained over time, generates uncertainty and fears, etc., which could lead to mental disorders in the population. This study evaluated the perceived threat from COVID-19 in the Spanish population. The study design was cross-sectional and observational. The sample of 1014 participants recruited in Spain had a mean age of 40.87 (*SD* = 12.42). The gender distribution was 67.2% (n = 681) women and 32.8% (n = 333) men. Data were collected with an online survey. The instrument used was the Perception of Threat from COVID-19 Questionnaire, validated for the Spanish population. Our data showed a clear correlation between perceived threat with female gender, having children in one's care and level of education. However, no association was observed with age or marital status. Finally, we concluded that there is a greater perception of threat from COVID-19 by women with a lower education who have children in their care, and that they are also more sensitive to minor mental disorders, such as anxiety or stress, appearing.

Keywords: coronavirus; COVID-19; public mental health; quarantine

Citation: Pérez-Fuentes, M.d.C.; Herrera-Peco, I.; Jurado, M.d.M.M.; Oropesa, N.F.; Gázquez Linares, J.J. Predictors of Threat from COVID-19: A Cross-Sectional Study in the Spanish Population. *J. Clin. Med.* **2021**, *10*, 692. https://doi.org/10.3390/jcm10040692

Academic Editor: Michele Roccella
Received: 12 January 2021
Accepted: 4 February 2021
Published: 10 February 2021

1. Introduction

When pneumonia was detected in December 2019 in Wuhan, Hubei Province, China, its origin was unknown. However, by the beginning of January 2020, it was identified as the novel SARS-CoV-2 virus which causes the disease known as COVID-19 [1–3]. Its course goes through a series of systemic physical symptoms, such as fever, cough, fatigue, headache and diarrhea, and also respiratory affections that could include rhinorrhea, pneumonia or acute respiratory distress syndrome [3–5].

COVID-19 characteristics facilitated its rapid expansion, leading the World Health Organization to define it as a global pandemic on 31 January 2020 [6]. Its incubation period is about 5.2 days [7], with symptoms appearing in an average of 14 days [8]. In addition, a high percentage of virus carriers are asymptomatic, but they are nevertheless infective and can infect others if not detected in time [9], which, along with the enormous stream of transportation, could amplify its spread [10,11] and the danger it represents to public health [12].

Due to the spread of the virus and the disease it causes, as well as the inexistence at the present time of effective treatments or vaccination against SARS-CoV-2 [13,14], a number of measures have been taken to reduce its spread and protect the population. These may be grouped in two main measures: limiting movement of the population and home confinement [15,16]. These measures, in addition to the pandemic itself, can have effects, not only on particular individuals but also on the physical and mental health of the entire population [17–22], and especially frontline professionals, such as healthcare workers [23,24]. With respect to the COVID-19 disease itself, as described in other infectious disease epidemics [25–28], some people have negative emotions causing behavior and attitudes that cause them to avoid contact with disease [29]. This defensive reaction to perceived threat from the disease can cause severe psychological maladjustments such as stress, depression and anxiety [17,20,26,30].

The confinement due to the COVID-19 pandemic has been described by some authors as a possible cause of collective hysteria [31–33], a situation which, if it worsens and measures are hardened to mass quarantine, could generate anxiety [18]. It has been observed that people subjected to isolation may experience feelings of loneliness and anger in addition to problems in relating to others person-to-person and even in group social relations when isolation ends [33,34].

The unpredictability of information received from authorities on control of the disease or severity of risk of contagion, and disinformation from both traditional communication media [18,35] and on social networks such as Twitter, YouTube, Instagram or Facebook, among others [36–38] combine with the situation above, generating stress, fear, guilt, displeasure [18,34,35,38] and so forth. Although they may not be considered mental illnesses in themselves, they can lead to situations compromising mental health [35]. Therefore, one's perception of the disease depends on the interpretation of experiences, how that interpretation is transferred to active behavior, the response to social reactions and the personal meaning attributed to the experience [39]. In the situation of imminent alarm in which society around the world now finds itself with COVID-19 and its effect on health [16,17,24], the perception adults have of the disease as government measures change their habits, becomes very important. Perhaps one of the most significant changes is in the care of children or other dependents [40], as women, who traditionally care for the most vulnerable members of the family [41–43], could find their situation worsened under conditions such as those generated by the current pandemic.

The significant role of healthcare professionals as guarantors of both physical and mental health of the population [44], even in situations of public health conflict [45] should also be mentioned. At the present time, there is not much information on the psychological impact and mental health of the general population [6]. A large number of scientific publications have focused on analysis and identification of epidemiological and clinical characteristics of infected patients, genome identification and morphology of the virus and situations related to the logistics and political and healthcare policy decision-making [5,32,46]. The the psychological state of the Spanish population has not yet been defined, although there are such studies on specific groups in the Spanish population, like nurses [47] or university students [48].

The objective of this study was to explore the threat perceived by Spanish society from the lockdown imposed because of the COVID-19 epidemic. We think that uncertainty and lack of information about COVID-19 could affect cognitive and emotional health [7]. An evaluation of perceived threat by COVID-19 [39] that would provide information on which groups are the most sensitive to the pernicious effects on mental health of both COVID-19 and the measures taken to slow down its contagion would be useful for healthcare authorities as well as primary care professionals in attending patients.

2. Method

2.1. Participants

The study sample was made up of a total of 1043 Spanish adults residing in 19 autonomous regions of which Andalusia was most represented with 37.9% of the participants, followed by Madrid with 27.5%. Of these 29 were eliminated because of random or incongruent answers on control questions included in the questionnaire, leaving 1014 participants in the study.

Ethical research standards were complied with, providing information on the project and requesting consent to participate. The study was approved by the University of Almería Bioethics Committee.

2.2. Design and Data Collection

A cross-sectional observational study planned was carried out as an online survey due to the state of emergency decreed in Spain last 14 March and the restriction of movement, making a person-to-person format impossible.

The sample was acquired by snowball sampling by spreading the link to the questionnaire on social networking sites. Data was acquired from 18 March through 23 March 2020.

2.3. Instruments and Variables

This study used the Perception of Threat from COVID-19 Questionnaire validated for an adult Spanish population [39]. The questionnaire consists of five items focused on the perception of threat from COVID-19 (Table 1), where the participants rate their agreement with the statements on a Likert-type scale of 0 to 10. The test offers an overall score on the representation of the disease, where the highest scores indicate greater perception of COVID-19 as a threat. This questionnaire showed acceptable internal consistency ($\alpha = 0.66$).

Table 1. Items measured by the Perception of Threat from COVID-19 instrument (by author).

Items	Range	M	SD
How much is coronavirus infection affecting your life?	1–10	7.62	2.13
How long do you think the coronavirus infection alert will last?	1–10	6.84	1.60
To what extent do you feel symptoms due to infection by coronavirus?	1–10	2.03	1.85
How much are you worried about infection by coronavirus?	1–10	7.65	2.15
How much are you affected emotionally by infection by coronavirus? (That is, do you feel furious, afraid, angry, depressed?)	1–10	6.58	2.41

In addition, an ad hoc questionnaire on the following socio descriptive variables was included: Gender (man or woman), age, marital status (married, single, widowed or divorced), education (no education, primary school, high school and higher education), autonomous region, "Do you have any minor children?" (yes, no), "Is anyone close to you COVID-19 positive?" (yes, no).

2.4. Data Analysis

First, relative and absolute frequencies were calculated in a descriptive analysis of the sociodemographic variables.

Then, relationships between the quantitative variables were explored by correlation analysis, and categorical variables by Student's *t*-test and ANOVA. In the hypothesis comparisons, 0.05 was considered statistical significance and the confidence intervals were calculated at 95%.

After that, a binary logistic regression was performed using the enter method. The dependent variable for this was perceived threat, previously dichotomized into medium-low/medium high. The predictor variables, based on the results of preliminary analyses, were sex, having minor children in one's care and education.

SPSS version 23.0 for Windows was used for data processing and analysis.

3. Results

3.1. Descriptive Analysis

The mean age was 40.87 (SD = 12.42) in a range of 18 to 76. The gender distribution was 67.2% (n = 681) women and 32.8% (n = 333) men, with a mean age of 39.88 (SD = 12.35) and 42.92 (SD = 12.33), respectively. Over 90% of the sample was single (30.9%) or married (60.1%). Over 90% had a secondary or higher education (16% and 78.7%, respectively). When asked if they had minor children, 35.9% (364) answered affirmatively (see Table 2). And finally, only 16.4% (n = 166) had someone COVID-19 positive close to them.

Table 2. Sociodemographic characteristics of the participants.

Variables	%	n
Sex		
Men	32.8%	333
Women	67.2%	681
Marital status		
Single	30.9%	313
Married	60.1%	609
Divorced	8.1%	82
Widowed	1%	10
Education		
No education	0.3%	3
Primary school	5%	51
High school	16%	162
Higher education	78.7%	798
Do you have any minor children?		
No	64.1%	650
Yes	35.9%	364
Is anyone close to you COVID-19 positive?		
No	82.6%	848
Yes	16.4%	166

Potential explanatory variables were selected by descriptive analysis of their relationships with perceived threat. The quantitative variables were examined with bivariate correlations, in which no correlation with perceived threat was found for age: $r = 0.05$, $p = 0.092$, 95% CI (−0.009; 0.114). Education, coded on a scale in ascending order from 0 = "no education" to 3 = "higher education", correlated negatively to perceived threat: $r = -0.08$, $p < 0.01$; 95% CI (−0.149; −0.027). No statistically significant between-group differences were observed by marital status ($F = 2.03$; $p = 0.108$) in the analysis of perceived threat.

However, differences were detected (t1012 = −5.15; p < 0,001; d = 0.34) by gender (Figure 1a), in which women perceived higher threat (M = 31.47; SD = 6.29) than men (M = 29.21; SD = 7.03). Furthermore, those with minor children in their care (M = 31.50; SD = 6.63) differed significantly (t1012 = −2.77; p < 0,01; d = 0.18) from those who did not (M = 30.30; SD = 6.59), where the first scored higher in perceived threat from COVID-19 (Figure 1b).

3.2. Logistic Regression Model

Based on the above descriptive analyses, the independent variables entered in the logistic regression model for predicting perceived threat were gender, having minor children and education. In this case, the total score for the variable on the questionnaire was previously dichotomized by visual grouping and percentiles based on the cases explored.

The cutoff point was set at 31.5, forming two intervals or groups, one medium-low threat with scores equal to or lower, and medium-high threat, with higher scores. Later recording of the variable (once the cutoff points had been found by visual grouping) was done manually.

Table 3 shows the results of the logistic regression analysis: regression coefficients, standard error of the estimate, Wald statistic, degrees of freedom and associated probability, partial correlation coefficient and cross-product.

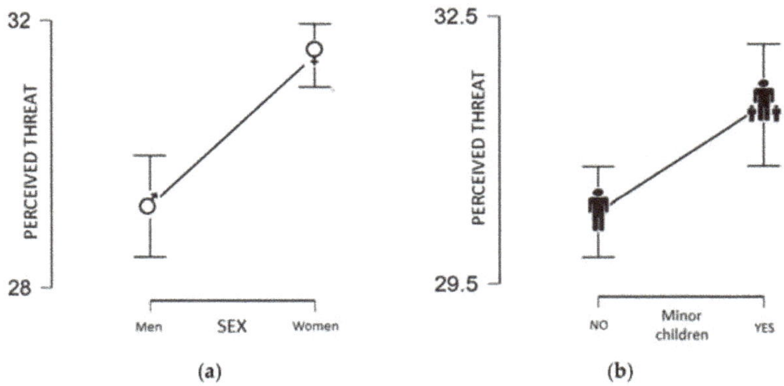

Figure 1. (**a**) Perceived threat by gender. (**b**) Perceived threat by whether there were minor children in their care.

Table 3. Results derived from the logistic regression for probability of perceived threat.

Variables	β	St. Error	Wald	df	Sig.	Exp(β)	CI 95%
Sex (a)	0.633	0.137	21.224	1	0.000	1.884	1.439–2.467
Minor children (b)	0.355	0.134	6.980	1	0.008	1.426	1.096–1.857
Education	−0.261	0.116	5.031	1	0.025	0.770	0.613–0.968
Constant	0.159	0.341	0.217	1	0.641	1.172	

Note. (a) Women; (b) With minors in their care.

The odds ratio found for each variable indicates that risk of perceiving strong threat is higher among women with minor children in their care and with low education.

Overall fit of the model ($\chi^2 = 32.57$; df = 3; $p < 0.001$), was confirmed by Hosmer–Lemeshow test ($\chi^2 = 1.54$; df = 5; $p = 0.908$). In addition, the Nagelkerke R2 indicated that 4.2% of the variability in the response variable would be explained by the logistic regression model.

4. Discussion

The novel results of this study found possible psychological problems related to perceived threat from the infectious disease COVID-19.

In the first place, analysis of the threat perceived by the population showed that neither participant age nor marital status influenced perception of threat. However, gender did influence that perception. It was observed that women were particularly more prone to perceive the COVID-19 disease as a threat. This might be attributed to a woman's traditional role in society as planner and caregiver of the family unit [41–43], related to a feeling of moral and affective obligation [40]. Although men have become more involved with childcare since the economic crisis of 2008, or when they are unemployed, it seems that this trend is not maintained when they are employed, devoting less time to caring for children than mothers [40]. This is not the case of women, who care for the family regardless of whether they are otherwise employed.

Another factor found to be positively related to perception of threat was having children in one's care, which could be associated with fear that the children would be infected by the disease or even lost [23,28,49].

A lower level of education was associated with perceived threat from COVID-19, perhaps related to access to sources of information and to understanding based on previous knowledge [47,48,50]. Thus, a higher level of education would be associated with a greater critical capacity of information consumed and processed and the tendency to seek other sources of information to corroborate or refute information acquired [51].

It is worth mentioning that information sources, whether communication media or social networking sites, may generate uncertainty [18,35,36,38] because of the way the news is explained, providing incoherent data which could generate anxiety or fear in an epidemic, or by way of "false experts" who generate biased and erroneous interpretations of data, causing confusion and unease.

A clear example that social networks can generate a high percentage of untrustworthy information if one does not know how to filter it is YouTube, where during the Zika pandemic, it was found that 25% of the videos published on that subject contained unreliable and biased information [38]. This was also true during the Ebola pandemic, where 63.5% of the videos analyzed contained unreliable information [37], and also at other social networking sites [36]. This situation of uncertainty due to access to unclear and even biased information can generate a high level of uncertainty associated in turn with anxiety and depressive symptoms [20].

In addition, it was found that women without an education and with minor children in their care had a stronger feeling of threat from COVID-19. This could explain the association in the sample studied, as they did not have enough knowledge to enable them to filter information received from the communication media or social networks, thus generating anxiety and stress, a normal response of fear and protection for loved ones [19,49] in the traditional caregiver role of women [40,42,43].

Even though the COVID-19 pandemic is considered a public health emergency [12] understood as a binomial made up of physical and mental health [21], it should be highlighted that there are no studies on the analysis of threat perceived by the population and the possible importance of this perception on development of alterations in mental health during crisis situations, such as the COVID-19 pandemic. In this regard, the increase in minor mental disorders in the Spanish population during the economic crisis of 2008 should be emphasized [44]. This situation and experiences in countries where the fight against the disease has been longer, such as China, makes intervention for possible psychological affectation necessary in the population as a public health response [18,22,25].

In spite of the contributions made in this study, it is important to emphasize its limitations. The study sample, due to the nonprobability sampling used, was not representative. In this respect, it should be mentioned that a high percentage of participants were women, and that most of the participants had a higher education, which also affects the representativeness of the results. Moreover, there may have been social desirability biases associated with the self-reports used for data collection. Lastly, (although it might not be considered a real limitation, it should be noted that) due to the sudden occurrence of the pandemic, we were unable to assess the mental health burden in a Spanish population beforehand. Therefore, future research should improve the sampling technique to avoid possible biases.

Finally, while our original research goal was to analyze the perception of the threat associated with the COVID-19 pandemic and control strategies for reducing the spread of the virus, we realize that previous studies have also been done in countries like Italy [52], Greece [53] or Canada [54] that suggest a relationship between the COVID-19 pandemic and control strategies, with the appearance of anxiety and depression disorders in these populations. Therefore as a future line of research, we will delve more deeply into the relationship of anxiety and depression to the Spanish population's mental health during the COVID-19 pandemic.

5. Conclusions

In conclusion, the results of this study show that in a situation such as the one we are now experiencing, there is a feeling of threat from COVID-19, which is worsened by isolation during lockdown. Some groups in the sample had a greater perception of threat, especially women with lower education who have children in their care, and they were more sensitive to minor mental disorders appearing, such as anxiety or stress.

We believe this situation may be similar to past economic crises which have caused a significant increase in burnout [54] and mental disorders in Spain. Therefore, healthcare authorities should evaluate the implementation of policies directed at providing the material and human resources for healthcare professional teams in community care, so these professionals can detect and act quickly against any minor mental health disorder derived from the stress and fear from perceived threat of COVID-19 and daily abnormal situations through community activities and even educational intervention.

Author Contributions: M.d.C.P.-F. contributed to the concept, design, and analysis and interpretation of the data. I.H.-P. contributed to collecting the data, to the concept and design, and manuscript preparation. M.d.M.M.J. contributed to the concept, design, and analysis and interpretation of the data. N.F.O. contributed to the technical details and manuscript preparation. J.J.G.L. contributed to critically revising the manuscript for important intellectual content and the final approval of the version to be published. All authors have read and agreed to the published version of the manuscript.

Funding: This research received no external funding.

Institutional Review Board Statement: The study was conducted according to the guidelines of the Declaration of Helsinki, and approved by the Ethics Committee of University of Almería (protocol code UALBIO2020/021 25/06/2020).

Informed Consent Statement: Informed consent was obtained from all subjects involved in the study.

Data Availability Statement: The data presented in this study are available on request from the corresponding author.

Acknowledgments: The present study was undertaken in collaboration with Excma. Diputación Provincial.

Conflicts of Interest: The authors declare no conflict of interest.

References

1. Lai, C.C.; Shih, T.P.; Ko, W.C.; Tang, H.J.; Hsueh, P.R. Severe acute respiratory syndrome coronavirus 2 (SARS-CoV-2) and coronavirus disease-2019 (COVID-19): The epidemic and the challenges. *Int. J. Antimicrob. Agents* **2020**, *55*, 105924. [CrossRef]
2. Rodríguez-Morales, A.J.; MacGregor, K.; Kanagarajah, S.; Patel, D.; Schlagenhauf, P. Going global–Travel and the 2019 novel coronavirus. *Travel Med. Infect. Dis.* **2020**, *33*, 101578. [CrossRef]
3. Rothan, H.A.; Byrareddy, S.N. The epidemiology and pathogenesis of coronavirus disease (COVID-19) outbreak. *J. Autoimmun.* **2020**, *109*, 102433. [CrossRef]
4. Lake, A.M. What we know so far: COVID-19 current clinical knowledge and research. *Clin. Med.* **2020**, *20*, 124–127. [CrossRef] [PubMed]
5. Chen, N.; Zhou, M.; Dong, X.; Qu, J.; Gong, F.; Han, Y.; Qiu, Y.; Wang, J.; Liu, Y.; Wei, Y.; et al. Epidemiological and clinical characteristics of 99 cases of 2019 novel coronavirus pneumonia in Wuhan, China: A descriptive study. *Lancet* **2020**, *395*, 507–513. [CrossRef]
6. Wang, F.-S.; Zhang, C. What to do next to control the 2019-nCoV epidemic? *Lancet* **2020**, *395*, 391–393. [CrossRef]
7. Li, Q.; Guan, X.; Wu, P.; Wang, X.; Zhou, L.; Tong, Y.; Ren, R.; Leung, K.S.M.; Lau, E.H.Y.; Wong, J.Y.; et al. Early transmission dynamics in Wuhan, China, of Novel Coronavirus–infected pneumonia. *N. Engl. J. Med.* **2020**, *382*, 1199–1207. [CrossRef] [PubMed]
8. Wang, W.; Tang, J.; Wei, F. Updated understanding of the outbreak of 2019 novel coronavirus (2019-nCoV) in Wuhan, China. *J. Med. Virol.* **2020**, *92*, 441–447. [CrossRef] [PubMed]
9. Rothe, C.; Schunk, M.; Seilmaier, M.; Drosten, C.; Vollmar, P.; Zwirglmaier, K.; Zange, S.; Wölfel, R.; Hoelscher, M.; Sothmann, P.; et al. Transmission of 2019-nCoV infection from an asymptomatic contact in Germany. *N. Engl. J. Med.* **2020**, *382*, 970–971. [CrossRef]
10. Balcan, D.; Gonçalves, B.; Hu, H.; Ramasco, J.J.; Colizza, V.; Vespignani, A. Modeling the spatial spread of infectious diseases: The gLobal Epidemic and mobility computational model. *J. Comput. Sci.* **2010**, *1*, 132–145. [CrossRef]
11. Chinazzi, M.; Davis, J.T.; Ajelli, M.; Gioannini, C.; Litvinova, M.; Merler, S.; Piontti, A.P.Y.; Mu, K.; Rossi, L.; Sun, K.; et al. The effect of travel restrictions on the spread of the 2019 novel coronavirus (COVID-19) outbreak. *Science* **2020**, *368*, 395–400. [CrossRef]
12. Cruz, M.P.; Santos, E.; Cervantes, M.V.; Juárez, M.L. COVID-19, una emergencia de salud pública mundial. *Rev. Clín. Esp.* **2021**, *221*, 55–61. [CrossRef] [PubMed]
13. Abdelhafiz, A.S.; Mohammed, Z.; Ibrahim, M.E.; Ziady, H.H.; Alorabi, M.; Ayyad, M.; Sultan, E.A. Knowledge, perceptions, and attitude of egyptians towards the novel coronavirus disease (Covid-19). *J. Commun. Health* **2020**, *45*, 881–890. [CrossRef]
14. Li, J.-Y.; You, Z.; Wang, Q.; Zhou, Z.-J.; Qiu, Y.; Luo, R.; Ge, X.-Y. The epidemic of 2019-novel-coronavirus (2019-nCoV) pneumonia and insights for emerging infectious diseases in the future. *Microbes Infect.* **2020**, *22*, 80–85. [CrossRef] [PubMed]

15. Lau, H.; Khosrawipour, V.; Kocbach, P.; Mikolajczyk, A.; Schubert, J.; Bania, J.; Khosrawipour, T. The positive impact of lockdown in Wuhan on containing the COVID-19 outbreak in China. *J. Travel Med.* **2020**, *27*, taaa037. [CrossRef] [PubMed]
16. Zhu, W.; Li, X.; Wu, Y.; Xu, C.; Li, L.; Yang, J.; Fang, S. Community quarantine strategy against coronavirus disease 2019 in Anhui: An evaluation based on trauma center patients. *Int. J. Infect. Dis.* **2020**, *96*, 417–421. [CrossRef]
17. Ho, C.S.; Chee, C.Y.; Ho, R.C. Mental health strategies to combat the psychological impact of COVID-19 beyond paranoia and panic. *Ann. Acad. Med. Singap.* **2020**, *49*, 1–3.
18. Rubin, G.J.; Wessely, S. The psychological effects of quarantining a city. *BMJ* **2020**, *368*, m313. [CrossRef]
19. Berggren, N.; Curtis, H.; Derakshan, N. Interactions of emotion and anxiety on visual working memory performance. *Psychon. Bull. Rev.* **2016**, *24*, 1274–1281. [CrossRef]
20. Dar, K.A.; Iqbal, N.; Mushtaq, A. Intolerance of uncertainty, depression, and anxiety: Examining the indirect and moderating effects of worry. *Asian J. Psychiatry* **2017**, *29*, 129–133. [CrossRef]
21. Ohrnberger, J.; Fichera, E.; Sutton, M. The relationship between physical and mental health: A mediation analysis. *Soc. Sci. Med.* **2017**, *195*, 42–49. [CrossRef] [PubMed]
22. Dong, L.; Bouey, J. Public mental health crisis during COVID-19 pandemic, China. *Emerg. Infect. Dis.* **2020**, *26*, 1616–1618. [CrossRef] [PubMed]
23. Hernández, B.C.; Rugarcía, Y.T. Attitudes toward the risk prevention in health professionals in cases of epidemiological alert. *Med. Segur. Trab.* **2015**, *61*, 254–272.
24. Greenberg, N.; Docherty, M.; Gnanapragasam, S.; Wessely, S. Managing mental health challenges faced by healthcare workers during covid-19 pandemic. *BMJ* **2020**, *368*, m1211. [CrossRef]
25. Tucci, V.; Moukaddam, N.; Meadows, J.; Shah, S.; Galwankar, S.C.; Kapur, G.B. The forgotten plague: Psychiatric manifestations of ebola, zika, and emerging infectious diseases. *J. Glob. Infect. Dis.* **2017**, *9*, 151–156. [CrossRef]
26. Lai, J.; Ma, S.; Tan, H.; Kang, L.; Yao, L.; Huang, M.; Wang, H.; Wang, G.; Liu, Z.; Hu, S.; et al. Factors associated with mental health outcomes among health care workers exposed to coronavirus disease 2019. *JAMA Netw. Open* **2020**, *3*, e203976. [CrossRef]
27. Cosic, K.; Popovic, S.; Sarlija, M.; Kesedzic, I. Impact of human disasters and COVID-19 pandemic on mental health: Potential of digital psychiatry. *Psychiatr. Danub.* **2020**, *32*, 25–31. [CrossRef]
28. Maunder, R.; Hunter, J.; Vincent, L.; Bennett, J.; Peladeau, N.; Leszcz, M.; Sadavoy, J.; Verhaeghe, L.M.; Steinberg, R.; Mazzulli, T. The immediate psychological and occupational impact of the 2003 SARS outbreak in a teaching hospital. *CMAJ* **2003**, *168*, 1245–1251.
29. Li, S.; Wang, Y.; Xue, J.; Zhao, N.; Zhu, T. The impact of COVID-19 epidemic declaration on psychological consequences: A study on active weibo users. *Int. J. Environ. Res. Public Health* **2020**, *17*, 2032. [CrossRef]
30. Broadbent, E.; Wilkes, C.; Koschwanez, H.; Weinman, J.; Norton, S.; Petrie, K.J. A systematic review and meta-analysis of the Brief Illness Perception Questionnaire. *Psychol. Health* **2015**, *30*, 1361–1385. [CrossRef] [PubMed]
31. Barbisch, D.; Koenig, K.L.; Shih, F.-Y. Is there a case for quarantine? Perspectives from SARS to Ebola. *Disaster Med. Public Health Prep.* **2015**, *9*, 547–553. [CrossRef] [PubMed]
32. Wang, C.; Pan, R.; Wan, X.; Tan, Y.; Xu, L.; Ho, C.; Ho, R. Immediate psychological responses and associated factors during the initial stage of the 2019 coronavirus disease (Covid-19) Epidemic among the general population in China. *Int. J. Environ. Res. Public Health* **2020**, *17*, 1729. [CrossRef]
33. Xiang, Y.-T.; Yang, Y.; Li, W.; Zhang, L.; Zhang, Q.; Cheung, T.; Ng, C.H. Timely mental health care for the 2019 novel coronavirus outbreak is urgently needed. *Lancet Psychiatry* **2020**, *7*, 228–229. [CrossRef]
34. Zhang, J.; Wu, W.; Zhao, X.; Zhang, W. Recommended psychological crisis intervention response to the 2019 novel coronavirus pneumonia outbreak in China: A model of West China Hospital. *Precis. Clin. Med.* **2020**, *3*, 3–8. [CrossRef]
35. Bao, Y.; Sun, Y.; Meng, S.; Shi, J.; Lu, L. 2019-nCoV epidemic: Address mental health care to empower society. *Lancet* **2020**, *395*, e37–e38. [CrossRef]
36. Gao, J.; Zheng, P.; Jia, Y.; Chen, H.; Mao, Y.; Chen, S.; Wang, Y.; Fu, H.; Dai, J. Mental health problems and social media exposure during COVID-19 outbreak. *PLoS ONE* **2020**, *15*, e0231924. [CrossRef]
37. Fung, I.C.-H.; Fu, K.-W.; Chan, C.-H.; Chan, B.S.B.; Cheung, C.-N.; Abraham, T.; Tse, Z.T.H. Social media's initial reaction to information and misinformation on Ebola, August 2014: Facts and rumors. *Public Health Rep.* **2016**, *131*, 461–473. [CrossRef] [PubMed]
38. Bora, K.; Das, D.; Barman, B.; Borah, P. Are internet videos useful sources of information during global public health emergencies? A case study of YouTube videos during the 2015–16 Zika virus pandemic. *Pathog. Glob. Health* **2018**, *112*, 320–328. [CrossRef]
39. Pérez-Fuentes, M.D.C.; Molero Jurado, M.D.M.; Ruiz Oropesa, N.F.; Marto Martínez, Á.; Simon Márquez, M.D.M.; Herrera-Peco, I.; Gázquez Linares, J.J. Questionnaire on perception of threat from COVID-19. *J. Clin. Med.* **2020**, *9*, 1196. [CrossRef]
40. Calasanti, T.; King, N. Taking 'women's work' 'like a man': Husbands' experiences of care work. *Gerontologist* **2007**, *47*, 516–527. [CrossRef]
41. Guberman, M.N.; Maheu, M.P.; Maillé, C. Women as family caregivers: Why do they care? *Gerontologist* **1992**, *32*, 607–617. [CrossRef] [PubMed]
42. Benson, R.; Glaser, K.; Corna, L.M.; Platts, L.G.; Di Gessa, G.; Worts, D.; Price, D.; McDonough, P.; Sacker, A. Do work and family care histories predict health in older women? *Eur. J. Public Health* **2017**, *27*, 1010–1015. [CrossRef]

43. Halper, L.R.; Cowgill, C.M.; Rios, K. Gender bias in caregiving professions: The role of perceived warmth. *J. Appl. Soc. Psychol.* **2019**, *49*, 549–562. [CrossRef]
44. Gómez, R.A.; Reina, L.L.; Méndez, I.F.; García, J.M.; Briñol, L.G. El psicólogo clínico en los centros de salud. Un trabajo conjunto entre atención primaria y salud mental. *Atención Primaria* **2019**, *51*, 310–313. [CrossRef] [PubMed]
45. Gené-Badia, J.; Comice, P.; Belchín, A.; Erdozain, M. Ángeles; Cáliz, L.; Torres, S.; Rodríguez, R. Perfiles de soledad y aislamiento social en población urbana. *Aten. Prim.* **2020**, *52*, 224–232. [CrossRef]
46. Phan, T. Genetic diversity and evolution of SARS-CoV-2. *Infect. Genet. Evol.* **2020**, *81*, 104260. [CrossRef]
47. Blanco-Donoso, L.M.; Moreno-Jiménez, J.; Amutio, A.; Gallego-Alberto, L.; Moreno-Jiménez, B.; Garrosa, E. Stressors, job resources, fear of contagion, and secondary traumatic stress among nursing home workers in face of the COVID-19: The case of Spain. *J. Appl. Gerontol.* **2020**. [CrossRef]
48. Martínez-Lorca, M.; Martínez-Lorca, A.; Criado-Álvarez, J.J.; Armesilla, M.D.C.; Latorre, J.M. The fear of COVID-19 scale: Validation in Spanish university students. *Psychiatry Res.* **2020**, *293*, 113350. [CrossRef] [PubMed]
49. Cuan-Baltazar, J.Y.; Muñoz-Perez, M.J.; Robledo-Vega, C.; Pérez-Zepeda, M.F.; Soto-Vega, E. Misinformation of COVID-19 on the internet: Infodemiology study. *JMIR Public Health Surveill.* **2020**, *6*, e18444. [CrossRef]
50. Singh, D.R.; Sunuwar, D.R.; Karki, K.; Ghimire, S.; Shrestha, N. Knowledge and perception towards universal safety precautions during early phase of the COVID-19 outbreak in Nepal. *J. Community Health* **2020**, *45*, 1116–1122. [CrossRef] [PubMed]
51. Epifanio, M.S.; Andrei, F.; Mancini, G.; Agostini, F.; Piombo, M.A.; Spicuzza, V.; Riolo, M.; Lavanco, G.; Trombini, E.; La Grutta, S. The impact of COVID-19 pandemic and lockdown measures on quality of life among Italian general population. *J. Clin. Med.* **2021**, *10*, 289. [CrossRef] [PubMed]
52. Skapinakis, P.; Bellos, S.; Oikonomou, A.; Dimitradis, G.; Gkikas, P.; Perdikari, E.; Mavreas, V. Depression and its relationship with copping strategies and illness perceptions during the COVID-19 lockdown in Greece: A croos-sectional survey of the population. *Depress. Res. Treat.* **2020**, *2020*, 3158954. [CrossRef] [PubMed]
53. Liu, S.; Lithopoulos, A.; Zhang, C.-Q.; Garcia-Barrera, M.A.; Rhodes, R.E. Personality and perceived stress during COVID-19 pandemic: Testing the mediating role of perceived threat and efficacy. *Pers. Individ. Differ.* **2021**, *168*, 110351. [CrossRef] [PubMed]
54. Pérez-Fuentes, M.D.C.; Molero-Jurado, M.D.M.; Gázquez-Linares, J.J.; Simón-Márquez, M.D.M. Analysis of Burnout Predictors in Nursing: Risk and Protective Psychological Factors. *Eur. J. Psychol. Appl. Leg. Context* **2019**, *11*, 33–40. [CrossRef]

Journal of *Clinical Medicine*

MDPI

Article

The Effect of COVID-19 Lockdown Measures on Physical Activity Levels and Sedentary Behaviour in a Relatively Young Population Living in Kosovo

Masar Gjaka [1,†], Kaltrina Feka [2,3,4,†], Antonino Bianco [2,3], Faton Tishukaj [5], Valerio Giustino [2,3,4], Anna Maria Parroco [2], Antonio Palma [2,3,6] and Giuseppe Battaglia [2,3,6,*]

1 Department of Sport and Movement Science, University for Business and Technology, 10000 Pristina, Kosovo; masar.gjaka@ubt-uni.net
2 Department of Psychology, Educational Science and Human Movement, University of Palermo, 90128 Palermo, Italy; kaltrina.feka@unipa.it (K.F.); antonino.bianco@unipa.it (A.B.); valerio.giustino@unipa.it (V.G.); annamaria.parroco@unipa.it (A.M.P.); antonio.palma@unipa.it (A.P.)
3 Sport and Exercise Science Research Unit, University of Palermo, 90144 Palermo, Italy
4 PhD Program in Health Promotion and Cognitive Sciences, University of Palermo, 90128 Palermo, Italy
5 Faculty of Physical Education and Sport, University of Pristina, 10000 Pristina, Kosovo; faton.tishukaj@uni-pr.edu
6 Regional Sports School of CONI Sicilia, 90141 Sicily, Italy
* Correspondence: giuseppe.battaglia@unipa.it; Tel.: +39-09123899616
† Share the first authorship.

Citation: Gjaka, M.; Feka, K.; Bianco, A.; Tishukaj, F.; Giustino, V.; Parroco, A.M.; Palma, A.; Battaglia, G. The Effect of COVID-19 Lockdown Measures on Physical Activity Levels and Sedentary Behaviour in a Relatively Young Population Living in Kosovo. *J. Clin. Med.* **2021**, *10*, 763. https://doi.org/10.3390/jcm10040763

Academic Editor: Michele Roccella

Received: 28 January 2021
Accepted: 11 February 2021
Published: 14 February 2021

Publisher's Note: MDPI stays neutral with regard to jurisdictional claims in published maps and institutional affiliations.

Abstract: To abate the spread of the COVID-19 virus, different restriction measures were imperative, limiting the possibility to be engaged in physical activity. Therefore, this study aimed to evaluate the effect of COVID-19 lockdown on physical activity (PA) levels expressed as energy expenditure (MET-min/week) and sedentary behaviour in Kosovo. The possible association between PA levels and other factors was analyzed. 1633 participants (age range: 13 to 63 years; mean: 24.70 ± 9.33 years; body height: 172 ± 10.57 cm; body mass: 69.10 ± 13.80 kg; BMI: 23.09 ± 3.63 kg/m^2) participated in the study, categorized by age, gender, BMI, and living area. An online survey, including an adapted version of the IPAQ-SF, was administered once during lockdown to assess PA levels and sedentary behaviour both before and during COVID-19 lockdown. The Wilcoxon signed-rank, Mann–Whitney U and Kruskal–Wallis rank of sum tests were used for statistical analysis. COVID-19 restrictions had a negative impact on the types of and overall PA levels MET-min/week ($p < 0.001$). Sedentary behaviour significantly increased during COVID-19 restrictions ($p < 0.001$). Higher decreases in MET-min/week during lockdown were observed among males, young and young adults, overweight, and urban-living participants. Finally, COVID-19 restrictions decreased the PA levels and MET-min/week, and increased sedentary behaviour also in a relatively young cohort. Such differences were dependent on several factors.

Keywords: physical activity; COVID-19; Kosovo; restrictions; public health

1. Introduction

In the last decades, the literature has extensively described the numerous benefits of physical activity (PA) on health, including aspects directly associated with the amelioration of general health as well as the prevention of cardiovascular diseases, type II diabetes, colon cancer, immune function, and obesity [1–4]. The ability of different types of exercise to respond also to bone, muscle, and joint pathologies as well as degenerative diseases has been very well established [5–10].

Conversely, sedentary behaviour and a lack of daily PA might lead to health-related problems such as dyslipidaemia [11], microvascular dysfunction, and problems associated with peripheral insulin resistance [12], which are related to increased odds of weight gain and an accompanying increased risk of indicators for cardiometabolic health-related risks [13]. Studies regarding health-related adverse effects of physical inactivity have defined it as the fourth leading risk factor, accounting for 6% of global deaths [14].

Since the beginning of 2020, humankind is globally fighting against a deadly virus (COVID-19) which is a very serious public health concern, initially detected in Wuhan (China) at the end of December 2019 [15,16]; it is now spread out worldwide, having infected over 48 million people and causing over 1.2 million deaths to date [17]. Due to its fast human-to-human transmission and the damage the virus causes to human beings—in serious cases, resulting in death—the World Health Organization (WHO) has declared the COVID-19 virus a pandemic (11 March 2020) [18]. In view of all the facts mentioned above, the WHO and other relevant national bodies, including also their respective governments, have implemented different kinds of lockdown strategies relative to the severity of the COVID-19 outbreak [19] including isolation, home confinement, and also social distancing [20]. In addition, due to the precaution measures imposed by the respective countries, restricted access to PA spaces (e.g., gyms) has limited PA possibilities, especially for activities usually performed outdoors and/or in groups [19].

After the first COVID-19 positive case was detected (March 13), the precaution measures were also taken in Kosovo by closing universities, schools, and borders, and also by suspending social gatherings and sports competitions at amateur and professional levels [21,22].

Yet, although social distancing and self-isolation are acknowledged as effective measures to flatten the spreading curve of COVID-19, these measures are also considered to increase the burden among humans [23,24]. In fact, home confinement and other imposed safety measures have negatively influenced PA levels, which has already been reported in other studies in countries such as Italy [25], Croatia [26], Spain [27], Canada [28], and also in large-scale surveys including countries from all over the world [20]. Furthermore, the negative impact of prolonged isolation on psychological well-being, causing post-traumatic stress symptoms, confusion, and anxiety, has been reported [29]. Moreover, studies have shown an increased time spent in sedentary behaviour (sitting time) during the COVID-19 pandemic compared to pre-pandemic time [20], which might be an increased concern for public health. Indeed, Hossain and his colleagues (2020) highlighted that there might be an association between regional anti-COVID-19 policies and socio-economic factors with differences in PA levels during COVID-19 lockdown [30]. Additionally, COVID-19 lockdown consequences on behavioural outcomes, including PA, affect all inhabitants regardless of age, sex, and ethnicity [10]. On the contrary, the living area was found to be an important factor related to the PA levels during COVID-19 lockdown [31].

In light of these facts, besides noticeable and severe changes, to the best of the authors' knowledge, no scientific data have been reported regarding the effect of COVID-19 lockdown measures on PA levels and sedentary behaviour in the Kosovo population.

Therefore, this exploratory study aimed to evaluate the effect of COVID-19 lockdown in PA levels expressed as energy expenditure (MET-minutes/week) and sedentary behaviour among the Kosovo population. Additionally, the potential link between factors such as age, gender, anthropometrics, and living area and the level and frequency of PA has been investigated.

We hypothesized that the COVID-19 lockdown would have a negative impact on the Kosovan population by decreasing the PA level and increasing the exposure time to sedentary behaviour. Additionally, it is hypothesized that the PA level and MET-minutes/week changes during COVID-19 lockdown depend on age, gender, anthropometrics, and living area.

2. Materials and Methods

2.1. Study Design and Procedure

The current study is a cross-sectional study design implemented using an online survey, including an adapted version of the International Physical Activity Questionnaire-

Short Form (IPAQ-SF), created on the Google Forms platform (Google LLC, Mountain View, CA, USA) during the COVID-19 pandemic outbreak in Kosovo. During the period this study was conducted, Kosovo inhabitants were exposed to the government anti-COVID-19 restriction measures.

Approximately four weeks after the lockdown measures started (13 March 2020), the online survey was launched and randomly dispersed to as many people as possible. Initially, an official email including the link of the online survey was sent to all students and academic and non-academic staff of the University for Business and Technology. Afterwards, in order to increase the number of participants, the snowball sampling recruitment approach was used, spreading the online survey link via e-mailing channels and social media such as Instagram, Facebook, WhatsApp and Viber, encouraging participants to enroll in the study [20,25,27,28,32].

The study was conducted in accordance with the principles of the Declaration of Helsinki and received ethical clearance from the Ethics Committees of the University of Palermo (Protocol Number: 14/2020).

2.2. Participants

Participants who completed the online survey launched on 8 April until 21 April 2020 (during the government restriction measures) were considered eligible for the current study.

An overall total of 1928 of participants representing the country participated in the study by filling out the online survey. In order to minimize the effect of errors, a data cleaning process was adopted comprised of the following steps: exclusion of ineligible respondents including participants who did not complete the entire survey and of multiple submissions from the same participant; identification and management of meaningless data (e.g., duration expressed in hours, not in minutes; duration reported as weekly, not daily; duration reported as text, not as a number etc.).

Yet, after the cleaning process, a total of 1633 participants were included in the study.

2.3. Internal Consistency of the Questionnaire

The questionnaire used within the current study was built from IPAQ-SF. The questionnaire focused on two different moments, relating to before and during COVID-19 confinement restrictions. Specifically, it consisted of 31 items, assessing demographics (question 2 and 3), anthropometrics (question 4 and 5), PA before COVID-19 (question 7), employment status and residence during COVID-19 confinement (questions 8 to 13), the frequency and duration of vigorous-intensity PA before and during COVID-19 confinement (questions 14 to 17), the frequency and duration of moderate-intensity PA before and during COVID-19 confinement (questions 18 to 21), the frequency and duration of walking before and during COVID-19 confinement (questions 22 to 25), sedentary behaviour before and during COVID-19 confinement (question 26 and 27), and information related to PA during COVID-19 confinement. The introductory page of the questionnaire provided a concise description of the study and its main purposes, as well as the declarations of anonymity and confidentiality, and the personal data protection policy.

Since the questionnaire collected information of two different moments, to assess the validity of the obtained answers relating to past behaviour, question 7—"Before COVID-19 quarantine, how many days/week did you train regularly?" (with options ranging from 0 to 7 days per week)—was categorized into a dichotomous variable; according to the American College of Sports Medicine (ACSM) physical activity guidelines, people are considered sedentary if they train from 0 to 2 days per week, while they are considered physically active if they train from 3 to 7 days per week [33]. Therefore, a new variable, "physically active", with possible answers "Yes" or "No" was derived from the previous question.

Afterwards, to check if people where honest in their answers, a Mann–Whitney test was performed comparing the level of PA intensity (vigorous, moderate, walking) between sedentary and physically active individuals before the quarantine. If the respondents were honest in their answers, and the questionnaire was sensitive in detecting the amount of

PA prior to the COVID-19 lockdown, sedentary people should also have reported less pre-confinement PA than active people. From the results reported in Table 1, sedentary respondents reported an amount of the three intensities of PA that is significantly lower than physically active respondents, indicating that they were honest in indicating their PA before quarantine.

Table 1. Internal consistency of the questionnaire: types of PA before COVID-19 quarantine declared by sedentary and physically active respondents (According to the ACSM Physical Activity Guidelines 2018).

	Sedentary (n = 704)			**Physically Active (n = 929)**			
	Mean	**SD**	**Median**	**Mean**	**SD**	**Median**	p
VPA							
Days	1.40	1.52	1.00	3.41	1.64	4.00	<0.001
Minutes	26.19	30.09	20.00	53.37	30.86	60.00	<0.001
MET	533.35	685.96	240.00	1673.20	1195.64	1140.00	<0.001
MPA							
Days	3.20	2.02	3.00	4.07	1.66	4.00	<0.001
Minutes	50.65	36.86	45.00	64.62	35.13	60.00	<0.001
MET	986.27	727.92	792.00	1119.14	753.18	990.00	<0.001
Walking							
Days	5.32	1.79	5.00	5.70	1.60	6.00	<0.001
Minutes	53.63	32.53	45.00	57.79	33.33	60.00	0.01
MET	986.27	727.92	792.00	1119.14	753.18	990.00	<0.001

VPA: vigorous physical activity; MPA: moderate physical activity.

2.4. Scoring Protocol

Based on the well-known concept of metabolic equivalent (MET), the total weekly PA level, expressed as energy expenditure (MET-min/week), was calculated [34]. Consequently, the total weekly energy expenditure (MET-min/week) was estimated according to the specific metabolic equivalent (MET) values for each category of PA (3.3 MET for walking, 4 MET for moderate-intensity PA, and 8 MET for vigorous-intensity PA) [35–37]. The following formula was used to calculate the total weekly energy expenditure (MET-min/week): *total weekly energy expenditure (MET-min/week) = MET x duration of PA type (minutes) x frequency.* All calculations were performed in accordance with the specifications provided elsewhere [35–37], and also following the "Guidelines for Data Processing and Analysis of the International Physical Activity Questionnaire (IPAQ)—Short and Long Forms" (http://www.ipaq.ki.se (accessed on 15 September 2020)) [38].

Furthermore, following the IPAQ guidelines for scoring protocol (http://www.ipaq.ki.se (accessed on 15 September 2020)) [38], according to the total weekly energy expenditure (MET-min/week) from all types of PA, participants were assigned to one of the following categories: (1) low activity (<600 MET-min/week), (2) moderate activity (≥600 MET-min/week), and (3) high activity (≥3000 MET-min/week).

2.5. Statistical Analysis

Several variables derived from the online survey were re-coded for further statistical analyses. The following categories were used to categorize participants based on their body mass index (BMI) levels: underweight (UW) (BMI < 18.5), normal weight (NW) (18.5 < BMI < 25), and overweight (OW) (BMI > 25) [25,39]. Participants were grouped into five different age categories: young (≤ 25 years), young adults (25 < years ≤ 35), adults (35 < years ≤ 55), senior adults (55 < years ≤ 65), and elderly (>65 years) [25,40]. The Shapiro–Wilk test was used to test the normality of the distribution for all variables. Data are computed and presented as means, standard deviation, and percentages.

To test the difference in the total energy expenditure (MET-min/week) before and during COVID-19 confinement, the Wilcoxon signed-rank test for dependent groups was used. The Mann–Whitney U test was chosen to analyze the differences in responses before and during for type of PA, gender, and living area (urban vs. rural living environment). To assess pre- and during COVID-19 confinement differences between categories assigned based on BMI and age, the Kruskal–Wallis rank-sum test was employed, with the Mann–Whitney U test chosen for pairwise comparisons. Non-parametric tests have been used because the normality assumption of the distribution, tested by the Shapiro–Wilks test, was violated.

The level of significance was set at $p < 0.05$. All of the statistical analyses were performed using the Statistical Package for Social Sciences (SPSS), version 21.0 (SPSS Inc., Chicago, IL, USA). GraphPad Prism version 8.4.3 was used to design graphs and figures.

3. Results

3.1. Descriptive Analysis

Participants

A total of 1633 (812 males and 823 females) Kosovan participants (age range: 13 to 63 years; mean: 24.70 ± 9.33 years; body height: 172 ± 10.57 cm; body mass: 69.10 ± 13.80 kg; BMI: 23.09 ± 3.63 kg/m^2) who all voluntarily participated in the study. All of the demographic characteristics of participants including gender, age, BMI category, and living area are presented in Table 2.

Table 2. Demographic characteristics of the participants.

Variables		N	%
Sample			
	Participants	1633	
	Female	823	50.4
	Male	810	49.6
Age Categories			
	Young	1130	69.2
	Young adults	299	18.3
	Adults	176	10.8
	Senior adults	28	1.7
BMI Category			
	Underweight	123	7.5
	Normal weight	1129	69.1
	Overweight	381	23.3
Living Area			
	Urban	1032	63.2
	Rural	601	36.8

N: number; %: percentage; BMI: Body Mass Index.

3.2. Physical Activity before and during the COVID-19 Confinement Period

All PA results derived from the questionnaire, registered before and during home confinement, are presented in detail in Table 3.

3.2.1. Vigorous Intensity Physical Activity

The number of days/week and minutes/day of vigorous intensity PA during compared to before home confinement declined significantly by 25.7% ($p < 0.001$) and 36.2% ($p < 0.001$), respectively. Moreover, the energy expenditure (MET-min/week) of vigorous intensity PA decreased by 45.7% during compared to before home confinement ($p < 0.001$).

3.2.2. Moderate Intensity Physical Activity

A statistically significant reduction in the number of days/week (17.1%) and minutes/week (27.5%) of moderate intensity PA during home confinement was found. Likewise, significantly lower MET-min/week values were found during compared to before home confinement (36.4%; $p < 0.001$).

Table 3. Physical activity responses recorded pre- and during confinement.

		Pre-Confinement	During Confinement	Δ (Δ%)	*p* Value
VPA	Days/week	2.54 ± 1.87	1.89 ± 1.76	0.65 (25.7%)	<0.001
	min/week	41.7 ± 33.7	26.6 ± 25.3	15.09 (36.2%)	<0.001
	MET/week	1181.8 ± 1155.2	641.9 ± 794.4	539.94 (45.7%)	<0.001
MPA	Days/week	3.7 ± 1.9	3.1 ± 1.9	0.63 (17.1%)	<0.001
	min/week	58.6 ± 36.54	42.5 ± 29.6	16.11 (27.5%)	<0.001
	MET/week	967.3±765.4	615.5 ± 578	351.78 (36.4%)	<0.001
Walking	Days/week	5.54 ± 1.69	3.98 ± 2.44	1.58 (28.5%)	<0.001
	min/week	56 ± 33.04	32.9 ± 22.6	23.12 (41.3%)	<0.001
	MET/week	1061.9 ± 745	500.8 ± 478.9	561.1 (52.9%)	<0.001
All PA	Days/week	3.92 ± 1.23	2.96 ± 1.43	0.95 (24.32%)	<0.001
	min/week	52.1 ± 23.4	33.9 ± 18.7	18.11 (34.8%)	<0.001
	MET/week	3211 ± 1880	1756.5 ± 1387.2	493.45 (26.2%)	<0.001
Sitting	hours/week	5.33 ± 1.7	8.13 ± 2.2	2.8 (34%)	<0.001

VPA: vigorous physical activity; MPA: moderate physical activity; Δ: difference before vs. during confinement; Δ%: percentage of difference before vs. during confinement.

3.2.3. Walking

The number of days/week of walking declined significantly by 28.5% during home confinement ($p < 0.001$). Similarly, the number of minutes/week and the MET-min/week of walking significantly decreased ($p < 0.001$) by 41.3% and 52.9%, respectively.

3.2.4. All Physical Activity

Likewise, the number of days/week, minutes/week, and MET-min/week of all PA was significantly lower during home confinement by 24.32%, 34.8%, and 26.2%, respectively.

3.2.5. Sitting Time

The statistical analysis indicated a significant increase in the number of sitting hours/day by 34% during home confinement ($p < 0.001$).

As depicted in Figure 1, significant differences were reported in the energy expenditure expressed as (MET-min/week) before and during home confinement ($p < 0.001$).

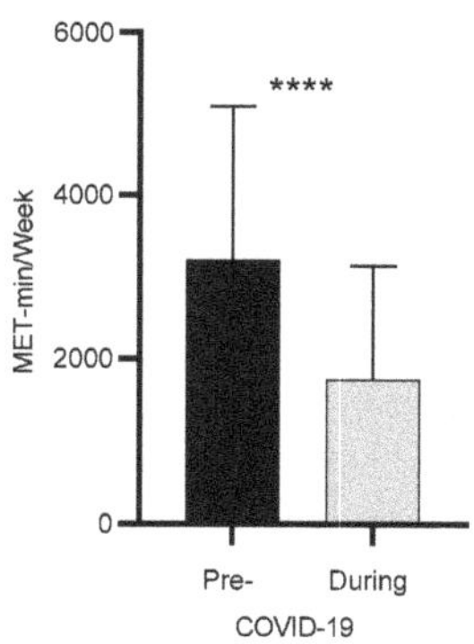

Figure 1. Overall MET-min/week (pre and during COVID-19). Total weekly energy expenditure (MET-min/week) pre-home confinement, during home confinement, and the difference between pre- and during home confinement. Legend: ****: ($p < 0.001$).

Following the IPAQ recommendations for scoring protocol, participants were assigned to one of the three PA categories (i.e., < 600; ≥ 600; ≥ 3000 MET–min/week). For the pre-home confinement condition, results revealed that 49 participants belonged to the low activity category (3%), 801 were moderately active (49.1%), and 783 (47.9%) participants were highly active. In this regard, results for during the home confinement condition revealed an increase in the low activity category ($n = 311$; 19%) and in the moderate activity category ($n = 1069$; 65.5%), while a decline in the number of high activity participants was found ($n = 253$; 15.5%).

3.3. Energy Expenditure in Relation to Gender, Age Category, BMI Classification

Significant gender differences in MET-min/week were found ($p < 0.001$), with male participants expressing higher values of energy expenditure in the pre-confinement condition compared to the female participants (Figure 2a). On the other hand, no significant gender differences were found during the confinement condition in MET-min/week ($p = 0.53$) (Figure 2b). The difference between pre- and during confinement showed a higher decrease in MET-min/week among male participants (Figure 2c).

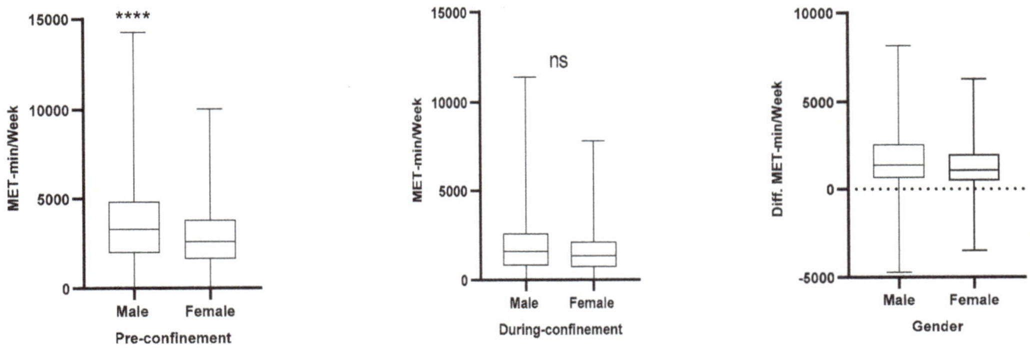

(a) (b) (c)

Figure 2. Gender differences in MET-min/week (pre and during COVID-19). (**a**) Total weekly energy expenditure (MET-min/week) pre home confinement condition in relation to gender category. (**b**) Total weekly energy expenditure (MET-min/week) during home confinement condition in relation to gender category. (**c**) Total weekly energy expenditure (MET-min/week) difference between pre and during home confinement in relation to gender category. Legend: ****: ($p < 0.001$); ns: non-significant difference.

Analysis of the age categories showed a significant difference in MET-min/week between pre and during home confinement condition ($p < 0.001$), except for senior adults, where the difference was ($p = 0.006$). Pairwise comparison analysis revealed a significant difference between the young and adults ($p < 0.001$), young and senior adults ($p < 0.001$), young adults and adults ($p < 0.001$), and young adults and senior adults ($p = 0.002$) in MET-min/week pre confinement condition (Figure 3a). Likewise, the during-confinement condition pairwise analysis showed the same significant differences between the young and adults ($p < 0.001$), young and senior adults ($p = 0.005$), young adults and adults ($p = 0.001$), and young adults and senior adults ($p = 0.02$) in MET-min/week for the during-confinement condition (Figure 3b). As depicted in Figure 3c, the highest MET-min/week difference between pre- and during confinement was found among the young and young adult categories.

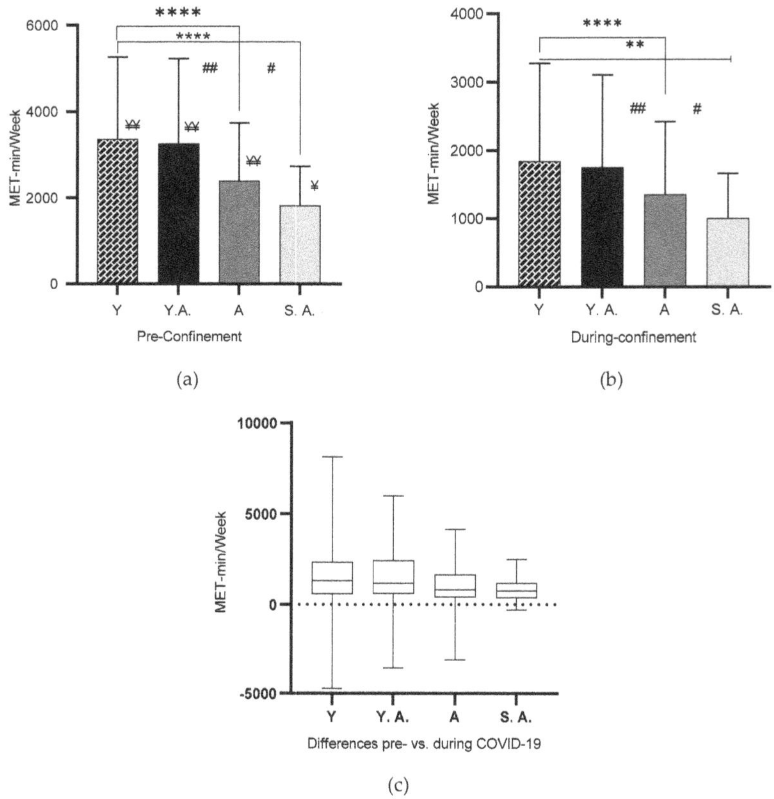

Figure 3. Age category differences in MET-min/week (pre and during COVID-19). (**a**) Total weekly energy expenditure (MET-min/week) pre-home confinement condition in relation to age categories. Legend: Y: young; Y. A.: young adult; A: adult; S. A: senior adult; ****: ($p < 0.001$); ##: ($p < 0.001$); #: ($p = 0.002$); ¥¥: differences between pre and during confinement ($p < 0.001$); ¥: differences between pre- and during confinement ($p = 0.006$). (**b**) Total weekly energy expenditure (MET-min/week) during home confinement condition in relation to age categories. Legend: Y: young; Y. A.: young adult; A: adult; S. A.: senior adult; ****: ($p < 0.001$); **: ($p = 0.005$); ##: ($p = 0.001$); #: ($p = 0.02$). (**c**) Total weekly energy expenditure (MET-min/week) difference between the pre- and during-confinement condition in relation to age categories. Legend: Y: young; Y. A.: young adult; A: adult; S. A.: senior adult.

Analysis regarding the differences between BMI categories revealed that during the pre-confinement condition the NW category showed a higher MET-min/week value compared to the UW ($p = 0.006$) and OW ($p < 0.001$) categories (Figure 4a). Likewise, in the during-confinement condition, the NW category showed a higher MET-min/week value compared to both UW and OW ($p = 0.04$) and ($p < 0.001$), respectively. On the other hand, when comparing MET-min/week between pre- and during-confinement conditions, statistically significant differences were found for all BMI categories ($p < 0.001$). Moreover, the analysis of MET-min/week differences between the pre- and during-confinement condition revealed that the NW was the category with the highest difference (Figure 4b).

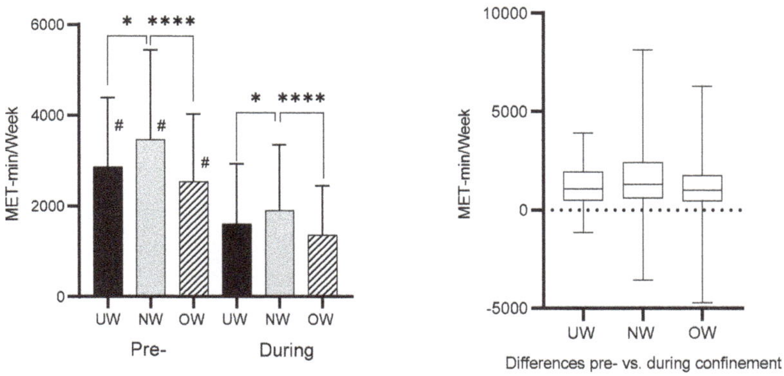

(a) (b)

Figure 4. BMI category differences in MET-min/week (pre and during COVID-19). (**a**) Total weekly energy expenditure (MET-min/week) pre and during home confinement condition in relation to BMI category. (**b**) Total weekly energy expenditure (MET-min/week) difference between pre and during home confinement in relation to BMI category. Legend: UW—underweight; NW—normal weight; OW—overweight; *—($p < 0.05$); ****—($p < 0.001$); #—($p < 0.001$).

3.4. Urban vs. Rural Living Environment

Statistical analysis showed significant differences in MET/min/week for the pre-confinement condition between participants living in urban and rural environments ($p = 0.002$). Additionally, significant differences in the total weekly energy expenditure (MET-min/week) were depicted for the during-confinement condition ($p < 0.001$), with participants living in rural environments reporting higher values (Figure 5a). On the other hand, the analysis revealed significant changes in MET-min/week between the pre- and during-confinement condition, for both participants living in urban and rural environments ($p < 0.001$) and ($p < 0.001$), respectively (Figure 5a). Likewise, significant differences were recorded in the MET-min/week difference between urban and rural living environments, with a higher decrease among urban living participants ($p < 0.001$) (Figure 5b).

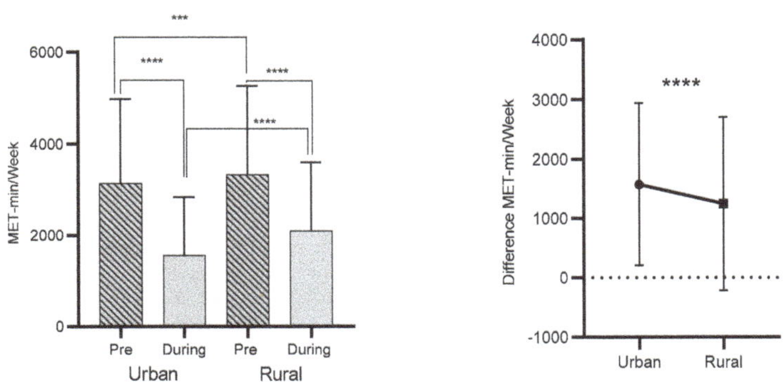

(a) (b)

Figure 5. Living environment differences in MET-min/week (pre and during COVID-19). (**a**) Total weekly energy expenditure (MET-min/week) pre- and during home confinement in relation to urban and rural living environment. (**b**) Total weekly energy expenditure (MET-min/week) difference between pre- and during home confinement in relation to urban and rural living environment. Legend: ****: ($p < 0.001$); ***: ($p = 0.002$).

4. Discussion

The purpose of this study was to evaluate the effect of COVID-19 lockdown in PA levels expressed as energy expenditure (MET-minutes/week) and sedentary behaviour among the Kosovo population. Additionally, this study analysed the possible effect of covariates such as age, gender, anthropometrics, and living area on the PA levels of the Kosovan population.

This study has provided several important findings. The main finding of the present study showed a negative effect of COVID-19 home confinement on PA levels, leading to a significant decrease in days, minutes/day, and energy expenditure (MET-minutes/week) for three types of PA (vigorous intensity, moderate intensity, and walking activity) compared to the pre-home-confinement condition, as well as on overall PA level expressed as energy expenditure (MET-minutes/week).

Similarly, decreased PA levels during home confinement were reported also in other similar recent studies in people with and without disabilities [20,25–28,41–43]. Unsurprisingly, current results have demonstrated a significant negative effect of home confinement on PA intensity, causing an increased proportion of participants in the low and moderate activity category (16% and 17.6%, respectively), and a decrease in the high activity cohort of 32.4%. Further, this study strengthens the findings reported in comparable recent research, in which the authors reported the same pattern of PA reduction in active Sicilian adults due to home confinement restrictions [25].

As previously reported, sport clubs play a massive role in maintaining higher PA levels [44]. Particularly for Kosovo, the proportion of young individuals doing sports or other types of PA is relatively high as compared to older ones. Taking this into consideration, closing gyms, sports clubs and other public and private spaces has had the most detrimental impact on PA levels in the majority of the Kosovo population, taking into account the population demography. In addition, the lack of technical knowledge of the population on appropriate training routines has been reported as a factor leading to lower PA levels [45]. While other countries during COVID-19 lockdown were encouraging and stimulating their inhabitants to get enrolled in non-intensive indoor and outdoor PA to stimulate their mental and physical well-being [46], in Kosovo, no such governmental campaigns were organized.

Sitting behaviour (hours/day) was significantly higher during home confinement compared to pre-home-confinement. Results indicated a 34% increase in sitting behaviour (hours/day) during home confinement, most likely because participants were ordered to stay inside their homes to avoid infection. These results are in accordance with results reported in a recent large-scale research representing a multi-national and multi-continental sample, where a significant increase in sitting behaviour during home confinement was reported [20].

The amount of decrease in the PA level might be affected by different factors. In this regard, when our results were stratified by gender, significant differences were found between genders in PA levels pre-home-confinement, but such differences were not present during COVID-19 home confinement. A decrease in PA levels due to COVID-19 home confinement was noticed among both genders, with a higher drop among males. These findings are not in accordance with the results observed in a previous research, where gender differences in PA level during home confinement were reported [25]. This fact could be explained by the cultural context in which Kosovan people live in. In general, females living in Kosovo are more involved in household activities compared to males, which has helped the female participants to prevent as much of a decrease in PA levels as among males. This fact is supported by scientific evidence where household chores were reported to be the most prevalent PA type during home confinement [27].

For the age category variable, our results have revealed significant differences between pre- and during COVID-19 home confinement in PA levels. The highest PA level for both pre- and during home confinement conditions was reported from the young and young adult categories, while senior adults reported the lowest PA level. These findings are in complete agreement with the results published showing a similar trend of PA levels pre- and during home confinement [25,47]. Indeed, it has been previously reported that younger people are more physically active than the older ones [48] and the PA level progressively decreases with aging [43]. These results could have possibly been affected by such a high number of young and young adult participants. Nevertheless, this high number of young and young adult participants could be considered as representative for Kosovo, since the majority of the people belong to these two categories [49]. Considering the increased mortality rate of COVID-19 among older individuals, it might be speculated that this has prevented them from moving outside their living environments, resulting in higher levels of inactivity. Nevertheless, a recent study has shown that older adults who met the WHO physical activity guidelines during home confinement had better mental well-being [23]. Bearing this in mind, despite the restrictions, it is recommended that older adults engage in physical activity, even in their houses.

Furthermore, results of the current study have revealed significant differences in energy expenditure (MET-min/week) between BMI categories, with, as generally expected, the normal weight category expressing the highest values before and during COVID-19 home confinement. In fact, significant differences in energy expenditure between pre- and during home confinement existed for all three categories (underweight, normal weight, and overweight), with the normal weight category reporting the highest MET-min/week difference between pre- and during COVID-19 home confinement. This is not supported by the results of a similar study recently published, where no significant differences between BMI categories in energy expenditure were reported pre-confinement, but differences were reported to be present among the overweight category during COVID-19 home confinement [25]. Indeed, a higher decrease of PA during home confinement has been reported among participants with lower BMI compared to their counterparts with higher BMI [50].

Living area has been reported as an important factor influencing PA levels and fitness [51–53]. In this regard, our results demonstrated that the decrease in PA levels of Kosovan people during lockdown living in rural areas was smaller compared to the urban living ones, which showed a larger decrease in their PA levels. Such differences could be explained by the fact that people who live in rural areas of Kosovo usually have plenty of outdoor spaces and most of them are involved in farming and householding activities, which might have helped them to preserve their PA levels during the COVID-19 restrictions. These results are in line with the findings reported for Croatian adolescents, in which the authors found a larger decrease in PA levels during lockdown among urban living adolescents compared to their rural living counterparts [31].

Strengths and Limitations of the Study

To the best of our knowledge, this is the first study with a relatively large number of participants to assess the impact of the COVID-19 pandemic and associated public health restrictions on the PA behaviour of Kosovan population.

As a strength, it is worth noting that, besides having a representative sample form the entire country, in this study, the participants' living environment was also included. Taking into consideration the importance of PA and the maintenance of its levels during COVID-19 home confinement, we think that these results could be of importance to plan and develop proper strategies and policies when facing situations such as a pandemic.

Beside its strengths, this study also had some limitations that should be acknowledged. PA was not objectively measured, but was assessed by a self-reported questionnaire, increasing the risk of self-reporting bias. Nevertheless, since the questionnaire was administered both before and during COVID-19 home confinement, this bias does not influence our results to a great extent.

Another limitation is the comparability with the other studies, which, for their purposes, have used different methodologies and instruments.

A limitation that must be highlighted is the fact that it was not possible to demonstrate the validity of the questionnaire through the common analysis methods (i.e., using objective measures of PA from movement devices such as accelerometers or pedometers for comparison with the self-reported measures) [54]. In fact, the common analysis methods used for the validation are:

(1) correlation of the self-reported PA data with data from a relative measure of an objective measurement device
(2) computation of the absolute differences between self-reported and objective measurements [54].

However, we were unable to perform either the first or second method due to government restrictive measures which limited the possibilities of PA and therefore the consequent objective measure of PA practiced.

However, although the instrument used has detected the PA levels related to two different periods (i.e., pre- and during COVID-19 confinement measures) in a single administration, it should be noted that:

(1) The IPAQ is an instrument allows to evaluate the physical activity levels for either the last seven days (in the present study, the period during COVID-19 confinement) or the usual week (that we can consider for the questions related to the pre-COVID-19 confinement) [35];
(2) The results related to the PA levels of the week before COVID-19 confinement were compared and resulted consistent with those already published in the literature [55,56];
(3) The items related to the PA levels of the week during COVID-19 confinement refer to the classic IPAQ procedure in which the level of PA of the previous seven days is assessed.

5. Conclusions

Finally, based on the results, it can be concluded that COVID-19 home-confinement measures have had a negative impact on PA levels and energy expenditure (MET-min/week), especially among males, overweight participants, and those participants living in an urban area. The results of this study indicated also a significant increase in sitting behaviour among the Kosovan population during the COVID-19 lockdown.

Moreover, significant differences between age categories in MET-min/week were detected, with higher MET-min/week values among young and young adult categories for both pre- and during COVID-19 home confinement conditions. A high number of participants in the young and young adult age categories might have affected the decreased amount of PA levels compared to the latter, which represents the real demographics of the Kosovo population. Nevertheless, MET-min/week values in these two categories were affected the most due to COVID-19 restrictions. The lower number of adult and older adult participants has prevented us from drawing general conclusions regarding the decrease of PA levels for the entire population.

Currently, we are facing the second wave of COVID-19 infections, and these results could have potential important implications to help the decision-making bodies to implement strategies keeping in mind the maintenance of PA levels as crucial part of the public health sector.

Author Contributions: Conceptualization, M.G.; K.F. and G.B.; methodology, M.G.; K.F.; G.B.; A.B.; V.G. and A.P.; software, M.G. and K.F.; validation, M.G.; K.F. and F.T.; formal analysis, M.G.; K.F.; V.G. and A.M.P.; investigation, M.G.,K.F., F.T. and G.B.; data curation, M.G., K.F.; F.T. and A.M.P.; writing—original draft preparation, M.G., K.F.; A.B. and G.B.; visualization, M.G.; K.F. and A.P.; supervision, G.B.; A.B. and A.P.; project administration, M.G., K.F. and G.B. All authors have read and agreed to the published version of the manuscript.

Funding: This research received no external funding.

Institutional Review Board Statement: The study was conducted according to the guidelines of the Declaration of Helsinki, and approved by the Institutional Review Board (or Ethics Committee) of University of Palermo (Protocol Number: 14/2020).

Informed Consent Statement: Informed consent was obtained from all subjects involved in the study.

Data Availability Statement: The raw data will be made available by the authors, without undue reservations, upon request to the first author of this article.

Acknowledgments: The authors of the manuscript deeply thank all participants for being part of this research during a very stressful situation.

Conflicts of Interest: The authors declared no conflict of interest.

References

1. Haskell, W.L.; Blair, S.N.; Hill, J.O. Physical activity: Health outcomes and importance for public health policy. *Prev. Med.* **2009**, *49*, 280–282. [CrossRef] [PubMed]
2. Zinman, B.; Ruderman, N.; Campaigne, B.N.; Devlin, J.T.; Schneider, S.H.; American Diabetes, A. Physical activity/exercise and diabetes mellitus. *Diabetes Care* **2003**, *26* (Suppl. 1), S73–S77. [CrossRef]
3. Romeo, J.; Warnberg, J.; Pozo, T.; Marcos, A. Physical activity, immunity and infection. *Proc. Nutr. Soc.* **2010**, *69*, 390–399. [CrossRef]
4. Wu, N.; Bredin, S.S.D.; Guan, Y.; Dickinson, K.; Kim, D.D.; Chua, Z.; Kaufman, K.; Warburton, D.E.R. Cardiovascular Health Benefits of Exercise Training in Persons Living with Type 1 Diabetes: A Systematic Review and Meta-Analysis. *J. Clin. Med.* **2019**, *8*, 253. [CrossRef]
5. Musumeci, G. Effects of exercise on physical limitations and fatigue in rheumatic diseases. *World J. Orthop.* **2015**, *6*, 762–769. [CrossRef]
6. Castrogiovanni, P.; Trovato, F.M.; Szychlinska, M.A.; Nsir, H.; Imbesi, R.; Musumeci, G. The importance of physical activity in osteoporosis. From the molecular pathways to the clinical evidence. *Histol. Histopathol.* **2016**, *31*, 1183–1194. [CrossRef] [PubMed]
7. Pedersen, B.K.; Saltin, B. Evidence for prescribing exercise as therapy in chronic disease. *Scand. J. Med. Sci. Sports* **2006**, *16* (Suppl. 1), 3–63. [CrossRef]
8. Szychlinska, M.A.; Castrogiovanni, P.; Trovato, F.M.; Nsir, H.; Zarrouk, M.; Lo Furno, D.; Di Rosa, M.; Imbesi, R.; Musumeci, G. Physical activity and Mediterranean diet based on olive tree phenolic compounds from two different geographical areas have protective effects on early osteoarthritis, muscle atrophy and hepatic steatosis. *Eur. J. Nutr.* **2019**, *58*, 565–581. [CrossRef]
9. Warburton, D.E.; Nicol, C.W.; Bredin, S.S. Health benefits of physical activity: The evidence. *CMAJ* **2006**, *174*, 801–809. [CrossRef]
10. Narici, M.; De Vito, G.; Franchi, M.; Paoli, A.; Moro, T.; Marcolin, G.; Grassi, B.; Baldassarre, G.; Zuccarelli, L.; Biolo, G.; et al. Impact of sedentarism due to the COVID-19 home confinement on neuromuscular, cardiovascular and metabolic health: Physiological and pathophysiological implications and recommendations for physical and nutritional countermeasures. *Eur. J. Sport Sci.* **2020**, 1–22. [CrossRef] [PubMed]
11. Homer, A.R.; Owen, N.; Dunstan, D.W. Too much sitting and dysglycemia: Mechanistic links and implications for obesity. *Curr. Opin. Endocr. Metab. Res.* **2019**, *4*, 42–49. [CrossRef]
12. Hamburg, N.M.; McMackin, C.J.; Huang, A.L.; Shenouda, S.M.; Widlansky, M.E.; Schulz, E.; Gokce, N.; Ruderman, N.B.; Keaney, J.F., Jr.; Vita, J.A. Physical inactivity rapidly induces insulin resistance and microvascular dysfunction in healthy volunteers. *Arterioscler. Thromb. Vasc. Biol.* **2007**, *27*, 2650–2656. [CrossRef]
13. King, A.J.; Burke, L.M.; Halson, S.L.; Hawley, J.A. The Challenge of Maintaining Metabolic Health During a Global Pandemic. *Sports Med.* **2020**, *50*, 1233–1241. [CrossRef] [PubMed]
14. World Health Organization. *Global Recommendations on Physical Activity for Health*; World Health Organization: Geneva, Switzerland, 2010.
15. Guo, Y.R.; Cao, Q.D.; Hong, Z.S.; Tan, Y.Y.; Chen, S.D.; Jin, H.J.; Tan, K.S.; Wang, D.Y.; Yan, Y. The origin, transmission and clinical therapies on coronavirus disease 2019 (COVID-19) outbreak—An update on the status. *Mil. Med. Res.* **2020**, *7*, 11. [CrossRef]
16. Nishiura, H.; Jung, S.M.; Linton, N.M.; Kinoshita, R.; Yang, Y.; Hayashi, K.; Kobayashi, T.; Yuan, B.; Akhmetzhanov, A.R. The Extent of Transmission of Novel Coronavirus in Wuhan, China, 2020. *J. Clin. Med.* **2020**, *9*, 330. [CrossRef] [PubMed]
17. World Health Organization. WHO Coronavirus Disease (COVID-19) Dashboard. Available online: https://covid19.who.int/ (accessed on 6 November 2020).
18. World Health Organization. Coronavirus Disease 2019 (COVID-19). Situation Report-51. Available online: https://www.who.int/docs/default-source/coronaviruse/situation-reports/20200311-sitrep-51-covid-19.pdf (accessed on 2 September 2020).
19. Burtscher, J.; Burtscher, M.; Millet, G.P. (Indoor) isolation, stress, and physical inactivity: Vicious circles accelerated by COVID-19? *Scand. J. Med. Sci. Sports* **2020**, *30*, 1544–1545. [CrossRef]
20. Ammar, A.; Brach, M.; Trabelsi, K.; Chtourou, H.; Boukhris, O.; Masmoudi, L.; Bouaziz, B.; Bentlage, E.; How, D.; Ahmed, M.; et al. Effects of COVID-19 Home Confinement on Eating Behaviour and Physical Activity: Results of the ECLB-COVID19 International Online Survey. *Nutrients* **2020**, *12*, 1583. [CrossRef] [PubMed]

21. Qeveria e Kosovës. Vendim. 2020. Available online: https://kryeministri-ks.net/wp-content/uploads/2020/03/Vendimet-e-Mbledhjes-së-15-të-të-Qeverisë-së-Republikës-së-Kosovës.pdf (accessed on 18 October 2020).
22. Qeveria e Kosovës. Vendim. 2020. Available online: https://kryeministri-ks.net/wp-content/uploads/2020/05/Vendimet-e-mbledhjes-s%C3%AB-9-t%C3%AB.pdf (accessed on 21 October 2020).
23. Carriedo, A.; Cecchini, J.A.; Fernandez-Rio, J.; Mendez-Gimenez, A. COVID-19, Psychological Well-being and Physical Activity Levels in Older Adults During the Nationwide Lockdown in Spain. *Am. J. Geriatr. Psychiatry* **2020**, *28*, 1146–1155. [CrossRef]
24. Zhang, Y.; Zhang, H.; Ma, X.; Di, Q. Mental health problems during the COVID-19 pandemics and the mitigation effects of exercise: A longitudinal study of college students in China. *Int. J. Environ. Res. Public Health* **2020**, *17*, 3722. [CrossRef]
25. Giustino, V.; Parroco, A.M.; Gennaro, A.; Musumeci, G.; Palma, A.; Battaglia, G. Physical Activity Levels and Related Energy Expenditure during COVID-19 Quarantine among the Sicilian Active Population: A Cross-Sectional Online Survey Study. *Sustainability* **2020**, *12*, 4356. [CrossRef]
26. Sekulic, D.; Blazevic, M.; Gilic, B.; Kvesic, I.; Zenic, N. Prospective Analysis of Levels and Correlates of Physical Activity During COVID-19 Pandemic and Imposed Rules of Social Distancing; Gender Specific Study Among Adolescents from Southern Croatia. *Sustainability* **2020**, *12*, 4072. [CrossRef]
27. López-Bueno, R.; Calatayud, J.; Andersen, L.L.; Balsalobre-Fernández, C.; Casaña, J.; Casajús, J.A.; Smith, L.; López-Sánchez, G.F. Immediate impact of the COVID-19 confinement on physical activity levels in Spanish adults. *Sustainability* **2020**, *12*, 5708. [CrossRef]
28. Lesser, I.A.; Nienhuis, C.P. The Impact of COVID-19 on Physical Activity Behavior and Well-Being of Canadians. *Int. J. Environ. Res. Public Health* **2020**, *17*, 3899. [CrossRef] [PubMed]
29. Brooks, S.K.; Webster, R.K.; Smith, L.E.; Woodland, L.; Wessely, S.; Greenberg, N.; Rubin, G.J. The psychological impact of quarantine and how to reduce it: Rapid review of the evidence. *Lancet* **2020**. [CrossRef]
30. Hossain, M.M.; Sultana, A.; Purohit, N. Mental health outcomes of quarantine and isolation for infection prevention: A systematic umbrella review of the global evidence. *Epidemiol. Health* **2020**, *42*, e2020038. [CrossRef]
31. Zenic, N.; Taiar, R.; Gilic, B.; Blazevic, M.; Maric, D.; Pojskic, H.; Sekulic, D. Levels and Changes of Physical Activity in Adolescents during the COVID-19 Pandemic: Contextualizing Urban vs. Rural Living Environment. *Appl. Sci.* **2020**, *10*, 3997. [CrossRef]
32. Constandt, B.; Thibaut, E.; De Bosscher, V.; Scheerder, J.; Ricour, M.; Willem, A. Exercising in Times of Lockdown: An Analysis of the Impact of COVID-19 on Levels and Patterns of Exercise among Adults in Belgium. *Int. J. Environ. Res. Public Health* **2020**, *17*, 4144. [CrossRef]
33. American College of Sports Medicine. Physical Activity Guidelines for Americans. Available online: https://health.gov/sites/default/files/2019-09/Physical_Activity_Guidelines_2nd_edition.pdf (accessed on 28 January 2021).
34. Byrne, N.M.; Hills, A.P.; Hunter, G.R.; Weinsier, R.L.; Schutz, Y. Metabolic equivalent: One size does not fit all. *J. Appl. Physiol. (1985)* **2005**, *99*, 1112–1119. [CrossRef]
35. Ainsworth, B.E.; Haskell, W.L.; Whitt, M.C.; Irwin, M.L.; Swartz, A.M.; Strath, S.J.; O'Brien, W.L.; Bassett, D.R., Jr.; Schmitz, K.H.; Emplaincourt, P.O.; et al. Compendium of physical activities: An update of activity codes and MET intensities. *Med. Sci. Sports Exerc.* **2000**, *32*, S498–S504. [CrossRef]
36. Ainsworth, B.E.; Haskell, W.L.; Leon, A.S.; Jacobs, D.R., Jr.; Montoye, H.J.; Sallis, J.F.; Paffenbarger, R.S., Jr. Compendium of physical activities: Classification of energy costs of human physical activities. *Med. Sci. Sports Exerc.* **1993**, *25*, 71–80. [CrossRef]
37. Ainsworth, B.E.; Haskell, W.L.; Herrmann, S.D.; Meckes, N.; Bassett, D.R., Jr.; Tudor-Locke, C.; Greer, J.L.; Vezina, J.; Whitt-Glover, M.C.; Leon, A.S. 2011 Compendium of Physical Activities: A second update of codes and MET values. *Med. Sci. Sports Exerc.* **2011**, *43*, 1575–1581. [CrossRef]
38. IPAQ. *Guidelines for the Data Processing and Analysis of the International Physical Activity Questionnaire*; Available online: https://sites.google.com/site/theipaq/ (accessed on 15 September 2020).
39. Willet, W.; Dietz, W.; Colditz, G. Primary care: Guidelines for weight. *N. Engl. J. Med.* **1999**, *341*, 427–434. [CrossRef]
40. Paroli, R.; Consonni, G.; Rosina, A. The Measure of Population Aging in Different Welfare Regimes: A Bayesian Dynamic Modeling Approach. *Eur. J. Popul.* **2020**, *36*, 363–385. [CrossRef]
41. Di Stefano, V.; Battaglia, G.; Giustino, V.; Gagliardo, A.; D'Aleo, M.; Giannini, O.; Palma, A.; Brighina, F. Significant reduction of physical activity in patients with neuromuscular disease during COVID-19 pandemic: The long-term consequences of quarantine. *J. Neurol.* **2020**. [CrossRef] [PubMed]
42. Maugeri, G.; Castrogiovanni, P.; Battaglia, G.; Pippi, R.; D'Agata, V.; Palma, A.; Di Rosa, M.; Musumeci, G. The impact of physical activity on psychological health during Covid-19 pandemic in Italy. *Heliyon* **2020**, *6*, e04315. [CrossRef] [PubMed]
43. Li, W.; Procter-Gray, E.; Churchill, L.; Crouter, S.E.; Kane, K.; Tian, J.; Franklin, P.D.; Ockene, J.K.; Gurwitz, J. Gender and Age Differences in Levels, Types and Locations of Physical Activity among Older Adults Living in Car-Dependent Neighborhoods. *J. Frailty Aging* **2017**, *6*, 129–135. [CrossRef] [PubMed]
44. Kokko, S.; Martin, L.; Geidne, S.; Van Hoye, A.; Lane, A.; Meganck, J.; Scheerder, J.; Seghers, J.; Villberg, J.; Kudlacek, M.; et al. Does sports club participation contribute to physical activity among children and adolescents? A comparison across six European countries. *Scand. J. Public Health* **2019**, *47*, 851–858. [CrossRef] [PubMed]
45. Martinez-Ferran, M.; de la Guia-Galipienso, F.; Sanchis-Gomar, F.; Pareja-Galeano, H. Metabolic Impacts of Confinement during the COVID-19 Pandemic Due to Modified Diet and Physical Activity Habits. *Nutrients* **2020**, *12*, 1549. [CrossRef] [PubMed]

46. Hammami, A.; Harrabi, B.; Mohr, M.; Krustrup, P. Physical activity and coronavirus disease 2019 (COVID-19): Specific recommendations for home-based physical training. *Manag. Sport Leis.* **2020**, 1–6. [CrossRef]
47. Ammar, A.; Trabelsi, K.; Brach, M.; Chtourou, H.; Boukhris, O.; Masmoudi, L.; Bouaziz, B.; Bentlage, E.; How, D.; Ahmed, M. Effects of home confinement on mental health and lifestyle behaviours during the COVID-19 outbreak: Insight from the "ECLB-COVID19" multi countries survey. *medRxiv* **2020**.
48. Hallal, P.C.; Andersen, L.B.; Bull, F.C.; Guthold, R.; Haskell, W.; Ekelund, U.; Lancet Physical Activity Series Working, G. Global physical activity levels: Surveillance progress, pitfalls, and prospects. *Lancet* **2012**, *380*, 247–257. [CrossRef]
49. Kosovo Agency of Statistics. Seria 1: Statistikat e Përgjithshme. 2020. Available online: https://ask.rks-gov.net/media/5624/kosova-n%C3%AB-shifra-2019.pdf (accessed on 28 January 2021).
50. He, M.; Xian, Y.; Lv, X.; He, J.; Ren, Y. Changes in Body Weight, Physical Activity, and Lifestyle During the Semi-lockdown Period After the Outbreak of COVID-19 in China: An Online Survey. *Disaster Med. Public Health Prep.* **2020**, 1–6. [CrossRef]
51. Donatiello, E.; Dello Russo, M.; Formisano, A.; Lauria, F.; Nappo, A.; Reineke, A.; Sparano, S.; Barba, G.; Russo, P.; Siani, A. Physical activity, adiposity and urbanization level in children: Results for the Italian cohort of the IDEFICS study. *Public Health* **2013**, *127*, 761–765. [CrossRef]
52. Regis, M.F.; Oliveira, L.M.F.T.D.; Santos, A.R.M.D.; Leonidio, A.d.C.R.; Diniz, P.R.B.; Freitas, C.M.S.M.d. Urban versus rural lifestyle in adolescents: Associations between environment, physical activity levels and sedentary behavior. *Einstein (São Paulo)* **2016**, *14*, 461–467. [CrossRef] [PubMed]
53. Tishukaj, F.; Shalaj, I.; Gjaka, M.; Ademi, B.; Ahmetxhekaj, R.; Bachl, N.; Tschan, H.; Wessner, B. Physical fitness and anthropometric characteristics among adolescents living in urban or rural areas of Kosovo. *BMC Public Health* **2017**, *17*, 711. [CrossRef] [PubMed]
54. Lee, P.H.; Macfarlane, D.J.; Lam, T.H.; Stewart, S.M. Validity of the International Physical Activity Questionnaire Short Form (IPAQ-SF): A systematic review. *Int. J. Behav. Nutr. Phys. Act.* **2011**, *8*, 115. [CrossRef]
55. Kalvenas, A.; Burlacu, I.; Abu-Omar, K. Reliability and Validity of the International Physical Activity Questionnaire in Lithuania. *Baltic J. Health Phys. Act. J. Gdan. Univ. Phys. Educ. Sport* **2016**, *8*. [CrossRef]
56. Riviere, F.; Widad, F.Z.; Speyer, E.; Erpelding, M.L.; Escalon, H.; Vuillemin, A. Reliability and validity of the French version of the global physical activity questionnaire. *J. Sport Health Sci.* **2018**, *7*, 339–345. [CrossRef] [PubMed]

Journal of
Clinical Medicine

MDPI

Article

Influence of COVID-19 on Health-Related Quality of Life and the Perception of Being Vaccinated to Prevent COVID-19: An Approach for Community Pharmacists from Romania and Bulgaria

Adina Turcu-Stiolica [1,†], Maria Bogdan [2,*], Mihaela-Simona Subtirelu [1,†], Andreea-Daniela Meca [2,†], Adriana-Elena Taerel [3], Irina Iaru [4], Maria Kamusheva [5,*] and Guenka Petrova [5]

1 Department of Pharmacoeconomics, University of Medicine and Pharmacy of Craiova, 200349 Craiova, Romania; adina.turcu@gmail.com (A.T.-S.); mihaela.subtirelu@yahoo.com (M.-S.S.)
2 Department of Pharmacology, University of Medicine and Pharmacy of Craiova, 200349 Craiova, Romania; andreea_mdc@yahoo.com
3 Department of Pharmaceutical Management, University of Medicine and Pharmacy "Carol Davila", 020021 Bucharest, Romania; adriana.taerel@yahoo.com
4 Department of Pharmacology, Physiology and Pathophysiology, Iuliu Hatieganu University of Medicine and Pharmacy, 400012 Cluj-Napoca, Romania; cazacuirina@yahoo.com
5 Department of Organization and Economics of Pharmacy, Medical University-Sofia, 1000 Sofia, Bulgaria; gpetrova@pharmfac.mu-sofia.bg
* Correspondence: bogdanfmaria81@yahoo.com (M.B.); mkamusheva@pharmfac.mu-sofia.bg (M.K.)
† All these authors have contributed equally to this work.

Citation: Turcu-Stiolica, A.; Bogdan, M.; Subtirelu, M.-S.; Meca, A.-D.; Taerel, A.-E.; Iaru, I.; Kamusheva, M.; Petrova, G. Influence of COVID-19 on Health-Related Quality of Life and the Perception of Being Vaccinated to Prevent COVID-19: An Approach for Community Pharmacists from Romania and Bulgaria. *J. Clin. Med.* **2021**, *10*, 864. https://doi.org/10.3390/jcm10040864

Academic Editor: Mauro Giovanni Carta

Received: 22 January 2021
Accepted: 17 February 2021
Published: 19 February 2021

Abstract: Community pharmacists are essential front-line health workers, involved in relieving the COVID-19 burden. Their health-related quality of life status needs to be assessed, as lower levels could affect their functioning. In order to evaluate the current status of community pharmacists' quality of life from Romania and Bulgaria during the COVID-19 pandemic, and to identify factors associated with their decision on being vaccinated to prevent COVID-19, an online survey involving 395 community pharmacists was conducted from 15th July 2020 to 15th August 2020. The 15D instrument was used for quality-of-life assessment. The pharmacists' recommendations for vitamin C and D intake during the COVID-19 pandemic were also analyzed in order to promote future training programs for community pharmacists. Descriptive statistics, comparative analyses between pharmacists from Romania and Bulgaria, and multiple correlation analyses were performed on the collected data. Significant differences were observed for the level of quality of life between the two groups of pharmacists according to their age; smaller values, directly correlated with their age (total 15D score and age: Spearman $r = 0.168$, $p = 0.022$), were obtained for Bulgarian pharmacists regarding sleeping, usual activities, mental function, discomfort and symptoms, depression, distress. The perception of being vaccinated did not differ between Romanian and Bulgarian pharmacists, as almost 50% agreed to vaccination ($p = 0.7542$). Their willingness to vaccinate was correlated with vitamin D usage ($p = 0.0134$), rather than with vitamin C ($p = 0.4157$). No other significant associations were found between willingness to get vaccinated to prevent COVID-19 and other characteristics (age, gender, income, quality-of-life markers). Evidence-based interventions are required to enhance the health-related quality of life of community pharmacists involved in the first line of the COVID-19 pandemic.

Keywords: quality of life; 15D; COVID-19; vaccination; community pharmacists

1. Introduction

Over a year has passed since the first declared case of COVID-19, a life-threatening infection, on 31st of December 2019, and all of our socio-economic life aspects have been affected while facing this worldwide pandemic [1–4]. Frontline health workers have reached unprecedented anxiety levels, as information regarding contagiousness and pharmacotherapeutic management remains uncertain [1]. Long-lasting immense stress and panic, as well as physical exhaustion, could lead to post-traumatic disorders or depression, with a higher prevalence among healthcare workers [1]. Moreover, the performance of health care professionals could also be affected due to increased workload and fear of self-infection, social rejection, or even transmission to family members [5,6].

Inter-professional collaboration among healthcare settings, including community pharmacies, is highly recommended in order to face and manage the COVID-19 pandemic [2]. During the Ebola epidemics, for example, effective communication between physicians and community pharmacists was noted as a good control measure in avoiding the infection spread [7]. Pharmacists are exposed daily through face-to-face interactions with individuals [3], but are often neglected as frontline health care providers, although they represent accessible, essential health care workers [6–9]. Although pharmaceutical services cannot be offered from a remote location, little information about COVID-19 exposure and prevalence among community pharmacists is noted [9,10], which could be underestimated [7,10]. However, a higher risk of exposure to COVID-19-infected individuals involves a greater psychological impact [11]. Permanent fear of infection due to insufficient social distancing in pharmacies, aggressive patient behavior and higher stress levels could affect cognitive functioning in pharmacists and could weaken their attention [1,12]. Community pharmacists have also been involved in the screening and triage of COVID-19 patients (Figure 1), as well as in ensuring continuity of care for non-COVID-19 illnesses and promoting pharmacological adherence, which further increased the negative impact on their well-being [2,9]. However, pharmacists have shown a trustworthy attitude regarding the adoption of protective measures (Figure 1), despite the increased risk of burnout [8,10,12]. They even provided surveillance of suspicious cases, symptoms-related counselling and advice to patients on whether they should be quarantined or not, depending on their clinical manifestations (Figure 1) [7]. Community pharmacists also improved medical education among their patients by using telehealth consulting and new technologies [2]. Moreover, pharmacists maintained contact, through different and accessible smart mobile applications, e-mails, video calls and written text messages, with all individuals who requested pharmaceutical assistance (Figure 1) [2]. Continuous pharmaceutical monitoring and communication with patients not only supported rational medicine use, but also ensured constant clarification of various misconceptions regarding prophylactic or long-term curative treatments (Figure 1) [2]. Thereby, community pharmacists helped reduce unnecessary visits to health departments, which were already overwhelmed, ensuring a cost-effective approach to the COVID-19 pandemic [7]. A systematic review conducted in July 2019 underlined the importance and involvement of pharmacists in public threat recovery [6]; therefore, their proper mental health and quality of life are highly needed.

Community pharmacists are involved in pharmacovigilance activities and are able to educate and counsel individuals regarding both the pharmacotherapeutic approach of the COVID-19 infection and the proper use of personal protective equipment and sanitizers (Figure 1) [2,7,12]. Pharmacists are also able to communicate effectively in order to combat the flood of misinformation regarding COVID-19 and discourage dangerous self-medication [7,8,11–13]. Moreover, pharmacists could play a key role in the prevention and containment of COVID-19 pandemic, promoting patients' adherence to prophylactic immunomodulatory treatment (such as vitamins C and D); they could also promote vaccination and support vaccinovigilance (Figure 1) [2,7,8,13].

The European Medicines Agency (EMA) authorized Cominarty (developed by BioNTech and Pfizer) as the first vaccine used for prevention of COVID-19, in people aged over 16 years, in European countries, on 21st December 2020 [14]. Another conditional marketing authorization was given on 6th January 2021 for COVID-10 vaccine Moderna, recommended in individuals from 18 years of age [14]. The first two approved vaccines are based on the mRNA technique, preparing the human body to generate a proper immune response in case of infection. The most recent recommended vaccine for European authorization was the one from AstraZeneca, on 29th January 2021, based on modified adenovirus. All three vaccines will be monitored in both European countries (Romania [15] and Bulgaria [16]) through pharmacovigilance online systems, and intensively supported and promoted by pharmacists.

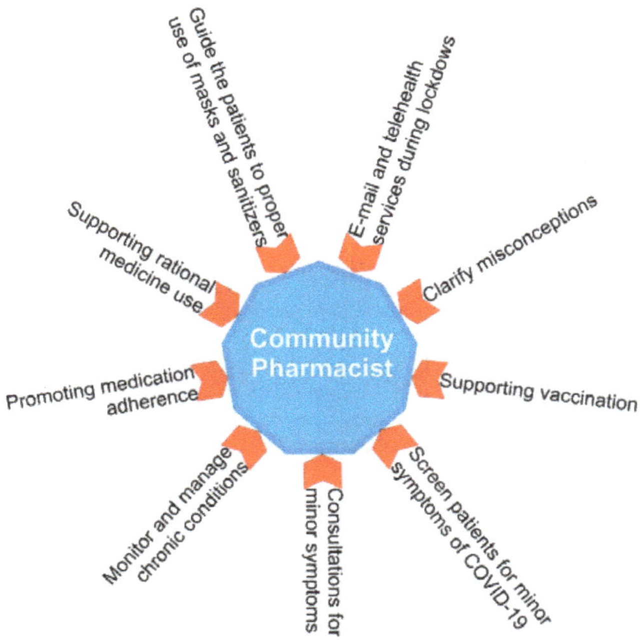
Community Pharmacist
Guide the patients to proper use of masks and sanitizers
E-mail and telehealth services during lockdows
Clarify misconceptions
Supporting vaccination
Screen patients for minor symptoms of COVID-19
Consultations for minor symptoms
Monitor and manage chronic conditions
Promoting medication adherence
Supporting rational medicine use

Figure 1. Community pharmacy services during COVID-19 pandemic.

Vitamin C (ascorbic acid) cannot be synthesized by the human organism, but it is found in many fruits and vegetables [17–19] and is used as a supplement, alone or in combination with other vitamins and minerals [20]. Vitamin D exists in two forms: vitamin D2 (found in plants) and vitamin D3 (found in food and synthesized in the skin under sunlight ultraviolet-B ray exposure), both of which are available in dietary supplements [21,22]. An indoor lifestyle, sun avoidance for health or cultural reasons, and a modern diet based on highly processed food are significant contributors to the evolution of global vitamin D deficiency [23]. Even more, due to the long period of lockdown and following limitation of activities outside the home, vitamin D intake is beneficial during the pandemic. Both vitamin C and vitamin D supplementation has demonstrated positive effects on the immune system and on respiratory tract infections [24,25].

Pharmacists represent the first point of contact with individuals who need psychiatric assistance [12]. Robinson et al. emphasizes that in order to assist patients with behavioural health conditions (such as concern, fear, insomnia, fatigue, anger, frustration, intense anxiety, panic attacks, depression) and to help relieve the pandemic pressure, community pharmacists should be trained to first manage their own psychological disorders [3–6,9,12]. Nevertheless, self-care (physical activity, proper eating and sleep hygiene, mindfulness techniques) and resilience need greater promotion among pharmacists [11,12]. Multidisciplinary mental health services, such as training programs and careful evaluation of the pharmacy staff, should be initiated and provided for pharmacists as soon as possible [9,12].

Romania declared a COVID-19 lockdown from 16th March 2020 to 15th May 2020, whereas in Bulgaria the state of emergency was between 13th March 2020 and 13th May 2020. In both countries, it was followed by an alert period with many limitations and restrictions, which still continues. The reason we choose these two countries for the study was because both are from the Central and Eastern European region and have similar drug policies and health legislation [26].

Our aim was to analyze the health-related quality of life (HRQoL) of community pharmacists from Romania and Bulgaria during the COVID-19 pandemic and to identify factors associated with perception of being vaccinated against COVID-19, in order to provide evidence-based interventions to community pharmacists to improve vaccine use. Associations between HRQoL, demographics, pharmacists' recommendations for vitamin C and D intake during the pandemic, and perception of being vaccinated against COVID-19 were evaluated. At the same time, based on multiple clinical trials about the vitamin C/vitamin D relation with COVID- 19, we aimed to assess the insight of the community pharmacists regarding the recommendation of over-the-counter drugs with vitamin C and D during the COVID-19 pandemic.

2. Materials and Methods

2.1. Study Design

The cross-sectional study was conducted from 15th July 2020 to 15th August 2020. The online survey was developed using Google Forms and included three main sections: socio-demographic characteristics, 15D instrument and perception towards COVID-19 vaccination (Supplementary file_Questionnaire). The online survey was anonymous and confidential. As dissemination channels, we used pharmacist groups from social media, such as Facebook, and emails to our former students.

The socio-demographic section was composed of items exploring age, gender, marital status, experience as a pharmacist, income working as a pharmacist, and pharmacy specialization. Monthly income working as a pharmacist was stratified into low (less than 600 Euro), medium (600–1000 Euro), or high (more than 1000 Euro).

The second section of the questionnaire assessed the HRQoL using the 15D instrument [27,28]. The 15D questionnaire comprises 15 dimensions (mobility, vision, hearing, breathing, sleeping, eating, speech, excretion, usual activities, mental function, discomfort and symptoms, depression, distress, vitality, and sexual activity), with each dimension being divided into five levels that range from no problems to severe difficulties. The single index score (15D score), representing the overall HRQoL on a 0–1 scale (1 = full health, 0 = being dead) and the dimension level values, reflecting the goodness of the levels relative to no problems on the dimension (=1) and to being dead (=0), are calculated from the questionnaire by using a set of population-based preference or utility weights.

The third section included five items specifically developed for the purpose of the study, which were related to vitamin C or D supplementation (self or recommended to others) during the COVID-19 pandemic and to vaccination against COVID-19.

2.2. Participants

The survey was addressed to pharmacists working in community pharmacies from Romania and Bulgaria.

To calculate an appropriate representative sample from the targeted population, convenience sampling was used [29]. Power analysis was conducted using G*Power 3 (alpha equal to 0.05) and a sample size of 176 pharmacists was calculated to demonstrate statistically significant results for the study [30]. Ethical approval for this study was obtained from the Ethics Committee of the University of Medicine and Pharmacy of Craiova (Registration no. 54/08.07.2020) according to the Declaration of Helsinki. All pharmacists provided electronic informed consent, starting with the first question of the survey.

2.3. Data Analysis

Continuous variables were summarized as mean ± standard deviation (SD) or median with interquartile range (IQR). Statistical differences were analyzed by Student's *t*-test or Mann–Whitney test. Categorical variables were summarized as frequencies and percentages. Chi-squared test was performed to compare categorical variables as appropriate. We further assessed the association of continuous variables with 15D scores by Spearman's correlation test. ANCOVA was used to capture association between continuous and categorical variables. We did not have missing data. Data were analyzed using GraphPad Prism 9.0 software (GraphPad Software, LLC, San Diego, CA, USA). The significance level was 0.05.

3. Results

The sample included 395 pharmacists working in community pharmacies with possible contacts with COVID-19 patients: 241 from Romania and 154 from Bulgaria. The results are shown in Table 1.

Table 1. Baseline characteristics of pharmacists from Romania and Bulgaria.

	Romania (n = 241)	Bulgaria (n = 154)	p-Value
Gender			
Men	18 (7%)	33 (21%)	<0.0001 *
Women	223 (93%)	121 (79%)	
Age ^, years	30 (26–37)	26 (25–32)	<0.0001 *
Marital status			
Married	117 (49%)	49 (32%)	0.0010 *
Not married	113 (47%)	100 (65%)	
Divorced	9 (4%)	4 (3%)	
Widower	2 (1%)	1 (1%)	
Professional experience ^, years	7.36 ± 8.3	6.2 ± 7.8	0.0124 *
Income working as pharmacist			
Low (less than 600 Euro)	95 (39%)	29 (19%)	<0.0001 *
High (more than 1000 Euro)	18 (7%)	33 (21%)	
Specialist pharmacists			
Yes	108 (45%)	24 (16%)	<0.0001 *
No	133 (55%)	130 (84%)	

*, significantly different (p < 0.05); ^, did not pass normality test.

The characteristics of the two groups of pharmacists showed that the Romanian pharmacists were older, with a higher percentage of women, married people and specialists. When considering the income working as a pharmacist, there are statistically significant differences between the two groups; Bulgarian pharmacists have a higher income, even if they are less experienced.

Different pharmacy specialties exist in Romania and Bulgaria. Of the 108 specialist pharmacists from Romania, 47 (44%) were specialists in Clinical Pharmacy, 51 (47%) were specialists in General Pharmacy, and 10 (9%) were specialists in Pharmaceutical Laboratory. In Bulgaria, most pharmacists were specialists in Clinical Pharmacy (46%).

Table 2 shows the differences between the levels of quality of life of pharmacists from Romania and Bulgaria. We observed statistically significant differences regarding sleeping, usual activities, mental function, discomfort and symptoms, depression, distress and total 15D score, with low values for distress. The smaller values for Bulgarian pharmacists were directly correlated with age (for the association between total 15D score and age: Spearman $r = 0.168$, $p = 0.022$). A strong correlation was also observed between mental function and discomfort and symptoms (Spearman $r = -0.81$, $p = 0.028$).

We assessed whether gender had a significant effect on HRQoL outcomes and no associations were found: breathing (p-value = 0.060), sleeping (p-value = 0.302), speech (p-value = 0.191), excretion (p-value = 0.582), usual activities (p-value = 0.887), mental function (p-value = 0.065), discomfort and symptoms (p-value = 0.322), depression (p-value = 0.677), distress (p-value = 0.622), vitality (p-value = 0.809), sexual activities (p-value = 0.077) and HRQoL score (p-value = 0.661).

Table 2. Health-related quality of lige (HRQoL) results.

Mean ± SD	Romania (n = 241)	Bulgaria (n = 154)	p-value
Mobility	1	1	>0.999
Vision	1	1	>0.999
Hearing	1	1	>0.999
Breathing	0.903 ± 0.143	0.928 ± 0.132	0.0702
Sleeping	0.896 ± 0.161	0.848 ± 0.207	0.0494 *
Eating	1	1	>0.999
Speech	0.982 ± 0.084	0.975 ± 0.083	0.1778
Excretion	0.976 ± 0.094	0.961 ± 0.104	0.0786
Usual activities	0.975 ± 0.113	0.961 ± 0.114	0.041 *
Mental function	0.979 ± 0.087	0.943 ± 0.136	0.0007 *
Discomfort and symptoms	0.921 ± 0.141	0.979 ± 0.094	<0.0001 *
Depression	0.933 ± 0.130	0.853 ± 0.197	<0.0001 *
Distress	0.844 ± 0.187	0.765 ± 0.217	0.0002 *
Vitality	0.881 ± 0.139	0.844 ± 0.185	0.1305
Sexual activities	0.925 ± 0.155	0.930 ± 0.141	0.14
Total 15D score	0.956 ± 0.051	0.936 ± 0.063	0.0024 *

*, significantly different ($p < 0.05$); SD, Standard Deviation.

To determine whether community pharmacists used and recommended supplements with vitamin C and D, their answers were assessed and presented in Figure 2. We observed statistical differences between the two groups in the case of using supplements with vitamin C and D: the pharmacists from Bulgaria used them more. The same trend was not maintained in terms of recommending these supplements to their family/friends/patients: the percentage of pharmacists that recommend was higher than the percentage of pharmacists that used these products, without differences between Romania and Bulgaria.

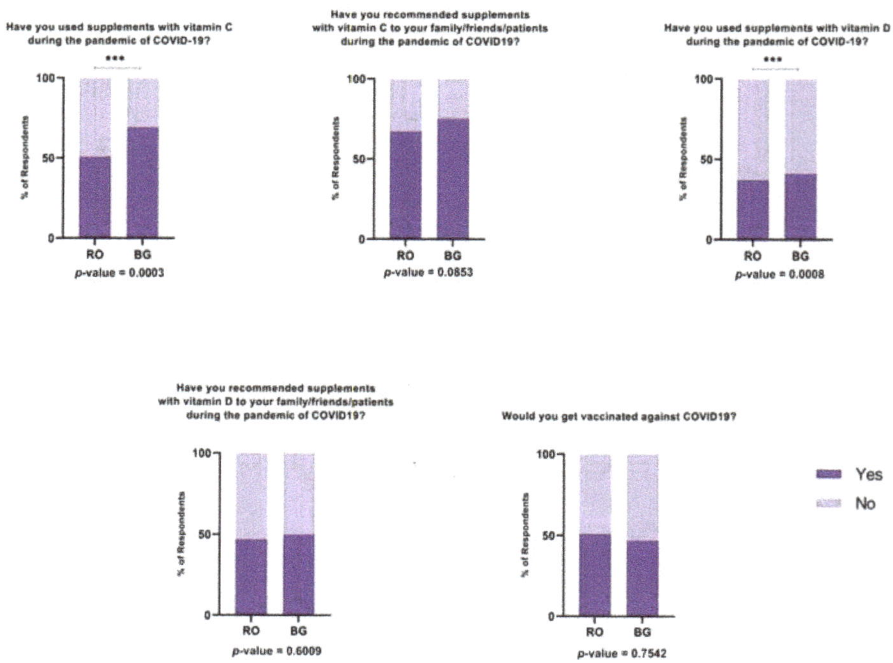

Figure 2. Perception towards COVID-19 vaccination and vitamin recommendation. *** p-value < 0.001.

The community pharmacists from the two countries reported willingness to get vaccinated to prevent COVID-19 in almost the same percentage: 50% (p = 0.7542). A statistically significant association was found between the willingness to get vaccinated and the use of vitamin D during the COVID-19 pandemic (p = 0.0134). However, no association was found between the willingness to get vaccinated and the use of vitamin C during the COVID-19 pandemic (p = 0.4157). No other significant associations were found between the willingness to get vaccinated to prevent COVID-19 and other characteristics (age, gender, income, quality-of-life markers).

4. Discussion

The extreme psychological pressure felt by health care providers in the last year could affect not only patients, but also entire public healthcare systems [11,12]. However, pharmacists were required during this challenging pandemic to enlarge their traditional pharmaceutical activities and to ensure a primary point of care and triage for many patients [31–33].

A strong statistical correlation was found between discomfort and specific symptoms and mental functions among the pharmacists who participated in our study. Our study did not underline the higher vulnerability to psychological impact during the COVID-19 pandemic among female pharmacists, as other studies [34]. Batra et al. reported higher levels of depression, distress and behavioral dysfunctionalities among female health workers who have prolonged contact with patients [5]. The mental health impact of COVID-19 pandemic has been noticed in more than 50% of pharmacists, and some studies even highlighted higher rates of burnout among pharmacists in comparison with nurses and physicians [35]. Another study, conducted by Lange et al. [36], showed that approximately 35% of community pharmacists reported mental health disturbances (anxiety, stress, insomnia, sense of losing control, fear, hopelessness [37]), with females being more affected [36]. These results, coming from the very first studies analyzing the psychological impact of COVID-19 pandemic among community pharmacists, in the French region of Normandy [37], are not consistent with our results because of the different period of the studies. The same results about the level of quality of life of Romanian young physicians during COVID-19 pandemic were obtained, with no association between gender and distress [38].

Furthermore, our study included more specialists and older pharmacists from Romania, which could be characterized by better ability to assist, emergency preparedness and probable stress coping mechanisms due to longer experience [35]. Thereby, we noticed that Romanian pharmacists reported a better quality of life, whereas Bulgarian pharmacists reported more sleeping disturbances, distress and depression. Our statistical correlations proved that Bulgarian pharmacists had more difficulties in coping with usual activities, also underlining the mental pandemic burden.

Dror et al. [39] mentioned that first-line medical staff have less hesitancy towards vaccination against COVID-19 and its efficacy, while medical workers who have less or no contact with infected patients are more skeptical [39]. Vaccine acceptance could be increased not only by recommendations and proper information transmitted to patients by community pharmacists, who play an essential educational role, but also by pharmacists considering themselves eligible for vaccine acquiescence [39,40]. Although conditional marketing authorization for COVID-19 preventive vaccines is used in case of benefits outweighing risks for patients [14], clarifications regarding importance of vaccination are still needed among general population. Pharmacists are important pawns in the immunization campaign in both European countries included in our study, relieving the COVID-19 burden [9,41,42]. Most individuals are still skeptical and have misconceptions about receiving vaccines, even though more than 2.5 million deaths are prevented annually worldwide through vaccination programs [42]. Community pharmacists are not only able to increase vaccination rates through direct recommendations, but also by receiving approval to administer vaccines to patients [42]. One of the most important predictive factors for vaccine acceptance is the self-perception of a high risk for COVID-19, which could be achieved through medical education [39,41]. On the other hand, females are less likely to accept vaccination [39], a result consistent with our statistic, due to the higher prevalence of female pharmacists from both countries in our study.

This study offers an important insight into the quality of life of community pharmacists during COVID-19 pandemic and their perception towards vaccination. A limitation could be the lower age category for the community pharmacists who answered to this survey, which could be due to the dissemination channels we used. More professional experience accumulated over the years could have influenced the pharmacists' answers to this survey. Additionally, the timeline for the survey dissemination may have influenced the pharmacists' opinion about COVID-19 impact and, therefore, their responses may differ over time.

Another limitation of the study could be the comparison between the pharmacists' income in the two countries, since the World Bank Country classification by income sets Bulgaria and Romania in different groups (Bulgaria is upper middle income and Romania is high income) [42]. Moreover, even if the World Bank Country sets Romania in the high-income group, the actual income for community pharmacists is still very low.

Our study represents one of the first published studies that, to our knowledge, analyzes COVID-19's impact on quality of life among pharmacists in Romania and Bulgaria. We found only one study that underlined the pressure that community pharmacists are subjected to during lockdown [36]. Our work also stands as a comparison between two neighboring countries regarding psychological disturbance in community pharmacists, as front-line health-care workers. Moreover, our study is a first attempt to evaluate the consumption and recommendation of vitamin C and D among pharmacists during the pandemic.

For the European countries, an inverse correlation was described between national estimates of vitamin D levels and COVID-19 incidence [43,44] and mortality [43–45]. There is evidence that vitamin D is correlated with diminished risk and severity of COVID-19 infection through different mechanisms (decreasing the production of inflammatory cytokine, decreasing the survival and replication of viruses, preserving endothelial integrity, and augmenting angiotensin-converting enzyme 2 concentrations) [46]. The prophylactic vitamin D administration in the COVID-19 management was underscored [47]. Various studies were revised and the recommended daily dose by consensus during the COVID-19 pandemic, 2000 IU for teenagers and adults, is 20 times lower than the amount which must be taken for many months to cause toxicity [48].

Vitamin C and D supplements are easily available on the pharmaceutical market in each country, have a low risk of adverse effects, and are inexpensive. Both vitamins are recommended with precise doses for prophylaxis and treatment as part of the COVID-19 management protocol [49]. However, the results of ongoing clinical trials are expected to elucidate various aspects of the vitamin C/vitamin D relationship with COVID-19 (52 [50] and 71 [51], respectively of clinical trials registered at present on ClinicalTrials.gov). The outcomes of these clinical trials could also contribute to future training programs for community pharmacists in order to recommend vitamin C and D supplementation during the pandemic to better manage the COVID-19 burden.

Both Bulgaria and Romania are countries where a large-scale peak in COVID-19 infection would lead to overcrowded health facilities and a shortage of medical specialists. Reliability of information and control of fear and disinformation are important issues during the spread of the disease. Community pharmacies are one of the few places that are kept open for public service even during strict safety measures. They have a unique, credible role with ease of accessibility [2].

In Romania, reducing the program or patients' access to it, the installation of protective panels or air purifiers, and disinfection of surfaces and personal objects at regular intervals (less than one hour), were measures adopted in order to ease the pandemic burden for both pharmacists and patients [52]. A survey conducted by Padureanu et al. between April and May 2020, in Romania, underlined that 52% of pharmacists were satisfied with the provided protection measures [53]. However, the same survey mentioned that 57% of pharmacists were afraid of COVID-19 exposure and infection, consistent with our results. Community pharmacists from Romania were allowed to release over-the-counter antibiotics for a correct and complete treatment of dental abscess during lockdown or whenever dental health services were blocked [52]. Elbeddini et al. showed that the increased distress was also caused by verbal abuse and harassment from patients demanding COVID-19 protocol drugs even if they did not have a prescription or were not diagnosed [9].

During the pandemic, pharmacists in Bulgaria were also in charge of additional administrative issues regarding the reporting of new paperless prescription forms, so-called "S blanks", for patients who were treated with medication prescribed with special protocols and paid by the National Health Insurance Fund (NHIF) [54]. The purpose of this was for chronically ill patients to avoid visiting their general practitioners and specialists for the issuing of a new protocol [54]. This led to an extra workload for pharmacies.

The pharmacy owners from both European countries were obliged to ensure protective gloves, safety goggles and masks for all pharmacists [52,54]. However, the Bulgarian Pharmaceutical Union (BPU) and other non-profit associations, such as the Bulgarian Medicines Verification Organization, provided some quantity of protective equipment for BPU members [54]. No governmental help was ensured, since pharmacists work in the private sector.

Further follow-up studies conducted in both countries would be informative for the society and their results could be compared with the period analyzed in the current study. The inclusion of further neighboring countries in such a comparison might bring added value and could present a broader picture of how the COVID-19 pandemic has affected community pharmacists' quality of life.

5. Conclusions

Evaluation of the health-related quality of life of pharmacists and assessment of the psychological impact of the COVID-19 pandemic leads to better recognition of their work and implicitly better management of community public health. The present study offers an important perspective regarding the perception of community pharmacists from Romania and Bulgaria towards vaccination and vitamins C and D recommendation. Our results could also support further strategies enhancing resilience during the COVID-19 pandemic among essential front-line healthcare workers such as pharmacists, which are often neglected.

Supplementary Materials: The following are available online at https://www.mdpi.com/2077-0383/10/4/864/s1, Supplementary file_Questionnaire.

Author Contributions: Conceptualization, A.T.-S., M.B. and M.K.; methodology, A.T.-S. and M.B.; formal analysis, A.T.-S.; investigation, M.-S.S. and A.-D.M.; data curation, M.-S.S., A.-D.M., A.-E.T. and I.I.; writing—original draft preparation, A.T.-S., M.B., M.-S.S. and A.-D.M.; writing—review and editing, I.I., M.K. and G.P.; supervision, A.T.-S. and G.P. All authors have read and agreed to the published version of the manuscript.

Funding: This research received no external funding.

Institutional Review Board Statement: The study was conducted according to the guidelines of the Declaration of Helsinki and approved by the Ethics Committee of the University of Medicine and Pharmacy of Craiova (Registration no. 54/08.07.2020).

Informed Consent Statement: Informed consent was obtained from all subjects involved in the study.

Data Availability Statement: Data supporting reported results can be asked from the corresponding author.

Acknowledgments: We are grateful to the pharmacists who participated in this study by responding to our survey.

Conflicts of Interest: The authors declare no conflict of interest.

References

1. Temsah, M.-H.; Al-Sohime, F.; Alamro, N.; Al-Eyadhy, A.; Al-Hasan, K.; Jamal, A.; Al-Maglouth, I.; Aljamaan, F.; Amri, M.A.; Barry, M.; et al. The psychological impact of COVID-19 pandemic on health care workers in a MERS-CoV endemic country. *J. Infect. Public Health* **2020**, *13*, 877–882. [CrossRef]
2. Bragazzi, N.L.; Mansour, M.; Bonsignore, A.; Ciliberti, R. The role of hospital and community pharmacists in the management of COVID-19: Towards an expanded definition of the roles, responsibilities, and duties of the pharmacist. *Pharmacy* **2020**, *8*, 140. [CrossRef] [PubMed]
3. Robinson, J.D.; Johnson, N.; Brand-Eubanks, D.C.; Kim, A.P. A call to action: Community pharmacists to address COVID-19 related behavioral health concerns. *J. Am. Pharm. Assoc.* **2020**, 1–3. [CrossRef]
4. Rolling Updates on Coronavirus Disease (COVID-19). Available online: https://www.who.int/emergencies/diseases/novel-coronavirus-2019/events-as-they-happen (accessed on 4 February 2021).
5. Batra, K.; Singh, T.P.; Sharma, M.; Batra, R.; Schvaneveldt, N. Investigating the psychological impact of COVID-19 among healthcare workers: A meta-analysis. *Int. J. Environ. Res. Public Health* **2020**, *17*, 9096. [CrossRef]
6. Aburas, W.; Alshammari, T.M. Pharmacists' roles in emergency and disasters: COVID-19 as an example. *Saudi Pharm. J.* **2020**, *28*, 1797–1816. [CrossRef] [PubMed]
7. Mallhi, T.H.; Liaqat, A.; Abid, A.; Khan, Y.H.; Alotaibi, N.H.; Alzarea, A.I.; Tanveer, N.; Khan, T.M. Multilevel engagements of pharmacists during the COVID-19 pandemic: The way forward. *Front. Public Health* **2020**, *8*, 561924. [CrossRef]
8. Hedima, E.W.; Adeyemi, M.S.; Ikunaiye, N.Y. Community Pharmacists: On the frontline of health service against COVID-19 in LMICs. *Res. Soc. Adm. Pharm.* **2021**, *17*, 1964–1966. [CrossRef]
9. Elbeddini, A.; Wen, C.X.; Tayefehchamani, Y.; To, A. Mental health issues impacting pharmacists during COVID-19. *J. Pharm. Policy Pract.* **2020**, *13*, 46. [CrossRef]
10. Cabas, P.; Bella, S.D.; Giuffre, M.; Rizzo, M.; Trombetta, C.; Luzzati, R.; Antonello, R.M.; Parenzan, K.; Liguori, G. Community pharmacists' exposure to COVID-19. *Res. Soc. Adm. Pharm.* **2021**, *17*, 1882–1887. [CrossRef] [PubMed]
11. Blake, H.; Bermingham, F.; Johson, G.; Tabner, A. Mitigating the psychological impact of COVID-19 on healthcare workers: A digital learning package. *Int. J. Environ. Res. Public Health* **2020**, *17*, 2997. [CrossRef]
12. Hayden, J.C.; Parkin, R. The challenges of COVID-19 for community pharmacists and opportunities for the future. *Ir. J. Psychol. Med.* **2020**, 1–6. [CrossRef]
13. Carico, R., Jr.; Sheppard, J.; Thomas, C.B. Community pharmacists and communication in the time of COVID-19: Applying the health belief model. *Res. Soc. Adm. Pharm.* **2021**, *17*, 1984–1987. [CrossRef]
14. Treatments and Vaccines for COVID-19: Authorised Medicines by European Medicines Agency. Available online: https://www.ema.europa.eu/en/human-regulatory/overview/public-health-threats/coronavirus-disease-covid-19/treatments-vaccines/treatments-vaccines-covid-19-authorised-medicines#covid-19-vaccines-section (accessed on 3 February 2021).
15. Report a COVID-19 Vaccine's Adverse Reaction at National Agency for Medicines and Medical Devices of Romania. Available online: https://www.anm.ro/medicamente-de-uz-uman/farmacovigilenta/raportarea-reactiilor-adverse-suspectate-vaccin-covid-19/ (accessed on 3 February 2021). (In Romanian).
16. Bulgarian Drug Agency. Available online: https://www.bda.bg/bg/ (accessed on 3 February 2021). (In Bulgarian)
17. Carr, A.C.; Rosengrave, P.C.; Bayer, S.; Chambers, S.; Mehrtens, J.; Shaw, G.M. Hypovitaminosis C and vitamin C deficiency in critically ill patients despite recommended enteral and parenteral in takes. *Crit. Care* **2017**, *21*, 300. [CrossRef] [PubMed]
18. Carr, A.C.; Maggini, S. Vitamin C and immune function. *Nutrients* **2017**, *9*, 1211. [CrossRef] [PubMed]
19. Mousavi, S.; Bereswill, S.; Heimesaat, M.M. Immunomodulatory and antimicrobial effects of vitamin C. *Eur. J. Microbiol. Immunol.* **2019**, *9*, 73–79. [CrossRef]
20. Bogdan, M.; Meca, A.D.; Boldeanu, M.V.; Gheorghe, D.N.; Turcu-Stiolica, A.; Subtirelu, M.S.; Boldeanu, L.; Blaj, M.; Botnariu, G.E.; Vlad, C.E.; et al. Possible involvement of vitamin C in periodontal disease-diabetes mellitus association. *Nutrients* **2020**, *12*, 553. [CrossRef]
21. Courbebaisse, M.; Cavalier, E. Vitamin D in 2020: An old pro-hormone with potential effects beyond mineral metabolism. *Nutrients* **2020**, *12*, 3378. [CrossRef] [PubMed]
22. Saponaro, F.; Saba, A.; Zucchi, R. An update on vitamin D metabolism. *Int. J. Mol. Sci.* **2020**, *21*, 6573. [CrossRef] [PubMed]
23. Zittermann, A.; Pilz, S.; Hoffmann, H.; Marz, W. Vitamin D and airway infections: A European perspective. *Eur. J. Med. Res.* **2016**, *21*, 14. [CrossRef]
24. Zmijewski, M.A. Vitamin D and human health. *Int. J. Mol. Sci.* **2019**, *20*, 145. [CrossRef]
25. Infusino, F.; Marazzato, M.; Mancone, M.; Fedele, F.; Mastroianni, C.M.; Severino, P.; Ceccarelli, G.; Santinelli, L.; Cavarretta, E.; Marullo, A.G.M.; et al. Diet Supplementation, probiotics, and nutraceuticals in SARS-CoV-2 infection: A scoping review. *Nutrients* **2020**, *12*, 1718. [CrossRef]
26. Kawalec, P.; Tesar, T.; Vostalova, L.; Draganic, P.; Manova, M.; Savova, A.; Petrova, G.; Rugaja, Z.; Männik, A.; Sowada, C.; et al. Pharmaceutical Regulation in Central and Eastern European Countries: A Current Review. *Front. Pharmacol.* **2017**, *8*, 892. [CrossRef]

27. Sintonen, H. The 15D instrument of health-related quality of life: Properties and applications. *Ann. Med.* **2001**, *33*, 328–336. [CrossRef] [PubMed]
28. Subtirelu, M.S.; Turcu-Stiolica, A.; Sintonen, H. Translation and cultural adaptation of 15D quality of life questionnaire from English to Romanian language. *Value Health* **2019**, *22*, S731. [CrossRef]
29. Cochran, W.G. *Sampling Techniques*, 3rd ed.; Wiley: New York, NY, USA, 1977.
30. Faul, F.; Erdfelder, E.; Lang, A.G.; Buchner, A. G*Power 3: A flexible statistical power analysis program for the social, behavioral, and biomedical sciences. *Behav. Res. Methods* **2007**, *39*, 175–191. [CrossRef] [PubMed]
31. Austin, Z.; Gregory, P. Resilience in the time of pandemic: The experience of community pharmacists during COVID-19. *Res. Soc. Adm. Pharm.* **2021**, *17*, 1867–1875. [CrossRef]
32. Merks, P.; Jakubowska, M.; Drelich, E.; Swieczkowski, D.; Bogusz, J.; Bilmin, K.; Sola, K.F.; May, A.; Majchrowska, A.; Koziol, M.; et al. The legal extension of the role of pharmacists in light of the COVID-19 global pandemic. *Res. Soc. Adm. Pharm.* **2021**, *17*, 1807–1812. [CrossRef] [PubMed]
33. Goff, D.A.; Ashiru-Oredope, D.; Cairns, K.A.; Eljaaly, K.; Gauthier, T.P.; Langford, B.J.; Mahmoud, S.F.; Messina, A.P.; Michael, U.C.; Saad, T.; et al. Global contributions of pharmacists during the COVID-19 pandemic. *J. Am. Coll. Clin. Pharm.* **2020**. [CrossRef]
34. Moccia, L.; Janiri, D.; Pepe, M.; Dattoli, L.; Molinaro, M.; De Martin, V.; Chieffo, D.; Janiri, L.; Fiorillo, A.; Sani, G.; et al. Affective temperament, attachment style, and the psychological impact of the COVID-19 outbreak: An early report on the Italian general population. *Brain Behav. Immun.* **2020**, *87*, 75–79. [CrossRef]
35. Johnston, K.; O'Reilly, C.L.; Cooper, G.; Mitchell, I. The burden of COVID-19 on pharmacists. *J. Am. Pharm. Assoc.* **2020**. [CrossRef]
36. Lange, M.; Joo, S.; Couette, P.A.; de Jaegher, S.; Joly, F.; Humbert, X. Impact on mental health of the COVID-19 outbreak among community pharmacists during the sanitary lockdown period. *Ann. Pharm. Fr.* **2020**, *78*, 459–463. [CrossRef]
37. Ardebili, M.E.; Naserbakht, M.; Bernstein, C.; Alazmani-Noodeh, F.; Hakimi, H.; Ranjbar, H. Healthcare providers experience of working during the COVID-19 pandemic: A qualitative study. *Am. J. Infect. Control* **2020**, *000*, 1–8. [CrossRef]
38. Ungureanu, B.S.; Vladut, C.; Bende, F.; Sandru, V.; Tocia, V.; Turcu-Stiolica, R.-V.; Groza, A.; Balan, G.G.; Turcu-Stiolica, A. Impact of the COVID-19 Pandemic on Health-Related Quality of Life, Anxiety, and Training Among Young Gastroenterologists in Romania. *Front. Psychol.* **2020**, *11*, 579177. [CrossRef]
39. Dror, A.A.; Eisenbach, N.; Taiber, S.; Morozov, N.G.; Mizrachi, M.; Zigron, A.; Srouji, S.; Sela, E. Vaccine hesitancy: The next challenge in the fight against COVID-19. *Eur. J. Epidemiol.* **2020**, *35*, 775–779. [CrossRef]
40. Lee, L.; Peterson, G.M.; Naunton, M.; Jackson, S.; Bushell, M. Protecting the herd: Why pharmacists matter in mass vaccination. *Pharmacy* **2020**, *8*, 199. [CrossRef]
41. Poudel, A.; Lau, E.T.L.; Deldot, M.; Campbell, C.; Waite, N.M.; Nissen, L. M, Pharmacist role in vaccination: Evidence and challenges. *Vaccine* **2019**, *37*, 5939–5945. [CrossRef] [PubMed]
42. World Bank Country and Lending Groups. Available online: https://datahelpdesk.worldbank.org/knowledgebase/articles/906519 (accessed on 4 February 2021).
43. Ilie, P.C.; Stefanescu, S.; Smith, L. The role of vitamin D in the prevention of coronavirus disease 2019 infection and mortality. *Aging Clin. Exp. Res.* **2020**, *32*, 7–1195. [CrossRef] [PubMed]
44. Singh, S.; Kaur, R.; Singh, R.K. Revisiting the role of vitamin D levels in the prevention of COVID-19 infection and mortality in European countries post infections peak. *Aging Clin. Exp. Res.* **2020**, *32*, 1609–1612. [CrossRef] [PubMed]
45. Jain, A.; Chaurasia, R.; Sengar, N.S.; Singh, M.; Mahor, S.; Narain, S. Analysis of vitamin D level among asymptomatic and critically ill COVID-19 patients and its correlation with inflammatory markers. *Sci. Rep.* **2020**, *10*, 20191. [CrossRef] [PubMed]
46. Mercola, J.; Grant, W.B.; Wagner, C.L. Evidence regarding vitamin D and risk of COVID-19 and its severity. *Nutrients* **2020**, *12*, 3361. [CrossRef] [PubMed]
47. Kumar, R.; Rathi, H.; Haq, A.; Wimalawansa, S.J.; Sharma, A. Putative roles of vitamin D in modulating immune response and immunopathology associated with COVID-19. *Virus Res.* **2021**, *292*, 198235. [CrossRef] [PubMed]
48. Benskin, L.L. A basic review of the preliminary evidence that COVID-19 risk and severity is increased in vitamin D deficiency. *Front. Public Health* **2020**, *8*, 513. [CrossRef] [PubMed]
49. Marik, P. EVMS COVID-19 Manage Protocol. An Overview of the MATH+ and I-MASK+ Protocols. Available online: https://www.evms.edu/media/evms_public/departments/internal_medicine/EVMS_Critical_Care_COVID-19_Protocol.pdf (accessed on 12 January 2021).
50. Clinical Trials. Available online: https://clinicaltrials.gov/ct2/results?cond=COVID-19&term=vitamin+c&cntry=&state=&city=&dist= (accessed on 13 January 2021).
51. Clinical Trials. Available online: https://clinicaltrials.gov/ct2/results?cond=COVID&term=vitamin+d&cntry=&state=&city=&dist= (accessed on 13 January 2021).
52. National Guide for Adaptation of Pharmaceutical Practice during Pandemic COVID-19. Available online: https://www.colegfarm.ro/userfiles/file/GHID%20orientativ%20de%20adaptare%20%20a%20practicii%20%20farmaceutice%20%20în%20cursul%20%20pandemiei%20%20COVID-19.pdf (accessed on 12 January 2021). (In Romanian)

53. Padureanu, V.; Bogdan, M.; Subtirelu, M.S.; Padureanu, R.; Turcu-Stiolica, A.; Petrescu, F.; Dumitrescu, F.; Mititelu-Tartau, L. Perceptions of COVID-19 vaccination among healthcare professionals in Romania. *Med. Surg. J.* **2020**, *124*, 454–460.
54. Terms and Conditions for Dispensing of Medicines, Medical Devices and Dietary Foods for Special Medical Purposes, Paid fully or Partially by the NHIF, Service, Extension of Validity of the Protocol Expensive Treatment for Chronically Ill Patients, in Connection with Emergency Declared by Decision of the National Essembly of 13.03.2020. Available online: https://www.nhif.bg/news_page?id=420414&page_id=422584 (accessed on 15 January 2021). (In Bulgarian)

Journal of
Clinical Medicine

MDPI

Article

The Outbreak of SARS-CoV-2 Pandemic and the Well-Being of Polish Students: The Risk Factors of the Emotional Distress during COVID-19 Lockdown

Dariusz Juchnowicz [1], Jacek Baj [2], Alicja Forma [3], Kaja Karakuła [4], Elżbieta Sitarz [5,*], Jacek Bogucki [6] and Hanna Karakula-Juchnowicz [5]

1 Department of Psychiatric Nursing, Medical University of Lublin, 20-093 Lublin, Poland; juchnowiczdariusz@wp.pl
2 Chair and Department of Anatomy, Medical University of Lublin, 20-090 Lublin, Poland; jacek.baj@umlub.pl
3 Student Research Group Department of Forensic Medicine, Medical University of Lublin, 20-090 Lublin, Poland; aforma@onet.pl
4 Psychiatry Student Research Group I Department of Psychiatry, Psychotherapy and Early Intervention, Medical University of Lublin, 20-439 Lublin, Poland; kaja.karakula@gmail.com
5 Chair and I Department of Psychiatry, Psychotherapy, and Early Intervention, Medical University of Lublin, 20-439 Lublin, Poland; hanna.karakula-juchnowicz@umlub.pl
6 Chair and Department of Organic Chemistry, Faculty of Pharmacy Medical University of Lublin, 20-093 Lublin, Poland; jacekbogucki@umlub.pl
* Correspondence: e.sitarz@hotmail.com

Citation: Juchnowicz, D.; Baj, J.; Forma, A.; Karakuła, K.; Sitarz, E.; Bogucki, J.; Karakula-Juchnowicz, H. The Outbreak of SARS-CoV-2 Pandemic and the Well-Being of Polish Students: The Risk Factors of the Emotional Distress during COVID-19 Lockdown. *J. Clin. Med.* **2021**, *10*, 944. https://doi.org/10.3390/jcm10050944

Academic Editors: Michele Roccella and Giacomo Mancini

Received: 2 January 2021
Accepted: 22 February 2021
Published: 1 March 2021

Abstract: The coronavirus disease 2019 (COVID-19) pandemic has a significant impact on both physical and mental health. The aim of this cross-sectional study was to (1) evaluate depression, anxiety, and stress levels among students from Polish universities during the first weeks of the COVID-19 pandemic and (2) assess the risk factors of the higher intensity of emotional distress. We conducted an online survey using the Depression, Anxiety, and Stress Scale-21 (DASS-21) to assess well-being. The study included 2172 respondents (73% female, 27% male) with a mean age of 22.1 ± 2.2. Moderate to extremely severe scores of depression, anxiety, and stress were reported by 43.4%, 27.3%, and 41.0% of the respondents, respectively. Higher scores of DASS-21 were related to female sex (odds ratio (OR) = 3.01), studying sciences (OR = 2.04), co-residence with the roommates (OR = 1.25), suffering from a mental disorder (OR = 5.88), loneliness (OR = 293.30), the usage of psychiatric support before pandemic (OR = 8.06), poor economic situation (OR = 13.49), and the lower scores were found for being currently employed (OR = 0.4). This study highlights an urgent need for (1) crisis-oriented psychological and psychiatric support for students during the outbreak of the COVID-19 pandemic and (2) preparing appropriate psychological interventions to improve the mental health of students for a possible similar situation in the future.

Keywords: COVID-19; SARS-CoV-2; pandemic; psychological well-being; DASS-21; depression; anxiety; stress; emotional distress

1. Introduction

A new viral disease due to the infection by the severe acute respiratory syndrome coronavirus-2 (SARS-CoV-2) has been named by the World Health Organization (WHO) as the coronavirus disease 2019 (COVID-19) and announced as a pandemic approximately five months after the 41 first reported cases of pneumonia in Wuhan, China [1–3]. Before it was officially reported as a pandemic, the spread of the SARS-CoV-2 has affected 114 countries, leading to nearly 188,000 infections, among which thousands of them included critical cases, as well as over 4000 deaths [4,5]. According to the most recent statistics, there are more than 100 million cases confirmed so far, and the number of new cases (confirmed or fatal) is continually increasing every other day.

Compared to the severe acute respiratory syndrome coronavirus (SARS-CoV) or the Middle East respiratory syndrome coronavirus (MERS-CoV), SARS-CoV-2 has affected a significantly greater number of people during the outbreak of the pandemic, mainly due to its higher transmission potential [6] and its efficient spread by various transmission routes including airborne, contact, or fecal-oral routes [7,8]. Several factors such as gender, age, or the presence of concomitant diseases have and an impact on the severity of SARS-CoV-2 infection that might range from the asymptomatic infection to the clinical conditions characterized by severe respiratory failure or death [5,8]. Factors that contribute to the higher risk of mortality rates of the infected patients include cardiovascular diseases, hypertension, respiratory diseases, diabetes, older age, obesity [6,8], or vitamin D deficiency [9].

According to the WHO, on 26 April 2020, which was the closing day of our survey, the course of events proceeded as follows—2,804,796 confirmed cases, 193,710 confirmed deaths [10]. From the date of the outbreak, in order to prevent the spread of the virus, many governments ordered the first recommendations regarding national lockdowns as well as traveling restrictions [11]. In Poland, on the same date (26 April 2020), there were 11,617 officially confirmed cases and 535 deaths already reported [12]. Numerous restrictions introduced by the governmental measures and public health recommendations during the COVID-19 pandemic have affected the daily living of the society, and those that primarily mattered were social distancing, social isolation, and home confinement. On 23 March, the Polish government announced a state of emergency due to the SARS-CoV-2 pandemic, and all schools and universities were closed [13]. From the 1 April till 26 April, people were not allowed to go out except in special cases such as work and going to the pharmacy, hospital, and grocery shops, besides, strict restrictions regarding the total number of customers who were allowed to be in the same room were introduced by the government. Moreover, the hours between 10 am and 12 am have been declared as 'the hours for seniors only' in all of the open institutions; parks, forests, and boulevards have been closed for all other citizens. Juveniles under 18 years old were not allowed to walk unsupervised by an adult [14]. People started to self-isolate, equipped with excess food, protective masks, and disinfectants. Incidences of shortages of masks and health equipment in numerous hospitals and pharmacies occurred [15]. Throughout the pandemic, information on the transmission dynamics, incubation time, basic reproductive frequency of COVID-19, or symptoms and clinical manifestations of the infection were unclear and continually changing. The absence of a specific cure or vaccine made the public more concerned about their health [16].

The risk of infection or death was not the only problem that was concerning society. Reports on the expansion of SARS-CoV-2 infection and new incidents of confirmed or fatal COVID-19 cases were more likely to be causing fear, anxiety, and distress [17]. The rapid spread of the virus, social isolation, changing of the command habits, many restrictions, postponing exams, reopening of schools and universities are pressuring the mental health of societies [10]. Moreover, the stigmatization or even discrimination of the individuals who might be associated with the area of spread of disease (e.g., healthcare workers) might be even more distressing [18]. In 2002, during the SARS pandemic, studies showed that the psychological impact on the non-infected community was higher in the younger population; besides, they presented with an increased self-blame, which could reflect frustration and guilt related to responsibility attribution [19]. There is an increasing number of studies that aim to assess the mental health of the general population during the COVID-19 pandemic; however, the long-term consequences remain questionable [20].

2. Psychological Consequences of the Pandemic

The outbreak of the SARS-CoV-2 pandemic has become an extremely pronounced stressor, which has extended to almost all of the countries worldwide. The fast spread of the pandemic was observed to affect all groups in society. At the current state of knowledge, it is believed that not only the pandemic alone but also the regulations and political measures that aim to prevent the spread of the virus have a significant impact on the mental health of societies. Researchers addressed the psychological and behavioral responses of people during the early stage of the COVID-19 pandemic and noticed higher depressive, anxiety, and stress symptoms in the general population [15,16,18,21–24]. Some researchers observed that particularly students' psychological health was more influenced by the pandemic crisis compared to the other groups but presented with similar stress and anxiety levels [15]. There is some evidence that youths have reported depressive symptoms at a higher prevalence than the older ones [23]. A systematic review by Xiong et al. showed that the major risk factors associated with mental distress during the COVID-19 pandemic primarily included the student status, female gender, age groups <40 years old, unemployment status, as well as the presence of either psychiatric or other chronic diseases [25]. In a study that combined the population of 113,285 individuals, it was demonstrated that the prevalence rate and intensity of depression, anxiety, and stress were significantly higher during the pandemic; besides, sleep disturbances and more intense psychological distress were also observed in a studied population [26]. During the first weeks of the pandemic outbreak, about half of the Chinese respondents' reported a moderate-to-severe psychological impact, whereas one-third of the studied group—moderate-to-severe anxiety [15]. Similar to the above-mentioned studies, student status and female gender were associated with greater levels of depression, anxiety, and stress. In the general population of Austria, depressive and anxiety symptoms were up to five and three times more prevalent, respectively, compared to the results obtained before the outbreak of the pandemic [27]. Unemployment, financial instability, and a lower income, in general, are major economic factors that might exaggerate both psychological and mental consequences during a pandemic [28–30]. Even though the outbreak began in China, a study comparing the distress between Poles and Chinese showed that Polish society tends to present significantly higher depression, anxiety, and stress levels [31]. Generally, younger individuals are more susceptible to depressive, anxiety, and stress symptoms related to the pandemic, comparing to the older population [32]. According to the most recent studies, the pandemic seems to affect individuals in all age groups. Several factors such as student status or female gender tend to additionally exaggerate psychological distress; however, there are also protective factors such as social support, proper relationships with family and friends, or the absence of any mental illnesses [33]. A study by Epifanio et al. performed in Italy during COVID-19 lockdown showed that younger adults (18–34 years old) presented with the lowest levels of psychological health, constituting the most vulnerable subjects in the general population at the same time [34]. Since numerous studies have already reported that students are most vulnerable to emotional distress during the pandemic, it is of great importance to find the risk and protective factors associated with the emotional distress in this group [35–39].

Therefore, the aim of this study was to (1) evaluate depression, anxiety, and stress levels among students from Polish universities during the first weeks of the COVID-19 pandemic, (2) assess the risk factors that increase the probability of the higher intensity of emotional distress, (3) create a portrait of a student who requires enhanced emotional support during the pandemic, (4) compare the results of our study with the results of research from other countries, that have also assessed the emotional well-being of the students during the first stages of COVID-19 lockdown with the usage of the same psychological tools.

3. Materials and Methods

3.1. Study Design and Survey Description

Before the survey preparation, the authors performed an independent review of the literature regarding the impact of the COVID-19 pandemic on mental health with a particular emphasis on the students. Subsequently, a structured questionnaire was created, including four parts: (1) sociodemographic data, (2) questions related to one's health condition, (3) economic situation, and (4) Polish adaptation of the Depression, Anxiety, and Stress Scale-21 (DASS-21) to assess depression, anxiety, and stress levels [40]. An anonymous online cross-sectional survey included the questionnaire that was distributed on 20 April 2020 via social media among Polish students from 87 universities, including all medical universities in Poland. The survey was prepared via a Google form and was posted on social media groups on Facebook that gather students from Poland. The questionnaire was also sent via e-mail to other universities in Poland with a request to distribute it to the private groups at universities as well. The survey was closed on 26 April. Therefore, it was conducted almost 6 weeks after applying the lockdown measures in Poland on 10 March. Hereby, the snowball sampling method was utilized. The respondents were completing the survey individually in an estimated average time of about 10 min. All the answers given by the respondents were confidential, and only those who were conducting the research had access to the answers.

3.2. Measures

The questionnaire was composed in such a way as to provide the most crucial information regarding the respondent's sociodemographic data, economic situation, and general, subjective knowledge about COVID-19. Sociodemographic data included (1) gender, (2) age, (3) field of study, (4) year of study, (5) place of residence, (6) place of residence during the COVID-19 pandemic, (7) marital status, (8) parental status, and (9) living situation and co-residence. Data related to student health conditions included questions regarding whether someone got COVID-19, cases of COVID-19 among family members and/or friends, deaths due to COVID-19 among family members and/or friends, active involvement in the fight against SARS-CoV-2, using the support of a psychologist/psychiatrist before the pandemic, taking medications or supplements that improve the immunity, and individual difficulties related to the current epidemiological situation. The section related to the economic situation included the following questions—(1) whether a respondent is currently working and (2) how the respondent assesses their economic situation during the pandemic.

3.3. DASS-21 Scale

The mental health status of the respondents was measured using the Depression, Anxiety, and Stress Scale-21 Items (DASS-21) [40]. In the following study, a polish adaptation of the DASS-21 scale was used [41]. The DASS-21 is a shortened version of the original 42-item DASS created by Lovibond and Lovibond, and both of them are self-report scales designed to estimate the overall emotional distress of a respondent, as well as to assess and evaluate the scores of the depression, anxiety, and stress levels [42,43]. It has been proved that both of the DASS scales show a high internal consistency [44]. The DASS-21 is composed of a hierarchical factor structure that includes the three first-order factors (depression, anxiety, and stress), as well as one second-order factor (emotional symptoms) [45]. Such a designated scale is suitable for both clinical and non-clinical purposes. An advantage is that compared to DASS-42, a shortened version (DASS-21) requires less time to be fulfilled by the respondents, providing similar outcomes at the same time. The main difference between these scales is the fact that the DASS-42 scale is preferably chosen for clinical purposes, whereas the DASS-21 is primarily chosen for research purposes. To compare the results with the normative data and scientific publications in which the DASS-42 scale was used, the statistical results obtained from the DASS-21 should be multiplied by 2. Such a conversion provides the possibility to obtain the validity of the statistical results that are comparable to those that are obtained while applying the DASS-42, however, being less time-consuming and more legible for the respondents at the same time [46].

The DASS-21 scale consists of three major scales (depression, anxiety, and stress), among which, each of them contains 7 items. The depression scale evaluates the lack of interest, devaluation of life, hopelessness, dysphoria, anhedonia, inertia, and self-deprecation. The anxiety scale evaluates the general autonomic agitation, situational anxiety, and a subjective experience of anxiety, whereas the stress scale assesses the chronic non-specific arousal such as tension, irritability, and nervousness. Responses were structured by a

4-point Likert scale ranging from 0 ('does not apply to me at all') to 3 ('applies to me very much or most of the time'), with higher scores indicating more negative experience in the past week. The total score of the DASS-21 ranges from 0 to 63, whereas the score for each of the subscales ranges from 0 to 21. After multiplication by 2 for further analysis of the results, we obtained a DASS-21 total maximum score of 126 and scores for every subscale equal to 42. The division of the total score multiplied by 2 of the depression, anxiety, and stress subscale is presented in Table 1 [42].

Table 1. The severity labels used to describe the range of scores in the population of the DASS-21 multiplied by 2.

	Depression	Anxiety	Stress
Normal	0–8	0–7	0–14
Mild	8–13	8–9	15–18
Moderate	14–20	10–14	19–25
Severe	21–27	15–19	26–33
Extremely severe	28+	20+	34+

In our study, the alpha coefficients for the reliability of the depression, anxiety, stress, and full scale in the entire group were 0.95, 0.89, 0.96, and 0.94, respectively. The calculated values of Cronbach's alpha for individual scales indicated the high reliability of the used scale.

3.4. Description of the Study Group

The final sample consisted of 2172 students of whom 73% (n = 1585) were women and 27% (n = 587) were men. The mean age of the sample was 22.1 ± 2.2. The majority of the respondents (60.5%) were medical students; other fields of study included students studying social sciences (19.2%), engineering (10%), arts and humanities (5%), and sciences (4.4%). The majority of students were in the first year of university (23.5%), and the least (4.9%), during the sixth year of university. The most prevalent place of residence of the students was the village (22.9%). In the studied group, most of the students were single (65.6%) or in an informal relationship (30.7%), whereas only 2.5% of the studied group was married. Regarding the place of residence during the COVID-19 pandemic, 48.3% of the respondents have answered that they are currently living with their parents. The smallest number of students answered that they lived with a partner and a child 1% (n = 21). The sociodemographic data of the respondents is presented in Table 2.

3.5. Characteristic of the Respondents' Health Status

The majority of the respondents (n = 2112; 97.2%) and their relatives and friends (n = 1943; 89.5%) did not suffer from COVID-19. Only 1.3% of the students, as well as 2.4% and 7.4% of students, either a family member or friend respectively, had gotten COVID-19. In this group, 0.6% of students suffered from a loss of a family member or friend due to COVID-19. Some students (20.2%) took part in an active fight against the spread of SARS-CoV-2 by sewing protective masks, helping elderly people with shopping, collecting money for hospital equipment, providing telephone consultations, and volunteering in hospitals. The majority of respondents (82.9%) did not get any psychological or psychiatric support before the outbreak of the pandemic, which led to the conclusion that 17.1% of the respondents had experienced some kind of mental disorder before. This data is consistent with the global data on the prevalence of mental disorders—about 17.6% of the population meets the criteria for common mental disorders [47]. With regards to the students who used such support, the psychological ones were most frequently chosen by the students (n = 162; 7.5%). The majority of the respondents (n = 1506; 69.3%) did not take any supplements or medicines to improve their immunity. From those who took supplements (n = 665; 30.6%), in most of the cases it was vitamin D (n = 157; 7.2%), vitamin C (n = 140; 6.5%), or a vitamin complex (n = 134; 6.2%), and the rest used other medications (n = 234; 10.8%), including magnesium, omega-3 fatty acids, herbs, and homeopathic remedies. Regarding the difficulties that were faced by the students during the pandemic, most of the students (n = 728; 33.5%) were afraid of infecting their relatives. Interestingly, the fear of being infected by oneself was the least prevalent fear amongst students (n = 66; 3.0%). In the case of chronic diseases, the majority of students denied the existence of any (n = 1837; 84.6%). However, 4.1% (n = 88) suffered from thyroid diseases, 2.5% (n = 54) from asthma, 1.9% (n = 41) from a mental disorder, 1.5% (n = 32) from an allergy, 0.7 (n = 15) from diabetes, and 4.8% (n = 105) from other diseases. The data of respondents' health status is provided in Table 3.

Table 2. Sociodemographic characteristics of the respondents included in the study.

Question	Answer	Number of Respondents	% of Respondents
Sex	Women	1585	73.0
	Men	587	27.0
Field of study	Arts and humanities	110	5.0
	Sciences	96	4.4
	Medicine	1314	60.5
	Engineering	219	10.0
	Social sciences	416	19.2
Year of study	I	511	23.5
	II	444	20.4
	III	507	23.3
	IV	322	14.8
	V	277	12.8
	VI	106	4.9
Place of residence (number of inhabitants) [in thousands]	Village	497	22.9
	Less than 20	219	10.1
	20–100	344	15.8
	100–300	276	12.7
	300–600	409	18.8
	More than 600	427	19.7
Marital status	Single	1426	65.6
	Informal relationship	667	30.7
	Married	54	2.5
Do you have children?	No	2130	98.1
	One child	20	0.9
I live with:	Alone	231	10.6
	Parents	1049	48.3
	Roommates	565	26.0
	Partner or spouse	301	13.9
	Partner/spouse and children	21	1.0

Table 3. Factors associated with the health status of respondents.

Question	Answer	Number of Respondents	% of Respondents
Did you get COVID-19?	No	2112	97.2
	Yes	28	1.3
Did any of your relatives/friends get COVID-19?	No	1943	89.5
	Yes, a family member	52	2.4
	Yes, a friend	161	7.4
Did any of your relatives/friends die because of COVID-19?	No	2142	98.6
	Yes, a family member	12	0.6
	Yes, a friend	14	0.6
Are you actively joining the fight against the COVID-19 epidemic?	No	1733	79.8
	Yes	439	20.2
Did you use psychological/psychiatric help before the beginning of the pandemic?	No	1800	82.9
	Yes, I used psychological support	162	7.5
	Yes, I used psychiatric support	80	3.7
	Yes, I used psychological and psychiatric support	130	6.0
Do you take any supplements/medicines that increase immunity?	No	1506	69.3
	Yes	665	30.6
What was most difficult for you during the pandemic?	Changes awaiting the world after the pandemic	440	20.3
	Change of the lifestyle	265	12.2
	Fear of being infected	66	3.0
	Fear of infection of the loved ones	728	33.5
	Financial instability	149	6.9
	Isolation	211	9.7
	Loneliness	149	6.9
Do you have any chronic disease?	No	1837	84.6
	Allergy	32	1.5
	Asthma	54	2.5
	Diabetes	15	0.7
	Mental disorders	41	1.9
	Thyroid diseases	88	4.1
	Other	105	4.8

3.6. Employment Status and Economic Situation of the Respondents

We asked the students if they were working before the pandemic broke out. Most of the respondents (n = 1469; 67.6%), answered that they did not work, whereas the smallest group of students (n = 30; 1.2%) answered that they ran their own business. During the pandemic, 15.2% of the students lost their job, which caused to rise in the unemployment group of students to 82.8% (n = 1799). We also asked how the students assessed their economic situation during the pandemic. Most of the respondents (n = 1278; 58.8%) answered that they have a stable family income, and nothing has changed for them. The smallest number of students (n = 21; 1%) answered that they had to start borrowing money from family or friends during the outbreak of the pandemic because they were not able to support themselves. The data related to respondents' economic situation is provided in Table 4.

Table 4. The economic situation of the respondents.

Question	Answer	Number of Respondents	% of Respondents
Did you work before the pandemic outbreak?	I did not work	1469	67.6
	I worked mentally	356	16.4
	I worked physically	316	14.5
	I ran my own business	30	1.2
Do you work currently?	No, I do not work	1799	82.8
	I work mentally	249	11.5
	I work physically	96	4.4
	I run my own business	28	1.3
How do you assess your economic situation during the pandemic?	I have a stable family income, nothing has changed	1278	58.8
	I have a stable family income, but the situation is worse than before	647	29.8
	I have to start using savings	191	8.8
	I have to borrow money from my family/friends during the outbreak of the pandemic because I do not have enough money to support myself	21	1.0
	I barely have enough money for living	27	1.2

4. Statistical Analysis

The statistical analysis of the results obtained in this study included descriptive statistics, distribution of the numbers with a percentage distribution, nonparametric tests (since data distribution obtained in a DASS test deviated from the normal distribution), U Mann–Whitney, as well as H Kruskal–Wallis tests with multiple comparisons test with Bonferroni correction. The distribution of the psychological variables was checked with the usage of analysis of histograms and the Shapiro–Wilk test in the Statistica program. The distribution in particular scales and the overall result deviated from the normal distribution, which was statistically significant. The effect size for the Kruskal-Wallis test was calculated as the eta squared based on the H-statistic: eta squared (H) = $(H - k + 1)/(n - k)$; where H is the value obtained in the Kruskal–Wallis test; k is the number of groups; n is the total number of observations. To check the reliability of the applied test, the values of the Cronbach's alpha test coefficient for individual scales of the tool were calculated (using the Statistica v.13 program; Statistica software—Polish version from StatSoft Corporation Poland, the partner of Tibco Corporation, Palo Alto, California, USA (licence for Medical University of Lublin)). To determine the risk factors for developing higher intensity of emotional distress, we standardized the scores of the DASS-21 total score, and then we distinguished two groups of subjects for further comparisons. The first group of subjects included the respondents with low scores (DASS 0; below mean (M)—standard deviation (SD)), whereas the second group—those with high scores (above M + SD). Afterward, odds ratio (OR) values along with the significance level were calculated using the MedCalc Odds Ratio Calculator program.

The control groups were allocated to the particular variable as follows—for 'sex'—men in the DASS 0 and DASS 2 groups; for 'field of study' and 'I live with'—the whole DASS 0 and DASS 2 groups; for 'Do you have any chronic disease'—the respondents who answered 'No' in the DASS 0 and DASS 2 groups; for 'Did you use psychological/psychiatric help before the beginning of the pandemics?' and 'Did you use psychological/psychiatric help during the pandemics'—the respondents who answered 'No' in the DASS 0 and DASS 2 groups; for 'What was the most difficult for you during pandemics?'—the respondents who answered 'I was not afraid' in the DASS 0 and DASS 2 groups; for 'Are you currently working'—the respondents who answered 'No, I do not work' in the DASS 0 and DASS 2 groups; for 'How do you assess your economic situation during pandemics?'—the respondents who answered 'I have a stable family income, nothing has changed' in the DASS 0 and DASS 2 groups.

5. Ethical Considerations

This study was approved by the Bioethical Commission of the Medical University of Lublin, Lublin, Poland, and was conducted in compliance with national legislation and the Declaration of Helsinki. Before fulfilling the questionnaire, all of the respondents had to sign a consent form declaring that they agree to take part in this study before the survey has started. Informed consent included information about the form and nature of the study along with its aim and information about the confidentiality and anonymity of data and the exploitation of the results only for scientific purposes. All of the data obtained in this study was gathered and analyzed anonymously.

6. Results

6.1. DASS-21

6.1.1. Total DASS Score

The total DASS score for the entire group of the respondents was 38.13 ± 26.51, which was lower than the cut-off score equal to 60, proposed by Lovibond and Lovibond [41]. The overall emotional distress was statistically higher ($p < 0.001$) in females (M = 40.54 ± 26.65) compared to males (M = 31.60 ± 25.02). The results showed that there was a relationship between the field of study and the DASS total score; the highest score was observed in science students (median (Me) = 42.00 ± 40.91), the second in turn was in the case of the participants studying arts and humanities (Me = 39.00 ± 28.98), social sciences (Me = 35.00 ± 28.14), and engineering (Me = 32.00 ± 26.79). The lowest score was obtained amongst the respondents who studied medicine (Me = 31.00 ± 25.48). Based on the Kruskal–Wallis test, the studied groups were statistically different (H = 16.16, $p = 0.0028$). The highest difference was noted between the medical and science students (z = 3.312, $p = 0.009$) (Supplementary Table S1). There were no statistical differences between the first-year students and the rest of the respondents in the DASS total score, as well as in none of the subscales (depression, anxiety, and stress).

6.1.2. Depression

The mean score for the depression subscale for the entire study group was 14.04 ± 10.44, which can be classified as a moderate level of depressive symptoms. The intensity of depression defined as normal in the DASS-21 subscale concerned 43.6% ($n = 948$) of the total group of students. The mild intensity of depression applied to 13% ($n = 282$) of the examined students, moderate to 19.9% ($n = 432$), severe to 10.2% ($n = 221$), and extremely severe to 13.3% ($n = 289$). The level of depression in the female group (M = 18.41 ± 14.05) was significantly higher ($p < 0.001$) than in males (M = 12.24 ± 14.37). The results obtained from the Kruskal–Wallis test showed no significant difference between the students' field of study and the level of depression (Supplementary Table S1.2).

6.1.3. Anxiety

In the anxiety subscale of DASS-21, the mean result for the entire group was 7.71 ± 8.29 (equivalent for mild anxiety). Among the examined students, the intensity of anxiety defined as normal in the DASS-21 subscale concerned 60.2% ($n = 1307$) of the respondents. Mild anxiety affected 12.5% ($n = 273$) of the respondents, moderate—9% ($n = 195$), severe—6.6% ($n = 144$), extremely severe—11.7% ($n = 253$). Again, as in the depression subscale women (M = 13.19 ± 11.54) reached ($p < 0.001$) a higher level of anxiety than male participants (M = 6.90 ± 9.92). Students of arts and humanities (Me = 6.00 ± 9.63), science (Me = 6.00 ± 9.2), social sciences (Me = 6.00 ± 8.63) reached the highest score, whereas medicine (Me = 4.00 ± 8.0) and engineering (Me = 4.00 ± 8.05) the lowest. The results did not vary significantly between different fields of studies (Supplementary Table S1.3).

6.1.4. Stress

The *mean* value for stress *intensity* for the whole group was 16.93 ± 10.98, which classifies as a mild level of stress. The stress level among the surveyed students, which is defined as normal in the DASS-21 subscale, concerned 47.2% (*n* = 1026) of the respondents, mild stress—11.8% (*n* = 255), moderate stress—15.3% (*n* = 333), severe stress—16.8% (*n* = 364), and the extremely severe stress—8.9% (*n* = 194) of the respondents. As previously, females (20.93 ± 15.45) scored statistically ($p < 0.001$) higher than males (12.58 ± 14.70). With regards to the anxiety subscale, the order was almost the same as in the case of the above-mentioned subgroups with science faculty (Me = 20.00 ± 11.12) in the highest place, then art and humanities (Me = 19.00 ± 11.62), and faculty of social sciences (Me = 16.00 ± 11.51), engineering (Me = 16.00 ± 10.82), and medicine (Me = 16.00 ± 10.73) with the lowest scores. The Kruskal–Wallis test showed no difference between the results of the stress subscale and the field of study (Supplementary Table S1.4).

The number of students with a particular degree of severity of depression, anxiety, and stress levels is presented in Table 5. Most of the students reached a normal level of depression (*n* = 948, 43.6%), anxiety (*n* = 1307, 60.2%), and stress (*n* = 1026, 47.2%). The highest level of depression symptoms was noted in 13.3% (*n* = 289) of the respondents. In the case of anxiety and stress, 11.7% (*n* = 253) and 8.9% (*n* = 194) of the students, respectively, were observed to have extremely severe symptoms (Table 5).

Table 5. The number of students presenting a severity ranges of overall emotional distress, depression, anxiety, and stress levels.

	Normal		Mild		Moderate		Severe		Extremely Severe	
	n	%	*n*	%	*n*	%	*n*	%	*n*	%
Depression	948	43.6	282	13	432	19.9	221	10.2	289	13.3
Anxiety	1307	60.2	273	12.5	195	9.0	144	6.6	253	11.7
Stress	1026	47.2	255	11.8	333	15.3	364	16.8	194	8.9

6.2. *Factors Correlating with the Emotional Distress in the Study Group*

6.2.1. Demographic Factors

One of the main goals of our study was to identify the factors that increase the probability of a higher intensity of emotional distress in the group of students (Supplementary Table S8).

Among the demographic factors associated with an increased intensity of the emotional response in the study group were female sex (OR = 3.01, 95% CI: 2.15–4.22) and science as a field of study (OR = 2.04, 95% CI: 0.99–4.19).

6.2.2. The Most Difficult Problem during the Pandemic

The respondents were asked to choose from the nine situations the only one that in the moment of the outbreak of the pandemic and through the first weeks was the most difficult for them. Students who choose 'loneliness' as the most difficult were observed to reach the highest level of overall emotional distress (Me = 52.00 ± 26.01), depression (Me = 20.00 ± 11.33), anxiety (Me = 8.00 ± 8.37), and stress (Me = 22.00 ± 10.41) measured by the DASS-21. Taking into consideration the intensity of the total DASS scores, the respondents who chose 'radical change in style and way of life' (Me = 35.00 ± 28.43) as the second one in ranking and the third as 'isolation' (Me = 34.00 ± 27.53) ex aequo with 'financial instability' (Me = 34.00 ± 27.64). In case of level of depression and stress, second were 'radical change in style and way of life' (depression: Me = 12.00 ± 11.27, stress: Me = 18.00 ± 11.25) and 'isolation' (depression: Me = 12.00 ± 10.24, stress: Me = 18.00 ± 11.33). With regards to the anxiety subscale, the 'fear of their own risk of infection illness, death' (Me = 6.00 ± 10.09), 'fear of infection of the loved ones' (Me = 6.00 ± 7.67), and "financial instability' (Me = 6.00 ± 8.31) were associated with the highest levels of anxiety. In total DASS and all subscales the differences between the groups were statistically significant—DASS-21 (H = 87.51, $p < 0.001$), depression (H = 106.68, $p < 0.001$), anxiety (H = 53.83, $p < 0.001$), stress (H = 74.58, $p < 0.001$) (Supplementary Tables S2, S2.2, S2.3, and S2.4). The increased feeling of loneliness was related to 292-fold higher odds of developing higher overall emotional distress (OR = 292, 95% CI: 15.77–5454.92).

6.2.3. Suffering from Chronic Diseases

In the case of the concomitant chronic diseases, the highest scores of overall emotional distress (Me = 58.00 ± 29.26), depression (Me = 20.00 ± 11.25), stress (Me = 24.00 ± 11.67), and anxiety (Me = 12.00 ± 11.68) were observed in people with mental disorders. The suffering from any chronic diseases was associated with the occurrence of overall emotional disorders in DASS-21 above the cut-off score. The presence of psychiatric disorders was significantly associated with a higher level of overall emotional distress (z = 4.831, $p < 0.001$), depression, (z = 4.424, $p < 0.001$) anxiety (z = 4.148, $p = 0.001$), and stress (z = 4.142, $p = 0.001$), compared to the respondents without any chronic diseases (Supplementary Tables S3, S3.2, S3.3, and S3.4). Students suffering from psychiatric disorders were almost six times more likely to exaggerate their emotional responses than those who had no mental health problems (OR = 5.89, 95% CI: 1.70–20.27). The usage of any supplements or medication to improve subject immunity did not correlate with the results of the DASS-21.

6.2.4. Psychological/Psychiatric Support before the Pandemic Broke-Out

Students who were using psychological and/or psychiatric help had the highest results in overall emotional distress (Me = 56.00 ± 29.53), depression (Me = 20.00 ± 10.43), anxiety (Me = 12.00 ± 10.43), and stress (Me = 24.00 ± 11.61). The use of the psychological and/or psychiatric support before the pandemic was associated with significantly higher levels of all the assessed variables of the DASS-21 (overall emotional distress (H = 102.21, $p < 0.001$); depression (H = 78.208, $p < 0.001$); anxiety (H = 92.198 $p < 0.001$); stress (H = 76.923, $p < 0.001$), and the total DASS scores were above the cut-off scores (Supplementary Tables S4, S4.2, S4.3, and S4.4). The respondents who had higher odds of emotional distress to the pandemic situation were those who used psychiatrist services before the outbreak of the pandemic (OR = 8.06, 95% CI: 2.79–23.28).

6.2.5. Economic Situation during a Pandemic

The self-assessment of students' economic situation in the time of pandemic was significantly related to overall emotional distress (H = 63.77, $p < 0.001$), depression (H = 51.86, $p < 0.001$), anxiety (H = 58.79, $p < 0.001$), and stress (H = 51.44, $p < 0.001$). Students who gave the answer 'stable family income, nothing has changed' had the lowest result in overall emotional distress (Me = 30.00 ± 25.43), depression (Me = 10.00 ± 10.09), anxiety (Me = 4.00 ± 7.80), and stress (Me = 14.00 ± 10.71) (Supplementary Tables S5, S5.2, S5.3, and S5.4). More than 13-fold higher odds (OR = 13.49, 95% CI: 1.71–106.33) of an increased emotional response was observed in the respondents who chose the answer that they had to start borrowing money from family or friends during the outbreak of the pandemic because they did not have sufficient funds to support themselves.

6.2.6. Employment Status during a Pandemic

The employment status during the pandemic was associated with the intensity of emotions measured with DASS-21—overall emotional distress (H = 17.76, $p < 0.001$) and depression (H = 30.49, $p < 0.001$). In total DASS scores and all subscales, the sequence was similar, reaching the highest levels in the group of students who were not working (overall emotional distress—Me = 34.00 ± 29.66, depression—Me = 12.00 ± 10.47, anxiety—

Me = 6.00 ± 8.41, stress—Me = 16.00 ± 10.92), in later order—in a group of the respondents that were working mentally, physically, and lastly—running their own businesses. The level of overall emotional distress (Me = 34.00 ± 26.66) observed in students who were currently not working reached above the cut-off score (Supplementary Tables S6, S6.2, S6.3, and S6.4). Currently working mentally (OR = 0.5, 95% CI: 0.34–0.85) and physically (OR = 0.4, 95% CI: 0.18–1.05) were related to a 0.5 and 0.4-fold lower odds of increased overall emotional distress respectively.

6.2.7. Living Situation

The living situation and the co-residence were observed to correlate with the results of the depression subscale (H = 37.22, $p < 0.001$). The highest levels of overall emotional distress (Me = 34.00 ± 25.82), depression (Me = 12.00 ± 10.32), anxiety (Me = 6.00 ± 8.18), and stress (Me = 16.00 ± 10.68) were found in a group of students living with roommates and students living with parents—overall emotional distress (Me = 34.00 ± 27.01), depression (Me = 12.00 ± 10.58), anxiety (Me = 6.00 ± 8.42), and stress (Me = 16.00 ± 11.08). People living with roommates and those living with their parents reached above the cut-off score in overall emotional distress results. The students who live with roommates presented 1.25-fold higher odds of depression, stress, and anxiety (OR = 1.25, 95% CI: 0.89–1.78) (Supplementary Tables S7, S7.2, S7.3, and S7.4).

6.3. Comparison with the Results of Other Authors' Studies

The results of our study have been compared with the ones conducted in Spain, China, India, and Bangladesh. The following countries were chosen by us since the other authors applied the same psychological instrument (DASS-21) and their studies were performed during the first stages of the pandemic, similarly to our research (Table 6).

Regarding the total DASS scores, higher emotional distress was noted among Polish students compared to Chinese students (t = 20.44, d = 0.76). Polish students also showed a greater severity of depression, anxiety, and stress in comparison to Spanish students (depression—t = 42.31, d = 1.04; anxiety—t = 27.40, d = 0.68; stress t = 10.12, d = 1.20). Statistically significant results were obtained between Poland and Bangladesh, where higher levels of depression, anxiety, and stress were shown by students from Bangladesh (depression—$t = -11.35$, d = 1.87; anxiety—$t = -23.66$, d = 1.07; stress $t = -14.23$, d = 1.91). Bangladeshi students also showed higher emotional intensity compared to Spanish students in all of the investigated subscales (depression—$t = -60.44$, d = 1.50; anxiety—$t = -59.69$, d = 0.69; stress $t = -72.65$, d = 1.40).

Table 6. The comparison of the results obtained applying the DASS-21 scale on a population of students in the studies performed in Poland, Spain, China, India, and Bangladesh.

Country	Poland	Spain	China	India	Bangladesh
Date of the start and closure of the survey	20 April–26 April	28 March–4 April	31 January–2 February	23 April–30 April	11 April–24 April
The time that has from the confinement till the start of the survey	6 weeks	2 weeks	3 days after the WHO announced COVID-19 as a public health emergency	One month	2 weeks
Number of the respondents	2172	3707	1210	500	3122
Females (%)	73	66.1	67.3	65	40.5
Males (%)	27	33.9	32.7	35	59.5
Mean age/age range	22.1 ± 2.2	27.9 ± 12.4	12–21.4—28.4% 21.4–30.8—53.2% 30.8–40.2—7.8% 40.2–49.6—7.4% 49.6–59—3.2%	21.2 ± 1.3	21.4 ± 2

Table 6. *Cont.*

Country			Poland	Spain	China	India	Bangladesh
Mean and SD of the DASS-21 total score **			38.13 ± 26.51	ND	20.16 ± 20.42	ND	ND
DASS-21 (mean and SD for each of the subscales) ***	Depression		14.04 ± 10.44	5.52 ± 4.92	ND	ND	17.4 ± 10.7
	Anxiety		7.71 ± 8.29	3.34 ± 3.87 *	ND	ND	13.8 ± 9.8
	Stress		16.93 ± 10.98	6.81 ± 4.72	ND	ND	21.3 ± 11
DASS-21 (% of the respondents with a particular degree of severity of depression, anxiety, and stress)	Depression	Normal	43.6	ND	69.7	57.5	23.9
		Mild	13.0		13.8	8.5	13.2
		Moderate	19.9		12.2	8.0	27.7
		Severe	10.2		4.3 *	8.0	15.5
		Extremely severe	13.3			18.0	19.7
	Anxiety	Normal	60.2		63.6	53.0	28.5
		Mild	12.5		7.5	5.0	7.9
		Moderate	9.0		20.4	10.5	23.3
		Severe	6.6		8.4 *	4.0	12.8
		Extremely severe	11.7			27.5	27.5
	Stress	Normal	47.2		67.9	68.0	29.9
		Mild	11.8		24.1	4.0	11.5
		Moderate	15.3		5.5	9.0	20.9
		Severe	16.8		2.6 *	6.5	21.2
		Extremely severe	8.9			12.5	16.5

ND—no data. * collectively for severe and extremely severe. ** the results of the analysis of the significance of the differences for DASS total score—Poland vs. China: t = 20,441, $p < 0.0001$, 95% CI: 19.69 to 16.246, Cohen's d = 0.759 (medium). *** the results of the analysis of the significance of the differences for DASS Depression—Poland vs. Spain: t = 42,313, $p < 0.0001$, 95% CI: 8.914–8.125, Cohen's d = 1.044 (large)—Poland vs. Bangladesh: t = −11.351, $p < 0.0001$, 95% CI: 2.779–3.94, Cohen's d = 1.868 (large) Spain vs. Bangladesh: t = −60,438, $p < 0.0001$, 95% CI: 11.494–12.265, Cohen's d = 1501 (large). *** the results of the analysis of the significance of the differences for DASS Anxiety—Poland vs. Spain: t = 27.402, $p < 0.0001$, 95% CI: 4.682–4.057, Cohen's d = 0.675 (medium)—Poland vs. Bangladesh: t = −23.664, $p < 0.0001$, 95% CI: 5.585–6.594, Cohen's d = 1.072 (large)—Spain vs. Bangladesh: t = −59.694, $p < 0.0001$, 95% CI: 10.116–10.803, Cohen's d = 0.694, (medium). *** the results of the analysis of the significance of the differences for DASS Stress—Poland vs. Spain: t = 10.120, $p < 0.0001$, 95% CI: 10.525–9.745, Cohen's d = 1.197 (large)—Poland vs. Bangladesh: t = −14.229, $p < 0.0001$, 95% CI: 3.767–4.972, Cohen's d = 1.906 (large)—Spain vs. Bangladesh: t = −72.654, $p < 0.0001$, 95% CI: 14.099–14.881, Cohen's d = 1.401 (large).

7. The Portrait of a Student who May Potentially Require Special Psychiatric and/or Psychological Support during the Pandemic

Based on the results of our study, the profile of a student who requires potential psychological or/and psychiatric support during the pandemic is a woman (OR = 3.01, 95% CI: 2.15–4.22), studying science (OR = 2.04, 95% CI: 0.99–4.19), living with her roommates (OR = 1.25, 95% CI: 0.89–1.78), suffering from mental disorders that appeared before the outbreak of the pandemic (OR = 5.88, 95% CI: 1.70–20.27), who was using psychiatric support before the outbreak of the pandemic (OR = 8.06, 95% CI: 2.79–23.28), complained of loneliness during the pandemic (OR = 293.31, 95% CI: 15.77–5454.92), and was in a difficult economic situation that forces her to borrow the money from the family or friends during the outbreak of the pandemic to support herself (OR = 13.49, 95% CI: 1.71–106.33).

8. Discussion

The rapid outbreak of the COVID-19 pandemic has forced many countries to introduce specific social distancing and lockdown measures. Such restrictions have a significant impact on the overall well-being and might develop and progress in the form of symptoms related to depression, anxiety, or stress [48]. The SARS-CoV-2 virus, as an unknown agent with undefined mortality and infectivity, undoubtedly had an impact on mental health. The contemporary world is not used to the situation that has arisen. Moreover, frequent media releases about new infection incidents and deaths could heighten the fear of the threat.

The main aim of this cross-sectional study, including a population of more than two thousand Polish students, was to assess depression, stress, and anxiety during the first weeks after the outbreak of the SARS-CoV-2 pandemic and the lockdown in Poland. We also searched for possible risk factors that may intensify students' emotional responses. Results of our study showed that moderate to extremely severe scores of depression, anxiety, and stress were reported by 43.4%, 27.3%, and 41.0% of the respondents, respectively.

After processing the results of our research, we decided to compare the DASS-21 results received in our study with those obtained by researchers in the period before the COVID-19 pandemic. The study was conducted in the winter semester 2018/2019 at the Jagiellonian University among Polish medicine students showed that the level of overall emotional distress was lower than those in our study. Unexpectedly, we noticed a lower severity of anxiety in comparison to the results obtained before the pandemic in the above-mentioned study. However, the authors of the study did not present the percentage distribution of the results achieved, making further comparisons in this matter impossible [49]. In a study by Martinotti et al. using an Italian population, the depression rate was lower (22.9%), whereas anxiety was greater (30.1%) compared to the results of our study. Besides, the authors also showed irritability (31.6%) and post-traumatic stress symptoms (5.4%) as one of the most prevalent during the quarantine period [50]. What is intriguing and might be interesting for further research is that negative emotions (fear, anxiety, and sadness) experienced less intensely but not less frequently could constitute a protective role of trait emotional intelligence during the COVID-19 pandemic, according to the Polish study performed by Moroń and Biolik-Moroń [51].

It seemed interesting to compare the intensity of the emotional distress presented by Polish students with the reaction of students from other countries during the coronavirus pandemic. We have reviewed the available literature and selected four countries from different parts of the world, including Spain, China, India, and Bangladesh, which also performed similar studies primarily on populations of students and used the DASS-21 scale (Figure 1).

Considering the time frames, China was the first to measure the intensity of the emotional response in the student population. The study in China was conducted three days after the WHO announced COVID-19 as a public health emergency [48]. Our study was conducted at the end of the lockdown in Poland, whereas the Chinese study—only after one week of the lockdown. Polish students presented significantly higher emotional distress compared to Chinese students. Compared to the other analyzed countries, China was the one with the lowest percentage of students with moderate to extremely severe depression. This result was consistent with Selye's Theory of Stress—General Adaptation Syndrome, in which anxiety and stress dominate in the initial alarm reaction stage, and depression appears only in the third phase—exhaustion stage [52]. In a meta-analysis conducted by Salari et al., which aimed to investigate the rates of depression, anxiety, and stress during the COVID-19 pandemic by particular continents, it turned out that Asia presented the highest prevalence of anxiety and depression, whereas the most intensified stress levels were observed in a population from Europe [24].

The researchers from India conducted a study on a date after the lockdown that was similar to ours since it was four and six weeks, respectively [53]. Surveys were distributed in both countries during the end of the lockdown period. The results showed that students from both countries differed significantly in terms of comparing the number of students experiencing the severity of emotional disorders from moderate to extremely severe. In the population of Polish students, depression and anxiety were mostly enhanced, while anxiety dominates in the profile of emotional distress in Indian students. Perhaps these differences can be explained by the large disparity in the rates of the number of infected and the number of deaths per million.

Researchers from Bangladesh achieved a surprising result, especially considering that Bangladesh had the lowest mortality and infection rates among all compared countries. Namely, Bangladeshi students reported the highest percentage level in the subscale from moderate to extremely severe stress [54]. Furthermore, students from Bangladesh showed significantly higher levels of depression, stress, and anxiety compared to Poland and Spain. DASS-21 scores were significantly higher among women aged 25 to 29 who live in urban areas, who were dissatisfied with their sleep, spent more hours browsing the Internet, were dissatisfied with academic studies in the current COVID-19 circumstances, and smoked. In each of the compared countries, women completed the survey more often than men. Only in the Bangladeshi population, the majority of respondents were men; nevertheless, female students showed higher levels of emotional distress similarly to all compared countries [53]. These results suggest that women, despite the country of origin, are more vulnerable to experience enhanced depressive, anxiety, and stress symptoms.

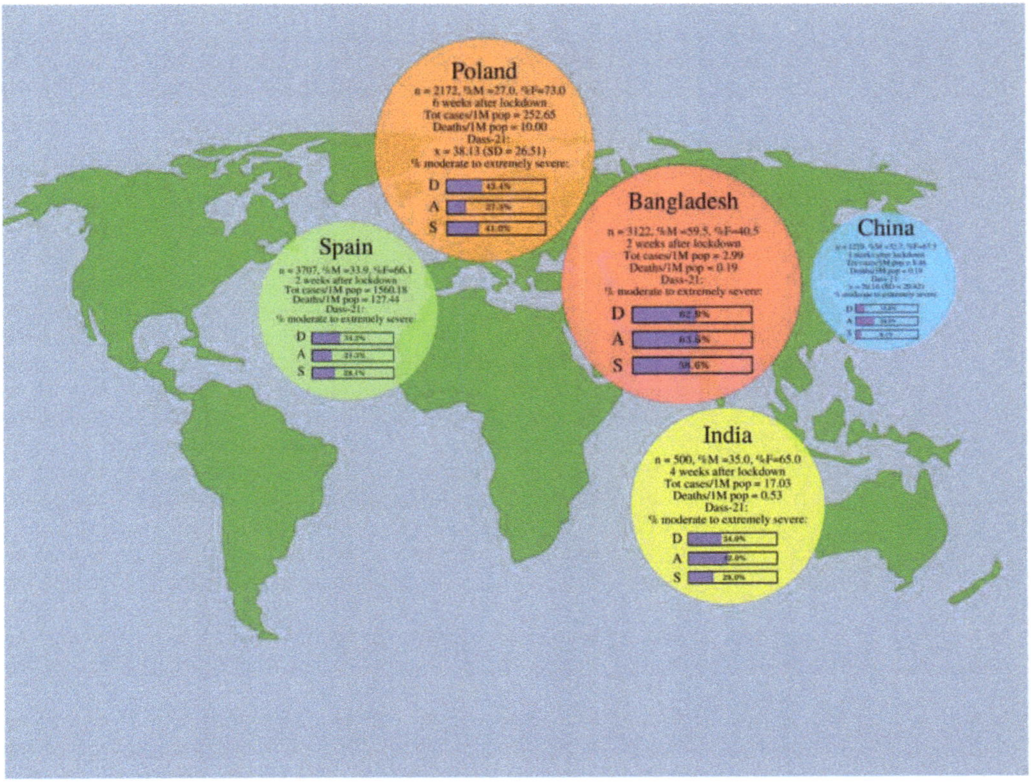

Figure 1. The results of the studies from Poland, Spain, China, India, and Bangladesh performed applying the DASS-21 scale. Legend: n = total number of the respondents, %M = percentage of male respondents, Tot cases/1M pop = total number of cases of COVID-19 per 1 million population on the first day of study, Tot deaths/1M pop = total number of deaths caused by COVID-19 per 1 million population on the first day of study, x = mean score of DASS-21, SD = standard deviation, % moderate to extremely severe = percentage of participants with Dass-21 score form moderate to extremely severe for depression (D), anxiety (A), and stress (S).

From all the above-analyzed countries, an unexpected situation was observed in Spain, where the highest rates of total confirmed cases and deaths of COVID-19 per 1 million population were noted. The percentage of students showing clinically significant levels of depression and stress was similar in the Spanish and Indian studies, although these countries significantly differed in terms of the mortality rates and the number of infections [38,53]. Comparing to Polish students, the respondents from Spain showed significantly lower results in all of the DASS-21 subscales (depression, anxiety, and stress). This observation indicates that there might be many different variables that may affect mental health except for the ones associated with COVID-19.

In our study, females showed statistically higher emotional distress levels compared to males. Generally, depressive [55] and anxiety [56,57] symptoms are more prevalently observed in females; therefore, increased levels of emotional distress in females compared to males seem not to be surprising.

Regarding the field of study, the greatest emotional response was shown by students of arts and humanities in both Poland and Spain; Spanish students who study either arts and humanities or social sciences and law presented the highest depression, anxiety, and stress levels [38]. In our study, we observed that being a science (OR = 2.04) or an art and humanities student (OR = 1.98) was associated with approximately 2-fold higher odds of more intensified total emotional distress. It is also worth emphasizing that the lowest intensity of the emotional response in both studies was observed among medical students, which is a very favorable phenomenon in the context of the nature of their future professional work and the potential risk of exposure to various stressors, including those related to the pandemic.

The results of our study showed that 'living with roommates' (OR = 1.25) constituted one of the risk factors that considerably intensifies the emotional distress among students. Such a high frequency of this chosen answer could be associated with numerous factors such as different emotional reactions of the roommates and their behaviors that could possibly cause negative thoughts and feelings in the respondents. Besides, it is worth noting that the students who were living with roommates could additionally worry about their family members or friends who were not living with them during the pandemic, contributing to the increased emotional distress of this group. Cao et al. pointed out that living with parents could potentially constitute a protective factor against anxiety symptoms [17]. Additionally, not living with a family during a pandemic has been associated with a greater risk of reporting at least one mental health outcome [58]. Isolation from family and friends and living with roommates during the lockdown could increase the emotional distress of participants, which was also confirmed in the studies by Wathelet et al. and Wang et al. [58,59]. Nevertheless, we do not have additional information about who the roommates actually were and whether they were rather a support or an emotional burden for the respondents. However, when we take into consideration the fact that amongst nine of the most stress-related situations, 'fear of infection of the loved ones' was one of the most strongly correlated with the general intensity of anxiety, then the isolation from the family due to lockdown and living with a roommate (other than family or any close relatives) might be an additional factor intensifying emotional distress.

In our study, loneliness turned out to be the greatest difficulty for Polish students during the outbreak of the COVID-19 pandemic (OR = 293.31), which is generally considered as a risk factor implicated in either development or progression of depression [60]. Due to the introduction of epidemiological restrictions, loneliness might significantly contribute to the higher intensity of depressive symptoms. Moreover, there is evidence that the feeling of loneliness because of the COVID-19 pandemic is more experienced in young people [61,62]. Interestingly, Sundarasen et al. showed that loneliness contributed to the increase in the anxiety levels in the group of students from Malaysia [36]. In a meta-analysis, Loades et al. pointed out that there was an association between loneliness and/or social isolation and exacerbation of depressive symptoms, especially in childhood/adolescence; the researchers observed that intensified depressive symptoms are more pronounced in females rather than males [63].

In the studied group, the co-occurrence of any mental disorder was associated with higher levels of emotional distress, depression, anxiety, as well as stress. However, we cannot completely assume whether such high levels of the above-mentioned variables were due to the pandemic itself or whether they were increased at baseline (before the outbreak of the pandemic); it was shown that generally, high levels of stress were related to numerous mental disorders, at the same time increasing the intensity of depressive and anxiety symptoms [64,65]. Those who used psychological and/or psychiatric support before the outbreak of the pandemic also showed significantly higher levels of emotional distress along with all of the DASS-21 subscales. Our results are consistent with those obtained by Vindegaard et al., who indicated that people who had preexisting psychiatric disorders are reported to experience worsening psychiatric symptoms during the COVID-19 pandemic [66]. Like the above-mentioned information, it is speculative whether it was associated with the pandemic or due to potentially increased depression and/or anxiety and/or stress symptoms at baseline of the possible psychological or psychiatric condition. Moreover, the observed relationship should be interpreted with caution; anxiety and depressive symptoms could be potentially intensified by the fear of illness and increased loneliness during the pandemic, respectively. It is extremely important for health workers to be aware of such associations, especially during the pandemic.

Regarding the economic situation, the respondents with stable family income presented the lowest emotional distress levels, contrary to those who had to start borrowing money during the pandemic. Low income is generally associated with greater psychological distress; therefore, the results of our study seem consistent [67]. Although the majority of the respondents were not working (neither physically nor mentally), the remaining (those who were working during the pandemic) mostly presented with increased depression levels. Working mentally or physically during the pandemic was related to a 0.5 and 0.4-fold lower odds of increased overall emotional distress, respectively. Therefore, it might be assumed that having a job by the students could be a potentially protective factor against increased overall emotional distress.

Already during the pandemic, Larionov and Mudło-Głagolska (2020) conducted a study on the Polish population and showed that females, families with a household of at least two persons, persons with children, unemployed individuals, and those with chronic diseases were at risk of a stronger emotional response during a pandemic [68]. The researchers presented percentage results that were quite close to those obtained in our study, although the average age of their respondents was 35.15 years (SD = 12.53). The DASS total score for this group was equal to 35.89 ± 33.74. In the depression subscale, the percentage of respondents ranging from moderate to extreme severe was 37.25%, whereas, in our study, it was 43.40%. On the anxiety subscale, 39.08% of respondents presented with moderate to extremely severe anxiety, and in our study, it was 27.3% of students. In the above-mentioned study, 34.12% of respondents ranged from moderate to extremely severe on the stress subscale, compared to 41% of the students in our study. The conclusion is that in the group with higher age, the intensity of anxiety was more intense than in the group of students.

Islam et al. (2020) showed that the male gender, living in the countryside, having satisfactory sleep (7–8 h per day), low Internet use (less than 2 h a day), and physical exercise might constitute potential protective factors against emotional distress. The authors also showed that tobacco smoking might be associated with higher levels of depression, anxiety, and/or stress and thus might constitute one of the potential risk factors. Besides, living in a nuclear family was assumed to be a potential risk factor for depression and stress [54]. It should be taken into consideration that the results of all of these studies differ due to several reasons. Firstly, it was because all of the surveys were launched on different dates and the time that had passed from the start of the lockdown in a particular country also differed, and the release of the survey was not standardized. Thus, the impact of SARS-CoV-2 spread on the mental health of the respondents might differ. What is more, the results might differ because of the restrictions introduced by a particular country that might be more or less strict and severe depending on both—the decisions of the government as well as the time when the survey was performed since the expansion of particular restrictions also differ in time. What could also affect the respondents' reactions and depression, anxiety, and stress levels could be the form of providing information for the societies that might differ between the local social media.

9. Limitations of the Study

One of the major limitations of this study is that the respondents involved in this study (n = 2172) were only Polish students; therefore, these results cannot be generalized to other nationalities, racial, or ethnic groups. Among them, the majority of the respondents were females (n = 1585) and medical students (n = 1314). Therefore, it is hard to establish the obtained results as generalizable because the group of students involved in this study was slightly limited.

The reliability of the results was also limited by the fact that the study was conducted in the form of an online survey where the researchers could not assess the reliability of the information provided by the respondents. Moreover, the other limitation is that the students who fulfilled our survey were only those who were interested in the potential consequences of the COVID-19 pandemic on mental health, had access to the Internet, and were simply interested in taking part in such an online questionnaire.

Besides, it should be taken into consideration that the comparison of our results with other countries (Spain, India, China, and Bangladesh) based on the DASS-21 scale should be analyzed with caution since there might be many potential reasons for any differences between those countries including cultural bias of reporting on mental health.

Another limitation is the fact that the results of the obtained study reflect the well-being of students only during the few days when the survey was conducted without any insight into longitudinal effects on students' mental health. On the other hand, the mental health status and psychological symptoms of the respondents before the COVID-19 pandemic were unknown to the researchers, which was associated with the potential difficulties in the interpretation of the obtained results as well.

Taking all the above facts into consideration, it must be stated that the obtained results cannot be assigned to the entire population of Polish students due to the profile of the student who most often completed the survey, the form of the survey which was carried out as an online questionnaire, and the time in which it was conducted that only reflect the well-being of Polish students in the short and particular period of the pandemic. It would be beneficial to perform further studies, especially longitudinal ones, which could provide a clearer understanding of the pandemic effect on students' depression, anxiety, and stress levels.

10. Conclusions

Our study was conducted six weeks after the lockdown in Poland when the restrictions were highly pronounced, the prevalence and the mortality rates were relatively low, and the knowledge about COVID-19 was still insufficient. The results of this study show that the severity of symptoms that range from moderate to extremely severe concerned the following groups of students—43.4% in the depression subscale, 27.3% in the anxiety subscale, and 41.0% in the stress subscale, indicating a high percentage of the students experienced significant clinical, emotional distress.

We tried to create a portrait of a Polish student who may potentially require specific psychological and/or psychiatric support during a pandemic. The results obtained in our study show that being a female science student, living with roommates, suffering from mental disorders, and using the support of a psychiatrist and/or psychologist before the pandemic predisposes a student to increased emotional response. Besides, additional aspects associated with the increased risk of enhanced emotional responses were a feeling of loneliness during the pandemic and a deterioration of the financial situation during the pandemic that required the need to borrow money to support oneself.

While comparing our results with other similar studies conducted during the lockdown with the usage of the same instrument—the DASS-21—it turned out that Polish students presented with higher depression, anxiety, and stress levels compared to Chinese and Spanish students, whereas they presented with lower levels compared to Bangladeshi students, indicating that socio-political factors might also potentially increase the emotional distress, and should be considered. Therefore, it must be taken into consideration that a particular nationality or culture might present different intensities of depression, anxiety, stress, or other emotional symptoms in response to the same agent. The understanding of this point is crucial to provide the right approach as well as proper potential psychological and/or psychiatric help for all of the students of different nationalities.

The social, economic, and health situations that are continually changing due to the ongoing COVID-19 pandemic in Poland and the world that require specific adaptive resources and social support might be a huge stressor to maintain the proper mental well-being of many students. Therefore, it is crucial to monitor the mental health status of students as well as to identify potential risk factors that might contribute to the induction of mental disorders to further provide the proper psychological and psychiatric help for those students who require it the most.

Supplementary Materials: The following are available online at https://www.mdpi.com/2077-0383/10/5/944/s1, Table S1: The results of the DASS total score for the field of study, Table S1.2: The results of the DASS depression scale for the field of study, Table S1.3: The results of the DASS anxiety scale for the field of study, Table S1.4: The results of the DASS stress scale for the field of study, Table S2: The results of the DASS total score for the most prevalent difficulties during pandemics, Table S2.2: The results of the DASS depression scale for the most prevalent difficulties during pandemics, Table S2.3: The results of the DASS anxiety scale for the most prevalent difficulties during pandemics, Table S2.4: The results of the DASS stress scale for the most prevalent difficulties during pandemics, Table S3: The results of the DASS total score for the most prevalent chronic diseases, Table S3.2: The results of the DASS depression scale for the most prevalent chronic diseases, Table S3.3: The results of the DASS anxiety scale for the most prevalent chronic diseases, Table S3.4: The results of the DASS stress scale for the most prevalent chronic diseases, Table S4: The results of the DASS total score for the usage of either psychological or psychiatric help before the pandemics outbreak, Table S4.2: The results of the DASS depression scale for the usage of either psychological or psychiatric help before the pandemics outbreak, Table S4.3: The results of the DASS anxiety scale for the usage of either psychological or psychiatric help before the pandemics outbreak, Table S4.4: The results of the DASS stress scale for the usage of either psychological or psychiatric help before the pandemics outbreak, Table S5: The results of the DASS total score for the economic situation during pandemics, Table S5.2: The results of the DASS depression scale for the economic situation during pandemics, Table S5.3: The results of the DASS anxiety scale for the economic situation during pandemics, Table S5.4: The results of the DASS stress scale for the economic situation during pandemics, Table S6: The results of the DASS total score for the current employment situation, Table S6.2: The results of the DASS depression scale for the current employment situation, Table S6.3: The results of the DASS anxiety scale for the current employment situation, Table S6.4: The results of the DASS stress scale for the current employment situation, Table S7: The results of the DASS total score for the current living situation, Table S7.2: The results of the DASS depression scale for the current living situation, Table S7.3: The results of the DASS anxiety scale for the current living situation, Table S7.4: The results of the DASS stress scale for the current living situation, Table S8: The sociodemographic data of the respondents.

Author Contributions: Conceptualization, H.K.-J., J.B. (Jacek Baj), and D.J.; methodology, E.S., K.K., J.B. (Jacek Bogucki), and A.F.; formal analysis, H.K.-J., D.J., and J.B. (Jacek Baj); investigation, E.S., K.K., and A.F.; resources, E.S., K.K., and A.F.; writing—original draft preparation, H.K.-J., E.S., K.K., and A.F.; writing—review and editing, H.K.-J., D.J., and J.B. (Jacek Baj); visualization, H.K.-J. and K.K.; supervision, H.K.-J. and D.J. All authors have read and agreed to the published version of the manuscript.

Funding: This research received no external funding.

Institutional Review Board Statement: The study was conducted according to the guidelines of the Declaration of Helsinki, and approved by the Ethics Committee of Medical University of Lublin (protocol code—KE-0254/91/2020; date of approval—30 April 2020).

Informed Consent Statement: Informed consent was obtained from all subjects involved in the study.

Conflicts of Interest: The authors declare no conflict of interest.

Abbreviations

COVID-19	Coronavirus disease 2019
DASS-21	Depression, Anxiety, and Stress Scale-21 Items
M	Mean
Me	Median
MERS-CoV	Middle East Respiratory Syndrome Coronavirus
OR	Odds ratio
SARS-CoV	Severe Acute Respiratory Syndrome Coronavirus
SARS-CoV-2	Severe Acute Respiratory Syndrome Coronavirus-2
WHO	World Health Organization

References

1. Lu, H.; Stratton, C.W.; Tang, Y.W. Outbreak of pneumonia of unknown etiology in Wuhan, China: The mystery and the miracle. *J. Med. Virol.* **2020**, *92*, 401–402. [CrossRef] [PubMed]
2. Huang, C.; Wang, Y.; Li, X.; Ren, L.; Zhao, J.; Hu, Y.; Zhang, L.; Fan, G.; Xu, J.; Gu, X.; et al. Clinical features of patients infected with 2019 novel coronavirus in Wuhan, China. *Lancet* **2020**, *395*, 497–506. [CrossRef]
3. World Health Organization. Rolling Updates On Coronavirus Disease (COVID-19) [Internet]. Available online: https://www.who.int/emergencies/diseases/novel-coronavirus-2019/events-as-they-happen (accessed on 27 April 2020).
4. World Health Organization. WHO Director-General's Opening Remarks at the Media Briefing on COVID-19–11 March 2020 [Internet]. Available online: https://www.who.int/dg/speeches/detail/who-director-general-s-opening-remarks-at-the-media-briefing-on-covid-19---11-march-2020 (accessed on 27 March 2020).
5. Di Gennaro, F.; Pizzol, D.; Marotta, C.; Antunes, M.; Racalbuto, V.; Veronese, N.; Smith, L. Coronavirus Diseases (COVID-19) Current Status and Future Perspectives: A Narrative Review. *Int. J. Environ. Res. Public Health.* **2020**, *17*, 2690. [CrossRef] [PubMed]
6. Nadeem, M.S.; Zamzami, M.A.; Choudhry, H.; Murtaza, B.N.; Kazmi, I.; Ahmad, H.; Shakoori, A.-R. Origin, Potential Therapeutic Targets and Treatment for Coronavirus Disease (COVID-19). *Pathogens* **2020**, *9*, 307. [CrossRef] [PubMed]
7. Mungroo, M.R.; Khan, N.A.; Siddiqui, R. Novel Coronavirus: Current Understanding of Clinical Features, Diagnosis, Pathogenesis, and Treatment Options. *Pathogens* **2020**, *9*, 297. [CrossRef]
8. Baj, J.; Karakuła-Juchnowicz, H.; Teresiński, G.; Buszewicz, G.; Ciesielka, M.; Sitarz, E.; Forma, A.; Karakuła, K.; Flieger, W.; Portincasa, P.; et al. COVID-19: Specific and Non-Specific Clinical Manifestations and Symptoms: The Current State of Knowledge. *J. Clin. Med.* **2020**, *9*, 1753. [CrossRef]
9. Grant, B.W.; Lahore, H.; McDonnell, L.S.; Baggerly, A.C.; French, B.C.; Aliano, L.J.; Bhattoa, H.P. Evidence that Vitamin D Supplementation Could Reduce Risk of Influenza and COVID-19 Infections and Deaths. *Nutrients* **2020**, *12*, 988. [CrossRef]
10. World Health Organization. Coronavirus Disease (COVID-19) Pandemic [Internet]. Available online: https://www.who.int/emergencies/diseases/novel-coronavirus-2019 (accessed on 27 April 2020).
11. British Broadcasting Company. Coronavirus: The World in Lockdown in Maps and Charts [Internet]. Available online: https://www.bbc.com/news/world-52103747 (accessed on 28 April 2020).
12. Government of Poland. Mapa Zarażeń Koronawirusem (SARS-CoV-2). [Map of coronavirus infection (SARS-CoV-2).] [Internet]. Available online: https://www.gov.pl/web/koronawirus/wykaz-zarazen-koronawirusem-sars-cov-2 (accessed on 26 April 2020).
13. Government of Poland. Wprowadzamy Stan Epidemii w Polsce [Introducing the Epidemic State in Poland] [Internet]. Available online: https://www.gov.pl/web/koronawirus/wprowadzamy-stan-epidemii-w-polsce (accessed on 28 April 2020).
14. Government of Poland. Kolejne Kroki W Walce Z Koronawirusem–W Sklepie Mniej Osób, Ograniczenia W Poruszaniu Nieletnich, a Parki, Plaże I Bulwary Zamknięte. [Next Steps in the Fight Against Coronavirus-fewer People in the Store, Restrictions on the Movement of Minors, and Parks, Beaches and Boulevards closed.] [Internet]. Available online: https://www.gov.pl/web/koronawirus/kolejne-kroki (accessed on 28 April 2020).
15. Wang, C.; Pan, R.; Wan, X.; Tan, Y.; Xu, L.; Ho, S.C.; Ho, R.C. Immediate Psychological Responses and Associated Factors during the Initial Stage of the 2019 Coronavirus Disease (COVID-19) Epidemic among the General Population in China. *Int. J. Environ. Res. Public Health* **2020**, *17*, 1729. [CrossRef] [PubMed]
16. Lee, M.; You, M. Psychological and Behavioral Responses in South Korea During the Early Stages of Coronavirus Disease 2019 (COVID-19). *Int. J. Environ. Res. Public Health* **2020**, *17*, 2977. [CrossRef]
17. Cao, W.; Fang, Z.; Guoqiang, H.; Han, M.; Xu, X.; Dong, J.; Zheng, J. The psychological impact of the COVID-19 epidemic on college students in China. *Psychiatry Res.* **2020**, *287*, 112934. [CrossRef] [PubMed]
18. He, J.; He, L.; Zhou, W.; Nie, X.; He, M. Discrimination and Social Exclusion in the Outbreak of COVID-19. *Int. J. Environ. Res. Public Health* **2020**, *17*, 2933. [CrossRef] [PubMed]
19. Sim, K.; Chan, Y.; Phui-Nah, C.; Chua, H.; Soon, S. Psychosocial and coping responses within the community health care setting towards a national outbreak of an infectious disease. *J. Psychosom. Res.* **2010**, *68*, 195–202. [CrossRef]

20. Saeed, S.A.; Hebishi, K. The psychiatric consequences of COVID-19: 8 Studies. *Curr. Psychiatry* **2020**, *19*, 22–24, 28–30, 32–35. [CrossRef]
21. Pérez-Fuentes, D.M.; Molero Jurado, D.M.; Oropesa Ruiz, F.N.; Martos Martínez, Á.; Simón Márquez, D.M.; Herrera-Peco, I.; Linares, J.J.G. Questionnaire on Perception of Threat from COVID-19. *J. Clin. Med.* **2020**, *9*, 1146. [CrossRef] [PubMed]
22. Nguyen, C.H.; Nguyen, H.M.; Do, N.B.; Tran, Q.C.; Nguyen, T.P.T.; Pham, M.K.; Pham, L.V.; Tran, K.V.; Duong, T.T.; Tran, T.V.; et al. People with Suspected COVID-19 Symptoms Were More Likely Depressed and Had Lower Health-Related Quality of Life: The Potential Benefit of Health Literacy. *J. Clin. Med.* **2020**, *9*, 965. [CrossRef] [PubMed]
23. Huang, Y.; Zhao, N. Generalized anxiety disorder, depressive symptoms and sleep quality during COVID-19 epidemic in China: A web-based cross-sectional survey. *Psychiatry Res.* **2020**, *288*, 112954. [CrossRef]
24. Salari, N.; Hosseinian-Far, A.; Jalali, R.; Vaisi-Raygani, A.; Rasoulpoor, S.; Mohammadi, M.; Rasoulpoor, S.; Khaledi-Paveh, B. Prevalence of stress, anxiety, depres- sion among the general population dur- ing the COVID-19 pandemic: A systematic review and meta-analysis. *Glob. Health.* **2020**, *16*, 57. [CrossRef]
25. Xiong, J.; Lipsitz, O.; Nasri, F.; Lui, L.M.W.; Gill, H.; Phan, L.; Chen-Li, D.; Iacobucci, M.; Ho, R.; Majeed, A.; et al. Impact of COVID-19 pandemic on mental health in the general population: A systematic review. *J. Affect. Disord.* **2020**, *277*, 55–64. [CrossRef]
26. Lakhan, R.; Agrawal, A.; Sharma, M. Prevalence of Depression, Anxiety, and Stress during COVID-19 Pandemic. *J. Neurosci. Rural. Pr.* **2020**, *11*, 519–525. [CrossRef]
27. Pieh, C.; Budimir, S.; Probst, T. The effect of age, gender, income, work, and physical activity on mental health during coronavirus disease (COVID-19) lockdown in Austria. *J. Psychosom. Res.* **2020**, *136*, 110186. [CrossRef]
28. García-Fernández, L.; Romero-Ferreiro, V.; López-Roldán, P.D.; Padilla, S.; Rodriguez-Jimenez, R. Mental Health in Elderly Spanish People in Times of COVID-19 Outbreak. *Am. J. Geriatr. Psychiatry* **2020**, *28*, 1040–1045. [CrossRef]
29. Mamun, M.A.; Akter, S.; Hossain, I.; Faisal, M.T.H.; Rahman, A.; Arefin, A.; Khan, I.; Hossain, L.; Haque, A.; Hossain, S.; et al. Financial threat, hardship and distress predict depression, anxiety and stress among the unemployed youths: A Bangladeshi multi-city study. *J. Affect. Disord.* **2020**, *276*, 1149–1158. [CrossRef]
30. Achdut, N.; Refaeli, T. Unemployment and Psychological Distress among Young People during the COVID-19 Pandemic: Psychological Resources and Risk Factors. *Int. J. Environ. Res. Public Health* **2020**, *17*, 7163. [CrossRef]
31. Wang, C.; Chudzicka-Czupała, A.; Grabowski, D.; Pan, R.; Adamus, K.; Wan, X.; Hetnał, M.; Tan, Y.; Olszewska-Guizzo, A.; Xu, L.; et al. The Association Between Physical and Mental Health and Face Mask Use During the COVID-19 Pandemic: A Comparison of Two Countries With Different Views and Practices. *Front. Psychiatry* **2020**, *11*, 569981. [CrossRef]
32. Kazmi, S.S.H.; Hasan, K.; Talib, S.; Saxena, S. COVID-19 and Lockdwon: A Study on the Impact on Mental Health. 2020. Available online: https://ssrn.com/abstract=3577515 (accessed on 8 November 2020).
33. Wu, M.; Xu, W.; Yao, Y.; Zhang, L.; Guo, L.; Fan, J.; Chen, J. Mental health status of students' parents during COVID-19 pandemic and its influence factors. *Gen Psychiatr.* **2020**, *33*, e100250. [CrossRef]
34. Epifanio, M.S.; Andrei, F.; Mancini, G.; Agostini, F.; Piombo, M.A.; Spicuzza, V.; Riolo, M.; Lavanco, G.; Trombini, E.; La Grutta, S. The Impact of COVID-19 Pandemic and Lockdown Measures on Quality of Life among Italian General Population. *J. Clin. Med.* **2021**, *10*, 289. [CrossRef] [PubMed]
35. Hoyt, L.T.; Cohen, A.K.; Dull, B.; Castro, E.M.; Yazdani, N. "Constant Stress Has Become the New Normal": Stress and Anxiety Inequalities Among, U.S. College Students in the Time of COVID-19. *J. Adolesc. Health* **2020**. [CrossRef]
36. Sundarasen, S.; Chinna, K.; Kamaludin, K.; Nurunnabi, M.; Baloch, G.M.; Khoshaim, H.B.; Hossain, S.F.A.; Sukayt, A. Psychological Impact of COVID-19 and Lockdown among University Students in Malaysia: Implications and Policy Recommendations. *Int. J. Environ. Res. Public Health.* **2020**, *17*, 6206. [CrossRef] [PubMed]
37. Li, Y.; Wang, Y.; Jiang, J.; Valdimarsdóttir, U.A.; Fall, K.; Fang, F.; Song, H.; Lu, D.; Zhang, W. Psychological distress among health professional students during the COVID-19 outbreak. *Psychol. Med.* **2020**, *11*, 1–3. [CrossRef] [PubMed]
38. Dratva, J.; Zysset, A.; Schlatter, N.; von Wyl, A.; Huber, M.; Volken, T. Swiss University Students' Risk Perception and General Anxiety during the COVID-19 Pandemic. *Int. J. Environ. Res. Public Health.* **2020**, *17*, 7433. [CrossRef] [PubMed]
39. Odriozola-González, P.; Planchuelo-Gómez, Á.; Irurtia, M.J.; de Luis-García, R. Psychological effects of the COVID-19 outbreak and lockdown among students and workers of a Spanish university. *Psychiatry Res.* **2020**, *290*, 113108. [CrossRef]
40. Polish Translation of DASS. Available online: http://www2.psy.unsw.edu.au/Groups/Dass/Polish/Polish.htm (accessed on 8 November 2020).
41. DASS Translations. Available online: http://www2.psy.unsw.edu.au/groups/dass/translations.htm (accessed on 8 November 2020).
42. Lovibond, S.H.; Lovibond, P.F. *Manual for the Depression Anxiety Stress Scales*; Sydney Psychology Foundation Australia: Sydney, Australia, 1995.
43. Antony, M.M.; Bieling, P.J.; Cox, B.J.; Enns, M.W.; Swinson, R.P. Psychometric properties of the 42-item and 21-item versions of the depression anxiety stress scales in clinical groups and a community sample. *Psychol. Assess.* **1998**, *10*, 176–181. [CrossRef]
44. Depression Anxiety Stress Scales–Short Form (DASS-21) [Internet]. NovoPsych Psychometrics. Available online: https://novopsych.com.au/assessments/depression-anxiety-stress-scales-short-form-dass-21/ (accessed on 19 June 2020).
45. Ruiz, F.; Garcia-Martin, M.; Suárez, F.; Juan, C.; Odriozola-González, P. The hierarchical factor structure of the Spanish version of the Depression Anxiety and Stress Scale-21 (DASS-21). *Int. J. Psychol. Psychol. Ther.* **2017**, *17*, 93–101.

46. Henry, J.D.; Crawford, J.R. The short-form version of the Depression Anxiety Stress Scales (DASS-21): Construct validity and normative data in a large non-clinical sample. *Br. J. Clin. Psychol.* **2005**, *44*, 227–239. [CrossRef]
47. Steel, Z.; Marnane, C.; Iranpour, C.; Chey, T.; Jackson, J.W.; Patel, V.; Silove, D. The global prevalence of common mental disorders: A systematic review and meta-analysis 1980–2013. *Int. J. Epidemiol.* **2014**, *43*, 476–493. [CrossRef] [PubMed]
48. Shah, S.M.A.; Mohammad, D.; Quereshi, M.F.H.; Abbas, M.Z.; Aleem, S. Prevalence, Psychological Responses and Associated Correlates of Depression, Anxiety and Stress in a Global Population, During the Coronavirus Disease (COVID-19) Pandemic. *Community Ment. Health J.* **2021**, *57*, 101–110. [CrossRef] [PubMed]
49. Zawislak, D.; Zur-Wyrozumska, K.; Habera, M.; Skrzypiec, K.; Pac, A.; Cebula, G. Evaluation of a Polish Version of the Depression Anxiety Stress Scales (DASS-21). *J. Neurosci. Cogn. Stud.* **2020**, *4*, 101.
50. Martinotti, G.; Alessi, M.C.; Di Natale, C.; Sociali, A.; Ceci, F.; Lucidi, L.; Picutti, E.; Di Carlo, F.; Corbo, M.; Vellante, F.; et al. Psychopathological Burden and Quality of Life in Substance Users During the COVID-19 Lockdown Period in Italy. *Front. Psychiatry* **2020**, *11*, 572245. [CrossRef] [PubMed]
51. Moroń, M.; Biolik-Moroń, M. Trait emotional intelligence and emotional experiences during the COVID-19 pandemic outbreak in Poland: A daily diary study. *Personal. Individ. Differ.* **2021**, *168*, 110348. [CrossRef]
52. Selye, I. The general adaptation syndrome and the diseases of adaptation. *J. Allergy.* **1946**, *17*, 289–323. [CrossRef]
53. Suryadevara, V.; Adusumalli, C.; Adusumilli, P.K.; Chalasani, S.H.; Radhakrishnan, R. Mental Health Status among the South Indian Pharmacy Students during Covid-19 Pandemic Quarantine Period: A Cross-Sectional Study. 2020. Available online: https://www.x-mol.com/paper/1260295362728624128 (accessed on 8 November 2020).
54. Islam, M.; Sujan, S.H.; Tasnim, R.; Sikder, T.; Potenza, M.N.; Os, J.V. Psychological Responses during the COVID-19 Outbreak among University Students in Bangladesh. 2020. Available online: https://psyarxiv.com/cndz7/ (accessed on 8 November 2020).
55. Lim, G.Y.; Tam, W.W.; Lu, Y.; Ho, C.S.; Zhang, M.W.; Ho, R.C. Prevalence of Depression in the Community from 30 Countries between 1994 and 2014. *Sci. Rep.* **2018**, *8*, 2861.
56. McLean, C.P.; Asnaani, A.; Litz, B.T.; Hofmann, S.G. Gender differences in anxiety disorders: Prevalence, course of illness, comorbidity and burden of illness. *J. Psychiatr. Res.* **2011**, *45*, 1027–1035.
57. Bahrami, F.; Yousefi, N. Females are more anxious than males: A metacognitive perspective. *Iran. J. Psychiatry Behav. Sci.* **2011**, *5*, 83–90. [PubMed]
58. Wathelet, M.; Duhem, S.; Vaiva, G.; Baubet, T.; Habran, E.; Veerapa, E.; Debien, C.; Molenda, S.; Horn, M.; Grandgenèvre, P.; et al. Factors Associated With Mental Health Disorders Among University Students in France Confined During the COVID-19 Pandemic. *JAMA Netw. Open* **2020**, *3*, e2025591.
59. Wang, X.; Hegde, S.; Son, C.; Keller, B.; Smith, A.; Sasangohar, F. Investigating Mental Health of US College Students During the COVID-19 Pandemic: Cross-Sectional Survey Study. *J. Med. Internet. Res.* **2020**, *22*, e22817. [CrossRef]
60. Hawkley, L.C.; Cacioppo, J.T. Loneliness matters: A theoretical and empirical review of consequences and mechanisms. *Ann. Behav. Med.* **2010**, *40*, 218–227. [PubMed]
61. Losda-Baltar, A.; Jiménez-Gonzalo, L.; Gallego-Alberto, L.; Pedroso-Chaparro, M.D.S.; Fernandes-Pires, J.; Márquez-González, M. "We're Staying at Home". Association of Self-Perceptions of Aging, Personal and Family Resources and Loneliness With Psychological Distress During the Lock-Down Period of COVID-19. *J. Gerontol. B Psychol. Sci. Soc. Sci.* **2021**, *76*, e10–e16.
62. Groarke, J.M.; Berry, E.; Graham-Wisener, L.; Mckenna-Plumley, P.E.; Mcglinchey, E.; Armour, C. Loneliness in the UK during the COVID-19 pandemic: Cross-sectional results from the COVID-19 Psychological Wellbeing Study. *PLoS ONE* **2020**, *15*, e0239698. [CrossRef]
63. Loades, M.E.; Chatburn, E.; Higson-Sweeney, N.; Reynolds, S.; Shafran, R.; Brigden, A.; Linney, C.; McManus, M.N.; Borwick, C.; Crawley, E. Rapid Systematic Review: The Impact of Social Isolation and Loneliness on the Mental Health of Children and Adolescents in the Context of COVID-19. *J. Am. Acad. Child Adolesc. Psychiatry* **2020**, *59*, 1218–1239.e3. [CrossRef]
64. Herbert, J. Stress, the brain, and mental illness. *BMJ* **1997**, *315*, 530–535. [CrossRef]
65. Cattaneo, A.; Riva, M.A. Stress-induced mechanisms in mental illness: A role for glucocorticoid signalling. *J. Steroid. Biochem. Mol. Biol.* **2016**, *160*, 169–174. [CrossRef] [PubMed]
66. Vindegaard, N.; Benros, M.E. COVID-19 pan-demic and mental health consequences: Sys-tematic review of the current evidence. *Brain. Behav. Immun.* **2020**, *89*, 531–542. [CrossRef] [PubMed]
67. Orpana, H.M.; Lemyre, L.; Gravel, R. Income and psychological distress: The role of the social environment. *Health Rep.* **2009**, *20*, 21–28. [PubMed]
68. Larionov, P.; Mudło-Głagolska, K. Mental Health Risk Factors during COVID-19 Pandemic in the Polish Population. 2020. Available online: https://psyarxiv.com/3ku8w/ (accessed on 8 November 2020).

Journal of
Clinical Medicine

MDPI

Article

The Impact of the COVID-19 Pandemic on Psychological Health and Insomnia among People with Chronic Diseases

Paweł Wańkowicz *, Aleksandra Szylińska and Iwona Rotter

Department of Medical Rehabilitation and Clinical Physiotherapy, Pomeranian Medical University in Szczecin, Żołnierska 48, 71-210 Szczecin, Poland; aleksandra.szylinska@gmail.com (A.S.); iwrot@wp.pl (I.R.)
* Correspondence: pawel.wankowicz@pum.edu.pl; Tel.: +48-91-48-00-914

Abstract: The outbreak of the severe acute respiratory syndrome coronavirus 2 (SARS-CoV-2) pandemic highlighted the serious problems of health care systems but also threatened the mental and physical health of patients worldwide. The goal of this study was to assess psychological health and insomnia in people with chronic diseases in the time of elevated stress associated with the pandemic. The study involved 879 people from Zachodniopomorskie province in Poland. Each participant provided basic demographic data, data on symptoms of insomnia, depression, anxiety and information on concomitant diseases such as hypertension, diabetes mellitus, coronary heart disease, heart failure, dyslipidemia, chronic obstructive pulmonary disease, Hashimoto's disease and smoking cigarettes. Chronic diseases included in this study showed a strong correlation between Hashimoto's disease and increase scores according to the Insomnia Severity Index (ISI, $r = 0.797$, $p < 0.001$), the Generalized Anxiety Disorder scale (GAD-7, $r = 0.766$, $p < 0.001$) and the Patient Health Questionnaire (PHQ-9, $r = 0.767$, $p < 0.001$). After the results were corrected for age, gender, diagnosed hypertension, dyslipidemia and cigarette smoking, it was confirmed that the diagnosis of Hashimoto's disease was associated with an increased risk of anxiety (odds ratio (OR) = 2.225; $p < 0.001$), depression (OR = 2.518; $p < 0.001$) and insomnia (OR = 3.530; $p < 0.001$). Our study showed that during the SARS-CoV-2 pandemic patients with Hashimoto's disease show a higher risk of insomnia, anxiety and depression.

Keywords: COVID-19; chronic diseases; Hashimoto's disease; GAD-7; PHQ-9; ISI

Citation: Wańkowicz, P.; Szylińska, A.; Rotter, I. The Impact of the COVID-19 Pandemic on Psychological Health and Insomnia among People with Chronic Diseases. *J. Clin. Med.* **2021**, *10*, 1206. https://doi.org/10.3390/jcm10061206

Academic Editor: Michele Roccella

Received: 26 January 2021
Accepted: 12 March 2021
Published: 14 March 2021

1. Introduction

In 2020, Poland was forced by the severe acute respiratory syndrome coronavirus 2 (SARS-CoV-2) pandemic to introduce its first-ever national lockdown. The disease, commonly referred to as Coronavirus Disease 2019 (COVID-19), was first observed at the end of 2019, while the first case of infection in Poland was recorded on 4 March 2020. A much more infectious SARS, and with a higher mortality rate than influenza, COVID-19 has resulted in more than 84 million confirmed cases and 1.8 million deaths worldwide [1]. In Poland, novel coronavirus has killed almost 28,000 people and more than 1.3 million have been infected.

During previous coronaviral epidemics, such as SARS and Middle East respiratory syndrome (MERS), symptoms were more severe in people with chronic diseases and were often associated with a poor prognosis [2]. The Centers for Disease Control and Prevention (CDC) continually updates the list of conditions that increase the risk of undergoing a severe course of COVID-19. This list is not definitive and currently only includes conditions for which there is adequate clinical evidence. It allows clinicians to identify the most at-risk groups of patients for individualized prevention, treatment or care strategies. Chronic diseases listed by the CDC as those that can lead to a severe course of COVID-19 include cancer, chronic kidney disease, chronic obstructive pulmonary disease, Down's syndrome, heart disease such as heart failure, coronary artery disease or cardiomyopathy, obesity, sickle cell anemia, smoking, diabetes, immune-weakening conditions due to blood or bone marrow transplantation, immune deficiencies such as in human immunodeficiency virus (HIV) and the use of corticosteroids or other immune-weakening drugs e.g., those for autoimmune diseases [3]. Autoimmune diseases, apart from cardiovascular diseases and cancer, are an increasing problem for the Western world. However, their exact causes are largely unknown and, moreover, are difficult to identify at the preclinical stage. It is likely that for this reason, they are not the most attractive topic for research in many countries, including Poland. Associated with abnormal functioning of the immune system, autoimmune diseases involve an undirected response against the body's own organs, tissues and cells [4]. Currently, more than 20 million people suffer from autoimmune diseases in the United States alone, while epidemiological data provide evidence of a steady increase in their incidence in Western societies over the past few decades. Incidence rates of autoimmune diseases vary from less than 5 per 100,000 for uveitis to over 350 per 100,000 for Hashimoto's disease [5]. Hashimoto's disease is one of the most common autoimmune diseases in the population. It is difficult to diagnose and diagnosis often occurs in the later stages of the disease. The most common biochemical abnormalities in Hashimoto's disease are elevated levels of thyrotropic hormone and low levels of free thyroxine combined with increased levels of antithyroid peroxidase antibodies. However, in the early stages of the disease, patients may be asymptomatic and biochemical test results may be normal which is associated with the periodic destruction of gland cells in this phase. This disease is most likely to affect young, active women [6]. Knowledge regarding autoimmune diseases appears to have a key role in the era of COVID-19. As the COVID-19 pandemic has progressed, there have been various reports on the development of autoimmune diseases in individuals infected with SARS-CoV-2. The mere entry of the SARS-CoV-2 virus into respiratory epithelial cells induces a severe inflammatory state known as a cytokine storm in some patients. Symptoms associated with autoimmune diseases such as fatigue, joint pain, muscle aches, and brain fog may appear during SARS-CoV-2 infection and persist even after infection. As well as this, autoimmune phenomena are supported by the presence of antinuclear antibodies, anti-DNA, or complement consumption in these patients [7]. In a study conducted by Bastard et al., it was observed that at least 101 of 987 patients with a life-threatening course of COVID-19 had neutralizing immunoglobulin G autoantibodies against interferon-ω, against interferon-α, or against both in the early stages of COVID-19. Several patients also had autoantibodies against the other three type I interferons [8].

The SARS-CoV-2 pandemic has seriously affected many aspect of human life and has dramatically threatened the mental and physical health of the general public. Ubiquitous information in the mass media about its high infectivity, mortality, diseases predisposing to the adverse course of SARS-CoV-2 infection, as well as social isolation, lack of targeted treatment, and limited access to medical care produce a huge mental burden which results in psychological distress and sleep disorders [9–13]. Patients with chronic conditions experience higher stress levels due to being at higher risk for worse outcome from COVID-19 [14]. In an analysis conducted by Addis et al., it was noted that older age, female sex, longer duration of illness, presence of respiratory symptoms and no social support were significantly associated with an abnormal psychological impact of COVID-19 on patients with chronic disease [15]. However, the analyses of mental health disorders refer mainly to health professionals, and rarely to people with chronic diseases [16]. To the best of our knowledge, until now, there has been no study on the psychological impact of COVID-19 among patients with chronic disease in Poland. Therefore, this study represents the first psychological impact of COVID-19 among high-risk groups, chronic disease patients in the West Pomerania region in Poland. Thus, this study aimed to assess the symptoms of insomnia, depression and anxiety, among people with chronic diseases during the COVID-19 pandemic in Zachodniopomorskie province in Poland. The result of our study may help the governmental and medical community in formulating comprehensive interventions to prevent psychological problems of chronic disease clients related to COVID-19.

2. Materials and Methods

We conducted a cross-sectional survey among the inhabitants with chronic diseases who attended the inpatient units and outpatient clinics of the West Pomerania region in Poland from 3 May to 17 May 2020. During this period at each inpatient units and outpatient clinics, all consecutive patients who corresponded to the inclusion criteria were invited to complete a 9-item Patient Health Questionnaire (PHQ-9), 7-item Insomnia Severity Index (ISI) and a 7-item Generalized Anxiety Disorder scale (GAD-7) in Polish followed by an interview with a structured socio-demographic questionnaire. The criteria for inclusion were as follows: (1) informed consent before the survey was conducted; (2) residence in the West Pomerania region; (3) age 18 years and older. Exclusion criteria: diagnosis of mental illness. Each participant provided details regarding their basic demographic data and chronic diseases such as hypertension, diabetes mellitus, heart failure, coronary heart disease, dyslipidemia, chronic obstructive pulmonary disease and nicotinism. Each patient was also asked about the presence of Hashimoto's disease, one of the most common, if not the most common, autoimmune disease. The survey involved 879 people. All participants gave their informed consent before the survey was conducted. These participants could interrupt the survey at any time. The full confidentiality of information was ensured. Prior to the survey, the opinion of the Bioethics Committee of the Pomeranian Medical University in Szczecin was received (KB-0012/26/04/2020/Z) which conformed to the ethical guidelines of the Declaration of Helsinki.

Insomnia symptoms were assessed using the 7-item Insomnia Severity Index (ISI; range 0–28) [17–19], depression symptoms using the 9-item Patient Health Questionnaire (PHQ-9; range 0–27) [20–22], and anxiety symptoms with the 7-item Generalized Anxiety Disorder scale (GAD-7; range 0–21) [23].

Statistical Analysis

Statistical analysis was conducted using Statistica 13.0 software (StatSoft, Tulsa, OK, USA). The Shapiro-Wilk test was used to assess the distribution of data. Mann–Whitney's U test was performed to analyze quantitative. X^2 test was applied for qualitative data; the Yates correction was used if the subgroup size was insufficient. Correlation analysis was performed using the Spearman's rank correlation coefficient. The multivariable logistic regression model analysis was used to evaluate the relationship between the analyzed parameters. It was corrected for potentially distorting data (gender, age, dyslipidemia, diagnosed hypertension, and cigarette smoking). Differences were deemed statistically significant at $p \leq 0.05$.

3. Results

3.1. Evaluation of Mean Scores on Generalized Anxiety Disorder (GAD-7), Patient Health Questionnaire (PHQ-9), and Insomnia Severity Index (ISI) Scales

Female subjects significantly more often presented symptoms of anxiety, depression and insomnia. Differences in mean scores on GAD-7 ($p = 0.004$), PHQ-9 ($p = 0.013$) and ISI ($p = 0.006$) were observed between patients with and without hypertension. Moreover, statistically significant differences in mean GAD-7, PHQ-9 and ISI scores were found between smoking and non-smoking patients ($p < 0.001$) and between patients with and without Hashimoto ($p < 0.001$). In addition, significant differences were found between patients with and without dyslipidemia in mean ISI scores ($p = 0.035$). The mean GAD-7, PHQ-9, and ISI scores are presented in Table 1.

Table 1. Mean GAD-7, PHQ-9, and ISI scores for selected parameters.

		GAD-7		PHQ-9		ISI	
		mean ± SD; Me	***p***	**mean ± SD; Me**	***p***	**mean ± SD; Me**	***p***
Gender	female	12.49 ± 5.89; 14.0	<0.001	14.25 ± 5.79; 16.0	<0.001	16.64 ± 6.47; 19.0	<0.001
	male	7.61 ± 5.28; 7.0		9.74 ± 5.19; 10.0		11.42 ± 6.15; 12.0	
Hypertension		9.32 ± 5.61; 9.0	0.004	11.51 ± 5.45; 11.0	0.013	13.55 ± 5.70; 13.0	0.006
Diabetes mellitus		10.00 ± 5.16; 11.0	0.580	11.80 ± 4.61; 10.0	0.392	13.95 ± 4.86; 13.0	0.384
Coronary heart disease		14.50 ± 4.95; 14.5	0.401	17.00 ± 4.24; 17.0	0.300	19.00 ± 2.83; 19.0	0.396
Heart failure		7.00 ± 2.83; 7.0	0.395	9.00 ± 4.24; 9.0	0.389	13.00 ± 2.83; 13.0	0.607
Dyslipidemia		10.12 ± 5.73; 11.0	0.157	12.08 ± 5.73; 12.0	0.142	13.89 ± 6.27; 15.0	0.035
Chronic obstructive pulmonary disease		8.67 ± 4.93; 11.0	0.568	9.00 ± 3.61; 10.00	0.280	9.33 ± 2.08; 10.0	0.126
Smoke cigarettes		7.27 ± 4.74; 7.0	<0.001	9.33 ± 5.01; 10.0	<0.001	11.31 ± 5.75; 13.0	<0.001
Hashimoto's disease		15.46 ± 2.33; 16.0	<0.001	17.34 ± 2.10; 17.0	<0.001	20.75 ± 2.19; 21.0	<0.001

Abbreviations: *p*–statistical significance; Me–median; SD–standard deviation; GAD-7–Generalized Anxiety Disorder scale; PHQ-9–Patient Health Questionnaire; ISI–Insomnia Severity Index.

3.2. Analysis of Correlation between Selected Parameters and GAD-7, PHQ-9, and ISI Scores

The correlation analysis showed a strong correlation between the occurrence of Hashimoto's disease and an increase in ISI score (r = 0.797, $p < 0.001$), GAD-7 scale (r = 0.766, $p < 0.001$) and PHQ-9 scale (r = 0.767, $p < 0.001$). A case comparison is presented in Table 2. Therefore, for further analysis, only Hashimoto's disease was included as a predictor of insomnia, anxiety, or depression.

Table 2. Analysis of correlations between selected parameters and GAD-7, PHQ-9, and ISI scores.

	GAD-7		PHQ-9		ISI	
	R	***p***	**R**	***p***	**R**	***p***
Age (years)	−0.082	0.009	−0.082	0.009	−0.077	0.015
Hypertension	−0.092	0.004	−0.079	0.013	−0.087	0.006
Diabetes mellitus	−0.018	0.579	−0.027	0.391	−0.028	0.384
Coronary heart disease	0.027	0.399	0.033	0.299	0.027	0.395
Heart failure	−0.027	0.394	−0.027	0.388	−0.016	0.606
Dyslipidemia	−0.045	0.156	−0.047	0.141	−0.067	0.035
Chronic obstructive pulmonary disease	−0.018	0.567	−0.034	0.279	−0.049	0.125
Smoke cigarettes	−0.350	<0.001	−0.347	<0.001	−0.327	<0.001
Hashimoto's disease	0.766	<0.001	0.767	<0.001	0.797	<0.001

Abbreviations: *p*–statistical significance; R–correlation coefficient; GAD-7–Generalized Anxiety Disorder scale; PHQ-9–Patient Health Questionnaire; ISI–Insomnia Severity Index.

3.3. Evaluation of Selected Parameters Depending on the Occurrence of Hashimoto's Disease

The analysis of the selected parameters depending showed statistically significant differences in gender ($p < 0.001$), age ($p < 0.001$), hypertension ($p < 0.001$), dyslipidemia ($p = 0.004$) and smoking cigarettes ($p < 0.001$) between participants with and without Hashimoto. The results are presented in Table 3.

Table 3. Evaluation of selected parameters depending on the occurrence of Hashimoto's disease.

		without Hashimoto ($n = 589$)	with Hashimoto ($n = 290$)	p
Gender (n, %)	female	275 (46.69%)	253 (87.24%)	<0.001
	male	314 (53.31%)	37 (12.76%)	
Age (years), mean ± SD; Me		39.71 ± 7.07; 39.0	37.97 ± 5.68; 37.0	<0.001
Hypertension (n, %)	no	487 (82.68%)	265 (91.38%)	<0.001
	yes	102 (17.32%)	25 (8.62%)	
Diabetes mellitus (n, %)	no	574 (97.45%)	286 (98.62%)	0.383
	yes	15 (2.55%)	4 (1.38%)	
Coronary heart disease (n, %)	no	588 (99.83%)	290 (100.00%)	0.717
	yes	1 (0.17%)	0 (0.00%)	
Heart failure (n, %)	no	587 (99.66%)	290 (100.00%)	0.809
	yes	2 (0.34%)	0 (0.00%)	
Dyslipidemia (n, %)	no	470 (79.80%)	255 (87.93%)	0.004
	yes	119 (20.20%)	35 (12.07%)	
Chronic obstructive pulmonary disease (n, %)	no	586 (99.49%)	290 (100.00%)	0.547
	yes	3 (0.51%)	0 (0.00%)	
Smoke cigarettes (n, %)	no	329 (55.86%)	277 (95.52%)	<0.001
	yes	260 (44.14%)	13 (4.48%)	

Abbreviations: p—statistical significance; n—number of patients; % percentage of patients.

3.4. Mental Health and Insomnia in Patients with Hashimoto's Disease

After the results were corrected for age, gender, diagnosed hypertension, dyslipidemia and cigarette smoking, it was confirmed that the diagnosis of Hashimoto's disease was associated with an increased risk of anxiety (GAD-7, OR = 2.225; $p < 0.001$), depression (PHQ-9, OR = 2.518; $p < 0.001$) and insomnia (ISI, OR = 3.530; $p < 0.001$). The results are presented in Table 4.

Table 4. Severity of mental health and insomnia in patients with Hashimoto's disease (multivariable logistic regression).

	Hashimoto's Disease (Adjusted by Potentially Distorting)			
	p	OR	CI −95%	CI+ 95%
GAD-7	<0.001	2.225	1.944	2.546
PHQ-9	<0.001	2.518	2.154	2.943
ISI	<0.001	3.530	2.721	4.581

Abbreviations: p–statistical significance; OR- odds ratio; CI-confidence interval; GAD-7–Generalized Anxiety Disorder scale; PHQ-9–Patient Health Questionnaire; ISI–Insomnia Severity Index. Notes: Potentially distorting data (age, gender, diagnosed hypertension, dyslipidemia and cigarette smoking).

4. Discussion

The COVID-19 pandemic has affected many aspects of human lives worldwide. Information about the diseases that predispose to severe and unfavorable course of COVID-19, the spectre of long-term quarantines, lack of targeted treatment or lack of medical support have been causing a huge psychological burden and generating psychological distress and sleep disorders.

Research on psychological distress and sleep disorders in patients with chronic diseases shows that they are particularly predisposed to mental health disorders [24]. The reported incidence of depression, anxiety or sleep disorders varies widely, depending on the population studied and diagnostic tools. In an analysis conducted by Pumar et al., it was noted that in patients with chronic obstructive pulmonary disease the prevalence of depression ranges from 10% to 57% and in the case of anxiety the prevalence ranges from 7% to 50% [25]. Budhiraja et al. noted sleep disorders in 27.3% of patients with chronic obstructive pulmonary diseases [26]. Other studies have confirmed the relationship between depression, anxiety and sleep disorders in patients with chronic pain, chronic neurological diseases, kidney diseases or autoimmune diseases [27–31].

The most important finding of the present study is the fact that among chronic diseases such as hypertension, diabetes, coronary artery disease, circulatory failure, dyslipidemia, chronic obstructive pulmonary disease, nicotinism, and Hashimoto's disease, it was the group of patients with Hashimoto's disease that showed a strong correlation with increased scores on ISI ($r = 0.797$, $p < 0.001$), GAD-7 ($r = 0.766$, $p < 0.001$) and PHQ-9 scales ($r = 0.767$, $p < 0.001$). The group of patients with Hashimoto's disease also showed significantly more frequent symptoms of anxiety, depression and insomnia compared to people without this condition ($p < 0.001$, $p < 0.001$, $p < 0.001$).

These individuals, also after the results were corrected for age, gender, hypertension, dyslipidemia and smoking, showed more than twice higher risk of aggravation of anxiety symptoms, more than 2.5 times greater increase in the severity of depression symptoms, and more than 3.5 times increase in the severity of insomnia.

Autoimmune thyroiditis often coexists with insomnia, depression and anxiety [32]. The prevalence of antithyroid autoantibodies in patients with depressive disorders is higher than in the general population. Carta et al. showed that the risk of depressive disorders in a group of patients with thyroid diseases was up to six times higher than in those without, regardless of thyroid dysfunction assessed by routine serological tests [33]. Similar results were obtained by Giynas et al. who confirmed an increased incidence of depressive disorders in a group of patients with thyroid diseases [34]. Kirim et al. pointed out an increased risk of depression in a group of patients with chronic inflammation of the thyroid gland even though its hormonal function was normal. In addition, they showed that an autoimmune inflammation of the thyroid gland can result in the failure of the thyroid gland, which in turn is a risk factor for the development of depression resistant to standard treatment [35]. Geracioti et al. described an interesting case of a patient with classic symptoms of emotionally unstable borderline personality, with co-occurring autoimmune thyroiditis, in whom mood swings and psychotic symptoms were directly related to the titer of antithyroid antibodies [36]. In a study by Huang et al., the severity of depression and insomnia were significantly correlated with low FT3 [37]. In anxiety disorders, the first symptom in patients with hypothyroidism is often generalized agitation [38]. Since this disorder commonly coexists with elevated blood pressure and tachycardia, it can be assumed that this condition leads to the development of generalized anxiety syndrome.

Suffering from an autoimmune disease can generate enormous stress, through a significant reduction in activity at home or at work, financial difficulties related to the cost of medical care and reduced income, lack of acceptance of its appearance resulting from, among other things, complications of the applied treatment, impaired interpersonal relations or loss of independence [39]. Even discreet intensification of everyday stress factors in people with autoimmune diseases affects the hypothalamic-pituitary-adrenal axis homeostasis, which leads to intensification of the disease symptoms or adversely affects its remission [40]. It seems that is why patients with Hashimoto's disease, who are aware of an increased risk of more severe symptoms of COVID-19, are most likely to develop anxiety, depression and insomnia among all chronic diseases, as confirmed by our study.

Our study had several limitations. Firstly, Hashimoto's disease was the only autoimmune disease that was included in this study, although there may be other autoimmune diseases which may induce similar psychological effects during the SARS-CoV-2 pandemic. Secondly, there is an interplay between depressive and anxiety symptoms on the one hand and the presence of insomnia symptoms on the other hand. Thirdly, as a cross-sectional study, it provided no information on any change in mental health of the respondents.

5. Conclusions

This study showed that patients with a diagnosis of Hashimoto's disease during the COVID-19 pandemic are at a higher risk of insomnia, depression and anxiety than patients with other chronic diseases. Therefore, people with Hashimoto's disease during the pandemic require appropriate medical support, information, stress reduction and rest.

The result of our study may help the governmental and medical community in formulating comprehensive interventions to prevent psychological problems among chronic disease clients related to COVID-19.

Author Contributions: Conceptualization, P.W.; Formal analysis, P.W., A.S. and I.R.; Investigation, P.W. and A.S.; Methodology, P.W.; Supervision, I.R.; Writing—original draft, P.W., A.S. and I.R.; Writing—review and editing, P.W., A.S. and I.R. All authors have read and agreed to the published version of the manuscript.

Funding: This research received no external funding.

Institutional Review Board Statement: The study was conducted according to the guidelines of the Declaration of Helsinki, and approved by the Bioethics Committee of the Pomeranian Medical University in Szczecin was received (KB-0012/26/04/2020/Z; 26.04.2020).

Informed Consent Statement: Informed consent was obtained from all subjects involved in the study.

Data Availability Statement: All data that support the findings of this study are available upon request from the corresponding author.

Conflicts of Interest: The authors have declared that no competing interests exist.

References

1. Yang, Y.; Peng, F.; Wang, R.; Guan, K.; Jiang, T.; Xu, G.; Sun, J.; Chang, C. The deadly coronaviruses: The 2003 SARS pandemic and the 2020 novel coronavirus epidemic in China. *J. Autoimmun.* **2020**, *109*, 102434. [CrossRef]
2. Yang, Y.M.; Hsu, C.Y.; Lai, C.C.; Yen, M.-F.; Wikramaratna, P.S.; Chen, H.-H.; Wang, T.-H. Impact of Comorbidity on Fatality Rate of Patients with Middle East Respiratory Syndrome. *Sci. Rep.* **2017**, *7*, 11307. [CrossRef] [PubMed]
3. CDC. *Coronavirus Disease 2019 (COVID-19)*; Department of Health and Human Services, CDC: Atlanta, GA, USA, 2020. Available online: https://www.cdc.gov/coronavirus/2019-ncov/index.html (accessed on 25 January 2021).
4. Wańkowicz, P.; Bobrowska-Snarska, D.; Nowacki, P.; Brzosko, M. Clinical manifestations of neuropsychiatric systemic lupus erythematosus: A single-center study from West Pomerania Province in Poland. *Pol. Arch. Intern. Med.* **2020**, *130*, 82–84.
5. Cooper, G.S.; Stroehla, B.C. The epidemiology of autoimmune diseases. *Autoimmun. Rev.* **2003**, *2*, 119–125. [CrossRef]
6. Mincer, D.L.; Jialal, I. Hashimoto Thyroiditis. In *StatPearls*; StatPearls Publishing: Treasure Island, FL, USA, 2020.
7. Cañas, C.A. The triggering of post-COVID-19 autoimmunity phenomena could be associated with both transient immunosuppression and an inappropriate form of immune reconstitution in susceptible individuals. *Med. Hypotheses* **2020**, *145*, 110345. [CrossRef]
8. Bastard, P.; Rosen, L.B.; Zhang, Q.; Michailidis, E.; Hoffmann, H.-H.; Zhang, Y.; Dorgham, K.; Philippot, Q.; Rosain, J.; Béziat, V.; et al. Auto-antibodies against type I IFNs in patients with life-threatening COVID-19. *Science* **2020**, *370*, eabd4585. [CrossRef] [PubMed]
9. Chen, Q.; Liang, M.; Li, Y.; Guo, J.; Fei, D.; Wang, L.; He, L.; Sheng, C.; Cai, Y.; Li, X.; et al. Mental health care for medical staff in China during the COVID-19 outbreak. *Lancet Psychiatry* **2020**, *7*, e15–e16. [CrossRef]
10. Zhang, C.; Yang, L.; Liu, S.; Ma, S.; Wang, Y.; Cai, Z.; Du, H.; Li, R.; Kang, L.; Su, M.; et al. Survey of Insomnia and Related Social Psychological Factors Among Medical Staff Involved in the 2019 Novel Coronavirus Disease Outbreak. *Front. Psychiatry* **2020**, *11*, 306. [CrossRef]
11. Lai, J.; Ma, S.; Wang, Y.; Cai, Z.; Hu, J.; Wei, N.; Wu, J.; Du, H.; Chen, T.; Li, R.; et al. Factors Associated with Mental Health Outcomes Among Health Care Workers Exposed to Coronavirus Disease 2019. *JAMA Netw. Open* **2020**, *3*, e203976. [CrossRef] [PubMed]
12. Bohlken, J.; Schömig, F.; Lemke, M.R.; Pumberger, M.; Riedel-Heller, S.G. COVID-19 Pandemic: Stress Exposure of Healthcare Workers [COVID-19 Pandemic: Stress Experience of Healthcare Workers—A Short Current Review]. *Psychiatry Pract.* **2020**, *47*, 190–197.
13. Bao, Y.; Sun, Y.; Meng, S.; Shi, J.; Lu, L. 2019-nCoV epidemic: Address mental health care to empower society. *Lancet* **2020**, *395*, e37–e38. [CrossRef]
14. Kendzerska, T.; Zhu, D.T.; Gershon, A.S.; Edwards, J.D.; Peixoto, C.; Robillard, R.; E Kendall, C. The Effects of the Health System Response to the COVID-19 Pandemic on Chronic Disease Management: A Narrative Review. *Risk Manag. Healthc. Policy* **2021**, *14*, 575–584. [CrossRef]

15. Addis, S.G.; Nega, A.D.; Miretu, D.G. Psychological impact of COVID-19 pandemic on chronic disease patients in Dessie town government and private hospitals, Northeast Ethiopia. *Diabetes Metab. Syndr. Clin. Res. Rev.* **2021**, *15*, 129–135. [CrossRef]
16. Wańkowicz, P.; Szylińska, A.; Rotter, I. Assessment of Mental Health Factors among Health Professionals Depending on Their Contact with COVID-19 Patients. *Int. J. Environ. Res. Public Health* **2020**, *17*, 5849. [CrossRef] [PubMed]
17. Morin, C.M. *Insomnia: Psychological Assessment and Management*; Guilford Press: New York, NY, USA, 1993.
18. Bastien, C.H.; Vallières, A.; Morin, C.M. Validation of the Insomnia Severity Index as an outcome measure for insomnia research. *Sleep Med.* **2001**, *2*, 297–307. [CrossRef]
19. Morin, C.M.; Belleville, G.; Bélanger, L.; Ivers, H. The Insomnia Severity Index: Psychometric Indicators to Detect Insomnia Cases and Evaluate Treatment Response. *Sleep* **2011**, *34*, 601–608. [CrossRef] [PubMed]
20. Spitzer, R.L.; Williams, J.B.; Kroenke, K.; Linzer, M.; Degruy, F.V.; Hahn, S.R.; Brody, D.; Johnson, J.G. Utility of a new procedure for diagnosing mental disorders in primary care. The PRIME-MD 1000 study. *JAMA* **1994**, *272*, 1749–1756. [CrossRef] [PubMed]
21. Kroenke, K.; Spitzer, R.L.; Williams, J.B.W. The PHQ-9: Validity of a brief depression severity measure. *J. Gen. Intern. Med.* **2001**, *16*, 606–613. [CrossRef] [PubMed]
22. Kroenke, K.; Spitzer, R.L. The PHQ-9: A new depression diagnostic and severity measure. *Psychiatr. Ann.* **2002**, *32*, 509–521. [CrossRef]
23. Spitzer, R.L.; Kroenke, K.; Williams, J.B.W.; Löwe, B. A brief measure for assessing generalized anxiety disorder: The GAD-7. *Arch. Intern. Med.* **2006**, *166*, 1092–1097. [CrossRef]
24. Koyanagi, A.; Garin, N.; Olaya, B.; Ayuso-Mateos, J.L.; Chatterji, S.; Leonardi, M.; Koskinen, S.; Tobiasz-Adamczyk, B.; Haro, J.M. Correction: Chronic Conditions and Sleep Problems among Adults Aged 50 years or over in Nine Countries: A Multi-Country Study. *PLoS ONE* **2015**, *10*, e0138261. [CrossRef] [PubMed]
25. Pumar, M.I.; Gray, C.R.; Walsh, J.R.; Yang, I.A.; Rolls, T.A.; Ward, D.L. Anxiety and depression—Important psychological comorbidities of COPD. *J. Thorac. Dis.* **2014**, *6*, 1615–1631. [PubMed]
26. Budhiraja, R.; Parthasarathy, S.; Budhiraja, P.; Habib, M.P.; Wendel, C.; Quan, S.F. Insomnia in Patients with COPD. *Sleep* **2012**, *35*, 369–375. [CrossRef] [PubMed]
27. Gerontoukou, E.I.; Michaelidoy, S.; Rekleiti, M.; Saridi, M.; Souliotis, K. Investigation of Anxiety and Depression in Patients with Chronic Diseases. *Health Psychol. Res.* **2015**, *3*, 2123. [CrossRef]
28. Wong, W.S.; Chen, P.P.; Yap, J.; Mak, K.H.; Tam, B.K.H.; Fielding, R. Chronic Pain and Psychiatric Morbidity: A Comparison between Patients Attending Specialist Orthopedics Clinic and Multidisciplinary Pain Clinic. *Pain Med.* **2011**, *12*, 246–259. [CrossRef]
29. Janowski, K.; Kurpas, D.; Kusz, J.; Mroczek, B.; Jedynak, T. Health-related behavior, profile of health locus of control and acceptance of illness in patients suffering from chronic somatic diseases. *PLoS ONE* **2013**, *8*, e63920. [CrossRef]
30. Theofilou, P. Quality of life and mental health in hemodialysis and peritoneal dialysis patients: The role of health beliefs. *Int. Urol. Nephrol.* **2011**, *44*, 245–253. [CrossRef]
31. Wańkowicz, P.; Szylińska, A.; Rotter, I. Evaluation of Mental Health Factors among People with Systemic Lupus Erythematosus during the SARS-CoV-2 Pandemic. *J. Clin. Med.* **2020**, *9*, 2872. [CrossRef] [PubMed]
32. Degner, D.; Meller, J.; Bleich, S.; Schlautmann, V.; Rüther, E. Affective Disorders Associated With Autoimmune Thyroiditis. *J. Neuropsychiatry Clin. Neurosci.* **2001**, *13*, 532–533. [CrossRef]
33. Carta, M.G.; Hardoy, M.C.; Carpiniello, B.; Murru, A.; Marci, A.R.; Carbone, F.; Deiana, L.; Cadeddu, M.; Mariottiet, S. A case control study on psychiatric disorders in Hashimoto disease and Euthyroid Goitre: Not only depressive but also anxiety disorders are associated with thyroid autoimmunity. *Clin Pract. Epidemiol. Ment Health* **2005**, *1*, 23. [CrossRef] [PubMed]
34. Giynas Ayhan, M.; Uguz, F.; Askin, R.; Gonen, M.S. The prevalence of depression and anxiety disorders in patients with euthyroid Hashimoto's thyroiditis: A comparative study. *Gen. Hosp. Psychiatry* **2014**, *36*, 95–98. [CrossRef] [PubMed]
35. Kirim, S.; Keskek, S.O.; Köksal, F.; Haydardedeoglu, F.E.; Bozkirli, E.; Toledano, Y. Depression in patients with euthyroid chronic autoimmune thyroiditis. *Endocr. J.* **2012**, *59*, 705–708. [CrossRef] [PubMed]
36. Geracioti, T.D., Jr.; Kling, M.A.; Post, R.M.; Gold, P.W. Antithyroid antibody-linked symptoms in borderline personality disorder. *Endocrine* **2003**, *21*, 153–158. [CrossRef]
37. Huang, X.; Zhang, H.; Qu, C.; Liu, Y.; Bian, C.; Xu, Y. Depression and Insomnia Are Closely Associated with Thyroid Hormone Levels in Chronic Hepatitis B. *Med. Sci. Monit.* **2019**, *25*, 2672–2678. [CrossRef] [PubMed]
38. Hall, R.C.; Hall, R.C. Anxiety and endocrine disease. *Semin. Clin. Neuropsychiatry* **1999**, *4*, 72–83. [PubMed]
39. Liang, M.H.; Rogers, M.; Larson, M.; Eaton, H.M.; Murawski, B.J.; Taylor, J.E.; Swafford, J.; Schur, P.H. The psychosocial impact of systemic lupus erythematosus and rheumatoid arthritis. *Arthritis Rheum.* **1984**, *27*, 13–19. [CrossRef]
40. Michelsen, B.; Kristianslund, E.K.; Sexton, J.; Hammer, H.B.; Fagerli, K.M.; Lie, E.; Wierød, A.; Kalstad, S.; Rødevand, E.; Krøll, F.; et al. Do depression and anxiety reduce the likelihood of remission in rheumatoid arthritis and psoriatic arthritis? Data from the prospective multicentre NOR-DMARD study. *Ann. Rheum. Dis.* **2017**, *76*, 1906–1910. [CrossRef] [PubMed]

Journal of
Clinical Medicine

MDPI

Article

Cardiovascular and Pre-Frailty Risk Assessment during Shelter-In-Place Measures Based on Multimodal Biomarkers Collected from Smart Telemedical Wearables

Eliasz Kańtoch [1,*] and Anna Kańtoch [2]

[1] AGH University of Science and Technology, 30-059 Krakow, Poland
[2] Jagiellonian University Medical College, Faculty of Medicine, Department of Internal Medicine and Gerontology, 30-688 Krakow, Poland; anna.kantoch@doctoral.uj.edu.pl
* Correspondence: kantoch@agh.edu.pl

Abstract: Wearable devices play a growing role in healthcare applications and disease prevention. We conducted a retrospective study to assess cardiovascular and pre-frailty risk during the Covid-19 shelter-in-place measures on human activity patterns based on multimodal biomarkers collected from smartwatch sensors. For methodology validation we enrolled five adult participants (age range: 32 to 84 years; mean 57 ± 22.38; BMI: 27.80 ± 2.95 kg/m^2) categorized by age who were smartwatch users and self-isolating at home during the Covid-19 pandemic. Resting heart rate, daily steps, and minutes asleep were recorded using smartwatch sensors. Overall, we created a dataset of 464 days of continuous measurement that included 50 days of self-isolation at home during the Covid-19 pandemic. Student's t-test was used to determine significant differences between the pre-Covid-19 and Covid-19 periods. Our findings suggest that there was a significant decrease in the number of daily steps (−57.21%; −4321; 95% CI, 3722 to 4920) and resting heart rate (−4.81%; −3.04; 95% CI, 2.59 to 3.51) during the period of self−isolation compared to the time before lockdown. We found that there was a significant decrease in the number of minutes asleep (−13.48%; −57.91; 95% CI, 16.33 to 99.49) among older adults. Finally, cardiovascular and pre-frailty risk scores were calculated based on biomarkers and evaluated from the clinical perspective.

Keywords: frailty; telemedicine; gerontechnology; wearable sensors; shelter-in-place measures; Covid-19; resting heart rate; sleep duration; activity pattern

Citation: Kańtoch, E.; Kańtoch, A. Cardiovascular and Pre-Frailty Risk Assessment during Shelter-In-Place Measures Based on Multimodal Biomarkers Collected from Smart Telemedical Wearables. *J. Clin. Med.* **2021**, *10*, 1997. https://doi.org/10.3390/jcm10091997

Academic Editors: Michele Roccella, Zan Gao and Marcel Blot-Chabaud

Received: 21 February 2021
Accepted: 27 April 2021
Published: 6 May 2021

1. Introduction

Coronavirus disease 2019 (Covid-19) lockdown polices were introduced worldwide during a global health crisis to combat the spread of the novel coronavirus (Severe Acute Respiratory Syndrome Coronavirus 2—SARS-CoV-2) pandemic, forcing people to change their behavior, daily habits, and routines which affected their activity level. However, the quantitative impact of these measures on older adults is unknown. Keesara et al. [1] reported that to face this crisis, we need an immediate digital revolution and the transformation of health care delivery into some telemedical solutions to protect against the spread of the pathogen to uninfected patients in a clinical and non-clinical settings. The Covid-19 pandemic has accelerated the paradigm shift in healthcare from traditional care to telemedical care. However, the procedures and methods for supporting healthcare professionals are not clearly defined, as well as there are challenges related to telemedical technologies. In 2019, Sim reported that major challenges for mobile health include the discovery and validation of digital biomarkers, and the regulation of mobile health technologies [2].

Interestingly, the Covid-19 pandemic has already disrupted health care and has accelerated the development of telemedical services. Over the past decade, many telemedical services are gaining traction, including teleconsultations, e-prescriptions, teleradiology, telecardiology. However, Keesara et al. reported that telemedical digital technologies had low penetration into the market [1].

During the pandemic, we observe a rapid shift from in-person doctor visits to teleconsultation based on information and telecommunication technologies, which becomes challenging for both patients and doctors. Teleconsultation, however, has several drawbacks and limitations. The major limitation is the lack of measured health parameters, which are often performed during a medical visit, such as auscultation, heart rate measurement, body temperature, etc., and the diagnosis is mainly based on the patient's medical interview.

Widespread mobile health technologies, especially wearable devices (e.g., smartphones, fitness trackers) may play a crucial role in the transition process and fill the missing category of home-based monitoring medical devices. We believe that data from wearable devices (such as smartwatches or fitness trackers) can be an auxiliary tool to assist teleconsultation with primary care physicians, especially in emergencies or health crises, because they may collect health data in the home setting, which can play an essential role in patient diagnosis or screening. Our previous work focused on investigating the desirable features and applications of telemedical services for the older adults delivered by wearable medical devices [3]. At present, smartwatches and fitness trackers are used to quantify physical activity and sleep quality with the primary goal of improving overall health. However, novel emerging applications include motion analysis and biomechanics, rehabilitation, active assistive living, and health parameters monitoring. Furthermore, wrist-worn activity trackers are now a validated tool to assess physical activity in chronic diseases such as atrial fibrillation [4].

Frailty syndrome is associated with a high incidence of adverse health outcomes in the geriatric population, including an increased risk of hospitalization, falls, disability, institutionalization, and mortality. Frailty can be reversed either spontaneously or through nutritional interventions and exercise [5]. Screening for frailty syndrome is recommended to identify older adults who would benefit most from a Comprehensive Geriatric Assessment [6]. There are many scales and questionnaires for assessing frailty syndrome. However, the most common is the frailty phenotype, also known as Linda Fried's Criteria, which includes five of the following criteria: exhaustion, unintentional weight loss, low physical activity, muscle weakness (handgrip strength), and slow gait speed. Frailty is defined as a clinical syndrome with at least three criteria, while pre-frailty is defined as the presence of one or two of these criteria [7]. It is estimated that the frailty syndrome affects 7–16.3% of the population aged 65 and over, and 25–40% of those aged $\geq$80 years, and the risk of frailty increases with age. Moreover, it is twice as high in women as in men [5,7–9]. Therefore, in our study, we tried to focus on octogenarians to create a useful prediction tool for Cardiovascular and Pre-Frailty Risk Assessment, as people 80 years of age and older are at increased risk of not only cardiovascular adverse events but also frailty due to their age.

The state of knowledge about the impact of Covid-19 restrictions on human activity is limited and is based mainly on online surveys. Recently, Gjaka et al. [10] published comprehensive research in which they investigated the effects of Covid-19 restrictions on physical activity based on online surveys. The authors showed that the restrictions had a negative impact on physical activity. It would be interesting how those results compare to the ground truth measured by movement sensors. Aggregate data from sports wristbands manufacturers are also available. Unfortunately, it is often difficult to analyze them because methodology is not clearly described and there is no information about population, data quality and consistency. Furthermore, the timetable for introducing the Covid-19 restrictions varied across countries and regions, which made data analysis difficult.

The aim of this paper was to propose a non-invasive triage methodology for the assessment of the cardiovascular and pre-frailty risk based on multimodal biomarkers collected from smartwatch sensors. For methodology validation we enrolled five adult participants (age range: 32 to 84 years; mean 57 $\pm$ 22.38; BMI: 27.80 $\pm$ 2.95 kg/m^2) categorized by age who were smartwatch users and self-isolating at home during the Covid-19 pandemic. Resting heart rate, daily steps, and minutes asleep were recorded using smartwatch sensors. Overall, we created a dataset of 5.68 person-years (464 days) of continuous measurement and clinical follow-up by a geriatric specialist that included 50 days of self-isolation at home during the Covid-19 pandemic. The novelty of research is twofold: first, the quantitative impact of shelter-in-place measures on biomarkers was investigated in two age groups and mapped to the cardiovascular and pre-frailty risk scale, secondly a non-invasive method to assess the cardiovascular and pre-frailty risk has been developed and validated during shelter-in-place measure in collaboration with a geriatric specialist to screen vulnerable patients. The significant advantage of this approach is the non-invasive measurement, continuous assessment, quantitative scale, and a telemedical interface. Study results might impact the clinical practice by providing easy to deploy, low-cost, and scalable tool for assessing cardiovascular and pre-frailty risk. In addition, the paper discusses the advantages of wearable telemedical devices as a future physician tool to screen the patient's overall health and improve the telehealth visit experience, especially during emergency scenarios (i.e., a pandemic).

We took advantage of global Covid-19 pandemic shelter-in-place measures to find a new perspective on human behavior during a pandemic. It is believed that people at home perform less physical activity, and their lifestyle is relatively sedentary, so the risk of frailty syndrome [11] and cardiovascular disease (CVD) increases [12]. Cardiovascular disease is a leading cause of death and many adverse outcomes among the elderly, including morbidity, disability, and the risk of hospitalization [13,14]. According to the 2016 European Guidelines on Cardiovascular Disease Prevention in Clinical Practice, healthy adults of all ages should exercise at least 150 min a week of moderate-intensity or 75 min of vigorous activity a week or in equivalent combinations [12]. What is more, the risk of frailty was significantly lower in older adults who walk at least 5000 steps a day [15].

However, during a period of self-isolation, these goals could be difficult to achieve due to limited possibilities of physical activity at home and a lack of motivation [16]. One of the solutions may be gamification, which may have a positive impact on health, wellbeing and motivation to exercise through interactive training programs [17]. Exergames were used in the population of long-term care residents to improve mobility [18]. Moreover, video games turned out to be an exciting option for motivating patients in the rehabilitation process [19].

We have organized the rest of this paper as follows. Section 2 is based on medical experience and provides an overview of the most critical parameters that can be measured with a smartwatch, and that can be useful during a medical teleconsultation. Section 3 describes the developed method to assess cardiovascular and pre-frailty risk and material. Section 4 presents the results. Section 5 discusses the results in the context of the Covid-19 pandemic. Finally, Section 6 concludes the article.

2. Clinical Point of View

One of the main risk factors for cardiovascular diseases is a sedentary lifestyle. It is believed that a sedentary lifestyle could easily be verified using a fitness tracker. However, physical activity, which could also be monitored by this device, has a positive effect on the frailty syndrome and many cardiovascular risk factors such as hypertension, cholesterol level, body weight and type 2 diabetes mellitus. What is more, regular physical activity could not only improve fitness and mental health but also reduce the risk of many adverse health outcomes [12].

2.1. Resting Heart Rate

Heart rate is the most common vital sign measured in clinical practice to assess cardiovascular health because it could be an excellent indicator of myocardial metabolism and cardiac output. The diagnosis of tachycardia, defined as an atrial and/or ventricular rate of >100 beats per minute (bpm), could be very dangerous because it could lead to many adverse events, including cardiomyopathy, myocardial ischemia, hypotension, low cardiac output, cardiac arrest, or even death [20].

Resting heart rate (RHR) is a determinant of prognostic value, indicating that elevated RHR values (RHR > 80 bpm) were associated with an increased incidence of cardiovascular disease and all-cause mortality compared to RHR < 60 bpm [21–24]. What is more, high RHRs were related to CVD complications and mortality among patients with type 2 diabetes mellitus [21]. Lower levels of RHR could be achieved through regular physical activity, which acts through the autonomic nervous system [21].

2.2. Sleep Duration and Quality

Sleep is a biological process that plays a crucial role in brain function and physiology, including metabolism, appetite regulation, and cardiovascular, hormonal, and immunological functions. According to the American Academy of Sleep Medicine classification, sleep could be divided into rapid eye movement (REM) and non-rapid eye movement (NREM) phases. NREM sleep consists of three stages: lighter (stages N1 and N2) and deeper sleep (stage N3) [25]. Sleep duration and quality are significant measures of sleep [26]. It is difficult to assess the perfect amount of sleep, which could be applied by everyone [27]. However, prolonged sleep time (>8 h/day) or shorter sleep times (<7 h/day) could be associated with many adverse health outcomes, including CVD, hypertension, type 2 diabetes, obesity, depression, and all-cause mortality [27–29]. Sleep quality is difficult to define and measure objectively, but it could be affected by many factors, such as environmental, psychological, or lifestyle behaviors: use of alcohol, caffeine, or stimulants, and use of phones or computers before sleep time [30,31]. Furthermore, poor quality of sleep could be associated with various adverse health outcomes [32].

2.3. Number of Daily Steps

A fitness tracker, which includes a pedometer, is a useful device to monitor the number of daily steps and provide feedback to promote walking [33]. Although 10,000 daily steps are widely recommended, evidence from previous prospective studies is still incomplete. According to the literature, a greater number of steps was associated with lower CVD, cancer, and all-cause mortality. Furthermore, a higher gait speed could also be associated with a reduced risk of death [34].

2.4. A Wearable Device for Health Tracking

Wearable devices are becoming more and more important in health tracking. A new category of medical wearable devices has emerged. Much recent research has shown that smartwatches can be widely used in healthcare. Smartwatches are used for monitoring activity or gait, chronic disease self-management, and nursing or home-based care. A systematic review by King et al. found that most studies used smartwatches to monitor Parkinson's disease or epilepsy [35]. Other possibilities of using smartwatches have found application in diabetes, dementia, asthma, and stroke, or in people with visual impairment [35,36]. Our previous study focused on assessing cardiovascular risk using machine learning based on the developed T-shirt equipped with wearable sensors [37]. Recent research indicates that smartwatches can detect Covid-19 before symptoms appear.

3. Materials and Methods

3.1. Cardiovascular and Pre-Frailty Risk Assessment (CFRA)

We developed a 4-point Cardiovascular and Pre-Frailty Risk Assessment (CFRA) method that provides a quantitative method for assessment of the cardiovascular and pre-frailty risk. We chose the following biomarkers: daily steps, resting heart rate, sleep duration, and age. The more points scored, the higher probability of developing cardiovascular health outcomes and frailty syndrome. The Cardiovascular and Pre-Frailty Risk Assessment 4-point method was exhibited in Table 1.

Table 1. Cardiovascular and Pre-Frailty Risk Assessment method.

Biomarker	Scores					Assumptions and References
	0	0.5	1.0	1.5	2.0	
Daily Steps	>12,500	10,000–12,500	7500–9999	5000–7499	<5000	[38,39]
Resting Heart Rate	<60 bpm	60–67 bpm	68–74 bpm	75–80 bpm	>80 bpm	[21–23,40]
Sleep Duration	7–8 h/day	-	-	-	<7 h/day or >8 h/day	[27–29]
Age	<70	70–74	75–79	80–84	85+	[41]

Table legend: bpm—beats per minute.

3.2. Study Design

We conducted a retrospective study to investigate the impact of shelter-in-place measures on human behavior, resting heart rate, sleep, and activity patterns in the context of telemedical services. We enrolled five adult volunteers of different age groups and backgrounds (three working participants and two octogenarians) who were smartwatch users and self-isolating at home during the Covid-19 pandemic. Eligible volunteers were those who met all of the following inclusion criteria for the study: 18 years of age or older, signed informed consent, stayed at home, and self-isolated during the lockdown period, and were Fitbit Versa users in the previous year. The last criterion was mandatory, as it was the only way to conduct a retrospective comparative analysis. Volunteers with dementia, stroke, and those who were not self-isolated at home were not eligible. The study protocol conformed to the guidelines set forth by the Declaration of Helsinki.

The self-isolate interval began on 10 March 2020 and ended on 30 April 2020 while the overall investigated interval began on 22 January 2019 and ended on 30 April 2020 (464 days).

To avoid bias in measurements among volunteers, we chose Fitbit Versa smartwatches, which allow for continuous recording of parameters: quality and duration of sleep, resting heart rate and the number of steps during the day. This choice was dictated by literature data which showed that the Fitbit Versa was 10 times more used in research projects and registered in ClinicalTrials than other brands [42].

Cardiovascular and Pre-Frailty Risk was assessed using a developed 4-point scale. The rationale for the selection of elements for the Cardiovascular and Pre-Frailty Risk Assessment is primarily the selection of available parameters measured with smartwatches and relating them to their suitability and usefulness for the elderly population, along with an appropriate justification of the selected parameters based on available literature data, cardiological (ESC) and geriatric guidelines and clinical experience. This scale could also be adapted in qualification for surgical procedures of the older adults. According to the ESC Guidelines (2016) [12], age is the dominant cardiovascular risk factor, but it should not be considered in isolation from other factors. Interestingly, Sergi et al. (2015) conducted a study with 1567 participants aged 65 to 96, which showed that pre-frailty is independently associated with a higher risk of developing cardiovascular disease in older adults [43]. The use of smartwatches to assess pre-frailty and cardiovascular risk is still unknown. We are the first to report the benefits of this type of measurement, especially among older adults. In our artificial intelligence-based approach to our Cardiovascular and Pre-Frailty Risk Assessment method, we mapped low physical activity (the component of frailty syndrome and cardiovascular risk) to fewer steps using the developed Python and Matlab scripts.

Aging is associated with a decreased ability not only to initiate but also to maintain sleep [44]. Deterioration of sleep in the older adults also correlates with deterioration of health and well-being. Sleep disturbances are very common in older patients with delirium. Delirium can be characterized by changes in the sleep-wake cycle and may be the first sign of deterioration in health, such as from infection [45–47].

In the Clinical point of view section, we emphasized the role of the resting heart rate as an important predictor of cardiovascular risk. Moreover, a recent study by Toosizadeh et al. (2021) suggested that measuring the dynamics of heart rate in response to daily activities could be a significant marker in screening for the frailty syndrome in older adults [48]. Our Cardiovascular and Pre-Frailty Risk Assessment method is a non-linear scale developed based on clinical practice. Reaching a high-risk state should be alarming and should prompt appropriate corrective action as it can still be reversible i.e., lifestyle change.

For validation we collected qualitative and narrative data from respondents using a proprietary questionnaire to verify the data collected by Fitbit Versa. The author's qualitative questionnaire covering sociodemographic status, self-assessment of changes in behavior, mood, sleep, physical activity, and daily activities was conducted by researchers using videoconferencing at the end of the shelter-in-place.

3.3. Methods

The analysis was performed on the basis of qualitative research and the descriptive statistics. Overall, we created a dataset consisting of 464 days of continuous measurements that included 50 days of self-isolation at home during the Covid-19 pandemic. We used Fitbit Versa (dimensions: $1.98 \times 3.98 \times 9.00$ inches) as a source of biomarkers, which is an advanced smartwatch featuring built-in wrist-based heart rate sensor, sleep tracker, accelerometer, 4 days battery life and Bluetooth wireless interface for Fitbit cloud communication. Data were extracted and analyzed from the Fitbit cloud application using developed Python and Matlab scripts. A quantitative and comparative study analysis was carried out using Python and Matlab.

The research was planned in such a way as to simultaneously compare changes in the measured physiological parameters, because the seasons have a large impact on the variability of human activity, e.g., in summer, human activity increases because it is warmer and there are more opportunities to spend time actively outdoors.

We believe that the comparison of physiological activity during hard lockdown with the same period in the preceding year is very reliable and reflects the real impact of the pandemic on human activity. A similar methodology was published by fitness tracker companies comparing the same periods to avoid confounding variables such as the seasons or holidays [49].

3.4. Statistical Analysis

For the purpose of statistical analysis, the study participants were divided into two groups: Group 1—professionally active participants (younger participants) and Group 2—octogenarians (participants aged $\geq$80 years). Descriptive statistics were based on the mean and standard deviation (SD). Student's t-test was used to determine significant differences between the pre-Covid-19 and Covid-19 dataset. $p < 0.05$ were considered statistically significant. Statistical analysis was performed using the Statistica 13 program.

3.5. Definitions

Throughout the text, the authors use the following terms: self-isolation and shelter-in-place to denote the period of the official policy of hard national lockdown, which was introduced in Poland on 10th March 2020, due to the Covid-19 pandemic and meant a total ban on leaving home, except for the necessity to make necessary purchases, going to work, church, with a dog or taking out the rubbish. The complete lockdown policy expired after the restrictions were relaxed on 30 April 2020. All study participants were self-isolated at home during the follow-up period. All working participants (three subjects) worked remotely from home.

4. Results

We analyzed the experimental dataset using dedicated scripts developed in Python and Matlab from five subjects of varying age, sex, marital, and occupational status. All study participants performed restrictive self-isolation at home during the lockdown period and wore a Fitbit Versa device during the self-isolation period. No study-related adverse events were reported during the study. The study showed that the lockdown policy affected the level of activity of all study participants compared to the same period of the previous year, as well as the appropriate period before self-isolation. However, the impact was less among participants aged 80 and older, whose activity before sheltering was moderate, according to data obtained by Fitbit Versa. The most significant impact of social distancing was observed among young, active adults, whose activity dropped dramatically during the lockdown. The comparison of the resting heart rate, number of steps, and sleep duration in the analyzed periods was showed in Table 2. General characteristics were presented in Table 3.

Table 2. The comparison of the resting heart rate, number of daily steps, sleep duration in the analyzed periods.

Variable		Pre-Covid-19		Covid-19		*p*-Value
		Mean	±SD	Mean	±SD	
Resting Heart Rate [bpm]	All	63.28	4.36	60.23	3.69	<0.001
	Group 1	65.17	3.28	61.80	2.18	<0.001
	Group 2	58.46	2.81	56.21	3.73	<0.001
Steps Count [results in thousands]	All	7550	4430	3230	1910	<0.001
	Group 1	9800	4570	3700	2160	<0.001
	Group 2	4750	2010	2640	1360	<0.001
Sleep Duration [min.]	All	423.79	81.84	416.97	97.12	0.499
	Group 1	422.02	86.07	430.67	86.21	0.441
	Group 2	429.64	66.80	371.73	117.19	0.008

Table legend: All—all participants, Group 1—professionally active participants (younger participants), Group 2—octogenarians (older participants), bpm—beats per minute, min—minutes, SD—standard deviation.

Table 3. General characteristics of the study participants.

Characteristic	Subject ID 1	Subject ID 2	Subject ID 3	Subject ID 4	Subject ID 5
Age	32	82	84	34	57
Gender	Female	Female	Male	Male	Female
Race	White	White	White	White	White
Marital Status	Single	Married	Married	Single	Divorced
Occupational Status	Employment	Pension	Pension	Employment	Employment
Number of Household Members	1	3	3	1	3
Current Smoker	No	No	No	No	No
Number of Diagnosed Chronic Diseases	0	8	9	1	1
Number of Chronic Medication Used	0	10	11	1	2
History of Cardiovascular Diseases:					
Hypertension	-	+	+	-	-
Chronic Heart Failure	-	+	+	-	-
Coronary Heart Disease	-	+	+	-	-
Atrial Fibrillation	-	-	+	-	-
Dyslipidemia	-	+	+	-	-
Type 2 Diabetes	-	+	-	-	-
Thyroid Disease	-	+	-	+	-
Functional Status:					
Uses Assistive Device for Ambulation	-	-	-	-	-
Able to Ambulate without Assistive Device	+	+	+	+	+

Table legend: + (yes), - (no).

4.1. Number of Daily Steps

We compared the number of daily steps taken during the self-isolation period with the number of daily steps taken in the same period of the year before without self-isolation. A good comparison of subject 1 is shown in Figure 1. In this comparison, we found a significant decline in the number of daily steps during lockdown (red color) in comparison to the same period in the previous year (blue color). In addition, we observed a significant decline in the number of daily steps during the lockdown in comparison to the period of 50 days prior to isolation (green color). In both cases, it was observed that self-isolation significantly disrupted the mobility of all study participants based on their number of daily steps.

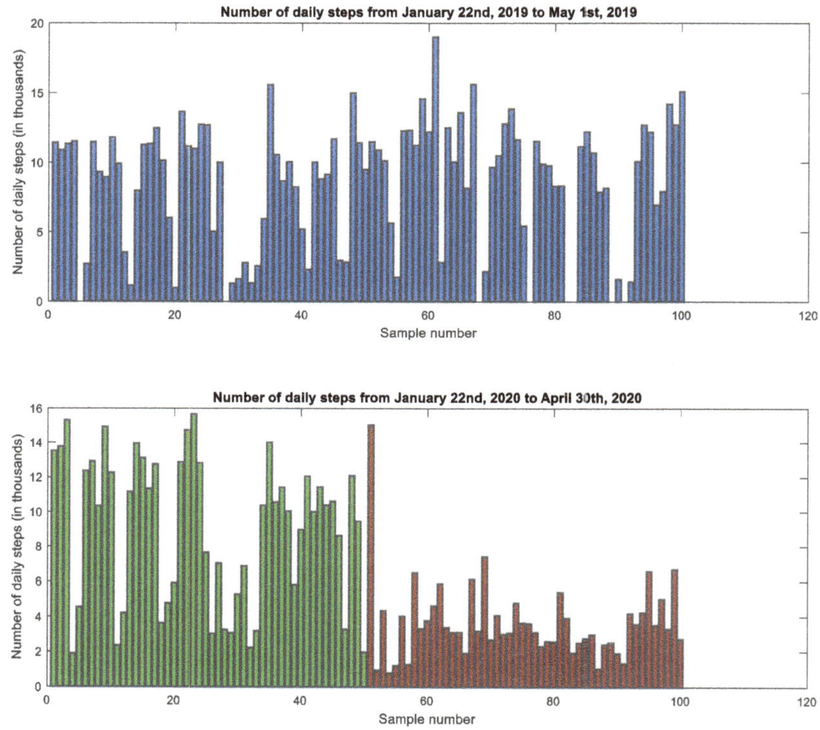

Figure 1. The number of daily steps in the analyzed intervals for Subject 1.

As can be seen in Figure 2, the total number of daily steps during the self-isolation period was significantly lower than the total number of daily steps in the control measures performed by all study participants in the previous year. Figures 3 and 4 show that both age groups had a significant ($p < 0.001$) decrease in the number of daily steps during the self-isolation period of Covid-19.

We found that in all study participants, the number of daily steps was lower in the self-isolation period compared to the time before sheltering in place (−57.21%; −4321; 95% CI, 3722 to 4920).

4.2. Resting Heart Rate

Resting heart rates (RHR) in the two analyzed intervals for Subject 4 are shown in Figure 5.

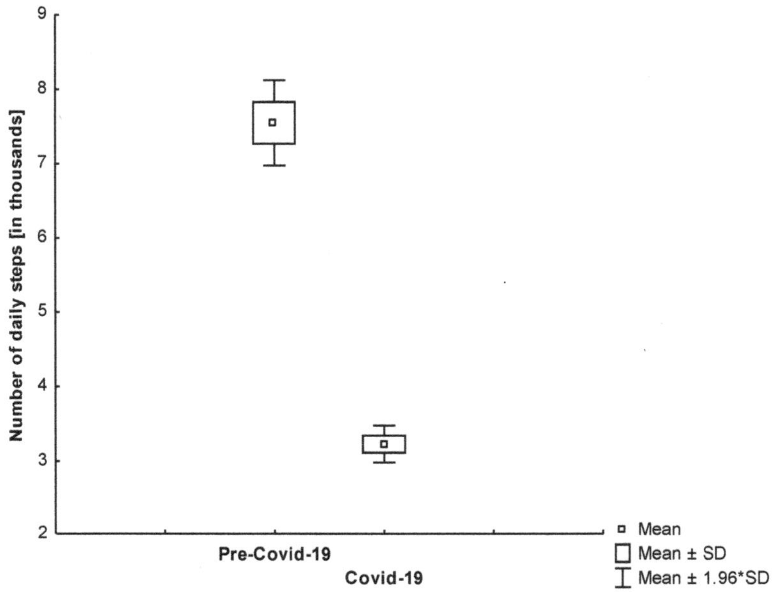

Figure 2. A comparison of the number of daily steps in the analyzed periods ($p < 0.001$).

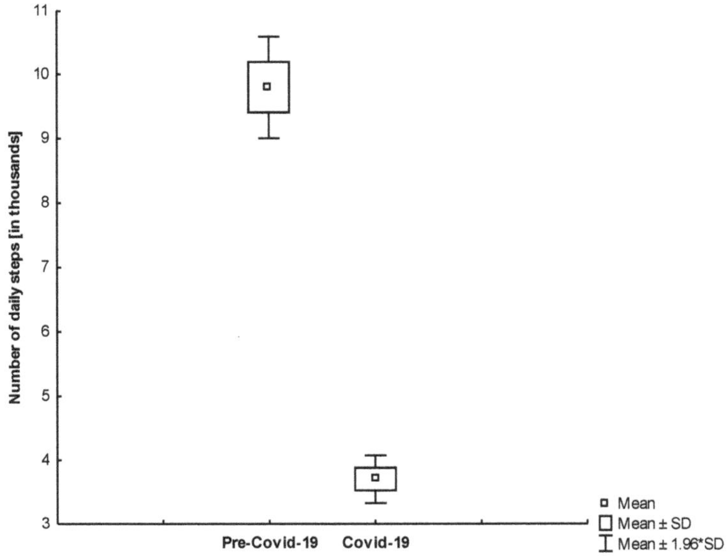

Figure 3. The comparison of the number of daily steps in the analyzed periods among young participants ($p < 0.001$).

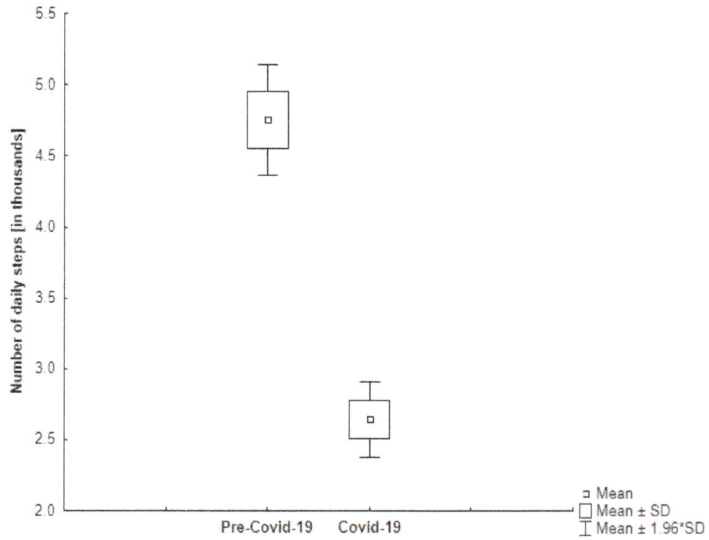

Figure 4. The comparison of the number of daily steps in the analyzed periods among older participants ($p < 0.001$).

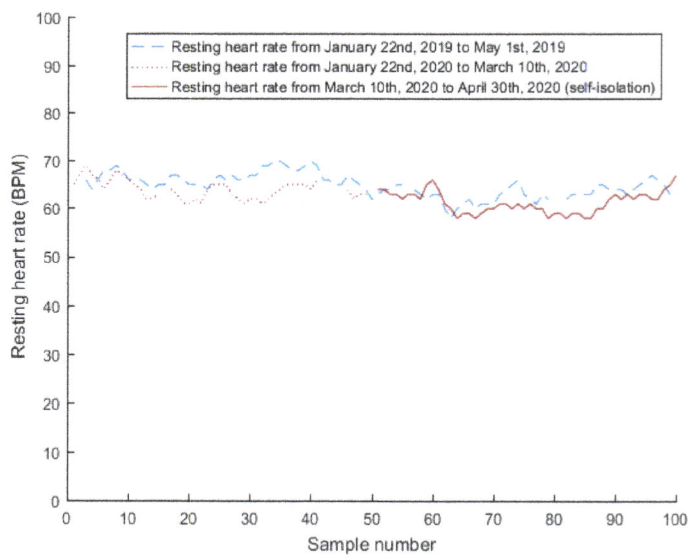

Figure 5. Resting heart rates (RHR) in the two analyzed intervals for Subject 4.

In our study, we observed that all participants in the study had a lower resting heart rate during self-isolation compared to the time before sheltering (−4.81%; −3.04; 95% CI, 2.59 to 3.51) which is shown in Figure 6. Interestingly, we found that the more active participants experienced a more significant decrease in their resting heart rate (Figure 7). However, we observed greater variability in resting heart rate in the elderly (Figure 8).

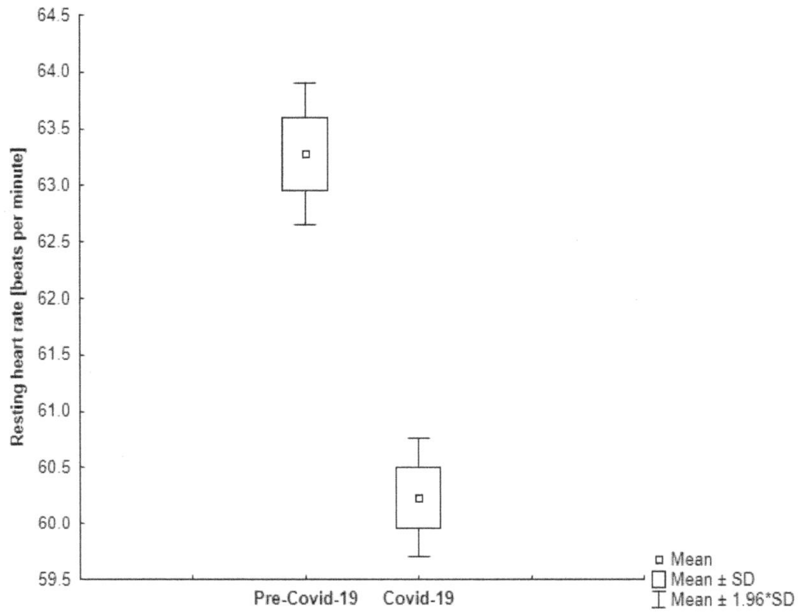

Figure 6. The comparison of the average resting heart rate in the analyzed periods ($p < 0.001$).

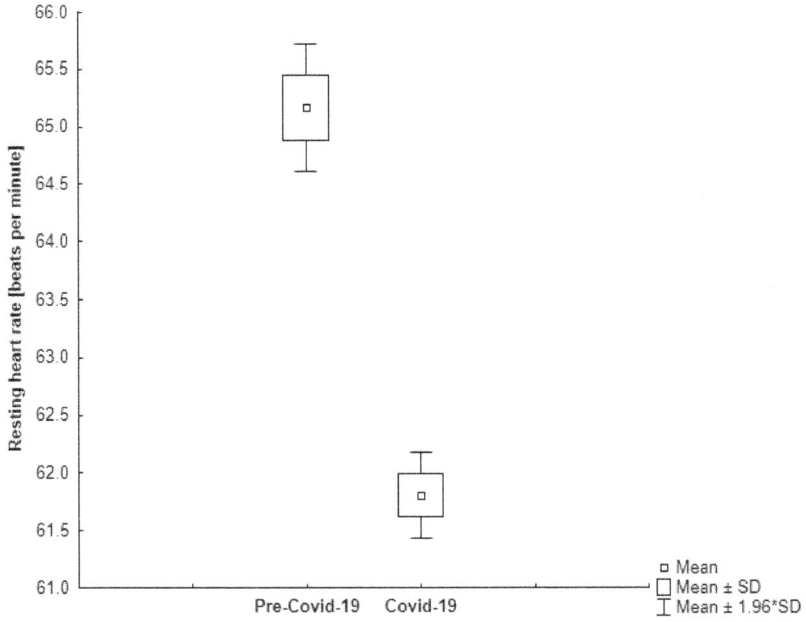

Figure 7. The comparison of the average resting heart rate in the analyzed periods among younger participants ($p < 0.001$).

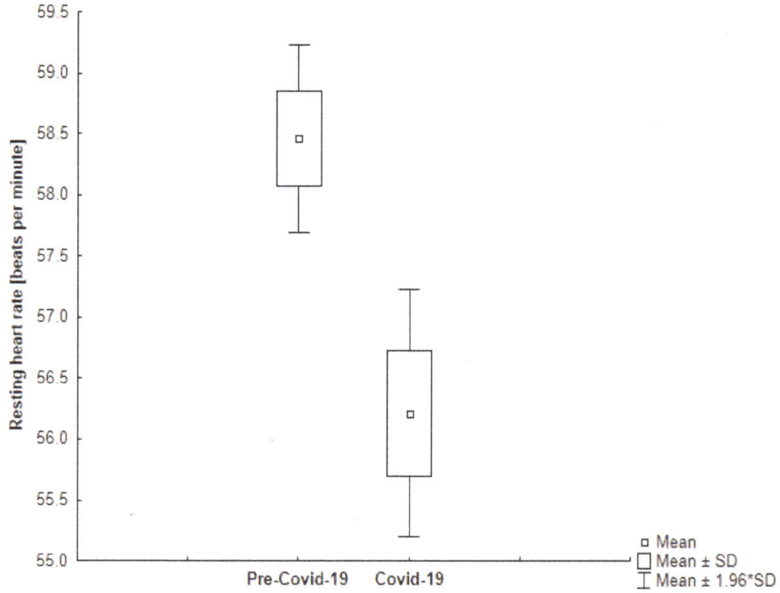

Figure 8. The comparison of the average resting heart rate in the analyzed periods among older participants ($p < 0.001$).

4.3. Sleep Duration and Quality

Our findings suggest that shelter-in-place measures a disrupted sleep duration. It turned out that the study participants went to bed later, and the results are challenging to interpret unequivocally.

We also found that the results differed by age group. Conversely, we noticed a significant drop in the average sleep time among octogenarians (−13.48%; −57.91; 95% CI, 16.33 to 99.49). The rest of the study participants did not significantly benefit from self-isolation in terms of sleep duration. Only one study participant had the same duration of sleep in both periods. We found that younger and active participants increased the length of sleep (Figure 9). The most physically and professionally active subject from our study group (Subject 1) had a significant increase in sleep time during the lockdown. The comparison of the average sleep time between reference and self-isolation for all study participants was shown in Figure 10. Interestingly, we found that the length of sleep in octogenarians decreased significantly during the Covid-19 period (Figure 11).

4.4. Cardiovascular and Pre-Frailty Risk Assessment Scores

We proposed the non-linear method to quantify the Cardiovascular and Pre-Frailty Risk based on the following digital biomarkers: daily steps, resting heart rate, sleep duration, and age. The method is based on scoring each parameter on a 2-point scale. The scores 5.5 and above are considered increased cardiovascular and pre-frailty risk. A specialist geriatrician was asked to assess the increased cardiovascular and pre-frailty risk. Our findings suggest that shelter-in-place measures increased cardiovascular and pre-frailty risk scores in the majority of participants. Cardiovascular and Pre-Frailty Risk Scores of subjects were shown in Table 4.

Table 4. Cardiovascular and Pre-Frailty Risk Assessment (reference versus self-isolation).

Biomarker	Subject ID 1		Subject ID 2		Subject ID 3		Subject ID 4		Subject ID 5	
	Reference	**Self-Isolation**	**Reference**	**Self-Isolation**	**Reference**	**Self-Isolation**	**Reference**	**Self-Isolation**	**Reference**	**Self-Isolation**
Daily steps	0.5	2	2	2	2	2	0.5	2	0.5	2
Resting heart rate	1	0.5	0	0	0.5	0.5	0.5	0.5	0.5	0.5
Sleep duration	0	0	2	2	0	2	0	2	0	0
Age	0	0	1.50	1.50	2	2	0	0	0	0
Cardiovascular and Pre-Frailty Risk score	1.5	2.5	5.5	5.5	4.5	6.5	1	4.5	1	2.5
Clinical validation–Cardiovascular and Pre-Frailty Risk	N	N	**Y**	**Y**	N	**Y**	N	N	N	N

Legend: N—no, Y—yes.

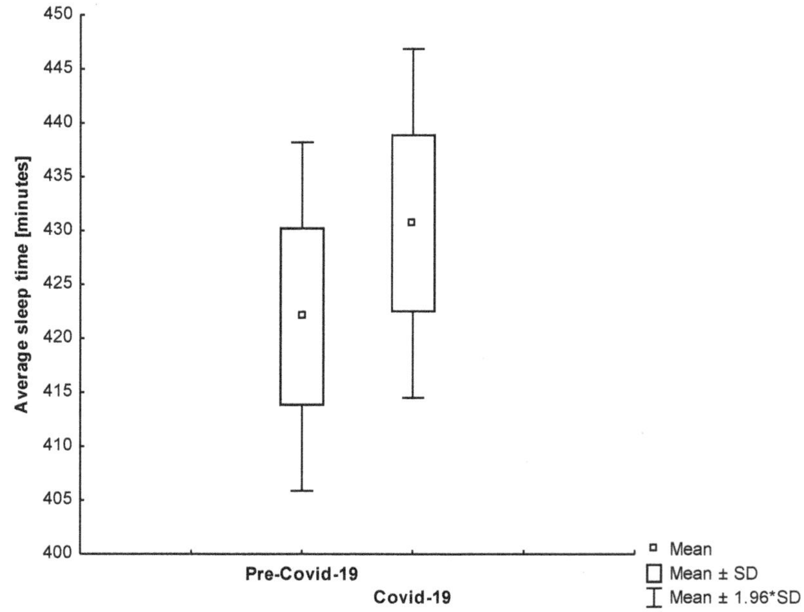

Figure 9. The comparison of the average sleep time in the analyzed periods among younger participants ($p = 0.441$).

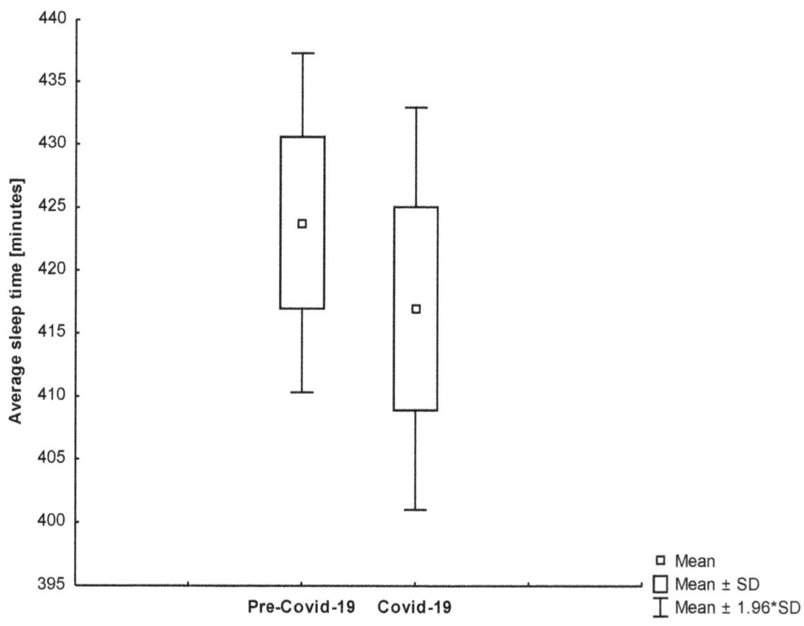

Figure 10. A comparison of the average sleep time between reference and self-isolation for all study participants ($p = 0.499$).

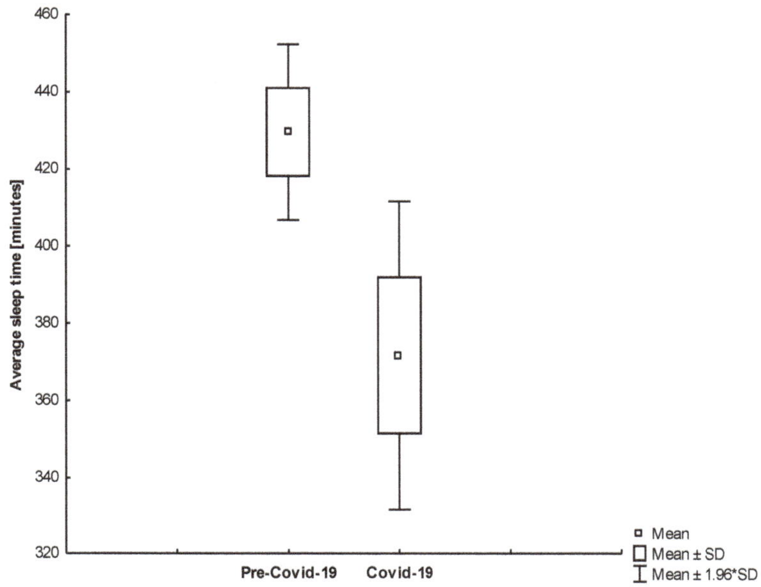

Figure 11. The comparison of the average sleep time in the analyzed periods among older participants ($p = 0.008$).

5. Discussion

Over the past decade, we witnessed the development of wearable devices equipped with biometric sensors, such as smartwatches or fitness trackers, which are ubiquitous in the lives of active people who focus on fitness and exercise. Smartwatches are able to measure heart rate, falls or number of steps accurately. We believe that these parameters contain important diagnostic or screening information that can be used in clinical practice, in particular as a basis for teleconsultation with a primary care physician and may indicate an early stage of the disease.

5.1. Smartwatch

The Covid-19 pandemic and lockdown policies revealed how important a tool the smartwatch could be during sheltering to monitor people's health and well-being. What is more, it could help doctors quickly diagnose and triage when healthcare systems are overwhelmed, and there is a shortage of medical personnel during a health crisis like the pandemic.

To the best of our knowledge, our study is the first to investigate the impact of a pandemic on activity levels measured using a smartwatch in the context of Cardiovascular and Pre-Frailty Risk Assessment. However, more research is needed to examine the safety and usefulness of this tool not only in diagnosing diseases but also in preventive strategies. The primary research contribution is information on how the complete lockdown at home affects the investigated parameters. Stay-at-home measures were shown be successful in limiting the spread of the infection, but it should not be forgotten that a sedentary lifestyle can lead to many cardiovascular complications [12]. Consequently, our results add to the state-of-the-art information about behavioral changes during a lockdown period and may help better support people by introducing an interactive exercise program in case of future lockdown policies.

Our findings reveal that self-isolation had an impact on health risk. Our results are consistent with the data provided by Fitbit, which conducted an analysis of the behavior of Fitbit users when shelter-in-place was ordered. The data showed that Fitbit users reacted to these policies and social distancing very quickly and thoughtfully, as a statistically significant decrease in the average number of steps was observed compared to the same period last year [49]. However, the severity of the decrease in the number of steps was found among European users, especially in Italy, Spain, Portugal, France, and Romania, in the range of a 7–38% decrease in the number of steps in the last week of March [49]. Interestingly, the largest decline was observed among users aged 18–29, with their steps between 16–23%, while users aged 65 and older had the lowest impact on activity levels (4–10%) [50]. A similar observation was also found in our study among octogenarians. This observation could be explained by the aging process and the tendency to decrease physical activity among older adults due to chronic diseases, frailty, sarcopenia, and disability [51]. Nowadays, the frailty syndrome in older adults—and its screening and diagnostic tools—are of great interest to many researchers [5].

Furthermore, it was observed that in locations with shelter-in-place mandates, the duration and quality of sleep shifted. People went to sleep later, but they had more sleep and quality rest. The quality of sleep was improved, which was visible in deep and REM sleep [52]. In contrast, in our study, we observed that most of the study participants experienced a significant reduction in sleep duration or did not improve sleep time during self-isolation, which could be due to poor sleep hygiene during the self-isolation period: lack of physical activity, eating or drinking before going to bed, working longer hours, or using a computer or smartphone before bedtime, which ultimately had a negative effect on sleep. Only one participant (subject 1) achieved the most significant benefit from the self-isolation period, which could be explained by fatigue and overwork before lockdown (it was the most active and working participant in the group). On the other hand, it could also be explained by the fact that Subject 1 regularly performed exercises during the self-isolation period, which had a positive impact on sleep. An interesting finding was also that most active people were affected to a greater extent by lockdown than those who were less active before. Octogenarians were less influenced by introduced measures because they had lower activity before. Our findings suggest that there was a significant reduction in the number of daily steps and resting heart rate for all study participants compared to the time before lockdown. We also believe that resting heart rate is an important indicator that plays a crucial role in managing anxiety and may be used as a metric for evaluating the stress level. This, apart from psychological surveys, can screen subjects with elevated stress levels or increased risk of medical condition e.g., fever.

Data provided by Fitbit demonstrated that social distancing and stay-at-home mandates affected all Fitbit users, but also proved that Fitbit users were actively involved in slowing the spread of the Covid-19. Contrary to the data published in the Fitbit study, in our study we carefully supervised study participants to ensure the proper study protocol and that our subject was completely isolated at home during the investigated period. However, in the Fitbit study, it was not possible to verify the quality of the data, as well as the correctness and coherence of the input data e.g., lack of information about wearing the device during all investigated period, obeying the lockdown, different lockdown dates and regulations in different countries, risk of sharing the device with family members, influence on results of unknown external factors, etc.

Our study had some limitations. The major limitation is the fact that our findings are based on a relatively small sample size. However, our study is rather a case study and could be an example of a restrictive lockdown policy, which was verified by researchers. What is more, our results are consistent with the results that were collectively presented by Fitbit globally and in different countries separately. Another limitation may be the selection of the time window for comparing lockdown state. The main limitation of our study was that researchers were unable to thoroughly verify that the participant was 100% adhering to the lockdown period. The developed pre-frailty risk assessment method is limited to five biomarkers and may be improved in the future if more health data can be harvested from the smartwatch i.e., glucose levels etc.

5.2. Telemedical Solutions during the Covid-19

Despite the many telemedical options available on the market that could offload hospitals and medical staff during the Covid-19 pandemic crisis, which dramatically hit many healthcare systems, especially in Italy, causing more than 24,000 deaths, there was no advocacy for using available telemedicine to provide continuity of care solutions for the chronically ill [39]. The only telemedical method used was a smartphone application for contact tracing. However, in a lockdown situation, an increase in the use of home telemonitoring systems to monitor vital signs was observed, which helped about half of the patients with chronic diseases to adjust the appropriate treatment [53]. Implemented remote patient-monitoring initiatives, such as Telehealth Intervention Programs for Seniors, that provide a weekly assessment of vital signs for low-income older people, can be an example of a successful program that reduces the number of hospital visits among older people [54].

One of the interesting telemedical solutions used in China during the Covid-19 pandemic was a mobile telehealth system, which was used to facilitate the presentation and discussion on the case study. This could help prevent the mobility of doctors in the hospital for consultation and decrease person-to-person contact to reduce the risk of transmission of infection between healthcare professionals [55].

According to the literature, the smartphone can be used as an adaptive physical activity smartphone intervention using a unique application supporting its positive effect on physical activity and a sedentary lifestyle [56]. However, during a pandemic and lockdown policy, smartphones do not seem to be such a useful tool to monitor the level of human activity because users do not wear them all the time at home.

The Covid-19 pandemic also had a significant impact on mental health. Isolation, social distancing, job loss, workload, and high exposure to coronavirus among healthcare professionals could lead to psychological distress and many adverse effects on mental health, including depressive symptoms, anxiety, burnout, and exacerbation of mental illness [57]. Telemental health services such as counseling, supervision, training, and psychoeducation via online platforms could provide adequate support to patients, family members, and health service providers during a pandemic [57].

5.3. The Post-Covid-19 Face of Telemedical Services

The pandemic redefined the use of primary care, healthcare services and the physical examination process. In the absence of data from physical examinations, the only source of information about the general health of the patient were smartwatches and home medical devices. We hypothesize that a novel category of medical devices is being introduced—a smartwatch or medical wearable device (certified in accordance with Regulation (EU) 2017/745 of the European Parliament and of the Council of 5 April 2017 on medical devices, PN-EN ISO 13485:2016 standards), which will focus on recording overall health on the basis of available data, which can be accurately recorded by wearable device sensors (e.g., smartwatch). These categories of devices may redefine the way primary care is delivered because physical examination can progress to remote examination, supported by data from a certified wearable medical device, which can improve diagnostic decisions and screening. The smartwatch already has the ability to synchronize health data with the cloud service, which allows easy remote sharing of health data with a primary care physician without additional cloud infrastructure. This allows for fast deployment of telemedical services based on wearable devices and scalability of solutions. Evaluation of the clinical effectiveness of wearable medical devices and mindset change of both healthcare professionals and patients are among important challenges in the adoption of wearable telemedical services. However, consideration should be given to ensuring the confidentiality, integrity, and security of sensitive medical data so as to prevent access by unauthorized persons. Other challenges include ensuring interoperability and supervision over the place where medical data is stored, along with compliance with related regulations and standards. Furthermore, there are wearable devices that are certified as medical devices and are FDA-approved for certain health indications, such as the Apple Watch and the Omron Health Guide Watch [58].

6. Conclusions

We presented a developed and validated methodology that we used to assess cardiovascular and pre-frailty risk during the Covid-19 shelter-in-place measures on human activity patterns based on multimodal biomarkers collected from smartwatch sensors. The developed method can be easily deployed in the software update of the smartwatches or other wearable devices and might be a useful health screening metric. We believe that in the future, smartwatches or novel wearable medical devices may play an essential role in telemedical services, especially during emergency scenarios or health crisis. However, the impact of long isolation on health is unknown and will be the subject of future research. Future research will also focus on human aspects during shelter-in-place measures. Our findings may be useful to policymakers and can be used to find solutions to support people, especially older adults, during the lockdown period and improve the quality of telemedical services.

Author Contributions: Conceptualization, E.K. and A.K. (clinical part); Data assessment, E.K.; Data processing, E.K. and A.K.; Analysis and interpretation, E.K. and A.K.; Writing—Original Draft Preparation, E.K. (lead) and A.K. Writing—Review & Editing, E.K.; A.K. Supervision, E.K.; Funding Acquisition, E.K. All authors have read and agreed to the published version of the manuscript.

Funding: This research was funded by AGH University of Science and Technology in 2019 as research project No. 16.16.120.773.

Institutional Review Board Statement: The study was conducted according to the guidelines of the Declaration of Helsinki, ethical review and approval were waived for this study, due to University guidelines for noninvasive retrospective studies.

Informed Consent Statement: Informed consent was obtained from all subjects involved in the study.

Data Availability Statement: The data presented in this study are available on request from the corresponding author.

Acknowledgments: Authors thank the anonymous reviewers for their valuable comments regarding the improvement of this manuscript.

Conflicts of Interest: The authors declare no conflict of interest. The funders had no role in the design of the study; in the collection, analyses, or interpretation of data; in the writing of the manuscript, or in the decision to publish the results.

References

1. Keesara, S.; Jonas, A.; Schulman, K. Covid-19 and Health Care's Digital Revolution. *N. Engl. J. Med.* **2020**, *382*, e82. [CrossRef]
2. Sim, I. Mobile Devices and Health. *N. Engl. J. Med.* **2019**, *381*, 956–968. [CrossRef]
3. Kańtoch, E.; Kańtoch, A. What Features and Functions Are Desired in Telemedical Services Targeted at Polish Older Adults Delivered by Wearable Medical Devices?—Pre-COVID-19 Flashback. *Sensors* **2020**, *20*, 5181. [CrossRef]
4. Semaan, S.; Dewland, T.A.; Tison, G.H.; Nah, G.; Vittinghoff, E.; Pletcher, M.J.; Olgin, J.E.; Marcus, G.M. Physical activity and atrial fibrillation: Data from wearable fitness trackers. *Heart Rhythm* **2020**, *17*, 842–846. [CrossRef] [PubMed]
5. Kańtoch, A.; Gryglewska, B.; Wizner, B.; Parnicka, A.; Grodzicki, T. Assumptions of the European FRAILTOOLS project and description of the recruitment process for this study in Poland. *Folia Med. Cracov.* **2020**, *60*, 15–23. [CrossRef] [PubMed]
6. Turner, G.; Clegg, A. Best practice guidelines for the management of frailty: A British Geriatrics Society, Age UK and Royal College of General Practitioners report. *Age Ageing* **2014**, *43*, 744–747. [CrossRef] [PubMed]
7. Fried, L.P.; Tangen, C.M.; Walston, J.; Newman, A.B.; Hirsch, C.; Gottdiener, J.; Seeman, T.; Tracy, R.; Kop, W.J.; Burke, G.; et al. Frailty in older adults: Evidence for a phenotype. *J. Gerontol. A Biol. Sci. Med. Sci.* **2001**, *56*, M146–M156. [CrossRef] [PubMed]
8. Bandeen-Roche, K.; Seplaki, C.L.; Huang, J.; Buta, B.; Kalyani, R.R.; Varadhan, R.; Xue, Q.L.; Walston, J.D.; Kasper, J.D. Frailty in Older Adults: A Nationally Representative Profile in the United States. *J. Gerontol. Ser. A Biol. Sci. Med. Sci.* **2015**, *70*, 1427–1434. [CrossRef]
9. Garcia-Garcia, F.J.; Gutierrez Avila, G.; Alfaro-Acha, A.; Amor Andres, M.S.; De Los Angeles De La Torre Lanza, M.; Escribano Aparicio, M.V.; Humanes Aparicio, S.; Larrion Zugasti, J.L.; Gomez-Serranillo Reus, M.; Rodriguez-Artalejo, F.; et al. The prevalence of frailty syndrome in an older population from Spain. The Toledo Study for Healthy Aging. *J. Nutr. Health Aging* **2011**, *15*, 852–856. [CrossRef]

10. Gjaka, M.; Feka, K.; Bianco, A.; Tishukaj, F.; Giustino, V.; Parroco, A.M.; Palma, A.; Battaglia, G. The Effect of COVID-19 Lockdown Measures on Physical Activity Levels and Sedentary Behaviour in a Relatively Young Population Living in Kosovo. *J. Clin. Med.* **2021**, *10*, 763. [CrossRef] [PubMed]
11. Kehler, D.S.; Hay, J.L.; Stammers, A.N.; Hamm, N.C.; Kimber, D.E.; Schultz, A.S.; Szwajcer, A.; Arora, R.C.; Tangri, N.; Duhamel, T.A. A systematic review of the association between sedentary behaviors with frailty. *Exp. Gerontol.* **2018**, *114*, 1–12. [CrossRef]
12. ESC Clinical Practice Guidelines: CVD Prevention in Clinical Practice (European Guidelines on) Guidelines. Available online: https://www.escardio.org/Guidelines/Clinical-Practice-Guidelines/CVD-Prevention-in-clinical-practice-European-Guidelines-on (accessed on 1 August 2020).
13. Kańtoch, A.; Gryglewska, B.; Wójkowska-Mach, J.; Heczko, P.; Grodzicki, T. Treatment of Cardiovascular Diseases among Elderly Residents of Long-term Care Facilities. *J. Am. Med. Dir. Assoc.* **2018**, *19*, 428–432. [CrossRef]
14. Yazdanyar, A.; Newman, A.B. The burden of cardiovascular disease in the elderly: Morbidity, mortality, and costs. *Clin. Geriatr. Med.* **2009**, *25*, 563–577. [CrossRef]
15. Yuki, A.; Otsuka, R.; Tange, C.; Nishita, Y.; Tomida, M.; Ando, F.; Shimokata, H.; Arai, H. Daily Physical Activity Predicts Frailty Development among Community-Dwelling Older Japanese Adults. *J. Am. Med. Dir. Assoc.* **2019**, *20*, 1032–1036. [CrossRef]
16. Trost, S.G.; Owen, N.; Bauman, A.E.; Sallis, J.F.; Brown, W. Correlates of adults' participation in physical activity: Review and update. *Med. Sci. Sports Exerc.* **2002**, *34*, 1996–2001. [CrossRef] [PubMed]
17. Johnson, D.; Deterding, S.; Kuhn, K.A.; Staneva, A.; Stoyanov, S.; Hides, L. Gamification for health and wellbeing: A systematic review of the literature. *Internet Interv.* **2016**, *6*, 89–106. [CrossRef] [PubMed]
18. Taylor, L.; Kerse, N.; Klenk, J.; Borotkanics, R.; Maddison, R. Exergames to Improve the Mobility of Long-Term Care Residents: A Cluster Randomized Controlled Trial. *Games Health J.* **2018**, *7*, 37–42. [CrossRef]
19. Bonnechere, B.; Van Vooren, M.; Jansen, B.; Van Sint, J.S.; Rahmoun, M.; Fourtassi, M. Patients' Acceptance of the Use of Serious Games in Physical Rehabilitation in Morocco. *Games Health J.* **2017**, *6*, 290–294. [CrossRef] [PubMed]
20. Gopinathannair, R.; Olshansky, B. Management of tachycardia. *F1000Prime Rep.* **2015**, *7*, 60. [CrossRef]
21. Saxena, A.; Minton, D.; Lee, D.C.; Sui, X.; Fayad, R.; Lavie, C.J.; Blair, S.N. Protective role of resting heart rate on all-cause and cardiovascular disease mortality. *Mayo Clin. Proc.* **2013**, *88*, 1420–1426. [CrossRef] [PubMed]
22. Zhang, D.; Shen, X.; Qi, X. Resting heart rate and all-cause and cardiovascular mortality in the general population: A meta-analysis. *CMAJ* **2016**, *188*, E53–E63. [CrossRef]
23. Arnold, J.M.; Fitchett, D.H.; Howlett, J.G.; Lonn, E.M.; Tardif, J.C. Resting heart rate: A modifiable prognostic indicator of cardiovascular risk and outcomes? *Can. J. Cardiol.* **2008**, *24* (Suppl. A), 3A–8A. [CrossRef]
24. Aune, D.; Sen, A.; o'Hartaigh, B.; Janszky, I.; Romundstad, P.R.; Tonstad, S.; Vatten, L.J. Resting heart rate and the risk of cardiovascular disease, total cancer, and all-cause mortality—A systematic review and dose-response meta-analysis of prospective studies. *Nutr. Metab. Cardiovasc. Dis.* **2017**, *27*, 504–517. [CrossRef] [PubMed]
25. Medic, G.; Wille, M.; Hemels, M.E. Short- and long-term health consequences of sleep disruption. *Nat. Sci. Sleep* **2017**, *9*, 151–161. [CrossRef] [PubMed]
26. Bin, Y.S. Is Sleep Quality More Important Than Sleep Duration for Public Health? *Sleep* **2016**, *39*, 1629–1630. [CrossRef] [PubMed]
27. Chaput, J.P.; Dutil, C.; Sampasa-Kanyinga, H. Sleeping hours: What is the ideal number and how does age impact this? *Nat. Sci. Sleep* **2018**, *10*, 421–430. [CrossRef] [PubMed]
28. Alvarez, G.G.; Ayas, N.T. The impact of daily sleep duration on health: A review of the literature. *Prog. Cardiovasc. Nurs.* **2004**, *19*, 56–59. [CrossRef]
29. Cappuccio, F.P.; D'Elia, L.; Strazzullo, P.; Miller, M.A. Sleep duration and all-cause mortality: A systematic review and meta-analysis of prospective studies. *Sleep* **2010**, *33*, 585–592. [CrossRef] [PubMed]
30. Rezaei, M.; Khormali, M.; Akbarpour, S.; Sadeghniiat-Hagighi, K.; Shamsipour, M. Sleep quality and its association with psychological distress and sleep hygiene: A cross-sectional study among pre-clinical medical students. *Sleep Sci.* **2018**, *11*, 274–280. [CrossRef] [PubMed]
31. Harvey, A.G.; Stinson, K.; Whitaker, K.L.; Moskovitz, D.; Virk, H. The subjective meaning of sleep quality: A comparison of individuals with and without insomnia. *Sleep* **2008**, *31*, 383–393. [CrossRef] [PubMed]
32. Chen, H.C.; Hsu, N.W.; Chou, P. Subgrouping Poor Sleep Quality in Community-Dwelling Older Adults with Latent Class Analysis—The Yilan Study, Taiwan. *Sci. Rep.* **2020**, *10*, 5432. [CrossRef] [PubMed]
33. Le Hello, C.; Trombert, B.; Morel, A.; Chieh, A.; Brouard, B.; Boissier, C. Performance analysis of walking of 10,000 regular users of a connected activity tracker. *J. Med. Vasc.* **2018**, *43*, 231–237. [CrossRef]
34. Saint-Maurice, P.F.; Troiano, R.P.; Bassett, D.R., Jr.; Graubard, B.I.; Carlson, S.A.; Shiroma, E.J.; Fulton, J.E.; Matthews, C.E. Association of Daily Step Count and Step Intensity with Mortality among US Adults. *JAMA* **2020**, *323*, 1151–1160. [CrossRef]
35. King, C.E.; Sarrafzadeh, M. A Survey of Smartwatches in Remote Health Monitoring. *J. Health Inf. Res.* **2018**, *2*, 1–24. [CrossRef]
36. Guk, K.; Han, G.; Lim, J.; Jeong, K.; Kang, T.; Lim, E.K.; Jung, J. Evolution of Wearable Devices with Real-Time Disease Monitoring for Personalized Healthcare. *Nanomaterials* **2019**, *9*, 813. [CrossRef]
37. Kańtoch, E. Recognition of Sedentary Behavior by Machine Learning Analysis of Wearable Sensors during Activities of Daily Living for Telemedical Assessment of Cardiovascular Risk. *Sensors* **2018**, *18*, 3219. [CrossRef] [PubMed]
38. Tudor-Locke, C.; Bassett, D.R., Jr. How many steps/day are enough? Preliminary pedometer indices for public health. *Sports Med.* **2004**, *34*, 1–8. [CrossRef]

39. Bassett, D.R., Jr.; Toth, L.P.; LaMunion, S.R.; Crouter, S.E. Step Counting: A Review of Measurement Considerations and Health-Related Applications. *Sports Med.* **2017**, *47*, 1303–1315. [CrossRef] [PubMed]
40. Kado, D.M.; Lui, L.Y.; Cummings, S.R.; Study of Osteoporotic Fractures Research Group. Rapid resting heart rate: A simple and powerful predictor of osteoporotic fractures and mortality in older women. *J. Am. Geriatr. Soc.* **2002**, *50*, 455–460. [CrossRef]
41. World Health Organization. *Men, Ageing and Health: Achieving Health Across the Life Span*; World Health Organization: Geneva, Switzerland, 2001; pp. 1–63. Available online: https://apps.who.int/iris/bitstream/handle/10665/66941/WHO_NMH_NPH_01.2.pdf;jsessioni (accessed on 22 March 2021).
42. Henriksen, A.; Haugen Mikalsen, M.; Woldaregay, A.Z.; Muzny, M.; Hartvigsen, G.; Hopstock, L.A.; Grimsgaard, S. Using Fitness Trackers and Smartwatches to Measure Physical Activity in Research: Analysis of Consumer Wrist-Worn Wearables. *J. Med. Internet. Res.* **2018**, *20*, e110. [CrossRef]
43. Sergi, G.; Veronese, N.; Fontana, L.; De Rui, M.; Bolzetta, F.; Zambon, S.; Corti, M.C.; Baggio, G.; Toffanello, E.D.; Crepaldi, G.; et al. Pre-frailty and risk of cardiovascular disease in elderly men and women: The Pro.V.A. study. *J. Am. Coll. Cardiol.* **2015**, *65*, 976–983. [CrossRef] [PubMed]
44. Mander, B.A.; Winer, J.R.; Walker, M.P. Sleep and Human Aging. *Neuron* **2017**, *94*, 19–36. [CrossRef] [PubMed]
45. Watson, P.L.; Ceriana, P.; Fanfulla, F. Delirium: Is sleep important? Best practice & research. *Clin. Anaesthesiol.* **2012**, *26*, 355–366. [CrossRef]
46. Kukreja, D.; Günther, U.; Popp, J. Delirium in the elderly: Current problems with increasing geriatric age. *Indian J. Med. Res.* **2015**, *142*, 655–662. [CrossRef] [PubMed]
47. Oh, E.S.; Fong, T.G.; Hshieh, T.T.; Inouye, S.K. Delirium in Older Persons: Advances in Diagnosis and Treatment. *JAMA* **2017**, *318*, 1161–1174. [CrossRef]
48. Toosizadeh, N.; Ehsani, H.; Parthasarathy, S.; Carpenter, B.; Ruberto, K.; Mohler, J.; Parvaneh, S. Frailty and heart response to physical activity. *Arch. Gerontol. Geriatr.* **2021**, *93*, 104323. [CrossRef] [PubMed]
49. The Impact of Coronavirus on Global Activity. Available online: https://blog.fitbit.com/covid-19-global-activity/ (accessed on 1 August 2020).
50. Are People Actually Sheltering-in-Place? Fitbit Looks at Steps to Find Out. Available online: https://blog.fitbit.com/social-distancing-mobility/ (accessed on 1 August 2020).
51. McPhee, J.S.; French, D.P.; Jackson, D.; Nazroo, J.; Pendleton, N.; Degens, H. Physical activity in older age: Perspectives for healthy ageing and frailty. *Biogerontology* **2016**, *17*, 567–580. [CrossRef] [PubMed]
52. The Impact of COVID-19 on Global Sleep Patterns. Available online: https://blog.fitbit.com/covid-19-sleep-patterns/?utm_source=ET&utm_medium=EM&utm_campaign=20200412_WB2_WW_FM_E_EI_FT_00_NA&utm_content=covidsleep+ (accessed on 1 August 2020).
53. Omboni, S. Telemedicine during the COVID-19 in Italy: A Missed Opportunity? *Telemed. J. e-Health* **2020**. [CrossRef]
54. Hamilton, T.; Johnson, L.; Quinn, B.T.; Coppola, J.; Sachs, D.; Migliaccio, J.; Phipps, C.; Schwartz, J.; Capasso, M.; Carpenter, M.; et al. Telehealth Intervention Programs for Seniors: An Observational Study of a Community-Embedded Health Monitoring Initiative. *Telemed. J. e-Health* **2020**, *26*, 438–445. [CrossRef] [PubMed]
55. Ren, X.; Zhai, Y.; Song, X.; Wang, Z.; Dou, D.; Li, Y. The Application of Mobile Telehealth System to Facilitate Patient Information Presentation and Case Discussion. *Telemed. J. e-Health* **2020**, *26*, 725–733. [CrossRef]
56. Direito, A.; Tooley, M.; Hinbarji, M.; Albatal, R.; Jiang, Y.; Whittaker, R.; Maddison, R. Tailored Daily Activity: An Adaptive Physical Activity Smartphone Intervention. *Telemed. J. e-Health* **2020**, *26*, 426–437. [CrossRef]
57. Zhou, X.; Snoswell, C.L.; Harding, L.E.; Bambling, M.; Edirippulige, S.; Bai, X.; Smith, A.C. The Role of Telehealth in Reducing the Mental Health Burden from COVID-19. *Telemed. J. e-Health* **2020**, *26*, 377–379. [CrossRef]
58. Omron Health Guide Watch. Available online: https://omronhealthcare.com/products/heartguide-wearable-blood-pressure-monitor-bp8000m/ (accessed on 1 August 2020).

Journal of
Clinical Medicine

MDPI

Article

A Well-Structured Follow-Up Program is Required after Recovery from Coronavirus Disease 2019 (COVID-19); Release from Quarantine is Not the End of Treatment

Keun-Mi Lee [1], Hae-Jin Ko [2,*], Geon Ho Lee [3], A-Sol Kim [4] and Dong-Wook Lee [5]

1 Yeungnam University Medical Center, Department of Family Medicine, School of Medicine, Yeungnam University, Daegu 42415, Korea; kmlee@yu.ac.kr
2 Department of Family Medicine, School of Medicine, Kyungpook National University, Kyungpook National University Hospital, Daegu 41944, Korea
3 Department of Family Medicine, Daegu Catholic University School of Medicine, Daegu 42472, Korea; totoslee@cu.ac.kr
4 Department of Family Medicine, School of Medicine, Kyungpook National University, Kyungpook National University Chilgok Hospital, Deagu 41404, Korea; deepai@knu.ac.kr
5 Department of Family Medicine, Dongguk University Gyeongju Hospital, Gyeongju 38067, Korea; fmleedu@dongguk.ac.kr
* Correspondence: liveforme@knu.ac.kr; Tel.: +82-53-200-6578

Citation: Lee, K.-M.; Ko, H.-J.; Lee, G.H.; Kim, A.-S.; Lee, D.-W. A Well-Structured Follow-Up Program is Required after Recovery from Coronavirus Disease 2019 (COVID-19); Release from Quarantine is Not the End of Treatment. *J. Clin. Med.* **2021**, *10*, 2329. https://doi.org/10.3390/jcm10112329

Academic Editor: Michele Roccella

Received: 2 April 2021
Accepted: 24 May 2021
Published: 26 May 2021

Publisher's Note: MDPI stays neutral with regard to jurisdictional claims in published maps and institutional affiliations.

Abstract: During the Coronavirus Infection Disease-19 (COVID-19) pandemic, the number of patients released from quarantine is exceeding the number of newly diagnosed cases. This study is a retrospective cohort study in which consultation data were collected from a COVID-19 follow-up health consultation program. The studied population was selected from patients who recovered after quarantine and treatment for COVID-19 in Daegu City and in Gyeongsangbukdo province, Korea, from March to June 2020. The healthcare providers comprised 20 family-medicine specialists who consulted and educated the patients through phone calls in accordance with structured guidelines. Physical and mental status before and after recovery were compared among patients who received a single consultation and those who received two or more consultations. A total of 1604 subjects were selected for the final analysis. Of these, 1145 (71.4%) had one consultation and 459 (28.6%) had two or more. The group that had two or more consultations reported significantly more physical symptoms, more psychological symptoms (including depression), and more psychological stress. Multivariate forward selection logistic regression analysis showed that re-confirmed cases of COVID-19, physical symptoms after quarantine, feelings of depression, and psychological stress had a significant effect on the number of consultations received. In conclusion, COVID-19 has various physical and mental sequelae after discharge from quarantine. Therefore, a well-structured follow-up program is needed after recovery.

Keywords: COVID-19; consultation; comprehensive health care; mental health; pandemics

1. Introduction

Coronavirus Infectious Disease-19 (hereafter referred to as COVID-19), is a respiratory syndrome caused by the SARS-CoV-2 virus that began with an outbreak in Wuhan City, China, in December 2019; since then, it has spread rapidly worldwide [1,2]. In Korea, the 31st patient with COVID-19 was confirmed in Daegu City on 19 February 2020; after that, the disease spread nationwide and prompted the Korean government to raise the infectious disease crisis alert to "serious" on 23 February 2020 [1]. On 12 March, the WHO declared COVID-19 to be a pandemic [3]. COVID-19 has a high basic reproduction number (R0) of 1.9–6.5; however, ~81% of patients are asymptomatic or have mild symptoms [4]. The most common symptoms are fever, fatigue, and a dry cough, although a considerable number of patients report anosmia (loss of the sense of smell) [5].

At the time of writing, Korea has reported >70,000 confirmed cases and >100 million infections; more than 2 million deaths have been reported worldwide and the numbers continue to rise. The number of confirmed cases and the number of people released from quarantine after full recovery is also increasing rapidly [1]. According to the Center for Disease Control and Prevention, release from quarantine is allowed under the following circumstances: absence of fever without the need for antipyretic drugs; improved clinical symptoms for a minimum period of 72 h at 10 days post-onset; and two negative COVID-19 (polymerase chain reaction, (PCR)) tests with an interval of at least 24 h [1]. Since March 2020, when the number of confirmed cases in Korea increased rapidly, the number of patients that recovered began to rise; as of 29 January 2021, the number of recovered patients had reached 66,503, which was seven times that in quarantine [1].

Patients who recover from an infectious disease may experience several sequelae. For example, severe acute respiratory syndrome (SARS) was prevalent in China from 2002 to 2004, and those who recovered had significant psychological problems lasting up to three months post-discharge. Problems included a marked deterioration in quality of life, post-traumatic stress disorder, depression, and anxiety [6]. Furthermore, 44.1% of patients complained of post-traumatic stress disorder even at four months post-discharge [7]. For patients hospitalized in an intensive care unit (ICU) due to severe disease, physical quality of life functions were significantly affected [6], Similarly, ~36% of patients with Middle East Respiratory Syndrome (MERS) reported sequelae such as pulmonary fibrosis even after successful discharge [8]. Therefore, data from patients who recovered from SARS and MERS suggest that COVID-19 is highly likely to have physical or psychological sequelae; indeed, COVID-19 leads to additional health problems such as respiratory symptoms, cognitive impairment, anxiety, depressive symptoms, insomnia, denial, anger, and post-traumatic stress [9,10]. Thus, patient care with psychological support after discharge is an important factor to consider.

An unusual aspect of COVID-19 is that people released from quarantine can test positive again. In China, several such cases have been reported [11,12]. In Korea, many people tested positive for COVID-19 within a short period after viral clearance. The Central Clinical Committee regards this phenomenon as being caused by genetic material from the remaining "dead virus" rather than by a live virus [13]. However, because the period of re-confirmation after a negative virus PCR test varies from 4 to 17 days [12], and re-infection, but not re-confirmation, after recovery is possible [14], there is no question that patients need appropriate care and screening for the recurrence of symptoms, even after discharge.

However, unlike programs designed to increase diagnosis and survival rates, care programs for recovered COVID-19 patients returning to the community are insufficient. Daegu Metropolitan city and Gyeongsangbukdo province had >75% of confirmed COVID-19 cases in Korea; this is because the virus spread via some local religious groups from February to April 2020, the initial period of disease spread in Korea. As mentioned above, the number of patients released from quarantine exceeds the number of new diagnoses; therefore, the proportion of recovered patients in Daegu city and Gyeongsangbukdo province was the highest in Korea [1]. Thus, the Daegu—Gyeongsangbukdo branch of the Korean Family Medicine Association developed a follow-up health consultation program for patients that recovered from COVID-19: 20 family-medicine faculties, in co-operation with Daegu and the Daegu Medical Association, volunteered to begin providing consultations for those who agreed to participate in the program. To the best of our knowledge, this program is the first of its kind in the world. This study investigated the need for, and the results of, a well-structured follow-up program for people who recovered from COVID-19.

2. Materials and Methods

2.1. Study Design and Subjects

This study is a retrospective cohort study in which consultation data were collected from the COVID-19 follow-up health consultation program and analyzed retrospectively. The program for recovered patients started on 9 March and ended on 5 June 2020. During this period, all patients who had been released from quarantine in Gyeongsangbukdo province were asked to participate in the consultation program in Daegu [15]. As of the date of approval of the research protocol, 1679 (26.9%) of 6247 recovered patients agreed to participate.

A diagnosis of COVID-19 was based upon the isolation of the SARS-CoV-2 virus from a nasopharyngeal sample or detection of a specific gene in a PCR test. A recovered patient was defined as an individual who had met the following clinical and test criteria: absence of fever, improvement in clinical symptoms without the need for antipyretic drugs, and negative results from two PCR tests conducted with an interval of at least 24 h [1]. Subjects who (i) withdrew consent for consultation, (ii) did not respond or could not be contacted by phone, and (iii) were under 18 years-of-age and did not have consent from the primary guardian were excluded. The study complied with the tenets of the Helsinki Declaration and was approved by the Institutional Review Board of the local hospital (protocol No. YUMC 2020-04-112).

Selected subjects were classified into two groups in accordance with the total number of consultations received during the study period: those who required or requested one consultation and those who required or requested more than one consultation.

2.2. Methods

2.2.1. A Follow-Up Health Consultation Program after Recovery from COVID-19

The follow-up health consultation program for recovered patients was developed by the Daegu-Gyeongsangbukdo branch of the Korean Family Medicine Association in co-operation with Metropolitan Daegu and the Daegu Medical Association to encourage the provision of health care for patients released from quarantine. The program is described in detail elsewhere [15]. The professional healthcare providers comprised 20 family-medicine specialists who were willing to volunteer for the program; these providers undertook consultations in accordance with structured guidelines published by the Daegu-Gyeongsangbukdo branch of the Korean Family Medicine Association. Using a mobile phone dedicated to individual patient consultations, they called all patients who agreed to participate and asked them about their physical and mental health status. Moreover, they provided emotional support, such as encouragement and reassurance, along with health education to minimize the risk of spreading the virus in the community and to make patients aware of the possibility of reactivation or re-infection of the disease. Each patient was able to call the cellphone of the doctor in charge at any time; if the phone was not answered, the patient received a call-back. In situations requiring further evaluation and treatment, doctors provided medical advice to enable the patient to visit a medical institution or hospital promptly. Patients were provided with a guide for self-care after discharge, the aim of which was to educate them about COVID-19.

2.2.2. General Characteristics of the Subjects and their Symptoms before Release from Quarantine

The general characteristics of the selected subjects included sex, age, underlying disease (past history), and drug use. Information related to COVID-19 included the dates of confirmation, hospitalization, and discharge, the status of hospitalization (inpatient facility or medical institution), and any period in an ICU. For those released from self-quarantine without having to be admitted to a medical institution, the date of diagnosis and the date of release from quarantine were recorded. Moreover, the primary clinical symptoms experienced during the 7 days prior to diagnosis were noted. Clinical symptoms included fever, cough, excess sputum, sore throat, rhinorrhea, nasal congestion, dysosmia, anosmia, dysgeusia, pressure or discomfort in the chest, dyspnea, myalgia, headache, fatigue and malaise, diarrhea, and abdominal discomfort. Asymptomatic cases were also recorded.

2.2.3. Evaluation of Physical Condition after Release from Quarantine

To evaluate the physical condition of patients released from quarantine, symptoms suggestive of recurrence were verified such as shortness of breath, a clinically possible sequela, cough, olfactory abnormality, and headache. Moreover, patients were asked to rate their general physical condition after release from quarantine using a five-point Likert scale: "much better", "slightly better", "similar", "slightly worse", and "much worse".

2.2.4. Evaluation of Psychological Status after Release from Quarantine

Psychological status after release from quarantine was verified with respect to anxiety, depression, insomnia, and mental stress. For anxiety and depression, questions to which responses were given on a four-point Likert scale: "never", "rarely", "sometimes", and "often". The criterion for "never" was the absence of any of the above symptoms. "Rarely" to "often" meant that symptoms affected daily life. Insomnia was rated on a three-point Likert scale: "never", "sometimes", and "often"; "often" means that it occurs so often that it affects daily life. Response to stress was rated on a five-point Likert scale: "never", "very rarely", "sometimes", "often", and "very often".

2.2.5. Evaluation of Family Relationships after Release from Quarantine

To evaluate changes in family relationships before and after COVID-19 infection, responses were rated on a three-point scale: "closer", "no change", and "more distant".

2.2.6. Positive Test after COVID-19 Viral Clearance

Subgroup analysis was conducted for patients that tested positive again during the consultation period to examine the presence of clinical factors associated with this phenomenon.

2.3. Statistical Analysis

Data were analyzed using an independent t-test, Pearson's Chi-square test, and Fisher's exact test to assess differences between those who received only one consultation and those who received two or more consultations. To confirm factors associated with the number of consultations, multivariate logistic regression analysis with the forward selection method (selection criterion: $p < 0.05$) was applied, using the demographic and clinical characteristics of the subjects as independent variables. All statistical analyses were performed using IBM SPSS statistics version 25.0 software (IBM Corp., Armonk, NY, USA). A value of $p < 0.05$ was considered statistically significant.

3. Results

3.1. The Participants in the Health Consultation Program

During the study period, 1679 recovered patients agreed to participate. Later, 72 subjects withdrew consent or refused to receive a consultation, and three were excluded for duplicate registration or registration errors; therefore, a total of 1604 subjects were selected for final analysis. Of these, 1145 (71.4%) completed the program with only one consultation, and 459 (28.6%) required two or more consultations. The average number of consultations was 1.38 ± 0.79, and each patient was offered a maximum number of 13 consultations.

3.2. General Characteristics of the Subjects, and Symptoms Prior to Release from Quarantine

The mean age of all subjects was 43.62 years, and 33% were male. Note that 1.7% had symptoms severe enough to require inpatient treatment in an ICU, whereas 22.8% had more than one underlying disease, the most common of which was hypertension (12.8%). Up to 7 days before a positive diagnosis of COVID-19, 74.6% of participants had symptoms, the most common being cough, excess sputum, fever, and myalgia. Although 25.4% of the subjects were asymptomatic, COVID-19 was confirmed through screening tests that were conducted for reasons such as a close contact with a positive case.

Compared with the group that received only one consultation, the group that received two or more had more ICU hospitalizations and more symptoms, including cough/sputum, chest tightness or shortness of breath, and fatigue or lethargy. There was no significant difference between the two groups with respect to age, sex, and underlying disease (Table 1).

Table 1. Clinical characteristics of the subjects during and before infection with COVID-19.

	Total (n = 1604)	No. of Consultations		p *
		Once (n = 1145)	Twice or More (n = 459)	
No. of consultations	1.38 ± 0.79	1.00	2.34 ± 0.95	<0.001
Age	43.62 ± 16.32	43.46 ± 16.40	44.02 ± 16.13	0.765
Sex, male	530 (33)	381 (33.3)	149 (32.5)	0.754
Quarantine period (days)	26.16 ± 9.99	26.32 ± 9.85	25.71 ± 10.33	0.376
ICU admission	28 (1.7)	15 (1.3)	13 (2.8)	0.035
Underlying disease	366 (22.8)	265 (23.1)	101 (22.0)	0.623
Hypertension	206 (12.8)	146 (12.8)	60 (13.1)	0.862
Diabetes	95 (5.9)	68 (5.9)	27 (5.9)	0.965
Dyslipidemia	25 (1.6)	20 (1.7)	5 (1.1)	0.337
Heart disease	26 (1.6)	16 (1.4)	10 (2.2)	0.263
Pulmonary disease	27 (1.7)	18 (1.6)	9 (2.0)	0.584
Allergic disease	29 (1.8)	22 (1.9)	7 (1.5)	0.590
Thyroid disease	12 (0.7)	8 (0.7)	4 (0.9)	0.751 †
Kidney disease	4 (0.2)	3 (0.3)	1 (0.2)	1.000 †
Any malignancies	20 (1.2)	17 (1.5)	3 (0.7)	0.175
Liver disease	12 (0.7)	7 (0.6)	5 (1.1)	0.341 †
Neurologic disease	17 (1.1)	13 (1.1)	4 (0.9)	0.791 †
Presence of symptoms before the diagnosis of COVID-19				
Asymptomatic	408 (25.4)	310 (27.1)	98 (21.4)	0.017
Any symptom	1196 (74.6)	835 (72.9)	361 (78.6)	
Fever	342 (21.3)	235 (20.5)	107 (23.3)	0.218
Cough, sputum	346 (21.6)	232 (20.3)	114 (24.8)	0.044
Sore throat, pharyngitis	180 (11.2)	126 (11.0)	54 (11.8)	0.663
Rhinorrhea, nasal congestion	96 (6.0)	71 (6.2)	25 (5.4)	0.565
Dysosmia, dysgeusia	212 (13.2)	150 (13.1)	62 (13.5)	0.828
Chest discomfort, dyspnea	73 (4.6)	40 (3.5)	33 (7.2)	0.001
Myalgia	308 (19.2)	223 (19.5)	85 (18.5)	0.660
Headache	122 (7.6)	86 (7.5)	36 (7.8)	0.821
Fatigue, malaise, lethargy	28 (1.7)	15 (1.3)	13 (2.8)	0.035
Diarrhea, abdominal discomfort	61 (3.8)	39 (3.4)	22 (4.8)	0.189

Data are presented as the mean ± standard deviation or as number (%). * Independent t-test for continuous variables, and Pearson's Chi-square test or † Fisher's exact test for discrete variables. COVID-19, coronavirus infectious disease-19; ICU, intensive care unit.

There were no significant differences in the number of consultations or the characteristics of assigned patients between the 20 physicians (Table S1).

3.3. Physical and Psychological Status and Family Relationships after Release from Quarantine

Table 2 shows the physical and psychological status of the subjects after release from quarantine. Overall, 27% said they had physical symptoms after release. The most common were cough/sputum, olfactory/taste disorders, sore throat, fatigue and weakness, and chest tightness. Moreover, 21.8% said their overall health status seemed worse; 33% reported anxiety; 19.3% reported depression; 23.5% reported insomnia; and 53.2% reported stress. In addition, 5.4% reported a deterioration in family relationships.

Table 2. Physical and psychological status after recovery from COVID-19.

	Total (n = 1604)	No. of Consultations: Once (n = 1145)	No. of Consultations: Twice or More (n = 459)	p *
Physical symptoms after recovering from COVID-19				
Asymptomatic	1171 (73.0)	874 (76.3)	297 (64.7)	<0.001
Any symptom	433 (27.0)	271 (23.7)	162 (35.3)	
Fever	10 (0.6)	5 (0.4)	5 (1.1)	
Cough, sputum	174 (10.9)	116 (10.1)	58 (12.6)	
Sore throat, pharyngitis	40 (2.5)	23 (2.0)	17 (3.7)	
Rhinorrhea, nasal congestion	33 (2.1)	26 (2.3)	7 (1.5)	
Dysosmia, dysgeusia	44 (2.7)	27 (2.4)	17 (3.7)	<0.001
Chest discomfort, dyspnea	38 (2.4)	23 (2.0)	15 (3.3)	
Myalgia	23 (1.4)	13 (1.1)	10 (2.2)	
Headache	23 (1.4)	16 (1.4)	7 (1.5)	
Fatigue, malaise, lethargy	40 (2.5)	18 (1.6)	22 (4.8)	
Diarrhea, abdominal discomfort	8 (0.5)	4 (0.3)	4 (0.9)	
General physical status after recovering from COVID-19				
Much better than before	31 (1.9)	25 (2.2)	6 (1.3)	
A little better than before	138 (8.6)	107 (9.3)	31 (6.8)	
Similar	1085 (67.6)	782 (68.3)	303 (66.0)	0.057
A little worse than before	314 (19.6)	208 (18.2)	106 (23.1)	
Much worse than before	36 (2.2)	23 (2.0)	13 (2.8)	
Anxiety after recovering from COVID-19				
Not at all	1075 (67.0)	813 (71.0)	262 (57.1)	
Mild	437 (27.2)	284 (24.8)	153 (33.3)	<0.001 †
Moderate	88 (5.5)	47 (4.1)	41 (8.9)	
Severe	4 (0.2)	1 (0.1)	3 (0.7)	
Depressive mood after recovering from COVID-19				
Not at all	1295 (80.7)	970 (84.7)	325 (70.8)	
Mild	244 (15.2)	143 (12.5)	101 (22.0)	<0.001 †
Moderate	61 (3.8)	30 (2.6)	31 (6.8)	
Severe	4 (0.2)	2 (0.2)	2 (0.4)	
Insomnia after recovering from COVID-19				
Not at all	1227 (76.5)	920 (80.3)	307 (66.9)	
Occasionally	199 (12.4)	125 (10.9)	74 (16.1)	<0.001
Frequently	178 (11.1)	100 (8.7)	78 (17.0)	
Psychological stress after recovering from COVID-19				
Not at all	751 (46.8)	585 (51.1)	166 (36.2)	
Rarely	417 (26.0)	287 (25.1)	130 (28.3)	
Occasionally	301 (18.8)	203 (17.7)	98 (21.4)	<0.001
Frequently	114 (7.1)	60 (5.2)	54 (11.8)	
Very often	21 (1.3)	10 (0.9)	11 (2.4)	
Family relationships after recovering from COVID-19				
Closer than before	97 (6.0)	74 (6.5)	23 (5.0)	
Unchanged	1421 (88.6)	1016 (88.7)	405 (88.2)	0.176
Deteriorated	86 (5.4)	55 (4.8)	31 (6.8)	
Re-positive result of COVID-19 test	35 (2.2)	9 (0.8)	26 (5.7)	<0.001

Data are presented as number (%). * Pearson's Chi-squared and † Fisher's exact tests.

After release from quarantine, the group that received two or more consultations had more physical symptoms than the group that received a single consultation (23.7% vs. 35.3%, $p < 0.001$). Symptoms included cough, fatigue, sore throat, and dysosmia/dysgeusia.

Compared with the group that received a single consultation, the group that received two or more consultations had more psychological symptoms, including anxiety (29.0% vs. 42.9%, $p < 0.001$) and depression (15.3% vs. 29.8%, $p < 0.001$). This included mild, moderate, or severe anxiety; and a mild, moderate or severe depressive mood. In addition, the group that received two or more consultations experienced more psychological stress: mild, moderate, or severe. There was no significant difference between the two groups with respect to changes in overall physical health status or family relationships.

3.4. Factors Affecting the Number of Consultations after Recovery from COVID-19

Multivariate forward-selection logistic regression analysis was conducted using relevant demographic and clinical characteristics as independent variables to identify factors that led to a requirement for two or more consultations with a doctor. Those with reconfirmed COVID-19 (adjusted odds ratio (aOR): 6.703), had more physical symptoms after quarantine (aOR: 1.558), felt depressed (aOR: 1.668 for mild depression, 1.922 for moderate depression), or felt psychological stress (aOR: 1.418 for rarely stressed, 2.029 for frequently stressed); and required more consultations (Table 3).

Table 3. Factors affecting the decision to request more than two consultations after recovering from COVID-19.

Factors	aOR	95% CI	p *
Re-confirmed COVID-19 test	6.703	3.062–14.674	<0.001
Presence of physical symptoms after recovering from COVID-19			
Asymptomatic	1.000		
Any symptom	1.558	1.220–1.989	<0.001
Depressive mood after recovering from COVID-19			
Not at all	1.000		
Mild	1.668	1.202–2.314	0.002
Moderate	1.922	1.034–3.573	0.039
Severe	1.961	0.268–14.374	0.508
Psychological stress after recovering from COVID-19			
Not at all	1.000		
Rarely	1.418	1.072–1.874	0.014
Occasionally	1.182	0.843–1.658	0.331
Frequently	2.029	1.248–3.299	0.004
Very often	1.963	0.751–5.130	0.169

* Multivariate forward selection logistic regression analysis using frequent (≥2) consultation as a dependent variable. aOR, adjusted odds ratio; CI, confidence interval.

3.5. Positive Cases after Clearance of Virus and a Negative Test Result

Subjects with no clinical symptoms were released from quarantine after two negative COVID-19 PCR test results (performed after an interval of 24 h or more). Nevertheless, 35 cases (2.2%) became positive again during the program: 5.7% in the two or more consultations group and 0.8% in the single consultation group (Table 2). Two of these 35 cases (5.7%) were hospitalized in an ICU after the first diagnosis and quarantined for a mean of 31.49 days. Twelve patients (34.3%) were tested again on the doctor's recommendation or at their own request due to residual symptoms. Twenty-three patients (65.7%) had no symptoms but were confirmed as positive by a mandatory screening test taken before returning to work or health care facilities (Table 4).

Table 4. Clinical characteristics of the patients with re-confirmed COVID-19 after viral clearance evidenced by a negative test result.

	Characteristics of Re-Confirmed Cases (n = 35)
Age, years	49.11 ± 15.35
Sex, male	8 (22.9)
Quarantine period (days)	31.49 ± 10.86
ICU admission	2 (5.7)
Underlying disease	8 (22.9)
Hypertension	7 (20.0)
Dyslipidemia	1 (2.9) *
Neurologic disease	1 (2.9) †
Purpose of COVID-19 re-test	
For their remaining symptoms	12 (34.3)
For returning to work or health care facilities	23 (65.7)

Data are presented as the mean ± standard deviation or as number (%). * One had both hypertension and dyslipidemia. † Meningitis. ICU, intensive care unit.

4. Discussion

This study was the first to conduct and analyze a follow-up health consultation program provided to patients who recovered from COVID-19 and lived in the region of Korea most severely affected by the outbreak. After the COVID-19 pandemic declaration, social distancing was strictly enforced in Korea, and all individuals with a confirmed infection were quarantined in a single hospitalization room until they recovered fully. Patients were discharged if they showed no physical symptoms and had two or more negative PCR tests. However, despite successful recovery, people reported marked physical and psychological sequelae, meaning that they required further medical advice. Moreover, 28.6% of these individuals required several consultations with doctors. Overall, 27% had physical symptoms; 33% had anxiety; 19.3% had depression; 23.5% had sleep problems, and 53.2% had mental stress. In particular, of the subjects that required two or more consultations, the number of re-confirmed cases was significantly higher among those who were hospitalized in the ICU, those who were symptomatic before hospitalization, or those who complained of physical symptoms after release from quarantine. Furthermore, a higher percentage of those who required multiple consultations reported mild anxiety, mild depression, and mild mental stress than those who required only a single consultation. These results strongly suggested that a follow-up health consultation program delivered by medical professionals and psychologists would play an important role in patient care after release from COVID-19 quarantine.

As mentioned above, patients who recovered from SARS and MERS also reported significant psychological problems after discharge [6,7]. However, the level of psychological distress reported for COVID-19 was much higher, principally because SARS-CoV-2 virus has neurological sequelae through both neuroinvasive and neurovirulent mechanisms. Studies show that SARS-CoV-2 can affect the central nervous system and infiltrate neurons [16]. In addition, unlike SARS or MERS, COVID-19 was declared a pandemic, after which countries implemented strict lockdowns. These lockdowns have had a negative effected on the mental health of the general population, as well as those infected with COVID-19 [17,18]. Also, and most importantly, if a person is infected or has been in close contact with someone who is, he or she has to self-isolate for several weeks. The average period of quarantine in this study was 26 days; patients spent ~4 weeks in an isolated space (hospital room or community treatment center). In particular, psychological distress was severe because patients were allowed no direct contact with others. The mental support provided by professional healthcare providers and psychologists was very important to patients isolated under such conditions. This notion is supported by the results of multivariate analysis, which identified depressive mood and psychological stress as factors that affected the decision to request more consultations.

COVID-19 has a spectrum of clinical symptoms ranging from asymptomatic to severe pneumonia and death [19]. Clinically, the most common symptoms are fever, cough, fatigue, and dyspnea (in that order) [20]. Analysis of 10,237 Korean patients with confirmed COVID-19 revealed that 62% were asymptomatic [21]. Among 40 confirmed patients in a city in Korea, 5% were asymptomatic [22], whereas in an Italian study it was 42.5% [23]. The proportion of asymptomatic patients infected with COVID-19 is thought to be ~40–45% [24]. Among the 1604 subjects examined in this study, 408 (25.4%) were asymptomatic. Common symptoms at diagnosis were cough, fever, myalgia, and dysosmia (in that order), a finding that was somewhat different from that reported in previous studies, probably because the numbers in the study cohorts varied from study to study. In addition, the policies and criteria used for screening tests to identify asymptomatic infections differed from country to country. Moreover, because this study included only those who agreed to participate in the consultation program, there was a possibility that relatively more symptomatic patients joined the program. We thought it interesting that, out of 408 subjects who stated that they were asymptomatic at the time of diagnosis, 29 (7.1%, data not shown) said that they had residual physical symptoms when asked. From March to April 2020, the outbreak in Daegu spread rapidly among a certain religious group [25]. They might not have answered honestly due to a fear of social stigma if they were infected because all their movements and relationships would be exposed [26]. Thus, they might have said they had no symptoms when in fact they did.

In general, according to WHO guidelines, patients can be hospitalized in a ICU if they show severe symptoms, ranging from severe disease to acute respiratory distress syndrome and sepsis [27]. Older age, diabetes, higher body temperature, and lower peripheral oxygen saturation all increase the possibility of ICU hospitalization [28]. Here, we found that subjects diagnosed with COVID-19 based on their symptoms, or those admitted to the ICU owing to the severity of COVID-19 symptoms, experienced more residual symptoms after discharge than those who were asymptomatic. This outcome is plausible because polyneuropathy, myopathy, and reduced pulmonary function are highly likely in patients who have severe disease [29–31]. Therefore, patients with symptomatic or severe COVID-19 infection required a more detailed follow-up program that allows close observation, even after discharge.

We found that 35 patients (2.2%) had re-confirmed COVID-19 after release from quarantine, and this group had the greatest effect on the number of consultations (aOR, 6.703). According to a report by the Korea Centers for Disease Control and Prevention, 292 re-confirmed cases (3.3% of 8922) were reported up until 29 April 2020; these were ascribed not to reactivation or re-infection, but to detection of genetic material from "dead virus" [13]. Similarly, the incidence of re-confirmed COVID-19 RT–PCR results in Italy was 13.7% on Day 14 post-discharge and 14.7% on Day 41 post-discharge [32]. The figure for China was 19% [33]. Here, 12 patients (34.3%) had re-confirmed infection after taking a test on the recommendation of a doctor during the follow-up consultation program because these patients showed residual symptoms that were considered minor but clinically important. Similar results were found in China, where 28% of re-confirmed patients complained of mild symptoms [33]. Re-confirmed cases are much less likely to transmit the disease than those with active infections [13]; however, the viral load is related to the clinical severity of COVID-19 [34], and concerns of infections driven by re-confirmed cases are increasing [14,35,36]. Therefore, physicians must verify whether recovered patients show symptoms; even mild symptoms. Accordingly, a well-structured follow-up program after recovery from COVID-19 (provided by healthcare professionals) will be an effective way to decide whether a patient requires another RT–PCR test.

This study has the following limitations. First, the results cannot be generalized over the general population because it was conducted on an ethnically homogeneous population in a single city. Second, because only patients who agreed to participate in the consultation program were enrolled, there is a possibility of selection bias and overestimation of the results. Third, even though the 20 consulting doctors had the same specialty, they are not professional psychiatrists, so the quality and quantity of consultation may vary. However, a general guideline was provided and a web-based communication site was set up to share information with the consulting doctors to minimize inter-physician variation. Fourth, standardized assessment tools were not applied to evaluate physical and psychological status. Further prospective cohort studies using validated assessment tools are needed.

Despite these limitations, this study has certain strengths. It is the first in which professional healthcare providers implemented a patient management program after discharge; moreover, because Daegu was in the region with the highest number of confirmed cases from February to April 2020, the results could be taken as a reflection of the Korean population during the early COVID-19 pandemic period.

5. Conclusions

This study showed that COVID-19 has various physical and mental sequelae after discharge, and that patients require follow-up medical consultations. COVID-19 is still prevalent and is still having adverse economic and social effects worldwide. It is necessary to develop and publicize a systematic follow-up care program to provide comprehensive health care for patients recovering from this highly contagious disease.

Supplementary Materials: The following are available online at https://www.mdpi.com/article/10.3390/jcm10112329/s1, Table S1: The characteristics of the subjects according to the physicians.

Author Contributions: Conceptualization, K.-M.L., H.-J.K. and G.H.L.; methodology, K.-M.L. and H.-J.K.; software, H.-J.K.; validation, G.H.L., A.-S.K. and D.-W.L.; formal analysis, H.-J.K.; investigation, K.-M.L., H.-J.K., G.H.L., A.-S.K. and D.-W.L.; resources, K.-M.L.; data curation, H.-J.K.; writing—original draft preparation, K.-M.L. and H.-J.K.; writing—review and editing, H.-J.K.; visualization, H.-J.K.; supervision, G.H.L. and A.-S.K.; project administration, K.-M.L.; funding acquisition, H.-J.K. All authors have read and agreed to the published version of the manuscript.

Funding: This study was supported by a research grant from the Daegu Medical Association COVID-19 scientific committee.

Institutional Review Board Statement: The study was conducted according to the guidelines of the Declaration of Helsinki, and approved by the Institutional Review Board of Yeungnam University Medical Center (Protocol No. YUMC 2020-04-112, APR-29-2020).

Informed Consent Statement: Not applicable due to retrospective study design.

Data Availability Statement: Please contact author for data requests.

Acknowledgments: This study was supported by a research grant from the Daegu Medical Association COVID-19 scientific committee. We thank the 20 family medicine specialists belonging to the Daegu-Gyeongbuk Branch of the Korean Family Medicine Association who volunteered to provide telephone consultations, and the Daegu Medical Association for providing the mobile phones used for consultation.

Conflicts of Interest: The authors declare no conflict of interest. The funders had no role in the design of the study; in the collection, analyses, or interpretation of data; in the writing of the manuscript, or in the decision to publish the results.

References

1. Korea Ministry of Health and Welfare and Centers for Disease Control and Prevention. Latest Updates. Available online: http://ncov.mohw.go.kr/en (accessed on 29 January 2021).
2. Lai, C.C.; Shih, T.P.; Ko, W.C.; Tang, H.J.; Hsueh, P.R. Severe acute respiratory syndrome coronavirus 2 (SARS-CoV-2) and coronavirus disease-2019 (COVID-19): The epidemic and the challenges. *Int. J. Antimicrob. Agents* **2020**, *55*, 105924. [CrossRef] [PubMed]
3. WHO Director-General's Opening Remarks at the Media Briefing on COVID-19—11 March 2020. Available online: https://www.who.int/dg/speeches/detail/who-director-general-s-opening-remarks-at-the-media-briefing-on-covid-19---11-march-2020 (accessed on 6 April 2020).
4. Park, M.; Cook, A.R.; Lim, J.T.; Sun, Y.; Dickens, B.L. A Systematic Review of COVID-19 Epidemiology Based on Current Evidence. *J. Clin. Med.* **2020**, *9*, 967. [CrossRef]
5. WHO. Q&A on Coronaviruses (COVID-19). Available online: https://www.who.int/news-room/q-a-detail/q-a-coronaviruses (accessed on 9 April 2020).

6. Kwek, S.K.; Chew, W.M.; Ong, K.C.; Ng, A.W.; Lee, L.S.; Kaw, G.; Leow, M.K. Quality of life and psychological status in survivors of severe acute respiratory syndrome at 3 months postdischarge. *J. Psychosom. Res.* **2006**, *60*, 513–519. [CrossRef] [PubMed]
7. Hong, X.; Currier, G.W.; Zhao, X.; Jiang, Y.; Zhou, W.; Wei, J. Posttraumatic stress disorder in convalescent severe acute respiratory syndrome patients: A 4-year follow-up study. *Gen. Hosp. Psychiatry* **2009**, *31*, 546–554. [CrossRef] [PubMed]
8. Das, K.M.; Lee, E.Y.; Singh, R.; Enani, M.A.; Al Dossari, K.; Van Gorkom, K.; Larsson, S.G.; Langer, R.D. Follow-up chest radiographic findings in patients with MERS-CoV after recovery. *Indian J. Radiol. Imaging* **2017**, *27*, 342–349. [CrossRef] [PubMed]
9. Torales, J.; O'Higgins, M.; Castaldelli-Maia, J.M.; Ventriglio, A. The outbreak of COVID-19 coronavirus and its impact on global mental health. *Int. J. Soc. Psychiatry* **2020**, *66*, 317–320. [CrossRef] [PubMed]
10. Carda, S.; Invernizzi, M.; Bavikatte, G.; Bensmaïl, D.; Bianchi, F.; Deltombe, T.; Draulans, N.; Esquenazi, A.; Francisco, G.E.; Gross, R.; et al. COVID-19 pandemic. What should Physical and Rehabilitation Medicine specialists do? A clinician's perspective. *Eur. J. Phys. Rehabil. Med.* **2020**, *56*, 515–524. [CrossRef]
11. Xing, Y.; Mo, P.; Xiao, Y.; Zhao, O.; Zhang, Y.; Wang, F. Post-discharge surveillance and positive virus detection in two medical staff recovered from coronavirus disease 2019 (COVID-19), China, January to February 2020. *Eurosurveillance* **2020**, *25*. [CrossRef]
12. Ye, G.; Pan, Z.; Pan, Y.; Deng, Q.; Chen, L.; Li, J.; Li, Y.; Wang, X. Clinical characteristics of severe acute respiratory syndrome coronavirus 2 reactivation. *J. Infect.* **2020**. [CrossRef]
13. Kang, Y.J. South Korea's COVID-19 Infection Status: From the Perspective of Re-positive Test Results After Viral Clearance Evidenced by Negative Test Results. *Disaster Med. Public Health Prep.* **2020**, 1–3. [CrossRef]
14. To, K.K.-W.; Hung, I.F.-N.; Ip, J.D.; Chu, A.W.-H.; Chan, W.-M.; Tam, A.R.; Fong, C.H.-Y.; Yuan, S.; Tsoi, H.-W.; Ng, A.C.-K.; et al. COVID-19 re-infection by a phylogenetically distinct SARS-coronavirus-2 strain confirmed by whole genome sequencing. *Clin. Infect. Dis.* **2020**. [CrossRef]
15. Kim, Y.A.; Lee, G.H.; Lee, K.M.; Ko, H.J.; Lee, D.; Kim, A.S. Communication and Cooperation Between the Medical Academy, Medical Association, and Local Government: Health Counseling Program After Recovery From Coronavirus Disease 2019 (COVID-19) in Daegu. *Front. Public Health* **2020**, *8*, 563757. [CrossRef]
16. Rabinovitz, B.; Jaywant, A.; Fridman, C.B. Neuropsychological functioning in severe acute respiratory disorders caused by the coronavirus: Implications for the current COVID-19 pandemic. *Clin. Neuropsychol.* **2020**, *34*, 1453–1479. [CrossRef]
17. Schnell, T.; Krampe, H. Meaning in Life and Self-Control Buffer Stress in Times of COVID-19: Moderating and Mediating Effects With Regard to Mental Distress. *Front. Psychiatry* **2020**, *11*, 582352. [CrossRef]
18. Grover, S.; Sahoo, S.; Mehra, A.; Avasthi, A.; Tripathi, A.; Subramanyan, A.; Pattojoshi, A.; Rao, G.P.; Saha, G.; Mishra, K.K.; et al. Psychological impact of COVID-19 lockdown: An online survey from India. *Indian J. Psychiatry* **2020**, *62*, 354–362. [CrossRef]
19. Kannan, S.; Shaik Syed Ali, P.; Sheeza, A.; Hemalatha, K. COVID-19 (Novel Coronavirus 2019)—Recent trends. *Eur. Rev. Med. Pharmacol. Sci.* **2020**, *24*, 2006–2011. [CrossRef]
20. Sheleme, T.; Bekele, F.; Ayela, T. Clinical Presentation of Patients Infected with Coronavirus Disease 19: A Systematic Review. *Infect. Dis.* **2020**, *13*, 1178633720952076. [CrossRef]
21. Jung, C.Y.; Park, H.; Kim, D.W.; Choi, Y.J.; Kim, S.W.; Chang, T.I. Clinical Characteristics of Asymptomatic Patients with COVID-19: A Nationwide Cohort Study in South Korea. *Int. J. Infect. Dis. IJID Off. Publ. Int. Soc. Infect. Dis.* **2020**, *99*, 266–268. [CrossRef]
22. Jeong, T.H.; Pak, C.; Ock, M.; Lee, S.H.; Son, J.S.; Jeon, Y.J. Real Asymptomatic SARS-CoV-2 Infection Might Be Rare: Importance of Careful Interviews and Follow-up. *J. Korean Med. Sci.* **2020**, *35*. [CrossRef]
23. Lavezzo, E.; Franchin, E.; Ciavarella, C.; Cuomo-Dannenburg, G.; Barzon, L.; Del Vecchio, C.; Rossi, L.; Manganelli, R.; Loregian, A.; Navarin, N.; et al. Suppression of a SARS-CoV-2 outbreak in the Italian municipality of Vo'. *Nature* **2020**, *584*, 425–429. [CrossRef]
24. Oran, D.P.; Topol, E.J. Prevalence of Asymptomatic SARS-CoV-2 Infection : A Narrative Review. *Ann. Intern. Med.* **2020**, *173*, 362–367. [CrossRef] [PubMed]
25. Kim, H.J.; Hwang, H.S.; Choi, Y.H.; Song, H.Y.; Park, J.S.; Yun, C.Y.; Ryu, S. The Delay in Confirming COVID-19 Cases Linked to a Religious Group in Korea. *J. Prev. Med. Public Health* **2020**, *53*, 164–167. [CrossRef] [PubMed]
26. Jung, G.; Lee, H.; Kim, A.; Lee, U. Too Much Information: Assessing Privacy Risks of Contact Trace Data Disclosure on People With COVID-19 in South Korea. *Front. Public Health* **2020**, *8*, 305. [CrossRef] [PubMed]
27. World Health Organization. Clinical Management of COVID-19: Interim Guidance. Available online: https://apps.who.int/iris/handle/10665/332196 (accessed on 18 September 2020).
28. Jang, J.G.; Hur, J.; Choi, E.Y.; Hong, K.S.; Lee, W.; Ahn, J.H. Prognostic Factors for Severe Coronavirus Disease 2019 in Daegu, Korea. *J. Korean Med. Sci.* **2020**, *35*, e209. [CrossRef]
29. Herridge, M.S.; Moss, M.; Hough, C.L.; Hopkins, R.O.; Rice, T.W.; Bienvenu, O.J.; Azoulay, E. Recovery and outcomes after the acute respiratory distress syndrome (ARDS) in patients and their family caregivers. *Intensive Care Med.* **2016**, *42*, 725–738. [CrossRef]
30. Shepherd, S.; Batra, A.; Lerner, D.P. Review of Critical Illness Myopathy and Neuropathy. *Neurohospitalist* **2017**, *7*, 41–48. [CrossRef]
31. Ohtake, P.J.; Lee, A.C.; Scott, J.C.; Hinman, R.S.; Ali, N.A.; Hinkson, C.R.; Needham, D.M.; Shutter, L.; Smith-Gabai, H.; Spires, M.C.; et al. Physical Impairments Associated With Post-Intensive Care Syndrome: Systematic Review Based on the World Health Organization's International Classification of Functioning, Disability and Health Framework. *Phys. Ther.* **2018**, *98*, 631–645. [CrossRef]

32. Cento, V.; Colagrossi, L.; Nava, A.; Lamberti, A.; Senatore, S.; Travi, G.; Rossotti, R.; Vecchi, M.; Casati, O.; Matarazzo, E.; et al. Persistent positivity and fluctuations of SARS-CoV-2 RNA in clinically-recovered COVID-19 patients. *J. Infect.* **2020**, *81*, e90–e92. [CrossRef]
33. Yang, C.; Jiang, M.; Wang, X.; Tang, X.; Fang, S.; Li, H.; Zuo, L.; Jiang, Y.; Zhong, Y.; Chen, Q.; et al. Viral RNA level, serum antibody responses, and transmission risk in recovered COVID-19 patients with recurrent positive SARS-CoV-2 RNA test results: A population-based observational cohort study. *Emerg. Microbes Infect.* **2020**, *9*, 2368–2378. [CrossRef]
34. Shi, F.; Wu, T.; Zhu, X.; Ge, Y.; Zeng, X.; Chi, Y.; Du, X.; Zhu, L.; Zhu, F.; Zhu, B.; et al. Association of viral load with serum biomakers among COVID-19 cases. *Virology* **2020**, *546*, 122–126. [CrossRef]
35. Torres, D.A.; Ribeiro, L.; Riello, A.; Horovitz, D.D.G.; Pinto, L.F.R.; Croda, J. Reinfection of COVID-19 after 3 months with a distinct and more aggressive clinical presentation: Case report. *J. Med. Virol.* **2020**. [CrossRef]
36. AlFehaidi, A.; Ahmad, S.A.; Hamed, E. SARS-CoV-2 re-infection: A case report from Qatar. *J. Infect.* **2020**. [CrossRef]

Journal of
Clinical Medicine

MDPI

Article

The Relationship between Fear of Infection and Insomnia among Dentists from Oradea Metropolitan Area during the Outbreak of Sars-CoV-2 Pandemic

Magdalena Iorga [1,2,*], Raluca Iurcov [3,*] and Lavinia-Maria Pop [2]

1 Behavioral Sciences Department, "Grigore T. Popa" University of Medicine and Pharmacy, 700115 Iasi, Romania
2 Faculty of Psychology and Education Sciences, "Alexandru Ioan Cuza" University, 700111 Iasi, Romania; lavinia.pop@student.uaic.ro
3 Dentistry Department, Faculty of Medicine, University of Oradea, 410073 Oradea, Romania
* Correspondence: magdalena.iorga@umfiasi.ro (M.I.); riurcov@uoradea.ro (R.I.)

Abstract: Various studies have shown the impact of COVID-19 pandemic on mental health, identifying that people with a strong fear of getting infected are more prone to become stressed, depressed, anxious and to experience sleeping disturbance. The present study focuses on the impact of fear of COVID-19 and its relationship with insomnia among dentists. 83 dentists from public and private clinics were included in the research. A questionnaire was especially constructed for this study, consisting of three parts: the first part gathered socio-demographic and medical data, and a succession of self-rated items collected opinions about lockdown and preventive behaviors; the second part evaluated the level of fear of infection with Coronavirus-19 using the Fear of Covid 19 Scale; the third part investigated the presence of insomnia using the Athens Insomnia Scale. Collected data were processed using SPSS (v. 25). The total scores for fear of COVID 19 and insomnia were assessed. A strong positive correlation was identified between the total score of AIS and the total score of FCV-19S. The fear of COVID-19 had a significant positive correlation with the practice of several preventive behaviors. Dentists with chronic diseases were found to be more prone to suffer from insomnia than healthy dentists. Significant differences between women and men in terms of night symptoms were discussed. The findings are useful for dentists and policy makers to evaluate the impact of fear of infection on mental health status.

Keywords: pandemic; dentist; stress; anxiety; fear; insomnia; mental health; preventive behavior; fear of Covid-19; Athens Insomnia Scale

Citation: Iorga, M.; Iurcov, R.; Pop, L.-M. The Relationship between Fear of Infection and Insomnia among Dentists from Oradea Metropolitan Area during the Outbreak of Sars-CoV-2 Pandemic. *J. Clin. Med.* **2021**, *10*, 2494. https://doi.org/10.3390/jcm10112494

Academic Editor: Michele Roccella

Received: 10 April 2021
Accepted: 29 May 2021
Published: 4 June 2021

1. Introduction

Since March 2020, when the World Health Organization (WHO) declared infection with COVID-19 as a pandemic [1] dentists have had to deal with many challenges: the COVID-19 pandemic has influenced the physical and mental health of dentists and impacted their family relationships and financial status, and has led to changes in professional practice [2–5].

From the beginning of the COVID-19 pandemic, doctors have been considered a hotspot for infection, with a high risk of bidirectional transmission—from doctor to patient and vice versa. The risk of contagion was extremely high, especially in the context of dental medical services: blood droplets and saliva that are deposited on the surfaces or aerosol inhalation generated by rotating instruments and ultrasound hand pieces put both doctors and patients at high risk [2,3].

Tysiąc-Miśta and Dziedzic [4] showed that one of the most important challenges for Polish dentists was that of medical protective equipment. Their study pointed out that 71.2% of dentists decided to suspend their clinical practice during the onset of the pandemic. Dentists who continued their clinical work during the first months of the pandemic were four and a half times more likely to have access to PPE than those who closed their dental offices. The same results were highlighted by Chamorro-Petronacci et al. [5] among Spanish dentists. The authors found that only 12.3% of participants could obtain personal protective equipment (PPE) including FFP2 masks, and dentists registered important economic losses due to the interruption of their activity. Casillas Santana et al. [6] showed that only a small percentage of Mexican dentists used protective masks and a large majority had to change disinfection rules between appointments to ensure a safe environment for patients. Consolo et al. [7] found that dentists from northern Italy reported feelings of concern (70.2%), anxiety (46.4%) and fear (42.4%) and most of them (89.6%) mentioned increased concerns about their professional future. Ahmed et al. [8] conducted a survey among dentists from thirty countries and found that 90% were anxious while treating a coughing patient or a patient suspected of being infected with COVID-19. More than 72% of the participants felt nervous when talking to patients in close proximity, and most of them (92%) were afraid of carrying the virus from workplace to their families. The authors also found that 73% were anxious about the cost of the treatment if they got infected, and 86% about the mortality rates presented by the media. More than half of the dentists recommended the closure of private and public dental clinics until the number of COVID-19 cases started to decline [8].

Shacham et al. [9] conducted a cross-sectional survey among Israeli dentists and dental hygienists and found higher psychological distress among those with history of illness, with an increased level of fear of contracting COVID-19 from their patients, and with those who self-rated their work as overloaded. Vergara-Buenaventura et al. [10] showed that there were important health consequences of the coronavirus disease 2019 pandemic in dentistry, including physical and psychological pressure, depression, social anxiety, and other mental health concerns. Sarialioglu Gungor et al. [11] highlighted that Turkish dentists had to deal with a high risk of infection, isolation from their families, discrimination, and overwork with inadequate protection, developing frustration and exhaustion. In Egypt, Hanafy identified that 75.1% of dentists reported difficulties in finding Personal Protective Equipment and 97.6% of the questioned doctors reported worry about acquiring COVID-19 while working. When questioned about it, 44% of participants reported anxiety, 28.7% concern, and 16.4% fear [12]. In a study conducted by Moraes et al. [13] of Brazilian dentists it was shown that there were three major impacts of the pandemic on dentistry: increasing inequalities due to health coverage differences between public and private clinics, the adoption of new clinical daily practices (correlated with an economic burden for dentists), and associations of regional COVID-19 incidence/mortality with fear of contracting the disease in the working environment. All these studies revealed that the Coronavirus-19 pandemic has had, since the beginning, a great impact on dentists' personal and professional lives, with important psychological consequences. Fear, anxiety and stress should be further investigated, due to their consequences regarding general health status.

Identifying the level of fear has a dual scientific purpose. The positive aspect of fear is that it is an alarm signal; fear is a normal reaction and determines awareness about a situation, produces changes in behaviors, and stimulates adaptability [9]. In the early stages of previous pandemics, such as Ebola or MERS, fear was associated with increased vaccination rates and the practice of preventive behaviors like hand washing, distance, body hygiene, etc. [14]. The negative side of fear is that the presence of high scores for fear is associated with the appearance and persistence of psychological problems such as anxiety, depression, post-traumatic stress disorder, sleeping disorder, eating disorder, or somatization [9,10,14–16]. Authors have shown that a fear construct is expected to have a significant predictive power of posttraumatic stress symptomatology, anxiety, and insomnia, since the most common clinical manifestations of fear include these psychological problems [15]. Therefore, the presence of fear determines the sufferer to search for preventive behaviors but also has negative consequences on physical and mental health [8,14]. That is why, when analyzing fear in the context of COVID-19 pandemic, as Nikopoulou et al. highlighted in their study [16], it is extremely important to discriminate between adults with extreme COVID-19-related fear and those with normal fear reactions, to prevent psychological consequences and to maintain mental health. In the context of the coronavirus-19 pandemic, the impact on mental health is just at the beginning. Studies have identified the influence of the pandemic on the psychological, physical, social, and financial status as an acute reaction [6,8,14].

Compared to other countries of the European Community, Romania registered a lower risk of community transmission and a considerably lower number of deaths. The first case of infection was identified on 26 February 2020. By Presidential Decree, on 16 March a state of alarm was imposed; on 21 March, by Military Decree, a lockdown was imposed till 15 May [17,18]. Dental offices had to close and only emergency dental offices from public institutions (hospitals or clinics) continued to provide dental services. Due to the small number of emergency dental care offices (less than 5%) private dental clinics could accept patients in compliance with two rules: to provide only a limited amount of dental care (emergency cases) and to have the approval of Territorial Health Departments (after checking that the clinics had respected all the preventive measures to limit the spread of the infection). Only a very small number of private clinics could follow the imposed rules, first because of the difficulty in finding protective suits or protective materials and, second, because of their costs that negatively impacted their financial balance. The third important reason is not to be ignored, that at the beginning of the pandemic, information on the ways of transmitting the virus was relatively limited, which determined both patients and dentists being careful in carrying out activities related to dental services.

A small number of articles were published during the first year of the pandemic about the practice of dental services in Romania and how the restrictions, fear of infection and the new adopted preventives rules impacted dental services. The study of Pituru et al. [19] conducted among Romanian dentists identified that 87.1% of the respondents preferred a full set of personal protective equipment, including gloves, goggles, N95 mask, face shield, head cover, gown and shoe cover while treating asymptomatic patients with positive travel/contact history. Moreover, Petrescu et al. [20] showed that certain pathologies provided in emergency dental rooms in Romania considerably increased during 2020, compared to 2019. In April 2019, 160 patients had visited the Emergency Department of County General Hospital whereas in April 2020, one month after the State of Alarm, 2131 patients sought dental treatment in this department, as other dental emergency centers and private practices were closed by the State of Emergency dispositions. The number of patients increased more than 13 times. The main causes of attendance at emergency dental offices were acute apical periodontitis and acute pulpitis. However, no studies evaluated the impact of the COVID-19 pandemic on the mental health of Romanian dentists.

The goal of the present research is to evaluate the mental status of dentists after the first wave of the COVID-19 pandemic (November–December 2020) by identifying the presence of fear of Covid-19 and insomnia, and their relationship with dentists' preventive behaviors. As secondary purpose, we wanted to highlight the correlation analysis between fear and the practice of preventive behaviors (as a health-protective consequence of fear) and fear and insomnia (as a negative consequence on health status) among dentists during the first months of the pandemic. This study is part of a larger investigation among dentists; previous results have evaluated preventive behaviors and new preventive practices in dental clinics, adopted by dentists to diminish the risk of infection from and to their patients, and the impact of the pandemic on their family life and financial status [21].

2. Materials and Methods

This cross-sectional study was conducted in Oradea department situated in the northwestern part of the country, one of the regions that immediately applied restrictive rules even before the imposed State of Alarm, decided by Presidential Ordinance on 15 March 2020, especially due to its closeness to the Romanian border. The data for the present research was collected between 18 November and 5 December 2020, after the first wave of the pandemic, thus covering the first seven months of the pandemic.

2.1. Participants and Data Collection

The questionnaire was created and distributed with the Google Forms application (Alphabet, Mountain View, CA, USA). The survey was distributed online to dentists registered in the College of Dentists of Oradea. The respondents were informed about the purpose of the research and the use of the collected data. The continuation of the questionnaire was assumed as an agreement to take part to the survey. No incentives were offered to the voluntary respondents. The inclusion criteria were dentists registered at that time by the Romanian College of Dentists, Oradea Department, working in public or private dental clinics or Dental Emergency Units. The exclusion criteria were retired or unemployed dentists, incomplete questionnaires (not fully filled in) and questionnaires returned after the deadline. The survey was sent to 125 dentists who previously agreed to receive news or questionnaires; 93 of them filled in the surveys (response rate was 74.4%). We excluded ten questionnaires because the respondents were retired dentists. Finally, 83 forms were included in our databases and considered for the research. In November 2020, 457 dentists were registered at the Oradea College of Dentists (metropolitan area and other cities in the department) so the sample is relevant for dentists working in the region.

2.2. Instruments

A questionnaire was used to collect the data for the present research, and contained three parts:

- The first part collected (a) sociodemographic data such as age, gender, length of employment, number of children, marital status, length of employment, environment, type of institutions, level of specialization; (b) medical-related data such as the presence of a chronic disease or having a previous positive diagnosis of infection with the virus; (c) preventive behaviors adopted to diminish the risk of infection with answers rated on a 5-point Likert as following: 1 (never), 2 (rarely), 3 (sometimes), 4 (often) and 5 (always).
- The second part evaluated the fear of COVID-19. The psychological tool used for the present research was Fear of COVID-19 (FCV-19S) elaborated in 2020 by Ahorsu et al. [22]. The tool included seven items, and the respondents had to indicate their level of agreement with the statements using a five-item Likert-type scale. Answers included strongly disagree, disagree, neither agree nor disagree, agree, and strongly agree. The minimum score possible for each question was 1, and the maximum was 5. A total score was calculated by adding up each item score (ranging from 7 to 35). The higher the score, the greater the fear of Cororonavirus-19. The instrument was used worldwide in the first year of the pandemic. Chi et al. [23] (2021) also identified two factors: one was fear thoughts including items 1, 2, 4, and 5, i.e., subjective experience of fear. The other was physical response including items 3, 6, and 7, which represents physiological response [23]. The scale proved its good validity and reliability as psychometric characteristics and versions in many languages and countries were employed, including a Romanian version [16,22,24–34]. The cut-off score was established at 16.5 points
- The third part identified the presence of insomnia using the Athens Insomnia Scale (AIS) of Soldatos et al. [24]. The scale is an eight-item instrument that was designed for quantifying sleep difficulty based on the ICD-10 criteria. It consists of eight items: the first five pertain to sleep induction, awakening during the night, final awakening, total sleep duration, and sleep quality; while the last three refer to well-being, functioning capacity, and sleepiness during the day. The first five address the participant's night-time symptoms and the other three investigate the daytime impact due to any reported sleep disturbances. Each item was rated on an ordinal scale of 0 (no problem at all) to 3 (very serious problem). The dentists were required to rate the items if they had

experienced any sleep difficulty described in each question at least three times a week during the previous month. A maximum total score of 24 indicated the most severe symptoms of insomnia. For this scale, the cut-off point of ≥6 represented a minimum criterion for the confirmation of insomnia symptoms in our respondents.

2.3. Statistical Analysis

All analyses were performed using the IBM Statistical Package for Social Sciences (SPSS) Statistics for Windows, version 25(SPSS Inc., Chicago, IL, USA). The descriptive statistics of socio-demographic and medical data were expressed as means and standard deviations (SD), frequencies and percentages. Given that the distribution of data is not normal, nonparametric tests were used. The Mann Whitney test was performed for the comparative analysis among genders and professional categories, as well as for marital and parenthood status. The correlation analysis was done using Spearman correlations. The level of statistical significance was set at $p < 0.05$.

2.4. Ethical Approval

The present study was conducted in accordance with the Declaration of Helsinki, and the protocol was approved by the Ethical Committee of the Emergency County Hospital of Oradea, Romania, with the registration number No. 26214/18.11.2020.

3. Results

3.1. Sociodemographic and Medical Data

Sociodemographic and medical data were gathered, together with professional environment characteristics and family related information. Detailed information is presented in Table 1.

Table 1. Sociodemographic and medical characteristics [1].

Sociodemographic and Medical Characteristics	n (%)/M ± SD
Age	37.81 ± 8.45
Length of employment (years)	11.87 ± 8.62
Number of working hours per week	30.94 ± 11.76
Gender	
Male	29 (34.94)
Female	53 (63.86)
I prefer not to say	1 (1.20)
Marital status	
Single	11 (13.25)
In relationship	72 (86.75)
Having children	
yes	46 (55.42)
1 child	22 (26.51)
2 children	19 (2.89)
3 children	4 (4.82)
4 children or more	1 (1.20)
none	37 (44.58)
Level of specialization	
Dentists	38 (45.78)
Male	17 (20.48)
Female	21 (25.30)
Residents	16 (19.28)
Male	1 (1.20)
Female	15 (10.64)
Specialists	10 (12.05)
Male	6 (7.23)
Female	4 (4.82)

Table 1. *Cont.*

Sociodemographic and Medical Characteristics	*n* (%)/M ± SD
Consultants	19 (22.89)
Male	5 (6.02)
Female	13 (15.66)
I prefer not to say	1 (1.20)
Teaching activity	
yes	23 (27.71)
no	60 (72.29)
Type of institution	
only public sector	3 (3.61)
only private sector	50 (60.24)
both private and public sectors	30 (36.14)
Working environment	
urban	77 (92.77)
rural	6 (7.23)
Having a chronic disease	
yes	9 (10.80)
no	74 (89.20)
Confirmed infected with COVID-19	
yes	3 (3.60)
no	80 (96.40)
Having at least one family member confirmed positive with COVID-19	
yes	21 (25.30)
no	62 (74.70)
Having periods during lockdown when living away from family	
yes	20 (24.10)
no	63 (75.90)

[1] Number of answers (*n*) and percentage (%), Means and standard deviations (M ± SD).

3.2. Opinions of Dentists on Infection and Preventive Measures

A succession of items identified the dentists' opinion about preventive measures such as establishing shorter dental interventions. Two items investigated the respondents' opinions about the risk of infection in dental settings. Additionally, some items self-rated the fear of infection related to patients (they did not declare the truth about their health; they could transmit the infection to dentists; they did not wear medical masks during dental interventions which increased the risk of contagion) and related to preventive practices (fear of infection due to inappropriate use; the medical suit did not offer 100% protection).

Finally, dentists were asked to rate their state of anxiety when watching the news and reading stories related to COVID-19 pandemic. The answers were rated on a Likert-like scale from 1 (never) to 5 (always) and the results are presented in Table 2.

Table 2. Fear of infection with COVID 19—self-rated items [1].

Items	M ± SD
I am afraid that wearing the protective suit against COVID-19 does not protect me enough	2.55 ± 1.41
I am afraid that the patients do not tell the truth about their health	3.47 ± 1.40
I am afraid I can get infected when I take off my protective suit	2.51 ± 1.43
I am afraid I might get infected from co-workers	2.54 ± 1.30
I am afraid of getting infected from my patients	2.78 ± 1.38
I believe that dentists have a very high risk of COVID-19 infection from their patients	3.52 ± 1.51
Dental procedures can be a source of infection and spread of COVID-19	2.81 ± 1.26
The fact that patients cannot wear a mask during the medical treatment causes fear of infection	2.48 ± 1.35
I try to shorten the duration of procedures for not staying in contact with patients too long	2.76 ± 1.51
I feel anxious when I watch the news and stories about COVID 19 on social platforms	2.49 ± 1.39

[1] Means and standard deviations (M ± SD).

3.3. Fear of COVID-19 Scale (FCV-19S)

For the present research, for the Fear of COVID-19 scale, Cronbach Alpha was 0.89, which proved a good internal consistency.

The total score was 14.56 ± 6.90 (ranging from 7 to 35). No significant differences were identified considering gender (male/female—p = 0.311), marital status (single/in relationship—p = 0.613), diagnostic of a chronic disease (yes/no—p = 0.066), or setting of work (public/private—p = 0.196).

The analysis of data showed positive correlations between FCV-19S score and the practice of some preventive behaviors such as shortening the duration of dental consult (r = 0.488 **, $p < 0.001$). This means that participants who were more fearful of Covid-19 were more likely to engage in preventative behaviors, such as shortening the duration of dental consultations.

Strong correlation was also identified related to total score for fear of infection and dentists' opinions about the fact that dental procedures were a major source of infection (r = 0.415 **, $p < 0.001$), and dentists had an increased risk of infection from the new virus in their patients (r = 0.598 **, $p < 0.001$). Fear of getting the infection from colleagues (r = 0.452 **, $p < 0.001$), fear of infection while taking off the protective suit (r = 0.635 **, $p < 0.001$), and fear of infection since patients cannot wear a mask during a medical treatment (r = 0.370 **, p = 0.001) were also found positively correlate with total score for FCV-19S. We must notice here that using self-rated items, we identified a high level of fear of infection from others (dental procedures, colleagues, patients, protective suits) and not the fear of transmitting the infection to others. This aspect will be detailed in the Discussion section.

We found that the number of children influenced the level of fear of infection; the more children the dentists had (r = −0.301 **, p = 0.007), the less intense the fear of COVID-19.

A previous study presented that Fear measured with FCV-19S had a bi-factor structure that indicated two dimensions: (1) the first was explained by general fear which reflects cognitive fear or a subjective experience of fear and (2) the second was explained by physical response group factors which indicates somatic fear, the physiological response of the organism [23]. Considering this, the comparative analysis showed that dentists who were university teachers (Mdn1 = 4) scored higher on physical response (Fear of COVID-19 subscale) (z = −2.033, p = 0.042) due to having a more intense physical experience, as opposed to those who did not carry out teaching activities (Mdn2 = 3).

3.4. Athens Insomnia Scale (AIS)

For our study, the Cronbach's Alpha for the total group was 0.87. A total score equal or greater than 6 was considered as indicative of insomnia for AIS. Our analysis of data showed a total score of 11.37 ± 3.45, meaning that our respondents showed a high level on this scale. Results ranged from a minimum score of 8 (19.3%, n = 16) to a maximum of 24 points (1.2%, n = 1). Detailed results are presented in Table 3.

Table 3. Results for items of Athens Insomnia Scale (AIS) [1].

Items of the AIS	M ± SD
Sleep induction	1.40 ± 0.64
Awakenings during the night	1.55 ± 0.63
Final awakening earlier than desired	1.43 ± 0.49
Total sleep duration	1.47 ± 0.57
Overall quality of sleep	1.30 ± 0.55
Sense of well-being during the day	1.42 ± 0.64
Functioning (physically and mentally) during the day	1.29 ± 0.55
Sleepiness during the day	1.51 ± 0.59

[1] Means and standard deviations (M ± SD).

The comparative analysis showed that dentists suffering from chronic diseases (Mdn = 17) had insomnia (z = −2.892, $p = 0.004$) more often than healthy dentists (Mdn = 10). Results of the Mann Whitney test (z = −3.583, $p < 0.001$) showed that dentists with a higher level of fear (Mdn = 14) had a higher score on the questionnaire assessing the severity of insomnia than the dentists who had lower levels for FCV-19S (Mdn = 10). Dentists with a higher level of fear (Mdn = 6) had had fewer working weeks since the outbreak of the pandemic compared (z = −2.900, $p = 0.004$) to dentists with a lower level of fear (Mdn = 9).

There were significant gender differences in terms of symptoms during the night, namely sleep induction, sleep quality and total sleep duration (z = −2.090, $p = 0.037$) in the sense that men (Mdn = 4) scored higher at this subscale and had more problems with night-time symptoms, as opposed to women (Mdn = 3).

The comparative analysis also showed that dentists who had a family member infected with COVID-19 (Mdn = 13) had a higher score on the questionnaire assessing the severity of insomnia (z = −2.529, $p = 0.011$) than dentists who did not have a family member infected with COVID-19 (Mdn =10).

A significant positive correlation was identified between the total score of AIS and the total score for the FCV-19S questionnaire (r = 0.42 **, $p < 0.001$), indicated by the correlation coefficient which proved a medium effect size. This means that the more the dentists were afraid of COVID-19, the more they would suffer from insomnia.

Our results showed that there was a positive correlation between the total score of AIS and variables which refer to some of the doctors' fears. Thus, we identified that the more the dentists were afraid of the fact that the patients did not declare the truth about their health, the more their insomnia would be severe (r = 0.29 **, $p = 0.007$). The more the dentists were afraid of the fact that they might be infected by their co-workers (r = 0.33 **, $p = 0.002$) or while taking off their protective suit (r = 0.26 *, $p = 0.016$), the more severe their insomnia would be. A negative correlation was identified between the total score of AIS and the fact that the patients respected COVID-19 preventive measures. We found that the more the patients respected these measures, the less the dentists suffered from insomnia (r =−0.26 *, $p = 0.016$).

For some dentists, wearing a protective suit became a difficult task because it prevented visibility and medical procedures. Thus, the more the dentists were concerned about the fact that wearing a protective suit would impede them from carrying out medical procedures (r = 0.40 **, $p = 0.002$) or about the fact that wearing a protective suit impeded visibility (r = 0.30 *, $p = 0.020$), the more they would have severe insomnia.

The statistical analysis proved that there were strong correlations between the anxiety state when dentists watched the news about the pandemic and both scores for fear and AIS. The results showed that the more anxious the dentists were when they followed news related to COVID-19, the higher both scores were (0.43 **, $p < 0.001$ for AIS, and: r = 0.79 **, $p < 0.001$ for FCV-19S). Positive correlations were also identified between AIS and other variables. Results are detailed in Table 4.

Table 4. Correlation analysis between Fear of Covid-19 Scale, Athens Insomnia Scale and self-rated items.

Items	AIS	FCV19S
I am afraid that patients do not tell the truth about their health	r = 0.293 ** p = 0.007	r = 0.514 ** p = 0.000
I am afraid I can get infected when I take off my protective suit	r = 0.263 * p = 0.016	r = 0.635 ** p = 0.000
I am afraid I might get infected from colleagues	r = 0.334 ** p = 0.002	r = 0.603 ** p = 0.000
Wearing a protective suit impedes me from doing medical maneuvers	r = 0.409 ** p = 0.002	r = 0.142 p = 0.291
Wearing a protective suit impedes my visibility	r = 0.304 * p = 0.021	r = 0.210 p = 0.116
When I watch the news and stories about COVID-19 on social platforms, I feel anxious	r = 0.437 ** p = 0.000	r = 0.000 ** p = 0.799
Fear of COVID-19 Scale	r = 0.427 ** p = 0.000	1 -
Patients follow protective measures against COVID-19 infection	r = −0.265 * p = 0.016	r = −0.377 ** p = 0.000

* $p < 0.05$; ** $p < 0.001$.

4. Discussion

Numerous studies conducted during the first year of the pandemic triggered by the Coronavirus infection have shown that there are vulnerable groups: women, people with minimal education, the unemployed, low-income individuals, and people living in the environment with high risk of infection [9–11,15]. Applied to the general population, the tool used to measure fear of Coronavirus infection scored highly, with most studies showing higher cutoff levels than the 16.5 score [16,22,23].

Dental offices had been closed for a long time, in terms of weeks, or months. Similarly, the number of patients had decreased considerably, with most patients showing that both patients and dentists preferred to intervene soon in case of urgent dental problems. However, although the financial impact had been significant, this was not crucial in increasing the fear of Coronavirus-19 infection. Similar results were highlighted by Gasparro et al. [35]. Researchers indicated that perceived job insecurity and fear of COVID-19 had negative impact on mental health, both variables being positively associated with depressive symptoms. The authors found that the effect of perceived job insecurity on depressive symptoms was weaker among those with a low fear of COVID-19. In a study conducted on Italian dentists, De Stefani et al. [36] also showed that more than half of the respondents declared that they were afraid because they were not sufficiently trained to restart work after the lockdown. They considered the virus infection highly dangerous, and they were concerned about the future economic situation of their clinical practices.

The scale proposed by Ahorsu et al. has been taken up by many researchers. Many published studies have validated the scale for use in various languages and in various countries [22,23,26]. The scale has also identified the level of fear of COVID-19 in populations in different countries. Some authors have argued that a weak point of the scale is that it did not propose cutoff scores, which made it impossible to make comparisons between populations, cultures, or ethnic groups [27,29–31]. Other research identified that different scores were highlighted by using the scale at various times during the first year after the onset of the pandemic. This showed that a high level was identified at the initial peak of the pandemic, after which the population became accustomed to the new preventive rules imposed to limit the spread of the virus. This peak in scores for fear of COVID-19 infection was also explained by the fact that little scientific information was available during the first months of the state of emergency.

The scale was applied to various populations of different countries but also on specific groups: students, doctors, medical professionals. The scale is useful for identifying the level of fear of infection and the results are useful for identifying people at risk (vulnerable populations, people from low socio-economic backgrounds, professions at risk of illness, patients with chronic diseases, etc.), but cannot be used for clinical purposes [16,18,22]. Some researchers have used the scale to provide a cutoff score, which is important when using a psychological tool. As Nikopoulou et al. [16] sustained, establishing a cutoff score is a common and useful practice in the psychiatry and psychology research fields to enable classification of respondents into either cases or non-cases. The authors proposed a cutoff score of 16.5 to separate both categories after having studied the Greek population.

In our study, the total score was 14.56 $\pm$ 6.90, lower than in other studies conducted on general healthcare professionals or dentists. Compared to other studies, the total score for FCV-19S was similar to those obtained by other investigations focusing on health professionals [27–34]. Firstly, this research was conducted on dentists and the respondents had more knowledge about infection, the spread of a virus and the implementation of protective practices. Secondly, this low score could be related to the period when the research was conducted, seven months from the beginning of pandemic. Compared to other studies, it is possible that the scores were lower compared to studies that measured the fear of COVID-19 during the peak of the pandemic [31–34]. Thirdly, the low score could also be related to easier access to medical supplies (a source of anxiety and fear during the first seven months of the pandemic). The fourth explanation could be related to the epidemiologic context, because in Romania the number of cases was not so high compared to other European countries (such as Italy, or Spain, where the number of cases and deaths increased considerably during the first seven months of pandemic).

Consolo et al. [7] identified similar results regarding the lower score compared to the general population. Their survey found that fear, anxiety, concern, sadness, and anger were commonly reported by dentists, but fortunately only a minority group reported a mild level of anxiety (10.3%), while 8.7% showed a score indicative of a severe level of anxiety. When thinking about COVID-19, only 4.2% of the questioned doctors reported an intense experience of fear. These results are similar to another survey conducted in Israel by Shacham et al. [9], in which elevated psychological distress was found in 11.5% of dentists. Similar to our study, anxiety was related to the level of fear of being infected by the patients. However, in our study we did not identify differences according to gender in terms of fear of contagion, these results being congruent with many others identified in the literature [21].

We found a positive correlation between the level of fear and the practice of some protective behaviors, results that were congruent with some studies conducted during the MERS or Ebola pandemics that proved the positive effect of fear on adopting preventive measures [37,38]. Therefore, normal fear of infection was associated with the adoption of recommended protection measures. Moreover, the implication of institutions, medical organizations, governments, and social entities was found to increase public compliance. Media, as well as social networks have the power to rapidly spread the information. When people have trust in medical institutions and policy makers, the power of fake news is lower, and compliance is higher [37]. In the case of the pandemic, the line between fear and anxiety will become less strong. Fear is related to a known or impending threat, whereas anxiety is mainly related to an imprecise or unknown threat [39]. So, the line will be created by the amount of knowledge that scientists, doctors, policy makers, media, or educators transmit about the virus. The higher the trust, the stronger the compliance. When these actors are missing, when they are undecided, when they do not transmit information or they transmit information which is contradictory, anxiety arise. The results of several studies indicated that public compliance with preventive behaviors like social distance, wearing masks, or vaccination during the health crisis required the development of social and institutional trust [40]. In our research, we found that breaking news about the pandemic had a negative impact on the mental state of dentists. We found a positive and strong relationship between the self-rated fear when dentists watched TV news about infection and scores for both fear of COVID-19 and insomnia. This result was due to the information related to the impact of the pandemic on health, financial incomes, food supplies or daily social activity. Trnka and Lorencova (2020) showed also that pessimistic communications used by the mass media considerably increasing traumatic feelings, fears and psychological distress in the Czech population during the outbreak of the pandemic [41] and Ermolaev et al. (2020) revealed that news about the speed of the spread of the coronavirus in Russia influenced people not to go to hospitals with minor health problems, when infection with the virus was seen to be putting their lives in danger [42].

Our study showed that dentists changed their preventive behaviors due to fear of infection. The results are congruent with other studies. For example, in a study conducted in thirty countries, Ahmed et al. (2020) showed that, despite the high level of medical knowledge among dentists, important levels of anxiety and fear were identified while working. The authors identified that a number of dental practices had been modified according to the recommended guidelines for emergency treatment and many offices had closed for an uncertain period [8].

The correlation between the fear of infection and the practice of preventive behaviors was also discussed by Becker et al. [43] in a study that included experts in dentistry from 32 countries. The authors identified preventive measures that were adopted by dentists in different countries. For example, 80% of the experts included in the research recommended wearing protective masks by patients even if they were not (at that time when the research was developed) recommended by professional associations or the WHO. These preventive behaviors could be explained by the fact that dentists had knowledge of and experience with contagious disease in dental settings. On the other hand, the high risks and fear of infection during maneuvers determined doctors to adopt supplementary strategies to diminish the risk of spread, even if they were not (yet) recommended.

We identified that dentists obtained a high score for insomnia (11.37 ± 3.45). As Nikopoulouet et al. [16] showed when they evaluated insomnia in the Greek population, results similar to those published by Sirajudeen et al. [25], an increasing amount of evidence indicated that there was a bidirectional relationship between psychosomatic conditions and insomnia and that this relationship may have been exacerbated by stress. In our study, the fear of infection and the anxiety related to financial matters during the first seven months from the outbreak of pandemic were related to the increased level of insomnia among our respondents. Our study showed that there was a strong positive correlation between total score of AIS and total score for FCV-19S questionnaire, meaning that the more the dentists were afraid of COVID-19, the more they would suffer from insomnia. Our results are similar to the few studies conducted on front-line medical staff working with COVID-infected patients. Xiao et al. [44] found that sleep quality was negatively associated with the degree of anxiety and stress and the effect of stress and anxiety on sleep was pointed out by many researchers [45,46] who also proved the negative impact on physical and mental health and the risk of developing chronic diseases.

Similar to our results, Bohlken et al. [47] showed that 18% of German doctors (psychiatrists and neurologists) reported that the pandemic triggered anxiety, while 9% reported sleep problems and Lai et al. [48] conducted a study on Chinese health care workers exposed to COVID-19 and proved that front-line health care workers had a high risk of developing unfavorable mental health outcomes and may have needed psychological support or interventions. Mustafa et al. [49] also identified fear of infection among dentists in South-Arabia, the main cause being contagion from patients. The researchers showed an increased concern about their accessibility to materials provided by dental health care authorities, which was mentioned as the best and safest approach for dealing with patients during and after the outbreak of pandemic.

We found that men where more prone than women to have sleep-related problems and that there was a strong positive relationship between both fear of infection and insomnia with self-rated fear when watching media news. The results of our study are in congruence with those obtained by Léger et al. (2020) who conducted a study on a French population. The researchers showed that media overexposure was associated with sleeping disorders during the lockdown and men were more prone to be overexposed to media and social media during lockdown [50]. Dai et al. (2020) identified that men had difficulties in maintaining sleep patterns and lifestyle during social distance restrictions and Sinha et al. (2020) showed that an increased digital media duration was evident in all age groups, mainly in males [51,52].

More studies should prove the effect of the pandemic on the physical and mental health of dentists Additionally, the long-term consequences of the fear of infection and of the application of measures to limit the disease need to be identified.

4.1. Reflections and Planning

Sleep quality is an indicator of physical and mental health. For healthcare professionals, sleep is an indicator of stress and burnout and these factors are the main cause of professional mistakes especially among doctors who are working in the frontline and under permanent pressure. Many studies have proven that sleep quality was closely related to addictive behaviors, burnout, malpractice complaints, poor communication with patients, low level of medical practice and suicide [53–58]. Due to the fact that fear of infection is an important cause of stress for dentists that is added to the overloaded activity during the pandemic period, dentists 'mental health must be an extremely important priority for hospitals and clinics. Psychological counselling, individual psychotherapy or Balint meetings must be provided to medical staff in order to help dentists to cope with the stress determined by the COVID-19 pandemic.

4.2. Strengths and Limitations of the Study

The most important strength of the study is that the results covered a great gap in scientific information related to the impact of fear of COVID-19 on mental health of medical professionals, especially of dentists. One of the limitations of the research is that the present study did not identify personality traits (according to the Big Five model, for example, which associated the presence of insomnia with neuroticism). Insomnia was more present in people with sleep vulnerability and introversion because all these were found to be linked to low gray matter density in the orbitofrontal cortex. Therefore, as Dekker et al. showed [59], introverts may be more vulnerable to COVID-19 fear and score higher on the insomnia scale.

Another limitation of the research is given by the small number of subjects. Thus, although the results are interesting, they cannot be generalized to the entire population of dentists, together with the geographical context related to the impact of the pandemic. So results cannot be generalized, and no causality is provided.

A third limitation of the research which should not be ignored is related to the fact that this study was conducted during the first part of the pandemic, when stress was connected to the fact that dentists did not have satisfactory access to protective materials or to complete information about the transmission of the virus, and were financially affected due to the closure of medical offices and the drastic decrease in financial profits. Therefore, sleep disorders could be strongly influenced by a combination of factors and not just by the fear of virus infection, and can affect quality of life [60].

The fourth limitation of the study is caused by the fact that the respondents were considered mentally healthy, no psychological or psychiatric diagnostic was obtained, and no supplementary psychological scale was applied. The presence of mental chronic diseases or various comorbidities could lead to a more pronounced presence of insomnia.

5. Conclusions

The COVID-19 pandemic had an important impact on the psychological health of dentists, especially during the first wave of lockdown. The fear of contagion, the closure of dental offices or the severe reduction of dental services, the collapse of financial incomes and the expensive preventive measures that started to be applied in dental settings with an important pressure on the budget, and also difficulties in terms of the impediment of visibility and of medical maneuvers had consequences on general well-being among dentists. The results of the studies must be interpreted considering the geographical context and the epidemiological particularities of each country during the fight against the COVID-19 pandemic. Dentists and policymakers must recognize that the COVID-19 pandemic has an impact on the physical and mental health of health professionals and dentists alike.

Author Contributions: Conceptualization, R.I. and M.I.; Data curation, R.I. and M.I.; Formal analysis, L.-M.P. and M.I.; Investigation, R.I., L.-M.P. and M.I.; Methodology, L.-M.P. and M.I.; Supervision, M.I.; Writing—original draft, R.I., M.I. and L.-M.P.; Writing—review and editing, R.I., L.-M.P. and M.I. All authors equally contributed to this paper. All authors equally contributed to the work reported. All authors have read and agreed to the published version of the manuscript.

Funding: This research received no external funding.

Institutional Review Board Statement: The study was conducted according to the guidelines of the Declaration of Helsinki and approved by the Ethical Committee of the Emergency County Hospital of Oradea, Romania, with the registration number No. 26214/18.11.2020. and by the Ethics Committee of the Faculty of Medicine, University of Oradea, Romania, with the registration No. 12/20.11.2020.

Informed Consent Statement: Informed consent was obtained from all subjects involved in the study.

Data Availability Statement: The data presented in this study are available on request from the corresponding author.

Conflicts of Interest: The authors declare no conflict of interest.

References

1. World Health Organization. WHO Timeline–COVID-19. Available online: https://www.who.int/news-room/de-tail/27-04-2020-who-timeline---covid-19 (accessed on 20 December 2020).
2. Villani, F.A.; Aiuto, R.; Paglia, L.; Re, D. COVID-19 and Dentistry: Prevention in Dental Practice, a Literature Review. *Int. J. Environ. Res. Public Health* **2020**, *17*, 4609. [CrossRef]
3. Peditto, M.; Scapellato, S.; Marcianò, A.; Costa, P.; Oteri, G. Dentistry during the COVID-19 Epidemic: An Italian Workflow for the Management of Dental Practice. *Int. J. Environ. Res. Public Health* **2020**, *17*, 3325. [CrossRef]
4. Tysiąc-Miśta, M.; Dziedzic, A. The Attitudes and Professional Approaches of Dental Practitioners during the COVID-19 Outbreak in Poland: A Cross-Sectional Survey. *Int. J. Environ. Res. Public Health* **2020**, *17*, 4703. [CrossRef]
5. Chamorro-Petronacci, C.; Carreras-Presas, C.M.; Sanz-Marchena, A.; A Rodríguez-Fernández, M.; Suárez-Quintanilla, J.M.; Rivas-Mundiña, B.; Suárez-Quintanilla, J.; Pérez-Sayáns, M. Assessment of the Economic and Health-Care Impact of COVID-19 (SARS-CoV-2) on Public and Private Dental Surgeries in Spain: A Pilot Study. *Int. J. Environ. Res. Public Health* **2020**, *17*, 5139. [CrossRef] [PubMed]
6. Santana, M.C.; Zumarán, A.M.; Marín, N.P.; Silva, B.C.; Valencia, C.S.; Orozco, M.S. How Dentists Face the COVID-19 in Mexico: A Nationwide Cross-Sectional Study. *Int. J. Environ. Res. Public Health* **2021**, *18*, 1750. [CrossRef] [PubMed]
7. Consolo, U.; Bellini, P.; Bencivenni, D.; Iani, C.; Checchi, V. Epidemiological Aspects and Psychological Reactions to COVID-19 of Dental Practitioners in the Northern Italy Districts of Modena and Reggio Emilia. *Int. J. Environ. Res. Public Health* **2020**, *17*, 3459. [CrossRef] [PubMed]
8. Ahmed, M.A.; Jouhar, R.; Ahmed, N.; Adnan, S.; Aftab, M.; Zafar, M.S.; Khurshid, Z. Fear and Practice Modifications among Dentists to Combat Novel Coronavirus Disease (COVID-19) Outbreak. *Int. J. Environ. Res. Public Health* **2020**, *17*, 2821. [CrossRef]
9. Shacham, M.; Hamama-Raz, Y.; Kolerman, R.; Mijiritsky, O.; Ben-Ezra, M.; Mijiritsky, E. COVID-19 Factors and Psychological Factors Associated with Elevated Psychological Distress among Dentists and Dental Hygienists in Israel. *Int. J. Environ. Res. Public Health* **2020**, *17*, 2900. [CrossRef] [PubMed]
10. Vergara-Buenaventura, A.; Chavez-Tuñon, M.; Castro-Ruiz, C. The Mental Health Consequences of Coronavirus Disease 2019 Pandemic in Dentistry. *Disaster Med. Public Health Prep.* **2020**, 1–4. [CrossRef] [PubMed]
11. Gungor, A.S.; Donmez, N.; Uslu, Y.S. Knowledge, stress levels, and clinical practice modifications of Turkish dentists due to COVID-19: A survey study. *Braz. Oral Res.* **2021**, *35*, e048. [CrossRef] [PubMed]
12. Hanafy, R. Assessment of Practical and Emotional Consequences of Novel Coronavirus Emergence on Clinical Dental Practice in Egypt: A Cross Sectional Study. *Adv. Dent. J.* **2021**, *1*, 35–43.
13. Moraes, R.R.; Correa, M.B.; Queiroz, A.B.; Daneris, Â.; Lopes, J.P.; Pereira-Cenci, T.; D'Avila, O.P.; Cenci, M.; Lima, G.S.; Demarco, F.F. COVID-19 challenges to dentistry in the new pandemic epicenter: Brazil. *PLoS ONE* **2020**, *15*, e0242251. [CrossRef] [PubMed]
14. Heymann, D.L. Ebola: Transforming fear into appropriate action. *Lancet* **2017**, *390*, 219–220. [CrossRef]
15. Perogamvros, L.; Castelnovo, A.; Samson, D.; Dang-Vu, T.T. Failure of fear extinction in insomnia: An evolutionary perspec-tive. *Sleep Med. Rev.* **2020**, *51*, 101277. [CrossRef]

16. Nikopoulou, V.A.; Holeva, V.; Parlapani, E.; Karamouzi, P.; Voitsidis, P.; Porfyri, G.-N.; Blekas, A.; Papigkioti, K.; Patsiala, S.; Diakogiannis, I. Mental Health Screening for COVID-19: A Proposed Cutoff Score for the Greek Version of the Fear of COVID-19 Scale (FCV-19S). *Int. J. Ment. Health Addict.* **2020**, 1–14. [CrossRef] [PubMed]
17. Military Ordinance. Available online: https://www.mai.gov.ro/wp-content/uploads/2020%9Ba-militar%C4%83-nr.-1-2020-m%C4%83suri-de-prima-urgen%C8%9B%C4%83-Decret.pdf (accessed on 3 December 2020).
18. National Executive Office of the Romanian College of Dentists. Recommendations for Preventing the Spread of COVID-19 in Emergency Dental Activity. Available online: https://cmdr.ro/download-zone-preview/0/1585254764/3114/7c1a06790c87eb490b59e77515bababd (accessed on 8 December 2020).
19. Pituru, S.; Imre, M.; Totan, A.; Pantea, M.; Tancu, A.; Amza, O.; Bencze, A.; Ionescu, E. Study on the ethical and safety aspects among romanian dental healthcare professionals during Covid-19 pandemic. *Rom. J. Leg. Med.* **2020**, *28*, 322–330. [CrossRef]
20. Petrescu, N.; Aghiorghiesei, O.; Mesaros, A.; Lucaciu, O.; Dinu, C.; Campian, R.; Negucioiu, M. Impact of COVID-19 on Dental Emergency Services in Cluj-Napoca Metropolitan Area: A Cross-Sectional Study. *Int. J. Environ. Res. Public Health* **2020**, *17*, 7716. [CrossRef] [PubMed]
21. Iurcov, R.; Pop, L.; Ciavoi, G.; Iorga, M. Evaluating the Practice of Preventive Behaviors and the Fear of COVID-19 among Dentists in Oradea Metropolitan Area after the First Wave of Pandemic; a Cross-Sectional Study. *Health* **2021**, *9*, 443. [CrossRef]
22. Ahorsu, D.K.; Lin, C.-Y.; Imani, V.; Saffari, M.; Griffiths, M.D.; Pakpour, A.H. The Fear of COVID-19 Scale: Development and Initial Validation. *Int. J. Ment. Health Addict.* **2020**, *27*, 1–9. [CrossRef] [PubMed]
23. Chi, X.; Chen, S.; Chen, Y.; Chen, D.; Yu, Q.; Guo, T.; Cao, Q.; Zheng, X.; Huang, S.; Hossain, M.; et al. Psychometric Evaluation of the Fear of COVID-19 Scale Among Chinese Population. *Int. J. Ment. Health Addict.* **2021**, 1–16. [CrossRef]
24. Soldatos, C.R.; Dikeos, D.G.; Paparrigopoulos, T.J. The diagnostic validity of the Athens Insomnia Scale. *J. Psychosom. Res.* **2003**, *55*, 263–267. [CrossRef]
25. Sirajudeen, M.S.; Manzar, D.; Alqahtani, M.; Alzhrani, M.; Albougami, A.; Pillai, P.S.; Spence, D.W.; Pandi-Perumal, S.R. Psychometric Properties of the Athens Insomnia Scale in Occupational Computer Users. *Healthcare* **2020**, *8*, 89. [CrossRef]
26. Stănculescu, E. Fear of COVID-19 in Romania: Validation of the Romanian Version of the Fear of COVID-19 Scale Using Graded Response Model Analysis. *Int. J. Ment. Health Addict.* **2021**, 1–16. [CrossRef]
27. Bitan, D.T.; Grossman-Giron, A.; Bloch, Y.; Mayer, Y.; Shiffman, N.; Mendlovic, S. Fear of COVID-19 scale: Psychometric characteristics, reliability and validity in the Israeli population. *Psychiatry Res.* **2020**, *289*, 113100. [CrossRef] [PubMed]
28. Satici, B.; Gocet-Tekin, E.; Deniz, M.E.; Satici, S.A. Adaptation of the Fear of COVID-19 Scale: Its Association with Psychological Distress and Life Satisfaction in Turkey. *Int. J. Ment. Health Addict.* **2020**, 1–9. [CrossRef] [PubMed]
29. Cavalheiro, F.R.S.; Sticca, M.G. Adaptation and Validation of the Brazilian Version of the Fear of COVID-19 Scale. *Int. J. Ment. Health Addict.* **2020**, 1–9. [CrossRef]
30. Soraci, P.; Ferrari, A.; Abbiati, F.A.; Del Fante, E.; De Pace, R.; Urso, A.; Griffiths, M.D. Validation and Psychometric Evaluation of the Italian Version of the Fear of COVID-19 Scale. *Int. J. Ment. Health Addict.* **2020**, 1–10. [CrossRef]
31. Alyami, M.; Henning, M.; Krägeloh, C.U.; Alyami, H. Psychometric Evaluation of the Arabic Version of the Fear of COVID-19 Scale. *Int. J. Ment. Health Addict.* **2020**, 1–14. [CrossRef] [PubMed]
32. Reznik, A.; Gritsenko, V.; Konstantinov, V.; Khamenka, N.; Isralowitz, R. COVID-19 Fear in Eastern Europe: Validation of the Fear of COVID-19 Scale. *Int. J. Ment. Health Addict.* **2020**, 1–6. [CrossRef]
33. Mercado-Lara, M.F.; Campo-Arias, A.; Monterrosa-Castro, Á. Validity and Reliability of the Spanish Version of Fear of COVID-19 Scale in Colombian Physicians. *Int. J. Ment. Health Addict.* **2021**, 1–8. [CrossRef]
34. Caycho-Rodríguez, T.; Vilca, L.W.; Cervigni, M.; Gallegos, M.; Martino, P.; Portillo, N.; Barés, I.; Calandra, M.; Videla, C.B. Fear of COVID-19 scale: Validity, reliability and factorial invariance in Argentina's general population. *Death Stud.* **2020**, 1–10. [CrossRef] [PubMed]
35. Gasparro, R.; Scandurra, C.; Maldonato, N.M.; Dolce, P.; Bochicchio, V.; Valletta, A.; Sammartino, G.; Sammartino, P.; Mariniello, M.; Di Lauro, A.E.; et al. Perceived Job Insecurity and Depressive Symptoms Among Italian Dentists: The Moderating Role of Fear of COVID-19. *Int. J. Environ. Res. Public Health* **2020**, *17*, 5338. [CrossRef]
36. De Stefani, A.; Bruno, G.; Mutinelli, S.; Gracco, A. COVID-19 Outbreak Perception in Italian Dentists. *Int. J. Environ. Res. Public Health* **2020**, *17*, 3867. [CrossRef]
37. Lima, D.L.; Lopes, M.A.A.A.D.M.; Brito, A.M. Social media: Friend or foe in the COVID-19 pandemic? *Clinics* **2020**, *75*, 75. [CrossRef] [PubMed]
38. Newman, E.N. What are the challenges associated with testing for Ebola? A focus on the 2014 outbreak in West Africa. *Futur. Virol.* **2015**, *10*, 469–471. [CrossRef]
39. Shao, R.; Shi, Z.; Zhang, D. Social Media and Emotional Burnout Regulation During the COVID-19 Pandemic: Multilevel Approach. *J. Med. Internet Res.* **2021**, *23*, e27015. [CrossRef] [PubMed]
40. Mesch, G.S.; Schwirian, K.P. Social and political determinants of vaccine hesitancy: Lessons learned from the H1N1 pandemic of 2009–2010. *Am. J. Infect. Control.* **2015**, *43*, 1161–1165. [CrossRef]
41. Trnka, R.; Lorencova, R. Fear, anger, and media-induced trauma during the outbreak of COVID-19 in the Czech Republic. *Psychol. Trauma Theory Res. Pr. Policy* **2020**, *12*, 546–549. [CrossRef] [PubMed]
42. Ermolaev, V.V.; Sorokoumova, E.A.; Voroncova, J.; Nasonova, D.K.; Chetverikova, A.I. Psychological features of social fears associated with the COVID-19 content of news feed in Russia. *Eurasian J. Biosci.* **2020**, *14*, 2403–2409.

43. Becker, K.; Brunello, G.; Gurzawska-Comis, K.; Becker, J.; Sivolella, S.; Schwarz, F.; Klinge, B. Dental care during COVID-19 pandemic: Survey of experts' opinion. *Clin. Oral Implant. Res.* **2020**, *31*, 1253–1256. [CrossRef]
44. Xiao, H.; Zhang, Y.; Kong, D.; Li, S.; Yang, N. The Effects of Social Support on Sleep Quality of Medical Staff Treating Patients with Coronavirus Disease 2019 (COVID-19) in January and February 2020 in China. *Med. Sci. Monit.* **2020**, *26*, e923549-1. [CrossRef]
45. Dahlgren, A.; Kecklund, G.; Akerstedt, T. Different levels of work-related stress and the effects on sleep, fatigue and cortisol. *Scand. J. Work. Environ. Health* **2005**, *31*, 277–285. [CrossRef] [PubMed]
46. Oladunjoye, A.; Oladunjoye, O. An evolving problem—Mental health symptoms among health care workers during COVID-19 pandemic. *Asian J. Psychiatry* **2020**, *54*, 102257. [CrossRef] [PubMed]
47. Bohlken, J.; Schömig, F.; Seehagen, T.; Köhler, S.; Gehring, K.; Roth-Sackenheim, C.; Matschinger, H.; Riedel-Heller, S.G. Experience of practice-based psychiatrists and neurologists during the COVID-19 pandemic. *Psychiatr. Prax.* **2020**, *47*, 214–217. [CrossRef]
48. Lai, J.; Ma, S.; Wang, Y.; Cai, Z.; Hu, J.; Wei, N.; Wu, J.; Du, H.; Chen, T.; Li, R.; et al. Factors Associated With Mental Health Outcomes Among Health Care Workers Exposed to Coronavirus Disease 2019. *JAMA Netw. Open* **2020**, *3*, e203976. [CrossRef] [PubMed]
49. Mustafa, R.M.; AlShali, R.Z.; Bukhary, D.M. Dentists' Knowledge, Attitudes, and Awareness of Infection Control Measures during COVID-19 Outbreak: A Cross-Sectional Study in Saudi Arabia. *Int. J. Environ. Res. Public Health* **2020**, *17*, 9016. [CrossRef] [PubMed]
50. Léger, D.; Beck, F.; Fressard, L.; Verger, P.; Peretti-Watel, P.; Seror, V.; Cortaredona, S.; Launay, O.; Raude, J.; Legleye, S.; et al. Poor sleep associated with overuse of media during the COVID-19 lockdown. *Sleep* **2020**, *43*. [CrossRef]
51. Dai, W.; Zhou, J.; Li, G.; Zhang, B.; Ma, N. Maintaining normal sleep patterns, lifestyles and emotion during the COVID-19 pandemic: The stabilizing effect of daytime napping. *J. Sleep Res.* **2021**, e13259. [CrossRef]
52. Sinha, M.; Pande, B.; Sinha, R. Impact of COVID-19 lockdown on sleep-wake schedule and associated lifestyle related behavior: A national survey. *J. Public Health Res.* **2020**, *9*, 1826. [CrossRef] [PubMed]
53. Clough, B.A.; March, S.; Chan, R.J.; Casey, L.M.; Phillips, R.; Ireland, M.J. Psychosocial interventions for managing occupational stress and burnout among medical doctors: A systematic review. *Syst. Rev.* **2017**, *6*, 1–19. [CrossRef] [PubMed]
54. Chohan, L.; Dewa, C.S.; El-Badrawy, W.; Nainar, S.M.H. Occupational burnout and depression among paediatric dentists in the United States. *Int. J. Paediatr. Dent.* **2020**, *30*, 570–577. [CrossRef] [PubMed]
55. Chipchase, S.Y.; Chapman, H.R.; Bretherton, R. A study to explore if dentists' anxiety affects their clinical decision-making. *Br. Dent. J.* **2017**, *222*, 277–290. [CrossRef] [PubMed]
56. Song, K.-W.; Choi, W.-S.; Jee, H.-J.; Yuh, C.-S.; Kim, Y.-K.; Kim, L.; Lee, H.-J.; Cho, C.-H. Correlation of occupational stress with depression, anxiety, and sleep in Korean dentists: Cross-sectional study. *BMC Psychiatry* **2017**, *17*, 1–11. [CrossRef]
57. Keeter, S.C. People Financially Affected by COVID-19 Outbreak are Experiencing more Psychological Distress than Others. Pew Research Center. 30 March 2020. Available online: https://www.pewresearch.org/fact-tank/2020/03/30/people-financially-affected-by-covid-19-outbreak-are-experiencing-more-psychological-distress-than-others/ (accessed on 20 January 2021).
58. Wańkowicz, P.; Szylińska, A.; Rotter, I. The Impact of the COVID-19 Pandemic on Psychological Health and Insomnia among People with Chronic Diseases. *J. Clin. Med.* **2021**, *10*, 1206. [CrossRef] [PubMed]
59. Dekker, K.; Blanken, T.F.; Van Someren, E.J.W. Insomnia and Personality—A Network Approach. *Brain Sci.* **2017**, *7*, 28. [CrossRef]
60. Pacutova, V.; Geckova, A.M.; Kizek, P.; de Winter, A.F.; Reijneveld, S.A. The Impact of Pandemic Management on the Quality of Life of Slovak Dentists. *Int. J. Environ. Res. Public Health* **2021**, *18*, 5484. [CrossRef]

Journal of
Clinical Medicine

MDPI

Article

Coping Strategies by University Students in Response to COVID-19: Differences between Community and Clinical Groups

Víctor-María López-Ramos, Benito León-del-Barco *, Santiago Mendo-Lázaro * and María-Isabel Polo-del-Río

Psychological Counseling Services, Faculty of Teacher Training College, University of Extremadura, 10071 Cáceres, Spain; vmlopez@unex.es (V.-M.L.-R.); mabelpdrio@unex.es (M.-I.P.-d.-R.)
* Correspondence: bleon@unex.es (B.L.-d.-B.); smendo@unex.es (S.M.-L.)

Abstract: Last year, the COVID-19 pandemic had severe consequences on the health and well-being of millions of people. Different studies try to identify the main effects that the crisis and several lockdowns have had on the citizens' mental health. This research analyses the coping strategies generated by students from a community group and a clinical group in response to this crisis, using the Coping Responses Inventory—Adult Form (CRI-A) by Moos with a sample of 1074 students of Universidad de Extremadura. Multivariate analysis and receiver operating characteristic curve analysis have been carried out, revealing, amongst other things, a greater predisposition of the clinical sample towards factors such as seeking guidance and support, cognitive avoidance or emotional discharge. Results show that students with prior mental health problems perform an unhealthy coping response based on avoidance strategies. This group of students suffers a double source of distress and anxiety, one derived from their prior psychopathologic problems and the stress of the lockdown and another one originating from an inefficient coping response, which makes coping strategies raise levels of distress and anxiety.

Keywords: pandemic; lockdown; mental health; anxiety; stress; psychological coping

Citation: López-Ramos, V.-M.; León-del-Barco, B.; Mendo-Lázaro, S.; Polo-del-Río, M.-I. Coping Strategies by University Students in Response to COVID-19: Differences between Community and Clinical Groups. *J. Clin. Med.* **2021**, *10*, 2499. https://doi.org/10.3390/jcm10112499

Academic Editor: Michele Roccella

Received: 5 March 2021
Accepted: 31 May 2021
Published: 5 June 2021

1. Introduction

On 11 March 2020, the World Health Organisation (WHO) declared COVID-19 (acronym for "coronavirus disease 2019") a pandemic due to the high morbidity and mortality registered since this novel coronavirus was first detected in the city of Wuhan (China) in December 2019. The health, economic and social effects of the pandemic are currently extremely severe, and there is still no confirmation of how long they will last. Consequently, the Government of Spain approved a Royal Decree (RD 463/2020, on 14 March) that declared a state of alarm in order to manage the sanitary crisis caused by the pandemic. During the state of alarm, movement had to be individual and limited to first-need activities or commuting to workplace; passenger transport options were radically reduced; cultural, artistic and sporting venues were closed; working from home became a priority and face-to-face education was suspended at all levels, favouring online education.

The lockdown experienced by the Spanish society, as well as almost every country nearby, was an extraordinary situation as it was unfamiliar and has proved to have a strong impact on the psychological well-being of citizens, with various sources of stress.

A first study on the psychological impact of the COVID-19 quarantine in China [1] showed that psychosocial stress and the loss of habits and routines are the two main factors affecting physical and mental well-being during a period of confinement such as the one we have experienced. Studies on situations of risk, conflict and emergencies allow us to synthetise that the main variables implied in psychological impact are the following: fear of contracting diseases, feelings of frustration and boredom, not being able to meet basic needs and the lack of information and clear action guidelines [2], or the presence of previous mental health pathologies or economic hardships [3]. Additionally, stigma and social rejection of people infected or exposed to the disease are potential triggers for having difficulties when adapting to the situation [2]. The impact degree depends on several factors. According to Sprang and Silman's research [4], people who have already experienced a quarantine during a pandemic are more likely to develop acute stress, adaptation and pain disorders (30 percent of them presenting criteria of post-traumatic stress disorder).

Nonetheless, there is still scant evidence about the immediate psychological impact of the consequences of the pandemic on the general population, mainly through research studies carried out with Chinese individuals. In a first study with a sample of 1210 people, 53% valued the psychological impact of the situation as moderate to severe, 16% referred moderate to severe depression symptoms, 28% referred moderate to severe anxiety symptoms and 8% declared moderate to severe levels of stress. For 75% of the individuals studied, the main concern was their relatives becoming infected with the disease [1]. Another research carried out with inhabitants of Wuhan and neighbouring towns showed a prevalence of 7% for symptoms of post-traumatic stress [5]. Moreover, the same group considered a wider sample of 2091 people and got a prevalence of 4.6% for symptoms of acute post-traumatic stress one month after the COVID-19 outbreak [6].

The social–cultural and psychosocial reality in Spain may have elements of connection with the results obtained in these and other international research studies, although we could also anticipate important cultural, social and health particularities. During the months of April, May and June 2020, several surveys were carried out, most of them with reduced and not very representative samples, as well as polls that compiled basically descriptive data. Broadly, conclusive results on these kinds of studies are yet to be published, although we do have some works that are starting to offer valuable data, such as the study developed by Ozmiz-Etxeberria et al. [7] with a sample of 976 people, collected in Northern Spain, which indicates that severe and extremely severe levels of stress, anxiety and depression found in this sample were less than those collected in the study carried out in China by Wang et al. [1]. This is probably due to the fact that Spain had broader access to information about the virus since it got here one and a half month later. Otherwise, it is noteworthy that the study by Ozmiz-Etxeberria et al. [7] found higher averages for stress, anxiety and depression in people aged 18–25 years old, followed by those aged 26–60, the average in the three dimensions being lower in those over 60. This may imply that the younger group of the study mainly comprised students and that the stress generated was increased by added stress due to the need to adapt to the new educational context without on-site classes. Another study concluded that 89% of a sample composed by children presented behavioural or emotional alterations as a consequence of lockdown [8]. In this sense, the fact of resuming healthy routines and habits once lockdown was over, together with getting healthy support, must allow the affected individuals to recover to normal functioning [9]. Nevertheless, the need of some type of psychological support after a period of lockdown is to be expected, especially amongst those who presented previous psychological conditions, development disorders or other psychopathologies [10].

It is evident that the impact of lockdown measurements on the general population between the months of March and June, and even the consequences of the restrictive measures prevailing after the state of alarm, have differently affected the various populational sectors that compose Spain's social structure. We consider that, for university students, this impact requires a more detailed study since apart from being young—18 to 25—they were also forced to end the school year 2019–2020 in an online modality and to face final exams also virtually. Determining the extent of consequences for university students would significantly aid the proposals of improvement related to psychological orientation and counselling in this context, and it would also allow the definition of proceedings aimed to manage stress and anxiety in universities, especially in situations of crisis, with a particular approach to individuals with prior mental health issues or disorders.

The unusual, unpredictable nature of the lockdown imposed in Spain to control the spread of COVID-19 gives us an opportunity to reflect on the personalised support models that should be put in place for university students, especially in risk and conflict situations. In this regard, echoing Balluerka et al. [10], individuals who are predisposed to certain problems or who have displayed psychopathological symptoms in the past are likely to be at greater risk of these symptoms reappearing after lockdown. Therefore, in line with Balluerka et al. [10], two types of psychological effects are anticipated to have emerged during and after the lockdown among our sample of university students:

1. Specific effects that are directly linked to one or more stimuli caused by the COVID-19 pandemic: family and personal circumstances leading to moderate to severe suffering as a result of high levels of stress and emotional disturbance, with medical, social and economic repercussions.
2. Unspecific effects that are very difficult to attribute to a specific trigger beyond the contextual changes arising as a result of the pandemic and lockdown, which are linked to intense worry, fear of contagion, pessimism about the future, sense of vulnerability, uneasiness in the face of uncertainty, etc.

Situations such as the one generated by the COVID-19 pandemic force us more precisely define the conceptualisation of coping strategies as a fundamental element for adaptations made by people in every diverse critical situation they may face [11]. In this way, coping must be approached as a stabilising variable that helps people to keep their psychosocial adaptation in moments of high stress levels [12,13]. A number of studies have concluded that coping strategies focused on the problem itself reduce psychological distress, whereas strategies based on emotions increase it [14]. In this sense, active skills appear to be associated with health, while avoidance ones are linked to the development of a range of diseases [15,16].

The characteristics and nature of the events faced by people influence both the availability and mobilisation of resources, as well as the coping strategies for those [17] (Moos, 1993). From the coping model raised by this author, the characteristics specific to a crisis and the evaluation of the situation carried out by an individual contextualise the response choice specific to coping [11]. It has been observed that stressful situations tend to promote a higher amount of behavioural active coping responses, while those due to interpersonal relationships generate a higher amount of coping focused on emotion [18]. In this sense, it seems to be demonstrated that the more negative life situations and chronic stress sources are present, the less employment of responses focused on approach to the problem there are, and higher the use of responses focused on avoidance is [19]. In relation with evaluation of stressful life situations, it has been checked that, when stressors are evaluated as a challenge, they tend to provoke coping responses focused on approach more than on avoidance. This means that type, severeness and evaluation performed in moments of crisis influence the coping strategies used, which proves the need and pertinence of the interconnection established between the different coping responses and concretion of the situation [19].

Another element of key importance is the degree of controllability of the stressful situation itself. The perceived controllability of the stressful stimulus has an impact on the type of strategy used and on its effectivity for lowering the stress level [20]. In this sense, Moos and Schaefer [13] propose that coping responses focused on approach should be more effective in situations that are regarded as changeable and controllable. In this regard, studies by Mikulic and Crespi [21,22] carried out with people in situations of deprivation of liberty found a prevalence of coping responses focused on avoidance, which are related to the perception of not being able to operate in the imprisonment situation that generates discomfort because of the multiplicity of variables beyond the control of the individuals.

Along these lines, the Coping Responses Inventory—Adult Form (CRI-A) by Moos becomes an important tool for the study of coping responses in an adult population thanks to its psychometric inputs in multiple sociocultural contexts [11].

The Present Study

This study analyses the coping strategies adopted by university students in response to the COVID-19 pandemic. To do this, it uses the Coping Responses Inventory—Adult Form (CRI-A) by Moos [17].

Drawing on previous studies, the aim is to compare a community group with a clinical group to identify discriminative coping responses displayed by students in response to the Spanish lockdown lasting several months. Two key variables have been established for the study: the group to which the individual belongs, either community or clinical, and the coping response adopted by the individual according to the typology set out in the CRI-A (logical analysis; positive reappraisal; seeking guidance and support; problem solving; cognitive avoidance; acceptance or resignation; seeking alternative rewards; and emotional discharge).

2. Materials and Methods

2.1. Participants

In order to be included in the study, participants had to be enrolled at the University of Extremadura during the 2019–2020 academic year. The sample was made up of 1074 students. The average age was 23.07 years old (SD = 5.28; range 18–37); 56.4% (n = 606) were female and 43.6% (n = 468) were male. In all, 16.8% of the students were in their first year, 18.2% in their second year, 25.9% in their third year, 21.2% in their fourth year and 17.9% in their fifth, sixth or master's year on different degree courses at the University of Extremadura. The number of participants was calculated on the basis of the 20,000 students enrolled in the 2019–2020 academic year, considering a sample error of 3% and a confidence level of 96%. Students were selected from the faculties at the University of Extremadura using multistage cluster sampling and random selection by degree course and year of study. The sample from the psychopathological clinical population was made up of 135 individuals: 60% were male and 40% were female. The clinical group comprised students diagnosed with mental health disorders, predominantly anxiety and depression, by public and private mental health services.

Both the clinical and the community group were equivalent in age t (1063) = −0.478, p = 0.633, gender $\chi^2(1) = 0.197$, p = 0.657, and year $\chi^2(6) = 5.940$, p = 0.460.

2.2. Instruments

The adaptation by Kirchner and Forns [23] of the Coping Responses Inventory—Adult Form (CRI-A) by Moos [17] was used. The inventory consists of 48 items on a Likert scale of 0 to 3 (0 = never; 1 = rarely, 2 = occasionally; 3 = very frequently) evaluating eight factors (six items per factor; minimum score = 0; maximum score = 18) or coping responses: (1) Logical analysis (LA): cognitive attempts to understand and mentally prepare to cope with a stressor and its consequences. (2) Positive reappraisal (PR): cognitive attempts to construct and restructure a problem in a positive manner while accepting the reality of the situation. (3) Seeking guidance and support (SG): behavioural attempts to seek out information, support and guidance. (4) Problem solving (PS): behavioural attempts to carry out actions leading to the root of the problem. (5) Cognitive avoidance (CA): cognitive attempts to avoid thinking about the problem realistically. (6) Acceptance or resignation (AR): cognitive attempts to respond to the problem by accepting it. (7) Seeking alternative rewards (SR): behavioural attempts to engage in alternative activities and create new sources of satisfaction. (8) Emotional discharge (ED): behavioural attempts to reduce tension by expressing negative feelings. The LA, PR, CA and AR strategies relate to the cognitive dimension of coping, whereas SG, PS, SR and ED relate to the behavioural dimension. The LA, PR, SG and PS coping responses are considered approach strategies, while the CA, AR, SR and ED responses are considered avoidance strategies.

Kirchner and Forns [23] reviewed and validated the psychometric properties of the questionnaire in its Spanish version in line with the coping responses proposed by Moos [17], who notes that individuals tend to respond to a specific situation in either a cognitive or behavioural manner, with a focus on approach or avoidance strategies [24]. Table 1 summarises the response types in relation to the eight factors of the CRI-A:

Table 1. Coping responses according to Moos (source: Pujada [24]).

		Focus	
		Approach	**Avoidance**
Method	Cognitive	Logical analysis (LA) Positive reappraisal (PR)	Cognitive avoidance (CA) Acceptance or resignation (AR)
	Behavioural	Seeking guidance and support (SG) Problem solving (PS)	Seeking alternative rewards (SR) Emotional discharge (ED)

In relation to reliability, values are similar to those from the CRIA-A adaptation study [23]. Cronbach's alpha's values (α) of all eight strategies were between 0.61 and 0.73, presenting a lower value than expected for the AL factor ($\alpha = 0.61$). All four dimensions—cognitive ($\alpha = 0.72$), behavioural ($\alpha > 0.71$), approach ($\alpha = 0.83$) and avoidance ($\alpha = 0.71$)—obtained acceptable values.

2.3. Procedure

The CRI-A was administered online using the Google Forms application (a Google Drive tool, for the individuals of both the community and the clinical group. In accordance with the ethical guidelines issued by the American Psychological Association (APA, 2009), all participants gave their informed consent before completing the questionnaires. The questionnaires were anonymous, guaranteeing the confidentiality of the data obtained and the exclusive use of these data for research purposes. Data were collected between 10 May and 10 June 2020, during home lockdown decreed by Spain's government (from 14 March to 20 June 2020). When this research was carried out, in Spain there were 242,280 officially confirmed COVID-19 cases and 27,136 people had died from the disease.

At the time of the data collection, the clinical group was formed by 113 people who were being treated or had been previously treated at the Psychological Care Unit (UNAP, for its acronym in Spanish), reporting to the Research Group in Social and Personality Evolutive Psychology (GIPES-UEx). This counselling is available on request by the students and does not aim to be a clinical psychological intervention but an action based on psychological counselling and on strategy training and personal advice oriented towards studying the efficiency of this counselling and towards the improvement of their interpersonal relationships, taking into account the disorders and alterations suffered.

In this group, 46 individuals had a previous diagnosis performed by external professionals not related to UNAP, from both public and private mental health services, and 67 had been assessed within UNAP. The most diagnosed disorder was related to general anxiety episodes (52% of individuals from the clinical group), as wells as fears or specific phobias with continuous concern, exaggerated or unrealistic (43%). Diagnoses of depression (32%) and obsessive–compulsive disorder (14%) were also remarkable; as for the clinical assessments carried out by UNAP, the most relevant findings were those related to sleep (75%) and eating (60%) disorders, and also alterations in intimate relationships and in sexual behaviour and health, with special emphasis on aspects such as communication between intimate partners (26%), emotional climate in the relationship (24%) or a decreasingly satisfactory sex life (22%).

The study was conducted according to the guidelines of the Declaration of Helsinki and was approved by the Bioethics and Biosafety Committee of the University of Extremadura (21/001/UAP).

2.4. Data Analysis

SPSS 21.0 was used to perform statistical analysis on the collected data (IBM Corp., New York, NY, USA, 2012). The reliability of the instruments used was calculated using Cronbach's alpha. After checking the assumptions of normality and homoscedasticity, a multivariate analysis (MANOVA) and receiver operating characteristic curve analysis (ROC) were carried out.

3. Results

Firstly, multivariate comparisons of the mean scores for the CRI-A factors were carried out by group (community/clinical) and gender, as well as for the interaction between the two variables (Table 2).

Table 2. Descriptive analysis for the eight CRI-A factors and univariate analysis by group (community/clinical) and gender.

CRI-A Factors	Sample	Male		Female		Total		Between-Subject Effects Group and Gender		
		M	SD	M	SD	M	SD	F	p	η
(LA)	Community	10.71	2.79	10.15	3.39	10.28	3.26	1.678	0.195	0.002
	Clinical	11.50	4.02	10.29	3.05	10.56	3.32			
	Total	10.80	2.96	10.16	3.35	10.32	3.27	6.079	0.014	0.006
(PR)	Community	10.72	3.86	11.13	3.81	11.03	3.83	0.951	0.330	0.001
	Clinical	10.40	4.37	10.63	3.36	10.58	3.59			
	Total	10.68	3.92	11.06	3.76	10.97	3.80	0.573	0.449	0.001
(SG)	Community	8.36	3.28	8.85	3.27	8.73	3.28	4.621	0.032	0.004
	Clinical	9.80	5.24	9.03	3.98	9.20	4.28			
	Total	8.53	3.59	8.87	3.37	8.79	3.42	0.141	0.708	0.000
(PS)	Community	11.53	3.62	11.18	3.64	11.27	3.63	6.531	0.011	0.006
	Clinical	10.50	5.13	10.14	3.61	10.22	3.98			
	Total	11.41	3.83	11.05	3.65	11.14	3.69	0.755	0.385	0.001
(CA)	Community	10.09	3.70	10.75	3.29	10.59	3.40	23.881	0.000	0.022
	Clinical	12.60	4.41	11.91	3.14	12.07	3.45			
	Total	10.39	3.86	10.90	3.29	10.78	3.44	0.001	0.971	0.000
(AR)	Community	8.45	3.43	8.95	3.21	8.83	3.27	64.611	0.000	0.057
	Clinical	12.10	3.51	11.03	2.80	11.27	2.99			
	Total	8.88	3.63	9.22	3.23	9.14	3.33	0.652	0.420	0.001
(SR)	Community	8.35	3.13	8.76	3.35	8.66	3.30	4.183	0.041	0.004
	Clinical	9.70	2.28	8.89	3.21	9.07	3.04			
	Total	8.51	3.07	8.78	3.33	8.72	3.27	0.302	0.583	0.000
(ED)	Community	7.63	2.91	8.75	3.07	8.48	3.07	72.025	0.000	0.063
	Clinical	11.10	3.07	10.91	2.76	10.96	2.82			
	Total	8.04	3.13	9.03	3.12	8.79	3.15	1.982	0.159	0.002

LA = logical analysis; PR = positive reappraisal; SG = seeking guidance and support; PS = problem solving; CA = cognitive avoidance; AR = acceptance or resignation; SR = seeking alternative rewards; ED = emotional discharge.

The multivariate analysis (MANOVA) gave a significant main effect by group (community/clinical), Wilks' $\lambda = 0.901$, F (8, 1063) = 14.594 $p < 0.001$, $\eta = 0.099$, and by gender, Wilks' $\lambda = 0.982$, F (8, 1063) = 2.372, $p = 0.016$, $\eta = 0.018$), although no significant main effect was found for the group–gender interaction, Wilks' $\lambda = 0.988$, F (8, 1063) = 1.555, $p = 0.134$, $\eta = 0.012$.

As for the univariate contrasts, the tests for between-individual effects (Table 2) revealed significantly higher scores in the clinical group ($p < 0.05$) than in the community group in the seeking guidance and support, problem solving, cognitive avoidance, acceptance or resignation, seeking alternative rewards and emotional discharge factors. Male participants obtained significantly higher scores ($p = 0.014$) in the logical analysis factor than female participants did.

Multivariate comparison of the average scores in the CRI-A dimensions was carried out by group (community/clinical) and gender, as well as for the interaction between the two variables (Table 3).

Table 3. Descriptive analysis for the four CRI-A dimensions and univariate analysis by group (community/clinical) and group-gender interaction.

CRI-A Dimensions	Sample	Male		Female		Total		Between-Subject Effects Sample and Group-Gender Interaction		
		M	SD	M	SD	M	SD	F	p	η
Cognitive	Community	39.97	7.82	40.97	8.94	40.73	8.69	24.332	0.000	0.022
	Clinical	46.60	12.70	43.86	7.76	44.47	9.11			
	Total	40.75	8.77	41.34	8.85	41.20	8.83	2.773	0.082	0.004
Behavioural	Community	35.87	8.39	37.55	8.80	37.14	8.73	11.796	0.001	0.011
	Clinical	41.10	10.84	38.97	8.89	39.44	9.36			
	Total	36.48	8.86	37.73	8.82	37.43	8.84	3.858	0.050	0.004
Approach	Community	41.32	10.05	41.31	10.73	41.31	10.57	0.021	0.885	0.000
	Clinical	42.20	12.73	40.09	10.97	40.56	11.37			
	Total	41.42	10.38	41.15	10.76	41.22	10.67	0.795	0.373	0.001
Avoidance	Community	34.52	7.53	37.21	8.26	36.57	8.17	88.033	0.000	0.076
	Clinical	45.50	7.96	42.74	6.85	43.36	7.17			
	Total	35.81	8.35	37.92	8.30	37.42	8.35	9.599	0.002	0.009

The multivariate analysis (MANOVA) gave a significant main effect by group (community/clinical), Wilks' $\lambda = 0.905$, F (8, 1063) = 33.095 $p < 0.001$, $\eta = 0.085$, and by group–gender interaction, Wilks' $\lambda = 0.990$, $F(8, 1063) = 3.430$, $p = 0.017$, $\eta = 0.010$, although no significant main effect was found for gender, Wilks' $\lambda = 0.998$, F (8, 1063) = 0.593, $p = 0.620$, $\eta = 0.002$.

As for the univariate contrasts, the tests for between-subject effects (Table 3) show that the clinical group obtained significantly higher scores ($p \leq 0.001$) than the community group in the cognitive, behavioural and avoidance dimensions. They also revealed a significant group–gender interaction ($p < 0.05$) in the behavioural and avoidance dimensions.

The pairwise comparisons for interaction effects showed, on the one hand, that the difference between the groups (clinical/community) in the behavioural dimension was only significant ($p = 0.002$) between men, and, on the other hand, that men obtained significantly higher scores in the behavioural ($p = 0.013$) and avoidance ($p \leq 0.001$) dimensions in the community sample.

To analyse differences in the most commonly adopted strategies between the community and clinical groups, a repeated-measures ANOVA was performed between the scores for the cognitive, behavioural, approach and avoidance dimensions for the community and clinical groups (Table 4).

Table 4. Repeated-measures analysis between the four CRI-A dimensions by group (community/clinical).

Sample	CRI-A Dimensions								Within-Subject Effects		
	Cognitive		Behavioural		Approach		Avoidance				
	M	SD	M	SD	M	SD	M	SD	F	p	η
Community	40.73	8.69	37.14	8.73	41.31	10.57	36.57	8.17	457.050	0.000	0.328
Clinical	44.47	9.11	39.44	9.36	40.56	11.37	43.36	7.17	5.140	0.025	0.037

The repeated-measures analysis showed significant differences ($p < 0.05$) between the scores obtained in the four dimensions of the CRI-A in both groups (Table 4). The pairwise comparisons indicated the following: (1) In the community group, significantly higher scores ($p < 0.001$) were obtained in the cognitive and approach dimensions than in the behavioural and avoidance dimensions, with the score ($p < 0.001$) for the approach dimension being significantly higher than for the cognitive dimension. (2) In the clinical group, significantly higher scores ($p < 0.05$) were obtained in the cognitive and avoidance dimensions than in the behavioural and approach dimensions.

In order to evaluate the discriminative accuracy of the coping responses, a receiver operating characteristic curve analysis (ROC) was carried out to identify the cut-off points for the scores in the dimensions of the CRI-A (cognitive, behavioural, approach, avoidance), after which behavioural disorders become more likely.

In the nonparametric ROC analysis (Figure 1), the area beneath the curve for the cognitive dimension is 0.609 ($p < 0.001$; confidence interval 95%; min. = 0.555; max. = 0.622), the area beneath the curve for the behavioural dimension is 0.582 ($p = 0.002$; confidence interval 95%; min. = 0.529; max. = 0.635), the area beneath the curve for the approach dimension is 0.496 ($p = 0.875$; confidence interval 95%; min. = 0.444; max. = 0.547) and provides no significant information, and finally, the area beneath the curve for the avoidance dimension is 0.724 ($p < 0.001$; confidence interval 95%; min. = 0.683; max. = 0.765).

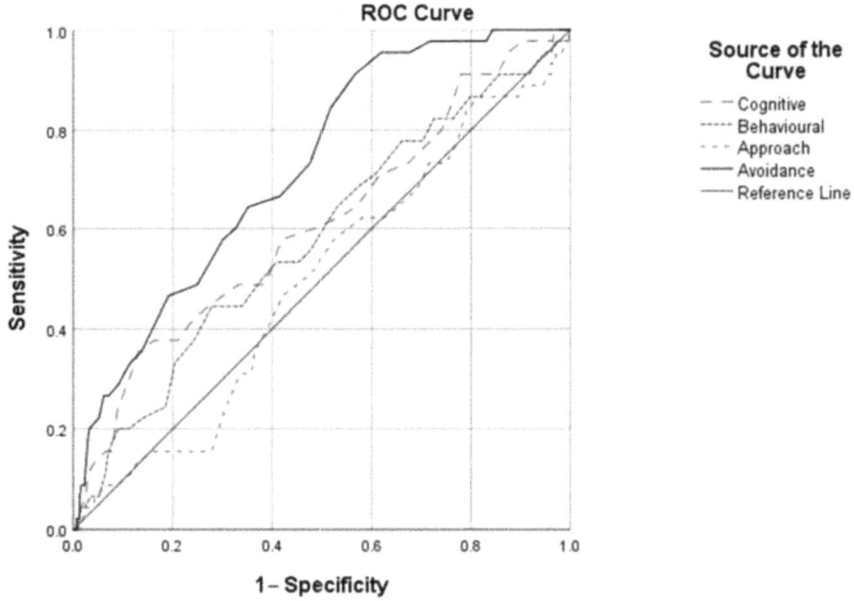

Figure 1. ROC curve for the CRI-A dimensions predicting the presence of psychopathological disorders.

Table 5 shows the cut-off points maximising both sensitivity and specificity and the cut-off points maximising sensitivity and specificity for the dimensions providing significant information ($p \leq 0.05$).

With regard to the presence of psychopathological disorders, a score of $\geq$42.5 in the cognitive dimension maximised both sensitivity (58%) and specificity (58%) (Youden's index = 0.159), a score of 41.5 maximised sensitivity (60%) while maintaining specificity higher than random, and a score of 43 maximised specificity (60%) while maintaining sensitivity higher than random. In the behavioural dimension, a score of $\geq$39.5 maximised both sensitivity (53%) and specificity (59%) (Youden's index = 0.124), a score of 37.5 maximised sensitivity (56%) while maintaining specificity higher than random, and a score of 40.0 maximised specificity (61%) while maintaining sensitivity higher than random. Finally, in the avoidance dimension, a score of $\geq$39.5 maximised both sensitivity (64%) and specificity (65%) (Youden's index = 0.293), a score of 36.0 maximised sensitivity (79%)

while maintaining specificity higher than random, and a score of 42.0 maximised specificity (73%) while maintaining sensitivity higher than random.

Table 5. Sensitivity, specificity and Youden's index for scores in the cognitive, behavioural and avoidance dimensions of the CRI-A to identify the presence of psychopathological disorders.

CRI-A	Cut-Off Point	Sensitivity	Specificity	Youden's Index
Cognitive dimension	41.5 *	0.600	0.514	0.114
	42.0	0.589	0.548	0.137
	42.5 ***	0.578	0.581	0.159
	43.0 **	0.533	0.597	0.131
Behavioural dimension	37.5 *	0.556	0.524	0.081
	38.0	0.545	0.535	0.080
	38.5	0.533	0.546	0.079
	39.0	0.533	0.569	0.102
	39.5 ***	0.533	0.591	0.124
	40.0 **	0.511	0.610	0.121
Avoidance dimension	36.0 *	0.789	0.503	0.291
	37.5	0.733	0.524	0.257
	38.0	0.700	0.555	0.255
	38.5	0.667	0.585	0.252
	39.0	0.655	0.617	0.273
	39.5 ***	0.644	0.649	0.293
	40.0	0.622	0.662	0.284
	40.5	0.600	0.674	0.274
	41.0	0.589	0.687	0.276
	41.5	0.578	0.700	0.278
	42.0 **	0.533	0.726	0.259

* Score maximising sensitivity. ** Score maximising specificity. *** Score maximising sensitivity and specificity.

4. Discussion

The lockdown restrictions imposed in Spain and across Europe gave rise to a unique and unprecedented situation that had a serious impact on the population's psychological well-being, generating a number of sources of stress. The aim of this study was to ascertain discriminative coping responses to lockdown by university students, divided into a community group and a clinical group.

Firstly, the results of the multivariate comparisons of the average scores for the factors and dimensions of the CRI-A by group (community/clinical) and gender showed that the clinical sample obtained significantly higher scores than the community group in the seeking guidance and support, cognitive avoidance, acceptance or resignation, seeking alternative rewards and emotional discharge factors. The effect size tests indicated a medium–high effect in the cognitive avoidance (η = 0.022), acceptance or resignation (η = 0.057) and emotional discharge (η = 0.063) factors, which are typical of an avoidance response. Coping using cognitive avoidance and acceptance or resignation strategies, as displayed by the clinical group, represents a more cognitive response. Meanwhile, coping using seeking guidance and support and seeking alternative rewards is suggestive of a more behavioural response. The community group obtained significantly higher scores in the problem solving factor.

Secondly, the repeated-measures analysis and the pairwise comparisons corroborated the results set out above, showing significantly higher scores for the clinical group in the cognitive and avoidance dimensions than in the behavioural and approach dimensions, whereas the community group obtained significantly higher scores in the cognitive and approach dimensions than in the behavioural and avoidance dimensions.

In short, the clinical group adopted an unhealthy coping response based on primarily cognitive avoidance strategies (cognitive avoidance and acceptance or resignation). These strategies have a limited effect and are associated with poorer life satisfaction and more severe psychopathological symptoms [25,26]. The clinical group only displayed one healthier, more active strategy: seeking guidance and support. These results raise several questions: (1) Why does the clinical group adopt a pattern of avoidance coping? (2) Why does the clinical group report more extensive use of one approach strategy, seeking guidance and support? (3) What was the influence of gender?

With regard to the first question, the clinical group uses avoidance coping strategies (cognitive avoidance, acceptance or resignation and emotional discharge) and the community group tends to use approach strategies (problem solving). Active or approach strategies appear to be associated with health, while avoidance strategies are linked to the development of a range of diseases [15,16]. It has been demonstrated that the more chronic stressors are present, the less likely individuals will be to adopt approach responses and the more likely they will be to adopt avoidance responses [16]. Other studies show a positive association between avoidance coping strategies and stress, anxiety, anger, sadness and loneliness [27]. The clinical group experienced distress and anxiety as a result of their prior mental health issues and the stress of the lockdown (loss of habits and routines, fear of contagion, concern for classes and exams, etc.).

The clinical group in this study is a sample of a psychopathological clinical population with a large number of pathologies, predominantly anxiety and depression. In general, people with a psychopathological clinical profile (depression, anxiety, eating disorders, addictions, etc.) tend to use ineffective coping strategies and struggle to adopt a healthy coping response [28]. Some studies have shown an association between avoidance strategies and eating disorders [29]. Other longitudinal studies on mood psychopathology found a significant association between depressive symptoms and avoidance coping responses [30–32]. In a similar vein, research has shown that lower use and inhibition of problem solving as a coping strategy is a consequence of depressive states [33].

In answer to the second question, the clinical group obtained significantly higher scores than the community group in the seeking guidance and support factor, which we consider an approach strategy as it represents a behavioural effort to manage or address stressors. Guidance and support may be understood as behavioural attempts to seek information, advice or assistance through social relations with people and groups. According to Yu et al. [34], guidance and support can influence people's physical and mental health as it is beneficial for all individuals and acts to mitigate stress. A number of studies have shown that seeking guidance and support protects people from developing symptoms of depression and anxiety [35–37]. Most existing research indicates that guidance and support have a positive impact on psychological well-being and act as a protective factor against stress [34,38–40]. Support from friends and family plays a crucial role in helping individuals to manage stressful situations such as infectious disease outbreaks [41]. It is possible that the differences observed between the clinical group and the community group in terms of seeking guidance and support lie in the fact that the clinical group is more accustomed to seeking support from friends and family due to their existing mental health issues.

In relation to the third question, male participants obtained significantly higher scores than female participants in the logical analysis factor. Logical analysis refers to cognitive attempts to cope with a stressful situation and its consequences and is closely linked to problem solving. Mataud [42] studied gender differences in coping strategies in Spain and found that women obtained lower scores than men in more rational coping strategies and higher scores than men in more emotional strategies. These results coincide with the meta-analysis conducted by Tamres et al. [43] and research by Rose and Rudolph [44], which found that women scored higher on emotional strategies, avoidance and seeking support. More recently, several studies have confirmed that women report greater use of the strategy of seeking guidance and support than men [45,46].

Finally, to evaluate the discriminative accuracy of the coping responses, a receiver operating characteristic curve analysis (ROC) was carried out to identify the cut-off scores on the CRI-A dimensions after which the probability of behavioural disorders rises. The results of this analysis showed that the highest scores for sensitivity and specificity were obtained by avoidance coping strategies. Certain coping strategies can increase the risk of psychopathological disorders and psychopathology can also determine the use of a specific type of coping strategy [47].

Limitations

This study has several limitations. The use of self-reports as a data collection method is an important limitation. Other limitations include the cross-sectional design, which makes it difficult to establish further inferences about the relationship between the study variables. Finally, cultural influences and differences in the measures adopted between countries during lockdown mean that any attempts to extrapolate the results of this study to other contexts should be approached with caution. Although we obtained group data of the participants enrolled at the University of Extremadura, the generalisation of our findings needs to be considered. The results cannot be generalised to other population groups.

5. Conclusions

The study of coping strategies adopted by individuals in response to stressful situations is a crucially important topic due to its association with mental health and psychological well-being. Mental health problems are a matter of significant social concern and lead to high economic costs for public health [48]. This study has advanced our understanding of coping strategies and shown that a stressful situation such as lockdown prompts students with existing health problems to adopt an unhealthy coping response based largely on cognitive avoidance strategies (cognitive avoidance and acceptance or resignation). The clinical group experienced a dual spiral of distress and anxiety due to their psychopathological issues and the stress of the lockdown, as well as their ineffective coping responses. In this case, rather than acting as a protective factor, coping strategies became a risk factor that increased levels of distress and anxiety.

In conclusion, it is important to design interventions to ensure that this clinical group develops active, effective coping strategies in response to stressful situations and learns to manage the anxiety caused by the pandemic. Urgent action must be taken to provide this group with medical and social support.

Author Contributions: V.-M.L.-R., B.L.-d.-B., S.M.-L., and M.-I.P.-d.-R. designed the study and had full access to all the data in the study, performed all statistical analyses and the interpretation of the data and contributed to manuscript preparation. All authors have read and agreed to the published version of the manuscript.

Funding: This work has been funded by the support to Research Groups of the Junta de Extremadura (SEJO14 GR15079).

Institutional Review Board Statement: The study was conducted according to the guidelines of the Declaration of Helsinki and was approved by the Bioethics and Biosafety Committee of the University of Extremadura.

Informed Consent Statement: Informed consent was obtained from all individuals involved in the study.

Data Availability Statement: Data is contained within the article.

Conflicts of Interest: The authors declare no conflict of interest.

References

1. Wang, C.; Pan, R.; Wan, X.; Tan, Y.; Xu, L.; Ho, C.S.; Ho, R.C. Immediate psychological responses and associated factors during the initial stage of the 2019 coronavirus disease (COVID-19) epidemic among the general population in China. *Int. J. Environ. Res. Public Health* **2020**, *17*, 1729. [CrossRef] [PubMed]
2. Brooks, S.K.; Webster, R.K.; Smith, L.E.; Woodland, L.; Wessely, S.; Greenberg, N.; Rubin, G.J. The psychological impact of quarantine and how to reduce it: Rapid review of the evidence. *Lancet* **2020**, *395*, 912–920. [CrossRef]

3. Wang, Y.; Zhang, D.; Du, G.; Du, R.; Zhao, J.; Jin, Y.; Fu, S.; Gao, L.; Cheng, Z.; Lu, Q.; et al. Remdesivir in adults with severe COVID-19: A randomised, double-blind, placebo-controlled, multicentre trial. *Lancet* **2020**, *395*, 1569–1578. [CrossRef]
4. Sprang, G.; Silman, M. Posttraumatic stress disorder in parents and youth after health-related disasters. *Disaster Med. Public Health Prep.* **2013**, *7*, 105–110. [CrossRef]
5. Liu, J.J.; Bao, Y.; Huang, X.; Shi, J.; Lu, L. Mental health considerations for children quarantine because of COVID-19. *Lancet Child. Adolesc. Health* **2020**, *4*, 347–349. [CrossRef]
6. Sun, L.; Sun, Z.; Wu, L.; Zhu, Z.; Zhang, F.; Shang, Z.; Jia, Y.; Gu, J.; Zhou, Y.; Wang, Y.; et al. Prevalence and risk factors of acute posttraumatic stress symptoms during the COVID-19 outbreak in Wuhan, China. *medRxiv* **2020**, 20032425. [CrossRef]
7. Ozmiz-Etxeberria, N.; Dosil-Santamaria, M.; Picaza-Gorrochategui, M.; Idoiaga-Mondragon, N. Niveles de estrés, ansiedad y depresión en la primera fase del brote del COVID-19 en una muestra recogida en el norte de España. *Cad. Saúde Pública* **2020**, *36*, e00054020. [CrossRef] [PubMed]
8. Orgilés, M.; Morales, A.; Delvecchio, E.; Mazzeschi, C.; Espada, J.P. Immediate psychological effects of the COVID-19 quarantine in youth from Italy and Spain. *Front. Psychol.* **2020**, *11*, 2986. [CrossRef]
9. Bartlett, J.D.; Griffin, J.; Thomson, D. Resources for supporting children's emotional well-being during the COVID-19 pandemic. *Child. Trends* **2020**, *12*, 1–8.
10. Balluerka Lasa, N.; Gómez Benito, J.; Hidalgo Montesinos, M.D.; Gorostiaga Manterola, A.; Espada Sánchez, J.P.; Padilla García, J.L.; Santed Germán, M.A. Las consecuencias psicológicas de la COVID-19 y el confinamiento. *Inf. Investig.* **2020**, *1*, 5–209. Available online: https://canal.ugr.es/wp-content/uploads/2020/05/Consecuencias-psicologicas-COVID-19.pdf (accessed on 15 January 2021).
11. Mikulic, I.M.; Crespi, M.C. Adaptación y validación del inventario de respuestas de afrontamiento de moos (CRI-A) para adultos. *Anu. Investig.* **2008**, *15*, 305–3012.
12. Lazarus, R.S.; Folkman, S. *Estrés y Procesos Cognitivos (Tress and Cognitive Processes)*; Martínez Roca: Barcelona, Spain, 1986.
13. Moos, R.H.; Schaefer, J.A. Coping resources and processes: Current concepts and measures. In *Handbook of Stress: Theoretical and Clinical Aspects*, 2nd ed.; Free Press: New York, NY, USA, 1993; pp. 234–257.
14. Griffith, M.A.; Dubow, E.C.; Ippolito, M.F. Developmental and cross-situational differences in adolescents coping strategies. *J. Youth Adolesc.* **2000**, *29*, 183–204. [CrossRef]
15. Törestad, B.; Magnusson, D.; Oláh, A. Coping, Control, and experience of anxiety: An interactional perspective. *Anxiety Res.* **1990**, *3*, 1–16. [CrossRef]
16. Billings, A.G.; Moos, R.H. Copig, stress, and social resources among adults with unipolar depression. *J. Personal. Soc. Psychol.* **1984**, *94*, 140–153.
17. Moos, R.H. *Coping Responses Inventory*; Psychological Assessment Resources: Washington, DC, USA, 1993.
18. Moos, R.H. *Coping with Life Crises: An Integrated Apporoach*; Plenum: New York, NY, USA, 1986.
19. Holahan, C.; Moos, R.; Brennan, P. Social context, coping strategies, and depressive symptoms: An expanded model with cardiac patients. *J. Personal. Soc. Psychol.* **1997**, *72*, 918–928. [CrossRef]
20. Mattlin, J.; Wethington, E.; Kessler, R.C. Situational determinants of coping and coping effectiveness. *J. Health Soc. Behav.* **1990**, *31*, 103–122. [CrossRef] [PubMed]
21. Mikulic, I.M.; Crespi, M.C. Resiliencia y calidad de vida: Nuevos aportes para la evaluación psicológica en contexto carcelario. *Anu. Investig. Fac. Psicol. Univ. B. Aires* **2004**, *2*, 381–390.
22. Mikulic, I.M.; Crespi, M.C. Contexto carcelario: Un estudio de los estresores y las respuestas de afrontamiento en detenidos primarios y reincidentes. *Anu. Investig. Fac. Psicol. Univ. B. Aires* **2004**, *2*, 381–391.
23. Kirchner, T.; Forns, M. *Adaptación Española del Inventario de Respuestas de Afrontamiento de R. Moos*; TEA: Madrid, Spain, 2010.
24. Pujada, M.D. Diseño de un Programa de Evaluación e Intervención de Variables Emocionales Conductuales y Personales para Personal de Emergencias. Ph.D. Thesis, Universitat de les Illes Balears, Palma de Mallorca, Spain, 2015.
25. Dörfel, D.; Rabe, S.; Karl, A. Coping strategies in daily life as protective and risk factors for post traumatic stress in motor vehicle accident survivors. *J. Loss Trauma* **2008**, *13*, 422–440. [CrossRef]
26. Tsay, S.L.; Halstead, M.T.; McCrone, S. Predictors of coping efficacy, negative moods and post-traumatic stress syndrome following major trauma. *Int. J. Nurs. Pract.* **2001**, *7*, 74–83. [CrossRef]
27. MacIntyre, P.D.; Gregersen, T.; Mercer, S. Language teachers' coping strategies during the Covid-19 conversion to online teaching: Correlations with stress, wellbeing and negative emotions. *System* **2020**, *94*. [CrossRef]
28. Zimmer-Gembeck, M.; Skinner, E. The development of coping: Implications for psychopathology and resilience. In *Developmental Psychopathology, Risk, Resilience, and Intervention*; Cicchetti, D., Ed.; John Wiley and Sons: Hoboken, NJ, USA, 2016; Volume 4, pp. 485–545.
29. Schmidt, U.; Treasure, J. Anorexia nervosa: Valued and visible. A cognitive-interpersonal maintenance model and its implications for research and practice. *Br. J. Clin. Psychol.* **2006**, *45*, 343–366. [CrossRef] [PubMed]
30. Herman-Stabl, M.; Stemmler, M.; Petersen, A. Approach and avoidant coping: Implications for adolescent mental health. *J. Youth Adolesc.* **1995**, *24*, 649–665. [CrossRef]
31. Sawyer, M.; Pfeiffer, S.; Spence, S. Life events, coping and depressive symptoms among young adolescents: A one-year prospective study. *J. Affect. Disord.* **2009**, *117*, 48–54. [CrossRef]

32. Seiffge-Krenke, I.; Klessinger, N. Long-Term effects of avoidant coping on adolescents' depressive symptoms. *J. Youth Adolesc.* **2000**, *29*, 617–630. [CrossRef]
33. Nrugham, L.; Holen, A.; Sund, A. Suicide attempters and repeaters: Depression and coping: A prospective study of early adolescents followed up as young adults. *J. Nerv. Ment. Dis.* **2012**, *200*, 197–203. [CrossRef] [PubMed]
34. Yu, H.; Li, M.; Li, Z.; Xiang, W.; Yuan, Y.; Liu, Y.; Li, Z.; Xion, Z. Coping style, social support and psychological distress in the general Chinese population in the early stages of the COVID-19 epidemic. *BMC Psychiatry* **2020**, *20*, 2–11. [CrossRef]
35. Burton, E.; Stice, E.; Seeley, J. A prospective test of the stress-buffering model of depression in adolescent girls: No support once again. *J. Consult. Clin. Psychol.* **2004**, *72*, 689. [CrossRef]
36. DuBois, D.; Felner, R.; Brand, S.; Adan, A.; Evans, E. Aprospective study of life stress, social support, and adaptation in early adolescence. *Child. Dev.* **1992**, *63*, 542–557. [CrossRef]
37. Zimmerman, M.; Ramirez-Valles, J.; Zapert, K.; Maton, K. A longitudinal study of stress-buffering effects for urban African-American male adolescent problem behaviors and mental health. *J. Community Psychol.* **2000**, *28*, 17–33. [CrossRef]
38. Turner, S.B. Resilience of nurses in the face of disaster. *Disaster Med. Public Health Prep.* **2015**, *9*, 601–604. [CrossRef]
39. Labrague, L.J.; Yboa, B.C.; McEnroe-Petitte, D.M.; Lobrino, L.R.; Brennan, M.G.B. Disaster preparedness in Philippine nurses. *J. Nurs. Scholarsh.* **2016**, *48*, 98–105. [CrossRef] [PubMed]
40. Xiao, H.; Zhang, Y.; Kong, D.; Li, S.; Yang, N. The effects of social support on sleep quality of medical staff treating patients with coronavirus disease 2019 (COVID-19) in January and February 2020 in China. *Med. Sci. Monit.* **2020**, *26*, e923549.
41. Langan, J.C.; Lavin, R.; Wolgast, K.A.; Veenema, T.G. Education for developing and sustaining a health care workforce for disaster readiness. *Nurs. Adm. Q.* **2017**, *41*, 118–127. [CrossRef]
42. Mataud, M.P. Gender differences in stress and coping styles. *Personal. Individ. Differ.* **2004**, *37*, 1401–1415. [CrossRef]
43. Tamres, L.K.; Janicki, D.; Helgeson, V.S. Sex differences in coping behavior: A meta-analytic review and an examination of relative coping. *Personal. Soc. Psychol. Rev.* **2002**, *6*, 2–30. [CrossRef]
44. Rose, A.J.; Rudolph, K.D. A review of sex differences in peer relationship processes: Potential trade-offs for the emotional and behavioral development of girls and boys. *Psychol. Bull.* **2006**, *132*, 98–131. [CrossRef] [PubMed]
45. Eschenbeck, H.; Schmid, S.; Schröder, I.; Wasserfall, N.; Kohlmann, C.-W. Development of coping strategies from childhood to adolescence. *Eur. J. Health Psychol.* **2018**, *25*, 18–30. [CrossRef]
46. Malooly, A.; Flannery, K.; Ohannessian, C. Coping mediates the association between gender and depressive symptomatology in adolescence. *Int. J. Behav. Dev.* **2017**, *41*, 185–197. [CrossRef] [PubMed]
47. Compas, B.; Jaser, S.; Bettis, A.; Watson, K.; Gruhn, M.; Dunbar, J.; Thigpen, J. Coping, emotion regulation, and psychopathology in childhood and adolescence: A meta-analysis and narrative review. *Psychol. Bull.* **2017**, *143*, 939. [CrossRef] [PubMed]
48. Belfer, M.L. Child and adolescent mental disorders: The magnitude of the problem across the globe. *J. Child Psychol. Psychiatry Allied Discipl.* **2008**, *49*, 226–236. [CrossRef] [PubMed]

Journal of
Clinical Medicine

MDPI

Article

A Comparison of Depression and Anxiety among University Students in Nine Countries during the COVID-19 Pandemic

Dominika Ochnik [1,*], Aleksandra M. Rogowska [2], Cezary Kuśnierz [3], Monika Jakubiak [4], Astrid Schütz [5], Marco J. Held [5], Ana Arzenšek [6], Joy Benatov [7], Rony Berger [8,9], Elena V. Korchagina [10], Iuliia Pavlova [11], Ivana Blažková [12], Zdeňka Konečná [13], Imran Aslan [14], Orhan Çınar [15,16], Yonni Angel Cuero-Acosta [17] and Magdalena Wierzbik-Strońska [1]

1. Faculty of Medicine, University of Technology, 40-555 Katowice, Poland; rektorat@wst.com.pl
2. Institute of Psychology, University of Opole, 45-052 Opole, Poland; arogowska@uni.opole.pl
3. Faculty of Physical Education and Physiotherapy, Opole University of Technology, 45-758 Opole, Poland; c.kusnierz@po.edu.pl
4. Faculty of Economics, Maria Curie-Sklodowska University in Lublin, 20-031 Lublin, Poland; monika.jakubiak@poczta.umcs.lublin.pl
5. Department of Psychology, University of Bamberg, 96047 Bamberg, Germany; astrid.schuetz@uni-bamberg.de (A.S.); marco.held@uni-bamberg.de (M.J.H.)
6. Faculty of Management, University of Primorska, 6101 Koper, Slovenia; ana.arzensek@fm-kp.si
7. Department of Special Education, University of Haifa, Haifa 3498838, Israel; jbentov2@gmail.com
8. The Center for Compassionate Mindful Education, Tel Aviv 69106, Israel; bergerrony@gmail.com
9. Bob Shapell School of Social Work, Tel-Aviv University, Tel Aviv 69978, Israel
10. Institute of Industrial Management, Economics and Trade, Peter the Great St. Petersburg Polytechnic University, 195251 St. Petersburg, Russia; elena.korchagina@mail.ru
11. Department of Theory and Methods of Physical Culture, Lviv State University of Physical Culture, 79007 Lviv, Ukraine; pavlova.j.o@gmail.com
12. Department of Regional and Business Economics, Mendel University in Brno, 613 00 Brno, Czech Republic; blazkova@mendelu.cz
13. Faculty of Business and Management, Brno University of Technology, 612 00 Brno, Czech Republic; konecna@fbm.vutbr.cz
14. Health Management Department, Bingöl University, Bingöl 12000, Turkey; imranaslan@gmail.com
15. Faculty of Economics and Administrative Sciences, Ataturk University, Erzurum 25240, Turkey; orhanar@gmail.com
16. Faculty of Economics and Administrative Sciences, Ağrı İbrahim Çeçen University, Ağrı 04000, Turkey
17. School of Management, Universidad del Rosario, Bogotá 111711, Colombia; yonnia.cuero@urosario.edu.co

* Correspondence: dominika.ochnik@wst.pl

Citation: Ochnik, D.; Rogowska, A.M.; Kuśnierz, C.; Jakubiak, M.; Schütz, A.; Held, M.J.; Arzenšek, A.; Benatov, J.; Berger, R.; Korchagina, E.V.; et al. A Comparison of Depression and Anxiety among University Students in Nine Countries during the COVID-19 Pandemic. *J. Clin. Med.* **2021**, *10*, 2882. https://doi.org/10.3390/jcm10132882

Academic Editor: Michele Roccella

Received: 20 April 2021
Accepted: 27 June 2021
Published: 29 June 2021

Abstract: The mental health of young adults, particularly students, is at high risk during the COVID-19 pandemic. The purpose of this study was to examine differences in mental health between university students in nine countries during the pandemic. The study encompassed 2349 university students (69% female) from Colombia, the Czech Republic (Czechia), Germany, Israel, Poland, Russia, Slovenia, Turkey, and Ukraine. Participants underwent the following tests: Patient Health Questionnaire (PHQ-8), Generalized Anxiety Disorder (GAD-7), Exposure to COVID-19 (EC-19), Perceived Impact of Coronavirus (PIC) on students' well-being, Physical Activity (PA), and General Self-Reported Health (GSRH). The one-way ANOVA showed significant differences between countries. The highest depression and anxiety risk occurred in Turkey, the lowest depression in the Czech Republic and the lowest anxiety in Germany. The χ^2 independence test showed that EC-19, PIC, and GSRH were associated with anxiety and depression in most of the countries, whereas PA was associated in less than half of the countries. Logistic regression showed distinct risk factors for each country. Gender and EC-19 were the most frequent predictors of depression and anxiety across the countries. The role of gender and PA for depression and anxiety is not universal and depends on cross-cultural differences. Students' mental health should be addressed from a cross-cultural perspective.

Keywords: mental health; anxiety; depression; students; COVID-19; general self-reported health; physical activity; gender; cross-national study

1. Introduction

The newly-emerged coronavirus is responsible for a highly viral and infectious disease resulting in a severe acute respiratory syndrome (SARS-Cov-2). The pandemic began in December 2019 and has subsequently spread rapidly worldwide [1].

The first wave of the coronavirus disease (COVID-19) pandemic entered a global stage in the spring of 2020 and prevailed until the summer [2]. The COVID-19 pandemic has forced the introduction of preventive restrictions. Due to the restrictions, social isolation was experienced on an unprecedented scale globally. This contributed to the deterioration of mental health [3–7]. The COVID-19 pandemic is also perceived as the deepest global economic recession in the past eight decades [8]. Considering increased levels of anxiety and depression during previous economic crises [9], the financial instability caused by the pandemic can become a crucial risk factor in relation to mental health deterioration. Research has also shown a linkage between lower social status and mental health issues [10,11]. Therefore, due to financial instability, the current pandemic can affect the mental health of individuals who are not at a serious risk of becoming infected with COVID-19. Recent cross-national studies revealed that mental health deterioration associated with the pandemic is not exclusively limited to individuals who have been infected but extends to the general population [12].

Young adults are highly vulnerable to mental health deterioration during the COVID-19 pandemic [13–15] even though they are the least susceptible to the COVID-19 infection [16]. Young age is one of the key risk factors as the prevalence of depressive symptoms in early adulthood is high and dynamic and mediated by several environmental and biological factors [17]. Mental health issues are common in the student population—more than one-third of students experienced some form of mental health problem in the pre-pandemic period [18]. Despite the fact that students are a socially privileged population, they have been at a higher depression risk compared to the general population, even in the pre-pandemic period [19,20]. Students' physical health status is also relatively poor when compared to their non-studying working peers or the overall population [21,22]. Based on the meta-analysis of studies conducted between 1990 and 2010, the prevalence of depression among students amounted to 30.6% on average [19] compared to 12.9% in the global population based on data from 30 countries collected between 1994 and 2014 [20]. Financial difficulties constitute a risk factor for the increase of anxiety and depression levels. They can also lead to poor academic performance [23]. Financial concerns are not the only factor affecting students' mental health issues. They can also be influenced by [24] academic pressure and demanding workloads [25], student mistreatment and abuse [26] and worries about health [27]. Students are particularly susceptible to affective disorders due to high social expectations as they are deemed to represent the future of a community [28]. Research showed that during the ongoing pandemic, student status (particularly being a student on the first-cycle of studies) is a relevant risk factor for mental health issues [29–32]. Social isolation during the COVID-19 pandemic revealed a higher experience of insecurity concerning housing and employment opportunities [33], smaller living space and lower levels of social interaction in young adults compared to adults [4,34]. Academic stress and virtual learning are also crucial risk factors [35,36]. According to the International Labor Organization [37], the education sector has been strongly affected by the COVID-19 pandemic. Therefore, the student population is at a high risk of mental health deterioration during the COVID-19 pandemic and special attention should be paid to research encompassing this cohort.

There are several additional risk factors for mental health deterioration during the ongoing pandemic, such as female gender and lower income [12,31,32,38–41], place of residence [42,43], financial and learning-related concerns [44,45] or physical inactivity [39]. Concerns regarding loved ones, own health, or academic performance were pronounced during the pandemic [45] and contributed to an increase in anxiety and depression levels [44]. Students also shifted their main concerns from learning-related to financial and/or health-related matters [46]. Recent studies showed that exposure to COVID-19-related matters may increase the risk of anxiety symptoms in students (particularly among men) [47]. Physical activity constitutes the next key predictor of mental health problems. People who spent more time outside during mobility restrictions reported lower stress and higher positive mental health [48]. International research showed that social isolation during the COVID-19 pandemic was linked to lower PA intensity. Additionally, eating patterns were less healthy [49]. Students who were physically inactive (less than 150 min of activity a week) during the COVID-19 pandemic reported higher anxiety and depression compared to the physically active group [39]. Physical activity turned out to be a stronger predictor of depression than anxiety in students [39]. An additional issue related to reactions to the pandemic is mixed media coverage and rapid changes in official messages regarding protective behaviors. Misinformation is one of the crucial factors in anxiety response during the pandemic [50]. Regular searching for additional information concerning the coronavirus turned out to be a risk factor related to the fear of the coronavirus [51].

The number of research papers dedicated to the COVID-19 pandemic has already exceeded the number of studies dedicated to Ebola and H1N1. However, few studies were created via international collaboration [52]. Additionally, cross-national research regarding mental health during the COVID-19 pandemic frequently refers to the general population [12,29–31,53–57] rather than the student population [45,58,59]. Additionally, in articles related to students' mental health, a binational, rather than cross-national perspective appears more frequently [45,58,59]. Cross-national studies concerning mental health during the COVID-19 pandemic indicate that mental health differentiates the general population at a country level [12,29–31,53–57]. Analyses from 78 countries showed a slightly higher depression in Poland compared to the overall mean and an even stronger effect in Turkey [30]. The Polish general population manifested the highest anxiety and depression rate during the COVID-19 pandemic compared to the sample from China, Spain, Iran, United States of America, Pakistan, and Vietnam [57].

The main aim of this study is to compare depression and anxiety levels among university students in nine countries: Colombia, the Czech Republic (Czechia), Germany, Israel, Poland, Russia, Slovenia, Turkey, and Ukraine during the first wave of the COVID-19 pandemic. Risk factors for depression and anxiety will also be examined separately in each country, including gender, place of residence, level of study, exposure to COVID-19, the perceived impact of COVID-19 on students' well-being (including qualifications, economic status, and social relationships), physical activity and physical health.

2. Materials and Methods

2.1. Participants

The required sample size for each country group was computed a priori by means of G*Power software (Düsseldorf, Germany) [60]. In order to obtain a medium effect size of Cohen's $W = 0.03$ with given 95% power in a $2 \times 2\ \chi^2$ contingency table, $df = 1$ (two groups in two categories each, two tailed), $\alpha = 0.05$, G*Power suggests 145 participants are required in each country group (non-centrality parameter $\lambda = 13.05$, critical $\chi^2 = 3.84$, power = 0.95). Initially, the total sample consisted of 2453 respondents. However, 104 persons (4.24% of the initial total sample) declined participation (responded "No" to the informed consent). Therefore, the final total sample encompassed 2349 university students from nine countries: Colombia ($n = 155$), Czechia ($n = 310$), Germany ($n = 270$), Israel ($n = 199$), Poland ($n = 301$), Russia ($n = 285$), Slovenia ($n = 209$), Turkey ($n = 310$), and Ukraine ($n = 310$). The present number of university students in each country exceed the required sample size. This may lead to an increase in the power of 0.95 for the statistical analysis. All the respondents were eligible for the study and confirmed their student status. Additionally, respondents who decided not to reveal their gender were excluded from statistical analyses concerning gender ($n = 6$).

Colombian students ($n = 155$) were recruited from Bogota universities: Del Rosario University ($n = 142$, 92%) and El Bosque University ($n = 13$, 8%). The total sample in Czechia was comprised of students recruited from Mendel University in Brno ($n = 310$, 100%), and in Germany from the University of Bamberg (*n* = 270, 100%). The Israeli sample represented the University of Haifa (*n* = 199, 100%). The Polish sample consisted of 301 students recruited from Maria Curie-Sklodowska University (UMCS) in eastern Poland (*n* = 149, 48%) and from the University of Opole in the south of Poland (*n* = 152, 51%). Russian students were recruited from universities located in Sankt Petersburg: Peter the Great St. Petersburg Polytechnic University (*n* = 155, 54%), Higher School of Economics (HSE) University (*n* = 90, 31%), and St. Petersburg State University of Economics and Finance (*n* = 42, 15%). The total sample in Slovenia was comprised of students recruited from the University of Primorska in Koper (*n* = 209, 100%). Turkish students were from eleven Turkish universities mostly located in eastern Turkey: Bingol University, Bingöl (*n* = 148, 48%); Atatürk University, Erzurum (*n* = 110, 35%); Muğla Sıtkı Koçman University, Muğla (*n* = 35, 11%); Ağrı İbrahim Çeçen University, Ağrı (*n* = 6, 2%); Fırat University, Elazığ (*n* = 3, 0.8%); Kırıkkale University, Kırıkkale (*n* = 1, 0.3%); Adnan Menderes University, Aydın (*n* = 1, 0.3%); Başkent University, (*n* = 3, 1%); Boğaziçi University (*n* = 1, 0.3%), Dicle University, Diyarbakır (*n* = 1, 0.3%), and Istanbul University (*n* = 1, 0.3%). Ukrainian students represented the Lviv State University of Physical Culture (*n* = 310, 100%).

Female students constituted 69% of the sample (*n* = 1627). Over half of respondents lived in rural areas and small towns (*n* = 1248; 54%). First cycle studies (Bachelor) were represented by the highest number of students (*n* = 1843; 78%) compared to the second cycle or higher (*n* = 506; 22%). The majority of participants studied in the full-time mode (*n* = 2007; 85%). The mean age of participants was 23 (*SD* = 4.66). The mean values for depression and anxiety in the total sample were 7.16 (*SD* = 5.52) and 8.85 (*SD* = 6.05), respectively. Detailed descriptive statistics for each country are presented in Table S1.

All questions included in the Google Forms questionnaire were designated as mandatory. Therefore, participants were unable to omit any response. However, hot-deck imputation was introduced to deal with a low number of missing data (*n* = 5, 0.02%) in the German sample (study conducted via SoSci Survey [61]).

2.2. Study Design

The cross-national study was conducted during the first wave of the COVID-19 pandemic (May–July 2020). The sample consisted of 2349 university students from Colombia, Czechia, Germany, Israel, Poland, Russia, Slovenia, Turkey, and Ukraine. The survey study was conducted via Google Forms in all countries except Germany. This country exploited the SoSci Survey [61]. The invitation to participate in the survey was sent to students by researchers via a variety of means, e.g., Moodle e-learning platform, student offices, email, or social media. The average time of data collection was 23.26 min (*SD* = 44.03). No form of compensation was offered as an incentive to participate in eight countries. In Germany, students were offered a possibility to enter into a lottery for a €20 Amazon gift card as an incentive to participate. In Israel, the participants were eligible to win NIS 300 gift cards. To minimize bias sources, the student sample was highly diversified as regards its key characteristics: the type of university, field of study and the cycle of study. Sampling was purposive. The selection criterion was university student status.

Ethics Statement: The study protocol was approved by the ethics committee of the University Research Committee at the University of Opole, Poland, decision no. 1/2020. The study followed the ethical requirements of the anonymity and voluntariness of participation. Each person answered the informed consent question. Following the Helsinki Declaration, a written informed consent was obtained from each student before inclusion.

2.3. Measurements

The Patient Health Questionnaire (PHQ-8) [62] was used to measure depression symptoms. The PHQ-8 consists of eight items, conforming with DSM-V diagnostic criteria [48]. The symptoms include depressed mood, loss of interest in most or all activities, loss of energy, or feeling of worthlessness [62]. Participants use a Likert-type response scale ranging from 0 = not at all, to 3 = nearly every day. The range of PHQ-8 scores is from 0 to 24, severe. A cut-off score of 10 or above is recommended to screen for major depressive disorder risk [62]. Due to the requirements of a further statistical analysis with the use of the χ^2 independence test and logistic regression, the PHQ-8 was dichotomized as follows: 0 = No risk (PHQ-8 < 10), 1 = Risk (PHQ-8 $\geq$ 10). The internal consistency reliability of the original version measured by Cronbach's α equals 0.86. The value of 0.88 for the total sample was recorded in this study.

In order to measure anxiety risk, the 7-item Generalized Anxiety Disorder (GAD-7) scale [63] was exploited. GAD-7 is a self-reported measure designed to screen for symptoms following Diagnostic and Statistical Manual of Mental Disorders, fifth edition (DSM-V) criteria [64]. The Generalized Anxiety Disorder (GAD) is characterized by a persistent and excessive worry about various issues. It relates to anxiety as a state [63]. People rate how often they experienced anxiety symptoms in the course of two weeks preceding the study on a 4-point Likert scale (0 = not at all, 1 = several days, 2 = more than half the days, and 3 = nearly every day). The GAD-7 ranges from 0 to 21. Scores above 10 points indicate an anxiety disorder risk [63]. Due to the requirements of the χ^2 independence test and logistic regression, GAD-7 was dichotomized as follows: 0 = No risk (GAD-7 < 10), 1 = Risk (GAD-7 $\geq$ 10). The Cronbach's α for the GAD-7 in this study was 0.92 in the total sample.

Exposure to COVID-19 [39] was assessed based on eight questions regarding the coronavirus consequences: (1) Have you experienced symptoms that could indicate the coronavirus infection?; (2) Have you been tested for the coronavirus?; (3) Were you hospitalized for the coronavirus?; (4) Did you have to be in strict quarantine for at least 14 days, in isolation from loved ones because of the coronavirus infection?; (5) Has anyone in your family, among friends, or relatives been infected with the coronavirus?; (6) Have any of your relatives died of the coronavirus?; (7) Have you or a loved one lost their job because of the coronavirus?; and (8) Are you currently experiencing a worsening of your functioning or economic status due to the coronavirus pandemic's effects? Individuals answered each of these questions (0 = No, 1 = Yes) The total score was a sum of eight items, where a higher score indicated stronger coronavirus exposure. The results were divided into two categories for the χ^2 independence test and logistic regression: 0 = Low exposure (score 0), 1 = High exposure (scores 1–8).

The Perceived Impact of Coronavirus (PIC) on students' well-being [39] was measured using five statements Participants used a 5-item Likert scale (from 1 = I strongly disagree, to 5 = I definitely agree) to express how much they are afraid that the current situation associated with the coronavirus pandemic (COVID-19) may negatively affect their lives in each of the following five aspects: (1) Completing the semester and obtaining qualifications; (2) Finding a job and professional development; (3) Financial situation (e.g., subsistence during studies); (4) Relationships with loved ones, family, (5) Relations with colleagues, friends. Next, scores obtained from the five items were summarized to a total score of the perceived coronavirus impact on students' well-being (PCI). The higher the scores, the more significant the coronavirus-related concerns were. We have used the median to dichotomize the total score of the PIC and its three subscales: Qualifications (Graduation), Economic Status, and Social Relationships. The total PIC was coded as follows (for the χ^2 independence test and logistic regression): 0 = Lower (PIC $\leq$ 15), 1 = Higher (PIC $\geq$ 16). We added scores of items PIC1 and PIC2 for the Qualifications scale and then coded as 0 = Low (scores 2–6), 1 = High (scores 7–10). Social Relationships scale consisted of items PIC4 and PIC5 coded as 0 = Low (scores 2–4), 1 = High (scores 5–10). Single item PIC3 concerning Economic Status scale was coded as 0 = Low (scores 1–3), 1 = High (scores 4–5). The Cronbach's α (indicating the internal reliability of the scale) amounted to 0.71 in the present study (in the total sample).

Physical activity (PA) during the coronavirus-related lockdown was assessed using the following question: "How many days a week did you exercise physically or pursued sports activities at home or away from home, at the university, in clubs, or at the gym, in the last month?" [39]. Participants answered this question on an eight-point scale (from 0 = Not one day to 7 = Seven days a week). Next, the students responded to the question:

"How many minutes a day (on average) did you practice?" indicating the average number of minutes of PA per day. The number of days was multiplied by the number of minutes per day to calculate the previous week's PA level. We divided the total sample into two groups: 0 = Sufficient (PA $\geq$ 150 min weekly) and 1 = Insufficient (PA < 150 min weekly), in line with the WHO recommendation [65].

The General Self-Rated Health (GSRH) status was assessed using two single-item questions as a shorter alternative to the standard general physical health (PH) survey (SF-12V) [66,67]. The first question GSRH-1 concerns an overall physical health (GSRH) assessment (i.e., "In general, would you say your health is . . . ?"), while the second GSRH-2, compares self-health with other people (i.e., "Compared to others your age, would you say your health is . . . ?") (GSRH Comparative). Both GSRH items are rated on a 5-point Likert scale (1 = Excellent, 2 = Very Good, 3 = Good, 4 = Fair, and 5 = Poor). Therefore, higher scores denote worse health status. Research indicates that poorly self-rated health in the single-item GSRH has a strong association with mortality [66]. We spilt the GSRH as follows (due to the χ^2 independence test and logistic regression requirements): 0 = Better health (GSRH $\leq$ 3), 1 = Worse health (GSRH $\geq$ 4). In the present study, the Cronbach's α for GSRH was 0.88 (N = 2349).

Demographic data included questions regarding age (in years), gender (0 = Men, 1 = Women), place of residence (Village, Town, City, Agglomeration/Metropolis), and the current level of study (Bachelor, Master, Postgraduate, Doctoral). We divided answers regarding the place of residence into two categories (for the χ^2 independence test and logistic regression) coded as: 0 = village and town, 1 = city, agglomeration, or metropolis. Additionally, we have incorporated 4% of participants who studied at a doctoral or postgraduate level into the category Master. Therefore, for further analysis, the level of study is comprised of two categories: 0 = Bachelor and 1 = Master (for Master or higher).

2.4. Statistical Analysis

The statistical analysis included descriptive statistics: mean (M), standard deviation (SD), 95% of confidence interval (CI) with lower limit (LL) and upper limit (UL). Subsequently, a one-way analysis of variance (ANOVA) was performed to test the differences in the mean scores of depression and anxiety between university students from the nine countries: Slovenia, Czechia, Germany, Poland, Ukraine, Russia, Turkey, Israel, and Colombia. The effect size for ANOVA was assessed using $\eta_p{}^2$ (a value of $\eta_p{}^2$ = 0.01 is considered to be a small effect size, 0.09 a medium effect, and 0.25 a large effect). Tukey's honest significant difference (HSD) test was used to find means that are significantly different from each other. Furthermore, Pearson's χ^2 independence test was conducted to examine relationships between depression and anxiety and other variables in each of the nine countries. A 2 $\times$ 2 contingency table was provided in each country separately, for depression and anxiety as independent variables, as well as such predictor variables as gender, place of residence, level of study, physical activity, exposure to the COVID-19 pandemic, the total impact of COVID-19 on students' well-being, as well as impact in the domain of qualifications, economic status, and social relationships, self-rated physical health, and comparative self-rated physical health (Comparative PH). However, all Colombian students (100%) were assigned to the Town/City category, and 97% (n = 155) to the first cycle study. Therefore, place of residence and level of study were excluded from the statistical analysis in the Colombian sample. The effect size for Pearson's χ^2 independence test was assessed using φ statistic (a value of φ = 0.1 is considered to be a small effect, 0.3 a medium effect, and 0.5 a large effect). Next, multivariate logistic regression analysis was performed in each country separately to test the adjusted odds ratio (AOR), in order to assess potential risk factors (gender, place of residence, exposure to COVID-19, PIC, PA, PH, Comparative PH) as predictors of depression and anxiety in each country. All predictors were entered into the model simultaneously. The following statistics were calculated for estimation: coefficient estimates, 95% confidence intervals (CI) for the regression coefficient, standard errors of the regression coefficient, odds ratio, z-values, and their corresponding p-values.

The bias-corrected accelerated bootstrapping (BCa) method of estimating regression coefficient was also applied, with the number of replications set to 5000 (if the bias-corrected 95% confidence intervals (CI_B) did not include the null value, then a statistically significant effect was considered). Goodness of fit of the regression model was assessed using pseudo R^2, including Cox and Snell R^2_{CS}, McFadden R^2_{McF}, and Nagelkerke R^2_N. All analyses were performed using Statistica Version 13.1, StatSoft Polska (Cracow, Poland) [68] and the open-source statistical software JASP Version 014.1 [69].

3. Results

3.1. Country Differences in Depression and Anxiety

A one-way between subjects ANOVA was conducted to compare the effect of country on depression and anxiety (see Figures 1 and 2, for more details). There was a significant effect of country on depression with a large effect size, $F(8, 2340) = 31.02$, $p < 0.001$, $\eta_p^2 = 0.09$. Post hoc comparisons using the Tukey HSD test indicated that the mean score of the PHQ-8 in Poland was significantly higher than in Slovenia ($p < 0.01$), Czechia ($p < 0.001$), Ukraine ($p < 0.001$), and Germany ($p < 0.05$), and was significantly lower than in Turkey ($p < 0.001$). In addition, Slovenia demonstrated higher depression than Czechia ($p < 0.01$), but lower than Turkey ($p < 0.001$) and Colombia ($p < 0.05$). Among all of the nine countries, the lowest scores in depression emerged in Czechia, where it was significantly lower than that of Russia ($p < 0.001$), Germany ($p < 0.001$), Turkey ($p < 0.001$), Israel ($p < 0.001$), and Colombia ($p < 0.001$). Depression in Ukraine was found as being significantly lower than in Russia ($p < 0.05$), Turkey ($p < 0.001$), and Colombia ($p < 0.001$). Turkey scored the highest in depression, when compared to other countries, including Russia ($p < 0.001$), Germany ($p < 0.001$), Israel ($p < 0.001$), and Colombia ($p < 0.01$). The mean scores for depression are shown in Figure 1.

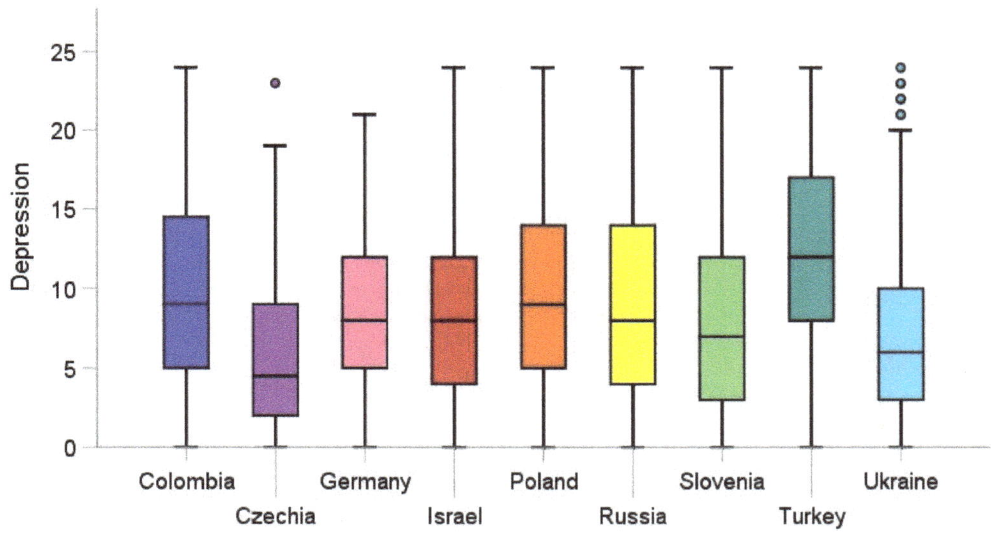

Figure 1. Mean scores of depression (PHQ-8) among university students across the nine countries during the first wave of the COVID-19 pandemic. The dots in the figure represent outliers.

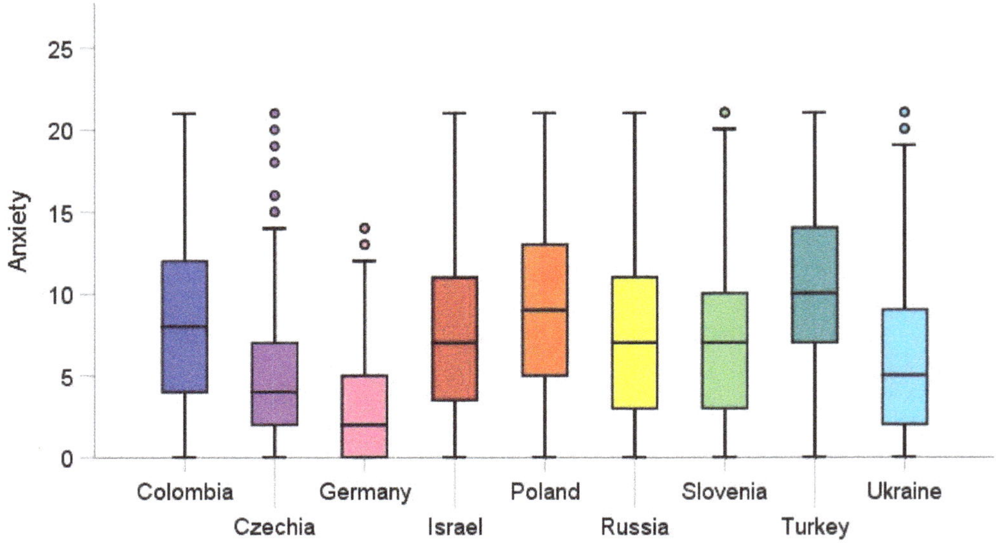

Figure 2. Mean scores for anxiety (GAD-7) among university students across the nine countries during the first wave of the COVID-19 pandemic. The dots in the figure represent outliers.

A significant effect of country on anxiety was also revealed, with a large effect size, $F(8, 2340) = 57.78$, $p < 0.001$, $\eta_p{}^2 = 0.15$. As Tukey's HSD test indicates, the mean score of the GAD-7 in Poland was significantly higher than in Slovenia ($p < 0.01$), Czechia ($p < 0.001$), Ukraine ($p < 0.001$), Russia ($p < 0.01$), and Germany ($p < 0.001$). Slovenia showed significantly higher scores in anxiety than Czechia ($p < 0.001$) and Germany ($p < 0.001$), and lower than Turkey ($p < 0.001$). Czechia demonstrated significantly lower anxiety than Ukraine ($p < 0.05$), Russia ($p < 0.001$), Turkey ($p < 0.001$), Israel ($p < 0.001$), and Colombia ($p < 0.001$), and significantly higher anxiety than Germany ($p < 0.001$). Anxiety level in Ukraine was found as being significantly lower than in Russia ($p < 0.05$), Turkey ($p < 0.001$), Israel ($p < 0.01$), and Colombia ($p < 0.001$), and higher than in Germany ($p < 0.01$). As far as anxiety is concerned, Russia significantly differed from Germany ($p < 0.001$) and Turkey ($p < 0.01$). Among the nine countries, Germany showed the lowest scores in anxiety, significantly lower than Turkey ($p < 0.001$), Israel ($p < 0.001$), and Colombia ($p < 0.001$). In contrast, Turkey demonstrated the highest anxiety, significantly higher than Israel ($p < 0.001$), and Colombia ($p < 0.01$). The mean scores of anxiety are shown in Figure 2.

3.2. *Association of Depression and Anxiety with Other Variables*

A Pearson's χ^2 test of independence was performed separately for each country to examine 2 × 2 association between mental health indices, such as depression and anxiety, and such variables as gender, place of residence, level of study, exposure to COVID-19, the perceived impact of COVID-19 on students' well-being (PIC), including qualifications (graduation), economic status, and relationships, physical activity, and physical health as rated independently and compared with people of the same age. As shown in Tables S1 and S2, numerous associations were found for the nine countries for depression and anxiety, respectively.

The relationship between depression and gender was significant in Colombia ($\chi^2(1) = 4.44$, $p < 0.05$, $\phi = 0.17$), Poland ($\chi^2(1) = 7.28$, $p < 0.01$, $\phi = 0.16$), Russia ($\chi^2(1) = 10.24$, $p < 0.01$, $\phi = 0.19$), Turkey ($\chi^2(1) = 15.40$, $p < 0.001$, $\phi = 0.22$), and Ukraine ($\chi^2(1) = 9.02$, $p < 0.01$, $\phi = 0.17$). Place of residence was not significantly associated with depression at all in any country. The level of study was significantly related to depression in Colombia ($\chi^2(1) = 4.16$,

$p < 0.05$, $\phi = -0.16$), Czechia ($\chi^2(1) = 5.71$, $p < 0.05$, $\phi = -0.13$), and Slovenia ($\chi^2(1) = 8.24$, $p < 0.01$, $\phi = -0.19$), while it was of no importance in the other countries. The relationship between depression and exposure to COVID-19 was significant in most countries (except Turkey and Colombia), including Slovenia ($\chi^2(1) = 0.23$, $p < 0.001$, $\phi = 0.33$), Czechia ($\chi^2(1) = 11.44$, $p < 0.001$, $\phi = 0.19$), Germany ($\chi^2(1) = 4.16$, $p < 0.05$, $\phi = 0.12$), Poland, ($\chi^2(1) = 7.60$, $p < 0.01$, $\phi = 0.16$), Ukraine ($\chi^2(1) = 6.65$, $p < 0.01$, $\phi = 0.15$), Russia ($\chi^2(1) = 10.39$, $p < 0.01$, $\phi = 0.19$), and Israel ($\chi^2(1) = 15.99$, $p < 0.001$, $\phi = 0.28$). Except Colombia, the total PIC was linked to depression in the following: Slovenia ($\chi^2(1) = 33.96$, $p < 0.001$, $\phi = 0.40$), Czechia ($\chi^2(1) = 16.10$, $p < 0.001$, $\phi = 0.23$), Germany ($\chi^2(1) = 39.80$, $p < 0.001$, $\phi = 0.39$), Poland, ($\chi^2(1) = 20.85$, $p < 0.001$, $\phi = 0.26$), Ukraine ($\chi^2(1) = 13.00$, $p < 0.001$, $\phi = 0.21$), Russia ($\chi^2(1) = 19.72$, $p < 0.001$, $\phi = 0.26$), Turkey ($\chi^2(1) = 9.26$, $p < 0.01$, $\phi = 0.17$), and Israel ($\chi^2(1) = 35.64$, $p < 0.001$, $\phi = 0.42$). Qualifications were insignificant in Czechia and Poland. However, they were of concern in Slovenia ($\chi^2(1) = 32.67$, $p < 0.001$, $\phi = 0.40$), Germany ($\chi^2(1) = 16.95$, $p < 0.001$, $\phi = 0.25$), Ukraine ($\chi^2(1) = 4.96$, $p < 0.05$, $\phi = 0.13$), Russia ($\chi^2(1) = 15.66$, $p < 0.001$, $\phi = 0.23$), Turkey $\chi^2(1) = 6.09$, $p < 0.05$, $\phi = 0.14$), Israel ($\chi^2(1) = 12.94$, $p < 0.001$, $\phi = 0.26$), and Colombia ($\chi^2(1) = 3.93$, $p < 0.05$, $\phi = 0.16$). Deterioration of economic status was a source of concern in most countries (except Poland): Slovenia ($\chi^2(1) = 10.10$, $p < 0.01$, $\phi = 0.22$), Czechia ($\chi^2(1) = 8.46$, $p < 0.01$, $\phi = 0.16$), Germany ($\chi^2(1) = 14.02$, $p < 0.001$, $\phi = 0.23$), Ukraine ($\chi^2(1) = 4.65$, $p < 0.05$, $\phi = 0.12$), Russia ($\chi^2(1) = 11.25$, $p < 0.001$, $\phi = 0.20$), Turkey $\chi^2(1) = 13.58$, $p < 0.001$, $\phi = 0.21$), Israel ($\chi^2(1) = 13.12$, $p < 0.001$, $\phi = 0.26$), and Colombia ($\chi^2(1) = 5.06$, $p < 0.05$, $\phi = 0.18$). Relationships with friends and family members were a source of concern in most countries during the COVID-10 pandemic (except Colombia): Slovenia ($\chi^2(1) = 13.70$, $p < 0.001$, $\phi = 0.27$), Czechia ($\chi^2(1) = 11.06$, $p < 0.001$, $\phi = 0.19$), Germany ($\chi^2(1) = 9.76$, $p < 0.01$, $\phi = 0.19$), Poland ($\chi^2(1) = 24.57$, $p < 0.05$, $\phi = 0.29$), Ukraine ($\chi^2(1) = 8.36$, $p < 0.01$, $\phi = 0.16$), Russia ($\chi^2(1) = 24.16$, $p < 0.001$, $\phi = 0.29$), Turkey $\chi^2(1) = 4.26$, $p < 0.05$, $\phi = 0.12$), and Israel ($\chi^2(1) = 14.38$, $p < 0.001$, $\phi = 0.27$). The relationship between high depression and insufficient physical activity (PA less than 150 min. per week) was revealed in Poland ($\chi^2(1) = -4.85$, $p < 0.05$, $\phi = -0.13$), Ukraine ($\chi^2(1) = -11.77$, $p < 0.001$, $\phi = -0.20$), Russia ($\chi^2(1) = -7.36$, $p < 0.01$, $\phi = -0.16$), and Israel ($\chi^2(1) = 3.89$, $p < 0.05$, $\phi = -0.14$). An association between high depression and worse physical health was significant in most countries (except Czechia and Ukraine): Slovenia ($\chi^2(1) = 15.16$, $p < 0.001$, $\phi = 0.27$), Germany ($\chi^2(1) = 21.71$, $p < 0.001$, $\phi = 0.29$), Poland ($\chi^2(1) = 13.14$, $p < 0.001$, $\phi = 0.21$), Russia ($\chi^2(1) = 10.00$, $p < 0.01$, $\phi = 0.19$), Turkey $\chi^2(1) = 5.89$, $p < 0.05$, $\phi = 0.14$), Israel ($\chi^2(1) = 4.89$, $p < 0.05$, $\phi = 0.16$), and Colombia ($\chi^2(1) = 5.14$, $p < 0.05$, $\phi = 0.18$). When students compared self-rated physical health to other people of the same age, the association between depression and comparative health was noted in most countries (except Russia): Slovenia ($\chi^2(1) = 20.88$, $p < 0.001$, $\phi = 0.32$), Czechia ($\chi^2(1) = 14.45$, $p < 0.001$, $\phi = 0.22$), Germany ($\chi^2(1) = 7.09$, $p < 0.01$, $\phi = 0.16$), Poland ($\chi^2(1) = 21.64$, $p < 0.001$, $\phi = 0.27$), Ukraine ($\chi^2(1) = 6.96$, $p < 0.01$, $\phi = 0.15$), Turkey $\chi^2(1) = 10.73$, $p < 0.001$, $\phi = 0.19$), Israel ($\chi^2(1) = 5.76$, $p < 0.05$, $\phi = 0.17$), and Colombia ($\chi^2(1) = 6.83$, $p < 0.01$, $\phi = 0.21$).

Anxiety was related to gender in Israel ($\chi^2(1) = 4.87$, $p < 0.05$, $\phi = 0.16$), Russia ($\chi^2(1) = 4.15$, $p < 0.05$, $\phi = 0.12$), Turkey ($\chi^2(1) = 9.15$, $p < 0.01$, $\phi = 0.17$) and Ukraine ($\chi^2(1) = 7.52$, $p < 0.01$, $\phi = 0.16$). An association between anxiety and place of residence was significant solely in Poland ($\chi^2(1) = 7.67$, $p < 0.01$, $\phi = 0.16$). The relationship between the level of study and anxiety was observed in Czechia ($\chi^2(1) = 6.80$ $p < 0.01$, $\phi = -0.15$) and Slovenia ($\chi^2(1) = 5.61$, $p < 0.05$, $\phi = -0.16$). Exposure to COVID-19 was significantly associated with anxiety in all countries, Slovenia ($\chi^2(1) = 13.25$, $p < 0.001$, $\phi = 0.25$), Czechia ($\chi^2(1) = 10.34$, $p < 0.01$, $\phi = 0.18$), Germany ($\chi^2(1) = 8.82$, $p < 0.01$, $\phi = 0.18$), Poland ($\chi^2(1) = 8.97$, $p < 0.01$, $\phi = 0.17$), Ukraine ($\chi^2(1) = 10.03$, $p < 0.01$, $\phi = 0.18$), Russia ($\chi^2(1) = 6.95$, $p < 0.01$, $\phi = 0.16$), Turkey $\chi^2(1) = 7.90$, $p < 0.01$, $\phi = 0.16$), Israel ($\chi^2(1) = 10.28$, $p < 0.01$, $\phi = 0.23$), and Colombia ($\chi^2(1) = 4.40$, $p < 0.05$, $\phi = 0.17$). The total PIC was significantly related to anxiety in all countries: Slovenia ($\chi^2(1) = 29.98$, $p < 0.001$, $\phi = 0.38$), Czechia ($\chi^2(1) = 13.01$, $p < 0.001$, $\phi = 0.20$), Germany ($\chi^2(1) = 9.36$, $p < 0.01$, $\phi = 0.18$), Poland ($\chi^2(1) = 12.74$, $p < 0.001$, $\phi = 0.21$), Ukraine ($\chi^2(1) = 17.48$, $p < 0.001$, $\phi = 0.24$), Russia ($\chi^2(1) = 5.34$, $p < 0.05$, $\phi = 0.14$), Turkey $\chi^2(1) = 11.92$, $p < 0.001$, $\phi = 0.20$), Israel ($\chi^2(1) = 32.27$, mboxemphp < 0.001, $\phi = 0.40$), and Colombia ($\chi^2(1) = 8.14$, $p < 0.01$, $\phi = 0.23$). Qualifications (graduation) were an important source of concern in most countries (except in Poland): Slovenia ($\chi^2(1) = 23.19$, $p < 0.001$, $\phi = 0.33$), Czechia ($\chi^2(1) = 17.80$, $p < 0.001$, $\phi = 0.24$), Germany ($\chi^2(1) = 11.62$, $p < 0.001$, $\phi = 0.21$), Ukraine ($\chi^2(1) = 11.31$, $p < 0.001$, $\phi = 0.19$), Russia ($\chi^2(1) = 7.37$, $p < 0.01$), Turkey $\chi^2(1) = 8.78$, $p < 0.01$, $\phi = 0.27$), Israel ($\chi^2(1) = 9.81$, $p < 0.01$, $\phi = 0.22$), and Colombia ($\chi^2(1) = 8.06$, $p < 0.01$, $\phi = 0.23$). Deterioration of economic status was important in Slovenia ($\chi^2(1) = 4.96$, $p < 0.05$, $\phi = 0.15$), Czechia ($\chi^2(1) = 15.81$, $p < 0.001$, $\phi = 0.23$), Germany ($\chi^2(1) = 4.27$, $p < 0.05$, $\phi = 0.13$), Russia ($\chi^2(1) = 4.47$, $p < 0.05$, $\phi = 0.13$), Turkey $\chi^2(1) = 15.00$, $p < 0.001$, $\phi = 0.22$), and Israel ($\chi^2(1) = 4.42$, $p < 0.05$, $\phi = 0.15$). Excluding Germany, social relationships were of importance in Slovenia ($\chi^2(1) = 13.39$, $p < 0.001$, $\phi = 0.25$), Czechia ($\chi^2(1) = 4.27$, $p < 0.05$, $\phi = 0.12$), Poland ($\chi^2(1) = 21.95$, $p < 0.001$, $\phi = 0.27$), Ukraine ($\chi^2(1) = 13.05$, $p < 0.001$, $\phi = 0.21$), Russia ($\chi^2(1) = 10.04$, $p < 0.01$, $\phi = 0.19$), Turkey $\chi^2(1) = 4.87$, $p < 0.05$, $\phi = 0.13$), Israel ($\chi^2(1) = 14.66$, $p < 0.001$, $\phi = 0.27$), and Colombia ($\chi^2(1) = 5.62$, $p < 0.01$, $\phi = 0.19$). The relationship between insufficient level of physical activity and high anxiety was statistically significant in Poland ($\chi^2(1) = -7.94$, $p < 0.01$, $\phi = 0.16$) and Ukraine ($\chi^2(1) = -4.80$, $p < 0.05$, $\phi = 0.12$). Poor physical health was related to high anxiety in most countries (except Czechia and Israel): Slovenia ($\chi^2(1) = 6.45$, $p < 0.05$, $\phi = 0.18$), Germany ($\chi^2(1) = 9.38$, $p < 0.01$, $\phi = 0.17$), Poland ($\chi^2(1) = 18.51$, $p < 0.001$, $\phi = 0.25$), Ukraine ($\chi^2(1) = 6.47$, $p < 0.05$, $\phi = 0.14$), Russia ($\chi^2(1) = 4.97$, $p < 0.05$, $\phi = 0.13$), Turkey $\chi^2(1) = 13.29$, $p < 0.001$, $\phi = 0.21$), and Colombia ($\chi^2(1) = 4.24$, $p < 0.05$, $\phi = 0.16$). Comparative physical health was linked to anxiety in most countries (except Ukraine, Israel): Slovenia ($\chi^2(1) = 10.75$, $p < 0.01$, $\phi = 0.23$), Czechia ($\chi^2(1) = 4.64$, $p < 0.05$, $\phi = 0.12$), Germany ($\chi^2(1) = 4.19$, $p < 0.05$, $\phi = 0.13$), Poland ($\chi^2(1) = 18.56$, $p < 0.001$, $\phi = 0.25$), Russia ($\chi^2(1) = 4.50$, $p < 0.05$, $\phi = 0.13$), Turkey $\chi^2(1) = 11.19$, $p < 0.001$, $\phi = 0.19$), and Colombia ($\chi^2(1) = 8.00$, $p < 0.01$, $\phi = 0.23$).

3.3. Predictors of Depression in the Nine Countries

Multivariate logistic regression was performed to explore significant predictors of depression among a set of variables that were previously included in the relationship analysis using Pearson's χ^2 test. An estimation was assessed separately for each country: Colombia (Table S3), Czechia (Table S4), Germany (Table S5), Israel (Table S6), Poland (Table S7), Russia (Table S8), Slovenia (Table S9), Turkey (Table S10), and Ukraine (Table S11). All estimates of the multivariate logistic regressions are shown in Figure 3.

The regression model performed for depression among Colombian university students showed a significant effect only for gender; estimate = 0.76, 95% CI = 0.004, 1.516, SE = 0.39, OR = 2.14, Z = 1.97, Wald's $\chi^2(1) = 3.88$, $p < 0.05$ (Table S3). However, the bias corrected accelerated bootstrapping (BCa) method did not confirm gender to be a significant predictor of depression in Colombian students; bootstrap BCa 95% $CI_B = -0.092$, 1.539. The regression model was found to be significant, $\chi^2(143) = 21.591$, $p < 0.01$, $R^2_{CS} = 0.13$, $R^2_{McF} = 0.10$, $R^2_N = 0.18$.

For Czech students (Table S4), logistic regression showed two predictors of depression, namely exposure to COVID-19 (estimate = 0.66, 95% CI = 0.052, 1.267, SE = 0.31, OR = 1.93, Z = 2.13, Wald's $\chi^2(1) = 4.53$, $p < 0.05$) and comparative health (estimate = 1.301, 95% CI = 0.396, 2.207, SE = 0.46, OR = 3.67, Z = 2.81, Wald's $\chi^2(1) = 7.93$, $p < 0.01$). On the other hand, bootstrap confirmed only comparative self-rated health as a significant predictor of depression among Czech students (BCa 95% CI_B = 0.119, 2.223). This model of regression was significant, $\chi^2(296) = 38.639$, $p < 0.001$, $R^2_{CS} = 0.12$, $R^2_{McF} = 0.12$, $R^2_N = 0.18$.

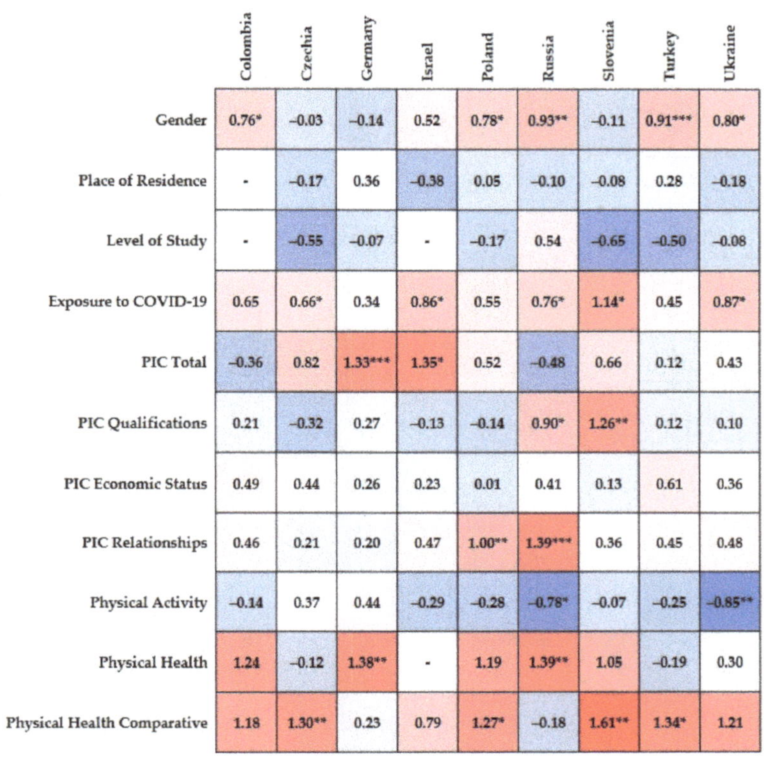

Figure 3. Logistic regression estimates heatmap for depression symptoms among university students from Colombia, Czechia, Germany, Israel, Poland, Russia, Slovenia, Turkey, and Ukraine. Positive estimates are marked in red, negative estimates are marked in blue. PIC = Perceived Impact of COVID-19 on Students' Well-being. * $p < 0.05$, ** $p < 0.01$, *** $p < 0.001$.

Among German students (Table S5), depression can be predicted by the total perceived impact of the coronavirus on daily life (estimate = 1.33, 95% *CI* = 0.483, 2.170, *SE* = 0.43, OR = 3.77, *Z* = 3.08, Wald's $\chi^2(1) = 9.51$, $p < 0.01$) and physical health (estimate = 1.38, 95% *CI* = 0.419, 0.2.345, *SE* = 49, OR = 3.98, *Z* = 2.81, Wald's $\chi^2(1) = 7.91$, $p < 0.01$). These findings were confirmed by the bootstrapping method for both variables, total PIC (BCa 95% CI_B = 0.351, 2.101) and PH (BCa 95% CI_B = 0.232, 2.395). The regression model showed adequate significance, $\chi^2(253) = 60.82$, $p < 0.001$, $R^2_{CS} = 21$, $R^2_{McF} = 0.17$, $R^2_N = 0.28$.

For Israeli participants (Table S6), excluding study level and physical health as predictors of depression, $\chi^2(189) = 49.79$, $p < 0.001$, $R^2_{CS} = 0.22$, $R^2_{McF} = 0.18$, $R^2_N = 0.30$, the regression model was found to be significant. Among two significant predictors of depression, namely, exposure to the coronavirus (estimate = 0.86, 95% *CI* = 0.092, 1.633, *SE* = 0.39, OR = 2.37, *Z* = 2.19, Wald's $\chi^2(1) = 4.81$, $p < 0.05$) and total PIC (estimate = 1.35, 95% *CI* = 0.302, 2.394, *SE* = 0.53, OR = 3.85, *Z* = 2.53, Wald's $\chi^2(1) = 6.39$, $p < 0.05$), only total PIC was confirmed by the bootstrapping procedure (BCa 95% CI_B = 0.147, 2.524).

When the regression was performed for Polish students (Table S7), three variables revealed sufficient significance level using both classical and bootstrapping methods, namely gender (estimate = 0.78, 95% *CI* = 0.190, 1.377, *SE* = 0.30, OR = 2.19, *Z* = 2.59, Wald's $\chi^2(1) = 6.70$, $p < 0.01$; BCa 95% CI_B = 0.115, 1.393), total PIC (estimate = 1.00, 95% *CI* = 0.299, 1.700, *SE* = 0.36, OR = 2.72, *Z* = 2.80, Wald's $\chi^2(1) = 7.82$, $p < 0.01$; BCa 95% CI_B = 0.197, 1.653), and comparative PH (estimate = 1.27, 95% *CI* = 0.286, 2.250, *SE* = 0.50, OR = 3.55,

$Z = 2.53$, Wald's $\chi^2(1) = 6.41$, $p < 0.05$; BCa 95% $CI_B = 0.126, 2.323$). The regression model was found to be significant, $\chi^2(288) = 62.46$, $p < 0.001$, $R^2_{CS} = 0.19$, $R^2_{McF} = 0.15$, $R^2_N = 0.25$.

In the Russian sample of university students (Table S8), the following predictors of depression were found: gender (estimate = 0.93, 95% $CI = 0.300, 1.560$, $SE = 0.32$, OR = 2.53, $Z = 2.89$, Wald's $\chi^2(1) = 8.37$, $p < 0.01$), exposure to the coronavirus (estimate = 0.76, 95% $CI = 0.080, 1.443$, $SE = 0.35$, OR = 2.14, $Z = 2.19$, Wald's $\chi^2(1) = 4.80$, $p < 0.05$), PIC-qualification (estimate = 0.90, 95% $CI = 0.175, 1.624$, $SE = 0.37$, OR = 2.46, $Z = 2.43$, Wald's $\chi^2(1) = 5.92$, $p < 0.05$), PIC-social relationships (estimate = 1.39, 95% $CI = 0.681, 2.100$, $SE = 0.36$, OR = 4.02, $Z = 3.84$, Wald's $\chi^2(1) = 14.76$, $p < 0.001$), physical activity (estimate = −0.78, 95% $CI = -1.375, -0.176$, $SE = 0.31$, OR = 0.46, $Z = -2.54$, Wald's $\chi^2(1) = 6.43$, $p < 0.05$), and physical health (estimate = 1.39, 95% $CI = 0.472, 2.304$, $SE = 0.48$, OR = 4.01, $Z = 2.97$, Wald's $\chi^2(1) = 8.83$, $p < 0.01$). In addition, bootstrap showed a significant effect for gender (BCa 95% $CI_B = 0.209, 1.590$), PIC-qualification (BCa 95% $CI_B = 0.102, 1.636$), PIC-social relationships (BCa 95% $CI_B = 0.195, 2.157$), and PH (BCa 95% $_B = 0.125, 2.305$). The regression model was significant, $\chi^2(271) = 69.38$, $p < 0.001$, $R^2_{CS} = 0.22$, $R^2_{McF} = 0.18$, $R^2_N = 0.29$.

The regression model conducted in the Slovenian sample of students (Table S9) showed a good fit, $\chi^2(197) = 77.13$, $p < 0.001$, $R^2_{CS} = 0.31$, $R^2_{McF} = 0.29$, $R^2_N = 0.43$. Among variables, exposure to COVID-19 (estimate = 1.14, 95% $CI = 0.258, 2.021$, $SE = 0.45$, OR = 3.125, $Z = 2.534$, Wald's $\chi^2(1) = 6.423$, $p < 0.05$), PIC-qualifications (estimate = 1.26, 95% $CI = 0.337, 2.183$, $SE = 0.47$, OR = 3.52, $Z = 2.68$, Wald's $\chi^2(1) = 7.154$, $p < 0.01$), and comparative PH (estimate = 1.61, 95% $CI = 0.402, 2.825$, $SE = 0.62$, OR = 5.02, $Z = 2.61$, Wald's $\chi^2(1) = 6.81$, $p < 0.01$) were found to be significant predictors of depression. The bootstrapping method confirmed the significance of all three variables, namely exposure to the coronavirus (BCa 95% $CI_B = 0.058, 2.114$), PIC-qualifications (BCa 95% $CI_B = 0.155, 2.076$), and comparative PH (BCa 95% $CI_B = 0.165, 2.916$).

Although three variables were shown as significant predictors of depression among Turkish students (Table S10), namely gender (estimate = 0.91, 95% $CI = 0.398, 1.413$, $SE = 0.26$, OR = 2.48, $Z = 3.50$, Wald's $\chi^2(1) = 12.24$, $p < 0.001$), PIC-social relationships (estimate = 0.61, 95% $CI = -0.001, 1.213$, $SE = 0.31$, OR = 1.83, $Z = 1.96$, Wald's $\chi^2(1) = 3.84$, $p < 0.05$), and comparative PH (estimate = 1.37, 95% $CI = 0.090, 2.583$, $SE = 0.64$, OR = 3.81, $Z = 2.10$, Wald's $\chi^2(1)$ 4.42, $p < 0.05$), only gender was confirmed using the bootstrapping method (BCa 95% $CI_B = 0.350, 1.429$). The model's fit for the Turkish sample was good, $\chi^2(294) = 42.17$, $p < 0.001$, $R^2_{CS} = 0.13$, $R^2_{McF} = 0.10$, $R^2_N = 0.18$. Among Ukrainian participants (Table S11), depression can be predicted by gender (estimate = 0.80, 95% $CI = 0.150$, 1,456, SE = 0.33, OR = 2.23, $Z = 2.41$, Wald's $\chi^2(1) = 5.81$, $p < 0.05$), exposure to COVID-19 (estimate = 0.87, 95% $CI = 0.060, 1.686$, SE = 0.42, OR = 2.39, $Z = 2.11$, Wald's $\chi^2(1) = 4.43$, $p < 0.05$), and PA (estimate = −0.85, 95% $CI = -1.413, -0.288$, SE = 0.29, OR = 0.427, $Z = -2.97$, Wald's $\chi^2(1) = 8.79$, $p < 0.01$). Gender (BCa 95% $CI_B = 0.070, 1.512$) and PA (BCa 95% $CI_B = -1.396, -0.218$) were also found to be significant predictors when the bootstrapping method was used. The regression model presented a good fit, $\chi^2(298) = 45.65$, $p < 0.001$, $R^2_{CS} = 0.14$, $R^2_{McF} = 0.12$, $R^2_N = 0.20$.

3.4. *Predictors of Anxiety in the Nine Countries*

Similarly to the previous analyses, the multiple logistic regression was conducted for anxiety to find predictors among demographic and health-related variables among university students in each country. In Colombian students (Table S12), only comparative PH was found to be a significant predictor of anxiety (estimate = 1.35, 95% $CI = 0.132, 2.560$, $SE = 0.46$, OR = 3.84, $Z = 2.17$, Wald's $\chi^2(1) = 4.72$, $p < 0.05$). However, the bootstrapping procedure did not confirm it (BCa 95% $CI_B = -0.266, 2.819$). The model's fit was sufficient, $\chi^2(143) = 25.58$, $p < 0.01$, $R^2_{CS} = 0.15$, $R^2_{McF} = 0.13$, $R^2_N = 0.21$. All estimates of the multivariate logistic regressions are shown in Figure 4.

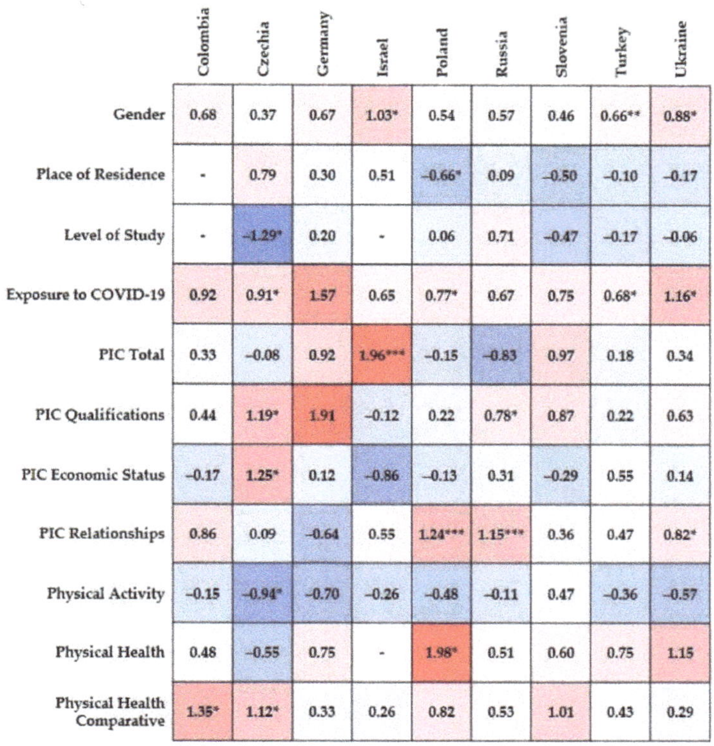

Figure 4. Logistic regression estimates heatmap for anxiety symptoms among university students from Colombia, Czechia, Germany, Israel, Poland, Russia, Slovenia, Turkey, and Ukraine. Positive estimates are marked in red, negative estimates are marked in blue. PIC = Perceived Impact of COVID-19 on Students' Well-being. * $p < 0.05$, ** $p < 0.01$, *** $p < 0.001$.

Among students in Czechia (Table S13), the following predictors of anxiety were found: study level (estimate = 1.35, 95% CI = 0.132, 2.560, SE = 0.46, OR = 3.84, Z = 2.17, Wald's $\chi^2(1) = 4.72$, $p < 0.05$), exposure to the coronavirus (estimate = 1.35, 95% CI = (0.132, 2.560), SE = 0.46, OR = 3.84, Z = 2.17, Wald's $\chi^2(1) = 4.72$, $p < 0.05$), PIC-qualifications (estimate = 1.35, 95% CI = 0.132, 2.560, SE = 0.46, OR = 3.84, Z = 2.17, Wald's $\chi^2(1) = 4.72$, $p < 0.05$), PIC-economic status, PA (estimate = 1.35, 95% CI = 0.132, 2.560, SE = 0.46, OR = 3.84, Z = 2.17, Wald's $\chi^2(1) = 4.72$, $p < 0.05$), and comparative PH (estimate = 1.35, 95% CI = 0.132, 2.560, SE = 0.46, OR = 3.84, Z = 2.17, Wald's $\chi^2(1) = 4.72$, $p < 0.05$). However, bootstrap showed a significant effect only for exposure to the coronavirus (BCa 95% CI_B = 0.024, 1.764) and PIC-social relationships (BCa 95% CI_B = 0.100, 2.533). The model presents a good fit, $\chi^2(296) = 48.69$, $p < 0.001$, $R^2_{CS} = 0.15$, $R^2_{McF} = 0.21$, $R^2_N = 0.27$.

The model of regression did not find any statistically significant predictors of anxiety in the sample of German university students (Table S14). Moreover, bootstrap did not show significance. However, the model's fit was satisfactory with $\chi^2(255) = 33.35$, $p < 0.001$, $R^2_{CS} = 0.12$, $R^2_{McF} = 0.30$, $R^2_N = 0.35$.

In the sample of students from Israel (Table S15), the following predictors of anxiety were revealed: gender (estimate = 1.03, 95% CI = 0.155, 1.901, SE = 0.45, OR = 2.80, Z = 2.31, Wald's $\chi^2(1) = 5.32$, $p < 0.05$; BCa 95% CI_B = 0.039, 2.007), and total PIC (estimate = 1.96, 95% CI = 0.757, 3.172) SE = 0.62, OR = 7.13, Z = 3.19, Wald's $\chi^2(1) = 10.17$, $p < 0.001$; BCa 95% CI_B = 0.471, 3.300), which was also confirmed using the bootstrap procedure. The level of study and PH were not included in the model because these variables did not sufficiently meet the criteria. The goodness of fit for the regression model was adequate, $\chi^2(189) = 48.23$, $p < 0.001$, $R^2_{CS} = 0.22$, $R^2_{McF} = 0.19$, $R^2_N = 0.30$.

Among Polish participants (Table S16), four predictors of anxiety were presented in the regression model: place of residence (estimate = −0.66, 95% *CI* = −1.271, −0.039, *SE* = 0.31, OR = 0.52, $Z = -2.09$, Wald's $\chi^2(1) = 4.35$, $p < 0.05$), exposure to the coronavirus (estimate = 0.77, 95% *CI* = 0.165, 1.365, *SE* = 0.31, OR = 2.15, $Z = 2.50$, Wald's $\chi^2(1) = 6.24$, $p < 0.05$), PIC-social relationships (estimate = 1.24, 95% *CI* = 0.513, 1.970, *SE* = 0.37, OR = 3.46, $Z = 3.40$, Wald's $\chi^2(1) = 11.15$, $p < 0.001$), and PH (estimate = 1.98, 95% *CI* = 0.297, 3.689, *SE* = 0.86, OR = 7.23, $Z = 2.31$, Wald's $\chi^2(1) = 5.32$, $p < 0.05$). However, only two of these were confirmed by the bootstrapping method: exposure (BCa 95% $CI_B = 0.069$, 1.403) and PIC-social relationships (BCa 95% $CI_B = 0.432$, 2.004). The model of regression presented a good fit, $\chi^2(288) = 64.78$, $p < 0.001$, $R^2_{CS} = 0.19$, $R^2_{McF} = 0.16$, $R^2_N = 0.26$.

The perceived impact of the coronavirus on social relationships was the sole predictor of anxiety for Russian university students (Table S17), estimate = 1.15, 95% *CI* = 0.446, 1.843, *SE* = 0.36, OR = 3.14, $Z = 3.21$, Wald's $\chi^2(1) = 10.32$, $p < 0.001$; BCa 95% $CI_B = 0.318$, 1.973. The regression model showed a sufficient fit, $\chi^2(271) = 34.05$, $p < 0.001$, $R^2_{CS} = 0.11$, $R^2_{McF} = 0.10$, $R^2_N = 0.16$.

Although the model's fit statistics were appropriate, $\chi^2(197) = 53.424$, $p < 0.001$, $R^2_{CS} = 0.23$, $R^2_{McF} = 0.22$, $R^2_N = 0.33$, the variables included into the regression model were not found to be predictors of anxiety in the sample of Slovenian students (Table S18).

In the Turkish group of students, gender (estimate = 0.66, 95% *CI* = 0.162, 1.151, *SE* = 0.25, OR = 1.93, $Z = 2.60$, Wald's $\chi^2(1) = 6.77$, $p < 0.01$) and exposure to the coronavirus (estimate = 0.68, 95% *CI* = 0.032, 1.319, *SE* = 0.33, OR = 1.97, $Z = 2.06$, Wald's $\chi^2(1) = 4.24$, $p < 0.05$) were found to be significant predictors of anxiety (Table S19). However, only gender was confirmed by the bootstrapping test (BCa 95% $CI_B = 0.111$, 1.175). The regression model's fit was adequate, $\chi^2(294) = 43.17$, $p < 0.001$, $R^2_{CS} = 0.13$, $R^2_{McF} = 0.10$, $R^2_N = 0.18$.

Both gender (estimate = 0.88, 95% *CI* = 0.148, 1.603, *SE* = 0.37, OR = 2.40, $Z = 2.36$, Wald's $\chi^2(1) = 5.57$, $p < 0.05$) and PIC-social relationships (estimate = 0.82, 95% *CI* = 037, 1.593, *SE* = 0.40, OR = 2.26, $Z = 2.05$, Wald's $\chi^2(1) = 4.21$, $p < 0.05$) were shown to be significant predictors of anxiety in the sample of Ukrainian university students (Table S20). However, when bootstrap was performed, only gender was a predictor of anxiety (BCa 95% $CI_B = 0.101$, 1.639).

4. Discussion

Our study showed the importance of a cross-national perspective in exploring university students' mental health during the first wave of the COVID-19 pandemic. The research revealed large differences in depression and anxiety rates in the nine countries. The highest rates of depression and anxiety were noted in Turkish students, whereas the lowest depression was reported in Czech students and the lowest anxiety in German students. We have also shown the associations of mental health with other variables in the nine countries. Physical activity turned out to be associated with mental health in less than half of the countries. However, the following factors proved to be associated with anxiety and depression in most of the countries: exposure to COVID-19, the perceived impact of COVID-19 on students' well-being, including graduation, economic status, and relationships quality, and general and comparative health.

The study revealed a variety of depression and anxiety risk factors in prediction models for each country. Even though certain variables, such as exposure to COVID-19, were significant among students across the nine countries, other key variables, e.g., gender or physical activity, were credible only in particular countries. Therefore, our results underline the necessity for the cultural context to be taken into account when exploring mental health in the student population.

4.1. Anxiety and Depression across the Nine Countries

Cross-national analyses allow for the obtained results to be analyzed from the global perspective. Previous cross-national research in European countries showed that a lower risk of depression is associated with socioeconomic factors [70]. In addition, a study using the Human Development Index (HDI) revealed that the highest depression prevalence was in medium HDI countries [20]. People in medium HDI countries might be subjected to more stressors compared to low HDI countries due to high expectations accompanied with high living costs and the cost of depression treatment [71]. However, in our research, all countries, except Ukraine and Colombia, are designated as very high HDI countries (HDI $\geq$ 0.800). Despite the above, large differences concerning depression in relation to the individual country were revealed. This suggests that other circumstances should be taken into account to explain the results of depression at a cross-national level. In certain cases, our results were in contrast to expectations, since e.g., Turkish students (very high HDI) exceeded all other students in the depression level, whereas Ukrainian students (high HDI) scored similarly to Czech students (very high HDI), thus presented the lowest level of depression in this study. Additionally, students from Czechia, which occupies 27th position in the HDI ranking, scored significantly lower in depression compared to students in Germany holding 6th position in this global ranking. Those inconsistent results may arise from the fact that the student population differs significantly from the general population. Moreover, the estimation of HDI change for 2020 globally shows an unprecedented shock to human development as all of HDI capabilities (long and healthy life, being knowledgeable, and having a decent standard of living) were severely affected indicating unparalleled acute decrease even compared to the post-2007 global financial crisis [72].

On the other hand, Turkish students, who reported the highest depressive symptoms among the nine countries, mostly live in eastern Turkey, where living standards are significantly lower compared to western Turkey [73]. The highest depression and anxiety levels in Turkey compared to the other nine countries may be explained by other significant factors. For example, in Turkey, the pandemic situation may affect student lifestyle by overlapping with other socioeconomic burdens, the current volatile economic situation [74], and high unemployment among young people, reaching 30% [75].

Nonetheless, when analyzing depression and anxiety levels in the nine countries from the global socioeconomic perspective, it appears that a country's financial situation and HDI may play a more prominent role in anxiety than depression. Students from Germany—the country with the highest HDI and the highest possible score in Standard & Poor's Global Ratings [76]—presented a minimal anxiety level, which notably, was the lowest among the nine countries. Among other predictors and associated variables, this may also be due to a more stable economy at the national level. Financial security may play a more significant role in decreasing anxiety than depression among students, as the German example shows.

4.2. Association of Depression and Anxiety Risk with Other Variables

Exposure to COVID-19, perceived impact of COVID-19 on students' well-being, including graduation, economic status, and relationships' quality, as well as general and comparative health, turned out to be associated with anxiety and depression in the majority of the surveyed countries. Therefore, these variables can be designated as key mental health risk factors from the cross-cultural perspective.

Even though previous research has shown the importance of physical activity for anxiety and depression in the student population [39], this study clearly manifests that the cultural context should be taken into account when analyzing this issue. Physical activity was associated with anxiety only in two (Poland and Ukraine) out of nine countries. The association with depression was revealed only in four countries (Poland, Ukraine, Russia and Israel). Therefore, in most countries, physical activity was not associated with mental health in students. One of the factors related to physical activity from the cross-cultural perspective is motivation to participate, as in individualistic cultures, like USA, the key motivation was competition, whereas in collectivistic cultures, like China, it was rather a social affiliation and wellness [77].

Living in a city or town/village turned out to be irrelevant for depression in the nine countries. This is in congruence with previous meta-analyses [20,78,79]. Students are quite a homogeneous group. Therefore, both groups living in rural and urban areas have common characteristics (i.e., young age) linked to depressive symptoms during the pandemic [13–15]. However, living in a small city or a village was associated with anxiety risk exclusively in Polish students. In all the remaining countries, it was an irrelevant factor. Previous research also showed inconsistent results. Living in an urban area was linked to lower anxiety in China [42] but higher anxiety in Bangladesh [43].

Our research showed that the association between gender and mental health risk is not clear when analyzed in different countries. Female students from Ukraine, Russia, and Turkey had a higher prevalence of anxiety and depression risk compared to male students in those countries. The highest rate of both depression and anxiety risk was revealed among Turkish female students. Furthermore, Polish and Israeli female students showed a higher prevalence of anxiety risk, whereas Colombian female students manifested the risk of depression. Previous research showed a gender effect on the prevalence of depression [20,70,79,80]. Additionally, a recent meta-analysis regarding students' mental health during the COVID-19 pandemic has revealed that female students were found to have a higher prevalence of anxiety and depression [81]. However, we have found no gender association with mental health issues among Slovenian, Czech, and German students. Therefore, the cultural context should be incorporated when exploring gender association with mental health issues.

4.3. Predictors of Depression and Anxiety in the Nine Countries

The multiple regression models are closer to actual psychological complexity, as they reveal risk factors in their simultaneous effect on mental health, compared to bivariate models where the particular factors predict mental health issues independently. The most frequent predictors of depression and anxiety in the nine countries were gender, exposure to COVID-19, and comparative physical health.

The multiple logistic regression proved gender to be a significant predictor of anxiety but only among Israeli, Ukrainian, and Turkish students. Gender was a more frequent predictor of depression among Colombian, Polish, Russian, Turkish, and Ukrainian students, but a less significant predictor in Colombia. Previous cross-national research in 23 European countries showed that the largest gender differences in depression were noted in certain former Soviet Union countries, and the lowest in Western and Nordic countries [70]. The results in our study partially conform with the aforementioned report. However, in our research, gender was not a risk factor for mental health issues among students in Slovenia and Czechia (former Soviet Union countries). This inconsistency can be partially explained by gender inequalities denoted by the the Gender Inequality Index (GII) [82], which in Slovenia (0.07) and Czechia (0.14) is relatively lower compared to Ukraine (0.29) and Russia (0.25). Therefore, the gender role hypothesis seems to be a more appropriate explanation, particularly for female gender as a risk factor for depression in five out of the nine countries.

The gender role hypothesis claims that the gender gap in the prevalence of mental health issues is due to specific differences in coping resources, stressors, or opportunities for expressing psychological distress distinctively for women and men [83]. Gender role (the concept of femininity and masculinity) affects major risk factors for internalizing and externalizing problems [84]. This hypothesis has found a partial confirmation as regards depression, but not anxiety [83]. Depression was revealed to be related to the changes in traditional female gender roles. Narrowing gender differences in depression was observed along with the declining gender role traditionality [83]. Our study also confirms the significance of gender as a predictor of depression in relation to the gender role hypothesis.

However, the results in Israel, Ukraine and Turkey also show the significance of gender in predicting anxiety in the student population during the COVID-19 pandemic.

Multiple regression models showed the importance of exposure to the COVID-19 infection in five countries (Slovenia, Czechia, Israel Russia, and Ukraine) for depression, and in four countries (Czechia, Poland, Turkey, and Ukraine) for anxiety, even though the stringency of restrictions index (ranging from 0 to 100) in those countries varied from 41 in Slovenia to 82 in Ukraine. Therefore, exposure to the infection as a risk factor of depression or/and anxiety appeared in several countries independently of restrictions introduced by the governments.

The perceived impact of COVID-19 on students' well-being was a risk factor for depression in Israel and Germany, and additionally, for anxiety in Israel. In other countries, this variable was insignificant in multivariate models. However, its subscales showed different patterns depending on the country. Worries about graduation were considered as risk factors for depression in Slovenia and Russia, and for anxiety in Czechia and Russia. The perceived impact of COVID-19 on students' economic status was significantly associated with depression and anxiety in the majority of the countries, as the above analysis showed. The deterioration of economic status as a risk factor for both depression and anxiety is in line with other studies [85,86]. However, when economic status was introduced in multiple models, it turned out to be a trivial predictor of depression, while being a significant predictor of anxiety only in one country (Czechia). Therefore, even though PIC Economic Status is relevant when analyzed as a singular risk factor for mental health, when combined with other risk factors for mental health, such as exposure to COVID-19 or female gender, it becomes insignificant.

Concern about relationship quality was the strongest predictor in the multivariate models of depression and anxiety in Poland and Russia. Therefore, in the countries with stronger traditional family values, the perceived impact of the COVID-19 pandemic on students' relationships with family was a significant risk factor for mental health issues. Insufficient physical activity in multivariate models was a risk factor for depression in Russia and Ukraine, and for anxiety in Czechia. Worse physical health played a different role than worse comparative physical health. General physical health was a strong predictor of depression in Germany and Russia and a weaker predictor of anxiety in Poland. Worse comparative health turned out to be a significant risk factor for depression in four countries (Czechia, Poland, Slovenia, and a weaker predictor in Turkey). For anxiety, this was true only for two countries. However, the results in Colombia and Czechia were not confirmed when the bias-corrected accelerated bootstrapping method was introduced. Therefore, comparative physical health was a more common predictor of depression than anxiety among students across the nine countries.

Although introduced variables allowed for the creation of multivariate models of depression in each country, anxiety was not explained by proposed predictors in Slovenia, Germany, and Colombia.

4.4. Limitations

There are several limitations to the present study. One is the cross-sectional character of the research. The longitudinal study could reveal the cause—effect relationship between the proposed indices and mental health issues. Direct comparisons among countries are also limited due to the different pace and extent of public health restrictions imposed by governments and due to the situation with COVID-19 related deaths in the observed period in each of the observed countries. Another limitation is a self-selected study sample and data collection via self-reported questionnaires. Therefore, the data can be subject to retrospective response bias. Previous research showed that more depressive symptoms can be elicited for milder forms of depression through self-reported measurements compared to clinician-rating methods (interview) [87]. More educated and younger people usually score higher on self-rated scales than on clinician-rating scales [88]. However, it should be noted that even though a milder form of depression may be elicited among young adults, depressive symptoms have increased during the pandemic [89,90]. Finally, generalizing the results may be hindered by the lack of random sampling and representation of the student population being limited to specific regions in each country.

Considering strengths and limitations of this study, future research ought to examine mental health using a longitudinal design from the cross-cultural perspective.

5. Conclusions

Our study has shown risk factors for depression and anxiety and differences in mental health among university students in the nine countries during the first wave of the COVID-19 pandemic. We have revealed that even so common a risk factor as gender does not predict anxiety or depression in all the countries. Moreover, physical inactivity as a risk factor strongly depends on the country, and in most of the nine countries was a significant predictor neither for anxiety nor depression.

This research underlines the necessity of interpreting data within the cross-cultural context and argues that presenting mental health results during the COVID-19 pandemic only in one country can be challenging in terms of generalization. We demonstrated that, even though there are several risk factors associated with mental health issues in all of the nine countries (i.e., exposure to COVID-19, perceived impact of COVID-19 on students' well-being, including graduation, economic status, and relationships quality, general and comparative health), the multivariate models differed drastically among the countries. Therefore, despite the globalization of a homogeneous student population, our study showed varied mental health predictors in relation to cultural, political and economic situation in a particular country. Planning and implementation of psychological intervention programs for students should include differentiation by country concerning mental health risk factors.

Supplementary Materials: The following are available online at https://www.mdpi.com/article/10.3390/jcm10132882/s1, Table S1: Association between depression risk and other variables among university students from Colombia, Czechia, Germany, Israel, Poland, Russia, Slovenia, Turkey, and Ukraine during the first wave of the COVID-19 pandemic. Table S2: Association between anxiety risk and other variables among university students from Colombia, Czechia, Germany, Israel, Poland, Russia, Slovenia, Turkey, and Ukraine during the first wave of the COVID-19 pandemic. Table S3: Logistic regression for depression symptoms among university students from Colombia during the first wave of the COVID-19 pandemic. Table S4: Logistic regression for depression symptoms among university students from Czechia during the first wave of the COVID-19 pandemic. Table S5: Logistic regression for depression symptoms among university students from Germany during the first wave of the COVID-19 pandemic. Table S6: Logistic regression for depression symptoms among university students from Israel during the first wave of the COVID-19 pandemic. Table S7: Logistic regression for depression symptoms among university students from Poland during the first wave of the COVID-19 pandemic. Table S8: Logistic regression for depression symptoms among university students from Russia during the first wave of the COVID-19 pandemic. Table S9: Logistic regression for depression symptoms among university students from Slovenia during the first wave of the COVID-19 pandemic. Table S10: Logistic regression for depression symptoms among university students from Turkey during the first wave of the COVID-19 pandemic. Table S11: Logistic regression for depression symptoms among university students from Ukraine during the first wave of the COVID-19 pandemic. Table S12: Logistic regression for anxiety symptoms among university students from Colombia during the first wave of the COVID-19 pandemic. Table S13: Logistic regression for anxiety symptoms among university students from Czechia during the first wave of the COVID-19 pandemic. Table S14: Logistic regression for anxiety symptoms among university students from Germany during the first wave of the COVID-19 pandemic. Table S15: Logistic regression for anxiety symptoms among university students from Israel during the first wave of the COVID-19 pandemic. Table S16: Logistic regression for anxiety symptoms among university students from Poland during the first wave of the COVID-19 pandemic. Table S17: Logistic regression for anxiety symptoms among university students from Russia during the first wave of the COVID-19 pandemic. Table S18: Logistic regression for anxiety symptoms among university students from Slovenia during the first wave of the COVID-19 pandemic. Table S19: Logistic regression for anxiety symptoms among university students from Turkey during the first wave of the COVID-19 pandemic. Table S20: Logistic regression for anxiety symptoms among university students from Ukraine during the first wave of the COVID-19 pandemic.

Author Contributions: Conceptualization, D.O., A.M.R., C.K.; data curation, D.O.; formal analysis, A.M.R., investigation, D.O., A.M.R., C.K., M.J., A.S., M.J.H., A.A., J.B., R.B., E.V.K., I.P., I.B., Z.K., I.A., O.Ç., Y.A.C.-A.; methodology, A.M.R., D.O.; project administration, D.O.; resources D.O., A.M.R., C.K., M.J., A.S., M.J.H., A.A., J.B., R.B., E.V.K., I.P., I.B., Z.K., I.A., O.Ç., Y.A.C.-A., M.W.-S.; supervision, D.O., A.M.R.; visualization, A.M.R.; writing—original draft preparation, D.O., A.M.R.; writing—review and editing, D.O., A.M.R., C.K., M.J., A.S., M.J.H., A.A., J.B., R.B., E.V.K., I.P., I.B., Z.K., I.A., O.Ç., Y.A.C.-A., M.W.-S. All authors have read and agreed to the published version of the manuscript.

Funding: This research received no external funding.

Institutional Review Board Statement: The study was conducted according to the guidelines of the Declaration of Helsinki, and approved by the local IRB: University Research Committee at the University of Opole, Poland, decision no. 1/2020.

Informed Consent Statement: Informed consent was obtained from all subjects involved in the study.

Data Availability Statement: The materials and methods are accessible at the Center for Open Science (OSF), titled: Well-being of undergraduates during the COVID-19 pandemic: International study [91]. The datasets generated during and/or analyzed during the current study are available from the corresponding author on reasonable request.

Conflicts of Interest: The authors declare no conflict of interest.

References

1. Baloch, S.; Baloch, M.A.; Zheng, T.; Pei, X. The coronavirus disease 2019 (COVID-19) pandemic. *Tohoku J. Exp. Med.* **2020**, *250*, 271–278. [CrossRef] [PubMed]
2. World Health Organization. Rolling Updates on Coronavirus Disease (COVID-19). Available online: https://www.who.int/emergencies/diseases/novel-coronavirus-2019/events-as-they-happen (accessed on 15 March 2021).
3. Rajkumar, R.P. Covid-19 and mental health: A review of the existing literature. *Asian J. Psychiatry* **2020**, *52*, 102066. [CrossRef] [PubMed]
4. Brooks, S.K.; Webster, R.K.; Smith, L.E.; Woodland, L.; Wessely, S.; Greenberg, N.; Rubin, G.J. The psychological impact of quarantine and how to reduce it: Rapid review of the evidence. *Lancet* **2020**, *395*, 912–920. [CrossRef]
5. Wang, X.; Lei, S.M.; Le, S.; Yang, Y.; Zhang, B.; Yao, W.; Gao, Z.; Cheng, S. Bidirectional influence of the covid-19 pandemic lockdowns on health behaviors and quality of life among Chinese adults. *Int. J. Environ. Res. Public Health* **2020**, *17*, 5575. [CrossRef]
6. Li, S.; Wang, Y.; Xue, J.; Zhao, N.; Zhu, T. The impact of Covid-19 epidemic declaration on psychological consequences: A study on active weibo users. *Int. J. Environ. Res. Public Health* **2020**, *17*, 2032. [CrossRef]
7. Troyer, E.A.; Kohn, J.N.; Hong, S. Are we facing a crashing wave of neuropsychiatric sequelae of COVID-19? Neuropsychiatric symptoms and potential immunologic mechanisms. *Brain Behav. Immun.* **2020**, *87*, 34–39. [CrossRef]
8. World Bank. *Global Economic Prospects, June 2020*; World Bank: Washington, DC, USA, 2020. [CrossRef]
9. Bartoll, X.; Palència, L.; Malmusi, D.; Suhrcke, M.; Borrell, C. The evolution of mental health in Spain during the economic crisis. *Eur. J. Public Health.* **2014**, *24*, 415–418. [CrossRef]
10. Williams, D.R.; Yu, Y.; Jackson, J.S.; Anderson, N.B. Racial differences in physical and mental health: Socio-economic status, stress and discrimination. *J. Health Psychol.* **1997**, *2*, 335–351. [CrossRef]
11. Murali, V.; Oyebode, F. Poverty, social inequality and mental health. *Adv. Psychiatr. Treat.* **2004**, *10*, 216–224. [CrossRef]
12. Bonsaksen, T.; Leung, J.; Schoultz, M.; Thygesen, H.; Price, D.; Ruffolo, M.; Geirdal, A.Ø. Cross-national study of worrying, loneliness, and mental health during the COVID-19 pandemic: A comparison between individuals with and without infection in the family. *Res. Sq.* **2020**. [CrossRef]
13. Fried, E.I.; Papanikolaou, F.; Epskamp, S. Mental Health and Social Contact during the COVID-19 Pandemic: An Ecological Momentary Assessment Study. 2020. Available online: psyarxiv.com/36xkp/ (accessed on 15 March 2021).
14. Elmer, T.; Mepham, K.; Stadtfeld, C. Students under lockdown: Comparisons of students' social networks and mental health before and during the covid-19 crisis in Switzerland. *PLoS ONE* **2020**, *15*, e0236337. [CrossRef]
15. Liang, L.; Ren, H.; Cao, R.; Hu, Y.; Qin, Z.; Li, C.; Mei, S. The effect of covid-19 on youth mental health. *Psychiatr. Q.* **2020**, *91*, 841–852. [CrossRef]
16. Vieira, C.M.; Franco, O.H.; Restrepo, C.G.; Abel, T. COVID-19: The forgotten priorities of the pandemic. *Maturitas* **2020**, *136*, 38–41. [CrossRef]
17. Schubert, K.O.; Clark, S.R.; Van, L.K.; Collinson, J.L.; Baune, B.T. Depressive symptom trajectories in late adolescence and early adulthood: A systematic review. *Aust. N. Z. J. Psychiatry* **2017**, *51*, 477–499. [CrossRef]

18. Zivin, K.; Eisenberg, D.; Gollust, S.E.; Golberstein, E. Persistence of mental health problems and needs in a college student population. *J. Affect. Disord.* **2009**, *117*, 180–185. [CrossRef]
19. Ibrahim, A.K.; Kelly, S.J.; Adams, C.E.; Glazebrook, C. A systematic review of studies of depression prevalence in university students. *J. Psychiatr. Res.* **2013**, *47*, 391–400. [CrossRef]
20. Lim, G.Y.; Tam, W.W.; Lu, Y.; Ho, C.S.; Zhang, M.W.; Ho, R.C. Prevalence of Depression in the Community from 30 Countries between 1994 and 2014. *Sci. Rep.* **2018**, *8*, 2861. [CrossRef]
21. Stewart-Brown, S.; Evans, J.; Patterson, J.; Petersen, S.; Doll, H.; Balding, J.; Regis, D. The health of students in institutes of higher education: An important and neglected public health problem? *J. Public Health Med.* **2000**, *22*, 492–499. [CrossRef]
22. Vaez, M.; Ponce de Leon, A.; Laflamme, L. Health-related determinants of perceived quality of life: A comparison between first-year university students and their working peers. *Work* **2006**, *26*, 167–177.
23. Andrews, B.; Wilding, J.M. The relation of depression and anxiety to life-stress and achievement in students. *Br. J. Psychol.* **2004**, *95*, 509–521. [CrossRef]
24. Wege, N.; Muth, T.; Li, J.; Angerer, P. Mental health among currently enrolled medical students in Germany. *Public Health* **2016**, *132*, 92–100. [CrossRef] [PubMed]
25. Elani, H.W.; Allison, P.J.; Kumar, R.A.; Mancini, L.; Lambrou, A.; Bedos, C. A systematic review of stress in dental students. *J. Dent. Educ.* **2014**, *78*, 226–242. [CrossRef] [PubMed]
26. Cook, A.F.; Arora, V.M.; Rasinski, K.A.; Curlin, F.A.; Yoon, J.D. The prevalence of medical student mistreatment and its association with burnout. *Acad. Med. J. Assoc. Am. Med. Coll.* **2014**, *89*, 749–754. [CrossRef] [PubMed]
27. Borst, J.M.; Frings-Dresen, M.H.W.; Sluiter, J.K. Prevalence and incidence of mental health problems among Dutch medical students and the study related and personal risk factors: A longitudinal study. *Int. J. Adolesc. Med. Health* **2016**, *28*, 349–355. [CrossRef]
28. El-Gendawy, S.; Hadhood, M.; Shams, R.; Ibrahim, A. Epidemiological aspects of depression among Assiut University students. *Assiut Med. J.* **2005**, *2*, 81–89.
29. Aristovnik, A.; Keržič, D.; Ravšelj, D.; Tomaževič, N.; Umek, L. Impacts of the COVID-19 Pandemic on Life of Higher Education Students: A Global Perspective. *Sustainability* **2020**, *12*, 8438. [CrossRef]
30. Gloster, A.T.; Lamnisos, D.; Lubenko, J.; Presti, G.; Squatrito, V.; Constantinou, M.; Nicolaou, C.; Papacostas, S.; Aydın, G.; Chong, Y.Y.; et al. Impact of COVID-19 pandemic on mental health: An international study. *PLoS ONE* **2020**, *15*, e0244809. [CrossRef]
31. Adamson, M.M.; Phillips, A.; Seenivasan, S.; Martinez, J.; Grewal, H.; Kang, X.; Coetzee, J.; Luttenbacher, I.; Jester, A.; Harris, O.A.; et al. International Prevalence and Correlates of Psychological Stress during the Global COVID-19 Pandemic. *Int. J. Environ. Res. Public Health* **2020**, *17*, 9248. [CrossRef]
32. Kavčič, T.; Avsec, A.; Kocjan, G.Z. Psychological Functioning of Slovene Adults during the COVID-19 Pandemic: Does Resilience Matter? *Psychiatr. Q.* **2020**, *92*, 207–216. [CrossRef]
33. Lee, S. Subjective well-being and mental health during the pandemic outbreak: Exploring the role of institutional trust. *Res. Aging* **2020**, *25*, 164027520975145. [CrossRef]
34. Tušl, M.; Brauchli, R.; Kerksieck, P.; Bauer, G.F. Impact of the COVID-19 crisis on work and private life, mental well-being and self-rated health in German and Swiss employees: A cross-sectional online survey. *BMC Public Health* **2021**, *21*, 741. [CrossRef] [PubMed]
35. Almarzooq, Z.I.; Lopes, M.; Kochar, A. Virtual Learning during the COVID-19 Pandemic: A Disruptive Technology in Graduate Medical Education. *J. Am. Coll. Cardiol.* **2020**, *75*, 2635–2638. [CrossRef] [PubMed]
36. Chaturvedi, K.; Vishwakarma, D.K.; Singh, N. COVID-19 and its impact on education, social life and mental health of students: A survey. *Child. Youth Serv. Rev.* **2021**, *121*, 105866. [CrossRef] [PubMed]
37. International Labour Organization. COVID-19 and the Education Sector. Available online: https://www.ilo.org/wcmsp5/groups/public/---ed_dialogue/---sector/documents/briefingnote/wcms_742025.pdf (accessed on 11 June 2021).
38. Zhang, Y.; Zhang, H.; Ma, X.; Di, Q. Mental health problems during the COVID-19 pandemics and the mitigation effects of exercise: A longitudinal study of college students in China. *Int. J. Environ. Res. Public Health* **2020**, *17*, 3722. [CrossRef]
39. Rogowska, A.M.; Pavlova, I.; Kuśnierz, C.; Ochnik, D.; Bodnar, I.; Petrytsa, P. Does Physical Activity Matter for the Mental Health of University Students during the COVID-19 Pandemic? *J. Clin. Med.* **2020**, *9*, 3494. [CrossRef]
40. Aslan, I.; Ochnik, D.; Çınar, O. Exploring Perceived Stress among Students in Turkey during the COVID-19 Pandemic. *Int. J. Environ. Res. Public Health* **2020**, *17*, 8961. [CrossRef]
41. Juchnowicz, D.; Baj, J.; Forma, A.; Karakuła, K.; Sitarz, E.; Bogucki, J.; Karakula-Juchnowicz, H. The Outbreak of SARS-CoV-2 Pandemic and the Well-Being of Polish Students: The Risk Factors of the Emotional Distress during COVID-19 Lockdown. *J. Clin. Med.* **2021**, *10*, 944. [CrossRef]
42. Cao, W.; Fang, Z.; Hou, G.; Han, M.; Xu, X.; Dong, J.; Zheng, J. The psychological impact of the covid-19 epidemic on college students in China. *Psychiatry Res.* **2020**, *287*, 112934. [CrossRef]
43. Islam, M.S.; Ferdous, M.Z.; Potenza, M.N. Panic and generalized anxiety during the covid-19 pandemic among Bangladeshi people: An online pilot survey early in the outbreak. *J. Affect. Disord.* **2020**, *276*, 30–37. [CrossRef]
44. Son, C.; Hegde, S.; Smith, A.; Wang, X.; Sasangohar, F. Effects of COVID-19 on college students' mental health in the United States: Interview survey study. *J. Med. Internet Res.* **2020**, *22*, e21279. [CrossRef]

45. Schiff, M.; Zasiekina, L.; Pat-Horenczyk, R.; Benbenishty, R. COVID-Related Functional Difficulties and Concerns Among University Students during COVID-19 Pandemic: A Binational Perspective. *J. Community Health* **2020**. [CrossRef]
46. Kecojevic, A.; Basch, C.H.; Sullivan, M.; Davi, N.K. The impact of the COVID-19 epidemic on mental health of undergraduate students in New Jersey, cross-sectional study. *PLoS ONE* **2020**, *15*, e0239696. [CrossRef]
47. Vigo, D.; Jones, L.; Munthali, R.; Pei, J.; Westenberg, J.; Munro, L.; Judkowicz, C.; Wang, A.Y.; Adel, B.V.D.; Dulai, J.; et al. Investigating the effect of COVID-19 dissemination on symptoms of anxiety and depression among university students. *BJPsych Open* **2021**, *7*, E69. [CrossRef]
48. Cindrich, S.L.; Lansing, J.E.; Brower, C.S.; McDowell, C.P.; Herring, M.P.; Meyer, J.D. Associations Between Change in Outside Time Pre- and Post-COVID-19 Public Health Restrictions and Mental Health: Brief Research Report. *Front. Public Health* **2021**, *9*, 619129. [CrossRef]
49. Ammar, A.; Brach, M.; Trabelsi, K.; Chtourou, H.; Boukhris, O.; Masmoudi, L.; Bouaziz, B.; Bentlage, E.; How, D.; Ahmed, M.; et al. Effects of COVID-19 Home Confinement on Eating Behaviour and Physical Activity: Results of the ECLB-COVID19 International Online Survey. *Nutrients* **2020**, *12*, 1583. [CrossRef]
50. Coelho, C.M.; Suttiwan, P.; Arato, N.; Zsido, A.N. On the nature of fear and anxiety triggered by COVID-19. *Front. Psychol.* **2020**, *11*, 3109. [CrossRef]
51. Mertens, G.; Gerritsen, L.; Duijndam, S.; Salemink, E.; Engelhard, I. Fear of the coronavirus (COVID-19): Predictors in an online study conducted in march 2020. *J. Anxiety Disord.* **2020**, *74*, 102258. [CrossRef]
52. Maalouf, F.T.; Mdawar, B.; Meho, L.I.; Akl, E.A. Mental health research in response to the COVID-19, Ebola, and H1N1 outbreaks: A comparative bibliometric analysis. *J. Psychiatr. Res.* **2021**, *132*, 198–206. [CrossRef]
53. Mækelæ, M.J.; Reggev, N.; Dutra, N.; Tamayo, R.M.; Silva-Sobrinho, R.A.; Klevjer, K.; Pfuhl, G. Perceived efficacy of COVID-19 restrictions, reactions and their impact on mental health during the early phase of the outbreak in six countries. *R. Soc. Open Sci.* **2020**, *7*, 200644. [CrossRef]
54. Margraf, J.; Brailovskaia, J.; Schneider, S. Behavioral measures to fight COVID-19: An 8-country study of perceived usefulness, adherence and their predictors. *PLoS ONE* **2020**, *15*, e0243523. [CrossRef]
55. Brailovskaia, J.; Cosci, F.; Mansueto, G.; Miragall, M.; Herrero, R.; Baños, R.M.; Krasavtseva, Y.; Kochetkov, Y.; Margraf, J. The association between depression symptoms, psychological burden caused by Covid-19 and physical activity: An investigation in Germany, Italy, Russia, and Spain. *Psychiatry Res.* **2021**, *295*, 113596. [CrossRef] [PubMed]
56. Ruffolo, M.; Price, D.; Schoultz, M.; Leung, J.; Bonsaksen, T.; Thygesen, H.; Geirdal, A.Ø. Employment Uncertainty and Mental Health during the COVID-19 Pandemic Initial Social Distancing Implementation: A Cross-national Study. *Glob. Soc. Welf.* **2021**, *8*, 141–150. [CrossRef] [PubMed]
57. Wang, C.; Chudzicka-Czupała, A.; Tee, M.L.; Núñez, M.I.L.; Tripp, C.; Fardin, M.A.; Habib, H.A.; Tran, B.X.; Adamus, K.; Anlacan, J.; et al. A chain mediation model on COVID-19 symptoms and mental health outcomes in Americans, Asians and Europeans. *Sci. Rep.* **2021**, *11*, 6481. [CrossRef]
58. Yehudai, M.; Bender, S.; Gritsenko, V.; Konstantinov, V.; Reznik, A.; Isralowitz, R. COVID-19 fear, mental health, and substance misuse conditions among university social work students in Israel and Russia. *Int. J. Ment. Health Addict.* **2020**, *6*, 1–8. [CrossRef]
59. Reznik, A.; Gritsenko, V.; Konstantinov, V.; Yehudai, M.; Bender, S.; Shilina, I.; Isralowitz, R. First and Second Wave COVID-19 Fear Impact: Israeli and Russian Social Work Student Fear, Mental Health and Substance Use. *Int. J. Ment. Health Addict.* **2021**, 1–8. [CrossRef]
60. Faul, F.; Erdfelder, E.; Lang, A.G.; Buchner, A. G*Power 3: A flexible statistical power analysis program for the social, behavioral, and biomedical sciences. *Behav. Res. Methods* **2007**, *39*, 175–191. [CrossRef]
61. Leiner, D.J. SoSci Survey (Version 3.1. 06) [Computer Software]. 2019. Available online: https://www.soscisurvey.de/ (accessed on 1 April 2020).
62. Kroenke, K.; Strine, T.W.; Spitzer, R.L.; Williams, J.B.; Berry, J.T.; Mokdad, A.H. The PHQ-8 as a measure of current depression in the general population. *J. Affect. Disord.* **2009**, *114*, 163–173. [CrossRef]
63. Spitzer, R.L.; Kroenke, K.; Williams, J.B.W.; Löwe, B.A. Brief Measure for Assessing Generalized Anxiety Disorder. *Arch. Intern. Med.* **2006**, *166*, 1092–1097. [CrossRef]
64. American Psychiatric Association. *Diagnostic and Statistical Manual of Mental Disorders (DSM-5®)*; American Psychiatric Pub.: Arlington, VA, USA, 2013.
65. WHO. Be Active during COVID-19. 2020. Available online: https://www.who.int/emergencies/diseases/novel-coronavirus-2019/question-and-answers-hub/q-a-detail/be-active-during-covid-19 (accessed on 15 March 2021).
66. DeSalvo, K.B.; Fan, V.S.; McDonell, M.B.; Fihn, S.D. Predicting mortality and healthcare utilization with a single question. *Health Serv. Res.* **2005**, *40*, 1234–1246. [CrossRef]
67. DeSalvo, K.B.; Fisher, W.P.; Tran, K.; Bloser, N.; Merrill, W.; Peabody, J. Assessing measurement properties of two single-item general health measures. *Qual. Life Res.* **2006**, *15*, 191–201. [CrossRef]
68. Statistica. *DELL Statistica (Version, 13.1) [Software for Windows]*; StatSoft Polska Sp.z o.o.: Krakow, Poland, 2019.
69. JASP. Team JASP (Version 0.14.1) [Computer Software]. 2020. Available online: https://jasp-stats.org/ (accessed on 15 March 2021).
70. Van de Velde, S.; Bracke, P.; Levecque, K. Gender differences in depression in 23 European countries. Cross-national variation in the gender gap in depression. *Soc. Sci. Med.* **2010**, *71*, 305–313. [CrossRef] [PubMed]

71. Ho, R.C.M.; Mak, K.-K.; Chua, A.N.C.; Ho, C.S.H.; Mak, A. The effect of severity of depressive disorder on economic burden in a university hospital in Singapore. *Expert Rev. Pharmacoecon. Outcomes Res.* **2013**, *13*, 549–559. [CrossRef] [PubMed]
72. Human Development and the Antropocene. Human Development Report 2020. The Next Frontier. Available online: http://hdr.undp.org/sites/default/files/hdr2020.pdf (accessed on 15 March 2021).
73. Erdin, C.; Ozkaya, G. Contribution of small and medium enterprises to economic development and quality of life in Turkey. *Heliyon* **2020**, *6*, e03215. [CrossRef] [PubMed]
74. TUİK. Labor Statistics. 2020. Available online: https://data.tuik.gov.tr/ (accessed on 15 March 2021).
75. TUİK. Consumer Price Index. 2021. Available online: https://data.tuik.gov.tr/ (accessed on 15 March 2021).
76. Standard & Poor's Global Ratings. Guide to Credit Rating Essentials: What Are Credit Ratings and How Do They Work? Available online: www.spglobal.com (accessed on 15 March 2021).
77. Yan, J.H.; McCullagh, P. Cultural influence on youth's motivation of participation in physical activity. *J. Sport Behav.* **2004**, *27*, 378–390.
78. Judd, F.K.; Jackson, H.J.; Komiti, A.; Murray, G.; Hodgins, G.; Fraser, C. High prevalence disorders in urban and rural communities. *Aust. N. Z. J. Psychiatry* **2002**, *36*, 104–113. [CrossRef]
79. Kim, H.J.; Park, E.; Storr, C.L.; Tran, K.; Juon, H.S. Depression among Asian-American Adults in the Community: Systematic Review and Meta-Analysis. *PLoS ONE* **2015**, *10*, e0127760. [CrossRef]
80. Cheng, H.G.; Shidhaye, R.; Charlson, F.; Deng, F.; Lyngdoh, T.; Chen, S.; Nanda, S.; Lacroix, K.; Baxter, A.; Whiteford, H. Social correlates of mental, neurological, and substance use disorders in China and India: A review. *Lancet Psychiatry* **2016**, *3*, 882–899. [CrossRef]
81. Deng, J.; Zhou, F.; Hou, W.; Silver, Z.; Wong, C.Y.; Chang, O.; Drakos, A.; Zuo, Q.K.; Huang, E. The prevalence of depressive symptoms, anxiety symptoms and sleep disturbance in higher education students during the COVID-19 pandemic: A systematic review and meta-analysis. *Psychiatry Res.* **2021**, *301*, 113863. [CrossRef]
82. Human Development Report 2020—Table 5: Gender Inequality Index. United Nations Development Programme. Available online: http://hdr.undp.org/en/content/table-5-gender-inequality-index-gii (accessed on 15 March 2021).
83. Seedat, S.; Scott, K.M.; Angermeyer, M.C.; Berglund, P.; Bromet, E.J.; Brugha, T.S.; Demyttenaere, K.; de Girolamo, G.; Haro, J.M.; Jin, R.; et al. Cross-national associations between gender and mental disorders in the World Health Organization World Mental Health Surveys. *Arch. Gen. Psychiatry* **2009**, *66*, 785–795. [CrossRef]
84. Rosenfield, S.; Mouzon, D. Gender and Mental Health. In *Handbook of the Sociology and Mental Health*; Aneshensel, C.S., Phelan, J.C., Bierman, A., Eds.; Springer: Dordrecht, The Netherlands, 2013.
85. Kerč, P.; Krohne, N.; Šraj Lebar, T.; Štirn, M. Izsledki Raziskave za Oceno Potreb po Psihosocialni Podpori med Epidemijo Covida-19 [Results of a Study to Assess the Need for Psychosocial Support during the Covid-19 Epidemic]. Slovenian Psychologists' Association. Available online: http://www.dps.si/wp-content/uploads/2021/03/Izsledki-raziskave-za-oceno-potreb.pdf (accessed on 19 April 2021).
86. Levkovich, I. The Impact of Age on Negative Emotional Reactions, Compliance with Health Guidelines, and Knowledge About the Virus during the COVID-19 Epidemic: A Longitudinal Study from Israel. *J. Prim. Care Community Health* **2020**, *11*, 1–10. [CrossRef]
87. Rush, A.J.; Hiser, W.; Giles, D.E. A comparison of self-reported versus clinician-related symptoms in depression. *J. Clin. Psychiatry* **1987**, *48*, 246–248.
88. Enns, M.W.; Larsen, D.K.; Cox, B.J. Discrepancies between self and observer ratings of depression—The relationship to demographic, clinical and personality variables. *J. Affect. Disord.* **2000**, *60*, 33–41. [CrossRef]
89. Li, Y.; Zhao, J.; Ma, Z.; McReynolds, L.S.; Lin, D.; Chen, Z.; Wang, T.; Wang, D.; Zhang, Y.; Zhang, J.; et al. Mental Health among College Students during the COVID-19 Pandemic in China: A 2-Wave Longitudinal Survey. *J. Affect. Disord.* **2021**, *281*, 597–604. [CrossRef]
90. Debowska, A.; Horeczy, B.; Boduszek, D.; Dolinski, D. A repeated cross-sectional survey assessing university students' stress, depression, anxiety, and suicidality in the early stages of the COVID-19 pandemic in Poland. *Psychol. Med.* **2020**, 1–4. [CrossRef]
91. Rogowska, A.M.; Kuśnierz, C.; Ochnik, D.; Schütz, A.; Kafetsios, K.; Aslan, I.; Pavlova, I.; Benatov, J.; Arzenšek, A.; Jakubiak, M.; et al. *Wellbeing of Undergraduates during the COVID-19 Pandemic: International Study*; OSF: Charlottesville, VA, USA, 2020; Available online: https://osf.io/q5f4e (accessed on 15 March 2021). [CrossRef]

Journal of
Clinical Medicine

MDPI

Article

The Quality of Medical Care in the Conditions of the COVID-19 Pandemic, with Particular Emphasis on the Access to Primary Healthcare and the Effectiveness of Treatment in Poland

Magdalena Kludacz-Alessandri [1,*], Renata Walczak [2,*], Liliana Hawrysz [3,*] and Piotr Korneta [3]

[1] College of Economics and Social Sciences, Warsaw University of Technology, 09-400 Plock, Poland
[2] Faculty of Civil Engineering, Mechanics and Petrochemistry, Warsaw University of Technology, 09-400 Plock, Poland
[3] Faculty of Management, Warsaw University of Technology, 02-524 Warsaw, Poland; piotr.korneta@pw.edu.pl
* Correspondence: magdalena.kludacz@pw.edu.pl (M.K.-A.); renata.walczak@pw.edu.pl (R.W.); liliana.hawrysz@pw.edu.pl (L.H.)

Abstract: Health has a significant influence on the quality of life of a society. The COVID-19 pandemic has forced many countries to implement restrictive measures to prevent its wider spread, including, inter alia, the introduction of remote healthcare in the form of teleconsultations. Therefore, there is the question of how such a change affects the quality of treatment and the primary healthcare of patients during the COVID-19 pandemic. The article aims to examine patient satisfaction with the access to primary healthcare and the effectiveness of treatment in a condition of remote medical care caused by the COVID-19 pandemic. We also analyse the impact of access to primary healthcare on the treatment effectiveness. Patient satisfaction was measured using a questionnaire assessing the quality of primary medical care. Of the 36 items studied, seven were related to the accessibility dimension and four were related to the treatment effectiveness dimension. Our results suggest that the treatment effectiveness and the access to primary healthcare services during the COVID-19 pandemic through telemedicine are quite highly rated by patients. Hence, further implementation of telemedicine in primary healthcare should improve the quality of lives of the wide society. We have also identified the access to primary healthcare has a considerable impact on the treatment effectiveness. Therefore, we recommend increasing the contact between patients and GPs via telemedicine under lockdown conditions.

Keywords: primary healthcare; COVID-19; access to healthcare; treatment effectiveness

Citation: Kludacz-Alessandri, M.; Walczak, R.; Hawrysz, L.; Korneta, P. The Quality of Medical Care in the Conditions of the COVID-19 Pandemic, with Particular Emphasis on the Access to Primary Healthcare and the Effectiveness of Treatment in Poland. *J. Clin. Med.* **2021**, *10*, 3502. https://doi.org/10.3390/jcm10163502

Academic Editor: Michele Roccella

Received: 2 July 2021
Accepted: 4 August 2021
Published: 9 August 2021

1. Introduction

Quality of life (QOL) can be defined as an individual's perception of his or her life status in terms of the cultural systems and values of life, and concerning personal goals, expectations, standards, and concerns [1]. Quality of life became established as a significant concept and target for research and practice in the fields of health and medicine. Understanding QOL is important for improving symptom relief, care and rehabilitation of patients. QOL is also used for identifying the range of problems that can affect patients. This kind of information can be communicated to future patients to help them anticipate and understand the consequences of their illness and its treatment. QOL is also important for medical decision-making because it is a predictor of treatment success and is therefore useful in diagnostics [2]. The studies carried out so far show that medical care significantly contributes to the improvement of patients' QOL [3,4].

QOL indicators, aimed at measuring progress in a society, should reflect its multidimensionality and cover aspects contributing to life satisfaction. One of the indicated aspects is health. Health has already been defined by the World Health Organization (WHO) as "a state of complete physical, mental and social well-being, and not merely the absence of disease or infirmity" [5,6]. Poor health not only has the potential to shorten people's life expectancy, but it can also worsen their quality of life. At the collective level, it hampers economic and social development, reducing the so-called "human capital" available to a society and generating additional costs. Thus, long and healthy life is an indicator of social prosperity and success and a QOL factor. This means that the improvement of the quality of life is very often seen as a desirable result of the provision of primary healthcare (PHC) [7].

Traditionally, the quality of life in the field of health sciences is also used as an outcome variable to evaluate treatment effectiveness [8]. Health-related indicators are also used in various studies to measure the quality of life, e.g., health and access to healthcare [9], deaths from cardiovascular diseases and government spending on healthcare [7]. On the other hand, some have suggested that the impact of health and medical care on the overall quality of life is rather small [10].

Health and well-being often depend on the quality of healthcare, which is defined as the degree to which health services for individuals and the population increase the likelihood of achieving desired health outcomes and are consistent with current professional knowledge [1]. The quality of healthcare is also defined as "the degree to which health services meet the needs, expectations and standards of medical care for patients, their families and other care recipients" [11]. These aspects are very often examined in patient satisfaction surveys [12–14]. Several terms are functioning interchangeably in the literature regarding healthcare quality, including health status, quality of life, quality of care and health-related quality of life (HRQoL) [5,15]. Most of the QOL research in medicine and healthcare is related to health, and HRQOL is becoming increasingly important in healthcare and clinical research [16].

The WHO suggests that quality of life covers several key areas known as "domains". In the domain defined as "environment", there is an area related to Health and social care, including the accessibility and quality dimension related to, inter alia, with effectiveness [17]. Overall, the goal of quality in healthcare is the continual improvement of the patient's condition. To decipher whether best practice on healthcare quality has been achieved, the concepts of access and effectiveness are systematically discussed in every healthcare environment [18,19]. For instance the studies that analyzed the impact of quality of care on patients' QoL have measured health and well-being in terms of access to health care, effective treatment and social care [20].

Health-related quality of life maximisation and to the pursuit to provide high-quality medical services are among the most important goals in the work of a family doctor and challenges for primary care organisations, especially in the context of limited treatment options during the COVID pandemic, where telemedicine is often the only possible form of patient care. The need to improve the quality of medical services also results from the legal and ethical obligations of the GP [1].

The scope of this study was deliberately narrowed to the primary healthcare. This was done due to the primary healthcare's fundamental role in many healthcare systems around the world [21] and in the Polish healthcare system [22]. It was already postulated that countries with developed primary healthcare enjoy fewer hospital admissions, better outcomes of patient treatments and, consequently, lower overall healthcare expenditure [23]. As a result, many scholars claim that the main objective of any governmental health policy should be the improvement of the primary healthcare quality [24]. The role of the primary healthcare is especially critical for the Polish healthcare system, mainly because of the following: ageing Polish society, substantial shortages in medical personnel (doctors and nurses) and lower expenditure compared to other EU countries on average.

Studies on the quality of primary healthcare during the COVID-19 pandemic in Poland are limited. On the other hand, researchers were dealing with this issue in the field of selected specialist services. This particularly included studies on access to medical care during pregnancy [25], bariatric care [26], cancer patients care [27], medical and non-medical services for the elderly [28]. Researchers agree that the COVID-19 pandemic situation leads to a growing problem of limited or complete lack of access to treatment for specific groups of patients who are in need of special care [29–31]. The perception of medical services during the COVID-19 pandemic was also studied in the context of cancer care [27]. However, no studies on patient satisfaction on the access to primary healthcare and treatment effectiveness in Poland could be found.

The core value of primary healthcare is that a well-organised and effective system of PHC is able to respond to the vast majority (even as much as 80%) of health needs with relatively small funds. Appreciation of the role of primary healthcare was the aftermath of analyses determining the impact of individual factors on healthy societies [32]. Barbara Starfield [33] has proven beyond any doubt that the quality of the entire healthcare system depends much more on the level of primary healthcare development than on the overall expenditure for the healthcare system.

Quality in primary healthcare is defined as the combination of access to healthcare, treatment effectiveness, while the improvement of the population's health and the access to medical care are considered as two important objectives related to the core activities of health systems [34,35]. QOL assessments related to primary healthcare access and effectiveness can benefit patients, clinicians, researchers, administrators, health organizations, and policymakers. As the effects of the COVID-19 pandemic are likely to persist, research into the accessibility and effectiveness of primary healthcare is becoming extremely important, particularly in the context of telemedicine and QOL [36]. To check if best practice on primary healthcare quality has been achieved, the concepts of access and effectiveness should be systematically discussed in every primary healthcare entity [18,19].

Access is critical to the functioning of primary healthcare systems around the world. However, access to primary healthcare remains a complex concept as exemplified by the concept's interpretations diversity by authors. In primary healthcare, access is often defined as access of a service, provider or institution, and is thus defined as the possibility or ease with which patients can use adequate medical services relative to their needs [37]. Some researchers tend to equate access to a delivery system (for example, distribution and volume regarding the medical workforce and medical facilities, availability of providers and health facilities). Others argue that access can best be assessed using performance indicators for a patient's passage through the system, such as utilisation rates or satisfaction scores [24,38,39].

In terms of remote medical appointments, access (accessibility) is considered as the patient's ability to receive primary healthcare [40]. Accessibility is also defined as a way of organising primary care resources to accommodate a wide range of patient opportunities to contact physicians and access to primary healthcare services. This includes the doctors' working hours, consultation times, telephone services and a flexible system enabling having an appointment for medical consultation [41].

Effectiveness was recognised as an important dimension of primary healthcare quality, but the literature emphasises the difficulty of characterising the definition of effectiveness for the primary healthcare sector. For example, in a 2004 study using the Delphi method to establish operational definitions for different dimensions of primary healthcare quality, despite repeated efforts, it was impossible to find a concise operational definition of effectiveness to which all experts could agree [41].

In real life, the concept of effectiveness is used interchangeably with the terms efficacy and efficiency, which is not correct from a scientific point of view. These three concepts have been originally distinguished by Drucker in management sciences [42] in which they bear the following meanings:

- efficacy—the ability to produce the desired amount of the desired effect, i.e., success in achieving a specific goal;
- effectiveness—the degree to which the planned results, objectives or tasks are achieved as a result of an action, intervention or initiative aimed at achieving the desired effect, in ordinary, uncontrolled circumstances;

- efficiency—doing things in the most economical way. It is the ratio of performance to the inputs of any system [43].

In the healthcare sector, efficacy is defined as the possibility of a beneficial change (or the therapeutic effect) as result of an intervention (e.g., drug, medical treatment, surgery, or public health intervention) under ideal or controlled conditions. Effectiveness is the ability of a [44] medical intervention (e.g., teleconsultation) to have a significant effect on patients under normal clinical conditions. In turn, efficiency must also clearly identify the inputs that are used to obtain the effect of interest (for example, hours of medical care, days when drugs are supplied or medical expenses) [45] Some authors define efficiency as achieving the desired results with the most profitable use of resources [41]. According to Głodziński, efficiency is the achievement of the highest level of satisfaction possible with the given inputs and technologies [46].

The dimensions of medical service effectiveness and efficacy were announced as quality dimensions in the PHC by the WHO Eastern Mediterranean Regional Office (EMRO) [47]. In turn, the efficiency and effectiveness dimensions were proposed by the US Agency for Healthcare Research and Quality (AHRQ) [48]. Effectiveness and efficiency were also used in the tools for quality assessment in Iran's PHC systems [44].

However, effectiveness is the most popular dimension among the tools for assessing the quality of primary healthcare. For instance, in the Iranian primary healthcare quality assessment framework, (QAF) out of 40 Quality Indicators (QIs), 33.5% were related to the effectiveness dimension. This dimension had the highest share among the quality dimensions [44]. The effectiveness dimension was also in common with the QAF of such countries as Australia, Canada and the United States in terms of the classification of dimensions and QIs [49,50].

Effectiveness plays an essential role in the tools for quality assessments designed for patient opinion surveys. The effectiveness of primary healthcare in regards to obtaining achievable health benefits based on an objective or subjective assessment stating that primary healthcare helped to improve the patient's health or well-being [51]. Effectiveness in primary healthcare facilities is a set of coordinated actions taken at various levels of reference, improving the patients' health through prevention and the provision of primary healthcare [52].

Testa and Simonson argue that any area of health can be measured objectively and subjectively [53]. There are therefore two main trends in the literature regarding the measurement of HRQoL. The first one concerns the measurement based on objective indicators, and the second one is based on subjective indicators. While the objective dimension is used to determine the patient's health status, the patient's subjective assessment is used to translate this condition into the patient's actual HRQoL. Hence, two patients with identical health status may have very different HRQoL depending on their subjective experiences, expectations and perceptions of health [5].

Today, most HRQoL tools are based on patient assessments and have a wide range of applications. A key distinguishing feature of HRQoL is the consideration of the patient's values, judgments and preferences [15,54]. Therefore, literature suggests the construction of social indicators to assess the quality of primary healthcare in a subjective manner [55].

A literature review clearly demonstrated that primary healthcare accessibility and treatment effectiveness are multidimensional constructs. They were taken into consideration in terms of many variables and indicators used to measure them.

In many studies, accessibility has been measured using quantitative indicators that can be objective measures of the availability of primary healthcare. Such objective indicators selected to measure the availability of primary healthcare concern, for instance, the waiting time for an appointment with a specific family doctor, with any family doctor, and for the initiation of consultations [34], the share of people who had or didn't have contact with the provider at a certain time, or the total number of services provided after contact. Such objective indicators also include the travel time, waiting time in the waiting room, the actual patient consultation time at the medical facility and the weighted sum of the difference between the ideal and the actual number of services, personnel and equipment in the community. In the scale of the entire primary healthcare system, patients' access to the system can also be measured by the number and availability of primary care physicians (the number of medical personnel, medical facilities per unit of population and per unit of geographic area) [56,57].

As already mentioned, literature suggests the construction of social indicators to assess the quality of medical care in a subjective manner [55]. Subjective accessibility indicators concern the patients' assessments of various aspects of their experience of being provided with care. Due to the fact that patients play a unique and important role as evaluators of quality of care, it can be concluded that the patients' opinions should also be taken into account by primary healthcare managers.

Therefore, our tested model provides an accessibility measurement that covers only more subjective indicators related to patients' opinions regarding access to a primary teleconsultation with a General Practitioner (GP), possibility of contacting a primary healthcare facility via telephone/Internet, possibility of obtaining help in emergency situations, convenient opening hours, punctuality of consultations. Such variable were also used in other studies [34,58,59]. This study did not take into account the accessibility dimensions adapted in terms of residential care, such as the location of the healthcare facility and the person's ability to access the facility [60], the ease and convenience of reaching a doctor, the availability of services at the place needed [56]. This study also ignores the more detailed accessibility dimensions adopted by Levesque et al. [61], which do not apply to the Polish conditions and the accessibility definition adopted for the purpose of the study. According to these authors, access to healthcare is affected by individual and environmental factors of the healthcare supply-side factors (e.g., approachability; accommodation; affordability) as well as demand-side factors (ability to perceive; ability to seek; ability to reach; ability to pay ability to engage).

The effectiveness is measured most often with indicators based on an objective or subjective assessment of whether primary healthcare has helped to improve the patient's health or well-being [51]. The most common measures of effectiveness are related to the quality of life, changes in health status, measures of health or well-being, the results reported by the patient, and the patient's knowledge [51]. Some authors recommend measuring effectiveness based on the skills and competencies of the medical personnel (physician's ability to make a proper diagnosis and treatment) [62].

The assessment of the treatment effectiveness of can be considered in three dimensions: (1) the health dimension assessed by the mortality and morbidity rates, (2) the satisfaction dimension, defined as the level of meeting the patient's expectations regarding primary healthcare, (3) the economic dimension regarding the cost of the services provided [63].

The paper is focused on the satisfaction dimension and examines the effectiveness of treatment as measured by patient satisfaction with improving health, solving a health problem and met expectations towards the treatment plan applied. It was assumed in the study that an effective GP helps to solve a health problem and improves the patient's health condition, and the treatment plan proposed by him or her meets the patient's expectations and does not require additional appointments with other specialists [62,64].

The study aims to describe patient satisfaction with the access to primary healthcare and treatment effectiveness in the conditions of remote medical care caused by the COVID-19 pandemic. The study is dealing with the subjective assessment of patient satisfaction in two dimensions: access to primary healthcare and treatment effectiveness. 98 patients of primary healthcare facilities participated in the survey. The other part of this paper is structured as follows. Section 2 includes the specification of the applied research methods. The Exploratory Factor Analysis (EFA) and Confirmatory Factor Analysis (CFA) are used to define the remote healthcare quality factors. Section 3 provides the results obtained in the study on patient satisfaction from access to primary healthcare and treatment effectiveness during the COVID-19 pandemic in Poland. It also includes comments on the impact of access to teleconsultations on the treatment effectiveness. Section 4 includes a discussion about the limitations of this study. Finally, the paper also provides conclusions and practical implications.

2. Materials and Methods

2.1. Methodology

The research methods used in this study included a subject literature analysis and an analysis of the results of own research carried out in Polish healthcare facilities in 2021. The analysis featured the use of descriptive statistics, the Exploratory Factor Analysis (EFA) and the Confirmatory Factor Analysis (CFA) for the development of the relationship between accessibility and effectiveness of telephone consultations. The extracted factors were used to perform a regression analysis to check the impact of accessibility to telehealth consultations on the treatment effectiveness.

According to Hair et al., the number of observations should be ten times higher than the number of variables in the factor analysis model. The minimum acceptable ratio of observations to variables is 5:1. Some researchers accept the ratio of 3:1. The absolute minimum number of observations in the factor model is 50 [65]. In this study, the number of observations is 98. Due to the fact that the 3:1 ratio requirement was met, an EFA analysis was conducted to indicate the variables loading onto two expected latent factors and indicate the initial structure of the factor model. The objective of the analysis was to prepare a questionnaire for a full-scale survey. After the initial EFA analysis, only eight variables were left since the 5:1 sample per item ratio has been satisfied. In addition, a regression analysis was used to evaluate the impact of accessibility on effectiveness.

2.1.1. Population and Data Collection

The study featured a survey conducted on the patients of the CortenMedic primary healthcare facilities. This preliminary study was aimed at preparing and checking the remote healthcare quality research tool—the structured questionnaire. It was important to explore the data structure and prepare a questionnaire for population studies [66]. The response rate meets all survey standards of at least 60% [67]. The questionnaire was assessed in terms of question comprehensibility and difficulty, clarity and ambiguity, length, completion time, and data collection manner [68].

The research was carried out in four primary healthcare facilities in Poland considering the limitations introduced during the pandemic. One of the facilities is located in Radom, a large district city in Poland. The remaining three (Warsaw 1, Warsaw 2, Warsaw 3) are located in Warsaw, the capital city of Poland. The total number of basic care patients registered in these facilities amounts to 46,700.

The data was collected during two sessions: on 25 February 2021–26 February 2021 and 11 March 2021–12 March 2021 through an anonymous survey with closed-ended questions. The randomly selected adult patients, who used telephone consultations during the pandemic, were surveyed using the computer-assisted telephone interviewing (CATI) method; an interviewer presented survey questions to the patients and collected their answers. All patients who agreed to take part in the survey were included in the study. Completed questionnaires were returned to the researchers who conducted the survey. One hundred five patients participated in the study, six patients declined and did not complete the questionnaire. One record was deleted due to more than 20% of missing data. Ninety-eight complete records were included in the study, representing a response rate of 93%. The survey structure presenting the place and date of data collection is shown in Table 1.

Table 1. Structure of the survey responses.

		Date and Type of the Survey		Total
		February 2021 CATI	March 2021 Paper-Based Survey	
		Number of Responses		
Facility	Warsaw 1	0	21	21
	Warsaw 2	19	0	19
	Warsaw 3	22	19	41
	Radom	24	0	24
Total		65	40	105

2.1.2. Patient Satisfaction Questionnaire

A research tool for patients' satisfaction survey was developed based on the previous research [69–73]. The survey instrument focused on relationships between variables consisting of two parts: biographical and methodological. The first part contained information about age, gender, marital status, education, place of residence, current occupation and professional activity, including the place and facility in which the survey was conducted. The methodological part consisted of 47 close-end questions pre-assigned to 7 categories. Each question was rated on the five-point Likert scale. The grade of each question scale was described verbally and numerically as follows: 1—I strongly disagree, 2—I disagree, 3—I am undecided, 4—I agree, 5—I strongly agree. The study only presents the accessibility and treatment effectiveness dimensions.

Accessibility variables were established based on the Haggerty et al. paper. The Authors define accessibility as the ease with which patients can obtain the needed care, support and advice from a selected (variable D2) or any (variable D3) primary care physician at a time (variables D4, D5) appropriate for the urgency of the problem (variable D1) [41].

Effectiveness is considered as a subjective assessment of whether primary care physician contributed to improving the patient's health. Variables E1 to E4 were selected based on the subject literature [35,52,74–77]. E1 is responsible for the well-being, E2 describes the doctor's ability to make an appropriate diagnosis, E4 states that this diagnosis could be made without additional consultations with specialists, E3 takes into account the patients' expectations (E4). The questions regarding both accessibility and treatment effectiveness are shown in Table 2.

Table 2. Questions concerning the accessibility and treatment effectiveness dimensions initially included in the questionnaire.

Variable Name		Question
Accessibility	D1	I can get medical help when I need it, even in case of emergency
	D2	I can easily make a telehealth consultation with a General Practitioner (GP) of my choice
	D3	I can easily make an appointment with a GP at the healthcare facility
	D4	The healthcare facility's working hours are convenient
	D5	Telehealth consultations take place at an agreed time
	D6	I can easily contact the healthcare facility via phone / Internet
	D7	I can easily ask questions after the telehealth consultation
Effectiveness	E1	The treatment helped me improve my health
	E2	The health problem with which I turned to the GP was solved
	E3	The treatment plan proposed by the GP meets my expectations
	E4	The health problem with which I turned to the doctor did not require additional medical consultations with other specialists

2.1.3. Ethics

The survey instrument was constructed based on the literature review. Literature-driven questions were slightly changed for this study. All questions were confirmed by the research team and by two experts from CortenMedic—a healthcare service provider. Detailed information on the purpose of the research and its course was prepared for respondents. During the first stage of the survey, an interviewer read the study rules out to the respondents. The survey was voluntary and completely anonymous. Only adult respondents took part in the survey. Each patient could withdraw from the study at any time or choose not answer all the questions. The completion of a single questionnaire required 20 min on average. The interviewer read all the questions and answers and marked the patients' responses in the database form one by one. The questionnaire form was anonymous. Patients completed the questionnaire voluntarily. The questionnaire was assessed from an ethical perspective by the Warsaw University of Technology Senate Committee for Professional Ethics.

3. Results

3.1. Data Analysis

The analysis was conducted using the SPSS v. 27 statistical package (Predictive Solution, Krakow, Poland) and Microsoft Excel 365 (Microsoft, Redmond, WA, USA). Prior to the questionnaires' statistical analysis, a database of responses was created. Data from the paper-based questionnaires were transferred to a spreadsheet. In the survey, the questions were not deliberately divided into dimensions. The next step was to sort the statements according to the dimensions: accessibility, coordination, comprehensiveness, effectiveness, continuity, communication and experience with the system; the analysis for the purpose of this study covered only two dimensions: accessibility and effectiveness.

The respondents were divided into six age groups (Figure 1): aged up to 25 (5 people, i.e., 5.1%), 25 to 34 years of age (12 people, i.e., 12.1%), 35 to 44 years of age (13 people, i.e., 13.1%), 45 to 54 years of age (14 people, i.e., 14.1%), 55 to 64 years of age (15 people, i.e., 15.2%) and aged above 65 (39 people, i.e., 39.4%). One person did not disclose his or her age (i.e., 1%). Eventually, this record was deleted due to many missing data.

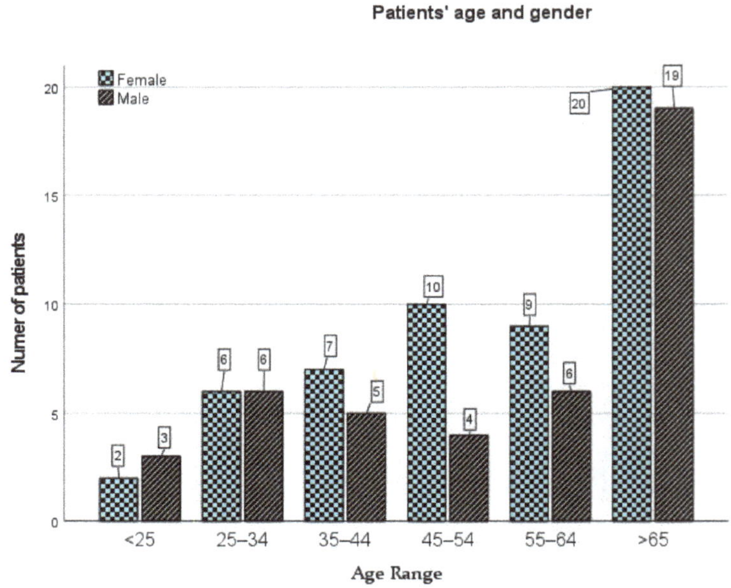

Figure 1. Patients' age structure by gender.

The most numerous group included married people (38 people; 38.4%); single persons constituted 28.3% of the respondents (28 persons). There were 20 (20.2%) widowed people and 13 (13.1%) were divorced. In addition, more than half of the respondents were people living in a very large city (with over 250,000 inhabitants)—72 people, i.e., 72.7%, residents of large cities (from 100,000 to 250,000 inhabitants) constituted 19.2% (19 people), medium-sized cities (from 20,000 to 100,000 inhabitants), 3.03% (three persons), rural areas—3.03% (three persons) and small towns (less than 20,000 inhabitants)—2.02% (two persons).

The biggest group included people with higher education—51 people (51.5%), then people with secondary education—26 people (26.3%), the minor groups included people with vocational education—15 people (15.2%) and primary or lower secondary school education—seven people (7.1%). Working people accounted for 44.4% of the population (44 people), retirees and pensioners, also 44.4% (44 people), five people were unemployed (5.1%), also three students were surveyed (3%). Two patients ran their own business (2%), while one person indicated a different economic activity (1%).

Patients who went to a given facility for the first visit (12 people) most often declared that their health condition required occasional visits (seven people); three people felt the need for rare visits, and two people—frequent visits. Control and periodic visits due to treatment continuation or chronic treatment took place once a quarter (10 people), once a month (nine people) or once a year (eight people). At the same time, remote consultations were used several times a month by three persons. The need to consult a GP for prevention and health promotion purposes (including vaccination) was revealed rarely (eight people), sporadically (five people) and often (three people). Twenty three patients asked for a prescription, referral to a specialist doctor or sick leave. The remaining patients met a doctor once a year (seven people), several times a month (six people) and once a month (four people). The surveyed patients most frequently visited the doctor once a quarter (45 people) and once a year (27 people), while the least numerous—once a month (18 people) and several times a month (nine people). During the COVID-19 pandemic, patients do not want to consult doctors unless they have urgent reasons [24].

Ninety four people consulted a doctor via telephone. Most patients were waiting for telephone consultation for more than 48 h (43 people); 28 people consulted a doctor the next day and 23 people—on the same day (including quick visits—11 people and waiting time exceeding 4 h—12 people). Two people used video calls via WhatsApp and Skype, their waiting time for consultation exceeded two days. Two people used Microsoft Teams and Zoom. The waiting time for a telephone consultation exceeding two days resulted in a poor evaluation of the healthcare facility.

3.1.1. Accessibility

The D1–D7 variables presented in Table 2 were used in the assessment of accessibility. The descriptive statistics of these dimension variables are shown in Table 3.

Table 3. Descriptive statistics of Accessibility variables.

Variable	Mean				Skewness		Kurtosis	
	Statistic	Std. Error	Std. Deviation	Variance	Statistic	Std. Error	Statistic	Std. Error
D1	3.8571	0.12049	1.19276	1.423	−0.983	0.244	0.202	0.483
D2	3.5816	0.13601	1.34642	1.813	−0.565	0.244	−0.966	0.483
D3	4.0306	0.11554	1.14382	1.308	−0.989	0.244	−0.023	0.483
D4	4.6735	0.08676	0.85886	0.738	−3.098	0.244	9.634	0.483
D5	4.3878	0.09359	0.92650	0.858	−1.807	0.244	3.223	0.483
D6	3.1122	0.17032	1.68610	2.843	−0.127	0.244	−1.703	0.483
D7	3.8469	0.11992	1.18715	1.409	−0.603	0.244	−0.505	0.483

Patients are most satisfied with the HC facility's working hours (D4: $\overline{x}$ = 4.68). 91.9% of the respondents claim that the facility's working hours (from 8:00 to 20:00) are convenient for them. 87.9% of patients are also satisfied with the punctuality of the visits (D5: $\overline{x}$ = 4.38). Unfortunately, 27.3% of respondents have a problem with making an appointment with a GP of their choice (D2: $\overline{x}$ = 3.57) and 13.1%—with booking an appointment with any GP (D3: $\overline{x}$ = 4.03). As many as 42.4% of patients reported that they had a problem with contacting the HC facility via telephone or Internet (D6: $\overline{x}$ = 3.12). 54.5% of the respondents believe that they can easily ask questions after the visit (D7: $\overline{x}$ = 3.85). 35.4% of respondents did not know how to answer question D7 because they have never used this form of contact after the consultation. If they had doubts or wanted to ask the GP additional questions, they made another appointment. 69.7% of the respondents stated that they could obtain medical aid whenever needed, even in an emergency (D1: $\overline{x}$ = 3.86). The distribution of answers is presented in Figure 2.

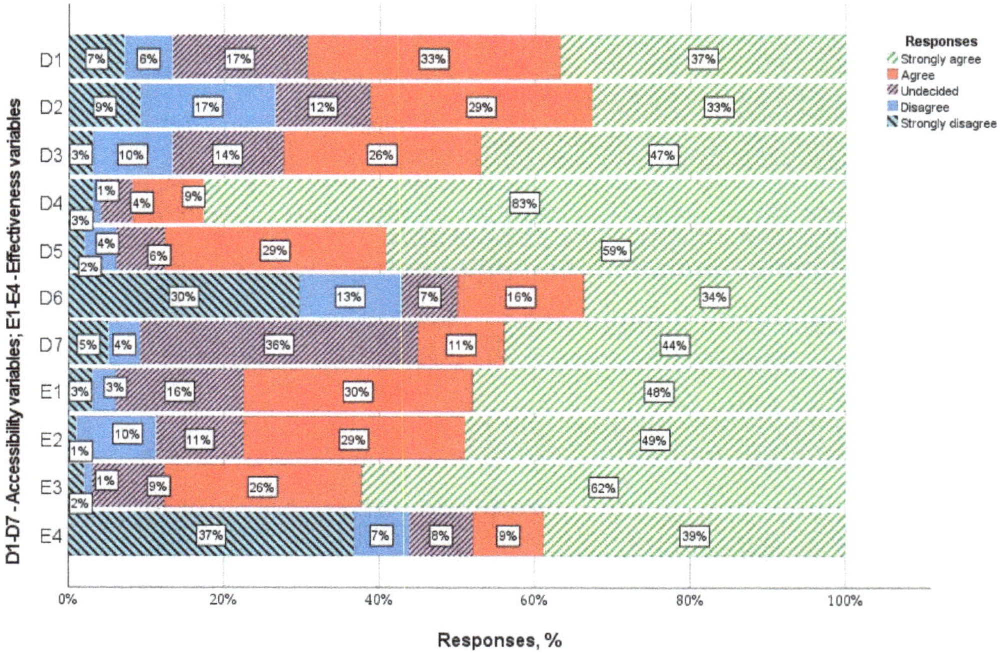

Figure 2. Distribution of accessibility and effectiveness responses.

3.1.2. Effectiveness

The E1–E4 variables presented in Table 2 were used in the assessment of effectiveness. The descriptive statistics of these dimension variables are shown in Table 4.

Table 4. Descriptive statistics of effectiveness variables.

Variable	Mean				Skewness		Kurtosis	
	Statistic	Std. Error	Std. Deviation	Variance	Statistic	Std. Error	Statistic	Std. Error
E1	4.1633	0.10225	1.01223	1.025	−1.249	0.244	1.276	0.483
E2	4.1429	0.10560	1.04536	1.093	−1.066	0.244	0.148	0.483
E3	4.4490	0.08718	0.86301	0.745	−1.902	0.244	4.127	0.483
E4	3.0612	0.18106	1.79240	3.213	−0.072	0.244	−1.817	0.483

The overall positive assessment of medical teleconsultations resulted from its high effectiveness. The applied treatment helped (29.3%) and definitely helped (47.47%) improve the respondents' health. The health problem addressed by 29.3% of patients was partially solved and solved for 48.5% of the respondents. The mean assessment of these variables was similar: (E1: $\bar{x} = 4.15$) and (E2: $\bar{x} = 4.14$). The treatment plan proposed by the doctor met the expectations of 26.3% of the patients and complied with the wishes of 61.6% of the respondents. The indications of primary care physicians largely took into account the expectations of patients—this was the best-assessed variable examining the effectiveness of remote consultations (E3: $\bar{x} = 4.44$). In the patients' opinion, their health problem did not require (9.1%) and definitely did not require (38.4%) additional medical consultations with other specialists. However, many patients believed otherwise—7.01% disagreed and 37.4% strongly disagreed with this statement. Hence, the health problems reported by half of the patients could be resolved during teleconsultation with a general practitioner (E4: $\bar{x} = 3.04$). Question E4 was assessed as average by all patients. The distribution of answers is presented in Figure 2.

3.2. *Factor Analysis*

3.2.1. Exploratory Factor Analysis

Exploratory factor analysis was conducted based on 98 observations for two dimensions: accessibility and effectiveness. Variables D4 and D5 did not meet the normality assumption. They were therefore removed from the EFA model. Variable D1 did not load correctly on the expected factors—accessibility. Eventually, eight variables: D2, D3, D6, D7, E1, E2, E3, and E4 were left. The principal component analysis (PCA) and promax rotation with Kaiser normalisation were used to extract two components (Table 5). The Kaiser-Meyer-Olkin measure of sampling adequacy (KMO) equalled 0.73 > 0.6. The KMO value considered as correct is 0.6. Bartlett's test of sphericity provided a significant result ($\chi^2 = 201.125$; df = 28, $p < 0.0001$). The probability p should be smaller than 0.05, thereby indicating that the values are correct and the sample size is sufficient for the factor analysis.

Table 5. Pattern matrix for the EFA model.

Variable	Component	
	Accessibility	Effectiveness
D3	0.804	
D6	0.795	
D2	0.777	
D7	0.686	
E2		0.837
E1		0.795
E3		0.645
E4		0.638

Extraction Method: Principal Component Analysis. Rotation Method: Promax with Kaiser Normalization, a. Rotation converged in 3 iterations.

PCA retained two factors with eigenvalues greater than 1. The total variance explained by the EFA model was equal to 56% (Table 6), which should be greater than 50% [78]. For eight variables, the factor loadings ranged from 0.638 to 0.837 and are greater than the recommended 0.35 cut-off point [79]. A reliability analysis showed that the extracted model was acceptable since the Cronbach's alpha coefficients for accessibility (0.666) and effectiveness (0.663) were greater than 0.6 [80]. Those values (Table 6) allowed for further factor analysis [65,81].

Table 6. Eigenvalues and total variance explained by the EFA model.

Component	Initial Eigenvalues			Extraction Sums of Squared Loadings			Rotation Sums of Squared Loadings
	Total	% of Variance	Cumulative %	Total	% of Variance	Cumulative %	Total
1	3.185	39.809	39.809	3.185	39.809	39.809	2.711
2	1.374	17.178	56.987	1.374	17.178	56.987	2.551
3	0.841	10.512	67.499				
4	0.725	9.069	76.568				
5	0.564	7.055	83.623				
6	0.527	6.594	90.216				
7	0.474	5.921	96.137				
8	0.309	3.863	100.000				

Extraction Method: Principal Component Analysis.

3.2.2. Confirmatory Factor Analysis

The CFA confirmed the EFA model with eight variables. Standardised and non-standardised solutions are presented respectively in Figures 3 and 4. A convergent validity—the strength of relationships of the model's factor variables is not supported by the average variance extracted (AVE), which has to be greater than 0.5. The AVE for accessibility equals 0.461 and AVE for effectiveness equals 0,401. This confirmed the low values of the Cronbach's alpha coefficients calculated during the EFA. Nevertheless, the convergent validity might be confirmed using the composite reliability (CR) index, which should be higher than 0.7. CR values for accessibility and effectiveness equal 0.771 and 0.722, respectively, which means that the convergent validity of the model is confirmed.

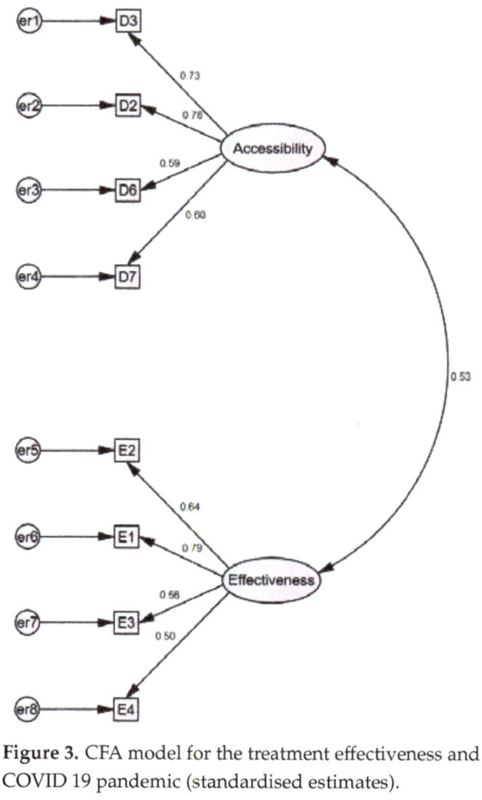

Figure 3. CFA model for the treatment effectiveness and the access to healthcare services during the COVID 19 pandemic (standardised estimates).

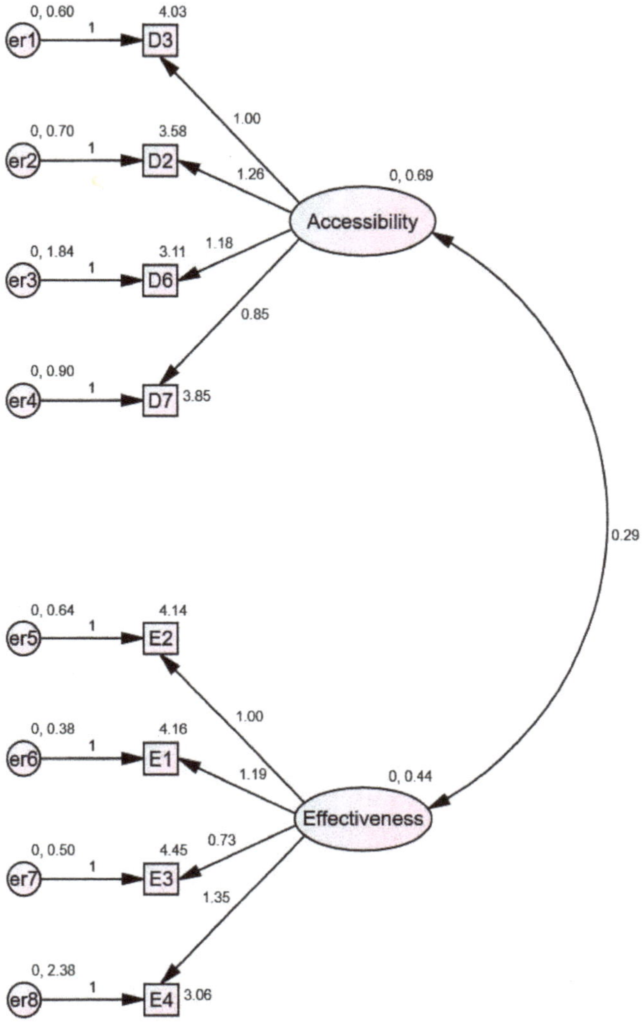

Figure 4. CFA model for the treatment effectiveness and the healthcare services accessibility during the COVID 19 pandemic (non-standardised estimates).

The model's discriminant validity is also confirmed using the Fornell Larker criterion, since the square root of the AVE for each factor is higher than the correlation between factors (Table 7). Also, the hetero trait – mono trait method points to a correlation between factors of 0.539, which should be smaller than 0.85. Taking into account the above results, it is possible to confirm the model's reliability and validity.

Table 7. Correlations between accessibility and effectiveness.

Correlations				
		D_Accessibility	E_Effectiveness	AVE
D_Accessibility	Pearson Correlation	1	0.390 **	0.461
	Sig. (2-tailed)		0.000	
	N	98	98	
E_Effectiveness	Pearson Correlation	0.390 **	1	0.401
	Sig. (2-tailed)	0.000		
	N	98	98	

**. Correlation is significant at the 0.01 level (2-tailed).

The model fit measures indicate that the model is correct. CMIN = 20.918; DF = 19.000. CMIN/DF = 1.101 (>1; <3), CFI = 0.989 (>0.95); SRMR = 0.054 (<0.08); RMSEA = 0.032 (<0.06); p-value = 0.605 (>0.05).

3.2.3. Regression Analysis

Aside from the CFA model, a regression analysis was also conducted. Two variables for effectiveness and accessibility were calculated based on the CFA model. Two hypotheses were formulated: null hypothesis H_0 stating that there is no statistical relationship between effectiveness and accessibility variables and H_1 hypothesis assuming that accessibility affects effectiveness.

Hypothesis H_0. *Accessibility does not affect effectiveness (null hypothesis).*

Hypothesis H_1. *Accessibility affects effectiveness (alternative hypothesis).*

The correlation analysis pointed to a relationship between the two variables. The Pearson Correlation equals 0.39 and is significant (Table 7), thereby allowing for regression analysis.

The ANOVA analysis showed that F coefficient equals is significant, $F (1; 96) = 17.23$; $p < 0.001$ (Table 8). The regression model points to the explanation of 14.3% of the variance, i.e., adjusted R-square equals 0.143 (Table 9). In the regression equation (Equation (1)), the constant is insignificant since the relationship between the variables can be described as follows:

$$\text{Accessibility } (\pm 0.93) = 0.39 \times \text{Effectiveness } (\pm 0.094) \quad (1)$$

Table 8. Correlation between accessibility and effectiveness.

ANOVA [a]						
Model		Sum of Squares	df	Mean Square	F	Sig.
1	Regression	14.762	1	14.762	17.233	0.000 [b]
	Residual	82.238	96	0.857		
	Total	97.000	97			

[a] Dependent Variable: E_Effectiveness. [b] Predictors: (Constant), D_Accessibility.

Table 9. Regression model summary.

Model Summary [b]				
Model	R	R Square	Adjusted R Square	Std. Error of the Estimate
1	0.390 [a]	0.152	0.143	0.92554997

[a] Predictors: (Constant), D. [b] Dependent Variable: E.

Based on the above regression analysis H_0 hypothesis was rejected in favor of the alternative hypothesis H_1.

4. Discussion

The quality of care in primary healthcare is a very important element of QOL and represents a combination of many dimensions, including access to healthcare and treatment effectiveness. Papers examining the full spectrum of dimensions of the quality of primary healthcare constitute important diagnostic tools in a health policy. As already mentioned, a well-organised and effective primary healthcare is able to respond to 80% of health needs, that is why it is so significant to medical care.

The first aim of the study was to identify variables for measuring access to primary healthcare and treatment effectiveness in primary healthcare units. The conducted literature analysis was aimed at suggesting appropriate initial sets of indicators for the assessment of access to primary healthcare and treatment effectiveness in remote conditions. The conducted statistical analyses were aimed at reducing and improving the critical empirical indicators used to measure the analysed constructs. Using various data reduction methodologies, the paper's objective was to identify a basic set of variables that could effectively measure the dimensions of remote primary healthcare accessibility and treatment effectiveness. The objective was achieved in the study. Referring to previous studies, seven variables were originally selected to measure the access do teleconsultations [34,41,58,59] and four variables to measure the treatment effectiveness [35,52,74–77]. As a result of a factor analysis, the number of variables to measure the access was reduced to four. The Exploratory Factor Analysis showed that the final model adopted for further research was correct.

The second aim was to study patients' satisfaction with these two dimensions of quality of primary healthcare and to analyse the impact of access to primary healthcare on the treatment effectiveness during the COVID-19 pandemic in Poland.

Most of the patients in this study positively assessed the access to primary healthcare and treatment effectiveness in the conditions of teleconsultation in primary healthcare facilities during the COVID-19 pandemic in Poland. This was the case even though telemedicine was never used in the Polish primary healthcare institutions before. 55.5% of the respondents believe that the medical care they received during teleconsultation was as good as meeting their GP face to face [82] The previous studies confirmed that, for some patients, telehealth can be as good as or even better than personal care, especially for those faced with problems concerning physical appointments, e.g., people living in rural areas [83].

According to the results, patients are rather satisfied with the access to remote primary healthcare. The vast majority of patients agree or strongly agree with all positive aspects of the care accessibility dimension. They are the least satisfied with the possibility of contacting the clinic via telephone/Internet (D6: $\overline{x} = 3.12$) and the possibility of making an appointment with the GP of their choice (D2: $\overline{x} = 3.57$). On the other hand, the clinic's working hours are rated the highest (D4: $\overline{x} = 4.68$). Majority of respondents stated that they could obtain medical help whenever needed, even in an emergency (D1: $\overline{x} = 3.86$). Quick access to GP appointments was assessed more positively in previous studies in which quick emergency care accessibility was rated the highest [84,85].

Systematic studies have shown that telemedicine has already been successfully used in other countries to provide routine and specialist medical services and has led to greater access to medical care. Moreover, telemedicine has shown similar, and in selected circumstances better, health effects compared to the conventional models of care [83,86], while demonstrating the ability to reduce unnecessary hospitalisations and costs [87].

In general, an analysis of other studies shows that telemedicine is actually pursuing its primary goal of improving access to care and it does so through innovative and constantly evolving tools. For instance, in Great Britain and Denmark, in order to ensure access to primary healthcare, teleconsultations take place in most primary care facilities as a standard procedure [88–90]. It is treated as "a strategic alternative to decentralisation and improving access to medical care, allowing to reduce costs and travel time for patients" [88].

Looking at the benefits, teleconsultations can reduce the patients' indirect costs in terms of time and money, and increase access to primary healthcare, especially if telehealth can be used to support routine or stable patient health problems [91]. The other benefits include less need for face-to-face consultations, the ability to manage physician workloads and allowing systems to be reorganised [88]. In addition, teleconsultation enable overcoming the distance barriers in a flexible and convenient way for patients, with the ability to contribute to the continuity of care, patient autonomy and resource savings. Other qualitative studies examining satisfaction with teleconsultation show that the main benefits commonly reported by patients are convenience, reduced travel time and precisely greater access to specialist care, as well as better appointment flexibility, enabling minimal disruption of everyday life [92,93].

Teleconsultations cannot replace personal medical care in all cases. Several studies have shown that patients were satisfied with the remote consultations, but would also like to be able to have face-to-face appointments [83]. The teleconsultations should not be used in rare or unstable conditions, or when a physical examination is needed. Some patients are more appreciative of direct contact with a physician (with direct examination if necessary) compared to the convenience of telehealth, which was also confirmed by previous studies [94–96]. Such direct contact is also necessary in the case of seriously ill patients. Unfortunately, this pilot study did not allow for the assessment of the quality of teleconsultation from the point of view of chronically ill people. Most of the respondents (40.4%) contacted a doctor for non-urgent reasons (administrative matters: prescription, referral to a specialist, sick leave) or for control reasons (30.3%). Only 12.1% of the respondents held a teleconsultation due to chronic treatment. The other studies show that it is important for the patients to have the choice and flexibility to use health services in the most appropriate way [97]. However, it should be remembered to enable personal appointments for people with more complex health needs [98].

The overall positive assessment of the quality of remote primary healthcare was also due to its high treatment effectiveness. Most patients participating in this study rated the treatment effectiveness quite high. The treatment applied helped or definitely helped most patients, as most of them have had their health problems solved (E1: $\overline{x} = 4.15$). The patients' expectations were taken into account by the GPs in the majority of cases (E3: $\overline{x} = 4.44$). Therefore, teleconsultations seem to be a safe and effective way of assessing and dealing with various clinical situations.

Also, other studies confirm that telemedicine maximises primary healthcare and offers the possibility of improving the treatment effectiveness [99]. The support for new communication technologies in the healthcare service provision is an important determinant of quality sought by all participants. Technological advances that are transforming traditional treatments and modern methods of care and diagnostics lead to positive changes in the form of better treatment outcomes for patients living in developing, rural areas or areas with limited healthcare options [100,101].

The correlation analysis and ANNOVA analysis conducted in this study pointed to a relationship between access to healthcare and treatment effectiveness in the primary healthcare. The regression model indicated that 14.3% of the variance is explained. The literature also consistently indicates that in the case of some diseases, telemedicine leads to the improvement of health outcomes. In areas such as type 2 diabetes, research shows that telemedicine intervention is comparable to the standards of traditional medical care and does not cause unnecessary risk or harm to patients [102]. Also, neurological and cardiological signs and simple ophthalmic symptoms such as strabismus can be safely diagnosed and treated through teleconsultation [83,88]. However, this study is the first one to show the impact of medical care accessibility on treatment effectiveness in primary healthcare in a crisis situation, such as the COVID pandemic.

There are some limitations to this study that need considering. Firstly, the indicators for measuring medical care accessibility and treatment effectiveness, despite their validation, have not been used in other populations, and therefore their external validity has not yet been confirmed. The same limitation can be attributed to the study population, which despite a large size is derived solely from four entities located in one region and therefore must be generalised conservatively. Although the sample size of the patients studied was varied, the extent to which they are representative of patients in other clinics is unknown. It would be interesting to repeat the study in other healthcare entities or organisations to see if these variables do indeed still determine the ultimate quality of care based on access to healthcare and treatment effectiveness. Otherwise, the studies conducted among primary care patients in Europe suggest that interpersonal aspects (e.g., communication with a physician, trust and respect [34] are more important dimensions of healthcare quality than accessibility and effectiveness, thereby making it necessary to include them in future studies. It is fair to say that research into these relationships requires further attention. However, the deliberations are limited solely to primary healthcare. Patients with severe diagnoses, e.g., cancer or unstable chronic diseases, would probably assess healthcare services differently than patients requiring stable follow-up appointments, thereby requiring more attention to be paid to groups of patients with unstable health conditions.

5. Conclusions

The COVID-19 pandemic has disrupted the provision of healthcare services, resulting in a considerable deterioration in patients' overall health, especially those with chronic diseases. Broad access to telemedicine could significantly reduce disruptions in the provision of healthcare services during the pandemic and prevent, at least to some extent, a deterioration in the patients' quality of life and careers. While remote healthcare solutions cannot completely replace face-to-face medical assessment, they can ensure the continuity of healthcare services and help protect patients, their families and healthcare professionals from disease transmission. The accessibility and effectiveness of medical care are considered key features of the care processes required to ensure high-quality outcomes. Sufficient documentation of the relationship between the accessibility and effectiveness of patient care is essential to support efforts to improve the outcomes of all types of disease treatment, especially chronic disease, and finally to improve the patients' quality of life. The purpose of this study was to examine patient satisfaction with the access to primary healthcare and the effectiveness of treatment in a condition of remote medical care caused by the COVID-19 pandemic. The model proposed in this study identified a positive and weak, but statistically significant, relationship between these factors. Although a better access to primary care has a positive effect on treatment effectiveness, there are undoubtedly other factors that affect this effectiveness to a greater extent and it would be worth investigating them in further studies.

Taking into account patients' views on the quality of medical services can help to improve overall healthcare delivery in the primary healthcare that is responsible for most health needs. Improving the quality of this care is of great clinical importance. It can positively impact the early detection of chronic diseases, rapid, effective and patient-centered delivery of medical care, adherence to treatment protocols and thus clinical outcomes. As a result, it can also lead to a better quality of life for patients. In addition, tools in the field of telemedicine, implemented at the primary healthcare level, can support clinical decision-making and thus improve the effectiveness of care by providing healthcare professionals with information and knowledge about a specific patient at the right time during interaction with the patient. According to the WHO, this can promote effective decision-making and enable different healthcare providers to understand and deal with the broad and complex health problems encountered in primary care.

To our knowledge, this is the first study in which access to this healthcare was examined on a sample of Polish primary care patients in the conditions of remote work caused by the COVID-19 pandemic. An analysis of the data from this study showed that patients positively assessed the accessibility of remote services and the treatment effectiveness in teleconsultation conditions. Future research should therefore be focused on patients with chronic diseases requiring coordinated healthcare and should also be extended to outpatient healthcare facilities. Health variables should also be considered as moderating variables in future studies.

Author Contributions: Conceptualization, M.K.-A. and L.H.; methodology, R.W., M.K.-A. and L.H.; validation, R.W.; formal analysis, R.W.; investigation, R.W., M.K.-A. and L.H.; resources, P.K.; data curation, R.W.; writing—original draft preparation, R.W., M.K.-A. and L.H.; writing—review and editing, R.W., M.K.-A., L.H. and P.K. visualization, R.W.; supervision, M.K.-A. and P.K.; project administration, M.K.-A. All authors have read and agreed to the published version of the manuscript. contributed substantially to the work reported.

Funding: This research was funded/by IDUB against the COVID-19 project granted by Warsaw University of Technology under the program Excellence Initiative: Research University (IDUB).

Institutional Review Board Statement: The study was conducted according to the guidelines of the Declaration of Helsinki, and approved by the Institutional Ethics Committee of Warsaw University of Technology (Certificate of Ethics approval—approved 15 Janaury 2021).

Informed Consent Statement: Informed consent was obtained from all subjects involved in the study.

Data Availability Statement: Data is contained within the article.

Conflicts of Interest: The authors declare no conflict of interest.

References

1. Kanecki, K.; Nitsch-Osuch, A.; Tyszko, P. Health-Related Quality of Life or Quality of Medical Service? Current challenges for family doctors. *Fam. Med. Prim. Care Rev.* **2016**, *18*, 382–386. [CrossRef]
2. Haraldstad, K.; Wahl, A.; Andenæs, R.; Andersen, J.; Andersen, M.; Beisland, E.; Borge, C.; Engebretsen, E.; Eisemann, M.; Halvorsrud, L.; et al. A systematic review of quality of life research in medicine and health sciences. *Qual. Life Res.* **2019**, *28*, 2641–2650. [CrossRef]
3. Van den Berg, J.P.; Kalmijn, S.; Lindeman, E.; Veldink, J.H.; de Visser, M.; Van der Graaff, M.M.; Wokke, J.H.J.; Van den Berg, L.H. Multidisciplinary ALS care improves quality of life in patients with ALS. *Neurology* **2005**, *65*, 1264–1267. [CrossRef]
4. Glimelius, B.; Hoffman, K.; Sjödén, P.O.; Jacobsson, G.; Sellström, H.; Enander, L.K.; Linné, T.; Svensson, C. Chemotherapy improves survival and quality of life in advanced pancreatic and biliary cancer. *Ann. Oncol.* **1996**, *7*, 593–600. [CrossRef] [PubMed]
5. Crosby, R.D.; Kolotkin, R.L.; Williams, G.R. Defining clinically meaningful change in health-related quality of life. *J. Clin. Epidemiol.* **2003**, *56*, 395–407. [CrossRef]
6. Constitution of the World Health Organization. *Chron. World Health Organ*; Constitution of the World Health Organization: Geneva, Switzerland, 1947; Volume 1.
7. Raphael, D.; Renwick, R.; Brown, I.; Rootman, I. Quality of life indicators and health: Current status and emerging conceptions. *Soc. Indic. Res.* **1996**, *39*, 65–88. [CrossRef]
8. Hollandsworth, J.G. Evaluating the impact of medical treatment on the quality of life: A 5-year update. *Soc. Sci. Med.* **1988**, *26*, 425–434. [CrossRef]
9. Erikson, R. Description of inequality: The Swedish approach to welfare research. In *The Quality of Life*; Oxford University Press: Oxford, UK, 1993.
10. Adler, N.E.; Boyce, W.T.; Chesney, M.A.; Folkman, S.; Syme, S.L. Socioeconomic Inequalities in Health: No Easy Solution. *JAMA J. Am. Med. Assoc.* **1993**, *269*, 3140–3145. [CrossRef]
11. Donabedian, A. Twenty years of research on the quality of medical care: 1964–1984. *Eval. Health Prof.* **1985**, *8*, 243–265. [CrossRef] [PubMed]
12. Pascoe, G.C. Patient satisfaction in primary health care: A literature review and analysis. *Eval. Program Plann.* **1983**, *6*, 185–210. [CrossRef]
13. Van Campen, C.; Sixma, H.; Friele, R.D.; Kerssens, J.J.; Peters, L. Quality of Care and Patient Satisfaction: A Review of Measuring Instruments. *Med. Care Res. Rev.* **1995**, *52*, 109–133. [CrossRef] [PubMed]
14. Strasser, S.; Aharony, L.; Greenberger, D. The Patient Satisfaction Process: Moving Toward a Comprehensive Model. *Med. Care Res. Rev.* **1993**, *50*, 219–248. [CrossRef] [PubMed]
15. Revicki, D.A.; Osoba, D.; Fairclough, D.; Barofsky, I.; Berzon, R.; Leidy, N.K.; Rothman, M. Recommendations on health-related quality of life research to support labeling and promotional claims in the United States. *Qual. Life Res.* **2000**, *9*, 887–900. [CrossRef] [PubMed]
16. Lin, X.J.; Lin, I.M.; Fan, S.Y. Methodological issues in measuring health-related quality of life. *Tzu Chi Med. J.* **2013**, *25*, 8–12. [CrossRef]
17. The World Health Organization. *WHOQOL-Measuring Quality of Life*; WHO: Geneva, Switzerland, 2012.
18. Campbell, S.M.; Roland, M.O.; Buetow, S.A. Defining quality of care. *Soc. Sci. Med.* **2000**, *51*, 1611–1625. [CrossRef]

19. Maxwell, R.J. Quality assessment in health. *Br. Med. J.* **1984**, *288*, 1470–1472. [CrossRef]
20. Alonazi, W.B.; Thomas, S.A. Quality of Care and Quality of Life: Convergence or Divergence? *Health Serv. Insights* **2014**, *7*, 13283. [CrossRef]
21. L'Esperance, V.; Sutton, M.; Schofield, P.; Round, T.; Malik, U.; White, P.; Ashworth, M. Impact of primary care funding on secondary care utilisation and patient outcomes: A retrospective cross-sectional study of English general practice. *Br. J. Gen. Pract.* **2017**, *67*, 792–799. [CrossRef]
22. Chmiel, M. Quality Attributes of Primary Health Care Services. *Sci. Pap. Silesian Univ. Technol. Organ. Manag. Ser.* **2019**, *2019*, 7–16. [CrossRef]
23. Korneta, P. Stakeholders and Performance Management Systems of Small and Medium-Sized Outpatient Clinics. *Found. Manag.* **2020**, *12*, 211–222. [CrossRef]
24. Korneta, P.; Kludacz-Alessandri, M.; Walczak, R. The impact of COVID-19 on the performance of primary health care service providers in a capitation payment system: A case study from Poland. *Int. J. Environ. Res. Public Health* **2021**, *18*, 1407. [CrossRef]
25. Jakubowski, D.; Sys, D.; Kajdy, A.; Lewandowska, R.; Kwiatkowska, E.; Cymbaluk-Płoska, A.; Rabijewski, M.; Torbé, A.; Kwiatkowski, S. Application of Telehealth in Prenatal Care during the COVID-19 Pandemic—A Cross-Sectional Survey of Polish Women. *J. Clin. Med.* **2021**, *10*, 2570. [CrossRef]
26. Major, P.; Stefura, T.; Wysocki, M.; Małczak, P.; Rzepa, A.; Proczko-Stepaniak, M.; Szeliga, J.; Pędziwiatr, M. Impact of SARS-CoV-2 pandemic on bariatric care in Poland: Results of national survey. *BMC Surg.* **2020**, *20*, 314. [CrossRef]
27. Konieczny, M.; Cipora, E.; Sawicka, J.; Fal, A. Patient satisfaction with oncological care during the SARS-CoV-2 virus pandemic. *Int. J. Environ. Res. Public Health* **2021**, *18*, 4122. [CrossRef] [PubMed]
28. Mazurek, J.; Biernat, K.; Kuciel, N.; Hap, K.; Sutkowska, E. The use of medical and non-medical services by the elderly during the SARS-CoV-2 pandemic differs between general and specialist practice: A one-center study in Poland. *Healthcare* **2021**, *9*, 8. [CrossRef]
29. Wysocki, P.J.; Kwinta, Ł.; Potocki, P.; Konopka, K.; Streb, J.; Wojtukiewicz, M.Z.; Radecka, B.; Tomczak, P.; Jarząb, M.; Kawecki, A.; et al. Systemic treatment of patients with solid tumors during the COVID-19 (SARS-CoV-2) pandemic-comprehensive recommendations of the Polish Society of Clinical Oncology. *Oncol. Clin. Pract.* **2020**, *16*, 41–52. [CrossRef]
30. Malicki, J.; Martenka, P.; Dyzmann-Sroka, A.; Paczkowska, K.; Leporowska, E.; Suchorska, W.; Lamperska, K.; Pieńkowski, P.; Chicheł, A.; Mocydlarz-Adamcewicz, M.; et al. Impact of COVID-19 on the performance of a radiation oncology department at a major comprehensive cancer centre in Poland during the first ten weeks of the epidemic. *Rep. Pract. Oncol. Radiother.* **2020**, *25*, 820–827. [CrossRef] [PubMed]
31. Maluchnik, M.; Podwójcic, K.; Więckowska, B. Decreasing access to cancer diagnosis and treatment during the COVID-19 pandemic in Poland. *Acta Oncol.* **2021**, *60*, 28–31. [CrossRef]
32. Zduńczyk, A.J.; Jakubiak, A.; Łuczak, J. *Raport Podstawowa Opieka Zdrowotna w Polsce-Diagnoza i Projekty Zmian*; Instytut Medycyny Wsi im: Lublin, Poland, 2018.
33. Starfield, B.; Shi, L.; Macinko, J. Contribution of primary care to health systems and health. *Milbank Q.* **2005**, *83*, 457–502. [CrossRef]
34. Bower, P.; Roland, M.; Campbell, J.; Mead, N. Setting standards based on patients' views on access and continuity: Secondary analysis of data from the general practice assessment survey. *Br. Med. J.* **2003**, *326*, 258–260. [CrossRef]
35. Campbell, S.M.; Hann, M.; Hacker, J.; Burns, C.; Oliver, D.; Thapar, A.; Mead, N.; Gelb Safran, D.; Roland, M.O. Identifying predictors of high quality care in English general practice: Observational study. *Br. Med. J.* **2001**, *323*, 784–787. [CrossRef]
36. Cankurtaran, D.; Tezel, N.; Yildiz, S.Y.; Celik, G.; Unlu Akyuz, E. Evaluation of the effects of the COVID-19 pandemic on children with cerebral palsy, caregivers' quality of life, and caregivers' fear of COVID-19 with telemedicine. *Ir. J. Med. Sci.* **2021**, 1–8. [CrossRef]
37. Whitehead, M. The concepts and principles of equity and health. *Int. J. Health Serv.* **1992**, *22*, 429–445. [CrossRef] [PubMed]
38. Andersen, R.M.; McCutcheon, A.; Aday, L.A.; Chiu, G.Y.; Bell, R. Exploring dimensions of access to medical care. *Health Serv. Res.* **1983**, *18*, 49–74. [PubMed]
39. Hawrysz, L.; Gierszewska, G.; Bitkowska, A. The research on patient satisfaction with remote healthcare prior to and during the COVID-19 pandemic. *Int. J. Environ. Res. Public Health* **2021**, *18*, 5338. [CrossRef] [PubMed]
40. Gordon, T.; Booysen, F.; Mbonigaba, J. Socio-economic inequalities in the multiple dimensions of access to healthcare: The case of South Africa. *BMC Public Health* **2020**, *20*, 289. [CrossRef] [PubMed]
41. Haggerty, J.; Burge, F.; Lévesque, J.F.; Gass, D.; Pineault, R.; Beaulieu, M.D.; Santor, D. Operational definitions of attributes of primary health care: Consensus among Canadian experts. *Ann. Fam. Med.* **2007**, *5*, 336–344. [CrossRef]
42. Drucker, P.F. *The Effective Executive*; Harper & Row: New York, NY, USA, 1967.
43. Palmer, S.; Torgerson, D.J. Economics notes: Definitions of efficiency. *BMJ Br. Med. J.* **1999**, *318*, 1136. [CrossRef]
44. Rezapour, R.; Tabrizi, J.S.; Farahbakhsh, M.; Saadati, M.; Abdolahi, H.M. Developing Iranian primary health care quality framework: A national study. *BMC Public Health* **2019**, *19*, 1–10. [CrossRef]
45. Burches, E.; Burches, M. Efficacy, Effectiveness and Efficiency in the Health Care: The Need for an Agreement to Clarify its Meaning. *Int. Arch. Public Health Community Med.* **2020**, *4*, 35. [CrossRef]

46. Głodziński, E. Efektywność Ekonomiczna—Dylematy Definiowania i Pomiaru Economic Efficiency—Dilemmas in Definition and Measurement; Zeszyty Naukowe. Organizacja i Zarządzanie/Politechnika Śląska. 2014; z. 73. pp. 155–167. Available online: https://yadda.icm.edu.pl/baztech/element/bwmeta1.element.baztech-9f73d895-2539-49fc-a3f4-5ccb3d7be1be (accessed on 15 June 2021).
47. World Health Organization. *Quality in Primary Health Care*; World Health Organization: Geneva, Switzerland, 2018.
48. Agency for Healthcare Research and Quality. *National Healthcare Quality and Disparities Reports*; Agency for Healthcare Research and Quality: Rockville, MD, USA, 2018.
49. (CIHI) Canadian Institute for Health Information. *Pan-Canadian Primary Health Care Indicator Update Report*. 2012, p. 186. Available online: https://secure.cihi.ca/estore/productFamily.htm?locale=en&pf=PFC2000 (accessed on 15 June 2021).
50. Australian Commission on Safety and Quality in Health Care. *Practice-Level Indicators of Safety and Quality for Primary Health Care*; Australian Commission on Safety and Quality in Health Care: Australia, 2012. Available online: https://www.safetyandquality.gov.au/publications-and-resources/resource-library/practice-level-indicators-safety-and-quality-primary-health-care-synthesis-submission-consultation-paper-and-recommended-national-indicator-set (accessed on 15 June 2021).
51. Langbecker, D.; Caffery, L.J.; Gillespie, N.; Smith, A.C. Using survey methods in telehealth research: A practical guide. *J. Telemed. Telecare* **2017**, *23*, 770–779. [CrossRef]
52. Raczyńska, E. Efektywność w ochronie zdrowaia jako wyzwanie dla zarządzania. *Przegląd Organ.* **2020**, *5*, 27–34. [CrossRef]
53. Testa, M.A.; Simonson, D.C. Assessment of Quality-of-Life Outcomes. *N. Engl. J. Med.* **1996**, *334*, 835–840. [CrossRef]
54. Gill, T.M.; Feinstein, A.R. A Critical Appraisal of the Quality of Quality-of-Life Measurements. *JAMA J. Am. Med. Assoc.* **1994**, *272*, 619–626. [CrossRef]
55. Wilcox, L.D.; Brooks, R.M.; Beal, G.M.; Klonglan, G.E. *Social Indicators and Societal Monitoring: An Annotated Bibliography*; Jossey-Bass Inc. Publishers: San Francisco, CA, USA, 1972.
56. Aday, L.A.; Andersen, R. A framework for the study of access to medical care. *Health Serv. Res.* **1974**, *9*, 208–220.
57. Gene-Badia, J.; Ascaso, C.; Escaramis-Babiano, G.; Sampietro-Colom, L.; Catalan-Ramos, A.; Sans-Corrales, M.; Pujol-Ribera, E. Personalised care, access, quality and team coordination are the main dimensions of family medicine output. *Fam. Pract.* **2006**, *24*, 41–47. [CrossRef] [PubMed]
58. Corscadden, L.; Levesque, J.-F.; Lewis, V.; Breton, M.; Sutherland, K.; Weenink, J.-W.; Haggerty, J.; Russell, G. Barriers to accessing primary health care: Comparing Australian experiences internationally. *Aust. J. Prim. Health* **2017**, *23*, 223. [CrossRef]
59. Engels, Y. Developing a framework of, and quality indicators for, general practice management in Europe. *Fam. Pract.* **2005**, *22*, 215–222. [CrossRef]
60. McIntyre, D.; Thiede, M.; Birch, S. Access as a policy-relevant concept in low- and middle-income countries. *Health Econ. Policy Law* **2009**, *4*, 179–193. [CrossRef]
61. Levesque, J.F.; Harris, M.F.; Russell, G. Patient-centred access to health care: Conceptualising access at the interface of health systems and populations. *Int. J. Equity Health* **2013**, *12*, 18. [CrossRef] [PubMed]
62. Hanson, K.; Yip, W.C.; Hsiao, W. The impact of quality on the demand for outpatient services in Cyprus. *Health Econ.* **2004**, *13*, 1167–1180. [CrossRef] [PubMed]
63. Sans-Corrales, M. Family medicine attributes related to satisfaction, health and costs. *Fam. Pract.* **2006**, *23*, 308–316. [CrossRef] [PubMed]
64. Zimmerman, B.S.; Seidman, D.; Berger, N.; Cascetta, K.P.; Nezolosky, M.; Trlica, K.; Ryncarz, A.; Keeton, C.; Moshier, E.; Tiersten, A. Patient perception of telehealth services for breast and gynecologic oncology care during the COVID-19 pandemic: A single center survey-based study. *J. Breast Cancer* **2020**, *23*, 542–552. [CrossRef] [PubMed]
65. Hair, J.F., Jr.; Black, W.C.; Babin, B.J.; Anderson, R.E. *Multivariate Data Analysis*; Pearson Education, Limited: London, UK, 2013.
66. Sapsford, R. *Survey Research*; SAGE Publications: New York, NY, USA, 2006.
67. Johnson, T.P. *Handbook of Health Survey Methods*; John Wiley & Sons, Incorporated: Hoboken, NJ, USA, 2014.
68. Punch, K.F. *Survey Research: The Basics*; Sage Publications: New York, NY, USA, 2003.
69. Davies, H.; Powell, A.; Rushmer, R. *Healthcare Professionals' Views on Clinician Engagement in Quality Improvement: A Literature Review*. 2007. Available online: https://www.health.org.uk/publications/healthcare-professionals%E2%80%99-views-on-clinician-engagement-in-quality-improvement (accessed on 15 June 2021).
70. Caccia-Bava, M.C.; Guimaraes, V.C.K.; Guimaraes, T. Important factors for success in hospital BPR project phases. *Int. J. Health Care Qual. Assur.* **2013**, *26*, 729–745. [CrossRef]
71. Hennington, A.; Janz, B.; Poston, R. I'm just burned out: Understanding information system compatibility with personal values and role-based stress in a nursing context. *Comput. Hum. Behav.* **2011**, *27*, 1238–1248. [CrossRef]
72. De Ryck, E.; Willems, S. Erratum: Measures of quality, costs and equity in primary healthcare: Instruments developed to analyse and compare primary healthcare in 35 countries (Quality in Primary Care (2013) 21:2 (67–79)). *Qual. Prim. Care* **2013**, *21*, 205.
73. Lai, H.; Gemming, L. Approaches to patient satisfaction measurement of the healthcare food services: A systematic review. *Clin. Nutr. ESPEN* **2021**, *42*, 61–72. [CrossRef]
74. European Patients Forum. Patients' Perceptions of Quality in Healthcare: Report of a survey conducted by EPF in 2016. Report in a Survey. 2017, p. 40. Available online: https://www.eu-patient.eu/globalassets/policy/quality-of-care/quality-survey-report.pdf (accessed on 15 June 2021).

75. Bargawi, A.A.; Rea, D.M. Quality in Primary Health Care. Health Policy Plan. 2015, pp. 37–40. Available online: https://www.who.int/docs/default-source/primary-health-care-conference/quality.pdf (accessed on 15 June 2021).
76. Shield, T.; Campbell, S.; Rogers, A.; Worrall, A.; Chew-Graham, C.; Gask, L. Quality indicators for primary care mental health services. *Qual. Saf. Health Care* **2003**, *12*, 100–106. [CrossRef]
77. Busse, R.; Klazinga, N.; Panteli, D.; Quentin, W. *Improving Healthcare Quality in Europe*; WHO: Geneva, Switzerland, 2019.
78. Tabachnick, B.; Fidell, L. *Using Multivariate Statistics*; Pearson Education: Upper Saddle River, NJ, USA, 2018; ISBN 9780134792859.
79. Horn, J.L. Factors in Factor Analysis. *Psychometrika* **1965**, *30*, 179–185. [CrossRef]
80. Zhang, X.; Xiang, S. *Learn About Reliability Analysis and Factor Analysis in SPSS With Online Shopping Data*; SAGE Publications: New York, NY, USA, 2019. [CrossRef]
81. Williams, B.; Onsman, A.; Brown, T. Exploratory factor analysis: A five-step guide for novices. *J. Emerg. Prim. Health Care* **2010**, *8*, 225–236. [CrossRef]
82. Kludacz-Alessandri, M.; Hawrysz, L.; Korneta, P.; Gierszewska, G.; Pomaranik, W.; Walczak, R. The impact of medical teleconsultations on general practitioner-patient communication during COVID- 19: A case study from Poland. *PLoS ONE* **2021**, *16*, e0254960. [CrossRef] [PubMed]
83. Barbosa, W.; Zhou, K.; Waddell, E.; Myers, T.; Dorsey, E.R. Improving Access to Care: Telemedicine across Medical Domains. In *Annual Review of Public Health*; Annual Reviews Inc.: Palo Alto, CA, USA, 2020; Volume 42, pp. 463–481.
84. Grol, R.; Wensing, M. Patients Evaluate General/Family Practice: The EUROPEP Instrument; 2000. Available online: https://equip.woncaeurope.org/sites/equip/files/documents/publications/resources/grolwensing2000theeuropepinstrumentequipwonca.pdf (accessed on 15 June 2021).
85. Smith, C.H.; Armstrong, D. Comparison of criteria derived by government and patients for evaluating general practitioner services. *Br. Med. J.* **1989**, *299*, 494–496. [CrossRef] [PubMed]
86. Ekeland, A.G.; Bowes, A.; Flottorp, S. Effectiveness of telemedicine: A systematic review of reviews. *Int. J. Med. Inform.* **2010**, *79*, 736–771. [CrossRef]
87. Champagne-Langabeer, T.; Langabeer, J.R.; Roberts, K.E.; Gross, J.S.; Gleisberg, G.R.; Gonzalez, M.G.; Persse, D. Telehealth Impact on Primary Care Related Ambulance Transports. *Prehospital Emerg. Care* **2019**, *23*, 712–717. [CrossRef] [PubMed]
88. de Catapan, S.C.; Calvo, M.C.M. Teleconsultation: An Integrative Review of the Doctor-Patient Interaction Mediated by Technology. *Rev. Bras. Educ. Med.* **2020**, *44*. [CrossRef]
89. Newbould, J.; Abel, G.; Ball, S.; Corbett, J.; Elliott, M.; Exley, J.; Martin, A.; Saunders, C.; Wilson, E.; Winpenny, E.; et al. Evaluation of telephone first approach to demand management in English general practice: Observational study. *BMJ* **2017**, *358*, 4197. [CrossRef]
90. Moth, G.; Huibers, L.; Christensen, M.B.; Vedsted, P. Drug prescription by telephone consultation in Danish out-of-hours primary care: A population-based study of frequency and associations with clinical severity and diagnosis. *BMC Fam. Pract.* **2014**, *15*, 142. [CrossRef]
91. Dawson, A.Z.; Walker, R.J.; Campbell, J.A.; Davidson, T.M.; Egede, L.E. Telehealth and indigenous populations around the world: A systematic review on current modalities for physical and mental health. *mHealth* **2020**, *6*, 30. [CrossRef]
92. Morris, J.; Campbell-Richards, D.; Wherton, J.; Sudra, R.; Vijayaraghavan, S.; Greenhalgh, T.; Collard, A.; Byrne, E.; O'Shea, T. Webcam consultations for diabetes: Findings from four years of experience in Newham. *Pract. Diabetes* **2017**, *34*, 45–50. [CrossRef]
93. Haig-Ferguson, A.; Loades, M.; Whittle, C.; Read, R.; Higson-Sweeney, N.; Beasant, L.; Starbuck, J.; Crawley, E. "It's not one size fits all"; the use of videoconferencing for delivering therapy in a Specialist Paediatric Chronic Fatigue Service. *Internet Interv.* **2019**, *15*, 43–51. [CrossRef]
94. Chwistek, M. "are You Wearing Your White Coat?": Telemedicine in the Time of Pandemic. *JAMA J. Am. Med. Assoc.* **2020**, *324*, 149–150. [CrossRef]
95. Sutherland, A.E.; Stickland, J.; Wee, B. Can video consultations replace face-to-face interviews? Palliative medicine and the COVID-19 pandemic: Rapid review. *BMJ Support Palliat. Care* **2020**, *26*, 26. [CrossRef]
96. Wade, V.A.; Karnon, J.; Elshaug, A.G.; Hiller, J.E. A systematic review of economic analyses of telehealth services using real time video communication. *BMC Health Serv. Res.* **2010**, *10*, 233. [CrossRef] [PubMed]
97. Imlach, F.; McKinlay, E.; Middleton, L.; Kennedy, J.; Pledger, M.; Russell, L.; Churchward, M.; Cumming, J.; McBride-Henry, K. Telehealth consultations in general practice during a pandemic lockdown: Survey and interviews on patient experiences and preferences. *BMC Fam. Pract.* **2020**, *21*, 269. [CrossRef]
98. Thornton, J. COVID-19: How coronavirus will change the face of general practice forever. *BMJ* **2020**, *368*, m1279. [CrossRef] [PubMed]
99. Raczkiewicz, D.; Kister, A.; Rzemek, C.; Tarkowski, K.; Dybciak, P.; Owoc, A.; Bojar, I. Telemedicine in the opinion of primary health care physicians. *Eur. J. Med. Technol.* **2018**, *2*, 43.
100. Ackerman, M.J.; Filart, R.; Burgess, L.P.; Lee, I.; Poropatich, R.K. Developing next-generation telehealth tools and technologies: Patients, systems, and data perspectives. In *Telemedicine and e-Health*; NCBI: Bethesda, MD, USA, 2010; Volume 16, pp. 93–95.

101. Zanaboni, P.; Wootton, R. Adoption of telemedicine: From pilot stage to routine delivery. *BMC Med. Inform. Decis. Mak.* **2012**, *12*, 1. [CrossRef]
102. Gomes Rodrigues, D.L.; Belber, G.S.; de Queiroz Padilha, F.V.; Spinel, L.F.; Moreira, F.R.; Maeyama, M.A.; Marques Pinho, A.P.N.; Júnior, Á.A. Impact of teleconsultation on patients with type 2 diabetes in the Brazilian public health system: Protocol for a randomized controlled trial (TELEconsulta diabetes trial). *JMIR Res. Protoc.* **2021**, *10*, e23679. [CrossRef] [PubMed]

Journal of
Clinical Medicine

MDPI

Article

Do Mental Health and Vitality Mediate the Relationship between Perceived Control over Time and Fear of COVID-19? A Survey in an Italian Sample

Silvana Miceli [1], Barbara Caci [1,*], Michele Roccella [1], Luigi Vetri [2], Giuseppe Quatrosi [2] and Maurizio Cardaci [1]

[1] Department of Psychology, Educational Science and Human Movement, University of Palermo, 90121 Palermo, Italy; silvana.miceli56@unipa.it (S.M.); michele.roccella@unipa.it (M.R.); maurizio.cardaci@unipa.it (M.C.)
[2] Department of Health Promotion, Mother and Child Care, Internal Medicine and Medical Specialties (ProMISE), University of Palermo, 90121 Palermo, Italy; luigi.vetri@gmail.com (L.V.); giuseppe.quatrosi01@community.unipa.it (G.Q.)
* Correspondence: barbara.caci@unipa.it; Tel.: +39-(0)91-23897739

Abstract: Several studies evidenced increased elevated symptomatology levels in anxiety, general stress, depression, and post-traumatic stress related to COVID-19. Real difficulties in the effective control of time that could be responsible for mental health issues and loss of vitality were also reported. Prior literature highlighted how perceived control over time significantly modulates anxiety disorders and promotes psychological well-being. To verify the hypothesis that perceived control over time predicts fear of COVID-19 and mental health and vitality mediate this relationship, we performed an online survey on a sample of 301 subjects (female = 68%; M_{age} = 22.12, SD = 6.29; age range = 18–57 years), testing a parallel mediation model using PROCESS macro (model 4). All participants responded to self-report measures of perceived control over time, COVID-19 fear, mental health, and vitality subscales of the Short-Form-36 Health Survey. Results corroborate the hypotheses of direct relationships between all the study variables and partially validate the mediation's indirect effect. Indeed, mental health (a1b1 = −0.06; CI: LL = −0.11; UL = −0.01; $p < 0.001$) rather than vitality (a2b2 = −0.06; CI: LL = −0.09; UL = 0.03; n.s.) emerges as a significant mediator between perceived control over time and fear of COVID-19. Practical implications of the study about treatment programs based on perceived control over time and emotional coping to prevent fear and anxiety toward the COVID-19 pandemic are discussed.

Keywords: perceived control over time; COVID-19; COVID-19 fear; mental health; vitality; health; quality of life; anxiety; emotion

Citation: Miceli, S.; Caci, B.; Roccella, M.; Vetri, L.; Quatrosi, G.; Cardaci, M. Do Mental Health and Vitality Mediate the Relationship between Perceived Control over Time and Fear of COVID-19? A Survey in an Italian Sample. *J. Clin. Med.* **2021**, *10*, 3516. https://doi.org/10.3390/jcm10163516

Academic Editor: Emmanuel Andrès

Received: 7 July 2021
Accepted: 9 August 2021
Published: 10 August 2021

1. Introduction

Since its first identification by the Wuhan Municipal Health Commission in China, the 2019 SARS-CoV-2 pandemic has now reached more than one year after its spread and assumed more dramatic proportions in the entire world ever. Most countries experienced second waves and perhaps prepared for even a third related to the SARS-CoV-2 virus mutations. As of March 2020, the excess mortality in Italy was 20.4%, lower than that of Spain (23.6%), Belgium (20.8%), and Poland (23.2%) but higher than that of France (13.2%), Germany (7%), Holland (14.7%), and Portugal (13.9%) (ISTAT: 2021). The world's social-economic system is in crisis, and the health system is overloaded. The latter must continuously deal with the coronavirus health emergency and is called upon to manage the increase in mental disorders deriving from the pandemic's living conditions. Several studies have analyzed the negative consequences of the coronavirus pandemic on people's mental health especially in patients with chronic or autoimmune diseases [1–3], evidencing elevated symptomatology levels in anxiety, general stress, depression, and post-traumatic stress related to COVID-19 [4]. Unpleasant emotions, anger, or vulnerability [5]; loss of vitality [6]; a lack of energy, an inability to start and carry out daily activities, or difficulty concentrating at work [7]; fatigue [8]; and social media addiction [9,10] are other negative consequences of the COVID-19 pandemic reported by the current literature. The coronavirus pandemic urgently forces people to live in the present moment, experiencing a sort of temporal disintegration in which time is stopped or slowed, the order of time and days confused. Even the future seems shortened, causing a real difficulty in the effective control of time in many cases. Therefore, this altered time control could be responsible for higher psychological distress and mental health issues [11]. Prior studies highlighted how perceived control over time significantly affects anxiety disorders [12]. It has also evidenced that it promotes psychological well-being [13] and coping strategies [14]. High levels of perceived control over time are associated with low levels of stress, high academic performance levels, problem-solving ability, and health [14].

Starting from these premises, we first aim to analyze the effect of perceived control over time on COVID-19 fear, a new form of situational anxiety [15]. We assume that higher levels of perceived control over time, which allow people to manage daily activities, are related to lower levels of COVID-19 fear. Therefore, Hypothesis 1 arises as follows:

Hypothesis 1 (H1). *Perceived control over time is negatively associated with COVID-19 fear.*

Another essential aspect of perceived control over time is the socio-cognitive-behavioral attribute of perceived control. Perceived control has been defined in the psychological literature as personal control, locus of control, self-efficacy, and sense of control, even if each term has distinct features [16–18]. In the framework of social learning theory [16], perceived control over time is a predictor of future health behavior and status. In general, socio-cognitive psychologists suggested that high levels of perceived control are related to proactive behaviors and the ability to feel healthy. In contrast, low levels are associated with depression, stress, and anxiety-related disorders [19]. Longitudinal and reciprocal relationships between perceived control over life circumstances and mental health have been suggested too [8]. In this sense, perceived control modulates affective responses to environmental stressors, enhances positive emotions, decreases negative ones, and sustains psychological vitality [20]. People with high vitality are more active and productive and have good coping strategies and greater well-being [21–24]. Vitality was also related to psychological distress [25], subjective happiness [23], and physical function and health-related quality of life [25,26].

Hence, the second aim of the current study is to explore the reciprocal relationships among perceived control over time, mental health, and vitality. In the framework of the coronavirus pandemic, we hypothesize that people with a high sense of control over their time, who can plan their working or studying tasks without procrastination, will be more able to manage their negative emotions and increase their sense of vitality compared to those with low control beliefs over time. Consequently, we state Hypotheses 2 and 3 as follows:

Hypothesis 2 (H2). *Perceived control over time is negatively associated with adverse mental health statuses.*

Hypothesis 3 (H3). *Perceived control over time is positively associated with vitality.*

Considering the linear relationships evidenced by literature for COVID-19 anxiety and mental health and vitality, as described above [4], we expect to find that people with both adverse mental health status and low vitality levels will present higher levels of COVID-19 fear as well.

We hypothesize then that

Hypothesis 4 (H4). *Adverse mental health statuses are positively associated with COVID-19 fear.*

Hypothesis 5 (H5). *Vitality is negatively associated with COVID-19 fear.*

Finally, in the current study, we tested a model assuming mental health and vitality as mediators in the relationship between perceived time control and COVID-19 fear. Prior psychological studies reported mental health effects on increasing well-being and performance [27], decreasing anxiety, heightening self-confidence, and improving individuals' self-control performance [28]. Scholars also showed that vitality contrasts with physical and mental fatigue, one of the pandemic's main psychological consequences [8]. Although the time available to us to carry out our activities has dramatically increased during the imposed restrictions, individuals often experienced a lack of energy, an inability to start and manage daily activities, and difficulty concentrating at work [7]. Such a state of fatigue can adversely affect a person's physical and mental well-being, but also, if prolonged, can, in the long term, predispose the individual to the onset of psychiatric diseases, especially depression. Morgul et al. [29], out of 4700 Turkish-nationality subjects, highlighted how fatigued individuals had more pessimistic attitudes toward the possibility that COVID-19 will finally be controlled, less satisfaction with the authorities' preventive measures, and less confidence that their country can overcome the COVID-19 pandemic. They also showed low compliance with safety protocols such as wearing masks, washing hands, and maintaining physical distance. Consequently, adverse mental health status and loss of vitality may decrease perceived control over time and increase anxiety toward COVID-19.

We then formulate Hypothesis 6:

Hypothesis 6 (H6). *Mental health and vitality mediate the relationship between perceived control over time and COVID-19 fear.*

In sum, the present study's results would contribute to studying the dramatic effects of the coronavirus pandemic state on people's anxiety levels, evidencing mental health and vitality as protective factors against anxiety toward SARS-Cov-2 infection.

2. Materials and Methods

2.1. Participants

A sample of 301 subjects (female = 68%; M_{age} = 22.12, SD = 6.29; age range = 18–57 years), coming almost all from southern Italy (85.7%), and having a diploma (79.1%) or a degree (16.3%) took part in the survey. According to the Declaration of Helsinki, all participants gave written consent about the anonymity of data handling, and the Bioethics Committee of the University of Palermo approved the study (n. 2/2020).

2.2. Procedure

Participants were recruited by responding voluntarily to the survey administered online via Google Forms on the researchers' distance learning university courses during Italy's lockdown phase. A snowballing procedure, asking subjects to recruit future participants from among their acquaintances, combined with respondent-driven sampling was used for acquiring a representative sample of the general population [30]. Google Forms presented the study information sheet in the first section. Data were automatically collected when participants filled the Google form online, reporting the electronic version of the assessment instrument consisting of demographic questions (i.e., gender, age, and education) and apposite measures of the studied variables. On average, the respondents completed the survey in 30 min.

2.3. Instruments

2.3.1. Perceived Control over Time

The perceived control over time subscale from the Time Management Behavior Scale of Macan et al. [31] was used in the current study to measure the individuals' perception of control over their time. It consists of five items scored on a five-point Likert scale with anchors from 1 = strongly disagree to 5 = strongly agree (example of item:" I feel in control of my time"; "I must spend much time on unimportant tasks"). The scale provides a total score by averaging the participants' scores for each scale item (Cronbach α = 0.70).

2.3.2. Fear of COVID-19

Fear of COVID-19 is a recent seven-item scale developed by Ahorsu et al. [15] to measure the fear of COVID-19 in the adult population (example of item: "I am most afraid of coronavirus-19"). Each item is scored on a five-point Likert scale having anchors from 1 = strongly disagree to 5 = strongly agree. We computed the total score by averaging the participants' scores for each scale item (Cronbach α = 0.86).

2.3.3. The Short-Form-36 Health Survey (SF-36)

We used both the five-item mental health and the four-item vitality subscale of the Italian version of the Short-Form-36 Health Survey [32], a general measure of population distress. One example of a mental health subscale item is "Have you felt so down in the dumps that nothing could cheer you up?". One item example of the vitality subscale is "Did you feel tired?". Each item is scored on a five-point Likert scale having anchors from 1 = strongly disagree to 5 = strongly agree. We computed the total score by averaging the participants' scores for the mental health scale (Cronbach α = 0.80) and for the vitality scale (Cronbach α = 0.75).

2.4. *The Parallel Mediation Model*

A parallel mediation model was used in the study to verify our assumptions. It is a basic mediation model (4) from Hayes PROCESS templates [33]. Our theoretical model (Figure 1) assumes that perceived control over time (X) would indirectly affect fear of COVID-19 (Y) through two mediators: mental health (m1) and vitality (m2). All the individual direct and indirect paths as the total indirect effect were calculated as described in Figure 1.

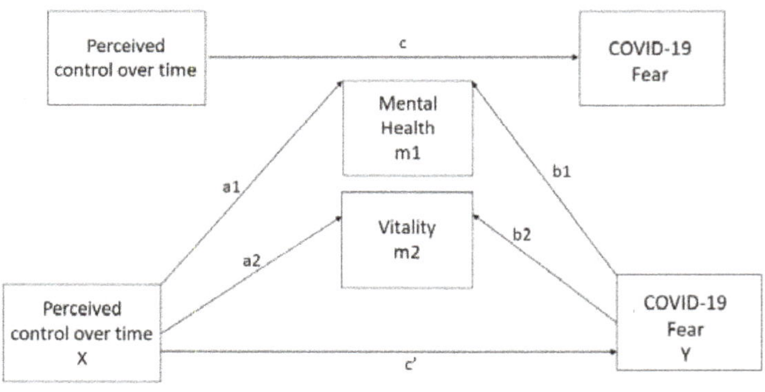

Figure 1. Hypothesized model. Note—perceived control over time: predictor variable; mental health: mediator 1; vitality: mediator 2; COVID-19 fear: outcome variable; a1b1: a specific indirect effect of perceived control over time on COVID-19 fear through mental health; a2b2: a specific indirect impact of perceived control over time on COVID-19 fear through vitality; c': direct effect of perceived control over time on COVID-19 fear; total indirect effect: a1b1 + a2b2.

2.5. *Data Analysis*

All the analyses were conducted through SPSS version 24 (IBM, Chicago, IL, USA). The first step was to calculate descriptive statistics and zero-order correlations. In the preliminary analysis, data were checked for accuracy. It was found that there were no missing values in the data. A correlation was used to see the relationship among all the included variables. The Hayes's PROCESS macro was used to test our mediational model since it is considered a more powerful and effective method than its alternatives [33]. Before testing the model, all variables were standardized. The parameters were estimated using the bootstrap method with 5000 samples and a 95% confidence interval (CI) using the percentile method bias corrected [31]. The parameters are significant if the CI does not include zero.

3. Results

3.1. Descriptive Statistics

Table 1 shows descriptive statistics, mean values, and standard deviations and a correlation matrix for the study variables.

Table 1. Descriptive statistics and zero-order correlation matrix.

	Mean (SD)	1	2	3	4	5	6
1. COVID-19 fear	1.76 (0.69)	1					
2. Perceived control over time	3.32 (0.70)	−0.12 *	1				
3. Vitality	3.00 (0.83)	−0.22 **	0.38 **	1			
4. Mental health	2.74 (0.84)	0.25 **	−0.33 **	−0.72 **	1		
5. Gender (dummy coded: male = 1; female = 0)		−0.26 **	−0.13 *	0.15 **	−0.15 **	1	
6. Age		−0.03	0.03	−0.00	−0.01	0.03	1

* Correlation is significant at $p < 0.05$ (two tiles). ** Correlation is significant at $p < 0.01$ (two tiles).

On average, participants reported medium–high scores in the perceived control over time scale ($M = 3.32$; SD = 0.70), low scores in the fear of COVID-19 scale ($M = 1.76$; SD = 0.69), and medium–low scores in SF-36 mental health ($M = 2.74$; SD = 0.84) and vitality subscales ($M = 3.0$; SD = 0.83). These results indicate that our sample can manage and control their time during the COVID-19 pandemic but are slightly scared by the SARS-CoV-2 virus. Participants also revealed that the COVID-19 pandemic has a medium impact on their mental health and vitality. A series of paired samples t-test indicated that there was a statistically significant difference, $t(298) = -2.27$, $p < 0.01$ on perceived control over time scores despite females ($M = 3.39$, SD = 0.70) obtaining higher scores than males ($M = 3.31$, SD = 0.60). Data also shows a statistically significant difference between COVID-19 scores, $t(298) = -4.77$, $p < 0.01$, with females ($M = 1.88$, SD = 0.70) reporting higher scores then males ($M = 1.49$, SD = 0.49) and depicting themselves as significantly more scared about SARS-CoV-2 infection. No significant differences between mental health and vitality scores in males and females were found.

3.2. Correlation and Regression Analyses

The correlation matrix exhibits a significant association between perceived control over time and fear of COVID-19 and the mediators under study—i.e., mental health and vitality. The correlation coefficient for perceived control over time and COVID-19 fear was −0.12 ($p < 0.05$), supporting our assumption H1 about the linear relationship between X and Y (X→Y) that perceived control over time is related to COVID-19 fear. Similarly, the correlation between perceived control over time and mental health (path a1) was significant with the coefficient $r = 0.33$ ($p < 0.01$) and that between perceived control over time and vitality (path a2) was $r = 0.38$ ($p < 0.01$), supporting hypotheses H2 and H3 of an association between our predictor (i.e., the perceived control over time) and mediators (i.e., mental health and vitality).

On the other hand, there was a positive relationship between mental health and COVID-19 fear (path b1) with $r = 0.25$ ($p < 0.01$), whereas vitality and COVID-19 fear (path b2) were negatively associated with $r = -0.22$ ($p < 0.01$), supporting H4 and H5 of significant linear relations between mediators and the dependent variable. Baron and

Kenny [34] recommended that mediators be significantly associated with independent and dependent variables.

It must be noted that we found a significant negative correlation among gender (dummy coded with 1 = male; 0 = female) and perceived control over time (r = −0.13, $p < 0.05$) or fear of COVID-19 (r = −0.26, $p < 0.01$), showing females reported higher scores on the scale measuring perceived control over time and had a higher fear of COVID-19 than males. Furthermore, a significant negative relationship was found between gender and adverse mental health (r = −0.15; $p < 0.01$), whereas a positive, significant one has emerged between gender and vitality (r = 0.15; $p < 0.01$). Therefore, females present higher adverse mental health statuses and lower vitality scores than males.

All data were then examined through regression to judge whether to include them in the path model or in order to establish the study variables' significance. After analyses, it was found that both mediators could be included in the path model. The independent variable explained 25% of the variance on its own, F = 7.09, R-square = 0.06, $p < 0.001$. Hence, all our assumptions (H1–H5) were supported.

3.3. *The Mediation Role of Mental Health and Vitality on the Relationship between Perceived Control over Time and Fear of COVID-19*

To test the model in which mental health and vitality mediate the relationship between perceived control over time and fear of COVID-19, a parallel mediation analysis using PROCESS model 4 was conducted on data from the whole sample.

Table 2 describes all the direct and indirect effects.

Table 2. Path coefficients for parallel mediation model.

Path	Effect	Boot LL-CI	Boot UL-CI	SE	T	*p*-Value
Total effect	−0.12	−0.23	−0.01	0.05	−2.20	0.028
Direct effect (c′)	−0.03	−0.15	0.08	0.05	−0.59	0.555
IV–m1 (a1)	−0.40	−0.53	−0.27	0.06	−6,.22	0.000
IV–m2 (a2)	0.44	0.32	0.57	0.06	7.17	0.000
M1–DV (b1)	0.15	0.01	0.28	0.06	4.13	0.000
M2–DP (b2)	−0.06	−0.19	0.07	0.06	4.13	0.000
Total indirect effect	−0.09	−0.15	−0.04	0.02		
IV–m1–DV (a1b1)	−0.06	−0.11	−0.01	0.03		
IV–m2–DV (a2b2)	−0.06	−0.09	0.03	0.03		

Note—These are the path coefficients for the parallel mediation model of Hayes process model 4, indirect effects and 95% confidence interval predicting fear of COVID-19 (n = 301), SE is standard error, IV: independent variable (perceived control over time), DV: dependent variable (fear of COVID-19), m1 and m2: parallel mediators (mental health and vitality); a1, a2, b1, and b2 are regression coefficients for X1 and X2, respectively; while b1 and b2 are the regression coefficients for m1 and m2, respectively. Boot LL-CI and Boot UL-CI are abbreviations for the lower limit bootstrap confidence interval and upper limit bootstrap confidence interval.

3.4. *Direct Effects*

Separate regression models were estimated for the entire path. First, as reported in Figure 2, mental health, the first mediator, was regressed on perceived control over time (path a1). Results show a significant negative association between perceived control over time and mental health, evidencing people with low perceived control over time having adverse mental health statuses. Secondly, the other mediator, vitality, was regressed on perceived control over time (path a2), and we found a significant positive path between perceived control over time and vitality. Thus, people with high perceived control over time also have an increased sense of vitality.

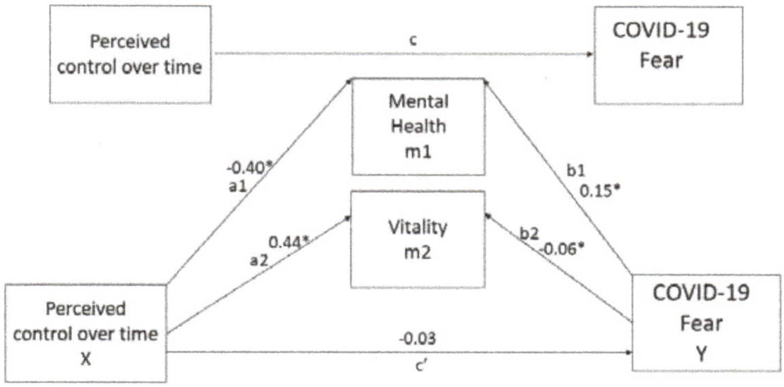

Figure 2. The mediating effect of mental health dimensions in the relationship between perceived control over time and fear of COVID-19. Note: * $p < 0.001$. All the presented effects are unstandardized.

Similarly, in the model, fear of COVID-19 was regressed on mental health (path b1). It was found that there was a significant positive effect, whereas, when fear of COVID-19 was regressed on vitality, we found a significant negative path (b2). The direct effect was explored by regressing the fear of COVID-19 on perceived control over time, which was not significant. This result allows us to verify for a total mediation.

3.5. Indirect Effects

The regression model predicts fear of COVID-19 from mental health, vitality, and perceived control over time. Through all the mediators, we can see a strong negative effect both for mental health (a1b1 = −0.06; CI: LL = −0.11; UL = −0.01) and for vitality (a2b2 = −0.06; CI: LL = −0.09; UL = 0.03). This result shows that only adverse mental health is significantly associated with perceived control over time and fear of COVID-19, considering that bootstrap CI is above zero while controlling for demographic variables.

3.6. Total Effects

The direct effect of perceived control over time on fear of COVID-19 (c′) was −0.03 (CI: LL = −0.15; UL = 0.08: p = n.s.) (see Figure 2). In contrast, the total indirect effect via both mediators (a1b1 + a2b2) was −0.12 (CI: LL = −0.23, UL = −0.01, $p < 0.001$). Consequently, the total effect (a1b1 + a2b2 + c′) of X on Y was −0.15. Therefore, the total effect (c = −0.12; CI: LL = −0.23, UL = −0.01, $p < 0.05$) of perceived control over time on fear of COVID-19 was due to a negative indirect path, as the coefficient for direct effect (c′ = −0.03) was higher than that of the total indirect effect (−0.15). Hence, results show that mental health is a significant mediator between perceived control over time and fear of COVID-19 whereas vitality is not.

4. Discussion

The present study has multiple aims: the first goal is to determine the predictive role of perceived control over time on COVID-19 fear; the second is to analyze the reciprocal linear associations among perceived control over time, mental health, and vitality as well those among mental health, vitality, and COVID-19 fear; the final aim is to understand the influence of perceived control over time on fear of COVID-19 by considering how mental health and vitality mediate this relationship.

The whole sample shows a significant negative association between perceived control over time and fear of COVID-19, corroborating H1 (path c). It should be noted that the subscale of perceived control over the time of the Time Management Behavior Scale of Macan et al. [18], which we used in the present study, explored how perceived control over time affects task completion within deadlines or procrastination. Thus, in line with prior literature reporting that perceived control may act as a protective factor buffering the psychological impact of the pandemic on general health and life satisfaction [35], we found that during the COVID-19 lockdown, when people feel confident in managing their time effectively, they also have less anxiety [36]. We could hypothesize that even if people are forced to remain at home by the lockdown restriction, they could be less pressured by the so-called deadline rush in completing their work, studying, or completing familiar tasks [37]. Thus, their belief in their ability to control their time prevents them from experiencing COVID-19 fear. The present study also evidences gender differences in perceived control over time and COVID-19 fear, showing females having higher scores than males. This outcome is not contradictory. Indeed, even if our data come from a sample composed chiefly of young undergraduate females (female = 68%), they reflect the prior findings in the literature on perceived control, usually depicting young and highly educated women as more able to manage their daily activities than men [34]. In addition, it is in line with psychological literature reporting that women having higher levels of chronic and daily stressors [20] and higher emotional vulnerability, particularly when responding to negative emotions in comparison with men [38]. It also must be noted that females did not differ from males in their scores for mediators.

We secondarily found that perceived control over time is significantly related to mental health and vitality, so data fully support H2 (path a1) and H3 (path a2). Research has demonstrated that people's ability/inability to control time is associated with well-being [13] and mental health complaints [39,40]. Our findings show a significant negative relationship between people's time management beliefs and mental health, indicating that individuals with higher perceived control over time had lower negative mental health statuses. Indeed, the recent literature on the COVID-19 pandemic assigned an essential role to perceived control in moderating the relationship between the perceived severity of COVID-19 and mental health problems. In particular, the more people perceive themselves to be in control of their lives (and time), the more satisfied and healthier they were [41].

Third, our results find strong evidence of the significant positive relationship between fear of COVID-19 and adverse mental health statuses and, conversely, of the significant negative relationship between fear of COVID-19 and vitality, fully corroborating H4 (path b1) and H5 (path b2). From this perspective, our results are consistent with recent outcomes showing that the COVID-19 fear represents a sort of chronic mental anxiety perceived by individuals under the current uncertain and ongoing pandemic [42–45]. This psychological distress leads people to be continuously worried about their health and future infection by SARS-CoV-2: depression, anxiety, boredom, loneliness, insomnia, or anger symptoms [46] are reported; in turn, adverse mental health statuses and loss of vitality enhance the fear toward COVID-19 infection.

Finally, we found partial support for H6 (path c') since the present study shows that only mental health but not vitality significantly mediates the relationship between perceived control over time and fear of COVID-19. We tested a parallel mediation model considering the effect of both mental health and vitality. We need to focus on the items' content measured by the SF-36 mental health and vitality subscales to understand this outcome. Indeed, on the one hand, the mental health subscale asks people to indicate what kind of emotions they feel, e.g., nervous, happy, peaceful, sad, or down in dumps; on the other hand, the vitality subscale requires people to indicate their level of energy, tiredness, and fatigue. Although the recent literature reported how fear of COVID-19 affects vitality [29] in line with the theory of perceived control, our results corroborate that ability to handle environmental stress is closely associated with emotional state. Controlling time alters individuals' perceptions regarding threats [47]. In turn, the crucial mediational role of mental health we found in the present study is supported by prior psychological literature about emotion regulation, demonstrating how emotions are critical factors for guiding individuals to avoid or cope with distressing situations, bringing about a positive outcome [48]. Therefore, we could argue that in managing such a negative situation as the COVID-19 pandemic, the loss of vitality represents more a physiological state related to inactivity and social isolation. Mental health statuses associated with emotions could, in contrast, vary during the day. Thus, even while experiencing exhaustion, positive or negative emotions are essential in modulating the relationship between perceived control over time and the fear of being infected. When people have favorable feelings, they also have a better perception of their time, manage their daily routines or working duties, and are less anxious toward the COVID-19 pandemic. Such a result has practical implications for developing treatment programs to enhance persons' capacity and competence to handle their daily activities, schedule their time, and use effective techniques based on emotional coping to prevent fear and anxiety toward the COVID-19 pandemic.

However, the present study has some limitations to report. First, the sample is based mainly on an Italian university population; thus, we cannot generalize to the entire general population. Further studies should be performed, for instance, on samples of workers or professionals to corroborate our results. A second limitation is the study's cross-sectional design, based on a sample mainly comprising women. Future studies should be based on a longitudinal design to compare the mental health and vitality statuses in the different lockdown phases and obtain a more balanced sample with regard to gender.

5. Conclusions

As suggested by the World Health Organization, mental health represents a public health priority [49], and it has become more significant nowadays due to the current COVID-19 pandemic. In sum, our study evidences the crucial mediating role of mental health between perceived control over time and COVID-19 anxiety. We measured mental health using the SF-36 mental health subscale assessing positive and adverse emotions. Hence, mental health could influence the perceived control over time, emotionally regulating people's behaviors in different life domains, such as for instance academic achievements [50], job performance [51], or social activities [52], improving well-being and quality of life. Thus, mental health also becomes a protective factor from psychopathological threats related to COVID-19 fear. Furthermore, our results have practical implications since they could help psychologists, psychiatrists, and educators define treatment programs and guide the states' governance measures combating psychological distress related to the COVID-19 pandemic.

Author Contributions: Conceptualization, S.M., B.C., and M.C.; methodology S.M. and B.C.; formal analysis, L.V. and G.Q.; data curation, L.V. and G.Q.; writing—original draft preparation, S.M., B.C., and M.C., writing—review and editing, S.M., B.C., M.R., and M.C.; supervision, S.M., M.R., and M.C. All authors have read and agreed to the published version of the manuscript.

Funding: This research received no external funding.

Institutional Review Board Statement: The study was conducted according to the guidelines of the Declaration of Helsinki and approved by the Bioethics Committee of the University of Palermo (n. 2/2020).

Informed Consent Statement: Informed consent was obtained from all subjects involved in the study.

Data Availability Statement: The data presented in this study are available on request from the corresponding author.

Conflicts of Interest: The authors declare no conflict of interest.

References

1. Wańkowicz, P.; Szylińska, A.; Rotter, I. Evaluation of Mental Health Factors among People with Systemic Lupus Erythematosus during the SARS-CoV-2 Pandemic. *J. Clin. Med.* **2020**, *9*, 2872. [CrossRef] [PubMed]
2. Wańkowicz, P.; Szylińska, A.; Rotter, I. The Impact of the COVID-19 Pandemic on Psychological Health and Insomnia among People with Chronic Diseases. *J. Clin. Med.* **2021**, *10*, 1206. [CrossRef] [PubMed]
3. Wańkowicz, P.; Szylińska, A.; Rotter, I. Insomnia, Anxiety, and Depression Symptoms during the COVID-19 Pandemic May Depend on the Pre-Existent Health Status Rather than the Profession. *Brain Sci.* **2021**, *11*, 1001. [CrossRef]
4. Qiu, J.; Shen, B.; Zhao, M.; Wang, Z.; Xie, B.; Xu, Y. A nationwide survey of psychological distress among Chinese people in the COVID-19 epidemic: Implications and policy recommendations. *Gen. Psychiatry* **2020**, *33*, e100213. [CrossRef]

5. Holmes, E.A.; O'Connor, R.C.; Perry, V.H.; Tracey, I.; Wessely, S.; Arseneault, L.; Ballard, C.; Christensen, H.; Silver, R.C.; Everall, I.; et al. Multidisciplinary research priorities for the COVID-19 pandemic: A call for action for mental health science. *Lancet Psychiatry* **2020**, *7*, 547–560. [CrossRef]
6. Favieri, F.; Forte, G.; Tambelli, R.; Casagrande, M. The Italians in the time of Coronavirus: Psychosocial aspects of unexpected COVID-19 pandemic. *Front. Psychol.* **2020**. [CrossRef]
7. Satici, B.; Gocet-Tekin, E.; Deniz, M.E.; Satici, S.A. Adaptation of the Fear of COVID-19 Scale: Its Association with Psychological Distress and Life Satisfaction in Turkey. *Int. J. Ment. Health Addict.* **2020**. [CrossRef]
8. Toyama, M.; Fuller, H.R. Longitudinal Associations Between Perceived Control and Health for American and Japanese Aging Adults. *Gerontologist* **2020**, 135. [CrossRef]
9. Caci, B.; Cardaci, M.; Miceli, S. Development and Maintenance of Self-Disclosure on Facebook: The Role of Personality Traits. *SAGE Open* **2019**, *9*, 1–14. [CrossRef]
10. Miceli, S.; Cardaci, M.; Scrima, F.; Caci, B. Time perspective and Facebook addiction: The moderating role of neuroticism. *Curr. Psychol.* **2021**. [CrossRef]
11. Holman, E.A.; Grisham, E.L. When time falls apart: The public health implications of distorted time perception in the age of COVID-19. *Psychol. Trauma: Theory Res. Pract. Policy* **2020**, *12*, S63–S65. [CrossRef] [PubMed]
12. Gallagher, R.P.; Borg, S.; Golin, A.; Kelleher, K. The personal, career, and learning skills needs of college students. *J. Coll. Stud. Dev.* **1992**, *33*, 301–310.
13. Chang, A.; Nguyen, L.T. The mediating effects of time structure on the relationships between time management behaviour, job satisfaction, and psychological well-being. *Aust. J. Psychol.* **2011**, *63*, 187–197. [CrossRef]
14. Nonis, S.A.; Hudson, G.I.; Logan, L.B.; Ford, C.W. Influence of Perceived Control over Time on College Students' Stress and Stress-Related Outcomes. *Res. High. Educ.* **1998**, *39*, 587–605. [CrossRef]
15. Ahorsu, D.K.; Lin, C.; Imani, V.; Saffari, M.; Griffiths, M.; Pakpour, A.H. The fear of COVID-19 scale: Development and initial validation. *Int. J. Ment. Health Addict.* **2020**. [CrossRef]
16. Bandura, A. *Social Learning Theory*; Prentice-Hall: Englewood Cliffs, NJ, USA, 1977.
17. Ross, C.E.; Sastry, J. The Sense of Personal Control. In *Handbook of the Sociology of Mental Health Handbooks of Sociology and Social, Research*; Aneshensel, C.S., Phelan, J.C., Eds.; Springer: Boston, MA, USA, 1999. [CrossRef]
18. Rotter, J.B. *Social Learning and Clinical Psychology*; Prentice-Hall, Inc.: Hoboken, NJ, USA, 1954.
19. Mirowsky, J.; Ross, C.E. Fundamental analysis in research on well-being: Distress and the sense of control. *Gerontologist* **1996**, *36*, 584–594. [CrossRef] [PubMed]
20. Hogan, J.M.; Carlson, J.G.; Dua, J. Stressors and stress reactions among university personnel. *Int. J. Stress Manag.* **2002**, *9*, 289–310. [CrossRef]
21. Kawabata, M.; Yamazaki, F.; Guo, D.W.; Chatzisarantis, N.L.D. Advancement of the Subjective Vitality Scale: Examining alternative measurement models for Japanese and Singaporeans. *Scand. J. Med. Sci. Sports* **2017**, *27*, 1793–1800. [CrossRef]
22. Ryan, R.M.; Deci, E.L. A self-determination theory approach to psychotherapy: The motivational basis for effective change. *Can. Psychol.* **2008**, *49*, 186–193. [CrossRef]
23. Uğur, E.; Kaya, Ç.; Özçelik, B. Subjective vitality mediates the relationship between respect toward partner and subjective happiness on teachers. *Univers. J. Educ. Res.* **2019**, *7*, 126–132. [CrossRef]
24. Arslan, G.; Yıldırım, M.; Tanhan, A.; Buluş, M.; Allen, K.-A. Coronavirus stress, optimism-pessimism, psychological inflexibility, and psychological health: Psychometric properties of the coronavirus stress measure. *Int. J. Ment. Health Addict.* **2020**. [CrossRef] [PubMed]
25. Rouse, P.C.; Van Zanten, J.J.V.; Ntoumanis, N.; Metsios, G.S.; Yu, C.; Kitas, G.D.; Duda, J.L. Measuring the positive psychological well-being of people with rheumatoid arthritis: A cross-sectional validation of the subjective vitality scale. *Arthritis Res. Ther.* **2015**, *17*, 312–318. [CrossRef]
26. Maniscalco, L.; Miceli, S.; Bono, F.; Matranga, D. Self-perceived health, objective health, and quality of life among people aged 50 and over: Interrelationship among health indicators in Italy, Spain, and Greece. *Int. J. Environ. Res. Public Health* **2020**, *17*, 2414. [CrossRef]
27. Lavrusheva, O. The concept of vitality. Review of the vitality-related research domain. *New Ideas Psychol.* **2020**, *56*, 100752. [CrossRef]
28. Muraven, M.; Gagné, M.; Rosman, H. Helpful self-control: Autonomy support, vitality, and depletion. *J. Exp. Soc. Psychol.* **2008**, *44*, 573–585. [CrossRef]
29. Morgul, E.; Bener, A.; Atak, M. COVID-19 pandemic and psychological fatigue in Turkey. *Int. J. Soc. Psychiatry* **2020**. [CrossRef]
30. Heckathorn, D.D. Respondent-Driven Sampling II: Deriving Valid Estimates from Chain-Referral Samples of Hidden Populations". In *Social Problems*; Oxford University Press: Oxford, UK, 2002; Volume 49, pp. 11–34. [CrossRef]
31. Macan, T.H.; Shahani, C.; Dipboye, R.L.; Phillips, A.P. College student's time management: Correlation with academic performance and stress. *J. Educ. Psychol.* **1990**, *82*, 760–768. [CrossRef]
32. Apolone, G.; Mosconi, P. The Italian SF-36 Health Survey: Translation, Validation, and Norming. *J. Clin. Epidemiol.* **1998**, *51*, 1025–1036. [CrossRef]
33. Hayes, A.F. Methodology in the social sciences. In *Introduction to Mediation, Moderation, and Conditional Process Analysis: A Regression-Based Approach*; Guilford Press: New York, NY, USA, 2013.

34. Baron, R.M.; Kenny, D.A. The moderator-mediator variable distinction in social psychological research: Conceptual, strategic, and statistical considerations. *J. Personal. Soc. Psychol.* **1986**, *51*, 1173–1182. [CrossRef]
35. Lei, Z.; Miao, M.; Yiqun, G. Perceived Control Buffers the Effects of the COVID-19 Pandemic on General Health and Life Satisfaction: The Mediating Role of Psychological Distance. *Appl. Psychol. Health Well-Being* **2020**, *12*, 1095–1114. [CrossRef]
36. Fritzsche, B.A.; Young, B.R.; Hickson, K.C. Individual differences in academic procrastination tendency and writing success. *Personal. Individ. Differ.* **2003**, *35*, 1549–1557. [CrossRef]
37. König, C.J.; Kleinmann, M. Deadline rush: A time management phenomenon and its mathematical description. *J. Psychol.* **2005**, *139*, 33–45. [CrossRef]
38. Ross, C.E.; Mirowsky, J. Age and the gender gap in the sense of personal control. *Soc. Psychol. Q.* **2002**, *65*, 125–145. [CrossRef]
39. Kret, M.E.; De Gelder, B. A review on sex differences in processing emotional signals. *Neuropsychologia* **2012**, *50*, 1211–1221. [CrossRef]
40. Elst, T.V.; Van den Broeck, A.; De Cuyper, N.; De Witte, H. On the reciprocal relationship between job insecurity and employee well-being: Mediation by perceived control? *J. Occup. Organ. Psychol.* **2014**, *87*, 671–693. [CrossRef]
41. Hofmann, W.; Luhmann, M.; Fisher, R.R.; Vohs, K.D.; Baumeister, R.F. Yes, but are they happy? Effects of trait self-control on affective well-being and life satisfaction. *J. Pers.* **2014**, *82*, 265–277. [CrossRef] [PubMed]
42. Caci, B.; Miceli, S.; Scrima, F.; Cardaci, M. Neuroticism and Fear of COVID-19, The Interplay Between Boredom, Fantasy Engagement, and Perceived Control Over Time. *Front. Psychol.* **2020**, *11*, 574393. [CrossRef] [PubMed]
43. Reznik, A.; Gritsenko, V.; Konstantinov, V.; Khamenka, N.; Isralowitz, R. COVID-19 Fear in Eastern Europe: Validation of the Fear of COVID-19 Scale. *Int. J. Ment. Health Addict.* **2020**, *12*, 1–6. [CrossRef]
44. Midorikawa, H.; Aiba, M.; Lebowitz, A.; Taguchi, T.; Shiratori, Y.; Ogawa, T.; Takahashi, A.; Takahashi, S.; Nemoto, K.; Arai, T.; et al. Confirming validity of The Fear of COVID-19 Scale in Japanese with a nationwide large-scale sample. *PLoS ONE* **2021**, *16*, e0246840. [CrossRef] [PubMed]
45. Lin, C.; Hou, W.; Mamun, M.A.; da Silva, J.A.; Broche-Pérez, Y.; Ullah, I.; Masuyama, A.; Wakashima, K.; Mailliez, M.; Carre, A.; et al. Fear of COVID-19 Scale (FCV-19S) across countries: Measurement invariance issues. *Nurs. Open* **2021**, *8*, 1892–1908. [CrossRef]
46. Fitzpatrick, K.M.; Harris, C.; Drawve, G. Fear of COVID-19 and the mental health consequences in America. *Psychol. Trauma* **2020**, *12*, S17–S21. [CrossRef]
47. Witt, J.K.; Proffitt, D.R.; Epstein, W. Tool use affects perceived distance but only when you intend to use it. *J. Exp. Psychol.* **2005**, *31*, 880–888. [CrossRef]
48. Hartley, C.; Phelps, E. Changing Fear: The Neurocircuitry of Emotion Regulation. *Neuropsychopharmacology* **2010**, *35*, 136–146. [CrossRef]
49. World Health Organization. *World Health Statistics 2013, World Health Organization*. 2013. Available online: https://apps.who.int/iris/handle/10665/81965 (accessed on 10 August 2021).
50. You, S.; Hong, S.; Ho, H.-Z. Longitudinal Effects of Perceived Control on Academic Achievement. *J. Educ. Res.* **2011**, *104*, 253–266. [CrossRef]
51. Brockner, J.; Spreitzer, G.; Mishra, A.K.; Hochwarter, W.; Pepper, L.; Weinberg, J. Perceived Control as an Antidote to the Negative Effects of Layoffs on Survivors' Organizational Commitment and Job Performance. *Adm. Sci. Q.* **2004**, *49*, 76–100. [CrossRef]
52. Miceli, S.; Maniscalco, L.; Matranga, D. Social networks and social activities promote cognitive functioning in both concurrent and prospective time: Evidence from the SHARE survey. *Eur. J. Ageing* **2019**, *16*, 145–154. [CrossRef]

Journal of
Clinical Medicine

MDPI

Article

The Assessment of the Severity of COVID-19-Related Anxiety Symptoms in Participants of the University of the Third Age in Poland: A Cross-Sectional Study among Internet Survey Respondents

Mateusz Cybulski [1,*], Urszula Cwalina [2], Dorota Sadowska [3] and Elżbieta Krajewska-Kułak [1]

1 Department of Integrated Medical Care, Faculty of Health Sciences, Medical University of Białystok, M. Skłodowskiej-Curie 7A str., 15-096 Białystok, Poland; elzbieta.krajewska-kulak@umb.edu.pl
2 Department of Medical Statistics and Health Informatics, Faculty of Health Sciences, Medical University of Białystok, Szpitalna 37 str., 15-295 Białystok, Poland; urszula.cwalina@umb.edu.pl
3 Department of Endocrinology, Diabetology and Internal Medicine, Faculty of Medicine, Medical University of Białystok, M. Skłodowskiej-Curie 24A str., 15-276 Białystok, Poland; dorotasad@gmail.com
* Correspondence: mateusz.cybulski@umb.edu.pl; Tel.: +48-(85)-686-51-08

Abstract: Introduction: Fear of infection with SARS-CoV-2 has become widespread. All over the world, since the very beginning of the pandemic, older adults have been considered one of the groups at highest risk of SARS-CoV-2 infection and death due to COVID-19. The aim of the study was to evaluate the severity of anxiety symptoms related to COVID-19 in the older adults who are participants of the Universities of the Third Age in Poland. Material and methods: The study included participants of the University of the Third Age in Poland. A total of 296 persons were enrolled, including 258 women and 38 men. The study was a diagnostic survey, conducted with the use of the following validated psychometric scales: General Anxiety Disorder-7 (GAD-7), Short Health Anxiety Inventory (SHAI), and State-Trait Anxiety Inventory (STAI). Results: In two scales (STAI and SHAI), the mean scores demonstrated mild symptoms indicative of anxiety disorders in the older respondents. Women and men did differ significantly in terms of the scores obtained in STAI X-1 and STAI X-2. Single respondents differed significantly from divorced ones in terms of STAI X-1 scores. Moreover, widows/widowers differed significantly from divorced ones in terms of STAI X-2, and GAD-7 scores. Respondents declaring their financial status as average differed significantly from those declaring their financial status as good in terms of: STAI X-1, STAI X-2, SHAI, and GAD-7 scores. Conclusions: The subjective experience of anxiety symptoms associated with fear of contracting COVID-19 was increased due to the ongoing pandemic, but was not significantly high in the analysed population of older people. COVID-19-related anxiety was significantly more common in lonely individuals and in those of worse financial status. Women and men differed significantly in terms of perceived state anxiety and trait anxiety measured by STAI. More studies addressing COVID-19-related anxiety in older people participating in the Polish Universities of the Third Age are needed to determine a more accurate distribution of this phenomenon in Poland.

Keywords: anxiety; COVID-19; fear; general anxiety disorder-7 (GAD-7); older adults; SARS-CoV-2; short health anxiety inventory (SHAI); state-trait anxiety inventory (STAI)

Citation: Cybulski, M.; Cwalina, U.; Sadowska, D.; Krajewska-Kułak, E. The Assessment of the Severity of COVID-19-Related Anxiety Symptoms in Participants of the University of the Third Age in Poland: A Cross-Sectional Study among Internet Survey Respondents. *J. Clin. Med.* **2021**, *10*, 3862. https://doi.org/10.3390/jcm10173862

Academic Editors: Michele Roccella and Allan H. Young

Received: 28 July 2021
Accepted: 26 August 2021
Published: 27 August 2021

1. Introduction

A series of cases of pneumonia of an unknown cause appeared at the end of 2019 in the Chinese province of Wuhan [1]. Several weeks later, in January 2020, the analysis of lab samples revealed a new virus, SARS-CoV-2, that induces an acute respiratory disease [2] which, on 11 February 2020, was referred to as COVID-19 by the World Health Organisation (WHO) Director-General, while on 11 March 2020, the WHO announced the pandemic [3].

On 27 July 2021, the number of all identified coronavirus infections in the world reached 194,995,684, of which 4,173,104 patients died due to the infection [4].

Fear of infection with SARS-CoV-2 has become widespread. It is constantly being enhanced by the media reports, where particular emphasis is put on the epidemiological data on mortality and incidence, dramatic information from intensive care units, and news about lacking healthcare resources. An additional factor that increases perceived anxiety is the so-called social distancing principle, which entails restrictions in interpersonal contact [5–7]. The estimated overall prevalence of anxiety in the general population during the COVID-19 pandemic is 25% [8]. In specific groups, the prevalence of fear of COVID-19 is varied, for example among medical students [9] and healthcare professionals [10] is also 25%, but among college students—36% [11].

All over the world, since the very beginning of the pandemic, older adults have been considered one of the groups at highest risk of SARS-CoV-2 infection and death due to COVID-19 [12]. The increased risk of contracting the disease and death depends on several factors. Firstly, Poland is one of the top European countries in terms of the number of confirmed COVID-19 cases. As of 27 July 2021, there have been 2,882,327 cases, of which 75,249 were fatal [13]. Moreover, the prevalence of chronic diseases, entailing multimorbidity, is high amongst the older adults all over the world, including in Poland, which increases the risk of severe health-related sequelae, including those related to COVID-19 [14]. The prevalence of multimorbidity in Poland is 38.7% [15].

Although, in principle, COVID-19 may evoke considerable fear among the older adults, there are no sufficient data about the perceived fear resulting from the ongoing COVID-19 pandemic in Poland, especially amongst actively ageing older people. The aim of the study was therefore to evaluate the severity of anxiety symptoms related to COVID-19 among the older adults who are participants of the Universities of the Third Age in Poland. In addition, it was evaluated how selected sociodemographic characteristics affect the level of anxiety symptoms in this subgroup of the older population from Poland. It was assumed that the level of anxiety symptoms among participants of the University of the Third Age will be relatively high. Additionally, we hypothesized that anxiety disorders related to the fear of COVID-19 would occur more frequently among women, single people, and people with lower education.

2. Materials and Methods

2.1. Participants

The study included participants of the University of the Third Age programme in Poland. A total of 296 persons were enrolled, including 258 women and 38 men. Over half of the respondents (54.73%) were in the age range from 60 to 69 years. A similar percentage of the respondents (51.35%) were married. Almost three-quarters of the University of the Third Age participants (71.96%) had higher education (Master's degree). Nearly one-third of the older adults lived in large cities (over 500,000 inhabitants). The vast majority of the respondents (91.55%) were retired. Eighteen respondents had a history of mental disorders. These were: depressive disorders (n = 13), bipolar disorder (n = 1) and anxiety disorder (n = 4).

Detailed sociodemographic characteristics of the respondents are shown in Table 1.

Table 1. Sociodemographic characteristics of the respondents.

Sociodemographic Feature		n	%
Sex	male	38	87.16%
	female	258	12.84%
Age	60–69 years	162	54.73%
	70–79 years	118	39.86%
	80–89 years	16	5.41%

Table 1. *Cont.*

Sociodemographic Feature		n	%
Marital status	married	152	51.35%
	widow/widower	75	25.34%
	separated	20	6.76%
	divorced	46	15.54%
	single	3	1.01%
Education	higher	213	71.96%
	secondary	76	25.68%
	technical	6	2.03%
	vocational	1	0.34%
Place of residence	village	24	8.11%
	town up to 50 thousand	84	28.38%
	town up to 200 thousand	37	12.50%
	city up to 500 thousand	48	16.22%
	city over 500 thousand	103	34.80%
Financial status	very bad	1	0.34%
	bad	2	0.68%
	average	114	38.51%
	good	153	51.69%
	very good	26	8.78%
Socio-professional status	retirement pensions	271	91.55%
	disability pensions	4	1.35%
	professionally active	21	7.09%
Voivodeship	Lower Silesian	32	10.81%
	Kuyavian-Pomeranian	2	0.68%
	Lublin	12	4.05%
	Lubusz	7	2.36%
	Łódź	1	0.34%
	Lesser Poland	67	22.64%
	Masovian	49	16.55%
	Opole	2	0.68%
	Subcarpathian	7	2.36%
	Podlaskie	61	20.61%
	Pomeranian	9	3.04%
	Silesian	23	7.77%
	Świętokrzyskie	4	1.35%
	Warmian-Masurian	16	5.41%
	Greater Poland	1	0.34%
	West Pomeranian	3	1.01%
History of mental disorders	yes	18	6.08%
	no	278	93.92%

2.2. Study Design and Data Collection

The cross-sectional study was conducted between 1 March and 10 May 2021. The invitations were sent to official e-mail addresses published on the websites of all University of the Third Age chapters in Poland. In this study, the snowball sampling method was employed; it is a non-random sample selection method consisting in recruiting participants by other participants (in our study by the Presidents of Universities of the Third Age or substantive coordinators the Universities that offer such forms of education for the older adults). We used this method in our study as we did not have a contact database for direct students of Universities of the Third Age.

The study involved an online survey created using dedicated software (Webankieta) (Get Feedback, Warsaw, Poland). A link to the survey was included in the invitation e-mails sent to the addresses available on the official University websites. The responses were recorded on the platform, and then downloaded as raw data prepared for a statistical analysis. The mean time to complete the survey was 29 min.

Apart from age and enrolment in the University of the Third Age programme, an additional inclusion criterion was written informed consent to participate in the study. The exclusion criteria were: (1) age ≤ 60 years; (2) illiteracy (a respondent who had completed at least primary school could participate in the study); and (3) lack of written consent to participate in the study. Each participant could withdraw from the study at any time.

The respondents were chosen by nonprobability sampling. Taking into account the total number of returned questionnaires, the rate of complete filling was 52.7%. The remaining questionnaires were incomplete (47.3%).

2.3. Measures

The study was a diagnostic survey, conducted with the use of the following validated psychometric scales: General Anxiety Disorder-7 (GAD-7), Short Health Anxiety Inventory (SHAI), and State-Trait Anxiety Inventory (STAI). The authors of the study asked respondents that questions from all standardized research tools used in the study should relate directly to fear of COVID-19.

2.3.1. State-Trait Anxiety Inventory (STAI)

The structure of the STAI tool is based on differentiating between anxiety understood as a transitory and situation-dependent state, and anxiety understood as a relatively constant personality trait. In his concept, Spielberger referred to other, earlier studies conducted by R.B. Cattell and I.H. Scheier [16]. They identified two different factors. The first, responsible for situation-dependent score variability, was called "state anxiety". The other, responsible for inter-individual differences, was termed "trait anxiety". The STAI questionnaire consists of two independent parts, each containing 20 statements. The first part, STAI X-1, can evaluate anxiety considered as the current emotional state. This part of the questionnaire is a very sensitive tool. It enables one to trace the dynamics of anxiety even in short time intervals. The other part, STAI X-2, concerns anxiety understood as a personality trait [17]. The patient responds to each statement by choosing one of 4 options. The level of anxiety is expressed as the score resulting from summing up the sub-scores obtained for all individual responses. The scores from each part of the questionnaire may vary from 20 to 80. The test is interpreted in the following way: the higher the score, the higher the level of perceived anxiety. The score range of 39–40 in state anxiety evaluation suggests the detection of clinical symptoms of anxiety disorder [18,19]. The psychometric value of the test makes it useful in group studies. The test reliability, based on the internal consistency coefficient, varies from 0.76 to 0.92 in adult women and men. The construct validity of the X-1 scale ranges from 0.51 for men to 0.57 for women [17].

2.3.2. Short Health Anxiety Inventory (SHAI)

The Short Health Anxiety Inventory (SHAI) is an 18-item scale designed to evaluate anxiety in two components of hypochondriasis: probability of disease and negative disease consequences. Each of the 18 items contains four statements of which respondents choose one that best describes their feelings over the past 6 months. The responses are scored on a 4-point scale where: 0—no symptoms, 1—mild symptoms, 2—severe symptoms, and 3—very severe symptoms. A cut-off score of 20 was optimal for detecting a severe form of health anxiety, providing the best balance between specificity and sensitivity [20,21].

2.3.3. Generalised Anxiety Disorder Assessment (GAD-7)

The GAD-7 is a 7-item scale that is based on the Likert scale. It can be used when evaluating the level of anxiety and the risk of generalised anxiety disorder (GAD). The questions included in the survey evaluate the respondent's feeling of anxiety, tension, nervousness, ability to control these feelings, how easily they appear and how problematic it is to relax. The respondent can obtain 0–3 points for each item, depending on the selected response, i.e., the frequency with which each problem occurs in the respondent (0—not at all; 1—several days; 2—more than half the days; 3—nearly every day). The evaluation concerns the past 14 days. The scores of 5, 10, and 15 indicate mild, moderate, and severe anxiety, respectively. The score of at least 10 indicates that generalised anxiety disorder is very likely [22].

2.4. *Procedure and Ethical Considerations*

The study was carried out in accordance with the recommendations, and was reviewed and approved by the Ethics Committee of the Medical University of Bialystok (No. R-I-002/592/2019). All subjects gave the written informed consent in accordance with the Declaration of Helsinki.

2.5. *Statistical Analysis*

The data were processed with Microsoft Excel 2020 spreadsheet and analysed with Statistica Data Miner C QC PL package. Normal distribution of quantitative variables was checked with the Shapiro–Wilk W-test. As none of the variables was distributed normally, they were analysed using non-parametric tests; the significance of the differences between two groups was verified with the Mann–Whitney U-test, and multiple groups were compared using Kruskal–Wallis ANOVA and appropriate post hoc tests. The associations between the pairs of quantitative variables were analysed based on the Spearman's coefficients of rank correlation. The results of all tests were considered significant at $p < 0.05$.

3. Results

Table 2 presents descriptive statistics of the standardised research tools applied in this study. In two scales (STAI and SHAI), the mean scores demonstrated mild symptoms indicative of anxiety disorders in the older respondents. In the remaining scale (GAD-7), the means scores were not sufficient to identify the presence of anxiety symptoms related to COVID-19. The detailed values for individual variables are listed in Table 2.

Table 2. Descriptive statistics for the scales applied in the study.

	$\bar{x}$	SD	Min.	Q_1	Me	Q_3	Max.
STAI X-1	44.48	11.38	20.00	37.00	43.00	53.00	77.00
STAI X-2	41.83	8.59	21.00	36.00	41.50	47.00	67.00
SHAI	14.62	7.23	1.00	9.00	14.00	19.00	41.00
GAD-7	4.51	4.66	0.00	1.00	3.00	7.00	21.00

Abbreviations: GAD-7—General Anxiety Disorder-7, Max.—maximum, Me—median, Min.—minimum, SD—standard deviation, SHAI—Short Health Anxiety Inventory, STAI—State-Trait Anxiety Inventory, Q_1—lower quartile, Q_3—upper quartile, and $\bar{x}$—mean.

Table 3 presents the prevalence of anxiety symptoms among students of University of the Third Age according to the standardized cut-off points. Most of the respondents showed anxiety symptoms measured by the STAI. Similarly, most older adults showed minimal or mild anxiety symptoms based on the GAD-7 scores. On the other hand, over 3/4 of the respondents did not show symptoms of anxiety disorders on the basis of the SHAI (Table 3).

Table 3. Prevalence of anxiety symptoms among students of University of the Third Age according to the standardized cut-off points.

	Cut-Off Points	n	%
STAI X-1	<40 (no symptoms)	103	34.7%
	≥40 (anxiety symptoms)	194	65.3%
STAI X-2	<40 (no symptoms)	119	40.1%
	≥40 (anxiety symptoms)	178	59.9%
SHAI	<20 (no symptoms)	226	76.1%
	≥20 (anxiety symptoms)	71	23.9%
GAD-7	0 (no symptoms)	66	22.2%
	1–4 (minimal symptoms)	109	36.7%
	5–9 (mild symptoms)	83	28.0%
	10–14 (moderate symptoms)	23	7.7%
	15–21 (severe symptoms)	16	5.4%

Abbreviations: GAD-7—General Anxiety Disorder-7, SHAI—Short Health Anxiety Inventory, and STAI—State-Trait Anxiety Inventory.

The analysis of the scores obtained using the applied scales in the study group, taking into account the individual sociodemographic variables, indicated that women and men did differ significantly in terms of the scores obtained in STAI X-1 ($p = 0.002$) and STAI X-2 ($p = 0.020$) (Table 4).

Table 4. Impact of sex on the scores obtained in the psychometric scales applied in the study.

	Women (n = 258)		Men (n = 38)		p
	$\bar{x} \pm$ SD	Me	$\bar{x} \pm$ SD	Me	
STAI X-1	45.26 ± 11.56	44	39.21 ± 8.39	39	0.002 *
STAI X-2	42.27 ± 8.73	42	38.84 ± 6.88	38	0.020 *
SHAI	14.84 ± 7.39	14	13.08 ± 5.92	12	0.205
GAD-7	4.69 ± 4.82	4	3.26 ± 3.23	2	0.195

Abbreviations: GAD-7—General Anxiety Disorder-7, Me—median, p—p-value, SD—standard deviation, SHAI—Short Health Anxiety Inventory, STAI—State-Trait Anxiety Inventory, $\bar{x}$—mean, and *—statistically significant.

There were no statistically significant differences between respondents with higher education and those with a different level of education. Nor were there any statistically significant differences between professionally active respondents and pensioners. A number of statistically significant differences were noted for the results of the applied scales in terms of the marital status. The analysis revealed that single respondents differed significantly from divorced ones in terms of STAI X-1 scores ($p = 0.046$). Moreover, widows/widowers differed significantly from divorced ones in terms of STAI X-2 ($p = 0.045$), and GAD-7 scores ($p = 0.032$) (Table 5).

Table 5. Impact of marital status on the scores obtained in the psychometric scales applied in the study *.

	Married (I) (n = 152)		Widow/Widower (II) (n = 75)		Separated (III) (n = 20)		Divorced (IV) (n = 46)		p	
	$\bar{x} \pm$ SD	Me	$\bar{x} \pm$ SD	Me	$\bar{x} \pm$ SD	Me	$\bar{x} \pm$ SD	Me	K-W	Post hoc
STAI X-1	44.68 ± 10.91	43	43.07 ± 11.44	42	39.8 ± 8.41	40.5	48.59 ± 12.91	48	0.046	III–IV: 0.046
STAI X-2	41.89 ± 7.54	42	40.41 ± 8.84	40	38.8 ± 8.68	39	45.39 ± 10.51	46	0.021	II–IV: 0.045
SHAI	14.01 ± 6.89	13	14.37 ± 7.12	13	14.6 ± 6.75	15	17.04 ± 8.5	16.5	0.1636	-
GAD-7	4.72 ± 4.64	4	3.41 ± 3.87	3	3.45 ± 3.9	2	6.24 ± 5.75	4.5	0.017	II–IV: 0.032

* The table also includes statistically significant results of the post hoc tests; for the remaining comparisons $p > 0.05$. Abbreviations: GAD-7—General Anxiety Disorder-7, K-W—Kruskal–Wallis test, Me—median, p—p-value, SD—standard deviation, SHAI—Short Health Anxiety Inventory, STAI—State-Trait Anxiety Inventory, and $\bar{x}$—mean.

Respondents declaring their financial status as average differed significantly from those declaring their financial status as good in terms of: STAI X-1, STAI X-2, SHAI, and GAD-7 scores. Details are included in Table 6.

Table 6. Impact of financial status on the scores obtained in the psychometric scales applied in the study *.

	Very Good (I) (n = 26)		Good (II) (n = 153)		Average (III) (n = 114)		p	
	$\bar{x} \pm$ SD	Me	$\bar{x} \pm$ SD	Me	$\bar{x} \pm$ SD	Me	K-W	Post hoc
STAI X-1	43 ± 11.85	41	42.84 ± 10.65	41	46.72 ± 11.83	47	0.010	II–III: 0.011
STAI X-2	39.5 ± 9.58	39	40.56 ± 7.68	40	43.82 ± 8.93	45	0.002	II–III: 0.005
SHAI	12.92 ± 7.21	11.5	13.71 ± 6.66	13	16.03 ± 7.49	15	0.017	II–III: 0.035
GAD-7	3.96 ± 4.46	3	3.85 ± 4.25	3	5.39 ± 5.01	4	0.023	II–III: 0.027

* The table also includes statistically significant results of the post hoc tests; for the remaining comparisons $p > 0.05$. Abbreviations: GAD-7—General Anxiety Disorder-7, K-W—Kruskal–Wallis test, Me—median, p—p-value, SD—standard deviation, SHAI—Short Health Anxiety Inventory, STAI—State-Trait Anxiety Inventory, and $\bar{x}$—mean.

When analysing the obtained data, no statistically significant association was found between age and scores of the individual scales. Moreover, the respondents were divided into subgroups by sex, marital status, level of education, and place of residence, and the associations between age and scale scores were also analysed within these individual subgroups. Taking into account the division by education, the significance was found for the correlation between age and STAI X-1 ($r = -0.140$, $p = 0.042$) in the group of people with higher education. As for the remaining divisions, the results obtained in the subgroups confirmed the results obtained in the full set analysis and, consequently, no significant correlation between age and scores of the applied scales was found.

The study also involved relationships between the values of all applied scales. It was found that each of the correlation coefficients was positive, high, and statistically significant (Table 7). Moreover, an analogous analysis was performed in subgroups, taking into account sex, marital status, education, and place of residence. All of the resultant correlation coefficients were positive, high, and statistically significant.

Table 7. Spearman's rank correlations between standardised psychometric scales used in the study.

		STAI X-1	STAI X-2	SHAI
STAI X-2	r	0.789	—	—
	p	<0.001 *		
SHAI	r	0.584	0.625	—
	p	<0.001 *	<0.001 *	
GAD-7	r	0.691	0.758	0.554
	p	<0.001 *	<0.001 *	<0.001 *

Abbreviations: GAD-7—General Anxiety Disorder-7, p—p-value, r—Spearman's rank correlation coefficient, SHAI—Short Health Anxiety Inventory, STAI—State-Trait Anxiety Inventory, and *—statistically significant.

4. Discussion

This study is one of the first to determine the correlation between various sociodemographic factors and perceived anxiety related to the ongoing COVID-19 pandemic in the older Polish population. It was shown that the actively ageing older people experience various levels of anxiety symptoms related to COVID-19, depending on the applied scales. However, none of the scales yielded sufficiently high results to identify high COVID-19-related anxiety, and the set research hypothesis was therefore not confirmed in this study.

Although the present study demonstrated only mild anxiety symptoms in STAI and SHAI scales, other studies among the older adults from other countries have revealed that COVID-19 contributes to the worsening of mental health in this age group, primarily due to anxiety related to death, which is a consequence of this disease [23,24].

In our study, the prevalence of anxiety symptoms as measured by GAD-7 was 41.1%, including 28% of mild, 7.7% of moderate, and 5.4% of severe anxiety symptoms. Another Polish study, conducted using the same tool among university students, found that the prevalence of anxiety was high and was 65%, including 32% of mild, 21% of moderate, and 14% cases of severe anxiety disorder [25]. It is worth noting that higher percentages were recorded among young adults, not seniors. These differences could have been influenced by the timing of the study (young people were examined at the beginning of the pandemic) and the size of the group (the group of students was much larger than the group of seniors).

The present study showed that age was not linked significantly with anxiety related to developing COVID-19. These results are in line with previous studies, both Polish [26] and conducted abroad [27–29], which have shown that age is negatively correlated with anxiety symptoms during the pandemic. The available literature contains publications that did confirm high anxiety in the oldest age groups, particularly in China [30,31].

The present study did not show any statistically significant differences between professionally active respondents and those that finished their career (receiving retirement or disability pensions). The reverse was observed by Mistry et al. [32]. These authors found that older people who were unemployed or retired felt anxious about contracting COVID-19, and about its negative consequences, significantly more often. The same study [32] also confirmed a similar relationship as in the present study, namely that subjects with a worse financial status experienced stronger COVID-19-related anxiety than people with a better financial status.

The present study demonstrated that women were characterised by a higher level of COVID-19-related anxiety than men. The obtained values are in line with evidence provided by other authors confirming that women more often complain about stronger anxiety symptoms compared to men [25,33,34]. Other authors have also observed this relationship in their studies; for instance, in the study involving the Chinese population, women reported stronger worries related to developing COVID-19 than men [35]. In the present study, the overrepresentation of women compared to men in the study population could have affected the resulting higher level of anxiety. The finding that female sex is a predictor of anxiety suggests (as does the report of Naharci et al. [36]) that older women are more susceptible to mental health risks associated with COVID-19. The previous COVID-19-related studies reported mixed results regarding the association between sex and anxiety disorders. Two population-based studies showed that women tend to worry more often and are more susceptible to mental problems [37,38]. A recent literature review suggested that women have a tendency to develop a more psychological anxiety experience [39]. Nonetheless, further studies are needed to reflect sex-based differences in stress exposure related to developing infectious diseases.

In the study conducted by Islam et al. [40], it was shown that generalised anxiety was not significantly correlated with respondents' education—a finding in line with the present study. Regarding educational level, the results revealed that older adults with higher education levels had lower levels of anxiety. This is consistent with the findings reported in Italy [41] and Egypt [42] which showed that lower level of education directly indicates the beginning of the increased pandemic stress. This may be attributed to the fact that education is the foundation for successful coping. On the other hand, some studies suggested that people with higher education tended to be more concerned, perhaps due to a high degree of self-awareness of their well-being [30]. The novel nature of coronavirus disease and changing perceptions about the disease are one of the main factors justifying these opposite results.

The current facts suggest that certain groups of people (for example, older adults) may be especially prone to experiencing generalised anxiety in the initial stages of the COVID-19 pandemic, and further investigations are needed to specify the causes and develop appropriate interventions to improve the public health of the entire population.

Limitations

The present study does have certain, potential limitations. First, it was a cross-sectional study, based only on a self-reportable survey. Although the applied scales are sensitive tools designed to detect anxiety symptoms, they all focus on subjective symptoms, rather than objective clinical criteria, which poses a risk of false-positive results. Second, the study group was too small to generalise the results to the whole population of Polish older people attending Universities of the Third Age. Third, the study group was overrepresented by women, and therefore the results should be also verified in a larger group of men. However, both the actual rate of University of the Third Age participants and the actual demographic trends in the Polish population distinguish a high rate of women in relation to men. Despite these limitations, the results of this research can be a starting point for further studies addressing anxiety symptoms caused by fear of developing COVID-19 and its sociodemographic determinants amongst participants of Universities of the Third Age. A longitudinal study could provide optimal answers to these questions.

5. Conclusions

1. The subjective experience of anxiety symptoms associated with fear of contracting COVID-19 was increased due to the ongoing pandemic, but was not significantly high in the analysed population of older people;
2. COVID-19-related anxiety was significantly more common in lonely individuals (widows/widowers, divorced individuals, and single persons) and in those of worse financial status;
3. Women and men differed significantly in terms of perceived state anxiety and trait anxiety measured by STAI;
4. More studies are needed addressing COVID-19-related anxiety in the older adults participating in the Polish Universities of the Third Age to determine a more accurate distribution of this phenomenon in Poland.

Author Contributions: Conceptualization, M.C.; Data curation, M.C., D.S. and E.K.-K.; Formal analysis, M.C. and U.C.; Funding acquisition, M.C.; Investigation, M.C., D.S. and E.K.-K.; Methodology, M.C. and U.C.; Project administration, M.C.; Writing—original draft, M.C. and U.C.; and

Writing—review and editing, M.C. and E.K.-K. All authors have read and agreed to the published version of the manuscript.

Funding: The research was financed by the funds from the Medical University of Białystok with a grant no. SUB/3/DN/21/001/3310 awarded by the Polish Ministry of Education and Science in the form of a subvention for maintaining and developing research potential in 2021. The APC was funded by Medical University of Białystok.

Institutional Review Board Statement: The study was conducted according to the guidelines of the Declaration of Helsinki, and approved by the Ethics Committee of the Medical University of Białystok, Poland (No. R-I-002/592/2019).

Informed Consent Statement: Informed consent was obtained from all the subjects involved in the study.

Data Availability Statement: Data are available upon reasonable request.

Acknowledgments: The authors thank the all respondents who participated in the study.

Conflicts of Interest: The authors declare no conflict of interest. The funders had no role in the design of the study; in the collection, analyses, or interpretation of data; in the writing of the manuscript, or in the decision to publish the results.

References

1. Lu, H.; Stratton, C.W.; Tang, Y.W. Outbreak of pneumonia of unknown etiology in Wuhan, China: The mystery and the miracle. *J. Med. Virol.* **2020**, *92*, 401–402. [CrossRef] [PubMed]
2. Huang, C.; Wang, Y.; Li, X.; Ren, L.; Zhao, J.; Hu, Y.; Zhang, L.; Fan, G.; Xu, J.; Gu, X.; et al. Clinical features of patients infected with 2019 novel coronavirus in Wuhan, China. *Lancet* **2020**, *395*, 497–506. [CrossRef]
3. World Health Organization: Coronavirus Disease (COVID-19) Pandemic. Available online: https://www.who.int/emergencies/diseases/novel-coronavirus-2019 (accessed on 27 July 2021).
4. COVID-19 Dashboard by the Center for Systems Science and Engineering (CSSE) at Johns Hopkins University (JHU). Available online: https://gisanddata.maps.arcgis.com/apps/dashboards/bda7594740fd40299423467b48e9ecf6 (accessed on 27 July 2021).
5. Chen, Q.; Liang, M.; Li, Y.; Guo, J.; Fei, D.; Wang, L.; He, L.; Sheng, C.; Cai, Y.; Li, X.; et al. Mental health care for medical staff in China during the COVID-19 outbreak. *Lancet Psychiatry* **2020**, *7*, e15–e16. [CrossRef]
6. Yang, Y.; Li, W.; Zhang, Q.; Zhang, L.; Cheung, T.; Xiang, Y.T. Mental health services for older adults in China during the COVID-19 outbreak. *Lancet Psychiatry* **2020**, *7*, e19. [CrossRef]
7. Smirni, P.; Lavanco, G.; Smirni, D. Anxiety in Older Adolescents at the Time of COVID-19. *J. Clin. Med.* **2020**, *9*, 3064. [CrossRef] [PubMed]
8. Santabárbara, J.; Lasheras, I.; Lipnicki, D.M.; Bueno-Notivol, J.; Pérez-Moreno, M.; López-Antón, R.; De la Cámara, C.; Lobo, A.; Gracia-García, P. Prevalence of anxiety in the COVID-19 pandemic: An updated meta-analysis of community-based studies. *Prog. Neuropsychopharmacol. Biol. Psychiatry* **2021**, *109*, 110207. [CrossRef]
9. Lasheras, I.; Gracia-García, P.; Lipnicki, D.M.; Bueno-Notivol, J.; López-Antón, R.; de la Cámara, C.; Lobo, A.; Santabárbara, J. Prevalence of Anxiety in Medical Students during the COVID-19 Pandemic: A Rapid Systematic Review with Meta-Analysis. *Int. J. Environ. Res. Public Health* **2020**, *17*, 6603. [CrossRef]
10. Santabárbara, J.; Bueno-Notivol, J.; Lipnicki, D.M.; Olaya, B.; Pérez-Moreno, M.; Gracia-García, P.; Idoiaga-Mondragon, N.; Ozamiz-Etxebarria, N. Prevalence of anxiety in health care professionals during the COVID-19 pandemic: A rapid systematic review (on published articles in Medline) with meta-analysis. *Prog. Neuropsychopharmacol. Biol. Psychiatry* **2021**, *107*, 110244. [CrossRef]
11. Li, Y.; Wang, A.; Wu, Y.; Han, N.; Huang, H. Impact of the COVID-19 Pandemic on the Mental Health of College Students: A Systematic Review and Meta-Analysis. *Front. Psychol.* **2021**, *12*, 669119. [CrossRef]
12. Xiang, Y.T.; Yang, Y.; Li, W.; Zhang, L.; Zhang, Q.; Cheung, T.; Ng, C.H. Timely mental health care for the 2019 novel coronavirus outbreak is urgently needed. *Lancet Psychiatry* **2020**, *7*, 228–229. [CrossRef]
13. Ministerstwo Zdrowia: Mapa Zarażeń Koronawirusem (SARS-CoV-2). Available online: https://www.gov.pl/web/koronawirus/wykaz-zarazen-koronawirusem-sars-cov-2 (accessed on 21 June 2021).
14. Souza, D.L.B.; Oliveras-Fabregas, A.; Minobes-Molina, E.; de Camargo Cancela, M.; Galbany-Estragués, P.; Jerez-Roig, J. Trends of multimorbidity in 15 European countries: A population-based study in community-dwelling adults aged 50 and over. *BMC Public Health* **2021**, *21*, 76. [CrossRef] [PubMed]
15. Bezerra de Souza, D.L.; Oliveras-Fabregas, A.; Espelt, A.; Bosque-Prous, M.; de Camargo Cancela, M.; Teixidó-Compañó, E.; Jerez-Roig, J. Multimorbidity and its associated factors among adults aged 50 and over: A cross-sectional study in 17 European countries. *PLoS ONE* **2021**, *16*, e0246623. [CrossRef]
16. Cattel, R.B. Anxiety and motivation: Theory and crucial experiments. In *Anxiety and Behavior*; Spielberger, C.D., Ed.; Academic Press: New York, NY, USA, 1966; pp. 23–62.

17. Wrześniewski, K.; Sosnowski, T.; Matusik, D. *Inwentarz Stanu i Cechy Leku STAI. Polska adaptacja STAI*; Pracownia Testów Psychologicznych Polskiego Towarzystwa Psychologicznego: Warsaw, Poland, 2002.
18. Knight, R.G.; Waal-Manning, H.J.; Spears, G.F. Some norms and reliability data for the State-Trait Anxiety Inventory and the Zung Self-Rating Depression scale. *Br. J. Clin. Psychol.* **1983**, *22*, 245–249. [CrossRef]
19. Addolorato, G.; Ancona, C.; Capristo, E.; Graziosetto, R.; Di Rienzo, L.; Maurizi, M.; Gasbarrini, G. State and trait anxiety in women affected by allergic and vasomotor rhinitis. *J. Psychosom. Res.* **1999**, *46*, 283–289. [CrossRef]
20. Kocjan, J. Short Health Anxiety Inventory (SHAI)-Polish version: Evaluation of psychometric properties and factor structure. *Arch. Psychiatry Psychother.* **2016**, *18*, 68–78. [CrossRef]
21. Abramowitz, J.S.; Deacon, B.J.; Valentiner, D.P. The Short Health Anxiety Inventory: Psychometric Properties and Construct Validity in a Non-clinical Sample. *Cognit. Ther. Res.* **2007**, *31*, 871–883. [CrossRef] [PubMed]
22. Spitzer, R.L.; Kroenke, K.; Williams, J.B.; Löwe, B. A brief measure for assessing generalized anxiety disorder: The GAD-7. *Arch. Intern. Med.* **2006**, *166*, 1092–1097. [CrossRef]
23. Banerjee, D. The impact of Covid-19 pandemic on elderly mental health. *Int. J. Geriatr. Psychiatry* **2020**, *35*, 1466–1467. [CrossRef] [PubMed]
24. Wu, B. Social isolation and loneliness among older adults in the context of COVID-19: A global challenge. *Glob. Health Res. Policy* **2020**, *5*, 27. [CrossRef]
25. Rogowska, A.M.; Kuśnierz, C.; Bokszczanin, A. Examining Anxiety, Life Satisfaction, General Health, Stress and Coping Styles During COVID-19 Pandemic in Polish Sample of University Students. *Psychol. Res. Behav. Manag.* **2020**, *13*, 797–811. [CrossRef] [PubMed]
26. Gambin, M.; Sękowski, M.; Woźniak-Prus, M.; Wnuk, A.; Oleksy, T.; Cudo, A.; Hansen, K.; Huflejt-Łukasik, M.; Kubicka, K.; Łyś, A.E.; et al. Generalized anxiety and depressive symptoms in various age groups during the COVID-19 lockdown in Poland. Specific predictors and differences in symptoms severity. *Compr. Psychiatry* **2021**, *105*, 152222. [CrossRef] [PubMed]
27. González-Sanguino, C.; Ausín, B.; Castellanos, M.Á.; Saiz, J.; López-Gómez, A.; Ugidos, C.; Muñoz, M. Mental health consequences during the initial stage of the 2020 coronavirus pandemic (COVID-19) in Spain. *Brain Behav. Immun.* **2020**, *87*, 172–176. [CrossRef]
28. Jia, R.; Ayling, K.; Chalder, T.; Massey, A.; Broadbent, E.; Coupland, C.; Vedhara, K. Mental health in the UK during the COVID-19 pandemic: Cross-sectional analyses from a community cohort study. *BMJ Open* **2020**, *10*, e040620. [CrossRef] [PubMed]
29. Traunmüller, C.; Stefitz, R.; Gaisbachgrabner, K.; Schwerdtfeger, A. Psychological correlates of COVID-19 pandemic in the Austrian population. *BMC Public Health* **2020**, *20*, 1395. [CrossRef]
30. Qiu, J.; Shen, B.; Zhao, M.; Wang, Z.; Xie, B.; Xu, Y. A nationwide survey of psychological distress among Chinese people in the COVID-19 epidemic: Implications and policy recommendations. *Gen. Psychiatry* **2020**, *33*, e100213. [CrossRef]
31. Tian, F.; Li, H.; Tian, S.; Yang, J.; Shao, J.; Tian, C. Psychological symptoms of ordinary Chinese citizens based on SCL-90 during the level I emergency response to COVID-19. *Psychiatry Res.* **2020**, *288*, 112992. [CrossRef]
32. Mistry, S.K.; Ali, A.R.M.M.; Akther, F.; Yadav, U.N.; Harris, M.F. Exploring fear of COVID-19 and its correlates among older adults in Bangladesh. *Global Health* **2021**, *17*, 47. [CrossRef]
33. Parlapani, E.; Holeva, V.; Voitsidis, P.; Blekas, A.; Gliatas, I.; Porfyri, G.N.; Golemis, A.; Papadopoulou, K.; Dimitriadou, A.; Chatzigeorgiou, A.F.; et al. Psychological and Behavioral Responses to the COVID-19 Pandemic in Greece. *Front. Psychiatry* **2020**, *11*, 821. [CrossRef]
34. McLean, C.P.; Anderson, E.R. Brave men and timid women? A review of the gender differences in fear and anxiety. *Clin. Psychol. Rev.* **2009**, *29*, 496–505. [CrossRef] [PubMed]
35. Wang, C.; Pan, R.; Wan, X.; Tan, Y.; Xu, L.; Ho, C.S.; Ho, R.C. Immediate Psychological Responses and Associated Factors during the Initial Stage of the 2019 Coronavirus Disease (COVID-19) Epidemic among the General Population in China. *Int. J. Environ. Res. Public Health* **2020**, *17*, 1729. [CrossRef] [PubMed]
36. Naharci, M.I.; Veizi, B.G.Y.; Katipoglu, B.; Tasci, I. Psychological Burden among Community-dwelling Older Adults with and without a History of a Recent Covid-19 Infection. *Clin. Gerontol.* **2021**, *31*. [CrossRef]
37. Bobes-Bascarán, T.; Sáiz, P.A.; Velasco, A.; Martínez-Cao, C.; Pedrosa, C.; Portilla, A.; de la Fuente-Tomas, L.; García-Alvarez, L.; García-Portilla, M.P.; Bobes, J. Early Psychological Correlates Associated With COVID-19 in A Spanish Older Adult Sample. *Am. J. Geriatr. Psychiatry* **2020**, *28*, 1287–1298. [CrossRef] [PubMed]
38. Sepúlveda-Loyola, W.; Rodríguez-Sánchez, I.; Pérez-Rodríguez, P.; Ganz, F.; Torralba, R.; Oliveira, D.V.; Rodríguez-Mañas, L. Impact of Social Isolation Due to COVID-19 on Health in Older People: Mental and Physical Effects and Recommendations. *J. Nutr. Health Aging* **2020**, *24*, 938–947. [CrossRef] [PubMed]
39. Robb, C.E.; de Jager, C.A.; Ahmadi-Abhari, S.; Giannakopoulou, P.; Udeh-Momoh, C.; McKeand, J.; Price, G.; Car, J.; Majeed, A.; Ward, H.; et al. Associations of Social Isolation with Anxiety and Depression During the Early COVID-19 Pandemic: A Survey of Older Adults in London, UK. *Front. Psychiatry* **2020**, *11*, 591120. [CrossRef] [PubMed]
40. Islam, M.S.; Ferdous, M.Z.; Potenza, M.N. Panic and generalized anxiety during the COVID-19 pandemic among Bangladeshi people: An online pilot survey early in the outbreak. *J. Affect. Disord.* **2020**, *276*, 30–37. [CrossRef]

41. Di Crosta, A.; Palumbo, R.; Marchetti, D.; Ceccato, I.; La Malva, P.; Maiella, R.; Cipi, M.; Roma, P.; Mammarella, N.; Verrocchio, M.C.; et al. Individual Differences, Economic Stability, and Fear of Contagion as Risk Factors for PTSD Symptoms in the COVID-19 Emergency. *Front. Psychol.* **2020**, *11*, 567367. [CrossRef]
42. Fadila, D.; Ibrahim, F.M.; El-Gilany, A.H. Psychological distress among older adults during COVID-19 pandemic: Prevalence and associated factors. *Geriatr. Nurs.* **2021**, *42*, 1077–1083. [CrossRef]

Journal of
Clinical Medicine

MDPI

Article

The Influence of the COVID-19 Pandemic on the Stress Levels and Occurrence of Stomatoghnatic System Disorders (SSDs) among Physiotherapy Students in Poland

Magdalena Gębska [1], Łukasz Kołodziej [1], Bartosz Dalewski [2], Łukasz Pałka [3,*] and Ewa Sobolewska [2]

1 Department of Rehabilitation Musculoskeletal System, Pomeranian Medical University, 70-204 Szczecin, Poland; mgebska@pum.edu.pl (M.G.); lukas@hot.pl (Ł.K.)
2 Department of Dental Prosthetics, Pomeranian Medical University, 70-204 Szczecin, Poland; bartosz.dalewski@pum.edu.pl (B.D.); rpsobolewski@wp.pl (E.S.)
3 Private Dental Practice, 68-200 Żary, Poland
* Correspondence: dr.lpalka@gmail.com; Tel.: +48-608882535

Abstract: Background: This study is a quantitative analysis examining the impact of the COVID-19 pandemic on the occurrence of stress and stomatognathic system disorders (SSDs) among students of physiotherapy. Objective: To assess stress severity, strategies of coping with stress and the presence of type D personality among physiotherapy students including those with symptoms of stomatognathic system disorders. Material and Methods: The research was conducted from October to December 2020 on a sample of 188 students of physiotherapy. The data were collected using a survey form related to the occurrence of SS disorders symptoms and standardized psychological questionnaires, such as the Perceived Stress Scale (PSS)-10, Mini-Cope, and the type-D Scale (DS14), developed for the purpose of this study. Results: Women experiencing at least one of the SS disorder-related symptoms were characterized by a significantly higher level of stress and a type D personality ($p < 0.05$). Among men, these differences were not statistically significant ($p > 0.05$). On the basis of the strategies of coping with stress, i.e., positive self-reevaluation, discharging and blaming oneself, and taking psychoactive substances, it is possible to predict the intensity of stress during the pandemic in the group of the examined students. Among the reported symptoms of SS, headache was a significant predictor of stress, which was accompanied by an increase in the intensity of stress by nearly 0.2 measurement points. Students with higher levels of stress showed more symptoms of type D personality, and those with more severe symptoms of SS showed higher levels of stress. Conclusions: People prone to stress and having type D personality traits should be assessed for the presence of SS disorders.

Keywords: COVID-19; stress; stomatognathic system; students

Citation: Gębska, M.; Kołodziej, Ł.; Dalewski, B.; Pałka, Ł.; Sobolewska, E. The Influence of the COVID-19 Pandemic on the Stress Levels and Occurrence of Stomatoghnatic System Disorders (SSDs) among Physiotherapy Students in Poland. *J. Clin. Med.* **2021**, *10*, 3872. https://doi.org/10.3390/jcm10173872

Academic Editor: Michele Roccella

Received: 2 July 2021
Accepted: 27 August 2021
Published: 28 August 2021

1. Introduction

The SARS-CoV-2 pandemic has significantly impacted the mental health of populations around the world [1]. As the pandemic-related threat developed, people were forced to change their lifestyle [1]. The economy and its mechanisms, tourism industry, the functioning of culture, and teaching methods at all levels of education have been transformed [1,2]. At medical universities in Poland, necessary recommendations were introduced, i.e., hybrid teaching, limited social and professional contacts, as well as restricted access to university hospitals. As medical college education is largely based on practical skills, students became concerned about their development. Moreover, the uncertainty accompanying senior-year students as to how to fill in the gaps in education could have influenced the level of stress they felt. The pandemic also had a negative impact on attention span and enhanced learning difficulties, which resulted in increased concerns about final exam results.

Social isolation resulting from the pandemic, fear for oneself and loved ones, and financial instability also had a negative impact on the psychophysical health of students. The everyday uncertainty created an environment of anxiety and depression, and the quarantines contributed to a loss of social ties, deepening the feeling of loneliness or anger [3]. These stress factors could lead to the development of health problems associated with the whole body. Psychological factors, especially stress and the ability to deal with it, play a significant role in the etiology of stomatognathic system disorders (SSDs). Coping with lockdown measures was also associated with increased alcohol intake in men [4,5].

Stress that accompanies our daily lives contributes not only to cardiovascular, digestive, and respiratory diseases, but also increases muscle tone of the SS. As a consequence, symptoms such as: bruxism, pain in the temporomandibular joints (TMJs), and headaches may appear. Long-term symptoms of SSDs may contribute to irreversible changes in this system, resulting in impaired chewing, swallowing, speech, and breathing functions [6–20]. Additionally, long-term reports about TMJ internal derangements were released [21–25]. Hypothalamus, limbic system and reticular formation are responsible for psychological processes in humans [26]. These centers, through gamma-efferent fibers, which supply the muscle spindles, influence the myogenic activity of the body. In long-term stressful situations, they cause an increase in muscle tonus, also in the facial part of the skull, contributing to the formation of myogenic dysfunctions of the SS [5].

In 1926, Hans Hugon Selye introduced the concept of stress to health sciences. In medical terms, it is defined as a disorder of the body's homeostasis caused by physical or psychological elements [6–8]. It can be caused by mental, physiological, anatomical [7,8], or physical factors [9–11,14]. Stressful situations lead to increased muscle tension, which is the body's natural response to threat. SS muscles, like other skeletal muscles in the human body, can react with increased tension, pain, and/or hypertrophy when strained [7].

People react differently to stressors, which may depend on the personality type of the individual [27]. At the end of the 1990s, the concept of distressed personality (type D) was introduced into the literature, which resulted in an increased interest in the problem of the relationship between personality and somatic diseases [28]. Type D consists of two main dimensions—negative affectivity and social inhibition. Negative emotionality is expressed as a tendency to experience strong negative emotions such as fear, anger, irritation, and hostility. On the other hand, social inhibition is associated with the tendency to refrain from expressing negative emotions and behavior consistent with these emotions. People with type D personalities tend to be worried, tense, and blamed [29]. They are characterized by a pessimistic way of looking at the world, low self-esteem, and low level of satisfaction with life [30]. Type D personality has been found to be a significant predictor of cardiovascular disease, gastric and duodenal ulcer, and skin diseases [31–34].

Medical college students may be particularly prone to the negative effects of the pandemic. This study is a quantitative analysis examining the impact of the psychological effects of the pandemic on the occurrence of stress and stomatognathic system disorders among students of physiotherapy. The results of this research may help in preparing appropriate future intervention programs and effective prevention strategies in crisis situations at universities [32,35–38].

The aim of this study was to assess stress severity, coping with stress strategies, and the presence of type D personality in students with symptomatic stomatognathic system disorders. We hypothesized that stress, the ability to cope with it, and the type D personality may influence the development of SS disorders.

2. Materials and Methods

The research was conducted from October to December 2020 among randomly selected students of physiotherapy at the Pomeranian Medical University in Szczecin. The sample consisted of 188 participants (125 female and 63 male) aged 20 to 35 years (mean =22.72). All participants agreed to voluntarily participate in the study by signing an informed consent. They were asked to fill in the survey consisting of two parts: the first part included a respondent's particulars (age, sex, year of study) and ten close-ended questions concerning the symptoms of SSDs and pain (Likert scale) [39–45]. The second part consisted of standardized psychological questionnaires, PSS10 (perceived stress scale), Mini-Cope (Inventory for measuring coping with stress), DS14 (Type-D scale) [46–54]. As a result of the activities performed, 150 participants (study group-P1) with SSD symptoms and pain were selected from the group. The remaining 38 participants who did not report any symptoms from SSD were enrolled into the control group P2.

The sample size was calculated based on the data on a specific population (finite population) and the formula for the minimum sample size was as follows:

$$N_{min} = \frac{P(1-P)}{\frac{e^2}{Z^2} + \frac{P(1-P)'}{N}}$$

where:

P—estimated fraction size,

Z—value resulting from the adopted significance level (α), calculated using the cumulative distribution function of the normal distribution,

N—size of the general population (in the case of a finite population),

e—maximum estimation error.

After entering the data, namely:

P—50%

Z—1% (0.01)

N—8017

e—10%

The finite population sample size equaled: 163

The inclusion and exclusion criteria were as follows:

Inclusion criteria:

- 1st or 2nd year student of physiotherapy learning in a hybrid system (stationary and remote),
- reported symptoms of US disorders (from 6 months),
- age: 20–35,
- a written consent to participate in the study.

Exclusion criteria:

- chronic diseases, including psychosomatic,
- people during or after the treatment of SS disorders,
- pregnancy.

The differentiating factor between the study group (P1) and the control group (P2) was the lack of symptoms of SS disorders in the control group.

Among 1st and 2nd year students of physiotherapy who met the inclusion and exclusion criteria, the study group (P1) and participants without symptoms of SSD (P2) were selected on the basis of the SSD symptom questionnaire.

The main goal of the present study was to compare the groups that are as homogeneous as possible in terms of everyday functioning and exposure to stressful situations while studying during the pandemic. Therefore, a small sample size resulted from the limited number of physiotherapy students.

2.1. Characteristics of the Studied Group

Table 1 contains information on the frequency of reported individual symptoms and the average intensity of pain. Descriptive statistics for the entire group and separate statistics for the P1 and P2 subgroups are given. The statistical comparison of these two groups was abandoned due to the lack of occurrence of the studied variables in the P2 group.

Table 1. Characteristics of the study group in terms of experienced SS symptoms.

Pain in the Region:	Whole Group, n = 188	P1, n = 150	P2, n = 38
Temporomandibular pain			
Occurrence *	27 (14.4%)	27 (18.0%)	0 (0.0%)
Intensity **	0.32 (0.82)	0.39 (0.90)	-
Headache			
Occurrence	102 (54.3%)	102 (68.0%)	0 (0.0%)
Intensity	1.39 (1.45)	1.73 (1.43)	-
Pain in the neck and pectoral girdle			
Occurrence	87 (46.3%)	87 (58.0%)	0 (0.0%)
Intensity	1.13 (1.35)	1.38 (136)	-
Facial pain			
Occurrence	18 (9.6%)	18 (12.0%)	0 (0.0%)
Intensity	0.20 (0.64)	0.25 (0.71)	-
Acoustic symptoms			
Occurrence	50 (26.6%)	50 (33.3%)	0 (0.0%)
Temporomandibular joint locking			
Occurrence	14 (7.4%)	14 (9.3%)	0 (0.0%)
Teeth clenching			
Occurrence	75 (39.9%)	75 (50.0%)	0 (0.0%)
Teeth grinding			
Occurrence	34 (18.1%)	34 (22.7%)	0 (0.0%)
Muscle tension			
Occurrence	45 (23.9%)	45 (30.0%)	0 (0.0%)

* the number (n) and percentage (%) for the occurrence of symptoms ** mean (M) and standard deviation (SD) for pain intensity.

As shown in Table 1, the most common symptoms of SS disorders reported by the participants included headaches (68.0%), pain in the neck and shoulder girdle (58.0%), teeth clenching (50.0%) and acoustic symptoms in the temporomandibular joints (33.3%).

2.2. Statistical Analysis

The results of the study were statistically analyzed using the IBM SPSS Statistics v. 25 package 9 (IBM, Armonk, NY, USA). To assess the compliance of the empirical distributions obtained in the study with the theoretical normal distribution, typical for general population, the Shapiro–Wilk test for small groups ($n < 50$) and the Kolmogorov–Smirnov test for large groups were implemented. The non-parametric Spearman correlation was used to analyze the relationships between the continuous variables, and the non-parametric Mann–Whitney U test was used to assess the differences between the two independent groups. After standardizing the selected variables, the hierarchical regression model was also used, and the statistical significance index was established at $p < 0.05$.

3. Results

Table 2 presents the effect of measuring the frequency of the intensity of stress in the studied groups. The participants scored the PSS-10 scale from low (four raw points, three sten) to very high (35 raw points, 10 sten), and the mean result in the group approaching 19 raw points was within the range of six sten, indicating average severity of stress. The median for the stress level in the P1 group was 20 points and this result was four points higher than in the P2 group—this difference was statistically significant (Z = −2.665;

$p = 0.008$). Differences in sten scores were also significant ($Z = -2.768$; $p = 0.006$). The stress level in the P1 group was higher than in the P2 group.

Table 2. Basic parameters of the distribution of stress measurement results in the study group ($n = 188$).

	PSS	Mean	SD	Median	Minimum	Maximum	Normality of Distribution
Whole group	Total score	18.82	6.19	18.00	4.00	35.00	0.061
	Sten score	6.27	1.83	6.00	3.00	10.00	<0.001
P1	Total score	19.43	6.18	20.00	4.00	35.00	0.232
	Sten score	6.45	1.83	7.00	3.00	10.00	<0.001
P2	Total score	16.45	5.75	16.00	4.00	29.00	0.751
	Sten score	5.53	1.66	5.00	3.00	9.00	0.036

Then, the correlation between the intensity of pain and stress in the P1 group ($n = 150$) was analyzed. The measurement data presented in Table 3 indicate that with the increase in the severity of the sense of stress, the severity of headache (rho = 0.359; $p < 0.001$) and pain in the neck and girdle (rho = 0.240; $p = 0.003$) increased as well.

Table 3. Analysis of the correlation between the intensity of stress and the intensity of pain in the P1 group.

PSS	TMD	Headache	Neck and Shoulder Girdle Pain	Facial Pain
Raw score	0.104	0.342 ***	0.241 **	0.139
Sten score	0.090	0.359 ***	0.240 **	0.149

** $p < 0.01$; *** $p < 0.001$.

Table 4 presents the results of measurements of two variables: stress intensity (according to PSS10) and type D personality (according to DS14) among participants who reported one symptom of SS disorders. The analyses were carried out separately for the group of females and males. Males and females differ in this respect; females experiencing at least one SS symptom were characterized by a significantly higher level of stress and a type D personality ($p < 0.05$) compared to P2 group. Among males, these differences were not statistically significant ($p > 0.05$).

Table 4. Comparison of the mean results of the measurement of stress and type D personality among people suffering from one SS symptom, taking into account gender.

Gender	Compared Variables	Symptoms Occurrence/Group		Group Comparison	
		P1	P2	Z	p
Female	PSS	20.63 (5.54)	18.18 (5.45)	−1.922	0.045
	DS14	14.89 (5.25)	11.36 (5.71)	−2.369	0.018
Male	PSS	16.79 (6.73)	12.53 (6.61)	−1.266	0.206
	DS14	14.06 (5.42)	8.75 (4.31)	−1.878	0.060

Table 5 summarizes the results of a hierarchical regression analysis explaining the intensity of stress experienced by the participants during the COVID-19 pandemic. In each of the five steps of the analysis, the model included successive groups of potential predictors of stress: coping strategies, occurrence of SS symptoms, pain intensity caused by these symptoms, type D personality index, and sociodemographic variables. Before the calculations were made, all data were standardized. It was assessed what percentage of the total variability (variance) in the observed stress intensity can be explained based on changes in individual potential predictors and which of the independent variables are statistically significant predictors. Ultimately, it was possible to explain more than half of the variability in the stress experienced by the participants during the pandemic.

Table 5. Hierarchical regression analysis explaining the intensity of stress among students during the pandemic.

Significant Predictors	Model 1, $R^2 = 0.328$		Model 2, $R^2 = 0.368$		Model 3, $R^2 = 0.375$		Model 4, $R^2 = 0.554$		Model 5, $R^2 = 0.579$	
	Beta	*p*	**Beta**	*p*	**Beta**	*p*	**Beta**	*p*	**Beta**	*p*
Positive evaluation	−0.17	0.034	−0.20	0.014	−0.22	0.007	−0.06	0.422	−0.06	0.349
Discharging	0.27	0.004	0.23	0.002	0.24	0.001	0.12	0.027	0.13	0.043
Taking psychoactive substances	0.13	0.041	0.12	0.047	0.11	0.094	0.13	0.027	0.15	0.007
Blaming oneself	0.26	<0.001	0.22	0.002	0.24	0.001	0.04	0.566	0.03	0.686
Headache	-	-	0.20	0.006	0.05	0.700	0.07	0.522	0.05	0.660
Intensified Neck pain	-	-	-	-	−0.31	0.022	−0.20	0.085	−0.23	0.040
DS14	-	-	-	-	-	-	0.56	<0.001	0.53	<0.001
Gender	-	-	-	-	-	-	-	-	−0.20	0.001

(1) In the first step, the possibility to predict the level of stress severity during the pandemic by applying the strategies of coping with stress among the participants was assessed. Out of 14 strategies, four were significant predictors, which accounted for 33% of the stress variance.

The analysis showed that the higher the level of positive evaluation, the lower the level of stress. The other three strategies: discharging, taking psychoactive substances, and blaming oneself were positively related to the stress level.

(2) In the second step, after adding the presence of SS symptoms alone to the model, the explained variance increased to almost 37%, which was a statistically significant change (X2 (10.163) = 2.087; $p = 0.002$). The occurrence of headaches alone became a significant predictor of stress and caused its intensification. All remedial strategies detected in Model 1 as significant maintained their statistical significance ($p < 0.05$).

(3) In the third model, the intensity of the symptoms of the SS was added as a pool of potential predictors. Including them in the model did not significantly increase the percentage of the explained stress variance (X2 (4.159) = 1.468; $p = 0.214$; up to 38% of variance). The severity of pain in the neck and shoulder girdle was a significant predictor—an increase in pain intensity in this area coexisted with a decrease in stress intensity. At the same time, after taking this predictor into account, the strategy of taking psychoactive substances and the occurrence of headaches became statistically insignificant.

(4) The fourth model included the results of measuring type D personality as a potential stress predictor, which resulted in a significant increase in the explained variance to 55% (X2 (1.158) = 64.591; $p < 0.001$). Of the temporary remedial strategies, only discharging and taking psychoactive substances remained relevant, and both previously diagnosed symptoms of SS lost their relevance. The result on the DS14 scale was the strongest predictor of stress, positively related to the explained variable. The increase in DS14 caused an increase in the level of stress.

(5) In the fifth model, additionally, a sociodemographic variable was introduced. The gender variable resulted in a significant increase in the explained variance of the stress intensity among students during the pandemic to 58% (X2 (3.155) = 4.109; $p = 0.008$). Among the implemented remedial strategies, the statistical significance was maintained by the discharging and taking psychoactive substances, and among the symptoms of SS, the increase in pain in the neck and shoulder girdle. The sum of type D personality indices was still the strongest predictor, while in the sociodemographic variable—gender—women were characterized by a greater intensity of stress than men.

Table 6 presents the results of the analysis of the correlation between the severity of stress and the styles of coping with it and DS14. It has been shown that the increase in type D personality manifestations was positively and moderately strongly associated with the overall intensity of stress (rho = 0.69; $p < 0.001$); participants with higher levels of stress were characterized by a greater number of type D personality symptoms. Moreover, this personality type was correlated with seven strategies for coping with stress. The severity of symptoms increased moderately with the increase in the tendency to blame oneself in problem situations (rho = 0.51; $p < 0.001$), and it also increased slightly with the increase in the tendency to denial (rho = 0.31; $p < 0.001$), discharging (rho = 0.27; $p < 0.001$), taking psychoactive substances (rho = 0.19; $p = 0.009$) and engaging in other activities (rho = 0.17; $p = 0.019$) and with a decrease in such constructive remedial strategies as positive reevaluation (rho = −0.29; $p < 0.001$) and sense of humor (rho = −0.19; $p = 0.0010$). The overall severity of stress moderately increased with the increase in tendency to blame oneself (rho = 0.46; $p < 0.001$) and weakly with the increase in ceasing activities (rho = 0.32; $p < 0.001$), discharging (rho = 0.31; $p < 0.001$), taking psychoactive substances (rho = 0.27; $p < 0.001$), denial (rho = 0.20; $p = 0.007$), engaging in other activities (rho = 0.15; $p = 0.042$), and with a decrease in the tendency to positively re-evaluate (rho = −0.27; $p < 0.001$), sense of humor (rho = −0.21; $p = 0.004$), active coping (rho = −0.17; $p = 0.018$), planning (rho = −0.16; $p = 0.028$), or seeking emotional support (rho = −0.14; $p = 0.047$).

Table 6. Spearman's correlation matrix.

Variables	1	2	3	4	5	6	7	8	9	10	11	12	13	14	15
1. DS14	-	-	-	-	-	-	-	-	-	-	-	-	-	-	-
2. PSS 10	0.69 ***	-	-	-	-	-	-	-	-	-	-	-	-	-	-
3. Active coping	−0.14	−0.17 *	-	-	-	-	-	-	-	-	-	-	-	-	-
4. Planning	−0.07	−0.16 *	0.51 ***	-	-	-	-	-	-	-	-	-	-	-	-
5. Positive evaluation	−0.29 ***	−0.27 ***	0.19 *	0.40 ***	-	-	-	-	-	-	-	-	-	-	-
6. Acceptance	−0.03	−0.13	0.21 **	0.29 ***	0.35 ***	-	-	-	-	-	-	-	-	-	-
7. Sense of humor	−0.19 *	−0.21 **	0.01	0.02	0.39 ***	0.40 ***	-	-	-	-	-	-	-	-	-
8. Turning to religion	−0.03	−0.02	0.07	0.15 *	0.18 *	0.12	0.07	-	-	-	-	-	-	-	-
9. Seeking emotional support	−0.12	−0.14 *	0.20 **	0.34 ***	0.35 ***	0.16 *	−0.02	0.11	-	-	-	-	-	-	-
10. Seeking instrumental support	−0.04	−0.04	0.18 *	0.27 ***	0.34 ***	0.19 *	−0.03	0.21 **	0.77 ***	-	-	-	-	-	-
11. Engaging in other activities	0.17 *	0.15 *	−0.01	0.11	0.11	0.15 *	0.15 *	0.03	0.16 *	0.17 *	-	-	-	-	-
12. Denial	0.14 *	0.20 **	−0.06	−0.06	0.05	−0.05	0.12	0.09	−0.17 *	−0.11	0.12	-	-	-	-
13. Discharging	0.26 ***	0.31 ***	−0.07	0.08	0.20 **	0.08	0.01	0.07	0.20 **	0.35 ***	0.26 ***	0.27 ***	-	-	-
14. Taking psychoactive substance	0.19 **	0.27 ***	−0.07	−0.02	−0.08	0.03	0.12	0.03	−0.12	−0.12	0.19 **	0.14	0.12	-	-
15. Ceasing activities	0.31 ***	0.32 ***	−0.45 ***	−0.29 ***	−0.19 **	−0.01	−0.01	−0.03	−0.24 **	−0.09	−0.06	0.27 ***	0.21 **	0.13	-
16. Blaming oneself	0.51 ***	0.46 ***	0.01	−0.09	−0.19 **	−0.10	−0.16 *	0.05	0.14 *	0.01	0.06	0.28 ***	0.25 ***	0.27 ***	0.26 ***

* $p < 0.05$; ** $p < 0.01$; *** $p < 0.001$.

4. Discussion

The outbreak of the COVID-19 pandemic generated a global public health emergency [55–58]. Taylor et al. reported that psychological responses to previous epidemics and pandemics depended on individual vulnerabilities such as intolerance, insecurity, disease susceptibility, and anxiety [59]. Therefore, the authors of the present study conducted research on the assessment of the level of stress, the method of coping with stress, and the occurrence of symptoms of SS disorders in students of physiotherapy during the COVID-19 pandemic.

Multiple researchers emphasized the importance of mental stress in shaping the pathology of the SS [17–20]. Stressors with somatic consequences are largely dependent on the patient's personality type and the ability to cope with stress. The long-term effects of stressors breaks the body's adaptive mechanisms and lead to the accumulation of various disorders, including SS disorders [60]. According to the authors' research on a group of 188 physiotherapy students, the symptoms of SS disorders were found in 150 participants (80%). Research conducted by Emodi-Perlaman et al. showed that the COVID-19 pandemic had a significant adverse effect on the psychoemotional state of Israeli and Polish populations, leading to an increase in bruxism and TMD symptoms [61]. In the author's own research, symptoms of bruxism, i.e., tooth clenching, were found in 75 participants and teeth grinding in 34 (50% and 22.7%, respectively). In studies by Przytańska et al., patients with high levels of stress reported parafunctional functions, i.e., awake bruxism, almost six times more often [62].

As it results from the conducted research, in the group of students with symptoms of SS disorders, higher scores were observed in the stress severity rating scale compared to the group without SS symptoms. The difference between the groups was statistically significant, which may indicate a significant role of stress in the development of SS disorders. De Medeiros et al. conducted research among Brazilian medical students and indicated that social isolation and stressful situations caused by the pandemic may increase the number of people with TMD symptoms [63].

It is generally accepted that mental stress causes increase in the muscular tension in different parts of the body [64,65]. The body posture adopted in stressful situations related to the so-called "fight or flight" reaction affects muscle contractions within the SS, leading to pain in the head and neck area. Therefore, muscle contractions in the body's upper quadrant may be a part of a stress-related defensive behavior [14–17]. In our study, the majority of physiotherapy students reported at least one symptom of SS and pain. The most common symptoms were headache (68%), neck and shoulder pain (58%), and teeth clenching (50%). Many clinical studies seem to confirm the relationship between the occurrence of SS disorders and severe stress, mostly in young people entering adulthood [66–69]. According to Quintiliani et al., as many as 89.4% of the respondents experienced an increase in perceived stress during the pandemic (66% reported moderate stress and 23.4% high stress) [70].

The authors of the study, by using the PSS 10 scale, found that the average stress intensity among physiotherapy students was in the range of six sten (19 raw points), indicating the average intensity of stress. Similar conclusions were drawn by other authors assessing the intensity of stress in emergency medical students, who also obtained an average value of six [70]. Importantly, in the present study, as many as 46.3% of the respondents obtained results in the range of 7–10 sten, which, according to the current interpretation of the research tool (PSS 10), qualifies them as high stress subjects. It is also worth noting that the maximum score on the PSS 10 scale in the group with symptoms of SSD was higher than in the control group.

The relationship between stress and neurological disorders, and tension headaches and migraines has been expensively described [71–74]. The results of our own research confirmed the existence of positive correlations between the intensity of stress and the symptoms of SS disorders, because with the increase in the intensity of the sense of stress, the intensity of headache and pain in the neck and shoulder girdle also increased. The above fact should prompt clinicians to evaluate the structures of SS in patients who report the above-mentioned pain symptoms in their history.

According to the literature, SS disorders and higher levels of stress are more common in women than in men [75–78]. Wang et al. found three times higher levels of depression and health anxiety in women than in men during the COVID-19 pandemic [79]. Moreover, in the research by Liu et al., women were stronger predictors of PTSS symptoms after the pandemic [80]. Our results are in accordance with the abovementioned findings, as we discovered that women with a symptom of SS disorders were characterized by a significantly higher level of stress and a type D personality ($p < 0.005$) compared to men ($p > 0.05$).

The analyses carried out by the authors of the publication with the use of the Mini-COPE test were aimed at examining the activity that students undertake in a stressful situation. These actions are known as "coping methods". Research conducted by Babicka-Wirkus et al. on a group of 577 students from 17 Polish universities showed that, during the COVID-19 pandemic, students most often used coping strategies such as acceptance, planning, and seeking emotional support [81]. The analysis of the authors' results did not bring similar conclusions, because out of 14 strategies, four were significant predictors, i.e., positive thinking strategies, discharge, taking psychoactive substances, and blaming oneself. The results also showed that the higher the level of perceived stress, the more frequently the remaining three strategies were used. The level of perceived stress most strongly influenced the frequency of using the discharge strategy, which is a strategy focusing on revealing negative emotions and is associated with a feeling of mental discomfort. The results obtained by the authors allow for the conclusion that maladaptive stress coping strategies in students, especially during the pandemic, may have long-term consequences for their psychophysiological health and academic achievement. According to the research, the presence of SS symptoms did not contribute to changes in the way of coping as all coping strategies retained their statistical significance ($p < 0.05$).

As it was shown in the study, the intensity of type D personality manifestations was positively and moderately strongly associated with the general intensity of stress (rho = 0.690; $p < 0.001$). Students experiencing higher levels of stress exhibited more symptoms of type D personality, and those with more severe symptoms showed higher levels of stress. In a study by Cho et al. conducted among Korean students, it was observed that type D personality is related to the level of perceived stress. Additionally, it has been concluded that there are gender differences in type D personality, stress, and coping strategies [82].

By analyzing the available scientific literature and the results of our own research, it can be determined with high probability that the COVID-19 pandemic increases the intensity of stress and may influence the development of SS disorders.

More research is required to better understand the impact of COVID-19 stressors on stomatognathic disorders.

The major limitation of the present study is the fact that it was carried out in a very specific population. Therefore, the results cannot be extrapolated convincingly to the general population.

5. Conclusions

1. The degree of stress intensity influences the occurrence symptoms of the stomatognathic system such as: headache, neck, and shoulder girdle pain.
2. It is important to develop and implement psychological support measures to deal with the COVID-19 pandemic for medical college students.
3. Dental care workers are encouraged to pay more attention to the occurrence of symptoms of SSDs in patients during the pandemic.

Author Contributions: Conceptualization: M.G., Ł.K.; Methodology: M.G., B.D.; Software: M.G., Ł.K.; Validation: M.G.; Formal analysis: M.G.; Investigation: M.G., Ł.K.; Resources: Ł.K.; Data curation: M.G., Ł.K.; Writing—original draft preparation: M.G., B.D., Ł.P.; Writing—review and editing: B.D., Ł.P., M.G.; Visualization: M.G.; Supervision: E.S., Ł.P.; Project administration: M.G.; Funding acquisition: E.S. All authors have read and agreed to the published version of the manuscript.

Funding: This research received no external funding.

Institutional Review Board Statement: Not applicable.

Informed Consent Statement: Informed consent was obtained from all subjects involved in the study.

Data Availability Statement: The data presented in this study are available on request from the corresponding author. The data are not publicly available due to sensitive information.

Conflicts of Interest: The authors declare no conflict of interest.

References

1. Hu, Z.; Lin, X.; Kaminga, A.C.; Xu, H. Impact of the COVID-19 Epidemic on Lifestyle Behaviors and Their Association With Subjective Well-Being Among the General Population in Mainland China: Cross-Sectional Study. *J. Med. Internet Res.* **2020**, *22*, e21176. [CrossRef]
2. Maqsood, A.; Abbas, J.; Rehman, G.; Mubeen, R. The paradigm shift for educational system continuance in the advent of COVID-19 pandemic: Mental health challenges and reflections. *Curr. Res. Behav. Sci.* **2021**, *2*, 100011. [CrossRef]
3. Brooks, S.K.; Webster, R.K.; Smith, L.E.; Woodland, L.; Wessely, S.; Greenberg, N.; Rubin, G.J. The psychological impact of quarantine and how to reduce it: Rapid review of the evidence. *Lancet* **2020**, *395*, 912–920. [CrossRef]
4. Dalewski, B.; Palka, L.; Kiczmer, P.; Sobolewska, E. The Impact of SARS-CoV-2 Outbreak on the Polish Dental Community's Standards of Care—A Six-Month Retrospective Survey-Based Study. *Int. J. Environ. Res. Public Health* **2021**, *18*, 1281. [CrossRef] [PubMed]
5. Fillingim, R.; Slade, G.D.; Greenspan, J.D.; Dubner, R.; Maixner, W.; Bair, E.; Ohrbach, R. Long-term changes in biopsychosocial characteristics related to temporomandibular disorder: Findings from the OPPERA study. *Pain* **2018**, *159*, 2403–2413. [CrossRef]
6. Neylan, T.C. Hans Selye and the Field of Stress Research. *J. Neuropsychiatry Clin. Neurosci.* **1998**, *10*, 230. [CrossRef]
7. Nagata, K.; Hori, S.; Mizuhashi, R.; Yokoe, T.; Atsumi, Y.; Nagai, W.; Goto, M. Efficacy of mandibular manipulation technique for temporomandibular disorders patients with mouth opening limitation: A randomized controlled trial for comparison with improved multimodal therapy. *J. Prosthodont. Res.* **2018**, *63*, 202–209. [CrossRef] [PubMed]
8. Kapos, F.P.; Look, J.O.; Zhang, L.; Hodges, J.S.; Schiffman, E.L. Predictors of Long-Term Temporomandibular Disorder Pain Intensity: An 8-Year Cohort Study. *J. Oral Facial Pain Headache* **2018**, *32*, 113–122. [CrossRef]
9. Polat, M.; Yanik, S. Efficiency of arthrocentesis treatment for different temporomandibular joint disorders. *Int. J. Oral Maxillofac. Surg.* **2020**, *49*, 621–627. [CrossRef]
10. Vrbanović, E.; Alajbeg, I.Z. Long-term Effectiveness of Occlusal Splint Therapy Compared to Placebo in Patients with Chronic Temporomandibular Disorders. *Acta Stomatol. Croat.* **2019**, *53*, 195–206. [CrossRef]
11. Guo, Y.-N.; Cui, S.-J.; Zhou, Y.-H.; Wang, X.-D. An Overview of Anterior Repositioning Splint Therapy for Disc Displacement-related Temporomandibular Disorders. *Curr. Med. Sci.* **2021**, *41*, 1–9. [CrossRef]
12. Nascimento, G.C.; De Paula, B.B.; Gerlach, R.F.; Leite-Panissi, C.R.A. Temporomandibular inflammation regulates the matrix metalloproteinases MMP-2 and MMP-9 in limbic structures. *J. Cell. Physiol.* **2021**, *236*, 6571–6580. [CrossRef]
13. Zhang, H.-Y.; Duan, J.; Wang, J.; Xie, M.-J.; Liu, Q.; Liu, J.-Q.; Yang, H.-X.; Wang, M.-Q. Masseter response to long-term experimentally induced anterior crossbite in Sprague-Dawley rats. *Arch. Oral Biol.* **2021**, *122*, 104985. [CrossRef]
14. Ploder, O.; Sigron, G.; Adekunle, A.; Burger-Krebes, L.; Haller, B.; Kolk, A. The Effect of Orthognathic Surgery on Temporomandibular Joint Function and Symptoms: What are the Risk Factors? A Longitudinal Analysis of 375 Patients. *J. Oral Maxillofac. Surg.* **2020**, *79*, 763–773. [CrossRef]
15. Fisch, G.; Finke, A.; Ragonese, J.; Dugas, L.; Wrzosek, M. Outcomes of physical therapy in patients with temporomandibular disorder: A retrospective review. *Br. J. Oral Maxillofac. Surg.* **2021**, *59*, 145–150. [CrossRef]
16. Kolk, A.; Scheunemann, L.-M.; Grill, F.; Stimmer, H.; Wolff, K.-D.; Neff, A. Prognostic factors for long-term results after condylar head fractures: A comparative study of non-surgical treatment versus open reduction and osteosynthesis. *J. Cranio-Maxillofac. Surg.* **2020**, *48*, 1138–1145. [CrossRef]
17. Braga, S.P.; Fiamengui, L.M.S.P.; Da Silveira, V.R.S.; Chaves, H.V.; Furquim, B.D.; Cunha, C.O.; Repeke, C.E.P.; Conti, P.C.R. Insights for temporomandibular disorders management: From psychosocial factors to genetics—A case report. *Spéc. Care Dent.* **2021**, *41*, 85–91. [CrossRef] [PubMed]
18. Seo, H.; Jung, B.; Yeo, J.; Kim, K.-W.; Cho, J.-H.; Lee, Y.J.; Ha, I.-H. Healthcare utilisation and costs for temporomandibular disorders: A descriptive, cross-sectional study. *BMJ Open* **2020**, *10*, e036768. [CrossRef] [PubMed]
19. Bergmann, A.; Edelhoff, D.; Schubert, O.; Erdelt, K.-J.; Duc, J.-M.P. Effect of treatment with a full-occlusion biofeedback splint on sleep bruxism and TMD pain: A randomized controlled clinical trial. *Clin. Oral Investig.* **2020**, *24*, 4005–4018. [CrossRef] [PubMed]

20. Wahlund, K.; Larsson, B. The course of pain intensity and frequency of adolescents treated because of temporomandibular disorders: A long-term follow-up. *Clin. Exp. Dent. Res.* **2020**, *6*, 407–414. [CrossRef] [PubMed]
21. Dalewski, B.; Kamińska, A.; Białkowska, K.; Jakubowska, A.; Sobolewska, E. Association of Estrogen Receptor 1 and Tumor Necrosis Factor α Polymorphisms with Temporomandibular Joint Anterior Disc Displacement without Reduction. *Dis. Markers* **2020**, *2020*, 6351817. [CrossRef] [PubMed]
22. Dalewski, B.; Kaczmarek, K.; Jakubowska, A.; Szczuchniak, K.; Pałka, Ł.; Sobolewska, E. *COL12A1* Single Nucleotide Polymorphisms rs240736 and rs970547 Are Not Associated with Temporomandibular Joint Disc Displacement without Reduction. *Genes* **2021**, *12*, 690. [CrossRef] [PubMed]
23. Checherita, L.E.; Stamatin, O.; Liana, A.; Luca, D.E. Parafunctions in dysfunctional syndrome of the stomatognathic system—literature review. *Rom. J. Med. Dent. Educ.* **2020**, *9*, 53–61.
24. Dalewski, B.; Kamińska, A.; Kiczmer, P.; Węgrzyn, K.; Pałka, Ł.; Janda, K.; Sobolewska, E. Pressure Algometry Evaluation of Two Occlusal Splint Designs in Bruxism Management-Randomized, Controlled Clinical Trial. *J. Clin. Med.* **2021**, *10*, 2342. [CrossRef] [PubMed]
25. Leketas, M. Stomatognathic Parafunctions and Their Etiology: Literature Review. Master's Thesis, Lithuanian University of Health Sciences Medical Academy Faculty of Medicine, Department of Oral and Maxillofacial Surgery, Kanuas, Lithuania, 2018.
26. Wolowski, A.; Eger, T.; Braas, R.; Gohr, J.; Weber, N.; Witanski, K.; Wörner, F. Long-term effects of splint therapy in patients with posttraumatic stress disease (PTSD). *Clin. Oral Investig.* **2020**, *24*, 1493–1497. [CrossRef] [PubMed]
27. Xin, Y.; Wu, J.; Yao, Z.; Guan, Q.; Aleman, A.; Luo, Y. The relationship between personality and the response to acute psychological stress. *Sci Rep.* **2017**, *7*, 16906. [CrossRef] [PubMed]
28. Bacon, S.L.; Moullec, G. Type-D Personality and Heart Disease: It Might Be 'One Small Step', but It Is Still Moving Forward: A Comment on Grande et al. *Ann. Behav. Med.* **2012**, *43*, 280–281. [CrossRef]
29. O'Riordan, A.; Howard, S.; Gallagher, S. Type D personality and life event stress: The mediating effects of social support and negative social relationships. *Anxiety Stress. Coping* **2020**, *33*, 452–465. [CrossRef]
30. Mols, F.; Denollet, J. Type D personality in the general population: A systematic review of health status, mechanisms of disease, and work-related problems. *Health Qual. Life Outcomes* **2010**, *8*, 9. [CrossRef]
31. Raykh, O.I.; Sumin, A.N.; Kokov, A.N.; Indukaeva, E.V.; Artamonova, G.V. Association of type D personality and level of coronary artery calcification. *J. Psychosom. Res.* **2020**, *139*, 110265. [CrossRef]
32. Chilicka, K.; Rogowska, A.M.; Szyguła, R.; Adamczyk, E. Association between Satisfaction with Life and Personality Types A and D in Young Women with Acne Vulgaris. *Int. J. Environ. Res. Public Health* **2020**, *17*, 8524. [CrossRef] [PubMed]
33. Raykh, O.I.; Sumin, A.N.; Korok, E.V. The Influence of Personality Type D on Cardiovascular Prognosis in Patients After Coronary Artery Bypass Grafting: Data from a 5-Year-Follow-up Study. *Int. J. Behav. Med.* **2021**, *6*, 1–11. [CrossRef]
34. Jordi, S.B.U.; Botte, F.; Lang, B.M.; Greuter, T.; Krupka, N.; Auschra, B.; Schreiner, P.; Sulz, M.C.; Biedermann, L.; von Känel, R.; et al. Type D personality is associated with depressive symptoms and clinical activity in inflammatory bowel disease. *Aliment. Pharmacol. Ther.* **2021**, *54*, 53–67. [CrossRef] [PubMed]
35. Zhan, H.; Zheng, C.; Zhang, X.; Yang, M.; Zhang, L.; Jia, X. Chinese College Students' Stress and Anxiety Levels Under COVID-19. *Front. Psychiatry* **2021**, *12*, 615390. [CrossRef] [PubMed]
36. Kim, E.-J.; Nho, J.-H.; Kim, H.-Y.; Park, S.-K. The Effects of Lifestyle Interventions on the Health-Promoting Behavior, Type D Personality, Cognitive Function and Body Composition of Low-Income Middle-Aged Korean Women. *Int. J. Environ. Res. Public Health* **2021**, *18*, 5637. [CrossRef] [PubMed]
37. O'Riordan, A.; Howard, S.; Brown, E.; Gallagher, S. Type D personality and cardiovascular reactivity to acute stress: The mediating effects of social support and negative social relationships. *Psychophysiology* **2020**, *57*, 13660. [CrossRef] [PubMed]
38. Köbling, T.; Váradi, Z.; Katona, É.; Somodi, S.; Kempler, P.; Páll, D.; Zrínyi, M. Predictors of dietary self-efficacy in high glycosylated hemoglobin A1c type 2 diabetic patients. *J. Int. Med. Res.* **2020**, *48*, 300060520931284. [CrossRef]
39. Kołtuniuk, A.; Kazimierska-Zając, M.; Cisek, K.; Chojdak-Łukasiewicz, J. The Role of Stress Perception and Coping with Stress and the Quality of Life Among Multiple Sclerosis Patients. *Psychol. Res. Behav. Manag.* **2021**, *14*, 805–815. [CrossRef]
40. Ali, H.; Ismail, A.A.; Abdalwahab, A. Mental Stress in Anesthesia and Intensive Care Physicians During COVID-19 Outbreak. *Anesthesiol. Pain Med.* **2020**, *10*, 106623. [CrossRef]
41. Avunduk, A.T.E.; Delikan, E. Satisfaction and stress levels of dentistry students relating to distance education. *Dent. Med. Probl.* **2021**, *58*, 58. [CrossRef]
42. Grabowski, J.; Stepien, J.; Waszak, P.; Michalski, T.; Meloni, R.; Grabkowska, M.; Macul, A.; Rojek, J.; Lorettu, L.; Sagan, I.; et al. Social Isolation During COVID-19 Pandemic. Perceived Stress and Containment Measures Compliance Among Polish and Italian Residents. *Front. Psychol.* **2021**, *12*, 673514. [CrossRef] [PubMed]
43. Ziarko, M.; Jasielska, A.; Stanisławska-Kubiak, M.; Daroszewski, P.; Samborski, W.; Mojs, E. Mental Health Outcomes Associated with COVID-19 Pandemic in a Group of Health Care Professionals. *J. Behav. Health Serv. Res.* **2021**, 1–10. [CrossRef]
44. Kowalczuk, K.; Krajewska-Kułak, E.; Sobolewski, M. Relationships Between Sleep Problems and Stress Coping Strategies Adopted by Nurses Including Socio-Occupational Factors. *Front. Psychiatry* **2021**, *12*, 660776. [CrossRef] [PubMed]
45. Betke, K.; Basińska, M.A.; Andruszkiewicz, A. Sense of coherence and strategies for coping with stress among nurses. *BMC Nurs.* **2021**, *20*, 1–10. [CrossRef]

46. Chodkiewicz, J.; Miniszewska, J.; Krajewska, E.; Biliński, P. Mental Health during the Second Wave of the COVID-19 Pandemic—Polish Studies. *Int. J. Environ. Res. Public Health* **2021**, *18*, 3423. [CrossRef] [PubMed]
47. Mocny-Pachońska, K.; Trzcionka, A.; Doniec, R.; Sieciński, S.; Tanasiewicz, M. The Influence of Gender and Year of Study on Stress Levels and Coping Strategies among Polish Dental. *Medicine* **2020**, *56*, 531. [CrossRef] [PubMed]
48. Unnithan, A.S.; Chidgey, B.A. Pre-visit education on pain management options prior to the first clinic visit improves chronic pain patient satisfaction with proposed treatment plans. *Pain Med.* **2021**. [CrossRef]
49. Dasukil, S.; Arora, G.; Shetty, S.K.; Degala, S. Impact of prolotherapy in temporomandibular joint disorder: A quality of life assessment. *Br. J. Oral Maxillofac. Surg.* **2020**, *59*, 599. [CrossRef] [PubMed]
50. Lindfors, E.; Arima, T.; Baad-Hansen, L.; Bakke, M.; De Laat, A.; Giannakopoulos, N.N.; Glaros, A.; Guimarães, A.S.; Johansson, A.; Le Bell, Y.; et al. Jaw Exercises in the Treatment of Temporomandibular Disorders—An International Modified Delphi Study. *J. Oral Facial Pain Headache* **2019**, *39*, 389–398. [CrossRef] [PubMed]
51. Lindfors, E.; Magnusson, T.; Ernberg, M. Patients' experiences of therapeutic jaw exercises in the treatment of masticatory myofascial pain—A postal questionnaire study. *J. Oral Rehabil.* **2019**, *46*, 800–806. [CrossRef]
52. Muzalev, K.; Van Selms, M.K.; Lobbezoo, F. No Dose-Response Association Between Self-Reported Bruxism and Pain-Related Temporomandibular Disorders: A Retrospective Study. *J. Oral Facial Pain Headache* **2018**, *32*, 375–380. [CrossRef]
53. Simma, I.; Simma, L.; Fleckenstein, J. Muscular Diagnostics and the Feasibility of Microsystem Acupuncture as a Potential Adjunct in the Treatment of Painful Temporomandibular Disorders: Results of a Retrospective Cohort Study. *Acupunct. Med.* **2018**, *36*, 415–421. [CrossRef] [PubMed]
54. Asquini, G.; Rushton, A.; Pitance, L.; Heneghan, N.; Falla, D. The effectiveness of manual therapy applied to craniomandibular structures in the treatment of temporomandibular disorders: Protocol for a systematic review. *Syst. Rev.* **2021**, *10*, 1–7. [CrossRef] [PubMed]
55. Peng, X.; Zhao, H.-Z.; Yang, Y.; Rao, Z.-L.; Hu, D.-Y.; He, Q. Post-traumatic Growth Level and Its Influencing Factors Among Frontline Nurses During the COVID-19 Pandemic. *Front. Psychiatry* **2021**, *12*, 632360. [CrossRef] [PubMed]
56. Yamaguchi, T. Neural circuit mechanisms of sex and fighting in males. *Neurosci. Res.* **2021**, 0168. [CrossRef]
57. Krupa, S.; Paweł, W.; Mędrzycka-Dąbrowska, W.; Lintowska, A.; Ozga, D. Sleep Disturbances in Individuals Quarantined Due to SARS-CoV-2 Pandemic in Poland: A Mixed Methods Design Study. *Glob. Adv. Health Med.* **2021**, *10*. [CrossRef] [PubMed]
58. Volkan, E. COVID-19: Structural Considerations for Virus Pathogenesis, Therapeutic Strategies and Vaccine Design in the Novel SARS-CoV-2 Variants Era. *Mol. Biotechnol.* **2021**, 1–13. [CrossRef]
59. Taylor, S. *The Psychology of Pandemics: Preparing for the Next Global Outbreak of Infectious Disease*; Cambridge Scholars Publishing: Cambridge, UK, 2019.
60. Dołoszycka, M.; Kulesa-Mrowiecka, M.; Kopański, Z.; Krzemiński, D.; Ptak, W.; Dyl, S.; Sklyarov, I. Behaviors leading to the occurrence of stomatognathic system disorders among students. *J. Publ. Health Nurs. Med. Rescue.* **2018**, *6*, 35–41.
61. Emodi-Perlman, A.; Eli, I.; Smardz, J.; Uziel, N.; Wieckiewicz, G.; Gilon, E.; Grychowska, N.; Wieckiewicz, M. Temporomandibular Disorders and Bruxism Outbreak as a Possible Factor of Orofacial Pain Worsening during the COVID-19 Pandemic—Concomitant Research in Two Countries. *J. Clin. Med.* **2020**, *9*, 3250. [CrossRef]
62. Przystańska, A.; Jasielska, A.; Ziarko, M.; Pobudek-Radzikowska, M.; Maciejewska-Szaniec, Z.; Prylińska-Czyżewska, A.; Czajka-Jakubowska, A. Psychosocialpredictors of bruxism. *BioMed Res. Int.* **2019**, *2019*, 2069716. [CrossRef]
63. Medeiros, R.A.D.; Vieira, D.L.; Silva, E.V.F.D.; Rezende, L.V.M.D.L.; Santos, R.W.D.; Tabata, L.F. Prevalence of symptoms of temporomandibular disorders, oral behaviors, anxiety, and depression in Dentistry students during the period of social isolation due to COVID-19. *J. Appl. Oral Sci.* **2020**, *28*, e20200445. [CrossRef]
64. Tassani, S.; Font-Llagunes, J.M.; Ballester, M.; Ángel, G.; Noailly, J. Muscular tension significantly affects stability in standing posture. *Gait Posture* **2019**, *68*, 220–226. [CrossRef] [PubMed]
65. Ekman, A.; Hagberg, M.; Wahlström, J.; Lindegård, A.; Ahlborg, G., Jr. Perceived muscular tension, emotional stress, psychological demands and physical load during VDU work. *Int. Arch. Occup. Environ. Health* **2003**, *76*, 584–590. [CrossRef]
66. Reissmann, D.R.; John, M.T.; Schierz, O.; Seedorf, H.; Doering, S. Stress-related adaptive versus maladaptive coping and temporomandibular disorder pain. *J. Orofac. Pain* **2012**, *26*, 181.
67. Schmitter, M.; Kares-Vrincianu, A.; Kares, H.; Bermejo, J.L.; Schindler, H.-J. Sleep-associated aspects of myofascial pain in the orofacial area among Temporomandibular Disorder patients and controls. *Sleep Med.* **2015**, *16*, 1056–1061. [CrossRef]
68. Staniszewski, K.; Lygre, H.; Bifulco, E.; Kvinnsland, S.; Willassen, L.; Helgeland, E.; Berge, T.; Rosén, A. Temporomandibular Disorders Related to Stress and HPA-Axis Regulation. *Pain Res. Manag.* **2018**, *2018*, 1–7. [CrossRef] [PubMed]
69. Augusto, V.G.; Perina, K.C.B.; Penha, D.S.G.; Dos Santos, D.C.A.; Oliveira, V.A.S. Temporomandibular Dysfunction, Stress and Common Mental Disorder in University Students. *Acta Ortopédica Bras.* **2016**, *24*, 330–333. [CrossRef]
70. Quintiliani, L.; Sisto, A.; Vicinanza, F.; Curcio, G.; Tambone, V. Resilience and psychological impact on Italian university students during COVID-19 pandemic. Distance learning and health. *Psychol. Health Med.* **2021**, *12*, 1–12. [CrossRef] [PubMed]
71. Bartczak, M.; Bartczak, M. Stress intensity and ways of coping with stress in paramedics and emergency medical students. *Sci. Yearb. Univ. Kujawsko-Pomor.* **2010**, *5*, 7–17.
72. Cathcart, S.; Winefield, A.H.; Lushington, K.; Rolan, P. Stress and tension-type headache mechanisms. *Cephalalgia* **2010**, *30*, 1250–1267. [CrossRef]

73. Maleki, N.; Becerra, L.; Borsook, D. Migraine: Maladaptive Brain Responses to Stress. *Headache J. Head Face Pain* **2012**, *52*, 102–106. [CrossRef] [PubMed]
74. Martin, P.R. Stress and Primary Headache: Review of the Research and Clinical Management. *Curr. Pain Headache Rep.* **2016**, *20*, 1–8. [CrossRef] [PubMed]
75. Warren, M.P.; Fried, J.L. Temporomandibular Disorders and Hormones in Women. *Cells Tissues Organs* **2001**, *169*, 187–192. [CrossRef] [PubMed]
76. Huang, J.Z.; Han, M.F.; Luo, T.D.; Ren, A.K.; Zhou, X.P. Mental health survey of 230 medical staff in a tertiary infectious disease hospital for COVID-19. *Zhonghua Lao Dong Wei Sheng Zhi Ye Bing Za Zhi* **2020**, *38*, 192–1951.
77. Özdin, S.; Özdin, S.B. Levels and predictors of anxiety, depression and health anxiety during COVID-19 pandemic in Turkish society: The importance of gender. *Int. J. Soc. Psychiatry.* **2020**, *66*, 504–511. [CrossRef]
78. Seo, D.; Ahluwalia, A.; Potenza, M.N.; Sinha, R. Gender differences in neural correlates of stress-induced anxiety. *J. Neurosci. Res.* **2017**, *95*, 115–125. [CrossRef] [PubMed]
79. Wang, Y.; Di, Y.; Ye, J.; Wei, W. Study on the public psychological states and its related factors during the outbreak of coronavirus disease 2019 (COVID-19) in some regions of China. *Psychol. Health Med.* **2021**, *26*, 13–22. [CrossRef] [PubMed]
80. Liu, N.; Zhang, F.; Wei, C.; Jia, Y.; Shang, Z.; Sun, L.; Wu, L.; Sun, Z.; Zhou, Y.; Wang, Y.; et al. Prevalence and predictors of PTSS during COVID-19 outbreak in China hardest-hit areas: Gender differences matter. *Psychiatry Res.* **2020**, *287*, 112921. [CrossRef]
81. Babicka-Wirkus, A.; Wirkus, L.; Stasiak, K.; Kozłowski, P. University students' strategies of coping with stress during the coronavirus pandemic: Data from Poland. *PLoS ONE* **2021**, *16*, e0255041. [CrossRef]
82. Cho, S.; Jeon, G.S. Gender Differences in Type D Personality and Mental Health among Korean College Entrants. *Korean J. Stress Res.* **2018**, *26*, 133. [CrossRef]

Journal of
Clinical Medicine

MDPI

Article

A Standardized Prospective Memory Evaluation of the Effects of COVID-19 Confinement on Young Students

Francesca Pisano [1], Giulia Torromino [1], Daniela Brachi [1], Agnese Quadrini [2], Chiara Incoccia [2] and Paola Marangolo [1,2,*]

[1] Department of Humanities Studies, University Federico II, 80133 Naples, Italy; francescapisano00@virgilio.it (F.P.); torromino.giulia@gmail.com (G.T.); daniela.brachi96@gmail.com (D.B.)
[2] IRCCS Santa Lucia Foundation, 00179 Rome, Italy; agnese.quadrini@gmail.com (A.Q.); c.incoccia@hsantalucia.it (C.I.)
* Correspondence: paola.marangolo@gmail.com

Abstract: The restriction imposed worldwide for limiting the spread of coronavirus disease 2019 (COVID-19) globally impacted our lives, decreasing people's wellbeing, causing increased anxiety, depression, and stress and affecting cognitive functions, such as memory. Recent studies reported decreased working memory (WM) and prospective memory (PM), which are pivotal for the ability to plan and perform future activities. Although the number of studies documenting the COVID-19 effects has recently blossomed, most of them employed self-reported questionnaires as the assessment method. The main aim of our study was to use standardized tests to evaluate WM and PM in a population of young students. A sample of 150 female psychology students was recruited online for the administration of two self-reported questionnaires that investigated psychological wellbeing (DASS-21), prospective, and retrospective memory (PRMQ). Subjects were also administered two standardized tests for WM (PASAT) and PM (MIST). We found increased anxiety, depression, and stress and decreased PM as measured by self-reports. The perceived memory failures agreed with the results from the standardized tests, which demonstrated a decrease in both WM and PM. Thus, COVID-19 restriction has strongly impacted on students' mental health and memory abilities, leaving an urgent need for psychological and cognitive recovery plans.

Keywords: COVID-19 confinement; prospective memory; working memory; psychological wellbeing

Citation: Pisano, F.; Torromino, G.; Brachi, D.; Quadrini, A.; Incoccia, C.; Marangolo, P. A Standardized Prospective Memory Evaluation of the Effects of COVID-19 Confinement on Young Students. *J. Clin. Med.* **2021**, *10*, 3919. https://doi.org/10.3390/jcm10173919

Academic Editor: Michele Roccella

Received: 29 July 2021
Accepted: 27 August 2021
Published: 30 August 2021

Publisher's Note: MDPI stays neutral with regard to jurisdictional claims in published maps and institutional affiliations.

1. Introduction

The coronavirus disease 2019 (COVID-19), caused by the novel severe acute respiratory syndrome coronavirus 2 (SARS-CoV-2), has become a global epidemic, posing a serious threat to public health throughout the world [1,2]. To contain and mitigate the speed of viral transmission, governments of many countries implemented extraordinary measures, including social isolation, limitation of mobility, and suspension of commercial, educational, and social activities [3]. Since then, the entire population has been forced to stay at home for long periods of time. Many adults have experienced changes in their work, financial, and personal situations. Children and adolescents have completely restricted social contacts with their peers and significantly limited their physical activities [4], causing major changes in their daily routine.

The social containment measures for which no one was prepared had a strong impact on mental and physical well-being [5,6]. The negative impact on mental health has been documented by a growing number of studies showing higher levels of anxiety, depression, and stress during the pandemic compared to the pre-COVID-19 emergency [7–9]. Social isolation, uncertainty due to prolonged school/academic closure, and lifestyle changes have also negatively affected young people [10–12]. Indeed, several studies have reported increased rates of anxiety, stress, and sleep disturbances in the young population [13–16]. Ahmed and colleagues [11] investigated through an online survey the mental health status of 1074 Chinese people due to the outbreak of the COVID-19 and the mass isolation. The authors showed that young people aged between 21 and 40 years were more psychologically vulnerable, with higher levels of anxiety and depression and a lower mental wellbeing compared to the pre-COVID-19 pandemic. Similarly, another cross-sectional and nationwide survey of college students in China confirmed these results, revealing the prevalence of acute stress, anxiety, and depressive symptoms during the COVID-19 emergency [15]. In line with this evidence, Wathelet and collaborators [16] demonstrated that university students seem to be particularly susceptible to mental health problems. Among risk factors, the authors have identified gender—with females being more affected—precariousness, social isolation, and low quality of social relations.

In addition to psychological variables, the distortion of temporal perception is another relevant aspect that emerged during the pandemic [17–20]. Recently, Ogden [17,18] reported a distortion in the perception of time in a large population of the UK. Indeed, 80% of people reported the feeling that time flew faster or slower during the lockdown with respect to pre-COVID-19 time. However, while during the first lockdown, a slowdown in the perception of time was associated with older age, increased stress, reduced workload, and lower levels of social interactions, during the second lockdown, age, gender, and workload did not influence the relative speed of time. A slower perception of time was associated with greater depression, shielding, and greater dissatisfaction with social interactions. Similarly, Cellini and colleagues [20] investigated the impact of the Italian restriction measures on young adults' daily habits, including sleep quality, digital media use, and the subjective experience of time perception. The results indicated a lower sleep quality associated with a higher level of depression, anxiety, and stress and a slower perception of time during the lockdown compared to prior the lockdown.

It is well known that the perception of time is related to prospective memory (PM) [21,22], which is the ability to remember and therefore to perform planned activities at some point in the future [23,24]. Remembering to collect laundry or remembering to switch off the stove after cooking are examples of PM tasks and illustrate the importance of this type of memory in daily activities. PM consists of two components: event-based and time-based intentions. In event-based tasks, the participants are engaged in an ongoing task, such as searching for words in a crossword puzzle, reading words, answering questions, or making lexical decisions. When a cue related to the intention appears (e.g., a face, an object), participants must remember the intention and therefore make some explicit and recordable response [25–27]. Thus, in the event-based memory, the planned activity is elicited by external environmental stimuli. For example, meeting the boss may serve as a reminder to ask to leave work early. These cues often promote automatic processing that facilitates remembering [28,29]. In contrast, a time-based PM task requires the intention to remember to perform a planned activity at a particular time or after a specific period of time has elapsed [25]. For example, remembering to attend a doctor's appointment at 13:00. As such, time-based tasks do not rely on external cues but require more conscious and intentional processing [25]. To date, many studies on age-related PM performance have been carried out in the laboratory, showing that young adults generally perform better than older adults in PM tasks (for a review, see [30]). Different theoretical models of PM have been proposed so far, some of which identify an interdependence between PM and working memory processes (WM). WM can be defined as the mental workspace responsible for the maintenance and temporary manipulation of information crucial for complex cognitive tasks, such as learning, language comprehension, reasoning, and also for planning future activities [31–34]. Most PM theoretical models argue that remembering to execute an intention requires an interaction between attention and WM. However, theoretical perspectives differ in their emphasis on top-down versus bottom-up processes, among which attention and WM may be involved proactively or reactively [35]. The Preparatory Attention and Memory Processes (PAM) proposes that strategic monitoring, including rehearsing an intention and trial-by-trial checking for cues, is always required to detect the occurrence of the PM cue in the environment [36–38]. Another prominent PM model is the Multiprocess Theory [29]. According to this view, spontaneous retrieval is characterized as a bottom-up, cue-triggered process that is introspectively experienced as a memory popping into mind. The Multiprocess Framework suggests that an intention is spontaneously retrieved when the PM cue is salient or focal. Recently, the Multiprocess Theory has evolved into the Dynamic Multiprocess View (DMPV, see [35,39–41]), according to which strategic monitoring and spontaneous retrieval are not mutually exclusive, but they might interplay dynamically to mediate performance on PM tasks. For instance, in the example "Karen has to remember to buy a bottle of milk on her way home from work", once Karen has formed this intention in the morning, she is unlikely to check the intention during her working day due to the lack of opportunity to buy milk. However, the event of getting into the car and starting the journey home could stimulate the recovery of the intention to stop at the supermarket and buy a bottle of milk. After recovering the intention in this context, Karen might start monitoring the supermarket on her way home. Thus, the DMPV model states that PM is accomplished via the flexible interplay of both top-down and bottom-up processes [35,39–41]. According to this dynamic view, WM capacity effectively engages monitoring at the appropriate moment and disengages it when the cues are unlikely to appear [35]. Indeed, WM processes are supposed to be necessary to support monitoring and to update the information relevant to the appropriate time point in which the intention has to be executed in PM tasks [30]. Accordingly, in a group of twenty-one young participants, Fronda et al. [42] found that failures in PM tasks were significantly associated with the highest load in WM tasks. Moreover, their ability to retrieve the information was less accurate in time-based than in event-based tasks. These findings are consistent with the assumptions that WM is more involved in self-controlled retrieval, which characterizes time-based PM tasks [42–44].

Given the importance of PM in everyday life [30], it is essential to understand the functioning of PM in acute stress situations. Several works have shown that high levels of stress lead to an uncontrolled production of cortisol, which affects cognitive functioning [45,46], also altering PM in different ways (for a review, see [47]). Some research revealed an enhancement of time-based PM performance in stressed participants compared to controls [48–51], while others revealed a negative effect of stress in event-based PM tasks [52].

Considering the COVID-19 pandemic as an undeniably stressful event, it is reasonable to think that the confinement required during the pandemic might have affected cognitive processes. Indeed, recently, in a group of 1215 participants, Fiorenzato and colleagues [53] found a deterioration of attention and executive abilities during the lockdown period, showing an improvement in PM and retrospective memory (RM) compared to the pre-COVID-19 period. Given that work stoppage is one factor of cognitive vulnerability, the authors hypothesized that the participants' memory skills did not deteriorate because most participants continued to work remotely from home.

In addition to PM, WM was also affected by the restrictive measures of the pandemic. As is well known, several studies have already shown that higher levels of anxiety are associated with poor WM performance [54,55]. In line with this evidence, during the first period of lockdown, Fellman and collaborators [56] confirmed a negative correlation between anxiety levels and WM performance, and Santangelo et al. [57] uncovered marked difficulties in memory and attention in a large sample of adults mainly constituted by non-workers.

To our knowledge, to date, most studies have used self-report questionnaires to assess the effects of COVID-19 on both psychological variables and cognitive skills. In the present study, we aimed at studying the impact of COVID-19 on psychological wellbeing, WM, and PM in a sample of 150 students by using standardized cognitive tests to reduce the effect of social desirability bias.

2. Materials and Methods

2.1. Participants

A total of 170 female students aged between 18 and 23 years old (mean = 19.8 years, SD = 1.37) with an educational level of 13 years were recruited for this study. All subjects attended the first year for their bachelor's degree in psychology. Inclusion criteria were: Italian language as mother tongue; right-handed [58]; and no history of chronic or acute neurologic, psychiatric, or medical disease. In terms of geographic distribution, all participants came from Campania, a southern Italian region. During the confinement, all participants lived in two-parent families. Among the study sample, nobody was diagnosed with COVID-19. Of the initial 170 participants, 20 students dropped out for personal reasons. The final sample was therefore made up of 150 students.

G*Power 3.1 [59] was used to calculate the sample size with $\alpha = 0.05$ and a power = 80%. The analysis indicated that a total sample size of $N \geq 34$ was necessary to detect a significant effect in our study. Our final sample comprised 150 students, which is a size well beyond this threshold.

2.2. Ethics Statement

The data analyzed in the current study were collected in accordance with the Helsinki Declaration and the Institutional Review Board of the IRCCS Fondazione Santa Lucia, Rome, Italy. Prior to participation, all participants signed an online informed consent form.

2.3. Materials

2.3.1. Self-Report Questionnaires

The materials included two psychometrically self-report questionnaires:

(1) Depression Anxiety Stress Scales (DASS-21), which consists of 21 questions with 7 items for each scale (e.g., for anxiety, "I feel I am close to panic"; for depression, "I cannot experience any positive feelings"; for stress, "I find hard to wind down"); all subscales are rated on a four-point Likert scale ranging from 0 (never) to 3 (almost always). Higher scores indicate more severe emotional distress (max–min total score: 21–0) [60];

(2) The Prospective and Retrospective Memory Questionnaire (PRMQ), which consists of 16 items on a five-point scale (e.g., for prospective memory, "Do you decide to do something in a few minutes and then forget to do it?"; for retrospective memory, "Do you forget something that someone told you a few minutes before?"). Higher total scores indicate more frequent self-reported memory difficulties (max–min total score: 80–16) [61].

2.3.2. Cognitive Tests

The Paced Auditory Serial Addition Task (PASAT) [62] and the Memory for Intentions Screening Test (MIST) [63] were used.

The PASAT measures WM performance. The test consists of a list of 60 numbers between 1 and 9. Subjects are asked to add up each auditorily presented number in the list with the next one and to give the response within 1.8 milliseconds. For example, if the first two numbers presented are 5 and 6, the subject must answer 11 (6 + 5) [62].

The MIST assesses the ability to remember and perform planned activities at some point in the future. It consists of 8 everyday PM activities that involve the individual in an assigned task at a specific time (i.e., after 2 min or 15 min from the assignment) or when a specific cue is given (i.e., an event cue or a time cue). For instance, for event-based tasks: "When I show you a red pen, write your name in the chatroom"; for time-based tasks: "In 15 min, please ask me to take a break". Within the time frame in which subjects are required to remember to perform the assigned tasks, they are involved in an ongoing task (i.e., word search puzzle) [63].

2.4. Procedure

Prior to performing the experiment, each participant received all the information on the research protocol via an online information sheet. Subjects who agreed to participate in the study signed and sent the online informed consent.

Each participant logged into Microsoft Teams platform, which allows to share the visual and auditory stimuli of the PASAT and MIST tests between the experimenter and the participant for a duration of one hour by using a personal access code. The examiner, after verifying the number code, shared the computer screen. For the PASAT test, subjects had to respond within 1.8 milliseconds, while for the MIST test, participants had to answer within 2 min for items 3, 5, 7, and 8 and within 15 min for items 1, 2, 4, and 6. The cognitive tests, PASAT and MIST, measured the participants' cognitive performance one month after the COVID-19 confinement (T1).

The two psychometrically self-reported questionnaires investigated the psychological factors (anxiety, depression, and stress) and prospective and retrospective memory by asking participants to compare their responses at two time-points: one month before (T0) and one month after (T1) the COVID-19 confinement. They were administered through a specific online platform (Google Forms, Google Inc., Mountain View, CA, USA).

The order of administration of the self-report questionnaires (DASS-21, PRMQ) and of the cognitive tests (PASAT, MIST) was randomized among participants.

2.5. Data Analysis

Data were analyzed with IBM SPSS Statistics 22 software. To verify the applicability of the parametric analysis, a Shapiro–Wilk normality test was applied, which did not reveal a normal distribution of the data.

For the self-report questionnaires, statistical analyses were performed on the mean percentage of responses with two separated Wilcoxon tests for DASS-21 and PRMQ to evaluate differences between T0 and T1 in anxiety, depression, and stress and in prospective and retrospective memory, respectively.

For the MIST and PASAT tests, we ran two separated Mann–Whitney U tests, which compared the mean number of incorrect—for the PASAT test—or correct responses—for the MIST test—at T1 with the normative data (T0) for the two tests. For the MIST test, the Wilcoxon signed-rank test for paired samples was also conducted to directly compare the results obtained in the event-based and time-based subtests at T1.

Finally, Spearman's correlations were calculated to examine possible relationships within the self-reported questionnaires (DASS-21 and PRMQ) and within the standardized tests (PASAT and MIST) at T1. Only significant correlations are reported in the Results section.

For all analyses, p-values < 0.05 were considered as statistically significant.

3. Results

3.1. Self-Report Questionnaires

For the DASS-21 test, the Wilcoxon signed-rank test revealed a significant increase in the mean percentage of anxiety (T0: mean = 19.5, SD = 7.2; T1: mean = 42.7, SD = 10.2; Z = −10.47; $p < 0.001$), depression (T0: mean = 23.6, SD = 8.5; T1: mean = 50.2, SD = 10.3; Z = −10.67; $p < 0.001$), and stress levels (T0: mean = 33.7, SD = 8.1; T1: mean = 79.1, SD = 10.2; Z = −10.65; $p < 0.001$) between T0 (pre-) and T1 (after confinement) (Figure 1). Moreover, the comparison of the mean score obtained at T1 for each domain of the DASS-21 to normative data confirmed an increased level of anxiety, depression, and stress, which reached the level of "severe" (Table 1).

In parallel, the Wilcoxon signed-rank test revealed a significant increase in the mean percentage of responses for both the prospective (T0: mean = 41.4, SD = 6.9; T1: mean = 51.6, SD = 6.8; Z = −9.96; $p < 0.001$) and the retrospective memory (T0: mean = 43.5, SD = 4.8; T1: mean = 52.4, SD = 7.4; Z = −10.02; $p < 0.001$) (Figure 2), which suggests an overall increase in the participants' self-reported failures in their memory abilities during the confinement. The comparison of the PM performance at T1 to normative data confirmed the above results (Table 2).

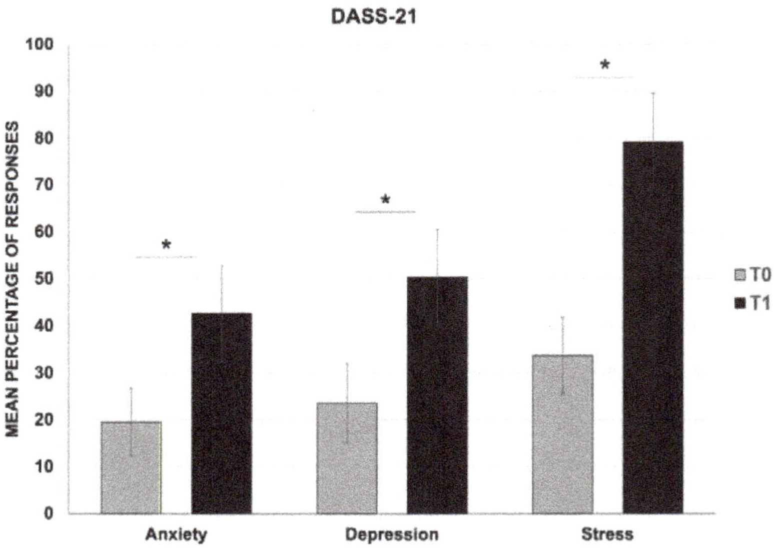

Figure 1. Mean percentage of responses for anxiety, depression, and stress scales (DASS-21) at two time-points: one month before (T0) and one month after the COVID-19 confinement (T1). * $p < 0.001$ T0 vs. T1.

Table 1. The mean scores of the anxiety, depression, and stress scale (DASS-21) at T1 compared to normative data [60].

Anxiety T1 Mean (SD)	Cut-Off
17.92 (4.3)	Normal 0–7 Mild 8–9 Moderate 10–14 **Severe 15–19** Extremely severe 20+
DEPRESSION T1 Mean (SD)	**Cut-Off**
21.08 (4.3)	Normal 0–9 Mild 10–13 Moderate 14–20 **Severe 21–27** Extremely severe 28+
STRESS T1 Mean (SD)	**Cut-Off**
33.21 (4.3)	Normal 0–14 Mild 15–18 Moderate 19–25 **Severe 26–33** Extremely severe 34+

SD, standard deviation.

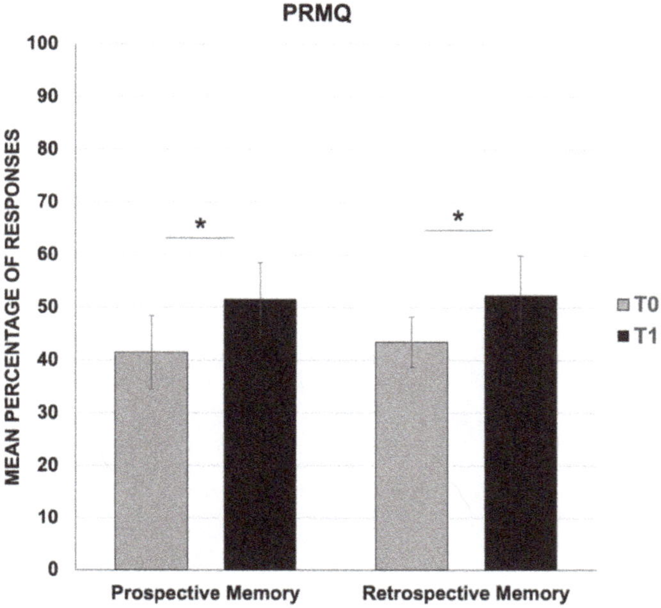

Figure 2. Mean percentage of responses for prospective and retrospective memory scales (PRMQ) at two time-points: one month before (T0) and one month after the COVID-19 confinement (T1). * $p < 0.001$ T0 vs. T1.

Table 2. The mean scores of the prospective memory scale (PRMQ) at T1 compared to normative data [64].

	Prospective Memory Mean (SD)	Retrospective Memory Mean (SD)
T1	20.7 (2.7) *	20.9 (3.0) *
ND	18.7 (5.5)	16.9 (5.0)

ND, normative data; SD, standard deviation. * $p < 0.001$.

3.2. Cognitive Tests

In the PASAT test, the Mann–Whitney U test revealed a significant decrease in the participants' performance (mean = 29.7, SD = 5.2; Z = −14.99; $p < 0.001$) at T1 compared to normative data (T0) [62] (Figure 3). Similarly, we found a significant decrease in PM (mean = 38.3, SD = 5.3; Z = −9.66; $p < 0.001$) by comparing the MIST results at T1 to its normative data (T0) [63] (Figure 4). In addition, the Wilcoxon signed-rank test showed a significant dissociation between event-based (mean = 7.1, SD = 1.2) and time-based (mean = 5.6, SD = 1.2) intentions in the MIST test, with lower scores in the time-based dimension with respect to the event-based tasks (Z = −8.12; $p < 0.001$) (Figure 5).

3.3. Correlation Analysis

A significant correlation between the anxiety levels, as measured by the DASS-21, and the participants' performance in the PRMQ scale was found at T1 (Table 3). A significant correlation was also observed at T1 between the participants' performance in the time-based tasks of the MIST and their WM performance measured through the PASAT (Table 4).

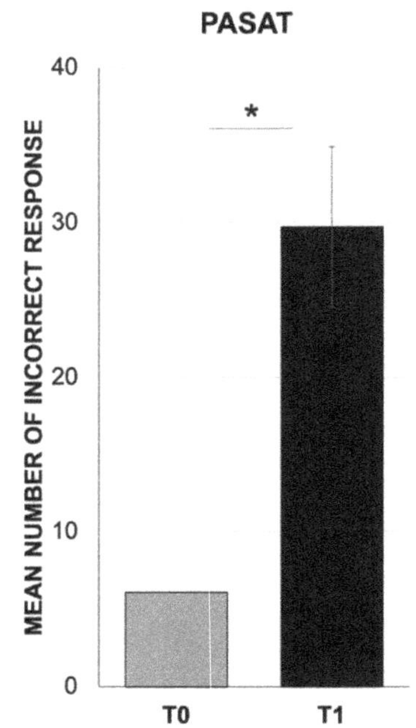

Figure 3. Mean number of incorrect responses for the working memory test (PASAT). The results collected at one month after the COVID-19 confinement (T1) compared to the normative data for the test (T0). * $p < 0.001$ T0 vs. T1.

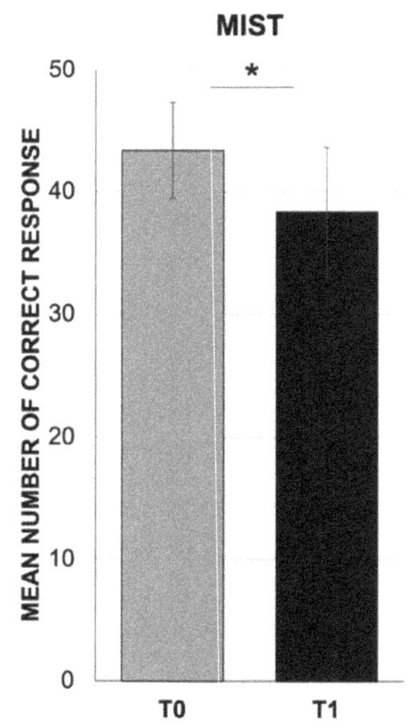

Figure 4. Mean number of correct responses for the prospective memory test (MIST). The results collected at one month after the COVID-19 confinement (T1) compared to the normative data for the test (T0). * $p < 0.001$ T0 vs. T1.

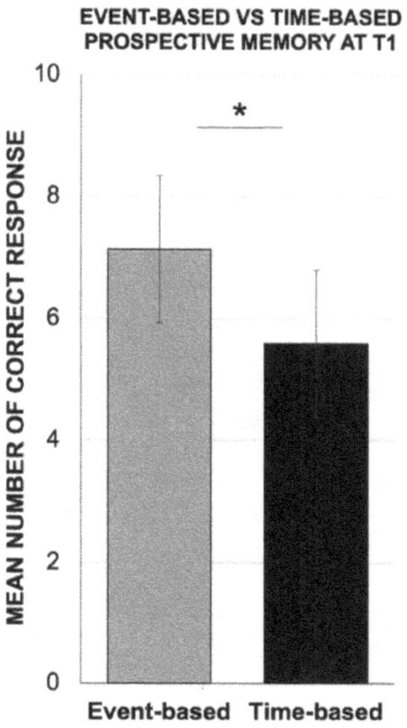

Figure 5. Mean number of correct responses for event-based and time-based tasks of the prospective memory test at T1. * $p < 0.001$ at T1.

Table 3. Spearman's correlation coefficients (ρ) and their significance levels (p) are reported between the anxiety levels in the DASS-21 and the PRMQ-Prospective (PM) and Retrospective Memory (RM) subtest scores.

Self-Reported Questionnaire	Anxiety (T1)
PRMQ-PM (T1)	ρ = 0.1974 (**p = 0.0154**)
PRMQ-RM (T1)	ρ = 0.2083 (**p = 0.0105**)

Table 4. Spearman's correlation coefficients (ρ) and their significance levels (p) are reported between the MIST total score, the event-based, and time-based tasks scores and the PASAT score.

Standardized Test	PASAT (T1)
MIST (T1)	ρ = −0.1139 (p = 0.1653)
Event-based MIST (T1)	ρ = 0.0112 (p = 0.8921)
Time-based MIST (T1)	ρ = −0.1970 (**p = 0.0157**)

4. Discussion

The main aim of the present study was to investigate the impact of COVID-19 on psychological wellbeing, PM, and WM in a large sample of young students. For this purpose, unlike most of the previous studies, we used not only self-reported questionnaires but also standardized cognitive tests, which are less susceptible to social desirability and recall biases.

In line with several recently published studies [10–16], our results showed that our sample of students experienced increased levels of anxiety, depression, and stress at one month after the COVID-19 confinement compared to the pre-COVID-19 condition. These results were also confirmed when comparing our results to normative data, which, for all dimensions, revealed that our sample reached the level of "severe". Thus, our data suggest that the pandemic has severely affected the mental health of our students, leading to social and emotional changes in their daily lives. Accordingly, to date, many studies have already pointed out that due to prolonged school/academic closure, lifestyle changes, and social distance, young people are more vulnerable to stress than older adults [65–67].

The findings from the self-reported PRMQ revealed that our sample perceived memory-domain failures during the confinement, both in the prospective and retrospective components, compared to the pre-lockdown period and to normative data. Thus, our findings are in line with previous suggestions, which proposed that lower rates of psychosocial well-being during the pandemic negatively affect the perception of time [17–20], a factor that is strongly related to PM processes [21,22]. In particular, some studies have identified stress as a detrimental factor for PM, suggesting that the psychological distress found in our students might have determined a distortion of time perception and, in turn, a PM disorder [52,68]. We also found a significant correlation at T1 between the score in the anxiety scale and the participant's performance in the PMRQ questionnaire. Thus, not surprisingly, the perceived worsening in PM found in our sample was also influenced by its increased levels in anxiety.

Interestingly, the results in the MIST test confirmed a decrease in the participants' PM performance compared to normative data, with a greater impact on time-based than on event-based tasks.

As reported in the introduction, PM involves two memory components: event-based and time-based intentions, which require different levels of cognitive demand and effort. Event-based tasks entail detecting cues or reminders in our environment related to previously established intentions (e.g., remembering to go to the supermarket for buying milk after work). These cues (e.g., a road sign referring to a supermarket) facilitate recall by promoting automatic processes [28,29]. Conversely, time-based intentions require the retrieval of previously formed plans (e.g., calling the doctor for a prescription) either at a specified time (e.g., at 6 p.m.) or after a certain time has elapsed (e.g., in 15 min). In this case, no external cues are provided that prompt the participant to initiate the performance. Thus, time-based intentions are cognitively more demanding than event-based intentions, as the former depend on implicit cues and require more self-initiation and monitoring [25,30]. Since confinement at home during the lockdown has significantly reduced the opportunity for students to take advantage of external cues to automatically recall future plans or intentions, a worsening in event-related memory was expected. However, we found that students had the worst performance in time-based tasks, which may be explained by the fact that these tasks require a greater cognitive load than event-based intentions, and they are known to depend upon WM engagement [42]. Indeed, together with a PM disorder, we found a decrease in WM performance, which was significantly correlated only with the time-based score of the MIST test. This latter evidence is in accordance with the most recent model of PM, the DMPV model, which posits that the ability to remember a planned intention depends upon the interplay between top-down and bottom-up processes, and it is influenced by WM capacity [35]. Accordingly, Fronda et al. [42] recently showed that time-based PM intentions are influenced by high cognitive load in WM tasks.

As far as we know, although previous studies have already shown a negative impact of the pandemic on different psychological and cognitive abilities [13,15,16,56,57], none of them measured the effects of the pandemic on PM tasks using standardized tests and their relationship with WM processes (but see [56] for WM). This constitutes the innovative and original aspect of our work with respect to most of the current studies conducted during the time of the pandemic, which included only subjective measurements. Indeed, in line with previous suggestions [69,70], we believe that the inclusion of standardized tests resulted advantageously since they are less influenced by response styles, social desirability, and self-report bias with respect to self-reported questionnaires. Accordingly, since the different tests rely on different ways to measure the subjects' performance, as in the study by Arnold et al. [70], we did not find any significant correlations between the self-report scales and the standardized tests.

Thus, we believe that our results point to the urgency of using standardized tests to investigate the effects of the pandemic in different populations. These tests, although they were not administered before the pandemic, as no one could have predicted what happened, can still be considered as valid and reliable measures by comparing the results obtained during the pandemic to their normative data from large reference populations of different ages and educational levels. In fact, it is highly unlikely that the use of normative data in a large sample such as ours could have biased the results. We also believe that, in the near future, a possible way to overcome the difficulty in collecting data before the pandemic might be the development of longitudinal studies. Indeed, this approach might detect a stabilization of the observed changes in the cognitive and psychological domains between the different waves of the pandemic or instead an ability of the people to adapt themselves following the prolonged time of exposure to stress.

A possible caveat of our study is that the sample consisted of only young women from the Southern Italy. In fact, it was not possible to make a gender comparison between males and females. In the literature, several studies have shown that women are more vulnerable to anxiety, depression, and stress with respect to men [71–73]. For example, in a repeated cross-sectional study, in the early stages of the COVID-19 pandemic, Debowska and colleagues [71] showed a significant decrease in psychological well-being in female students from Poland compared to males. Moreover, the authors reported that young adult students (aged between 18–24 years old) had more symptoms of depression, anxiety, and suicidality than adult students (>25 years old). Similarly, in Essadek and Rabeyron's work [72], female gender and younger age were identified as risk factors associated with mental distress during the COVID-19 pandemic. So far, no study has explored gender differences in PM tasks during the COVID-19 epidemic. To date, only the results of Fellman and colleagues [56] indicated that the impact of COVID-19 on WM cannot be explained by gender differences. It must also be considered that all of our students attended the first year for the bachelor's degree in psychology; thus, our results cannot be generalized to all university students.

In conclusion, our data highlight the need for strategic plans to improve wellbeing, mental health, and cognitive performance in different populations and above all, in young people. Although in our study, we compared an actual population of students to normative data as a strategy to overcome the difficulty in measuring their performance before the beginning of the pandemic, we believe that the inclusion of standardized tests gives strength to our results, and it represents an element of novelty compared to previous studies on COVID-19 restrictions. As stated above and confirmed by previous studies [69,70], we believe that standardized tests are more sensitive to cognitive changes and less vulnerable to social desirability and recall bias compared to self-reported measures.

Before the pandemic, we were not prepared to prevent the emotional and cognitive effects we are still experiencing. Young people are more vulnerable to these effects. Indeed, the COVID-19 crisis has severely affected labor markets around the world, hurting young people more than other age groups. Globally, youth employment has fallen. Thus, the development of different recovery strategies and their implementation in schools and academics is an urgent need for our societies.

Author Contributions: Conceptualization, F.P. and P.M.; methodology, F.P. and C.I.; software, F.P. and D.B.; formal analysis, F.P. and A.Q.; investigation, F.P. and D.B.; data curation, F.P. and A.Q.; writing—original draft preparation, F.P. and G.T.; writing—review and editing, G.T. and P.M.; supervision, P.M. All authors have read and agreed to the published version of the manuscript.

Funding: This research received no external funding.

Institutional Review Board Statement: The study was conducted according to the guidelines of the Declaration of Helsinki and approved by the Institutional Review Board of IRCCS Santa Lucia Foundation, Rome, Italy (CE/PROG.930, 26 July 2021).

Informed Consent Statement: Informed consent was obtained from all subjects involved in the study.

Data Availability Statement: The data presented in this study are available on request from the corresponding author. The data are not publicly available due to ethical and privacy restrictions.

Conflicts of Interest: The authors declare no conflict of interest.

References

1. Şencan, I.; Kuzi, S. Global threat of Covid 19 and evacuation of the citizens of different countries. *Turk. J. Med. Sci.* **2020**, *50*, 534–543. [CrossRef]
2. Peng, M. Outbreak of Covid-19: An emerging global pandemic threat. *Biomed. Pharmacother.* **2020**, *129*, 110499. [CrossRef]
3. Qiu, J.; Shen, B.; Zhao, M.; Wang, Z.; Xie, B.; Xu, Y. A nationwide survey of psychological distress among Chinese people in the Covid-19 epidemic: Implications and policy recommendations. *Gen. Psychiatry* **2020**, *33*, e100213. [CrossRef]
4. Danese, A.; Smith, P.; Chitsabesan, P.; Dubicka, B. Child and adolescent mental health amidst emergencies and disasters. *Br. J. Psychiatry* **2020**, *216*, 159–162. [CrossRef]
5. Brooks, S.K.; Webster, R.K.; Smith, L.E.; Woodland, L.; Wessely, S.; Greenberg, N.J.; Rubin, G.J. The psychological impact of quarantine and how to reduce it: Rapid review of the evidence. *Lancet* **2020**, *395*, 912–920. [CrossRef]
6. Hawryluck, L.; Gold, W.L.; Robinson, S.; Pogorski, S.; Galea, S.; Styra, R. SARS Control and psychological effects of quarantine, toronto, canada. *Emerg. Infect. Dis.* **2004**, *10*, 1206–1212. [CrossRef] [PubMed]
7. Pierce, M.; Hope, H.; Ford, T.; Hatch, S.; Hotopf, M.; John, A.; Kontopantelis, E.; Webb, R.; Wessely, S.; McManus, S.; et al. Mental health before and during the Covid-19 pandemic: A longitudinal probability sample survey of the UK population. *Lancet Psychiatry* **2020**, *7*, 883–892. [CrossRef]
8. Liu, K.; Chen, Y.; Lin, R.; Han, K. Clinical features of Covid-19 in elderly patients: A comparison with young and middle-aged patients. *J. Infect.* **2020**, *80*, e14–e18. [CrossRef]
9. Xiao, H.; Shu, W.; Li, M.; Li, Z.; Tao, F.; Wu, X.; Yu, Y.; Meng, H.; Vermund, S.H.; Hu, Y. Social distancing among medical students during the 2019 coronavirus disease pandemic in China: Disease awareness, anxiety disorder, depression, and behavioral activities. *Int. J. Environ. Res. Public Health* **2020**, *17*, 5047. [CrossRef]
10. Gualano, M.R.; Lo Moro, G.; Voglino, G.; Bert, F.; Siliquini, R. Effects of Covid-19 lockdown on mental health and sleep disturbances in Italy. *Int. J. Environ. Res. Public Health* **2020**, *17*, 4779. [CrossRef]
11. Ahmed, M.Z.; Ahmed, O.; Aibao, Z.; Hanbin, S.; Siyu, L.; Ahmad, A. Epidemic of Covid-19 in China and associated psychological problems. *Asian J. Psychiatry* **2020**, *51*, 102092. [CrossRef]
12. Yuan, S.; Liao, Z.; Huang, H.; Jiang, B.; Zhang, X.; Wang, Y.; Zhao, M. Comparison of the indicators of psychological stress in the population of hubei province and non-endemic provinces in china during two weeks during the coronavirus disease 2019 (Covid-19) outbreak in february 2020. *Med. Sci. Monit.* **2020**, *26*, e923767-1. [CrossRef]
13. Wang, C.; Pan, R.; Wan, X.; Tan, Y.; Xu, L.; McIntyre, R.S.; Choo, F.N.; Tran, B.; Ho, R.; Sharma, V.K.; et al. A longitudinal study on the mental health of general population during the Covid-19 epidemic in China. *Brain Behav. Immun.* **2020**, *87*, 40–48. [CrossRef]
14. Garfin, D.R.; Silver, R.C.; Holman, E.A. The novel coronavirus (COVID-2019) outbreak: Amplification of public health consequences by media exposure. *Health Psychol.* **2020**, *39*, 355–357. [CrossRef]
15. Ma, Z.; Zhao, J.; Li, Y.; Chen, D.; Wang, T.; Zhang, Z.; Chen, Z.; Yu, Q.; Jiang, J.; Fan, F.; et al. Mental health problems and correlates among 746 217 college students during the coronavirus disease 2019 outbreak in China. *Epidemiol. Psychiatr. Sci.* **2020**, *29*, e181. [CrossRef] [PubMed]
16. Wathelet, M.; Duhem, S.; Vaiva, G.; Baubet, T.; Habran, E.; Veerapa, E.; Debien, C.; Molenda, S.; Horn, M.; Grandgenèvre, P.; et al. Factors associated with mental health disorders among university students in France confined during the Covid-19 pandemic. *JAMA Netw. Open* **2020**, *3*, e2025591. [CrossRef]
17. Ogden, R.S. The passage of time during the UK Covid-19 lockdown. *PLoS ONE* **2020**, *15*, e0235871. [CrossRef]
18. Ogden, R. Distortions to the passage of time during England's second national lockdown: A role for depression. *PLoS ONE* **2021**, *16*, e0250412. [CrossRef]
19. Droit-Volet, S.; Gil, S.; Martinelli, N.; Andant, N.; Clinchamps, M.; Parreira, L.; Rouffiac, K.; Dambrun, M.; Huguet, P.; Dubuis, B.; et al. Time and Covid-19 stress in the lockdown situation: Time free, dying of boredom and sadness. *PLoS ONE* **2020**, *15*, e0236465. [CrossRef]

20. Cellini, N.; Canale, N.; Mioni, G.; Costa, S. Changes in sleep pattern, sense of time and digital media use during Covid-19 lockdown in Italy. *J. Sleep Res.* **2020**, *29*, e13074. [CrossRef]
21. Mioni, G.; Stablum, F. Monitoring behaviour in a time-based prospective memory task: The involvement of executive functions and time perception. *Memory* **2014**, *22*, 536–552. [CrossRef]
22. Mioni, G.; Grondin, S.; McLennan, S.N.; Stablum, F. The role of time-monitoring behaviour in time-based prospective memory performance in younger and older adults. *Memory* **2020**, *28*, 34–48. [CrossRef]
23. Brandimonte, M.A.; Einstein, G.O.; McDaniel, M.A. *Prospective Memory: Theory and Applications*; Erlbaum: Mahwah, NJ, USA, 1996.
24. Carlesimo, G.; Costa, A. An introduction to the special issue on the neuropsychology of prospective memory. *Neuropsychologia* **2011**, *49*, 2143–2146. [CrossRef]
25. Einstein, G.O.; McDaniel, M.A.; Richardson, S.L.; Guynn, M.J.; Cunfer, A.R. Aging and prospective memory: Examining the influences of self-initiated retrieval processes. *J. Exp. Psychol. Learn. Mem. Cogn.* **1995**, *21*, 996–1007. [CrossRef]
26. Ellis, J.; Kvavilashvili, L.; Milne, A. Experimental tests of prospective remembering: The influence of cue-event frequency on performance. *Br. J. Psychol.* **1999**, *90*, 9–23. [CrossRef]
27. McDaniel, M.A.; Robinson-Riegler, B.; Einstein, G.O. Prospective remembering: Perceptually driven or conceptually driven processes? *Mem. Cogn.* **1998**, *26*, 121–134. [CrossRef]
28. McDaniel, M.A.; Einstein, G.O. Strategic and automatic processes in prospective memory retrieval: A multiprocess framework. *Appl. Cogn. Psychol.* **2000**, *14*, S127–S144. [CrossRef]
29. McDaniel, M.A.; Einstein, G.O. *Prospective Memory: An Overview and Synthesis of an Emerging Field*; SAGE Publications Ltd.: London, UK, 2007.
30. Kliegel, M.; Jäger, T.; Phillips, L.H. Adult age differences in event-based prospective memory: A meta-analysis on the role of focal versus nonfocal cues. *Psychol. Aging* **2008**, *23*, 203–208. [CrossRef]
31. Baddeley, A.; Hitch, G. Working memory. In *The Psychology of Learning and Motivation*; Bower, G.H., Ed.; Academic Press: New York, NY, USA, 1974; pp. 47–89.
32. Baddeley, A. The episodic buffer: A new component of working memory? *Trends Cogn. Sci.* **2000**, *4*, 417–423. [CrossRef]
33. Baddeley, A. Working memory and language: An overview. *J. Commun. Disord.* **2003**, *36*, 189–208. [CrossRef]
34. Cowan, N.; Elliott, E.; Saults, J.S.; Morey, C.C.; Mattox, S.; Hismjatullina, A.; Conway, A.R. On the capacity of attention: Its estimation and its role in working memory and cognitive aptitudes. *Cogn. Psychol.* **2005**, *51*, 42–100. [CrossRef]
35. Shelton, J.T.; Scullin, M.K. The dynamic interplay between bottom-up and top-down processes supporting prospective memory. *Curr. Dir. Psychol. Sci.* **2017**, *26*, 352–358. [CrossRef]
36. Smith, R.E. The cost of remembering to remember in event-based prospective memory: Investigating the capacity demands of delayed intention performance. *J. Exp. Psychol. Learn. Mem. Cogn.* **2003**, *29*, 347–361. [CrossRef] [PubMed]
37. Smith, R.E.; Bayen, U.J. A multinomial model of event-based prospective memory. *J. Exp. Psychol. Learn. Mem. Cogn.* **2004**, *30*, 756–777. [CrossRef]
38. Smith, R.E.; Skinner, D.J. Prospective memory in context: Methods, findings, and future directions. In *Prospective Memory*; Routledge: Oxfordshire, UK, 2019.
39. Scullin, M.K.; McDaniel, M.A.; Shelton, J.T. The dynamic multiprocess framework: Evidence from prospective memory with contextual variability. *Cogn. Psychol.* **2013**, *67*, 55–71. [CrossRef]
40. Anderson, F.T.; Strube, M.J.; McDaniel, M.A. Toward a better understanding of costs in prospective memory: A meta-analytic review. *Psychol. Bull.* **2019**, *145*, 1053–1081. [CrossRef]
41. Shelton, J.; Scullin, K.M.; Hacker, Y.J. The multiprocess framework. Historical context and the "dynamic" extension. In *Prospective Memory*; Rummel, J., McDaniel, M.A., Eds.; Routledge: Oxfordshire, UK, 2019.
42. Fronda, G.; Monti, C.; Sozzi, M.; Corbo, M.; Balconi, M. Prospective memory and working memory in comparison. New experimental paradigms. *Int. J. Neurosci.* **2019**, *130*, 834–840. [CrossRef]
43. Kliegel, M.; Ramuschkat, G.; Martin, M. Exekutive funktionen und prospektive gedächtnisleistung im Alter. *Z. Gerontol. Geriatr.* **2003**, *36*, 35–41. [CrossRef]
44. Martin, M.; Kliegel, M.; McDaniel, M.A. The involvement of executive functions in prospective memory performance of adults. *Int. J. Psychol.* **2003**, *38*, 195–206. [CrossRef]
45. Liston, C.; McEwen, B.S.; Casey, B.J. Psychosocial stress reversibly disrupts prefrontal processing and attentional control. *Proc. Natl. Acad. Sci. USA* **2009**, *106*, 912–917. [CrossRef]
46. Qin, S.; Hermans, E.J.; van Marle, H.J.; Luo, J.; Fernandez, G. Acute psychological stress reduces working memory-related activity in the dorsolateral prefrontal cortex. *Biol. Psychiatry* **2009**, *66*, 25–32. [CrossRef]
47. Piefke, M.; Glienke, K. The effects of stress on prospective memory: A systematic review. *Psychol. Neurosci.* **2017**, *10*, 345–362. [CrossRef]
48. Möschl, M.; Walser, M.; Plessow, F.; Goschke, T.; Fischer, R. Acute stress shifts the balance between controlled and automatic processes in prospective memory. *Neurobiol. Learn. Mem.* **2017**, *144*, 53–67. [CrossRef]
49. Nater, U.; Okere, U.; Stallkamp, R.; Moor, C.; Ehlert, U.; Kliegel, M. Psychosocial stress enhances time-based prospective memory in healthy young men. *Neurobiol. Learn. Mem.* **2006**, *86*, 344–348. [CrossRef]

50. Szőllősi, Á.; Pajkossy, P.; Demeter, G.; Kéri, S.; Racsmány, M. Acute stress affects prospective memory functions via associative memory processes. *Acta Psychol.* **2018**, *182*, 82–90. [CrossRef]
51. Walser, M.; Fischer, R.; Goschke, T.; Kirschbaum, C.; Plessow, F. Intention retrieval and deactivation following an acute psychosocial stressor. *PLoS ONE* **2013**, *8*, e85685. [CrossRef]
52. Ihle, A.; Schnitzspahn, K.; Rendell, P.; Luong, C.; Kliegel, M. Age benefits in everyday prospective memory: The influence of personal task importance, use of reminders and everyday stress. *Aging Neuropsychol. Cogn.* **2012**, *19*, 84–101. [CrossRef]
53. Fiorenzato, E.; Zabberoni, S.; Costa, A.; Cona, G. Cognitive and mental health changes and their vulnerability factors related to Covid-19 lockdown in Italy. *PLoS ONE* **2021**, *16*, e0246204. [CrossRef]
54. Ashcraft, M.H.; Kirk, E.P. The relationships among working memory, math anxiety, and performance. *J. Exp. Psychol. Gen.* **2001**, *130*, 224–237. [CrossRef]
55. Andreotti, C.; Thigpen, J.E.; Dunn, M.J.; Watson, K.; Potts, J.; Reising, M.M.; Robinson, K.E.; Rodriguez, E.M.; Roubinov, D.; Luecken, L.; et al. Cognitive reappraisal and secondary control coping: Associations with working memory, positive and negative affect, and symptoms of anxiety/depression. *Anxiety Stress. Coping* **2013**, *26*, 20–35. [CrossRef]
56. Fellman, D.; Ritakallio, L.; Waris, O.; Jylkkä, J.; Laine, M. Beginning of the pandemic: Covid-19-elicited anxiety as a predictor of working memory performance. *Front. Psychol.* **2020**, *11*, 576466. [CrossRef]
57. Santangelo, G.; Baldassarre, I.; Barbaro, A.; Cavallo, N.D.; Cropano, M.; Maggi, G.; Nappo, R.; Trojano, L.; Raimo, S. Subjective cognitive failures and their psychological correlates in a large Italian sample during quarantine/self-isolation for Covid-19. *Neurol. Sci.* **2021**, *42*, 2625–2635. [CrossRef]
58. Oldfield, R.C. The assessment and analysis of handedness: The Edinburgh inventory. *Neuropsychologia* **1971**, *9*, 97–113. [CrossRef]
59. Faul, F.; Erdfelder, E.; Buchner, A.; Lang, A.-G. Statistical power analyses using G*Power 3.1: Tests for correlation and regression analyses. *Behav. Res. Methods* **2009**, *41*, 1149–1160. [CrossRef]
60. Bottesi, G.; Ghisi, M.; Altoè, G.; Conforti, E.; Melli, G.; Sica, C. The Italian version of the depression anxiety stress scales-21: Factor structure and psychometric properties on community and clinical samples. *Compr. Psychiatry* **2015**, *60*, 170–181. [CrossRef]
61. Crawford, J.; Smith, G.; Maylor, E.; Della Sala, S.; Logie, R. The prospective and retrospective memory questionnaire (PRMQ): Normative data and latent structure in a large non-clinical sample. *Memory* **2003**, *11*, 261–275. [CrossRef]
62. Ciaramelli, E.; Serino, A.; Benassi, M.; Bolzani, R. Paced auditory serial addition task (PASAT) standardizzazione di tre test di memoria di lavoro. *Giornale Italiano di Psicologia* **2006**, *33*, 607–624.
63. Raskin, S.A. Memory for intentions screening test: Psychometric properties and clinical evidence. *Brain Impair.* **2009**, *10*, 23–33. [CrossRef]
64. Crawford, J.R.; Henry, J.; Ward, A.L.; Blake, J. The prospective and retrospective memory questionnaire (PRMQ): Latent structure, normative data and discrepancy analysis for proxy-ratings. *Br. J. Clin. Psychol.* **2006**, *45*, 83–104. [CrossRef]
65. Kowal, M.; Coll-Martín, T.; Ikizer, G.; Rasmussen, J.; Eichel, K.; Studzińska, A.; Koszałkowska, K.; Karwowski, M.; Najmussaqib, A.; Pankowski, D.; et al. Who is the most stressed during the Covid-19 pandemic? Data from 26 countries and areas. *Appl. Psychol. Health Well Being* **2020**, *12*, 946–966. [CrossRef]
66. Birditt, K.S.; Turkelson, A.; Fingerman, K.L.; Polenick, C.A.; Oya, A. Age differences in stress, life changes, and social ties during the Covid-19 pandemic: Implications for psychological well-being. *Gerontologist* **2021**, *61*, 205–216. [CrossRef]
67. Varma, P.; Junge, M.; Meaklim, H.; Jackson, M.L. Younger people are more vulnerable to stress, anxiety and depression during Covid-19 pandemic: A global cross-sectional survey. *Prog. Neuro Psychopharmacol. Biol. Psychiatry* **2021**, *109*, 110236. [CrossRef]
68. Schnitzspahn, K.M.; Ihle, A.; Henry, J.; Rendell, P.; Kliegel, M. The age-prospective memory-paradox: An exploration of possible mechanisms. *Int. Psychogeriatr.* **2011**, *23*, 583–592. [CrossRef]
69. Althubaiti, A. Information bias in health research: Definition, pitfalls, and adjustment methods. *J. Multidiscip. Healthc.* **2016**, *9*, 211–217. [CrossRef]
70. Arnold, N.R.; Bayen, U.J. Prospective memory: Comparing self- and proxy-reports with cognitive modeling of task performance. *J. Appl. Res. Mem. Cogn.* **2019**, *8*, 244–254. [CrossRef]
71. Debowska, A.; Horeczy, B.; Boduszek, D.; Dolinski, D. A repeated cross-sectional survey assessing university students' stress, depression, anxiety, and suicidality in the early stages of the Covid-19 pandemic in Poland. *Psychol. Med.* **2020**, 3–6. [CrossRef]
72. Essadek, A.; Rabeyron, T. Mental health of French students during the Covid-19 pandemic. *J. Affect. Disord.* **2020**, *277*, 392–393. [CrossRef]
73. Pieh, C.; Budimir, S.; Probst, T. The effect of age, gender, income, work, and physical activity on mental health during coronavirus disease (Covid-19) lockdown in Austria. *J. Psychosom. Res. J.* **2020**, *136*, 110186. [CrossRef]

Journal of
Clinical Medicine

MDPI

Article

Assessment of Anxiety, Depression, Attitude, and Coping Strategies of the Egyptian Population during the COVID-19 Pandemic

Ghaydaa A. Shehata [1], Romany Gabra [2], Sara Eltellawy [3], Mohamed Elsayed [4], Dina Elsayed Gaber [5] and Hatem A. Elshabrawy [6,*]

1 Department of Neurology and Psychiatry, Assiut University Hospitals, Assiut 71511, Egypt; ghaidaa.abozaid@med.aun.edu.eg
2 Department of Psychiatry, Faculty of Medicine, Assiut University, Assiut 71511, Egypt; romanyhosny@med.aun.edu.eg
3 Department of Psychology, Faculty of Arts, Assiut University, Assiut 71511, Egypt; sara_hamdy@art.aun.edu.eg
4 Department of Psychiatry and Psychotherapy III, University of Ulm, Leimgrubenweg 12-14, 89075 Ulm, Germany; mohamed.elsayed@uni-ulm.de
5 Department of Neurology, Alexandria University Hospital, Alexandria University, Alexandria 21111, Egypt; Dina.gaber@alexmed.edu.eg
6 Department of Molecular and Cellular Biology, College of Osteopathic Medicine, Sam Houston State University, Conroe, TX 77304, USA
* Correspondence: hatem.elshabrawy@shsu.edu; Tel.: +1-(936)-202-5216; Fax: +1-(936)-202-5260

Citation: Shehata, G.A.; Gabra, R.; Eltellawy, S.; Elsayed, M.; Gaber, D.E.; Elshabrawy, H.A. Assessment of Anxiety, Depression, Attitude, and Coping Strategies of the Egyptian Population during the COVID-19 Pandemic. *J. Clin. Med.* **2021**, *10*, 3989. https://doi.org/10.3390/jcm10173989

Academic Editor: Michele Roccella

Received: 6 July 2021
Accepted: 31 August 2021
Published: 3 September 2021

Abstract: Background: The COVID-19 pandemic has imposed several challenges on different populations all around the world, with stress being identified as one of the major challenges. This study aims to investigate the impact of COVID-19-induced stress on the prevalence and severity of anxiety and/or depression, factors that predict the development of anxiety and/or depression, and coping strategies in the Egyptian population during the COVID 19 outbreak. Subjects and Methods: This is an observational cross-sectional online study. The questionnaire of our study included five sections: demographic and clinical data, attitude towards COVID-19, the State-Trait Anxiety Inventory (STAI), Beck Depression Inventory-II (BDI-II), and a specifically prepared and standardized Arabic version of a coping strategies scale. The questionnaire was uploaded on 20 May 2020 at 1 p.m. and closed on 7 July 2020 at 8 a.m. Results: The study questionnaire was completed by 283 Egyptians, with mean age 34.81 ± 11.36 years, of which 17% had been infected with COVID-19. The responses showed that 62.9% had moderate anxiety, whereas 12.4% had severe anxiety. Moreover, 13.8% had moderate depression, and 14.1% had severe depression. Our study demonstrated that age, mental status, and being infected with COVID-19 correlated with depression, whereas only age correlated with anxiety. Interestingly, our data showed that anxiety and depression were negatively correlated with some coping strategies during the COVID-19 pandemic. Conclusions: Pandemics, such as the COVID-19 pandemic, imposes stress on individuals, which leads to the development of anxiety and/or depression. Several factors, which could be population-dependent, may help predict the development of anxiety or depression. We show the factors correlated with depression and anxiety during the COVID-19 pandemic in the Egyptian population. Furthermore, certain personal coping strategies during the COVID-19 pandemic are negatively correlated with anxiety and depression. Therefore, our study sheds light on the importance of studying factors in each population that can lead to pandemic-induced psychological complications and those that can relieve such complications.

Keywords: coronavirus; SARS-CoV-2; COVID-19; stress; emotions; Egyptian; depression; anxiety; coping strategies; STAI; BDI-II

1. Introduction

In December 2019, a COVID-19 outbreak emerged in the city of Wuhan, China. SARS-CoV-2 was soon identified as the novel coronavirus (CoV) causative agent of this outbreak. COVID-19 then spread to all countries in the world, and the disease was declared a pandemic in March 2020 [1]. More than 159 million confirmed cases have been reported worldwide, with 3.4 million deaths as of 10 May 2021. In Egypt, from 3 January 2020 to 10 May 2021, there have been 239,740 confirmed COVID-19 cases and 14,033 deaths [2]. There are several serious impacts of pandemics on different populations, probably due to lack of information about the causative agent, disease progression, and infectious disease control measures [1].

Stress has been reported as a major challenge during the COVID-19 pandemic. Multiple factors that could contribute to stress include the ambiguity and novelty of the COVID-19 pandemic in addition to rapid transmission, high mortality, the unknown actual number of cases, and the unexpected outcome of infection. As a result of stress, levels of anxiety, depression, trauma, suicidal ideation, and panic have elevated during the COVID-19 pandemic. In addition, economic disturbances, community restriction, and uncertainty about the true numbers of COVID-19 cases have contributed to even more stress among the general population.

Reports in the year 2020 have shown that 80% of COVID-19 patients had mild symptoms, high recovery rates, and low mortality rates. However, in comparison to SARS-COV-1 and MERS-CoV combined, SARS-CoV-2 has shown higher transmissibility and mortality. The severe economic sanctions imposed by the governments of several countries, the doubts about the efficacy of personal protective equipment, and fears of shortages in medical supplies can all be reasons contributing to stress among individuals [3–7]. To our knowledge, few studies have investigated the coping strategies of general populations during pandemics. However, personality traits, such as optimism, resilience, and altruism, have previously been shown to have positive effects on reducing psychological stress. In addition, measures such as effective infection control, personal protective measures, clear institutional policies, and protocols have led to stress reduction among various populations [8].

This study aims to evaluate the impact of stress during the COVID-19 outbreak on the prevalence of anxiety and/or depression, predictive factors for the development of anxiety and/or depression, attitude towards COVID-19, and different coping strategies among the Egyptian population in response to the COVID 19 pandemic. Furthermore, we sought to correlate anxiety and depression with different coping strategies.

2. Subjects and Methods

This was an internet-based cross-sectional and observational study that was conducted among the Egyptian population. All Egyptian citizens above 18 years were eligible to be included in the study. Each subject was asked to agree to online written informed consent and to complete our questionnaire and submit the response.

2.1. *Study Participants and Method of Participation*

The online semi-structured questionnaire was developed in Arabic by using Google forms, with a consent form appended to it. The link for the questionnaire was sent through various social media platforms (emails, WhatsApp, Facebook, Instagram, Twitter, Reddit). Participants over 18 years old, who agreed to use the online application, were included in this study. Once the link was clicked, the participants were automatically transferred to the information related to the study. Informed consent and demographic details were obtained from all participants. The set of questions of the 15–20 min survey appeared in sequence, which the participants had to answer. The survey questions were designed to assess anxiety and depression in COVID-19 patients and coping strategies for dealing with COVID-19. At the end of the questionnaire, participants had the option to get their results via phone, email, WhatsApp, or other contact methods (optional). Participants also receive some personalized advice according to their results. The data collection was initiated on 20 May 2020 at 1 p.m. and closed on 7 July 2020 at 8 a.m. Data were collected from different governorates in Egypt.

Participants could withdraw from the survey at any moment without providing any justification, and no data was saved. Only data from complete responses to questionnaires were included in our study.

2.2. Study Questionnaire

The questionnaire for this study included five sections. All participants were required to understand the meaning of each question and to answer the questions on their own.

2.2.1. Section I

This section included sociodemographic and clinical questions related to age, gender, occupation, education, area of residence, marital status, and chronic illness (if applicable).

2.2.2. Section II

This section included questions about attitudes towards COVID-19, the reaction of the population to COVID-19 patients, and how to deal with others.

2.2.3. Section III. The State-Trait Anxiety Inventory (STAI)

The State-Trait Anxiety Inventory (STAI) is a commonly used measure of trait and state anxiety [9,10]. The standardized Arabic version of the state anxiety scale was used in this study [11] and included 20 items for assessing trait anxiety and 20 items for assessing state anxiety. State anxiety items included "I am tense; I am worried" and "I feel calm; I feel secure". Trait anxiety items included "I worry too much over something that really doesn't matter" and "I am content; I am a steady person". We assessed the state anxiety in the present study. All items were rated on a 4-point scale (e.g., from "almost never" to "almost always") [12,13]. Higher scores indicate greater anxiety. Internal consistency coefficients for the scale ranged from 0.550 to 0.751, and the value of Cronbach's alpha coefficient was 0.892.

2.2.4. Section IV. Beck's Depression Inventory II (BDI-II)

The BDI-II is a 21-item instrument that assesses the presence and severity of unipolar depressive symptoms. A standardized and validated Arabic version of the BDI-II was used [14]. In Beck's Depression Inventory, individuals rate each statement on a 0 to 3 scale according to how well it describes how they have felt over the past two weeks [15]. A sample item is as follows: "Sadness: 0 = I do not feel sad; 1 = I feel sad much of the time; 2 = I am sad all the time; 3 = I am so sad or unhappy that I can't stand it". Total scores were calculated by summing the score of each item. Higher scores indicated greater depression symptoms. In the current study, the value of Cronbach's alpha coefficient was excellent [14,16,17]. Depression was classified according to the BD-II score into mild, moderate, and severe [14].

2.2.5. Section V. Coping Strategies Scale

The scale was designed specifically for this study. The initial form of the scale included 43 questions to evaluate different coping strategies. The scale was evaluated by five referees to determine the suitability of its items (face validity). The percentage of agreement between the referees ranged from 80–100%. Accordingly, 20 items were deleted, resulting in 23 items in the final form of the scale, which were divided into five dimensions. The responses were graded according to three levels of the Likert scale (applies to me to a great extent = 3, applies to me to some extent = 2, does not apply = 1), and the statements were distributed randomly under different dimensions. The scores are calculated on each subscale. To estimate validity, reliability, and internal consistencies, the scale was applied in its initial form to a survey sample of 188 individuals (pilot study). The validity and reliability of the coping strategies questionnaire have been confirmed by national and international studies, and Cronbach's alpha coefficient was 0.84.

2.3. Statistical Analysis

Data were collected and analyzed using SPSS (Statistical Package for the Social Science, version 20, IBM, Armonk, NY, USA). Continuous data were expressed in the form of mean ± SD or median (range), while nominal data were expressed in the form of frequency (percentage). An independent sample *t*-test was used for continuous variables. A series of correlation coefficients and multiple linear regression analysis were used to examine the predictors for the occurrence of anxiety and depression. Additionally, the relation between different coping strategies and depression or anxiety was studied using Pearson's correlation. $p < 0.05$ was considered significant.

3. Results

3.1. Demographic and Clinical Characteristics of the Studied Group

A total of 283 responses from participants who were Egyptians over 18 years old were recorded, mostly from urban areas (90.1%). The mean age of the participants was 34.81 ± 11.36 years; 74.2% were females, and 25.8% were males. About 57.24% of participants exerted high levels of mental effort at work. Our data show that 17% of study participants had COVID-19, whereas 26.1% of participants had chronic illnesses. Our data show that 12.4% of respondents had severe anxiety, and 14.1% had severe depression (according to anxiety rating and Beck's depression scales; Table 1).

Table 1. Demographic and clinical data of the study population. Responses to the questionnaire, which included sociodemographic and clinical questions (section I), anxiety and depression assessment questions (sections III and IV, respectively), were recorded. Data are expressed as numbers (*N*) and percentages (%) or mean ± standard deviation (SD).

Variables		**Total *N* = 283**	
Age (mean ± SD)		34.81 ± 11.36	
		N	%
Gender	Male	73	25.8
	Female	210	74.2
Marital status	Single	108	38.2
	Married	158	55.8
	Divorced	10	3.5
	Widow	7	2.5
Nature of Work	Mental	162	57.2
	Manual	41	14.5
	No work	80	28.3
Residence Location	Urban	255	90.1
	Rural	28	9.9
Chronic Illness	Yes	74	26.1
	No	209	73.9
COVID-19	Yes	48	17
	No	235	83
Anxiety	Normal	70	24.7
	Moderate	178	62.9
	Severe	35	12.4
Depression	Normal	142	50.2
	Mild	62	21.9
	Moderate	39	13.8
	Severe	40	14.1

3.2. Attitude towards COVID-19

The responses to section II of the study questionnaire revealed the variable attitude of our sample population towards COVID-19. We found that 38.5% of our study population searched for treatment to strengthen their immune system. Moreover, 36.4% had the feeling that they were infected with COVID-19 once a week, whereas 10.6% had this feeling 3 times per week, and 3.9% had this feeling daily.

About one-fourth (N = 74; 26.1%) of the sample population had visited a doctor to assure themselves that they were infection-free, while 12% (N = 34) underwent a PCR or laboratory test to confirm the absence of infection. Seeking psychiatric consultation occurred in 2.8%, whereas 9.5% of our sample population used anxiolytics. Moreover, 17% of our study participants had a confirmed COVID-19 infection. Unfortunately, all of them reported that they were abused by others, whether by hints, looks, words (62.5%), or by avoidance of direct interaction (37.5%) (Table 2).

Table 2. Population attitude towards the COVID-19 pandemic. Responses to section II of the study questionnaire, which included questions about the attitudes and reactions of our sample Egyptian population towards COVID-19. Data are expressed as numbers (N) and percentages (%).

Variables		Total N = 283	
		N	%
Are you looking for treatments that may help cure or strengthen your immune system?	Yes	28	9.9
	Scarcely	48	17.0
	Sometimes	126	44.5
	Always	109	38.5
How many times have you felt you had symptoms like those of COVID-19?	Did not happen	122	43.1
	A few times (once per week)	103	36.4
	Many times (3 times per week)	30	10.6
	Most of the time (5 times per week)	17	6
	Most of the time (almost every day)	11	3.9
Have you performed any diagnostic medical tests to check on yourself?	Did not happen	249	88
	Yes, once a month	18	6.4
	Fortnightly	2	0.7
	Once a week	12	4.2
	More than once every two weeks	2	0.7
Have you consulted a doctor to check on your health?	Did not happen	209	73.9
	Once	42	14.8
	More than once	32	11.3
Did you go to a psychiatrist?	Yes	8	2.8
	No	275	97.2
Have you taken any medications for anxiety, depression, or sleep?	Yes	27	9.5
	No	256	90.5
The response of population towards you (if you had COVID-19 N = 48)	Some hints by looks or words	30/48	62.5
	Avoidance of direct interaction	18/48	37.5

3.3. Age, Work Nature, and COVID-19 Are Associated with Depression, Whereas Only Age Is Associated with Anxiety

A series of multiple linear regression tests were used to assess the effect of different demographic factors (age, gender, marital status, residence location, and nature of work), clinical factors (chronic illness or having COVID-19), and attitude towards COVID-19 in the development of depression or anxiety among our Egyptian population. We found that age had a significantly negative correlation with depression. However, mental effort at work and COVID-19 disease had significant positive correlations with depression. On the other hand, only age negatively correlated with anxiety (Table 3). These findings indicate that young age, high level of mental effort at work, and COVID-19 disease are significant predictors of depression in our study, whereas young age is the only significant predictor of anxiety in our population.

Table 3. Predictors of depression or anxiety in the Egyptian population. Linear regression tests were used to determine factors that significantly correlated with depression and anxiety. Linear-regression-dependent (dep.) variables included depression or anxiety, whereas the independent (indep.) variables included age, gender, mental effort at work, marital status, chronic illnesses, and COVID-19 disease.

Dep. Variables	Indep. Variables	Constant	R	R^2	F	B	SE	Beta	T	p-Value	CL 95%
Depression	Age	20.412	0.205	0.042	12.297	−2.09	0.597	−0.205	−3.51	0.001	{−3.269: −0.918}
	Mental effort at work	9.613	0.163	0.027	7.678	4.99	1.799	0.163	2.771	0.006	{1.444: 8.528}
	Gender	11.222	0.096	0.009	2.596	2.353	1.461	0.096	1.611	0.108	{−0.522: 5.228}
	Marital Status	18.304	0.106	0.011	3.219	−1.751	0.976	−0.106	−1.794	0.074	{−3.672: 0.170}
	Chronic Illnesses	13.777	0.05	0.002	0.702	1.228	1.466	0.05	0.838	0.403	{−1.657: 4.113}
	COVID-19	1.905	0.201	0.04	11.824	13.05	3.794	0.201	3.439	0.001	{5.578: 20.516}
Anxiety	Age	51.171	0.117	0.014	3.91	−1.16	0.587	−0.12	−1.976	0.049	{−2.316: −0.005}
	Mental effort at work	46.761	0.047	0.002	0.62	1.388	1.766	0.047	0.786	0.433	{−2.088: 4.863}
	Gender	45.856	0.060	0.004	1.02	1.43	1.42	0.06	1.01	0.31	{−1.363: 4.226}
	MaritalStatus	49.962	0.059	0.004	0.99	−0.95	0.95	−0.06	−0.997	0.32	{−2.816: 0.922}
	Chronic Illnesses	46.412	0.065	0.004	1.179	1.541	1.419	0.065	1.086	0.279	{−1.253: 4.334}
	COVID-19	48.029	0.030	0.001	0.26	0.24	0.476	0.03	0.51	0.61	{−0.696: 1.179}

3.4. Anxiety Management Is the Only Coping Strategy That Is Significantly Different between Males and Females

Our newly developed questionnaire was designed to identify the personal coping strategies used by the Egyptian population during COVID-19. Our questionnaire results indicated that anxiety management was the only coping strategy that was more significantly used by females than males (Table 4; $p = 0.037$). The use of personal coping strategies such as ignoring guidelines for disease prevention, following the guidelines of disease prevention, and rational handling of the problem was not significantly different between males and females.

Table 4. Coping strategies of males and females in the Egyptian population. A coping strategies questionnaire was used to identify coping strategies in the population. Respondents were given a score for each strategy based on their answers to the questionnaire. Data are expressed as mean ± SD, and an independent sample *t*-test was used to compare coping strategies between males ($N = 73$) and females ($N = 210$). Asterisk (*) indicates significant difference ($p = 0.037$).

Coping Strategies	Mean Score	Males (N = 73) Mean Score	Females (N = 210) Mean Score	p-Value
Ignore the Guidelines of Disease Prevention	9.31 ±2.66	9.68 ± 2.39	9.19 ± 2.73	0.171
Follow the Guidelines of Disease Prevention	13.34 ± 3.03	13.41 ± 3.07	13.31 ± 3.02	0.096
Religious Practices	12.77 ± 2.24	12.85 ± 2.26	12.75 ± 2.24	0.101
Anxiety Management	6.43 ± 1.53	6.11 ± 1.44	6.54 ± 1.55	0.037 *
Rational Handling of the Problem	7.25 ± 1.29	7.23 ± 1.31	7.26 ± 1.29	0.891

3.5. Coping Strategies during COVID-19 Negatively Correlated with Anxiety and Depression

Next, a series of Pearson correlations were performed to correlate coping strategies to the occurrence of depression or anxiety. Anxiety management had a significant positive correlation with anxiety and depression, whereas religious practices had a significant negative correlation with anxiety and depression. However, rational handling of the problem showed a significantly negative correlation only with depression (Table 5). These results indicate that certain coping strategies are effective in reducing the levels of anxiety and/or depression.

Table 5. Correlation between depression or anxiety and coping strategies in the Egyptian population. Pearson correlations were performed to correlate coping strategies to the occurrence of depression or anxiety. Asterisk (*) indicates a significant correlation ($p < 0.05$), whereas (**) indicate significant correlation ($p < 0.01$).

	Coping Strategies				
	Ignorethe Guidelines of Disease Prevention	**Follow the Guidelines of Disease Prevention**	**Religious Practices**	**Anxiety Management**	**Rational Handling of the Problem**
Depression	R: 0.065 (0.277)	R: −0.077 (0.198)	R: −0.305 (0.0001) **	R: 0.231 (0.0001) **	R: −0.191 (0.001) **
Anxiety	R: −0.081 (0.172)	R: 0.051 (0.390)	R: −0.141 (0.017) *	R: 0.277 (0.0001) **	R: −0.075 (0.210)

4. Discussion

The COVID-19 pandemic imposes many challenges that could lead to stress and depression. Different populations react differently to COVID-19-induced challenges. This study reports the prevalence of anxiety and depression due to COVID-19, factors that associate with anxiety and depression, and the coping strategies to deal with the pandemic in a sample of the Egyptian population.

Although our study is a cross-sectional study that does not represent the entire Egyptian population and is limited by the inability to assess incidence or make a causal inference, it provides insight into the reaction of the Egyptian population towards anxiety, depression, and coping strategies to overcome anxiety and depression. Three-quarters of our population had moderate anxiety (62.9%) to severe anxiety (12.4%). This is consistent with a study conducted in Iran, which revealed that approximately one-fifth of Iranians had experienced severe/very severe anxiety [3]. Depression was recorded among half of the studied sample. Most of them had mild (21.9%), moderate (13.8%), and severe depression (14.1%) according to scores of Beck's Depression Inventory II [18,19]. Another online study reported an increase in anxiety among the Indian population.

Anxiety and depression play a role in immune system dysfunctions and, consequently, increase the risk of viral infection [3]. Moreover, anxiety and depression may trigger public disruptive behaviors due to the attitude of people towards diseased individuals. Panic buying due to anxiety or depression leads to the exhaustion of resources, which could affect daily activities, whereas avoidance behavior causes limited socialization. Furthermore, anxious people can adopt various unwanted lifestyle and dietary modifications under the influence of their emotions.

In our study, 17% of the studied sample had COVID-19, and about 9.9% had direct contact with COVID-19 patients. High levels of anxiety were associated with a negative attitude towards COVID-19 patients. About 12% of our study population performed a laboratory test to check for COVID-19 infection, 26.1% consulted a doctor, 2.8% consulted a psychiatrist, and about 9.5% took medications for anxiety, depression, or sleep disturbance. These attitudes confirm the fear and panic among societies due to COVID-19 and can be attributed to lack of knowledge about the disease, deficiency of protective measures, and mistrusted social media news. To reduce stress, people resort to different strategies, including ignoring the guidelines for the prevention of disease spread, increased religious practices, anxiety management, and rational handling of the problem. All these methods are strategic in dealing with epidemics. In our study, the test to identify coping strategies was designed to be compatible with Egyptian society, with its various challenges. We found that the ability of women to adapt to this pandemic and to relieve emotions was significantly greater than that of men. This can be attributed to the ability of women to endure and adapt to surrounding conditions and the ability of women to better implement protective measures to reduce COVID-19 spread.

Our study showed that younger age, high mental effort at work, and getting infected with COVID-19 were significantly associated with higher levels of depression, whereas younger age was the only factor that was associated with higher levels of anxiety. As a result of increased rates of depression and/or anxiety, more patients sought medical advice and received medications. Next, we sought to determine the effectiveness of coping strategies that were used by our population. Our correlation studies showed that coping strategies such as anxiety management and religious practices were significantly correlated with anxiety and depression. However, rational handling of the problem had a significant negative correlation only with depression. Our results highlight the effectiveness of coping strategies in managing anxiety and/or depression. Therefore, identifying the coping strategies in any population is critical in order to determine which ones will be effective in dealing with stress-related anxiety or depression.

Author Contributions: Conceptualization, G.A.S., R.G., S.E., and H.A.E.; methodology, G.A.S., R.G., S.E., and H.A.E.; software, G.A.S., R.G., and S.E.; writing—original drafts, G.A.S., R.G., and S.E.; data collection, G.A.S., R.G., and S.E.; data analysis, G.A.S., R.G., S.E., M.E., D.E.G., and H.A.E.; writing—review and editing, G.A.S., R.G., S.E., M.E., D.E.G., and H.A.E.; investigation, G.A.S., and H.A.E.; validation, G.A.S., R.G., S.E., and H.A.E.; supervision, H.A.E.; project administration, H.A.E.; critical revisions and writing, H.A.E. All authors have read and agreed to the published version of the manuscript.

Funding: This research received no external funding.

Institutional Review Board Statement: The study was conducted according to the guidelines of the Declaration of Helsinki and approved by the Research and Ethics Committee of Assiut University (protocol code 173000433).

Informed Consent Statement: Informed consent was obtained from all subjects involved in the study.

Data Availability Statement: Not applicable.

Acknowledgments: Thanks to all who contributed to this study. We would like to thank Wafaa Farghaly for revising this paper.

Conflicts of Interest: The authors declare no conflict of interest.

References

1. Roy, D.; Tripathy, S.; Kar, S.K.; Sharma, N.; Verma, S.K.; Kaushal, V. Study of knowledge, attitude, anxiety & perceived mental healthcare need in Indian population during COVID-19 pandemic. *Asian J. Psychiatry* **2020**, *51*, 102083.
2. World Health Organization (WHO). Coronavirus Disease 2019 (COVID-19) Situation Report e 45. Mental Health and Psychosocial Considerations during the COVID-19 Outbreak 2020. Available online: https://www.who.int/docs/default-source/coronaviruse/situation-reports/20200305-sitrep-45-covid-19.pdf?sfvrsn\protect$\relax\protect{\begingroup1\endgroup\@@over4}$ed2ba78b_2 (accessed on 10 May 2021).
3. Moghanibashi-Mansourieh, A. Assessing the anxiety level of Iranian general population during COVID-19 outbreak. *Asian J. Psychiatry* **2020**, *51*, 102076. [CrossRef] [PubMed]
4. Dinakaran, D.; Manjunatha, N.; Kumar, C.N.; Suresh, B.M. Neuropsychiatric aspects of COVID-19 pandemic: A selective review. *Asian J. Psychiatry* **2020**, *53*, 102188. [CrossRef] [PubMed]
5. Kuroda, N. Mental health considerations for patients with epilepsy during COVID-19 crisis. *Epilepsy Behav.* **2020**, *111*, 107198. [CrossRef] [PubMed]
6. Leonardi, M.; Padovani, A.; McArthur, J.C. Neurological manifestations associated with COVID-19: A review and a call for action. *J. Neurol.* **2020**, *267*, 1573–1576. [CrossRef] [PubMed]
7. Zhou, Q.; Hu, Z.; Bian, G.; Yu, H.; Li, X.; Lu, Y.; Yu, C.; Li, X.; Yao, Q.; Zhou, W.; et al. Mental health and psychosocial function of general population during the COVID-19 epidemic in China. *Clin. Transl. Med.* **2020**, *10*, e103. [CrossRef] [PubMed]
8. Cai, H.; Tu, B.; Ma, J.; Chen, L.; Fu, L.; Jiang, Y.; Zhuang, Q. Psychological Impact and Coping Strategies of Frontline Medical Staff in Hunan Between January and March 2020 during the Outbreak of Coronavirus Disease 2019 (COVID19) in Hubei, China. *Med. Sci. Monit. Int. Med. J. Exp. Clin. Res.* **2020**, *26*, e924171.
9. Knight, R.G.; Waal-Manning, H.J.; Spears, G.F. Some norms and reliability data for the State–Trait Anxiety Inventory and the Zung Self-Rating Depression scale. *Br. J. Clin. Psychol.* **1983**, *22 Pt 4*, 245–249. [CrossRef]
10. Spielberger, C.D.; Gorsuch, R.L.; Lushene, R.; Vagg, P.R.; Jacobs, G.A. *Manual for the State-Trait Anxiety Inventory*; Consulting Psychologists Press: Palo Alto, CA, USA, 1983.
11. Abd El khalek, M.A. *Anxiety Inventory (Status and Trait) Instruction Manual*, 2nd ed.; Dar El Anglo Publishing: Cairo, Egypt, 1992.
12. Abdoli, N.; Farnia, V.; Salemi, S.; Davarinejad, O.; Jouybari, T.A.; Khanegi, M.; Alikhani, M.; Behrouz, B. Reliability and Validity of Persian Version of State-Trait Anxiety Inventory Among High School Students. *East Asian Arch. Psychiatry* **2020**, *30*, 44–47. [CrossRef]

13. Gustafson, L.W.; Gabel, P.; Hammer, A.; Lauridsen, H.; Petersen, L.K.; Andersen, B.; Bor, P.; Larsen, M.B. Validity and reliability of State-Trait Anxiety Inventory in Danish women aged 45 years and older with abnormal cervical screening results. *BMC Med. Res. Methodol.* **2020**, *20*, 89. [CrossRef]
14. Gharyb, A.G. *Beck Depression Inventory–II (BDI-II), Arabic Examiner's Handbook*; Dar El Anglo Publishing: Cairo, Egypt, 2000.
15. Byrne, B.M.; Baron, P.; Larsson, B.; Melin, L. Measuring depression for Swedish nonclinical adolescents: Factorial validity and equivalence of the Beck Depression Inventory across gender. *Scand. J. Psychol.* **1996**, *37*, 37–45. [CrossRef] [PubMed]
16. Giacomelli, A.; Pezzati, L.; Conti, F.; Bernacchia, D.; Siano, M.; Oreni, L.; Rusconi, S.; Gervasoni, C.; Ridolfo, A.L.; Rizzardini, G.; et al. Self-reported olfactory and taste disorders in SARS-CoV-2 patients: A cross-sectional study. *Clin. Infect. Dis. Off. Publ. Infect. Dis. Soc. Am.* **2020**, *71*, 889–890. [CrossRef] [PubMed]
17. Robinson, B.E.; Kelley, L. Concurrent validity of the Beck Depression Inventory as a measure of depression. *Psychol. Rep.* **1996**, *79 Pt 1*, 929–930. [CrossRef]
18. Madonna, S., Jr.; Philpot, V.D. Self-statements, self-esteem, and locus of control in discriminating college students' scores on the Beck Depression Inventory. *Psychol. Rep.* **1996**, *78*, 531–534. [CrossRef] [PubMed]
19. Forkmann, T.; Vehren, T.; Boecker, M.; Norra, C.; Wirtz, M.; Gauggel, S. Sensitivity and specificity of the Beck Depression Inventory in cardiologic inpatients: How useful is the conventional cut-off score? *J. Psychosom. Res.* **2009**, *67*, 347–352. [CrossRef] [PubMed]

Journal of
Clinical Medicine

MDPI

Article

Changes in Stress, Coping Styles, and Life Satisfaction between the First and Second Waves of the COVID-19 Pandemic: A Longitudinal Cross-Lagged Study in a Sample of University Students

Aleksandra Maria Rogowska [1,*], Cezary Kuśnierz [2] and Dominika Ochnik [3]

1 Institute of Psychology, Faculty of Social Sciences, University of Opole, 45-052 Opole, Poland
2 Faculty of Physical Education and Physiotherapy, Opole University of Technology, 45-758 Opole, Poland; c.kusnierz@po.edu.pl
3 Faculty of Medicine, University of Technology, 40-555 Katowice, Poland; dominika.ochnik@wst.pl
* Correspondence: arogowskas@uni.opole.pl

Abstract: In this study, we aimed to explain the interplay mechanism between stress, life satisfaction, and coping styles among university students. A cohort study was performed during the first (wave 1; W1) and second (wave 2; W2) waves of the Coronavirus disease 2019 (COVID-19) pandemic. The total sample included 231 university students, of which 59.31% were women. The Satisfaction with Life Scale (SWLS), Perceived Stress Scale (PSS), and Coping Inventory for Stressful Situations (CISS) were included in one online survey. Stress, emotion-oriented, and avoidance-oriented coping styles increased from W1 to W2 of the COVID-19 pandemic, while life satisfaction and task-oriented coping decreased. The partial mediation effect of all three coping styles during W1 and W2 (in a cross-sectional approach) on the relationship between perceived stress and life satisfaction was confirmed in this study. The task-oriented and emotion-oriented coping styles can play a mediating role in the reciprocal relationship between life satisfaction and perceived stress during W1 and W2 of the pandemic. There were no mutual interactions between stress and life satisfaction from a longitudinal approach. Coping styles changed subsequently due to stressful environmental changes related to lockdown during the COVID-19 pandemic. Having a wide range of coping strategies from which to choose during an unstable situation should help manage stress and well-being.

Keywords: avoidance-oriented coping; college students; coping styles; emotion-oriented coping; life satisfaction; perceived stress; task-oriented coping; satisfaction with life; university students

Citation: Rogowska, A.M.; Kuśnierz, C.; Ochnik, D. Changes in Stress, Coping Styles, and Life Satisfaction between the First and Second Waves of the COVID-19 Pandemic: A Longitudinal Cross-Lagged Study in a Sample of University Students. *J. Clin. Med.* **2021**, *10*, 4025. https://doi.org/10.3390/jcm10174025

Academic Editors: Michele Roccella and Emmanuel Andrès

Received: 19 May 2021
Accepted: 3 September 2021
Published: 6 September 2021
Corrected: 5 January 2022

1. Introduction

Satisfaction with life can be defined as the global cognitive self-judgment of well-being across a broad set of human activities at school, work, with family, and in social life [1]. Life satisfaction is considered a significant predictor of mental and physical health and successful adaptation to life [2–5]. Research indicates that higher levels of perceived stress are related to decreased levels of life satisfaction [4,6–14]. Numerous studies reported a decrease in well-being and increases in distress, loneliness, insomnia, anxiety, and depression during the coronavirus outbreak [15–36]. Physical and mental health was found to be a significant positive predictor of life satisfaction during the pandemic [37]. The most desirable skill in a pandemic situation seems to be coping strategies aimed at regulating and reducing negative emotions or pessimistic and unrealistic thinking, as well as solving current problems related to quarantine restrictions, isolation, job loss, deterioration of economic status, and countless lifestyle changes.

In Poland, lockdown started 10–12 March 2020 (with the closing of schools and universities), expanded on 25 March (to limiting non-family gatherings to two people and forbidding non-essential travel), and restrictions tightened on 31 March. Starting from 30

May 2020, wearing masks in outdoor places was no longer obligatory but was restored as of 10 October 2020 due to the increasing number of cases. Primary lockdown-related stress sources were as follows: isolation, restriction in moving, shopping, traveling, changes in daily lifestyle regards use of face masks, washing hands frequently, avoiding social contact and gatherings, restaurants, pubs, clubs, fitness clubs, limiting physical activity outdoors, and required remote online learning and work [17,38–43].

One of the largest sources of stress was an economic crisis due to prolonged lockdown, which increased concerns about future work-finding and financial stability [18,44]. Lee [45] showed that perceived employment and housing insecurity, deteriorating finances, and difficulties in paying for basic needs predicted life satisfaction, happiness, health self-esteem, mental health index, and mental stress among a large sample of European Union citizens. Remote online learning and academic stress were the risk factors for mental health and decreased well-being of university students before quarantine [46,47] as well as during the pandemic [48–51]. In the present study, university students were examined regarding perceived stress, coping styles, and life satisfaction during the Coronavirus disease 2019 (COVID-19) pandemic.

1.1. Association between Stress, Coping, and Subjective Well-Being

Coping strategies seem to play a pivotal role in physical and mental health, particularly during adaptation to stressful situations in life [52]. According to the transactional theory of stress [53], stress is understood as a relationship between an individual and their environment, which the person appraises as relevant to their well-being. Stress can emerge when an individual perceives an exceeding of their resources to cope. Lazarus [54] (p. 99) defined coping with stress as "constantly changing cognitive and behavioral efforts to manage specific external and/or internal demands that are appraised as taxing or exceeding the resources of the person". Coping has two main functions: regulating disturbing emotions (aimed at regulating emotional distress) and focusing cognition and behavior on solving the problem that causes distress (aimed at altering person–environment relationships).

Recent international research [55] performed in Russia, Kyrgyzstan, and Peru during the COVID-19 pandemic found that the coping responses related to problem-focused coping, socially supported coping, avoidance, and emotion-oriented coping explained 44% of the coping variability. Significant differences in religious coping and mental disengagement were found across the countries, suggesting that some coping behaviors may play distinct roles in responding to stressful events. Higher psychological distress was associated with more frequent use of passive (negative) coping, but less frequent use of an active (upbeat) coping style during the COVID-19 pandemic [56,57]. There was also an association between coping with stress and subjective well-being. In particular, task-oriented coping style was related positively to well-being, whereas emotion-oriented and avoidance-oriented coping strategies were related negatively [35,58–64].

1.2. The Theoretical Background of the Current Study

Studies from various regions of the world indicate that about 50% of people have experienced high stress levels during the coronavirus pandemic [65–68]. Khodami [24] found that younger people and individuals with a low quality of life were more likely to experience higher stress levels and more significant emotion regulation problems. With increasing quarantine time, quality of life decreased, and perceived stress and emotion regulation problems increased. From a biocultural perspective, financial crisis and prolonged emotional stress during the COVID-19 pandemic may substantially impact growth and development for the next generation, as suggested by Bogin and Varea [69]. Therefore, research on the factors that may decrease stress and elevate well-being in young adults is currently necessary to prepare adequate support, intervention strategies, and prevention programs.

In this study, we examined life satisfaction, stress, and coping style during the coronavirus-related lockdown, considering an intra-individual approach to coping across two stressful situations: the first and second waves of the COVID-19 pandemic. Previous research indicated that university students experience low life satisfaction, high levels of perceived stress, and emotion-oriented coping styles during the first wave of the COVID-19 pandemic [30,70,71]. Life events and coping are intertwined, as reported from studies on the mediating role of coping in the relationship between stress and imminent health consequences [72].

According to the cognitive-transactional model of stress [73], stress results from an interaction between a person and their environment and is subject to continuous change. The meaning of a particular stressful person–environment transaction is derived from the underlying context. Both coping and cognitive appraisals of demands and resources can play a mediating role in the association between experiencing stress and psychological well-being. Coping includes emotional (affective) components that cause physiological changes and have long-term effects concerning mental and somatic health and well-being, and social functioning. The coping strategy is selected as a result of the appraisal process. Lazarus and Folkman [53] suggested that the primary appraisal determines whether a situation is stressful, and a secondary appraisal is initiated to assess the situation, select an appropriate coping strategy, assess the likelihood that a coping option will achieve the expected effect, and whether the person can effectively apply the strategy. In the transactional process, people can continuously reappraise the situation as coping strategies are initiated and the person–environment relationship changes. The short- and long-term health-related outcomes of the process are determined by the selected coping strategy and may vary depending on the setting.

Lardier et al. [74] found a mediating effect of reflective (task-oriented) coping on the relationship between perceived stress and life satisfaction in a cross-sectional study among Hispanic undergraduate students. Reverse mediation analysis, with life satisfaction as a predictor of stress, was also performed [75]. The transactional model of stress [53,73] assumes a one-way relationship from stress (predictor) to life satisfaction (outcome). However, if adverse changes in the outcome (i.e., life satisfaction) are perceived as a stressor, this may trigger a primary appraisal and restart the complete transactional process. Therefore, the inverse model investigated by Gori et al. [75] seems to be equally likely. Here, we examined the interrelationship between stress and life satisfaction and coping styles as mediators of these relationships during the COVID-19 pandemic. Based on the previous studies described above, we formulated the following hypotheses:

Hypothesis 1 (H1): *Changes occurred between the first (W1) and second (W2) waves of the COVID-19 pandemic in perceived stress, life satisfaction, and coping styles, as a consequence of stressful person–environment transactional process* [53,73].

Hypothesis 2 (H2): *Life satisfaction at W2 may be explained by perceived stress and coping style during W1 and W2 and by life satisfaction measured during W1.*

Hypothesis 3 (H3): *Coping styles play a mediating role in the relationship between stress (predictor) and life satisfaction (outcome) during the first (W1) and second (W2) cross-sectional measurements* [74].

Hypothesis 4 (H4): *A reciprocal relationship exists between life satisfaction as a predictor and stress as an outcome, and coping styles as mediators, during the first (W1) and second (W2) cross-sectional measurements* [75].

Hypothesis 5 (H5): *Because the theory of transactional stress process [53,73] assumes continuous changes in stress and coping, the coping styles during W1 cannot predict either perceived stress during W2 or life satisfaction during W2 using a longitudinal approach.*

2. Materials and Methods

2.1. Study Design

A cohort study was performed in two waves. The first wave of cross-sectional study was conducted in spring 2020 and the second wave in autumn 2020, at a large public technical university in the south of Poland. The necessary sample size was determined using G*Power ver. 3.1.9.4. Software [76,77]. The sample size equaled 167 people, if calculated a priori for bivariate correlation with $r = 0.30$, $p < 0.01$, and 95% CI, and equaled 108 people for a linear multiple regression model with two independent variables, effect size $f^2 = 0.15$, $p < 0.01$, and 95% CI. University students were recruited through the online e-learning platform at a university. The invitation to participate in the study (with a link to the on-line survey) was provided on the Moodle platform from 3 March to 29 April 2020, during the first wave (W1) of the COVID-19 pandemic. The information about the study was provided and informed consent was obtained using the first page of the online questionnaire. Students were informed that participation was voluntary and they could refuse from the survey at any time. No form of compensation was offered as an incentive to participate. The average time for data collection was 20 min. The student sample was highly diverse to minimize sources of bias due to their key characteristics: field of study and study cycle. Among the university students, 986 people responded to the invitation during W1, but 12 refused to participate, and 60 presented more than 5% missing data, so they were excluded from further statistical analyses. Altogether, 914 students participated at measurement time one (W1) and completed all measures, including life satisfaction, perceived stress, and coping with stress (Figure 1).

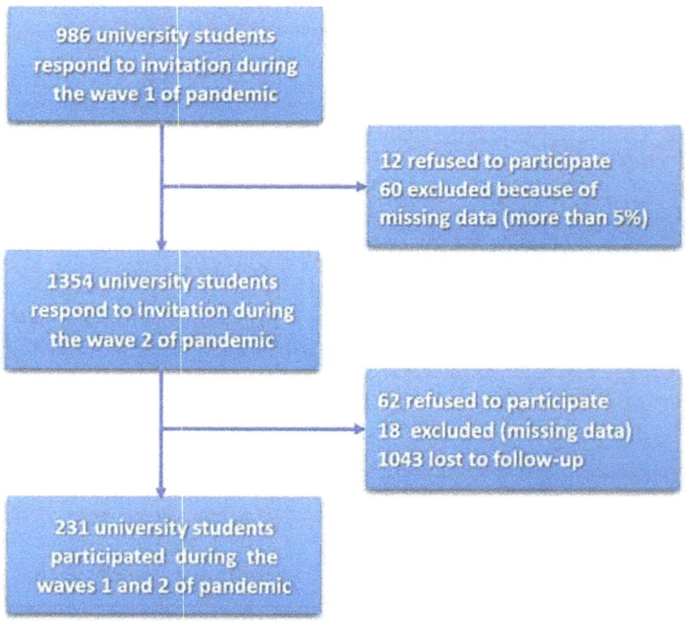

Figure 1. Flow chart of the study sample by recruitment strategy during each wave of the COVID-19 pandemic.

The same procedure was used during the second wave (W2) of the COVID-19 pandemic. The research was conducted from 3 November to 3 December 2020. Among university students, 1354 responded to the invitation. However, 62 refused to participate during W2, and 18 were excluded because more than 5% of their data was missing. Among the 1274 university students during W2, 231 participants matched the following demographic characteristics from W1: birth date, sex, place of residence, faculty, level, and year of the study (Figure 1). Therefore, 231 university students were included in the total sample that was examined using all statistical tests.

The Research Ethics Committee approved the study protocol at the University of Opole, Poland (1/2020). The study followed the ethical requirements of anonymity and voluntariness of participation. Following the Declaration of Helsinki, written informed consent was obtained from each student before inclusion. We received no specific funding for this work. This study is part of an international research project, "Well-being of undergraduates during the COVID-19 pandemic: International study", registered at the Center for Open Science (OSF) [78].

2.2. Participants

The participants in the study were 231 university students, aged between 21 and 37 years (M = 23.21, SD = 2.28), with a prevalence of women (n = 137, 59%), those living in villages (n = 107, 46%), studying physical education and physiotherapy (n = 72, 31%), in first level (Bachelor, n = 174, 75%), involved in full-time education (n = 200, 87%), and second-year of study (n = 102, 44%). More details about the demographic characteristics of the students during W2 of the COVID-19 pandemic are listed in Table 1.

Table 1. Demographic characteristics of the sample during the second wave of the COVID-19 pandemic.

Variable	Range	M	SD	n	%
Age	21–37	23.21	2.28	231	100
Gender					
Women				137	59.31
Men				92	39.83
Place of residence					
Village				107	46.32
Town				99	42.85
City				24	10.39
Agglomeration				1	0.43
Faculty of study					
Production Engineering and Logistics				45	19.48
Electrical Engineering, Automatics and Computer Science				65	28.14
Mechanical				40	17.32
Construction and Architecture				2	0.87
Economics and Management				7	3.03
Physical Education and Physiotherapy				72	31.17
Study level					
First level (Bachelor)				174	75.32
Second level (Master)				33	14.29
Five years' master study				23	9.96
Doctoral				1	0.43
Type of study					
Full-time				200	86.58
Part-time				31	13.42
Study Year	1–5	2.78	1.02		
First				11	4.76
Second				102	44.16
Third				61	26.41
Fourth				41	17.75
Fifth				16	6.93

2.3. Measurement

2.3.1. Perceived Stress

The Perceived Stress Scale (PSS) was developed for measuring psychological stress [79]. This is a self-report ten-item questionnaire, with a 5-point Likert scale (ranging from 0 = never to 4 = very often). The participant indicates how often they experienced a given type of behavior in the last month. Total scores range between 0 and 40, with higher scores indicating higher levels of perceived stress. The scores ranging between 5 and 11 indicate extremely low stress, 12–17 indicates low, 18–23 average, 24–28 high, and 29–35 extremely high stress. The internal consistency of the PSS-10 assessed by Cronbach's α was 0.88 during W1 and 0.90 during W2.2.3.2. Coping styles.

The Coping Inventory for Stressful Situations (CISS) was developed by Endler and Parker [80] on theoretical and empirical bases to provide a self-report measure of responses to stressful circumstances. The CISS consists of 48 items in three scales (16 items in each dimension): task-oriented, emotion-oriented, and avoidance-oriented coping styles. Task-oriented coping relies on restructuring and focusing on tasks, problem solving, altering the situation, and planning. An emotion-oriented coping style involves self-oriented emotional reactions in stressful situations (e.g., self-preoccupation, self-blaming, upset, getting angry, becoming tense, and fantasizing). Avoidance-oriented coping involves using distractions by other situations or tasks or social gatherings. Respondents rated on a 5-point Likert scale (1 = not at all to 5 = very much) the degree of engagement in various types of activity during a difficult, stressful, or upsetting situation. Higher scores are interpreted as greater use of the coping style. In the present study, the reliability (Cronbach's α) for task-, emotion-, and avoidance-oriented coping was 0.91, 0.91, and 0.80 during W1, and 0.93, 0.92, and 0.86 during W2, respectively.

2.3.2. Life Satisfaction

The Satisfaction With Life Scale (SWLS) is a short 5-item scale developed by Diener et al. [1] to assess global cognitive judgments of one's life satisfaction. An individual chooses how much they agree with a given item on a seven-point Likert scale (1 = strongly disagree to 7 = strongly agree). Higher scores indicate a higher level of life satisfaction, ranging from 5–9 = extremely dissatisfied, 10–14 = dissatisfied, 15–19 = slightly dissatisfied, 20 = neutral, 21–25 = slightly satisfied, 26–30 = satisfied, and 31–35 = extremely satisfied. The Satisfaction with Life Scale (SWLS) provides evidence of a stable one-factor structure, high reliability, validity, and invariance for sex [1,11,12,81–83]. The Cronbach's α for the SWLS in the present sample was 0.81 during W1 and 0.85 during W2.

2.4. Statistical Analysis

Missing data were handled by mean imputation, but if exceeding 5%, the case was removed from further statistical analysis. In the preliminary analysis, descriptive statistics were calculated for all measures, including the mean (M), 95% CI, standard deviation (SD), median, skewness, and kurtosis. All scores demonstrated good parametric properties. Therefore, further parametric analyses were conducted. The study hypotheses were tested in several ways. Repeated measures one-way ANOVA was used to examine changes in the mean scores of life satisfaction, perceived stress, and coping styles during the first and second waves of the COVID-19 pandemic. Effect sizes were calculated using the partial eta-squared statistic (η_p^2).

The Pearson's correlation matrix was used to test the bivariate correlations among the variables. Multiple linear regression was conducted to assess the association between life satisfaction during W2 as a dependent variable and perceived stress and coping styles during W1 and W2 of the COVID-29 pandemic as a predictor variable. The mediating role of coping styles in the relationship between perceived stress and life satisfaction was examined in a cross-sectional design, separately for the first and second pandemic waves, using structural equation modeling (SEM). Parallel mediation models (simultaneous analysis of all three coping styles as a mediator) were performed based on maximum likelihood (ML) estimation without missing values and including observed variables. The conditional effect was examined based on a bias-corrected bootstrapping procedure with 1000 samples. A bootstrap confidence interval (95% CI) not including 0 signaled a significant effect.

Next, a two-wave cross-lagged panel design with a time lag of a half-year between W1 and W2 was performed for testing the prospective effect of perceived stress and coping styles on life satisfaction [84]. Two waves of data collection are recommended as the optimal approach to longitudinal design because it curtails the cost of a study in terms of time and money [85]. Structural equation modeling (SEM) was used, based on maximum likelihood (ML) estimation, without missing values, including observed variables, and with the bootstrapping method to test the conditional effect. The parallel mediation model specified included ten observed variables. We decided not to use latent variables because of the problems related to measurement invariance for the total 126 items included in 10 variables (W1 and W2). Both cross-lag and autoregressive paths were used to examine stability and change simultaneously [86,87]. All latent structural models were evaluated using several goodness-of-fit criteria, including ML χ^2, df, and p-value (the ratio $\chi^2/df < 5$ representing a good fit), standardized root mean square residual (SRMR ≤ 0.08 indicates an acceptable fit), root mean square error of approximation (adequate fit if RMSEA ≤ 0.08), comparative fit index (CFI ≥ 0.90 meaning adequate fit), normed fit index (NFI ≥ 0.95 considering adequate fit), and the Tucker–Lewis index (TLI ≥ 0.90 indicating adequate fit) [88–90]. All statistical analyzes were conducted using SPSS 27 (for descriptive statistics, ANOVA, and correlation analysis) and AMOS 22 (for SEM).

3. Results

3.1. Differences between the First and Second Waves of the COVID-19 Pandemic

The repeated measures one-way ANOVA was performed separately for life satisfaction, perceived stress, and coping styles to examine differences between the first (W1) and second (W2) wave of the COVID-19 pandemic among university students. The results are presented in Table 2 and Figure 2. The sample of university students reported an average (neutral) level of life satisfaction during the second wave of the pandemic (range 5–34, M = 19.70, SD = 6.11). Among participants, 11 individuals (4.76%) were extremely dissatisfied, 41 (17.75%) were dissatisfied, 58 (25.11%) were slightly dissatisfied, 14 (6.06%) were neutral, 68 (29.44%) were slightly satisfied, 30 (12.99%) were satisfied, and 9 (3.90%) were extremely satisfied. Perceived stress was reported as average (range 2–39, M = 22.53, SD = 7.92). In the sample, 45 persons (8.66%) indicated extremely low stress, 55 (19.48%) low, 53 (23.81%) average, 58 (22.94%) high, and 20 (25.11%) reported extremely high stress. The mean results of coping styles are presented in Table 2.

Table 2. Differences in life satisfaction, perceived stress, and coping styles between the first and second waves of the COVID-19 pandemic.

Variable	Wave 1		Wave 2		F(1, 230)	p	η_p^2
	M	SD	M	SD			
Life satisfaction	21.75	5.28	19.70	6.11	32.97	<0.001	0.13
Perceived stress	20.56	8.66	22.52	7.92	11.65	<0.001	0.05
Coping style							
Task-oriented	52.54	10.82	48.63	12.44	22.07	<0.001	0.09
Emotion-oriented	40.90	12.91	41.94	13.54	1.34	0.248	0.00
Avoidance-oriented	43.74	9.78	42.35	11.00	5.06	0.025	0.02

Significant differences with a medium effect size were found in life satisfaction and task-oriented coping style, as well as in perceived stress and avoidance coping with a small effect size. However, considering the Bonferroni correction, the level of significance was above the threshold of $p < 0.01$ for the avoidance coping style, which means that the differences between the first and second waves of pandemic should be considered statistically non-significant. No differences were found in the emotional coping style between W1 and W2.

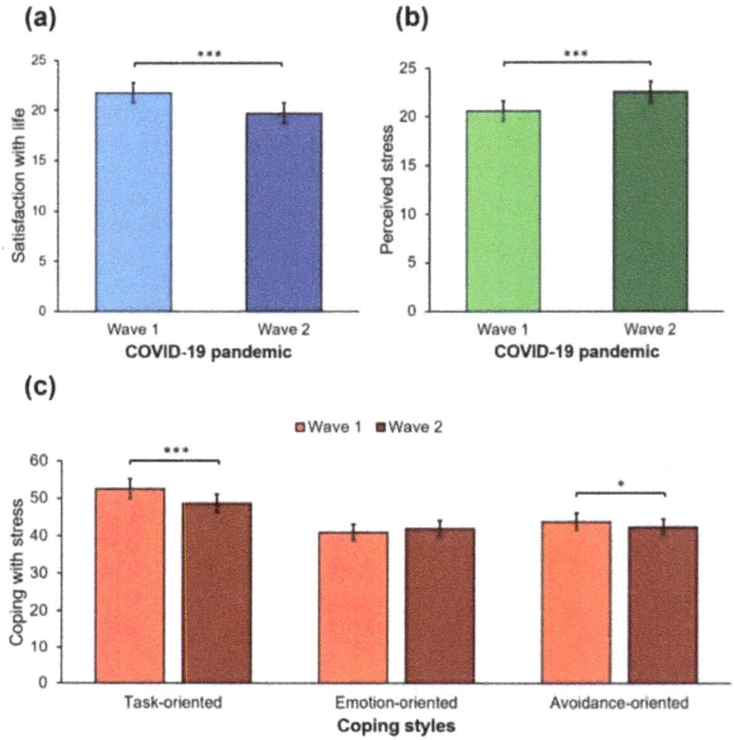

Figure 2. Differences between the first and second waves of the COVID-19 pandemic in (**a**) satisfaction with life; (**b**) perceived stress; and (**c**) task-oriented, emotion-oriented, and avoidance-oriented coping styles. * $p < 0.05$, *** $p < 0.001$.

3.2. Examining Predictors of Life Satisfaction at W2

In a preliminary analysis, Pearson's correlation was calculated to examine the association between satisfaction with life, perceived stress, and coping styles during the first and second waves of the COVID-19 pandemic. Almost all variables were related to each other, as shown in Table 3. The regression analysis was performed for life satisfaction during the second wave of the coronavirus pandemic (as a dependent variable) and predictor variables such as life satisfaction, perceived stress, and coping styles during the first and second wave.

Table 3. Correlations matrix for all variables in W1 and W2 of the COVID-19 pandemic.

	Variable	1	2	3	4	5	6	7	8	9
1	Life satisfaction W1									
2	Life satisfaction W2	0.56 ***								
3	Perceived stress W1	−0.38 ***	−0.21 **							
4	Perceived stress W2	−0.24 ***	−0.48 ***	0.45 ***						
				Coping style						
5	Task-oriented W1	0.25 ***	0.23 ***	−0.27 ***	−0.16 *					
6	Task-oriented W2	0.12	0.23 ***	−0.21 **	−0.27 ***	0.42 ***				
7	Emotion-oriented W1	−0.37 ***	−0.22 ***	0.61 ***	0.31 ***	−0.05	−0.01			
8	Emotion-oriented W2	−0.27 ***	−0.42 ***	0.38 ***	0.64 ***	−0.07	0.06	0.47 ***		
9	Avoidance-oriented W1	0.13 *	0.15 *	0.20 **	0.10	0.16 *	0.09	0.38 ***	0.16 *	
10	Avoidance-oriented W1	0.05	−0.03	0.22 ***	0.24 ***	0.02	0.20 **	0.27 ***	0.46 ***	0.60 ***

Notes. W1 = wave 1 of the COVID-19 pandemic; W2 = wave 2 of the COVID-19 pandemic. * $p < 0.05$, ** $p < 0.01$, *** $p < 0.001$.

Among all variables included in the regression model, the significant predictors were life satisfaction and perceived stress during the first wave of pandemic and perceived stress, task-oriented, and emotion-oriented coping styles during the second wave (Table 4). The model of regression explained 70% of the life satisfaction variance ($R^2 = 0.70$, $F(9, 221) = 24.09$, $p < 0.001$).

Table 4. Results of regression analysis for life satisfaction during the W2.

Variable	β	SE β	*b*	*SE b*	*t*(221)	*p*
Intercept			7.76	2.64	2.94	0.004
Life satisfaction W1	0.47	0.06	0.55	0.07	8.31	0.000
Perceived stress W1	0.20	0.07	0.14	0.05	2.99	0.003
Perceived stress W2	−0.32	0.07	−0.24	0.05	−4.49	0.000
Coping style						
Task-oriented W1	0.03	0.06	0.02	0.03	0.57	0.568
Task-oriented W2	0.12	0.06	0.06	0.03	2.01	0.046
Emotion-oriented W1	−0.03	0.07	−0.01	0.03	−0.38	0.705
Emotion-oriented W2	−0.16	0.08	−0.07	0.04	−2.01	0.046
Avoidance-oriented W1	0.12	0.07	0.08	0.04	1.80	0.072
Avoidance-oriented W1	−0.04	0.07	−0.02	0.04	−0.61	0.546

Notes. W1 = wave 1 of the COVID-19 pandemic; W2 = wave 2 of the COVID-19 pandemic.

3.3. The Indirect Effect of Perceived Stress on Life Satisfaction via Coping Styles

Cross-sectional parallel mediation analysis was conducted to examine the simultaneous mediation effect of all three coping styles on the relationship between perceived stress and life satisfaction (Figure 3). The analysis was performed separately for wave 1 (Model 1) and wave 2 (Model 2) of the COVID-19 pandemic. As shown in Table 5, all standardized estimates were statistically significant at both W1 and W2, which confirms the indirect effect of perceived stress on life satisfaction via task-oriented, emotion-oriented, and avoidance-oriented coping styles.

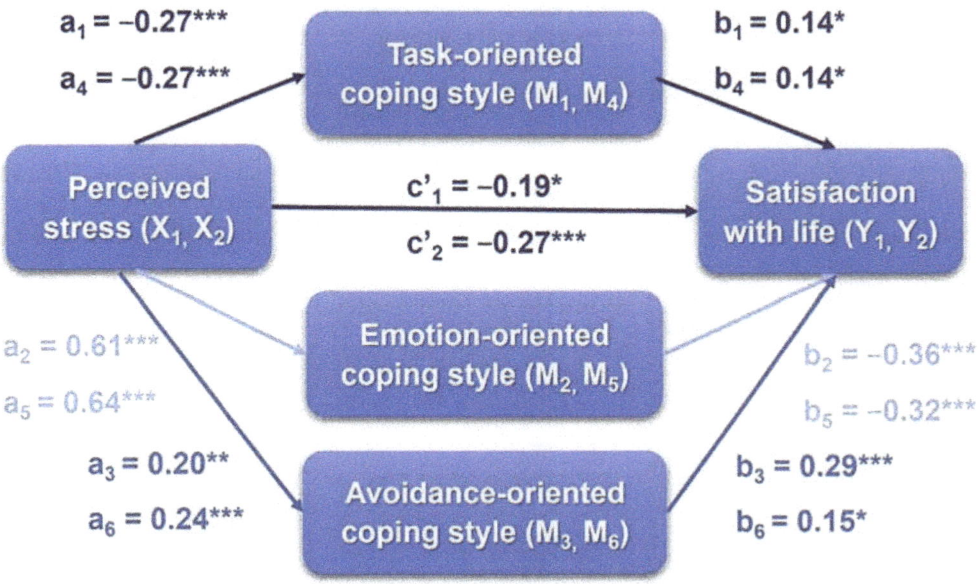

Figure 3. Path model of mediation of the effect of perceived stress on satisfaction with life, via coping styles; cross-sectional design (Model 1 and Model 2). * $p < 0.05$, ** $p < 0.01$, *** $p < 0.001$.

Table 5. Parameter estimates for latent structural mediation models in cross-sectional approach.

Antecedent	Consequent	Path	Model 1 W1	Path	Model 2 W2
Stress	Life satisfaction	c'_1	−0.185 *	c'_2	−0.272 ***
Stress	Task coping	a_1	−0.271 ***	a_4	−0.274 ***
Stress	Emotion coping	a_2	0.611 ***	a_5	0.638 ***
Stress	Avoidance coping	a_3	0.201 **	a_6	0.239 ***
Task coping	Life satisfation	b_1	0.136 *	b_4	0.140 *
Emotion coping	Life satisfation	b_2	−0.361 ***	b_5	−0.324 ***
Avoidance coping	Life satisfation	b_3	0.286 ***	b_6	0.152 *

Notes. W1 = wave 1 of the COVID-19 pandemic; W2 = wave 2 of the COVID-19 pandemic. The values in the table are standardized regression coefficients (β). * $p < 0.05$, ** $p < 0.01$, *** $p < 0.001$.

The goodness-of-fit indices for the cross-sectional parallel mediation during W1 (Model 1) and W2 (Model 2) are shown in Table 6. Some indices show good fit (i.e., SRMR, CFI, and NFI), whereas others are less acceptable (ML X^2/df, RMSEA, and TLI).

Table 6. Fit indices for alternative models.

Model	ML X^2	*df*	ML X^2/df	*p*	SRMR	RMSEA	95% CI	CFI	TLI	NFI
1	6.091	1	6.091	0.014	0.027	0.149	0.054–0.271	0.979	0.787	0.976
2	11.541	1	11.541	0.001	0.035	0.214	0.116–0.332	0.965	0.645	0.962
3	6.091	1	6.091	0.014	0.027	0.149	0.054–0.271	0.979	0.787	0.976
4	11.541	1	11.541	0.001	0.035	0.214	0.116–0.332	0.965	0.645	0.962
5	10.183	13	0.783	0.679	0.022	0.000	0.000–0.052	1.000	1.012	0.988
6	21.914	13	1.686	0.057	0.032	0.055	0.000–0.093	0.989	0.963	0.975
7	3.653	6	0.609	0.723	0.014	0.000	0.000–0.063	1.000	1.021	0.993

Notes. ML = maximum likelihood; SRMR = standardized root mean square residual; root mean square error of approximation = RMSEA; CI–confidence interval; CFI = comparative fit index; normed fit index = NFI; the Tucker–Lewis index = TLI.

3.4. The Indirect Effect of Life Satisfaction on Perceived Stress via Coping Styles

The cross-sectional parallel mediation analysis was performed separately for W1 and W2 to test the indirect effect of life satisfaction on perceived stress via coping styles (Figure 4). As is shown in Table 7, task-oriented and emotion-oriented coping (but not avoidance-oriented) were found as mediators in the association between life satisfaction and perceived stress for both W1 and W2. Table 6 demonstrates the goodness-of-fit indices for Model 3 (W1) and Model 4 (W2), which are the same as Model 1 and Model 2. According to the goodness-of-fit criteria, Model 3 and 4 (similar to Model 1 and 2) presents a satisfactory fit, taking into account SRMR (<0.08) CFI (>0.96), NFI (>0.95), and less acceptable for ML X^2/df (>5 is unacceptable), RMSEA (acceptable <0.08 in Model 1 and 3, but unacceptable >0.08 for Model 2 and 4), and TLI (<0.90 is unacceptable).

Table 7. Parameter estimates for latent structural mediation models in cross-sectional approach.

Antecedent	Consequent	Path	Model 3 W1	Path	Model 4 W2
Life satisfation	Stress	c'_1	−0.141 *	c'_2	−0.180 ***
Life satisfation	Task coping	a_1	0.248 ***	a_4	0.226 ***
Life satisfation	Emotion coping	a_2	−0.373 ***	a_5	−0.417 ***
Life satisfation	Avoidance coping	a_3	0.135 *	a_6	−0.031
Task coping	Stress	b_1	−0.222 ***	b_4	−0.274 ***
Emotion coping	Stress	b_2	0.527 ***	b_5	0.568 ***
Avoidance coping	Stress	b_3	0.057	b_6	0.025

Notes. W1 = wave 1 of the COVID-19 pandemic; W2 = wave 2 of the COVID-19 pandemic. The values in the table are standardized regression coefficients (β). * $p < 0.05$, *** $p < 0.001$.

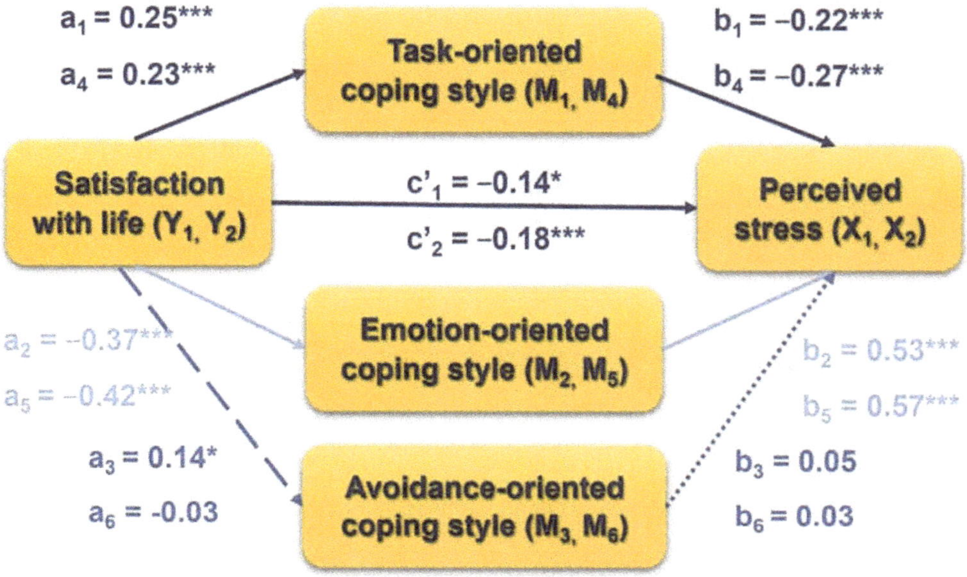

Figure 4. Path model of mediation for the effect of perceived stress on satisfaction with life, via coping styles; cross-sectional design (Model 3 and Model 4). * $p < 0.05$, *** $p < 0.001$.

3.5. Longitudinal Mediating Role of Coping Styles Using a Cross-Lagged Panel Model

The indirect effect of perceived stress on life satisfaction via coping styles was examined longitudinally across the two waves (W1 and W2) of the COVID-19 pandemic, using standard cross-lagged models (Figure 5a). Models 5 and 6 included cross-lagged (paths a and b) and autoregressive effects (paths x, m, and y). No mediation effect of all three coping styles was found in the parallel cross-lagged Model 5 (Table 8). Although the emotion-oriented coping style during W2 was predictable based on perceived stress during W1, no coping style at W1 was found as a significant predictor of life satisfaction at W2. Weak stability over time (i.e., across two waves of the COVID-19 pandemic) was found for perceived stress, life satisfaction, task-oriented coping, and emotion-oriented coping style, while moderate stability was found for avoidance-oriented coping style in Model 5. The cross-lagged parallel mediation Model 5 demonstrates a perfect fit, as shown in Table 6.

When the reverse order was examined, with life satisfaction as a predictor of perceived stress (Model 6, Figure 5b), coping style during W1 was not significantly related to stress at W2, nor was life satisfaction at W1 related to coping style during W2 (see Table 8 for more details). Therefore, the mediating effect of coping style on the relationship between life satisfaction and perceived stress was not confirmed in the longitudinal approach. The goodness-of-fit measures were acceptable for Model 6 (Table 6).

The last analysis considered the reciprocal relationships between stress and life satisfaction, including the coping styles as mediators (Model 7, Figure 6). As shown in Table 8, significant regression coefficients were found only for the autoregressive path. Each variable during W2 in Model 7 could be predicted by the same variable during W1. Weak stability was presented by stress, life satisfaction, task-oriented, and emotion-oriented coping styles, whereas moderate stability was found for avoidance coping with stress. However, none of the variables during W2 could be predicted from any variable at W1. Model 7 demonstrates a perfect fit, as shown in Table 5.

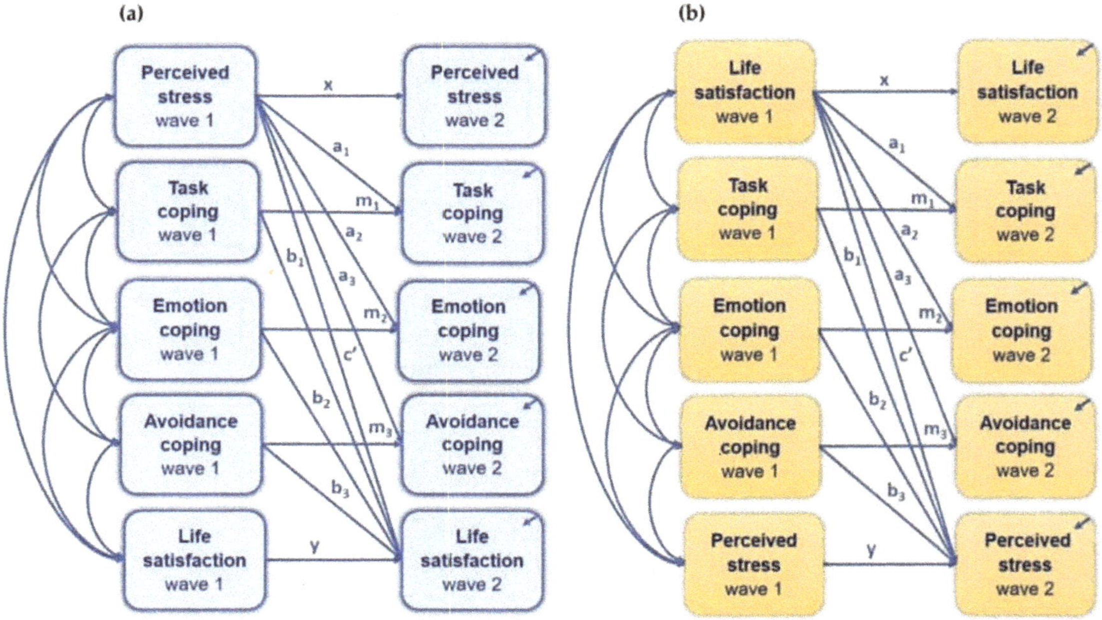

Figure 5. Conceptual cross-lagged path model for a prospective study on the parallel mediation role of coping styles in the relationship between perceived stress and satisfaction with life during the first and second waves of the COVID-19 pandemic: (**a**) perceived stress as a predictor of life satisfaction (Model 5); (**b**) life satisfaction as a predictor of perceived stress (Model 6).

Table 8. Parameter estimates for latent structural mediation models in the longitudinal approach.

Antecedent	Consequent	Model 5	Model 6	Model 7
Stress W1	Life satisfaction W2	0.018		0.054
Stress W1	Stress W2	0.450 ***	0.293 ***	0.357 ***
Stress W1	Task coping W2	−0.105		−0.107
Stress W1	Emotion coping W2	0.174 **		0.122
Stress W1	Avoidance coping W2	0.104		0.115
Task coping W1	Task coping W2	0.385 ***	0.410 ***	0.403 ***
Emotion coping W1	Emotion coping W2	0.337 ***	0.405 ***	0.363 ***
Avoidance coping W1	Avoidance coping W2	0.571 ***	0.591 ***	0.561 ***
Life satisfaction W1	Life satisfaction W2	0.479 ***	0.556 ***	0.499 ***
Task coping W1	Life satisfaction W2	0.075		−0.020
Emotion coping W1	Life satisfaction W2	−0.073		−0.086
Avoidance coping W1	Life satisfaction W2	0.101		0.022
Life satisfaction W1	Stress W2		−0.098	−0.057
Life satisfaction W1	Task coping W2		0.020	0.097
Life satisfaction W1	Emotion coping W2		−0.120	−0.110
Life satisfaction W1	Avoidance coping W2		−0.026	0.091
Task coping W1	Stress W2		−0.032	−0.056
Emotion coping W1	Stress W2		0.075	0.081
Avoidance coping W1	Stress W2		0.048	0.025

Notes. W1 = wave 1 of the COVID-19 pandemic; W2 = wave 2 of the COVID-19 pandemic. The values in the table are standardized regression coefficients (β). ** $p < 0.01$, *** $p < 0.001$.

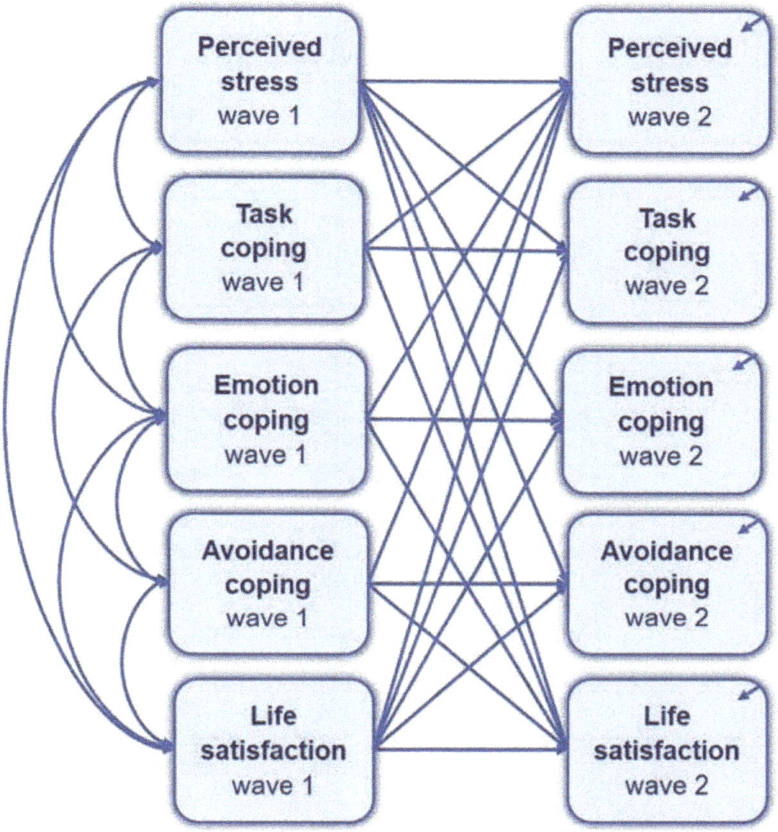

Figure 6. Conceptual reciprocal cross-lagged path model for a prospective study on the parallel mediation role of coping styles in the relationship between perceived stress and satisfaction with life.

4. Discussion

In this study, we examined for the first time the mediating effect of coping style on the relationship between perceived stress and life satisfaction in both cross-sectional and longitudinal models, in an extraordinary stressful situation such as the COVID-19 pandemic. Consistent with the transactional model of stress [53,73], we found significant changes between the first (W1) and second (W2) waves of the COVID-19 pandemic in perceived stress, life satisfaction, and some coping styles. The ANOVA showed that among the three coping styles, a larger change was reported for task-oriented coping. The frequency of using task-oriented and avoidance-oriented coping strategies significantly decreased, while the frequency of emotion-oriented coping slightly (but insignificantly) increased during W2 compared to W1. Furthermore, weak stability was noted in this study for stress, life satisfaction, and task- and emotion-oriented coping, whereas moderate stability was found for avoidance-oriented coping when the longitudinal cross-lagged model was examined. Both statistical methods (ANOVA and cross-lagged model) indicated that stress levels increased across pandemic waves, life satisfaction decreased, and the frequency of using selected coping strategies continuously changed over time.

The present results are consistent with previous research performed during the COVID-19 pandemic. A recent multi-cultural study showed that self-reported quality of life decreased over time, while perceived stress level and difficulty with emotion regulation increased significantly during the coronavirus pandemic [24]. Significant changes in stress and life satisfaction were found during the pandemic in various longitudinal studies [32–36]. Ruggieri et al. [32] performed a cross-lagged panel study during three waves (from one month before the lockdown), and they found increased levels of stress and decreased life satisfaction among Italian adults. A longitudinal study [34] on pre- and during-pandemic stressors and risk factors for distress changes showed that perceived stress during the pandemic was associated with pre-pandemic social stressors, stressful life events, low generalized trust, poor self-rated health, and some concurrent pandemic-related stressors and risk factors. Changes in lifestyle and economic disruptions, and loss of education or employment, were associated with greater increases in emotional distress. People who suffered high stress before the pandemic experienced increases in stress during the pandemic. During-pandemic stressors and hopelessness were found to be the strongest correlates of during-pandemic distress. Individuals distressed by the lockdown frequently used coping strategies such as seeking social support, engaging in distractions, and seeking professional help. Shanahan et al. [34] showed that several coping strategies significantly reduced distress during the pandemic, including keeping a daily routine, positive reappraisal/reframing, engaging in physical activity, acceptance, and keeping in contact with family and friends.

We found a 34% prevalence of high stress and 48% prevalence of low life satisfaction university students during W2 of the pandemic. In contrast, a systematic review found a 27% prevalence of high stress symptoms in the population during the COVID-19 pandemic [65]. However, a meta-analysis [66] indicated that very high stress was experienced by 45% of Chinese people during the crisis. Among Australian adults [67], 47% reported some degree of psychological distress during the first wave of the coronavirus pandemic, which was inversely related to coping strategies such as positive reframing, acceptance, and humor, and positively related to self-blame, venting, behavioral disengagement, and self-distraction. Research performed in Saudi Arabia found a 55.5% prevalence of high levels of stress during the quarantine, which was reduced by cognitive reappraisal and life satisfaction [68]. Numerous studies showed that the primary source of stress during the coronavirus pandemic was the significant lifestyle changes, related in particular to numerous restrictions and social isolation [17,38–43].

The partial mediating role of coping style in the relationship between stress and life satisfaction was confirmed in both cross-sectional studies during W1 (Model 1) and W2 (Model 2). A total of 70% of life satisfaction at W2 can be explained by predictor variables such as stress during W1 and W2, life satisfaction during W1, and by task-oriented and emotion-oriented coping styles during W2. However, among the three coping styles, emotion-oriented showed the strongest association with both stress and life satisfaction. In particular, a higher stress level was a predictor of the more frequent use of emotion-oriented coping strategies (positive association), which decreased life satisfaction (negative relation). This is consistent with previous studies [30,70,71], which indicated that university students reporting low life satisfaction, high stress, and most frequent use of emotion-oriented coping strategies during the pandemic. Marotta et al. [28] found an increase in negative and positive emotions, and a decrease in the quality of life among adult Italians during the first COVID-19 lockdown compared to reference data before the pandemic.

Higher stress levels were associated with a lower frequency of using task-oriented coping and a higher frequency of using avoidance-focused coping in the present study. This result is consistent with a previous study showing that people who experienced higher stress tended to use more passive rather than active coping strategies during pandemic [56,57]. When the environment is unpredictable and uncontrollable, task-oriented coping is perceived as less adaptive, whereas avoidance-focused coping strategies are more effective in reducing stress levels. This pattern was an adequate stress response in stressful life events or disasters [72].

The result of our mediation analysis is consistent to some extent with a previous study. Stapleton et al. [35] found that life satisfaction can be predicted by adaptive (positive association) and maladaptive (negative relation) coping, explaining 20% of the life satisfaction variance (R^2 = 0.20) among teachers. Lardier et al. [74] showed that life satisfaction is negatively related to perceived stress and both suppressive (avoidance-oriented) and reactive (task-oriented) coping and is positively correlated with reflective (task-oriented) coping among Hispanic undergraduate students. Mediation analysis [74] indicated that perceived stress is indirectly related to life satisfaction through a reflective coping style. Higher levels of stress were associated with lower levels of reflective coping, which were related to lower life satisfaction. Both suppressive and reactive coping were not mediators in the relationship between perceived stress and life satisfaction. In contrast, we found a mediating role among all three coping styles: task-, emotion-, and avoidance-oriented. The differences between the results of the previous and current studies may be due to the various measurement tools used to assess coping with stress and cross-cultural variance.

Our findings also directly link stress to life satisfaction (Models 1 and 2) and conversely from life satisfaction to stress (Models 3 and 4). A stronger negative association was noted in the second wave of the pandemic than during the first wave. The relationship between stress and life satisfaction or other indices of well-being was previously reported in numerous studies [4,6–14]. Subjective well-being depends on many environmental and person-centered factors, including school and work, family and social life, and individual differences in affective states and personality traits and dispositions [1–5,91]. All these well-being-related factors may increase stress if changes in environment and lifestyle are perceived as a threat. Many studies indicated that stress and risk of mental disorders increased during the COVID-19 pandemic, whereas life satisfaction and quality of life decreased [15–35]. Studies indicated an inverse relationship between stress and various measures of well-being, e.g., [4,14,20,32,35], where higher levels of well-being corelated with lower levels of stress.

The reciprocal relationship of how life satisfaction affects stress through coping style was also tested cross-sectionally during W1 and W2. The results confirmed the partial mediation effect of task- and emotion-oriented coping styles. A high level of life satisfaction was related to an increased likelihood of using task-oriented coping, leading to decreased stress. Conversely, higher life satisfaction was a predictor of less frequent emotion-oriented coping, which could predict higher levels of perceived stress. Avoidance-oriented coping was not found to be a significant predictor of stress. Therefore, this coping style cannot play a mediating role in the relationship between life satisfaction and stress. This pattern was demonstrated at both measurement times, W1 and W2, during the COVID-19 pandemic.

The positive relationship of well-being with task-oriented coping style and negative relationship with emotion-oriented and avoidance-oriented was reported previously [35,58–64]. Boysan [58] demonstrated that life satisfaction is positively related to task-oriented (0.18, $p < 0.01$) and avoidance-oriented coping (0.08, $p < 0.05$), whereas negatively related to emotion-oriented coping (−0.20, $p < 0.01$). Xu et al. [64] found a relationship of high life satisfaction with high levels of positive coping (i.e., problem-solving, seeking social support, and positively rationalized explanation) and low levels of negative coping (enduring, escape, emotion venting, and wishful thinking/denial). Well-being was significantly and positively associated with approach coping and inversely related to avoidant coping behavior among UK adults during the first wave of the COVID-19 pandemic [60]. Engagement-related coping such as problem-solving was positively related to well-being, whereas disengagement coping such as blaming was negatively related. However, distraction and denial as coping strategies were not significantly associated with well-being among a large sample of the German population [61].

Stapleton et al. [35] found a moderate negative correlation of life satisfaction with perceived stress and a weak correlation with maladaptive coping, and a very weak but significant positive correlation between life satisfaction and adaptive coping among teachers. A regression analysis [35] showed that maladaptive (emotion-focused) coping is a strong positive predictor of psychological distress, whereas adaptive coping (task-oriented coping) is a weak negative predictor, explaining 45% of stress variance (R^2 = 0.45). Problem-focused coping was considered an adaptive coping style since it was associated with better academic achievement among middle school students [92].

Another study showed that psychological well-being correlated negatively with avoidance strategy and positively with problem-solving coping among Italian university students [63]. Similarly, negative coping (i.e., high-stress perceptions, dysfunctional attitudes, and catastrophizing) showed a negative association with subjective well-being, whereas positive coping (hope, proactive coping style, and sense of humor) affected well-being positively [62]. Yan et al. [56] also showed that positive coping strategies are related to fewer symptoms of stress and mental health problems, whereas negative coping strategies aggravated emotional distress among a large sample of Chinese people during the first COVID-19 outbreak. Higher perceived adaptability to the COVID-19 pandemic was related to lower stress in a cross-sectional study in a sample of college students [93].

The result of this study is consistent to some extent with previous research on the mediating role of coping with stress [75]. Gori et al. [75] found a mediating effect of coping strategies on the relationship between life satisfaction and perceived stress in a cross-sectional study among Italian adults during the first wave of the COVID-19 pandemic. In particular, an indirect effect of life satisfaction on perceived stress was demonstrated via approach coping, positive attitude, and mature defenses, as indicated by a serial mediation model. Although Gori et al. [75] used a different tool to measure coping with stress (the Coping Orientations to Problems Experienced and the Forty-Item Defense Style Questionnaire), approach coping may be considered an alternative to task-oriented coping (in the CISS), positive attitude as an equivalent to inverse scores on the emotion-oriented coping scale, while mature defenses are similar (but only to some extend) to avoidance-oriented coping. Differences between previous [75] and the current study results in mediation analysis may be due to the various measurement methods used to assess coping styles and cross-cultural differences between the Italian adult population (with a mean age of 34 years old) and Polish university students (mean age of 23 years old).

Consistent with the hypothesis, longitudinal parallel mediation analysis across W1 and W2 during the pandemic was not confirmed. Although perceived stress during W1 was a significant positive predictor of emotion-oriented coping style during W2, no significant association was found between emotion-oriented coping style during W1 and life satisfaction during W2. Furthermore, neither task-oriented coping nor avoidance-oriented strategies were shown to be significantly related to stress or life satisfaction. When the reciprocal relationship between life satisfaction and stress via coping styles was examined, mediation was not found, and no coping style was associated with stress or life satisfaction. Notably, all autoregression pathways were significant in Models 5, 6 and 7. This means that all the variables at W2, included in Models 5 and 6, were predicted by the same variables at W1 (e.g., the perceived stress at W1 was a predictor of perceived stress at W2). Model 5, with perceived stress as a predictor of life satisfaction, received better fit indices than Model 6 with reciprocal relations. However, Model 7, with both paths from Model 5 and Model 6, showed a perfect and the best fit.

The results of this study indicate that a reciprocal association occurs between life satisfaction and stress, but it can only be observed at a given moment. We evidenced in cross-sectional studies during W1 and W2 that stress is a predictor of life satisfaction, and life satisfaction is a predictor of stress (Models 1 and 2, and Models 3 and 4, respectively). In addition, coping styles play a mediating role in the relationship between stress and life satisfaction, as well as in a reciprocal direction. In contrast, when the longitudinal design was examined, neither was perceived stress-related to life satisfaction (and vice versa), nor was coping style associated significantly with perceived stress or life satisfaction. As such, the mediation effect was not confirmed longitudinally. According to the transactional model of stress [53,73], stressful transactions between a person and their environment determines continuous changes in stress, coping, and well-being. Lifestyle changes and environmental stressful situations between W1 and W2 of the COVID-19 pandemic appear to be responsible for changes in the levels of the variables studied when comparing W1 to W2. This may explain why longitudinal mediation was not confirmed, although cross-sectional mediation was found twice during W1 and W2 of the pandemic. People adaptively change their coping strategies to the dynamic changes in stress levels and well-being as stressful events and lifestyle change during a pandemic. H5 was fully supported in this study.

Limitations of the Study

There are some limitations that do not allow for generalization of our study's results. First, the self-report measures of stress, life satisfaction, and coping styles may be biased to some extent. A future study can use experimental methods to assess the stress response. Although all measures were obtained during the COVID-19 pandemic, none include specific pandemic-related circumstances. Future studies may use more specific tools devoted to the stressful COVID-19 pandemic event. Although the sample size during the first and second cross-sectional studies was large, only 230 students participated in online surveys. The findings were collected at one technical university, so they may not represent all university students or the general population.

5. Conclusions

Perceived stress, life satisfaction, and coping styles significantly changed from the first to the second wave of the COVID-19 pandemic. University students considered changes in lifestyle and environment related to lockdown and adjusted their best coping strategies to these stressful events. As such, stress, and emotion-oriented and avoidance-oriented coping styles increased from W1 to W2, while life satisfaction and task-oriented coping decreased. These variables explained almost 70% of the variance in life satisfaction as stress and life satisfaction during W1, stress during W1 and W2, and emotion-oriented and task-oriented coping during W2. In the cross-sectional study, coping styles played a mediating role in the relationship between stress and life satisfaction at W1 and W2. However, in the longitudinal design, coping during W1 was not a useful predictor of life satisfaction or stress during W2. We found a reciprocal interrelation between stress and life satisfaction. Therefore, we found strong evidence aligned with the theory of the transactional model of stress. The findings provide new knowledge on our current understanding of stress and coping mechanisms concerning well-being. People try various coping strategies and choose the most effective at the moment and change them in response to the unstable environment. A vast repertoire of coping strategies, and flexibility in their selection, may be the best methods to effectively cope with stressful lockdowns during the COVID-19 pandemic and protect individuals against decreased well-being.

Author Contributions: Conceptualization, A.M.R., C.K. and D.O.; methodology, A.M.R. and D.O.; software, A.M.R.; validation, A.M.R., C.K. and D.O.; formal analysis, A.M.R.; investigation, C.K.; resources, A.M.R.; data curation, A.M.R.; writing—original draft preparation, A.M.R.; writing—review and editing, A.M.R., C.K., D.O.; visualization, A.M.R.; supervision, D.O.; project administration, C.K.; funding acquisition, C.K. and D.O. All authors have read and agreed to the published version of the manuscript.

Funding: The study was not financially supported by any grant or foundation. The APC was funded by the Opole University of Technology and University of Technology in Katowice.

Institutional Review Board Statement: The study was conducted according to the guidelines of the Declaration of Helsinki, and approved by the Ethics Committee of the University of Opole (protocol code 1/2020, date of approval 22 April 2020).

Informed Consent Statement: Informed consent was obtained from all subjects involved in the study.

Data Availability Statement: The datasets used and/or analysed during the current study are available from the corresponding author on reasonable request.

Conflicts of Interest: The authors declare no conflict of interest.

References

1. Diener, E.; Emmons, R.A.; Larsen, R.J.; Griffin, S. The Satisfaction with Life Scale. *J. Pers. Assess.* **1985**, *49*, 71–75. [CrossRef]
2. Diener, E. New findings and future directions for subjective well-being research. *Am. Psychol.* **2012**, *67*, 590–597. [CrossRef] [PubMed]
3. López-Ortega, M.; Torres-Castro, S.; Rosas-Carrasco, O. Psychometric properties of the Satisfaction with Life Scale (SWLS): Secondary analysis of the Mexican Health and Aging Study. *Health Qual. Life Outcomes* **2016**, *14*, 170. [CrossRef] [PubMed]
4. Yang, C.; Xia, M.; Han, M.; Liang, Y. Social support and resilience as mediators between stress and life satisfaction among people with substance use disorder in China. *Front. Psychiatry* **2018**, *9*, 436. [CrossRef] [PubMed]
5. Zhou, M.; Lin, W. Adaptability and life satisfaction: The moderating role of social support. *Front. Psychol.* **2016**, *7*, 1134. [CrossRef]
6. Coffman, D.L.; Gilligan, T.D. Social support, stress, and self-efficacy: Effects on students' satisfaction. *J. Coll. Stud. Ret.* **2002**, *4*, 53–66. [CrossRef]
7. Emanuel, F.; Molino, M.; Lo Presti, A.; Spagnoli, P.; Ghislieri, C. A crossover study from a gender perspective: The relationship between job insecurity, job satisfaction, and partners' family life satisfaction. *Front. Psychol.* **2018**, *9*, 1481. [CrossRef]
8. Gouveia, V.V.; Milfont, T.L.; da Fonseca, P.N.; de Miranda Coelho, J.A.P. Life satisfaction in Brazil: Testing the psychometric properties of the Satisfaction with Life Scale (SWLS) in Five Brazilian Samples. *Soc. Indic. Res.* **2009**, *90*, 267. [CrossRef]
9. Jovanović, V. The validity of the Satisfaction with Life Scale in adolescents and a comparison with single-item life satisfaction measures: A preliminary study. *Qual. Life Res.* **2016**, *25*, 3173–3180. [CrossRef]
10. Lee, J.; Kim, E.; Wachholtz, A. The effect of perceived stress on life satisfaction: The mediating effect of self-efficacy. *Chongsonyonhak Yongu* **2016**, *23*, 29–47. [PubMed]
11. Pavot, W.; Diener, E. The Satisfaction with Life Scale and the emerging construct of life satisfaction. *J. Posit. Psychol.* **2008**, *3*, 137–152. [CrossRef]
12. Pavot, W.; Diener, E. Review of the Satisfaction with Life Scale. In *Assessing Well-Being*; Social Indicators Research Series; Diener, E., Ed.; Springer: Dordrecht, Germany, 2009; Volume 39, pp. 101–117. [CrossRef]
13. Praharso, N.F.; Tear, M.J.; Cruwys, T. Stressful life transitions and well-being: A comparison of the stress-buffering hypothesis and the social identity model of identity change. *Psychiatry Res.* **2017**, *247*, 265–275. [CrossRef]
14. Rey, L.; Extremera, N. Core self-evaluations, perceived stress and life satisfaction in Spanish young and middle-aged adults: An examination of mediation and moderation effects. *Soc. Indic. Res.* **2015**, *120*, 515–524. [CrossRef]
15. Ahmed, Z.; Ahmed, O.; Aibao, Z.; Hanbin, S.; Siyu, L.; Ahmad, A. Epidemic of COVID −19 in China and associated psychological problems. *Asian J. Psychiatry* **2020**, *51*, 102092. [CrossRef] [PubMed]
16. Aslan, I.; Ochnik, D.; Çınar, O. Exploring Perceived Stress among Students in Turkey during the COVID-19 Pandemic. *Int. J. Environ. Res. Public Health* **2020**, *17*, 8961. [CrossRef] [PubMed]
17. Benke, C.; Autenrieth, L.K.; Asselmann, E.; Pané-Farré, C.A. Lockdown, quarantine measures, and social distancing: Associations with depression, anxiety and distress at the beginning of the COVID-19 pandemic among adults from Germany. *Psychiatry Res.* **2020**, *293*, 113462. [CrossRef]
18. Brooks, S.K.; Webster, R.K.; Smith, L.E.; Woodland, L.; Wessely, S.; Greenberg, N.; Rubin, G.J. The psychological impact of quarantine and how to reduce it: A rapid review of the evidence. *Lancet* **2020**, *395*, 912–920. [CrossRef]
19. Cao, W.; Fang, Z.; Hou, G.; Han, M.; Xu, X.; Dong, J.; Zheng, J. The psychological impact of the COVID-19 epidemic on college students in China. *Psychiatry Res.* **2020**, *287*, 112934. [CrossRef] [PubMed]
20. Dymecka, J.; Gerymski, R.; Machnik-Czerwik, A. How does stress affect life satisfaction during the COVID-19 pandemic? Moderated mediation analysis of sense of coherence and fear of coronavirus. *Psychol. Health Med.* **2021**, *31*, 1–9. [CrossRef]
21. Gao, J.; Zheng, P.; Jia, Y.; Chen, H.; Mao, Y.; Chen, S.; Wang, Y.; Fu, H.; Dai, J. Mental health problems and social media exposure during COVID-19 outbreak. *PLoS ONE* **2020**, *15*, e0231924. [CrossRef]
22. Gawrych, M.; Cichoń, E.; Kiejna, A. COVID-19 pandemic fear, life satisfaction and mental health at the initial stage of the pandemic in the largest cities in Poland. *Psychol. Health Med.* **2021**, *26*, 107–113. [CrossRef]
23. Huang, Y.; Zhao, N. Chinese mental health burden during the COVID-19 pandemic. *Asian J. Psychiatry* **2020**, *51*, 102052. [CrossRef]
24. Khodami, M.A. Perceived stress, emotion regulation and quality of life during the COVID-19 outbreak: A multi-cultural online survey. *Ann. Med. Psychol.* **2021**. [CrossRef]
25. Kobayashi, L.C.; O'Shea, B.Q.; Kler, J.S.; Nishimura, R.; Palavicino-Maggio, C.B.; Eastman, M.R.; Vinson, Y.R.; Finlay, J.M. Cohort profile: The COVID-19 Coping Study, a longitudinal mixed-methods study of middle-aged and older adults' mental health and well-being during the COVID-19 pandemic in the USA. *BMJ Open* **2021**, *11*, e044965. [CrossRef] [PubMed]
26. Lipskaya-Velikovsky, L. COVID-19 Isolation in healthy population in Israel: Challenges in daily life, mental health, resilience, and quality of life. *Int. J. Environ. Res. Public Health* **2021**, *18*, 999. [CrossRef] [PubMed]
27. Ma, Z.; Zhao, J.; Li, Y.; Chen, D.; Wang, T.; Zhang, Z.; Chen, Z.; Yu, Q.; Jiang, J.; Fan, F.; et al. Mental health problems and correlates among 746 217 college students during the coronavirus disease 2019 outbreak in China. *Epidemiol. Psychiatr. Sci.* **2020**, *29*, e181. [CrossRef]
28. Marotta, L.; Pesce, A.; Guazzini, A. Before and after the Quarantine: An Approximate Study on the Psychological Impact of COVID-19 on the Italian Population during the Lockdown Period. *Future Internet* **2020**, *12*, 229. [CrossRef]
29. Rajkumar, R.P. COVID-19 and mental health: A review of the existing literature. *Asian J. Psychiatry* **2020**, *52*, 102066. [CrossRef] [PubMed]

30. Rogowska, A.M.; Kuśnierz, C.; Bokszczanin, A. Examining anxiety, life satisfaction, general health, stress and coping styles during COVID-19 pandemic in Polish sample of university students. *Psychol. Res. Behav. Manag.* **2020**, *13*, 797–811. [CrossRef]
31. Rogowska, A.M.; Pavlova, I.; Kuśnierz, C.; Ochnik, D.; Bodnar, I.; Petrytsa, P. Does physical activity matter for the mental health of university students during the COVID-19 pandemic? *J. Clin. Med.* **2020**, *9*, 3494. [CrossRef]
32. Ruggieri, S.; Ingoglia, S.; Bonfanti, R.C.; Lo Coco, G. The role of on-line social comparison as a protective factor for psychological well-being: A longitudinal study during the COVID-19 quarantine. *Pers. Individ. Dif.* **2021**, *171*, 110486. [CrossRef]
33. Shi, L.; Lu, Z.A.; Que, J.Y.; Huang, X.L.; Liu, L.; Ran, M.S.; Gong, Y.M.; Yuan, K.; Yan, W.; Sun, Y.K.; et al. Prevalence of and risk factors associated with mental health symptoms among the general population in China during the coronavirus disease 2019 pandemic. *JAMA Netw. Open* **2020**, *3*, e2014053. [CrossRef] [PubMed]
34. Shanahan, L.; Steinhoff, A.; Bechtiger, L.; Murray, A.L.; Nivette, A.; Hepp, U.; Ribeaud, D.; Eisner, M. Emotional distress in young adults during the COVID-19 pandemic: Evidence of risk and resilience from a longitudinal cohort study. *Psychol. Med.* **2020**, 1–10. [CrossRef]
35. Stapleton, P.; Garby, S.; Sabot, D. Psychological distress and coping styles in teachers: A preliminary study. *Aust. J. Educ.* **2020**, *64*, 127–146. [CrossRef]
36. Wang, X.; Lei, S.M.; Le, S.; Yang, Y.; Zhang, B.; Yao, W.; Gao, Z.; Cheng, S. Bidirectional influence of the COVID-19 pandemic lockdowns on health behaviors and quality of life among Chinese adults. *Int. J. Environ. Res. Public Health* **2020**, *17*, 5575. [CrossRef] [PubMed]
37. Lee, C.-W.; Lin, L.-C.; Hung, H.-C. Art and cultural participation and life satisfaction in adults: The role of physical health, mental health, and interpersonal relationships. *Front. Public Health* **2021**, *8*, 582342. [CrossRef] [PubMed]
38. Chaturvedi, S.K. COVID −19, coronavirus, and mental health rehabilitation at times of crisis. *J. Psychosoc. Rehabil. Ment. Health* **2020**, *7*, 1–2. [CrossRef] [PubMed]
39. Dagnino, P.; Anguita, V.; Escobar, K.; Cifuentes, S. Psychological effects of social isolation due to quarantine in Chile: An exploratory study. *Front. Psychiatry* **2020**, *11*, 591142. [CrossRef]
40. Glowacz, F.; Schmits, E. Psychological distress during the COVID-19 lockdown: The young adults most at risk. *Psychiatry Res.* **2020**, *293*, 113486. [CrossRef]
41. Gonzalez-Bernal, J.J.; Rodríguez-Fernández, P.; Santamaría-Peláez, M.; González-Santos, J.; León-Del-Barco, B.; Minguez, L.A.; Soto-Cámara, R. Life satisfaction during forced social distancing and home confinement derived from the COVID-19 pandemic in Spain. *Int. J. Environ. Res. Public Health* **2021**, *18*, 1474. [CrossRef]
42. Zhang, S.X.; Wang, Y.; Rauch, A.; Wei, F. Unprecedented disruption of lives and work: Health, distress and life satisfaction of working adults in China one month into the COVID-19 outbreak. *Psychiatry Res.* **2020**, *288*, 112958. [CrossRef]
43. Zhang, Y.; Ma, Z.F. Impact of the COVID-19 Pandemic on Mental Health and Quality of Life among Local Residents in Liaoning Province, China: A Cross-Sectional Study. *Int. J. Environ. Res. Public Health* **2020**, *17*, 2381. [CrossRef] [PubMed]
44. Tušl, M.; Brauchli, R.; Kerksieck, P.; Bauer, G.F. Impact of the COVID-19 crisis on work and private life, mental well-being and self-rated health in German and Swiss employees: A cross-sectional on-line survey. *BMC Public Health* **2021**, *21*, 741. [CrossRef]
45. Lee, S. Subjective well-being and mental health during the pandemic outbreak: Exploring the role of institutional trust. *Res. Aging* **2020**. [CrossRef] [PubMed]
46. Liu, X.; Ping, S.; Gao, W. Changes in Undergraduate Students' Psychological Well-being as They Experience University Life. *Int. J. Environ. Res. Public Health* **2019**, *16*, 2864. [CrossRef]
47. Yoo, C. Stress coping and mental health among adolescents: Applying a multi-dimensional stress coping model. *Child. Youth Serv. Rev.* **2019**, *99*, 43–53. [CrossRef]
48. Almarzooq, Z.I.; Lopes, M.; Kochar, A. Virtual learning during the COVID-19 pandemic: A disruptive technology in graduate medical education. *J. Am. Coll. Cardiol.* **2020**, *75*, 2635–2638. [CrossRef]
49. Amir, L.R.; Tanti, I.; Maharani, D.A.; Wimardhani, Y.S.; Julia, V.; Sulijaya, B.; Puspitawati, R. Student perspective of classroom and distance learning during COVID-19 pandemic in the undergraduate dental study program Universitas Indonesia. *BMC Med. Educ.* **2020**, *20*, 392. [CrossRef]
50. Chaturvedi, K.; Vishwakarma, D.K.; Singh, N. COVID-19 and its impact on education, social life and mental health of students: A survey. *Child. Youth Serv. Rev.* **2021**, *121*, 105866. [CrossRef] [PubMed]
51. Gautam, R.; Sharma, M. 2019-nCoV pandemic: A disruptive and stressful atmosphere for Indian academic fraternity. *Brain Behav. Immun.* **2020**, *88*, 948–949. [CrossRef]
52. Endler, N.S.; Parker, J.D.A. Assessment of multidimensional coping: Task, Emotion, and avoidance strategies. *Psychol. Assess.* **1994**, *6*, 50–60. [CrossRef]
53. Lazarus, R.S.; Folkman, S. *Stress, Appraisal, and Coping*; Springer: New York, NY, USA, 1984.
54. Lazarus, R.S. Stress, coping and illness. In *Personality and Disease*; Friedman, H.S., Ed.; John Wiley & Sons: Chichester, NH, USA, 1990; pp. 97–120.
55. Voronin, I.A.; Manrique-Millones, D.; Vasin, G.D.; Millones-Rivalles, R.B.; Fernández-Ríos, N.; Marakshina, Y.A.; Lobaskova, M.M.; Symanyuk, E.E.; Pecherkina, A.A.; Ageeva, I.A.; et al. Coping Responses during the COVID-19Pandemic: A Cross-Cultural Comparison of Russia, Kyrgyzstan, and Peru. *Psychol. Russia* **2020**, *13*, 481. [CrossRef]
56. Yan, L.; Gan, Y.; Ding, X.; Wu, J.; Duan, H. The relationship between perceived stress and emotional distress during the COVID-19 outbreak: Effects of boredom proneness and coping style. *J. Anxiety Disord.* **2021**, *77*, 102328. [CrossRef]

57. Yu, H.; Li, M.; Li, Z.; Xiang, W.; Yuan, Y.; Liu, Y.; Li, Z.; Xiong, Z. Coping style, social support and psychological distress in the general Chinese population in the early stages of the COVID-19 epidemic. *BMC Psychiatry* **2020**, *20*, 426. [CrossRef] [PubMed]
58. Boysan, M. Validity of the Coping Inventory for Stressful Situations—Short Form (CISS-21) in a non-clinical Turkish sample. *Düşünen Adam* **2012**, *25*, 101–107. [CrossRef]
59. Cosway, R.; Endler, N.S.; Sadler, A.J.; Deary, I.J. The Coping Inventory for Stressful Situations: Factorial structure and associations with personality traits and psychological health. *J. Appl. Biobehav. Res.* **2000**, *5*, 121–143. [CrossRef]
60. Dawson, D.L.; Golijani-Moghaddam, N. COVID-19: Psychological flexibility, coping, mental health, and well-being in the UK during the pandemic. *J. Contextual. Behav. Sci.* **2020**, *17*, 126–134. [CrossRef] [PubMed]
61. Götmann, A.; Bechtoldt, M.N. Coping with COVID-19—Longitudinal analysis of coping strategies and the role of trait mindfulness in mental well-being. *Pers. Individ. Differ.* **2021**, *175*, 110695. [CrossRef]
62. Miller Smedema, S.; Catalano, D.; Ebener, D.J. The Relationship of Coping, Self-Worth, and Subjective Well-being: A Structural Equation Model. *Rehabil. Couns. Bull.* **2010**, *53*, 131–142. [CrossRef]
63. Sagone, E.; De Caroli, M.E. A Correlational study on dispositional resilience, psychological well-being, and coping strategies in university students. *Am. J. Educ. Res.* **2014**, *2*, 463–471. [CrossRef]
64. Xu, L.; Liu, R.-D.; Ding, Y.; Mou, X.; Wang, J.; Liu, Y. The Mediation Effect of Coping Style on the Relations between Personality and Life Satisfaction in Chinese Adolescents. *Front. Psychol.* **2017**, *8*, 1076. [CrossRef]
65. Arora, T.; Grey, I.; Östlundh, L.; Lam, K.B.H.; Omar, O.M.; Arnone, D. The prevalence of psychological consequences of COVID-19: A systematic review and meta-analysis of observational studies. *J. Health Psychol.* **2020**, *29*, 1359105320966639. [CrossRef]
66. Bareeqa, S.B.; Ahmed, S.I.; Samar, S.S.; Yasin, W.; Zehra, S.; Monese, G.M.; Gouthro, R.V. Prevalence of depression, anxiety and stress in china during COVID-19 pandemic: A systematic review with meta-analysis. *Int. J. Psychiatry Med.* **2021**, *56*, 210–227. [CrossRef] [PubMed]
67. Gurvich, C.; Thomas, N.; Thomas, E.H.; Hudaib, A.R.; Sood, L.; Fabiatos, K.; Sutton, K.; Isaacs, A.; Arunogiri, S.; Sharp, G.; et al. Coping styles and mental health in response to societal changes during the COVID-19 pandemic. *Int. J. Soc. Psychiatry* **2021**, *67*, 540–549. [CrossRef]
68. El Keshky, M.E.S.; Alsabban, A.M.; Basyouni, S.S. The psychological and social impacts on personal stress for residents quarantined for COVID-19 in Saudi Arabia. *Arch. Psychiatr. Nurs.* **2020**, *35*, 311–316. [CrossRef]
69. Bogin, B.; Varea, C. COVID-19, crisis, and emotional stress: A biocultural perspective of their impact on growth and development for the next generation. *Am. J. Hum. Biol.* **2020**, *32*, e23474. [CrossRef] [PubMed]
70. Agbaria, Q.; Mokh, A.A. Coping with Stress during the Coronavirus Outbreak: The Contribution of Big Five Personality Traits and Social Support. *Int. J. Ment. Health Addict.* **2021**, 1–19. [CrossRef]
71. Fu, W.; Wang, C.; Zou, L.; Guo, Y.; Lu, Z.; Yan, S.; Mao, J. Psychological health, sleep quality, and coping styles to stress facing the COVID-19 in Wuhan, China. *Transl. Psychiatry* **2020**, *10*, 225. [CrossRef] [PubMed]
72. Schwarzer, R.; Schulz, U. Stressful Life Events. In *Handbook of Psychology. Causal and Mediating Psychosocial Factors*; Weiner, I.B., Ed.; John Wiley & Sons, Inc.: New York, NY, USA, 2003; Part 2; pp. 27–49. [CrossRef]
73. Lazarus, R.S. *Emotion and Adaptation*; Oxford University Press: London, UK, 1991.
74. Lardier, D.T.; Lee, C.-Y.S.; Rodas, J.M.; Garcia-Reid, P.; Reid, R.J. The Effect of perceived college-related stress on depression, life satisfaction, and school satisfaction: The coping strategies of Hispanic college students from a Hispanic serving institution. *Educ. Urban Soc.* **2020**, *52*, 1204–1222. [CrossRef]
75. Gori, A.; Topino, E.; Di Fabio, A. The protective role of life satisfaction, coping strategies and defense mechanisms on perceived stress due to COVID-19 emergency: A chained mediation model. *PLoS ONE* **2020**, *15*, e0242402. [CrossRef] [PubMed]
76. Faul, F.; Erdfelder, E.; Lang, A.G.; Buchner, A. G*Power 3: A flexible statistical power analysis program for the social, behavioral, and biomedical sciences. *Behav. Res. Methods* **2007**, *39*, 175–191. [CrossRef]
77. Faul, F.; Erdfelder, E.; Buchner, A.; Lang, A.G. Statistical power analyses using G*Power 3.1: Tests for correlation and regression analyses. *Behav. Res. Methods* **2009**, *41*, 1149–1160. [CrossRef]
78. Rogowska, A.M.; Kuśnierz, C.; Ochnik, D.; Schütz, A.; Kafetsios, K.P.; Aslan, I.; Pavlova, I.; Benatov, J.; Arzenšek, A.; Jakubiak, M.; et al. Wellbeing of Undergraduates during the COVID-19 Pandemic: International Study. Available online: https://osf.io/q5f4e (accessed on 2 September 2021).
79. Cohen, S.; Kamarck, T.; Mermelstein, R. A global measure of perceived stress. *J. Health Soc. Behav.* **1983**, *24*, 385–396. [CrossRef]
80. Endler, N.S.; Parker, J.D. Multidimensional assessment of coping: A critical evaluation. *J. Pers. Soc. Psychol.* **1990**, *58*, 844–854. [CrossRef] [PubMed]
81. Clench-Aas, J.; Nes, R.B.; Dalgard, O.S.; Aarø, L.E. Dimensionality and measurement invariance in the Satisfaction with Life Scale in Norway. *Qual. Life Res.* **2011**, *20*, 1307–1317. [CrossRef]
82. Checa, I.; Perales, J.; Espejo, B. Measurement invariance of the Satisfaction with Life Scale by gender, age, marital status and educational level. *Qual. Life Res.* **2019**, *28*, 963–968. [CrossRef] [PubMed]
83. Shevlin, M.; Brunsden, V.; Miles, J.N.V. Satisfaction with Life Scale: Analysis of factorial invariance, mean structures and reliability. *Pers. Individ. Differ.* **1998**, *25*, 911–916. [CrossRef]
84. Lockhart, G.; MacKinnon, D.P.; Ohlrich, V. Mediation analysis in psychosomatic medicine research. *Psychosom. Med.* **2011**, *73*, 29–43. [CrossRef] [PubMed]

85. Little, T.D.; Preacher, K.J.; Selig, J.P.; Card, N.A. New developments in latent variable panel analyses of longitudinal data. *Int. J. Behav. Dev.* **2007**, *31*, 357–365. [CrossRef]
86. Cole, D.A.; Maxwell, S.E. Testing mediational models with longitudinal data: Questions and tips in the use of structural equation modeling. *J. Abnorm. Psychol.* **2003**, *112*, 558–577. [CrossRef]
87. Preacher, K.J. Advances in mediation analysis: A survey and synthesis of new developments. *Annu. Rev. Psychol.* **2015**, *66*, 825–852. [CrossRef] [PubMed]
88. Hooper, D.C.J.; Mullen, M. Structural equation modelling: Guidelines for determining model fit. *Electron. J. Bus. Res. Methods* **2008**, *6*, 53–60.
89. Hu, L.T.; Bentler, P.M. Cutoff criteria for fit indexes in covariance structure analysis: Conventional criteria versus new alternatives. *Struct. Equ. Model.* **1999**, *6*, 1–55. [CrossRef]
90. Kline, R.B. *Principles and Practice of Structural Equation Modeling*, 3rd ed.; The Guilford Press: New York, NY, USA, 2011.
91. Wu, C.-H.; Chen, L.H.; Tsai, Y.-M. Longitudinal invariance analysis of the satisfaction with life scale. *Pers. Individ. Differ.* **2009**, *46*, 396–401. [CrossRef]
92. MacCann, C.; Fogarty, G.J.; Zeidner, M.; Roberts, R.D. Coping mediates the relationship between emotional intelligence (EI) and academic achievement. *Contemp. Educ. Psychol.* **2011**, *36*, 60–70. [CrossRef]
93. Besser, A.; Flett, G.L.; Nepon, T.; Zeigler-Hill, V. Personality, cognition, and adaptability to the COVID-19 pandemic: Associations with loneliness, distress, and positive and negative mood states. *Int. J. Ment. Health Addict.* **2020**, 1–25. [CrossRef]

Journal of
Clinical Medicine

MDPI

Article

The Impact of the COVID-19 Emergency on Life Activities and Delivery of Healthcare Services in the Elderly Population

Siddarth Agrawal [1,2,*], Sebastian Makuch [2], Mateusz Dróżdż [3], Bartłomiej Strzelec [4], Małgorzata Sobieszczańska [5] and Grzegorz Mazur [1]

1 Department and Clinic of Internal Medicine, Occupational Diseases, Hypertension and Clinical Oncology, Wroclaw Medical University, Borowska St. 213, 50-556 Wrocław, Poland; grzegorz.mazur@umed.wroc.pl
2 Department of Pathology, Wroclaw Medical University, K. Marcinkowskiego St. 1, 50-368 Wrocław, Poland; sebastian.mk21@gmail.com
3 Laboratory of RNA Biochemistry, Institute of Chemistry and Biochemistry, Freie Universität Berlin, Takustraße 6, 14195 Berlin, Germany; m.drozdz@fu-berlin.de
4 Second Department and Clinic of General and Oncological Surgery, Wroclaw Medical University, Borowska St. 213, 50-556 Wrocław, Poland; b.strzelec94@interia.pl
5 Department of Geriatrics, Wroclaw Medical University, Marii Skłodowskiej-Curie St. 66, 50-369 Wroclaw, Poland; malgorzata.sobieszczanska@umed.wroc.pl
* Correspondence: siddarth@agrawal.pl; Tel.: +48-71-736-4000; Fax: +48-71-736-4009

Citation: Agrawal, S.; Makuch, S.; Dróżdż, M.; Strzelec, B.; Sobieszczańska, M.; Mazur, G. The Impact of the COVID-19 Emergency on Life Activities and Delivery of Healthcare Services in the Elderly Population. *J. Clin. Med.* **2021**, *10*, 4089. https://doi.org/10.3390/jcm10184089

Academic Editor: Michele Roccella

Received: 23 July 2021
Accepted: 7 September 2021
Published: 10 September 2021

Abstract: Due to the prevailing pandemic of the coronavirus disease COVID-19, we are experiencing emotional and social isolation, which negatively affects mental and physical health, particularly among the elderly population. In this study, we performed a cross-sectional analysis based on computer-assisted telephone interviews of 500 Polish adults aged 60 years or older in order to determine the impact of the SARS-CoV-2 pandemic on the older population's behavior, life activity, and delivery of healthcare services. According to our study, COVID-19 infection entailed a substantial change in older people's behavior. Over 50%, nearly 80%, and more than 25% of the surveyed participants reduced their social, recreational, and professional activities, respectively. The most significant change in senior's behavior due to the fear of COVID-19 infection was observed in patients (1) with cardiac and pulmonary problems, (2) being on multi-drug therapy, (3) vaccinated against influenza, and (4) with several mental difficulties including loneliness, social isolation, and depression. Furthermore, we demonstrated that 10% of participants canceled planned hospitalization due to the fear of COVID-19 infection. This was observed primarily in patients suffering from chronic heart and lung diseases, vaccinated against influenza, exhibiting the reluctance to carry out more complex daily activities, and with a higher level of anxiety, social loneliness, and malnutrition. Thus, these groups of seniors require more attention; hence, we propose telemedicine as a strategy directed to them that provides clinical healthcare and information regarding measurements, control, and protection against SARS-CoV-2 during the prevailing COVID-19 pandemic. We believe this strategy may improve treatment outcomes, reduce comorbidities-related complications and unnecessary hospitalizations.

Keywords: quality of life; fear of COVID-19; elderly population; telemedicine

1. Introduction

Severe acute respiratory syndrome coronavirus 2 (SARS-CoV-2), a novel virus responsible for COVID-19 infection, has caused a deadly pandemic worldwide. According to numerous independent studies, people of any age could be infected, but the number of older patients infected with COVID-19 has increased globally, causing a significant threat to the global population's life and health [1–3]. Therefore, patients in their 80s and older are the most likely to be hospitalized or die from COVID-19 [4]. The accumulating evidence indicates that infection in younger patients usually presents with mild symptoms, while in the older population, it is associated with a more severe course and a significantly higher mortality rate. The risk increases in particular in older adults with comorbidities such as hypertension, cardiovascular disease, diabetes mellitus, chronic respiratory disease, and chronic kidney disease [5–8]. A significant percentage of older Europeans and Americans suffer from one or more of these chronic diseases that put them at an increased risk of infection. Chronic diseases that lead to a severe course of COVID-19 have been classified by the Centers for Disease Control and Prevention and include cancer, chronic kidney disease, chronic lung diseases, dementia, diabetes, Down syndrome, heart conditions, obesity, sickle cell anemia, diabetes, immune-weakening conditions, and immune system disorders [9]. The disruption of health services in most countries during the pandemic has posed challenges for older adults suffering from chronic diseases [10]. According to a study conducted by Addis et al., older age, among other factors, was strongly associated with an abnormal psychological impact of COVID-19 on patients with chronic disease [11]. Moreover, several studies have reported higher rates of severe COVID-19 among patients with comorbid chronic medical conditions [12,13]. Given the fact that the aging population is one of the most significant problems around the world and that there is a higher prevalence of multimorbidity and lower resistance in older patients, there is an urgent need to examine the impact of the pandemic on health care and life activities of elderly people.

The pandemic has led to a significant limitation of physical activity in the global population. It exerts an enormous impact on global health in all age groups, but it seems that the most critical adverse influence could be observed predominantly in the older population, where physical and social activity is fundamental to maintain good health. Thus, in that age group, proper physical activity is correlated with the reduction of anxiety, depression, osteoporosis, sarcopenia, and metabolic syndrome [14–21]. Moreover, physical activity is also crucial in the prevention of many comorbidities, which are often presented in older patients, such as hypertension, diabetes, cardiovascular diseases, and respiratory diseases [22]. Therefore, it is assumed that the SARS-CoV-2 pandemic exerts an adverse influence on population health not only by developing complications and increasing mortality associated with COVID-19 but also by reducing physical activity, which significantly affects health outcomes. The objective of this cross-sectional analysis was to determine the impact of the SARS-CoV-2 pandemic on the older population's behavior, life activity, and delivery of healthcare services. Moreover, we attempted to identify the factors that influence seniors' behavior during the pandemic, such as socio-demographic factors, level of education, and the presence of diseases such as coronary heart disease, diabetes, asthma, chronic obstructive pulmonary disease (COPD), heart, and kidney failure.

2. Materials and Methods

2.1. Study Design

A cross-sectional study was carried out in November–December 2020 on a sample of 500 Polish adults aged 60 years or older using computer-assisted telephone interviews. The response rate was 40%. A stratified sampling per the demographic structure of voivodeship was used to obtain a representative sample of the elderly population. Target quotas were set for age and gender strata in each geographical region. The interviewers were properly trained and prepared to ensure the quality and accuracy of the interview. A data collection supervisor supervised all interviews, and a study coordinator randomly evaluated the recordings of the dialogue. The transcripts were not returned to participants for comment and/or correction, nor were repeat interviews carried out. The duration of the interview ranged from 15 to 20 min. Participants provided their consent at the beginning of the interview. No compensation was provided for participating in the study. The study was approved by the Bioethics Committee of Wroclaw Medical University.

2.2. Explanatory Variables

The questionnaire was designed in a way to provide the most crucial information regarding the respondent's socio-demographic data, economic situation, and general, subjective knowledge about COVID-19. Socio-demographic data included (1) gender (male/female), (2) age (categorized as 60–64; 65–69; 70 and more), (3) place of residence (village; town, less than 20,000 inhabitants; town, between 20,000 to 100,000 inhabitants; town, between 100,000 to 200,000 inhabitants; town, between 200,000 to 400,000 inhabitants; town, more than 400,000 inhabitants), (4) education (primary, vocational, secondary, higher), (5) body mass (kg), (6) body height (cm), and (7) BMI (kg/m^2). Patients were also asked for (8) household income per person per month (in Polish currency-PLN: less than 500 PLN; 501–1000 PLN; 1001–2000 PLN; 2001–3000 PLN; more than 3000 PLN; refusal to answer), (9) existing comorbidities (coronary heart disease, diabetes mellitus, asthma, COPD, heart failure, kidney failure, and gastroesophageal reflux disease) (10) the number of medications taken (1 to 3; 4 to 6; 7 to 10; more than 10), (11) type of class of currently taken medicines (cardiac drugs, antihypertensive drugs, analgesics, digestive ailments drugs, anticoagulants, antidepressants, and nootropics), and (12) the type of medications and/or supplements bought without a prescription (analgesics, drugs for heartburn, herbal drugs, vitamins, others). Surveyed patients were also asked about vaccination against influenza (Table 1).

Table 1. General, clinical and psychological characteristics of the surveyed people.

Feature (Variable)	**Statistics**
Gender	
Female	290 (58.0%)
Male	210 (42.0%)
Age	
60–64	141 (28.2%)
65–69	128 (25.6%)
70 and more	231 (46.2%)
Place of residence	
Village	110 (22.0%)
Town, less than 20,000 inhabitants	56 (11.2%)
Town, between 20,000 to 100,000 inhabitants	136 (27.2%)
Town, between 100,000 to 200,000 inhabitants	62 (12.4%)
Town, between 200,000 to 400,000 inhabitants	39 (7.8%)
Town, more than 400,000 inhabitants	97 (19.4%)
Housing situation	
Lives alone	108 (21.6%)
Lives with partner	202 (40.4%)
Lives with partner and children	117 (23.4%)
Lives alone with children	35 (7.0%)
Lives with family	29 (5.8%)
Other situation	9 (1.8%)
Education	
Primary	8 (1.6%)
Vocational	105 (21.0%)
Secondary	245 (49.0%)
Higher	142 (28.4%)
Body mass (kg)	
M ± SD	78.5 ± 15.7
Me (Q1–Q3)	76 (67–88)
Min–Max	48–140
Body height (cm)	
M ± SD	169 ± 9
Me (Q1–Q3)	168 (163–175)
Min–Max	141–210

Table 1. *Cont.*

Feature (Variable)	Statistics
BMI (kg/m^2)	
M ± SD	27.4 ± 4.6
Me (Q1–Q3)	27 (24–30)
Min–Max	19–46
Household income per person per month	
Less than 500 PLN	5 (1.0%)
501–1000 PLN	24 (4.8%)
1001–2000 PLN	188 (37.6%)
2001–3000 PLN	158 (31.6%)
More than 3000 PLN	110 (2.0%)
Refusal to answer	15 (3.0%)
Chronic diseases	
Coronary Heart Disease	63 (12.6%)
Diabetes Mellitus	74 (14.8%)
Asthma	43 (8.6%)
COPD	33 (6.6%)
Heart Failure	71 (14.2%)
Kidney Failure	20 (4.0%)
Gastroesophageal Reflux Disease	68 (13.6%)
Was vaccinated against influenza in 2019	62 (12.4%)
Was vaccinated against influenza in 2020	51 (10.2%)
Avoids vaccination because of possible complications	164 (32.8%)
Wants to be vaccinated against influenza but was unable due to lack of availability of vaccines	104 (20.8%)
The GP doctor recommended vaccination against influenza and pneumococci	81 (16.2%)
Number of drugs taken	
1 to 3	301 (60.2%)
4 to 6	151 (30.2%)
7 to 10	40 (8.0%)
More than 10	8 (1.6%)
Cardiac drugs	132 (26.4%)
Antihypertensive drugs	255 (51.0%)
Diuretics	78 (15.6%)
Analgesics	230 (46.0%)
Digestive ailments drugs	131 (26.2%)
Anticoagulants	87 (17.4%)
Antidepressants	78 (15.6%)
Nootropics	54 (10.8%)
All drugs are prescribed by the same doctor	352 (70.4%)
How many different doctors have prescribed your medications?	n = 148
2	82 (55.4%)
3	52 (35.1%)
4 and more	14 (9.4%)
Informs the GP about all new medications	391 (78.2%)
Buys drugs and/or supplements without a prescription	378 (75.6%)
Analgesics	305 (61.0%)
For heartburn	132 (26.4%)
Herbal	155 (31.0%)
Vitamins (C, B, D)	345 (69.0%)
Other	96 (19.2%)
Activities of Daily Living (ADL)	
M ± SD	5.9 ± 0.4
Me (Q1–Q3)	6 (6–6)
Min–Max	2–6

Table 1. *Cont.*

Feature (Variable)	Statistics
Fit people (5–6 pts.)	493 (98.6%)
Moderately disabled people (3–4 pts.)	6 (1.2%)
Disabled people (0–2 pts.)	1 (0.2%)
The Lawton Instrumental Activities of Daily Living (IADL)	
M ± SD	22.9 ± 2.3
Me (Q1–Q3)	24 (23–24)
Min–Max	11–24
Abbreviated Mental Test Score (AMTS)	
M ± SD	9.1 ± 1.0
Me (Q1–Q3)	9 (9–10)
Min–Max	5–10
Normal condition (7–10 pts.)	9.1 ± 1.0
Moderate disorder (4–6 pts.)	9 (9–10)
Geriatric depression scale (GDS-15)	
M ± SD	4.8 ± 4.0
Me (Q1–Q3)	4 (2–8)
Min–Max	0–15
Lack of depression (0–5 pts.)	324 (64.8%)
Depression (6–15 pts.)	176 (35.2%)
Gastric Anxiety Scale (GAS-10)	
M ± SD	7.2 ± 4.6
Me (Q1–Q3)	6 (4–10)
Min–Max	0–25
Lubben Social Network Scale (LSNS-6)	
M ± SD	14.2 ± 5.9
Me (Q1–Q3)	15 (10–18)
Min–Max	0–30
Social loneliness scale (Gierveld Scale)	
M ± SD	13.1 ± 1.8
Me (Q1–Q3)	13 (12–14)
Min–Max	6–18
Mini Nutritional Assessment (MNA)	
M ± SD	12.8 ± 1.5
Me (Q1–Q3)	13 (12–14)
Min–Max	6–14
Proper nutritional status (12–14 pts.)	418 (83.6%)
The danger of malnutrition (8–11 pts.)	78 (15.6%)
Malnutrition (0–7 pts.)	4 (0.8%)

2.3. Measures

Based on the obtained results, independent predictors affecting the life activities and delivery of healthcare services in elderly patients during the COVID-19 pandemic were determined using logit models. Data related to elderly health conditions were collected based on specified and validated scales such as (1) Activities of Daily Living scale (ADL), (2) the Lawton Instrumental Activities of Daily Living scale (IADL), (3) Abbreviated Mental Test Score (AMTS), (4) geriatric depression scale (GDS-15), (5) Gastric Anxiety Scale (GAS-10), (6) Lubben Social Network Scale (LSNS-6), (7) social loneliness scale (Gierveld Scale) and (8) Mini Nutritional Assessment (MNA) (Table 1). Furthermore, we distinguished patients who refused planned hospitalizations and/or resigned from admission to the Emergency Room due to a sudden deterioration of health because of the fear of COVID-19 infection. Finally, we presented groups of people who had difficulties with wearing masks and/or gloves during the COVID-19 pandemic.

2.4. Statistical Analysis

The distribution of the variables was assessed using descriptive statistics. Independent *t*-tests and ANOVA evaluated the mean differences using participants' characteristics. A multiple linear regression model was performed to outline the factors associated with fear and anxiety of COVID-19. Adjusted beta-coefficient (β) and 95% confidence interval (95% CI) are reported for regression analysis. All analyses were performed using the statistical software package Statistica. A *p*-value of <0.05 was considered to be statistically significant.

3. Results

3.1. Participants' Characteristics

The cross-sectional analysis included 500 patients (290 female, 58% and 210 male, 42%) aged 60 and more (mean M = 67.9 ± 4.2). Most of the participants suffered from one or more chronic diseases such as coronary heart disease (n = 63, 12.6%), diabetes mellitus (n = 74, 14.8%), asthma (n = 43, 8.6%), COPD (n = 33, 6.6%), heart failure (n = 71, 14.2%), kidney failure (n = 20, 4.0%) and gastroesophageal reflux disease (n = 68, 13.6%). Only 62 (12.4%) and 51 (10.2%) of patients underwent influenza vaccination in 2019 and 2020, respectively. The reason for such low interest in vaccination was the fear of possible vaccine adverse effects (n = 164, 32.8%), and lack of availability of vaccines (n = 104, 20.8%). Moreover, the GP doctor recommended vaccination against influenza and pneumococci only in 81 (16.2%) patients. All participants currently take medications. Most of them (n = 301, 60.2%) take 1 to 3 drugs. The most commonly used medications were antihypertensive (n = 255, 51.0%), and analgesics (n = 230, 46.0%). The majority of participants buy medication without prescription (n = 378, 75.6%), mostly analgesics (n = 305, 61.0%), and vitamins (n = 345, 69.0%). A significant number of patients suffer from depression (n = 176, 35.2%). Most of the participants are fit persons according to ADL (n = 493, 98.6%), and have proper nutritional status according to MNA (n = 418, 83.6%). A detailed data on the general, clinical and psychological characteristics of the surveyed people is presented in Table 1.

3.2. Reactions (Limitations) Related to the Fear of COVID-19 Infection

Fear of COVID-19 infection exerts a significant change in the surveyed population's behavior. A significant number of the participants have limited their professional (n = 133, 26.6%), social (n = 381, 76.2%), and recreational activities (n = 277, 55.4%). Furthermore, over 30% of patients stopped going out shopping (n = 162, 32.4%). Mainly, purchases are delivered by the family's members (n = 98, 60.5%). 39 patients try to eat less (n = 39, 24.1%) and 17 patients order food via internet (n = 17, 10.5%). Detailed data on the assessment of the behavior during the COVID-19 pandemic is presented in Table 2.

Anxiety and restriction of activity during the COVID-19 pandemic significantly more often occurred in patients who suffered from coronary heart disease (p < 0.001, Figure S1A in Supplementary Materials), COPD (p = 0.01, Figure S1B), and heart failure (p < 0.001, Figure S1C). Moreover, it occurred significantly more often in participants vaccinated against influenza in 2019 (p = 0.003, Figure S2A) and 2020 (p = 0.004, Figure S2B). This phenomenon was also observed among patients who were willing to be vaccinated against influenza but could not undergo vaccination due to the lack of availability of vaccines in pharmacies (p = 0.009, Figure S2C) and those advised by GP doctor to be vaccinated against influenza and pneumococci (p < 0.001, Figure S2D). Furthermore, the presence of anxiety and activity restriction during the COVID-19 pandemic was positively correlated with the number of medicines taken (p < 0.001, Figure S3A). This phenomenon was observed in patients who take cardiac drugs (p = 0.001, Figure S3B), antihypertensives (p = 0.009, Figure S3C), diuretics (p = 0.004, Figure S3D), drugs for digestive ailments (p = 0.037, Figure S3E) and anticoagulants (p < 0.001, Figure S3F), significantly more often. Moreover, anxiety and restriction of activity were significantly more often observed in less fit according to the IADL scale (p = 0.048, Figure S4A), with geriatric depression according to the GDS-15 scale ($p < 0.001$, Figure S4B), with a higher level of anxiety according to GAS-10 scale ($p < 0.001$, Figure S4C), with a higher level of social loneliness according to LSNS-6 scale ($p = 0.008$, Figure S4D), and with malnutrition according to MNA scale ($p = 0.011$, Figure S4E) participants.

Table 2. Assessment of the behavior during the COVID-19 pandemic.

Questionnaire Question, *n* (%)	**Statistics**
1. Have you limited your professional activity due to the fear of COVID-19 infection? (Yes = 1 pts., No = 0 pts.)	133 (26.6%)
2. Have you limited your social activities (family meetings, family and cultural events, meetings with friends) due to the fear of COVID-19 infection? (Yes = 1 pts., No = 0 pts.)	381 (76.2%)
3. Have you limited your recreational activities (walking, cycling, Nordic walking, swimming, etc.) due to the fear of COVID-19 infection? (Yes = 1 pts., No = 0 pts.)	277 (55.4%)
4. Have you limited shopping due to the fear of COVID-19 infection? (Yes = 1 pts., No = 0 pts.)	162 (32.4%)
If yes, how did you supply yourself with food?	$n = 162$
Through internet orders	17 (10.5%)
With the help of family	98 (60.5%)
With the help of neighbors	8 (4.9%)
I ate less	39 (24.1%)
5. Did you cancel your planned hospitalization due to the fear of COVID-19 infection? (Yes = 1 pts., No = 0 pts.)	50 (10.0%)
6. Have you resigned to report to the Emergency Room due to the sudden deterioration of your health due to the fear of COVID-19 infection? (Yes = 1 pts., No = 0 pts.)	32 (6.4%)
Total points:	
M ± SD	2.1 ± 1.4
Me (Q1–Q3)	2 (1–3)
Min–Max	0–6

Including all 500 surveyed patients, 50 (10.0%) of them canceled planned hospitalizations (Table 2, (question 5)). These cases occurred the most often in elderly patients who suffered from coronary heart disease ($p < 0.001$, Table S1). A slightly lower percentage of patients avoiding medical care was observed in those with asthma ($p = 0.026$, Table S1), COPD ($p < 0.001$, Table S1) and heart failure ($p < 0.001$, Table S1). Furthermore, patients vaccinated against influenza in 2019 ($p < 0.001$, Figure 1A, Table S1), and 2020 ($p = 0.008$, Table S1), also did not show up for an agreed medical examination. Moreover, we indicated that the likelihood of canceling planned hospitalizations was higher for patients being on current medication ($p < 0.001$, Table S1). These observations were the most visible in patients taking cardiac drugs ($p = 0.001$, Table S1) or nootropics ($p = 0.014$, Table S1). According to the IADL scale, GAS-10 scale, LSNS-6 scale, and MNA scale, planned hospitalizations were also canceled by less fit patients ($p < 0.001$, Figure 1B, Table S1), with a higher level of anxiety ($p = 0.002$, Table S1), social loneliness ($p = 0.004$, Table S1) and malnutrition ($p < 0.001$, Table S1), respectively.

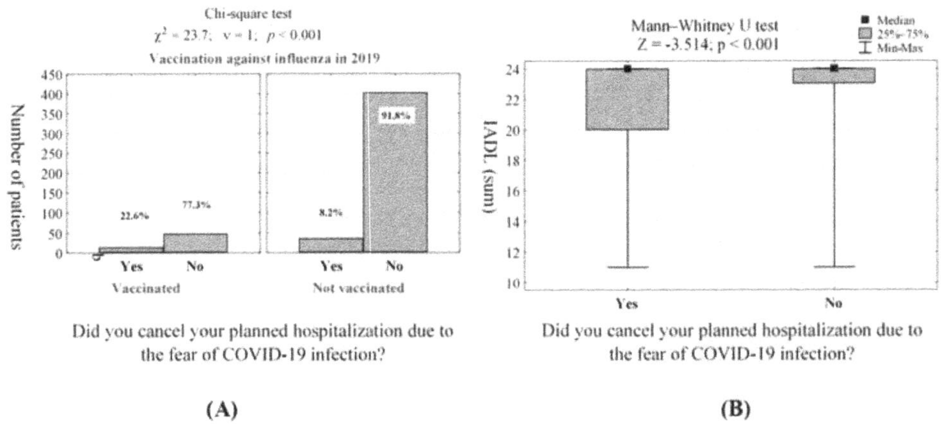

Figure 1. (**A**) Number (n) and percentage (%) of elderly patients in groups differing on those vaccinated against influenza or not in 2019, (**B**) Mann–Whitney U test showing the significant correlation between patients who are less fit (according to IADL scale) and canceled planned hospitalization due to the fear of COVID-19 infection.

The main individual predictors of avoiding medical care (manifested by canceling planned hospitalizations) due to the fear against COVID-19 infection in elderly patients are a vaccination against influenza in 2019, the number of drugs currently taken, and IADL score (Figure 1, Table S1). The chance of an affirmative answer to the question regarding the cancelation of planned hospitalizations was three times higher in elderly patients who were vaccinated against influenza in 2019 than those without vaccination (OR = 3, CI95% [1.46–6.16]). Furthermore, the risk of canceling planned hospitalization increased nearly twofold in elderly patients who take medications compared to those who do not (OR = 1.92, CI95% [1.33–2.78]). Moreover, performing more complex activities by elderly patients influences on higher likelihood to cancel planned hospitalization due to the fear of COVID-19 infection (OR = 0.87, CI95% [0.79–0.96]). Detailed data on analyzing elderly patients who avoid medical care due to the fear of COVID-19 infection, including the logit model, are presented in Table 3.

The generalized logit regression model leading to an estimate of the probability of affirmative answer to the question regarding canceling planned hospitalizations by elderly patients due to the fear of COVID-19 infection took the form:

$$\textbf{logit P} = -0.4 + 1.1 \times vaccination_{2019} + 0.65 \times \textit{the number of currently taken drugs} - 0.138 \times IADL$$

Out of a total of 500 participants, 32 (6.4%) resigned from admission to the Emergency Room due to the sudden deterioration of health (Table 2, question 6). Most of those patients suffered from coronary heart disease (p = 0.014, Table S2), COPD (p < 0.001, Figure 2A, Table S2) and heart failure (p = 0.009, Table S2). Similar to planned hospitalizations, patients did not show up in the Emergency Room after they were recommended by a GP doctor to be vaccinated against influenza and pneumococci (p = 0.032, Table S2). Furthermore, patients who take cardiac drugs (p = 0.012, Table S2) have difficulties with depression (according to GDS-15 scale, p < 0.001, Table S2), anxiety (according to GAS-10 scale, p < 0.001, Table S2), social loneliness (according to LSNS-6 scale, p < 0.001, Figure 2B, Table S2) and those with malnutrition (according to MNA scale, p < 0.001, Figure 2C, Table S2) also resigned to report to the Emergency Room more often compared to physically and mentally healthy patients.

Table 3. Results of univariate and multivariate logistic regression of the answer to the question regarding canceling planned hospitalization due to the fear of COVID-19 infection in elderly patients and socio-demographic and clinical factors as well as the odds ratio [OR] and its 95% confidence interval [CI] [the most statistically significant (p-value < 0.05) predictors of canceling planned hospitalizations in elderly patients].

Feature (Variable)	b	p	β	p	OR (95% CI)
Coronary Heart Disease	1.274	<0.001	-	>0.05	-
Asthma	0.988	0.016	-	>0.05	-
COPD	2.022	<0.001	-	>0.05	-
Heart Failure	1.546	<0.001	-	>0.05	-
Was vaccinated against influenza in 2019	**1.181**	**0.001**	**1.099**	**0.003**	**3.00 (1.46–6.16)**
Was vaccinated against influenza in 2020	1.062	0.005	-	>0.05	-
The GP doctor recommended vaccination against influenza and pneumococci	1.447	<0.001	-	>0.05	-
Number of drugs currently taken	**0.764**	**<0.001**	**0.652**	**0.001**	**1.92 (1.33–2.78)**
Cardiac drugs	1.073	<0.001	-	>0.05	-
Nootropics	0.982	0.009	-	>0.05	-
The number of different doctors prescribing currently taken drugs	0.567	0.023	-	>0.05	-
The Lawton Instrumental Activities of Daily Living (IADL)	**0.189**	**<0.001**	**−0.138**	**0.007**	**0.87 (0.79–0.96)**
Gastric Anxiety Scale (GAS-10)	0.089	0.003	-	>0.05	-
Lubben Social Network Scale (LSNS-6)	0.069	0.008	-	>0.05	-
Mini Nutritional Assessment (MNA)	0.311	<0.001	-	>0.05	-

b—linear regression coefficient, β—standardized multiple regression coefficients.

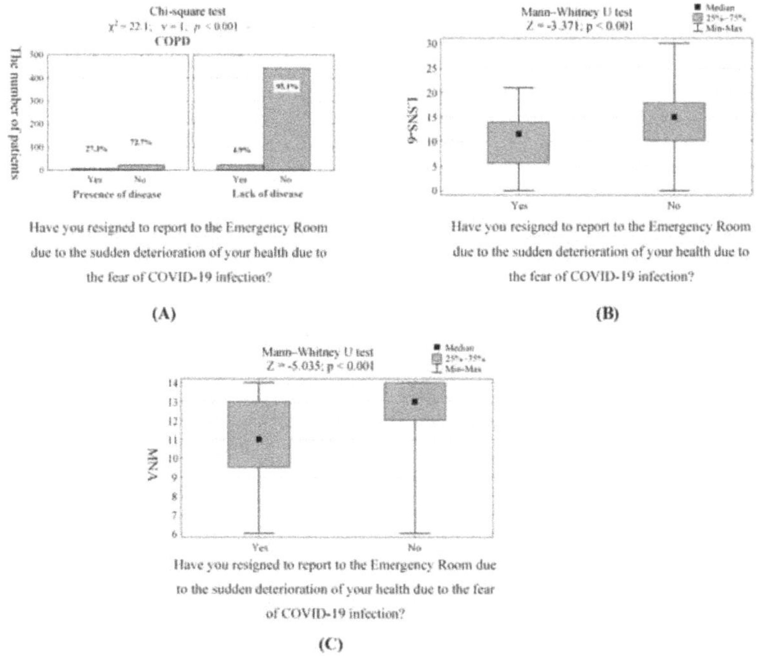

Figure 2. (**A**) Number (n) and percentage (%) of elderly patients who resigned to report to the Emergency Room due to the fear of COVID-19 infection in groups differing in those suffering from COPD or not; responses to the question regarding the resignation of reporting to the Emergency Room due to the fear of COVID-19 infection in feeling lonely patients (**B**) and patients with malnutrition (**C**) and the results of independent, non-parametric, significance tests.

Based on univariate and multivariate logistic regression analyses, we concluded that the main individual predictors of avoiding urgent medical care due to the fear against COVID-19 infection in elderly patients are: the presence of COPD, level of social loneliness (according to LSNS-6 scale), and malnutrition (according to MNA scale) (Figure 2, Table S2). The study showed statistical significance between patients suffering from COPD and healthy participants (OR = 5.77, CI95% [2.16–15.4]). Furthermore, the chance of an affirmative answer to the question regarding the resignation from going to the Emergency Room in elderly patients feeling lonely and/or those with malnutrition was approximately less than one time higher than in the groups of mentally healthy (OR = 0.91, [CI95% [0.84–0.98]) and with proper nutritional status (OR = 0.58, CI95% [0.47–0.71]) patients. Detailed data on analyzing those who avoid medical care, even during life-threatening conditions, due to the fear of COVID-19 infection are presented in Table 4.

Table 4. Results of univariate and multivariate logistic regression of the answer to the question regarding the resignation of the admission to the Emergency Room due to the fear of COVID-19 infection in elderly patients and socio-demographic and clinical factors as well as the odds ratio [OR] and its 95% confidence interval [CI] [the most statistically significant (p-value < 0.05) predictors of avoiding urgent medical care in elderly patients].

Feature (Variable)	b	p	β	p	OR (95% CI)
Coronary heart disease	1.099	0.009	-	>0.05	-
COPD	1.980	<0.001	1.753	<0.001	5.77 (2.16–15.4)
Heart Failure	1.109	0.006	-	>0.05	-
The GP doctor recommended vaccination against influenza and pneumococci	0.933	0.020	-	>0.05	-
Number of drugs currently taken	0.528	0.015	-	>0.05	-
Cardiac drugs	0.973	0.009	-	>0.05	-
The Lawton Instrumental Activities of Daily Living (IADL)	−0.202	<0.001	-	>0.05	-
Depression assessment (GDS-15)	0.197	<0.001	-	>0.05	-
Gastric Anxiety Scale (GAS-10)	0.137	<0.001	-	>0.05	-
Lubben Social Network Scale (LSNS-6)	−0.118	<0.001	−0.094	0.014	0.91 (0.84–0.98)
Mini Nutritional Assessment (MNA)	−0.602	<0.001	−0.553	<0.001	0.58 (0.47–0.71)

b—linear regression coefficient, β—standardized multiple regression coefficients.

The generalized logit regression model leading to estimate the probability of affirmative answer to question regarding resignation to report in Emergency Room due to the fear of COVID-19 infection in surveyed elderly patients took the form:

$$\textbf{logit P} = 4.92 - 0.094 \times \mathit{LSNS\text{-}6} + 1.753 \times \mathit{COPD} - 0.553 \times \mathit{MNA}$$

During the interviews, patients were also asked if wearing masks makes them feel uncomfortable. Thus, the difficulty of wearing masks was observed among 174 (34.8%) patients, mainly in those suffering from asthma ($p < 0.001$, Figure 3A, Table S3), COPD ($p = 0.008$, Table S3), and heart failure ($p < 0.001$, Table S3). Moreover, it occurred significantly more often in participants who are afraid of vaccination because of potential side effects ($p < 0.001$, Figure 3B, Table S3), those willing to be vaccinated against influenza but could not undergo vaccination due to the lack of vaccines in pharmacies ($p = 0.013$, Table S3) and those who take cardiac drugs ($p = 0.042$, Table S3) and analgesics ($p = 0.019$, Table S3). Moreover, difficulties with wearing masks and/or gloves were significantly more often observed in patients assessing more complex daily activities ($p = 0.005$, Figure 3C, Table S3), with depression according to GDS-15 ($p < 0.001$, Figure 3D, Table S3), with a higher level of anxiety according to GAS-10 ($p < 0.001$, Table S3), and with a higher level of social loneliness according to LSNS-6 ($p = 0.001$, Figure 3E, Table S3).

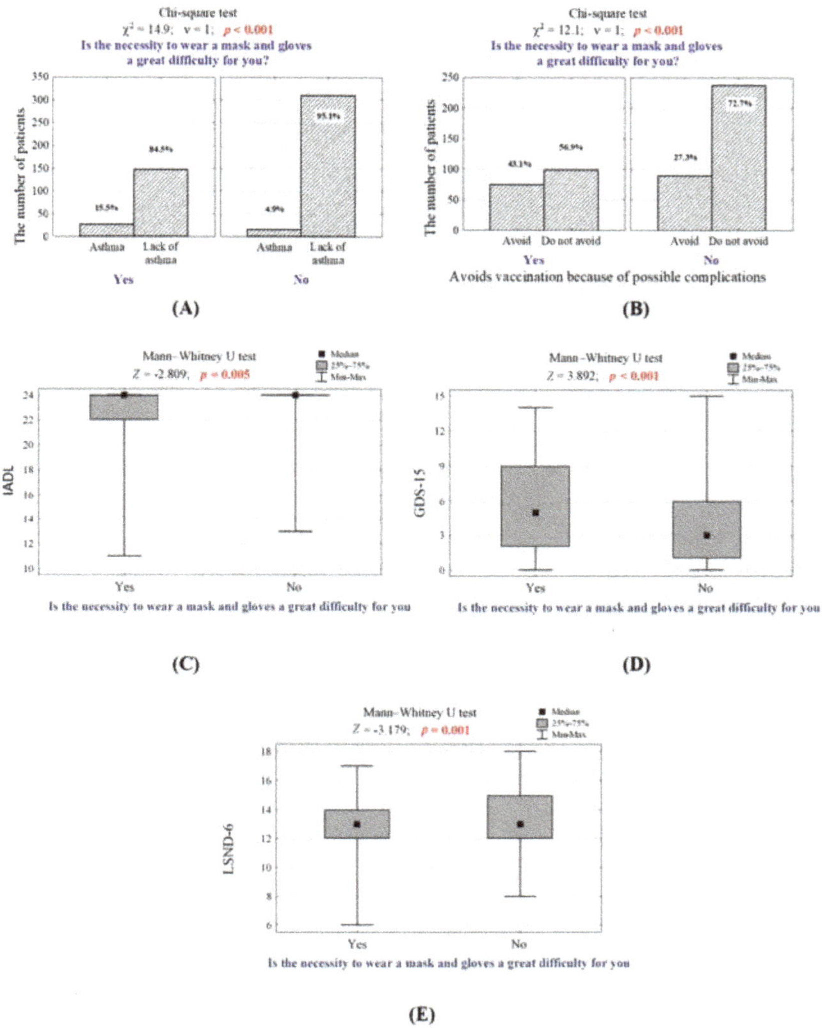

Figure 3. (**A**) Number (*n*) and percentage (%) of patients for whom wearing a mask and/or gloves is a great difficulty, differing in those suffering from asthma and healthy patients; (**B**) Number (*n*) and percentage (%) of patients avoiding vaccination due to potential side effects for whom wearing a mask and/or gloves is a great difficulty; responses/answers to the question regarding possible difficulties of wearing masks and/or gloves in less fit (**C**), depressed (**D**) and feeling lonely (**E**) patients and the number of independent, non-parametric, significance tests.

For instance, the chance of an affirmative answer to the question about the difficulty of wearing a mask and/or gloves in the group of people with asthma is almost three times higher in healthy patients (OR = 2.79, 95% CI [1.40–5.54]) and two times higher in those avoiding vaccinations due to potential side effects (OR = 2.00, 95% CI [1.33–2.99]). Difficulties with wearing a mask and/or gloves were also 0.91 times more common in patients assessing more complex activities (OR = 0.91, 95% CI [0.84–0.99]), 1.07 times more common in depressed patients (OR = 1.07, 95%CI [1.02–1.13]), and 0.86 more common in feeling lonely patients (OR = 0.86, 95%CI [0.77–0.96]) than physically and mentally healthy people. Detailed data on analyzing those having difficulties with wearing masks or gloves during the COVID-19 pandemic are presented in Table 5.

Table 5. Results of univariate and multivariate logistic regression of the answer to the question regarding difficulties with wearing a mask and/or gloves in elderly patients and socio-demographic and clinical factors as well as the odds ratio [OR] and its 95% confidence interval [CI] [the most statistically significant (p-value < 0.05) predictors of feeling difficulties in wearing a mask and/or gloves in elderly patients during COVID-19 pandemic].

Feature (Variable)	b	p	β	p	OR (95% CI)
Asthma	1.269	<0.001	1.025	0.003	2.79 (1.40–5.54)
COPD	1.005	0.006	-	>0.05	-
Heart failure	0.640	0.013	-	>0.05	-
Avoiding vaccination because of possible complications	0.702	<0.001	0.692	0.001	2.00 (1.33–2.99)
Willingness to be vaccinated against influenza, but it is difficult because there is no vaccine in pharmacies	−0.645	0.010	-	>0.05	-
Cardiac drugs	0.445	0.033	-	>0.05	-
Painkillers	0.460	0.015	-	>0.05	-
All medicines prescribed by the same doctor	−0.435	0.031	-	>0.05	-
The Lawton Instrumental Activities of Daily Living (IADL)	−0.124	0.002	−0.091	0.033	0.91 (0.84–0.99)
Depression assessment (GDS-15)	0.099	<0.001	0.071	0.006	1.07 (1.02–1.13)
Gastric Anxiety Scale (GAS-10)	0.083	<0.001	-	>0.05	-
Lubben Social Network Scale (LSNS-6)	−0.196	<0.001	−0.150	0.009	0.86 (0.77–0.96)
Status assessment nutrition (MNA)	−0.125	0.046	-	>0.05	-

b—linear regression coefficient, β—standardized multiple regression coefficients.

The generalized logit regression model leading to estimate the probability of an affirmative answer to the question is it difficult to wear a mask and/or gloves, by elderly patients took the form:

$$\textbf{logit P} = 2.72 + 1.025 \times \textit{asthma} - 0.091 \times \textit{IADL} - 0.15 \times \textit{LSNS-6} + 0.692 \times \textit{avoiding vaccination} + 0.071 \times \textit{GDS-15}$$

4. Discussion

4.1. The Impact of COVID-19 Pandemic on Everyday Activities of Elderly Population

Severe acute respiratory syndrome coronavirus 2 (SARS-CoV-2) may potentially lead to critical complications of the COVID-19 disease, especially in older adults. Many studies showed that the virus causes worse outcomes in the elderly, particularly in those with comorbidities such as hypertension, cardiovascular disease, diabetes, chronic respiratory disease, and chronic kidney disease [3,23]. Additional infection to older, ailing people suffering from many other health conditions results in a significant reduction in their quality of life and their lifespan [24]. According to our study, COVID-19 infection entails a substantial change in older people's behavior. Over 50% and nearly 80% of the surveyed group reduced their social and recreational activities, respectively. It is undoubtedly beneficial behavior for the limitation of virus transmission, but in contrast, physical activity is salutary for older people and significantly impacts the reduction of anxiety, depression, osteoporosis, sarcopenia, and metabolic syndrome [14–17,21]. The result from our analysis is in line with recent publications that have reported COVID-19-related fear, psychosocial effects, and uncertainty among the older population around the world [25–28]. For instance, in Japan, Takashima R interviewed 24 elderly participants (mean age, 78.2 ± 5.5 years) in order to examine their perceptions regarding how COVID-19 restricted their daily lives. The following points were touched: "difficulty of maintaining connections with people", "loss of activities for pleasure in life", "tightness that gradually built up", and "confusion due to the collapse of the schedule". Authors determined frequent changes in activity styles in surveyed participants, for example, reducing the number of shopping trips or shortening the time required for shopping. This result is consistent with our data showing that 162 participants limited doing shopping due to the fear of COVID-19 infection (162/500; 32.4%) [25].

Moreover, considering that interpersonal relations and social activity are particularly beneficial in seniors, reducing activity would decrease their quality of life [29–31]. Furthermore, more than 25% of participants reduced professional activity (133/500, 26.6%), which may produce substantial economic issues. Nowadays, although social distancing and isolation are beneficial to limit the number of potential cases of spreading the virus, this economic issue is still growing, especially in low-income countries and with a high percentage of COVID-19-infected inhabitants. Many businesses were shut down temporarily, leading, in consequence, to financial market turmoil, significant declines in revenue, insolvencies, and job losses in specific sectors [32]. Furthermore, because of travel bans, border closures, and quarantine measures, many workers could not move to their workplaces or carry out their jobs, leading to unbeneficial effects on their incomes [33]. Thus, government-imposed restrictions, together with the fear and anxiety of workers in different sectors about the COVID-19 infection, may lead to a further increase in the economic issue, especially in countries with low state budgets.

4.2. The Most Significant Findings of the Study

We noticed that the most significant change in surveyed seniors' behavior due to the fear of COVID-19 infection (an increase of anxiety and reduction of activity) was observed mainly in patients (1) with other comorbidities, (2) being on multi-drug therapy, (3) vaccinated against influenza, and (4) with several mental difficulties (inferred by specified and validated scales including ADL scale, IADL scale, GDS-15 scale, GAS-10 scale, LSNS-6 scale, MNA scale, and Gierveld scale). Firstly, we found that the change in senior's behavior was especially noticeable in participants suffering from coronary heart disease, COPD, and heart failure. It is already known that patients with at least one of these high-risk conditions suffer from a more severe course of COVID-19 infection and have increased mortality. For instance, according to data from the United States, approximately one-third of COVID-19-infected patients (2692, 38%) had at least one chronic disease or risk factor; the most common were cardiovascular diseases (647, 9%), chronic lung diseases (656, 9.2%), and diabetes (784, 11%) [34]. Furthermore, based on the meta-analysis including 22,148 patients from 40 studies, Liang et al. revealed the significant association between coronary heart disease and poor prognosis of COVID-19 (OR = 3.42, 95%CI [2.83, 4.13], $p < 0.001$); this correlation was affected mostly by hypertension ($p = 0.004$) [35]. Considering COPD patients, Gerayeli et al. examined the effects of this disease on COVID-19 outcomes as their primary endpoint. COPD was associated with increased odds of hospitalization (OR = 4.23, 95%CI [3.65–4.90], Intensive Care Unit (ICU) admission (OR = 1.35, 95% CI [1.02–1.78]), and mortality (OR = 2.47, 95% CI [2.18–2.79]) [36]. These introduced above results are in line with our cross-sectional study, explaining the increased fear and anxiety of COVID-19 infection in patients with cardiac and pulmonary problems. Moreover, we noticed that a significant change in behavior also exists in patients on multi-drug therapy. The reason is probably similar to mentioned before; thus, according to many studies, patients on multi-drug therapy recognize their state of health as worse compared to patients without medications or being on single-drug therapy. Fear and anxiety of COVID-19 infection in elderly patients increase, when cardiac drugs ($p = 0.001$, Figure S3B), antihypertensives ($p = 0.009$, Figure S3C), diuretics ($p = 0.004$, Figure S3D), drugs for digestive ailments ($p = 0.037$, Figure S3E) and anticoagulants ($p < 0.001$, Figure S3F) are taken simultaneously in different combinations. These findings confirm the fear of COVID-19 infection in patients with cardiac and pulmonary difficulties who take medicines as a treatment strategy.

Furthermore, our study revealed a substantial issue in the field of vaccination against influenza in the surveyed seniors' population. Only 62 (12.4%) and 51 (10.2%) of participants were vaccinated against influenza in 2019 and 2020, respectively. The reason for such behavior in 104 (20.8%) cases was the lack of vaccines in pharmacies, but in a substantial number of patients ($n = 164$, 32.8%), it was the fear of possible vaccination-related complications. Moreover, we also found that only in 81 (16.2%) cases, the GP advised on vaccination, which was probably the most stressful finding. Vaccination against influenza is especially beneficial in an older population and reduces influenza-related and comorbidities-related mortality [37,38]. In turn, due to the observed reduction of influenza cases during the COVID-19, the question arises if prior influenza vaccination may affect COVID-19 susceptibility and severity. To date, few studies have evaluated the effects of influenza on COVID-19. However, their results have been mostly conflicting. Massoudi et al. examined the role of the influenza vaccine in 261 healthcare workers, including 180 with a history of COVID-19 and 181 healthy controls. In the univariate analysis, the odds ratio of being vaccinated was 0.04 (95%CI [0.01–0.14]). The authors concluded that the influenza vaccine might have a protective effect in COVID-19 [39]. Furthermore, Zannetini et al. showed an inverse association of a greater influenza vaccination coverage in the elderly and mortality from COVID-19, suggesting a protective effect of the influenza vaccine [40]. Moreover, in patients who had received an influenza vaccination, there was a significant reduction in the odds of testing positive for COVID-19 (OR = 0.82, 95%CI [0.73–0.92], $p < 0.01$). In addition, influenza vaccinated patients were less likely to require hospitalization (OR = 0.58), mechanical ventilation (OR = 0.45) and had a shorter hospital stay (OR = 0.76). This result leads to the conclusion that the influenza vaccine is assumed to reduce the COVID-19 disease burden [41]. By contrast, in Italy, independently, Belingeri et al. and Pedote et al. found no evidence of a relationship between the influenza vaccine and either a COVID-19 diagnosis or a positive SARS-CoV-2 serology test in a group of healthcare workers and COVID-19 infected patients, respectively. Nevertheless, despite different evidence from independent studies, influenza vaccination must be promoted as a central public health measure because reducing the hospital burden can greatly benefit the management of COVID-19 patients [42,43]. It was not only information about vaccines but also routes of transmission, and updates on the number of infected cases and location (e.g., real-time, online tracking map) were associated with lower levels of anxiety [44]. It seems reasonable that educating the population leads to increased awareness about potential ways of protecting against the virus and eliminating COVID-19 cases. In this regard, the general public and social media seem to have a tremendous impact on people's awareness by promoting healthy behaviors and improving coping management strategies. This effect is seen mostly in seniors who tend to stay at home and watch media (radio, television, newspapers) more often than people of other ages. Therefore, we believe that the continuous process of education in influenza vaccination, routes of SARS-CoV-2 transmission, and protective strategies against the virus are crucial to maintain good health in the older population and reduce complications and the necessity of hospitalizations.

With the backdrop of high COVID-19 cases and the constantly evolving situation locally and globally, examining the psychological and mental health impacts, COVID-19 brings to individuals is imperative. One psychological response commonly reported is fear toward COVID-19 [45]. To date, several studies revealed a worsening of physical function after COVID-19 infection. This observation occurred mainly in COVID-19 infected older patients, especially those with dementia and psychiatric disorders, who were more likely to be burdened by the adverse effects of loneliness (i.e., perceived lack of meaningful relationships) and social isolation (i.e., lack of social interactions). The noticeable burden of disease resulting from physical and psychological sequelae of COVID-19 is one of the most important factors increasing the fear of COVID-19 infection. For instance, Zhu et al. conducted a multi-center retrospective cohort study in order to estimate the anxiety of COVID-19 survivors at discharge from hospital and analyze relative risk by exposures. Including a total of 432 survivors with laboratory-confirmed SARS-CoV-2 infection, they found a high prevalence of anxiety, accounting for 36.81% (95% CI [32.39–41.46]). Older age and severe disease course both independently increased the relative risk of IADL limitations and ADL dependence [46]. Furthermore, because one of the most common psychological reactions are symptoms of depression and anxiety, Han et al. examined the association between psychological factors and fear of COVID-19 among community-dwelling older adults during a COVID-19 lockdown in Singapore. The COVID-19 Fear Inventory scale, GDS-15 scale, and GAI-SF scale (Geriatric Anxiety Inventory—Short Form) revealed a strong interrelation between the fear of COVID-19 and affective symptoms suggesting the significant effect COVID-19 has on psychological well-being and mental health. Older age was associated with greater fear of COVID-19 [45]. However, due to the higher risks of cardiac and pulmonary problems in elderly patients (observed, for example, in our study), it is not surprising that higher fear levels were found in this subgroup of older adults.

Our study demonstrated that 10% of participants canceled planned hospitalization due to the fear of COVID-19 infection (50/500, 10%). Considering that hospitalized persons are more prone to COVID-19 infection, it could be paradoxically beneficial if the disease that would be the cause of hospitalization is not life-threatening at the moment. The most stressful finding was that over 5% of the surveyed population resigned to report to the Emergency room due to the sudden deterioration of health (32/500, 6.4%), despite, in many cases, the cause of health aggravation could be more dangerous than potential COVID-19 infection. Such behavior could produce an enormous number of complications, which would increase significant mortality in the older population. For instance, Vani et al. indicated that some patients suffering from breast cancer refused surgical treatment due to fear of COVID-19 contagion even at the risk of survival [47]. In likelihood, this behavior reported in Vani et al.'s study, as well as in our data, results from the fear that health care systems may be overrun and that adequate medical care will not be available for all COVID-19 infected and with other health difficulties [48].

4.3. Telemedicine as a Proposed Strategy against SARS-CoV-2

One of the proposed strategies providing clinical healthcare and information regarding measurements, control, and protection against SARS-CoV-2 during the prevailing COVID-19 pandemic is telemedicine. With this strategy, patients who need care for anxiety caused by COVID-19 infection can be assisted without the requirement for visiting a hospital, and therapy for psychological stabilization can be provided via the internet, without the need for an in-person consultation with the doctor. According to our study, patients suffering from coronary heart disease ($p < 0.001$, Table S1), asthma ($p = 0.026$, Table S1), COPD ($p < 0001$, Table S1), and heart failure ($p < 0.001$, Table S1), patients vaccinated against influenza in 2019 ($p < 0.001$, Figure 1A, Table S1) and in 2020 ($p = 0.008$, Table S1), patients being on multi-drug therapy ($p < 0.001$, Table S1), and patients exhibiting the reluctance to carry out more complex daily activities (IADL scale, $p < 0.001$, Figure 1B, Table S1), with a higher level of anxiety ($p = 0.002$, Table S1), social loneliness ($p = 0.004$, Table S1) and malnutrition ($p < 0.001$, Table S1), canceled planned hospitalizations due to the fear of COVID-19 infection. Thus, these groups of elderly patients require more attention, and hence telemedicine should be focused mostly on them. This strategy provides an alternative avenue to provide medical education for COVID-19 infected patients and avoid unnecessary mortality [49].

Due to the prevailing pandemic, numerous new platforms are projected to grow exponentially, allowing the older population to achieve sufficient knowledge to introduce precautionary measures against COVID-19 to protect themselves, their families, and the whole population while maintaining perfect harmony and peace of mind [50]. The positive effects of telemedicine providing psychological consultation, progress in educating patients as well as healthcare have been verified in many previous studies [50–52]. In one study, Tourkmani et al. found a significant positive effect of telemedicine care among high-risk patients with uncontrolled type 2 diabetes mellitus during the COVID-19 pandemic in Saudi Arabia [53]. Furthermore, Nan et al. proposed a telemedicine-based protocol to manage patients with ST-segment elevation myocardial infarction during the COVID-19 pandemic. Authors suggested that wearable medical devices with the proposed application can provide additional patient information, including heart rate, body weight, blood pressure, and others, that may be useful for doctors to make better decisions for their patients, especially when social distancing is necessary [37]. Thus, we believe that the reduction of activity during the pandemic is, in many cases, favorable and might possibly reduce the number of COVID-19-related complications and mortality, particularly in the susceptible, older population. However, it is worth noticing that physical and social activity is notably essential and beneficial in the senior population [18–20]. Another practical solution to utilize telemedicine more efficiently was proposed by Tolone et al. [54]. The authors proposed a simple and reproducible telephonic triage questionnaire that might be applicable before readmission of patients to hospitals for elective surgery to avoid unnecessary visits to the hospital and reduce healthcare costs and in-hospital positivity. We think that telemedicine's development in common with a continuous process of education and the process of vaccination against the SARS-CoV-2 virus would allow achieving a balance between cautious behavior and social, recreative, and professional activity. Moreover, it would facilitate a process of constant treatment of life-limiting and life-threatening comorbidities. We believe that such a proceeding could significantly impact patients' quality of life and economic and medical issues.

4.4. The Importance of COVID-19 Safety Measures

There is broad public health support for wearing face masks and face coverings in the community in order to fight against COVID-19 successfully. However, many people with secondary chronic diseases have questioned if it is safe for them to wear a mask. According to our study, 174 patients (34.8%) reported it is difficult for them to wear masks. It was observed mostly in patients with asthma ($p < 0.001$, Figure 3A, Table S3) and COPD ($p = 0.008$, Table S3). This finding is explainable due to possible occurring symptoms of these diseases, including difficulty breathing (shortness of breath) and wheezing. The physical barrier of the mask makes it harder to take in air; it also traps some carbon dioxide during exhaling, leading to breathing warmer and moister air [55]. However, it should be noted that according to the American Academy of Allergy, Asthma & Immunology (AAAAI), there is no evidence that wearing a face mask can worsen lung diseases [56]. Furthermore, we determined a subgroup of vaccine-hesitant individuals who both reported difficulties in wearing facemasks and refused the vaccination because of potential side effects ($p < 0.001$, Figure 3B, Table S3). This correlation was also observed in other studies. For instance, Latkin et al. examined the prevalence of COVID-19 vaccine hesitancy and factors associated with vaccine intentions in the US. From a total of 1056 respondents who completed a national panel survey, about half (53.6%) reported intending to be vaccinated, 16.7% did not intend, and 29.7% were unsure. Authors determined that compared to those who reported positive vaccine intentions, respondents with negative vaccine intentions were significantly less likely to report that they engaged in the COVID-19 prevention behaviors of wearing masks (OR = 0.53, 95% [CI 0.37–0.76]) and social distancing (OR = 0.22, 95% CI [0.12–0.42]) [57]. These results suggest that although COVID-19 vaccines are becoming more available, the continued communication and implementation of COVID-19 safety measures (e.g., face masks, personal hygiene, and social distancing) are still instrumental to effective pandemic control and containment [58]. These statements are currently even more necessary because masking can help to reduce the spread of new variants of SARS-CoV-2 while vaccines are rolling out [59].

5. Conclusions

In conclusion, COVID-19 infection is, particularly in the seniors' population, a dangerous and life-threatening disease, which leads to a significant change of behavior. Since the elderly population usually suffers from many medical conditions requiring a continuous treatment process, it is essential to provide proper medical care also during the pandemic. We believe that the development of modern telemedical solutions would improve treatment outcomes, reduce comorbidities-related complications and unnecessary hospitalizations. Moreover, considering that physical and social activity is essential to maintain good physical and psychical health in an older population, we think finding a balance between caution and activity is crucial, particularly in seniors. We believe that the equilibrium could be reached with the support of telemedicine, education, and COVID-19 vaccination.

Supplementary Materials: The following are available online at https://www.mdpi.com/article/10.3390/jcm10184089/s1, Figure S1: Responses to the question of the fear of COVID-19 infection in elderly patients who (A) suffer from coronary heart disease, (B) suffer from COPD, (C) suffer from heart failure and the results of independent non-parametric significance tests. Figure S2: Responses to the question of the fear of COVID-19 infection in elderly patients who (A) administrated the influenza vaccine in 2019, (B) administrated the influenza vaccine in 2020, (C) were willing to be vaccinated against influenza but could not undergo vaccination due to the lack of availability of vaccines in pharmacies, (D) were advised by GP doctor to be vaccinated against influenza and pneumococci and the results of the independent non-parametric significance tests. Figure S3: Responses to the question of the fear of COVID-19 infection in elderly patients who (A) take more than one medicine and the result of the analysis of variance and multiple comparisons (Kruskal–Wallis ANOVA, (B) take cardiac drugs, (C) take antihypertensives, (D) take diuretics, (E) take drugs for digestive ailments, (F) take anticoagulants and the results of independent non-parametric significance tests. Figure S4: Responses to the question of the fear of COVID-19 infection in elderly patients who (A) are less fit (according to IADL scale), (B) are depressed (according to GDS-15 scale), (C) with a higher level of anxiety (according to GAS-10 scale), (D) feel lonely (according to LSND-6 scale), and the results of independent non-parametric significance tests, (E) suffer from malnutrition and the result of the analysis of variance and multiple comparisons (Kruskal–Wallis ANOVA). Table S1: Responses to the questions regarding canceling planned hospitalizations due to the fear of COVID-19 infection in elderly patients and socio-demographic and clinical factors. Table S2: Responses to the questions regarding the resignation to report to the Emergency Room due to the fear of COVID-19 infection in elderly patients and socio-demographic and clinical factors. Table S3: Responses to the questions of whether wearing a mask and/or gloves is a great difficulty in elderly patients and socio-demographic and clinical factors.

Author Contributions: Conceptualization, S.A.; validation, M.S. and G.M.; investigation, S.M., M.D. and B.S.; writing—original draft preparation, S.A.; writing—review and editing, S.M., M.D. and B.S.; supervision, G.M.; project administration, G.M.; funding acquisition, S.A. All authors have read and agreed to the published version of the manuscript.

Funding: This research was funded by the Medical Research Agency Poland, grant number 2020/ABM/COVID19/0005 and National Center for Research and Development under the submeasure 1.1.1 Industrial research and development works, the Intelligent Development Operational Program 2014–2020, Co-financing Agreement No. POIR.01.01.01-00-0297/19-00 of 13 November 2019.

Institutional Review Board Statement: The study was approved by the Bioethics Committee of Wroclaw Medical University.

Informed Consent Statement: Participants provided their verbal consent at the beginning of the interview.

Data Availability Statement: The authors confirm that the data supporting the findings of this study are available within the article.

Conflicts of Interest: The authors declare no conflict of interest.

References

1. Meisner, B.A.; Boscart, V.; Gaudreau, P.; Stolee, P.; Ebert, P.; Heyer, M.; Kadowaki, L.; Kelly, C.; Levasseur, M.; Massie, A.S.; et al. Interdisciplinary and Collaborative Approaches Needed to Determine Impact of COVID-19 on Older Adults and Aging: CAG/ACG and CJA/RCV Joint Statement. *Can. J. Aging* **2020**, *39*, 333–343. [CrossRef]
2. Niu, S.; Tian, S.; Lou, J.; Kang, X.; Zhang, L.; Lian, H.; Zhang, J. Clinical characteristics of older patients infected with COVID-19: A descriptive study. *Arch. Gerontol. Geriatr.* **2020**, *89*, 104058. [CrossRef]
3. Lian, J.; Jin, X.; Hao, S.; Cai, H.; Zhang, S.; Zheng, L.; Jia, H.; Hu, J.; Gao, J.; Zhang, Y.; et al. Analysis of epidemiological and clinical features in older patients with coronavirus disease 2019 (COVID-19) outside Wuhan. *Clin. Infect. Dis.* **2020**, *71*, 740–747. [CrossRef]
4. Guan, W.; Ni, Z.; Hu, Y.; Liang, W.; Ou, C.; He, J.; Liu, L.; Shan, H.; Lei, C.; Hui, D.S.C.; et al. Clinical Characteristics of Coronavirus Disease 2019 in China. *N. Engl. J. Med.* **2020**, *382*, 1708–1720. [CrossRef] [PubMed]
5. Wu, J.; Liu, J.; Zhao, X.; Liu, C.; Wang, W.; Wang, D.; Xu, W.; Zhang, C.; Yu, J.; Jiang, B.; et al. Clinical characteristics of imported cases of coronavirus disease 2019 (COVID-19) in Jiangsu Province: A multicenter descriptive study. *Clin. Infect. Dis.* **2020**, *71*, 706–712. [CrossRef]

6. Shahid, Z.; Kalayanamitra, R.; McClafferty, B.; Kepko, D.; Ramgobin, D.; Patel, R.; Aggarwal, C.S.; Vunnam, R.; Sahu, N.; Bhatt, D.; et al. COVID-19 and Older Adults: What We Know. *J. Am. Geriatr. Soc.* **2020**, *68*, 926–929. [CrossRef] [PubMed]
7. Lithander, F.E.; Neumann, S.; Tenison, E.; Lloyd, K.; Welsh, T.J.; Rodrigues, J.C.L.; Higgins, J.P.T.; Scourfield, L.; Christensen, H.; Haunton, V.J.; et al. COVID-19 in older people: A rapid clinical review. *Age Ageing* **2020**, *49*, 501–515. [CrossRef] [PubMed]
8. Nanda, A.; Vura, N.V.R.K.; Gravenstein, S. COVID-19 in older adults. *Aging Clin. Exp. Res.* **2020**, *32*, 1199–1202. [CrossRef] [PubMed]
9. Wańkowicz, P.; Szylińska, A.; Rotter, I. The Impact of the COVID-19 Pandemic on Psychological Health and Insomnia among People with Chronic Diseases. *J. Clin. Med.* **2021**, *10*, 1206. [CrossRef] [PubMed]
10. Mistry, S.K.; Ali, A.M.; Yadav, U.N.; Ghimire, S.; Hossain, M.B.; Das Shuvo, S.; Saha, M.; Sarwar, S.; Nirob, M.M.H.; Sekaran, V.C.; et al. Older adults with non-communicable chronic conditions and their health care access amid COVID-19 pandemic in Bangladesh: Findings from a cross-sectional study. *PLoS ONE* **2021**, *16*, e0255534. [CrossRef]
11. Addis, S.G.; Nega, A.D.; Miretu, D.G. Psychological impact of COVID-19 pandemic on chronic disease patients in Dessie town government and private hospitals, Northeast Ethiopia. *Diabetes Metab. Syndr.* **2021**, *15*, 129. [CrossRef]
12. Mills, J.P.; Kaye, K.S.; Mody, L. COVID-19 in older adults: Clinical, psychosocial, and public health considerations. *JCI Insight* **2020**, *5*, e139292. [CrossRef]
13. Liu, H.; Chen, S.; Liu, M.; Nie, H.; Lu, H. Comorbid Chronic Diseases are Strongly Correlated with Disease Severity among COVID-19 Patients: A Systematic Review and Meta-Analysis. *Aging Dis.* **2020**, *11*, 668. [CrossRef]
14. Agrawal, S.; Gołębiowska, J.; Bartoszewicz, B.; Makuch, S.; Mazur, G. Clinical preventive services to reduce pandemic deaths. *Prev. Med. Rep.* **2020**, *20*, 101249. [CrossRef]
15. de Oliveira, L.D.S.S.C.B.; Souza, E.C.; Rodrigues, R.A.S.; Fett, C.A.; Piva, A.B. The effects of physical activity on anxiety, depression, and quality of life in elderly people living in the community. *Trends Psychiatry Psychother.* **2019**, *41*, 36–42. [CrossRef]
16. Dohrn, I.M.; Hagströmer, M.; Hellénius, M.L.; Ståhle, A. Short- and long-term effects of balance training on physical activity in older adults with osteoporosis: A randomized controlled trial. *J. Geriatr. Phys. Ther.* **2017**, *40*, 102–111. [CrossRef]
17. Steffl, M.; Bohannon, R.W.; Sontakova, L.; Tufano, J.J.; Shiells, K.; Holmerova, I. Relationship between sarcopenia and physical activity in older people: A systematic review and meta-analysis. *Clin. Interv. Aging* **2017**, *12*, 835–845. [CrossRef]
18. An, H.Y.; Chen, W.; Wang, C.W.; Yang, H.F.; Huang, W.T.; Fan, S.Y. The relationships between physical activity and life satisfaction and happiness among young, middle-aged, and older adults. *Int. J. Environ. Res. Public Health* **2020**, *17*, 4817. [CrossRef] [PubMed]
19. Lindsay Smith, G.; Banting, L.; Eime, R.; O'Sullivan, G.; van Uffelen, J.G.Z. The association between social support and physical activity in older adults: A systematic review. *Int. J. Behav. Nutr. Phys. Act.* **2017**, *14*, 56. [CrossRef] [PubMed]
20. De Labra, C.; Guimaraes-Pinheiro, C.; Maseda, A.; Lorenzo, T.; Millán-Calenti, J.C. Effects of physical exercise interventions in frail older adults: A systematic review of randomized controlled trials Physical functioning, physical health and activity. *BMC Geriatr.* **2015**, *15*, 154. [CrossRef] [PubMed]
21. Sun, F.; Norman, I.J.; While, A.E. Physical activity in older people: A systematic review. *BMC Public Health* **2013**, *13*, 449. [CrossRef]
22. Gallardo-Alfaro, L.; Bibiloni, M.D.M.; Mateos, D.; Ugarriza, L.; Tur, J.A. Leisure-time physical activity and metabolic syndrome in older adults. *Int. J. Environ. Res. Public Health* **2019**, *16*, 3358. [CrossRef]
23. McPhee, J.S.; French, D.P.; Jackson, D.; Nazroo, J.; Pendleton, N.; Degens, H. Physical activity in older age: Perspectives for healthy ageing and frailty. *Biogerontology* **2016**, *17*, 567–580. [CrossRef] [PubMed]
24. Moccia, F.; Gerbino, A.; Lionetti, V.; Miragoli, M.; Munaron, L.M.; Pagliaro, P.; Pasqua, T.; Penna, C.; Rocca, C.; Samaja, M.; et al. COVID-19-associated cardiovascular morbidity in older adults: A position paper from the Italian Society of Cardiovascular Researches. *GeroScience* **2020**, *42*, 1021–1049. [CrossRef] [PubMed]
25. Zhang, Y.; Ma, Z.F. Impact of the COVID-19 pandemic on mental health and quality of life among local residents in Liaoning Province, China: A cross-sectional study. *Int. J. Environ. Res. Public Health* **2020**, *17*, 2381. [CrossRef] [PubMed]
26. Takashima, R.; Onishi, R.; Saeki, K.; Hirano, M. Perception of COVID-19 restrictions on daily life among japanese older adults: A qualitative focus group study. *Healthcare* **2020**, *8*, 450. [CrossRef] [PubMed]
27. Goethals, L.; Barth, N.; Guyot, J.; Hupin, D.; Celarier, T.; Bongue, B. Impact of home quarantine on physical activity among older adults living at home during the COVID-19 pandemic: Qualitative interview study. *JMIR Aging* **2020**, *3*, e19007. [CrossRef]
28. Briguglio, M.; Giorgino, R.; Dell'Osso, B.; Cesari, M.; Porta, M.; Lattanzio, F.; Banfi, G.; Peretti, G.M. Consequences for the Elderly After COVID-19 Isolation: FEaR (Frail Elderly amid Restrictions). *Front. Psychol.* **2020**, *11*, 565052. [CrossRef]
29. Iorga, M.; Soponaru, C.; Socolov, R.V.; Cărăuleanu, A.; Socolov, D.G. How the sars-cov-2 pandemic period influenced the health status and determined changes in professional practice among obstetrics and gynecology doctors in Romania. *Medicina* **2021**, *57*, 325. [CrossRef] [PubMed]
30. Awick, E.A.; Ehlers, D.K.; Aguiñaga, S.; Daugherty, A.M.; Kramer, A.F.; McAuley, E. Effects of a randomized exercise trial on physical activity, psychological distress and quality of life in older adults. *Gen. Hosp. Psychiatry* **2017**, *49*, 44–50. [CrossRef]
31. Puciato, D.; Borysiuk, Z.; Rozpara, M. Quality of life and physical activity in an older working-age population. *Clin. Interv. Aging* **2017**, *12*, 1627–1634. [CrossRef]

32. Groessl, E.J.; Kaplan, R.M.; Rejeski, W.J.; Katula, J.A.; Glynn, N.W.; King, A.C.; Anton, S.D.; Walkup, M.; Lu, C.J.; Reid, K.; et al. Physical Activity and Performance Impact Long-term Quality of Life in Older Adults at Risk for Major Mobility Disability. *Am. J. Prev. Med.* **2019**, *56*, 141–146. [CrossRef] [PubMed]
33. OECD Evaluating the initial impact of COVID-19 containment measures on economic activity. In *Tackling Coronavirus (COVID-19) Contributing to a Global Effort*; OECD: Paris, France, 2020; pp. 1–5.
34. Kohler, H.; Bäuerle, A.; Schweda, A.; Weismüller, B.; Fink, M.; Musche, V.; Robitzsch, A.; Pfeiffer, C.; Benecke, A.V.; Dörrie, N.; et al. Increased COVID-19-related fear and subjective risk perception regarding COVID-19 affects behavior in individuals with internal high-risk diseases. *J. Prim. Care Community Health* **2021**, *12*, 2150132721996898. [CrossRef]
35. Liang, C.; Zhang, W.; Li, S.; Qin, G. Coronary heart disease and COVID-19: A meta-analysis. *Med. Clin.* **2021**, *156*, 547–554. [CrossRef]
36. Gerayeli, F.V.; Milne, S.; Cheung, C.; Li, X.; Yang, C.W.T.; Tam, A.; Choi, L.H.; Bae, A.; Sin, D.D. COPD and the risk of poor outcomes in COVID-19: A systematic review and meta-analysis. *EClinicalMedicine* **2021**, *33*, 100789. [CrossRef]
37. Nan, J.; Jia, R.; Meng, S.; Jin, Y.; Chen, W.; Hu, H. The Impact of the COVID-19 Pandemic and the Importance of Telemedicine in Managing Acute ST Segment Elevation Myocardial Infarction Patients: Preliminary Experience and Literature Review. *J. Med. Syst.* **2021**, *45*, 9. [CrossRef]
38. Gazibara, T.; Kovacevic, N.; Kisic-Tepavcevic, D.; Nurkovic, S.; Kurtagic, I.; Gazibara, T.; Pekmezovic, T. Flu vaccination among older persons: Study of knowledge and practices. *J. Health Popul. Nutr.* **2019**, *38*, 2. [CrossRef]
39. Demicheli, V.; Jefferson, T.; Di Pietrantonj, C.; Ferroni, E.; Thorning, S.; Thomas, R.E.; Rivetti, A. Vaccines for preventing influenza in the elderly. *Cochrane Database Syst. Rev.* **2018**, *2*, CD004876. [CrossRef] [PubMed]
40. Massoudi, N.; Mohit, B. A Case–Control Study of the 2019 Influenza Vaccine and Incidence of COVID-19 Among Healthcare Workers. *J. Clin. Immunol.* **2021**, *41*, 324–334. [CrossRef] [PubMed]
41. Zanettini, C.; Omar, M.; Dinalankara, W.; Imada, E.L.; Colantuoni, E.; Parmigiani, G.; Marchionni, L. Influenza vaccination and covid-19 mortality in the usa: An ecological study. *Vaccines* **2021**, *9*, 427. [CrossRef] [PubMed]
42. Conlon, A.; Ashur, C.; Washer, L.; Eagle, K.A.; Hofmann Bowman, M.A. Impact of the influenza vaccine on COVID-19 infection rates and severity. *Am. J. Infect. Control* **2021**, *49*, 694–700. [CrossRef] [PubMed]
43. Pedote, P.D.; Termite, S.; Gigliobianco, A.; Lopalco, P.L.; Bianchi, F.P. Influenza vaccination and health outcomes in COVID-19 patients: A retrospective cohort study. *Vaccines* **2021**, *9*, 358. [CrossRef] [PubMed]
44. Chow, N.; Fleming-Dutra, K.; Gierke, R.; Hall, A.; Hughes, M.; Pilishvili, T.; Ritchey, M.; Roguski, K.; Skoff, T.; Ussery, E. Preliminary Estimates of the Prevalence of Selected Underlying Health Conditions Among Patients with Coronavirus Disease 2019—United States, February 12–March 28, 2020. *MMWR. Morb. Mortal. Wkly. Rep.* **2020**, *69*, 382–386.
45. Han, M.F.Y.; Mahendran, R.; Yu, J. Associations Between Fear of COVID-19, Affective Symptoms and Risk Perception Among Community-Dwelling Older Adults During a COVID-19 Lockdown. *Front. Psychol.* **2021**, *12*, 961. [CrossRef]
46. Zhu, S.; Gao, Q.; Yang, L.; Yang, Y.; Xia, W.; Cai, X.; Hui, Y.; Zhu, D.; Zhang, Y.; Zhang, G.; et al. Prevalence and risk factors of disability and anxiety in a retrospective cohort of 432 survivors of Coronavirus Disease-2019 (COVID-19) from China. *PLoS ONE* **2020**, *15*, e0243883. [CrossRef]
47. International Labour Organization Global impact and policy recommendations. In *COVID-19 and the World of Work*, 1st ed.; ILO Monitor: Geneva, Switzerland, 2020; pp. 1–15.
48. Vanni, G.; Materazzo, M.; Pellicciaro, M.; Ingallinella, S.; Rho, M.; Santori, F.; Cotesta, M.; Caspi, J.; Makarova, A.; Pistolese, C.A.; et al. Breast cancer and COVID-19: The effect of fear on patients' decision-making process. *In Vivo* **2020**, *34*, 1651–1659. [CrossRef]
49. Lee, Y.R.; Lee, J.Y.; Park, I.H.; Kim, M.; Jhon, M.; Kim, J.W.; Ryu, S.; Kim, J.M.; Kim, S.W. The Relationships among Media Usage Regarding COVID-19, Knowledge about Infection, and Anxiety: Structural Model Analysis. *J. Korean Med. Sci.* **2020**, *35*, e426. [CrossRef]
50. De Bonis, S.; Salerno, N.; Bisignani, A.; Capristo, A.; Sosto, G.; Verta, A.; Borselli, R.; Capristo, C.; Bisignani, G. COVID-19 and STEMI: The role of telecardiology in the management of STEMI diagnosis during COVID 19 pandemic. *Int. J. Cardiol. Hear. Vasc.* **2021**, *32*, 100720.
51. Franklin, G.; Martin, C.; Ruszaj, M.; Matin, M.; Kataria, A.; Hu, J.; Brickman, A.; Elkin, P.L. How the COVID-19 pandemic impacted medical education during the last year of medical school: A class survey. *Life* **2021**, *11*, 294. [CrossRef]
52. Hau, Y.S.; Kim, J.K.; Hur, J.; Chang, M.C. How about actively using telemedicine during the COVID-19 pandemic? *J. Med. Syst.* **2020**, *44*, 108. [CrossRef] [PubMed]
53. Tourkmani, M.A.; Harbi, J.A.L.T.; Rsheed, A.M.B.; Alrasheedy, A.A.; ALMadani, W.; ALJuraisi, F.; AlOtaibi, A.F.; AlHarbi, M.; AlAbood, A.F.; Alshaikh, A.A.I. The impact of telemedicine on patients with uncontrolled type 2 diabetes mellitus during the COVID-19 pandemic in Saudi Arabia: Findings and implications. *J. Telemed. Telecare* **2021**. [CrossRef]
54. Tolone, S.; Gambardella, C.; Brusciano, L.; del Genio, G.; Lucido, F.S.; Docimo, L. Telephonic triage before surgical ward admission and telemedicine during COVID-19 outbreak in Italy. Effective and easy procedures to reduce in-hospital positivity. *Int. J. Surg.* **2020**, *78*, 123. [CrossRef]
55. Difficulty Breathing in a Face Mask? Advice for Asthma and Lung Disease. Available online: https://creakyjoints.org/living-with-arthritis/coronavirus/managing-symptoms/difficulty-breathing-face-mask-asthma-lung-disease/ (accessed on 1 September 2021).

56. AAAAI | American Academy of Allergy, Asthma & Immunology. Available online: https://www.aaaai.org/ (accessed on 1 September 2021).
57. Latkin, C.A.; Dayton, L.; Yi, G.; Colon, B.; Kong, X. Mask usage, social distancing, racial, and gender correlates of COVID-19 vaccine intentions among adults in the US. *PLoS ONE* **2021**, *16*, e0246970. [CrossRef]
58. Su, Z.; Wen, J.; McDonnell, D.; Goh, E.; Li, X.; Šegalo, S.; Ahmad, J.; Cheshmehzangi, A.; Xiang, Y.-T. Vaccines are not yet a silver bullet: The imperative of continued communication about the importance of COVID-19 safety measures. *Brain Behav. Immun.-Health* **2021**, *12*, 100204. [CrossRef] [PubMed]
59. SARS-CoV-2 Variant Classifications and Definitions. Available online: https://www.cdc.gov/coronavirus/2019-ncov/variants/variant-info.html (accessed on 1 September 2021).

Journal of
Clinical Medicine

MDPI

Article

Parental Distress and Perception of Children's Executive Functioning after the First COVID-19 Lockdown in Italy

Concetta Polizzi, Sofia Burgio *, Gioacchino Lavanco and Marianna Alesi

Department of Psychology, Educational Science and Human Movement, University of Palermo, 90128 Palermo, Italy; concetta.polizzi@unipa.it (C.P.); gioacchino.lavanco@unipa.it (G.L.); marianna.alesi@unipa.it (M.A.)
* Correspondence: sofia.burgio@unipa.it

Abstract: The spread of the novel coronavirus (COVID-19), and the consequential first italian lockdown to minimize viral transmission, have resulted in many significant changes in the every-day lives of families, with an increased risk of parental burnout. This study explores the impact of the first COVID-19 lockdown in Italy on parental distress and parental perceptions of children's executive functions (EFs). Participants were 308 Italian parents with children between 4 and 17 years of age; they were recruited through online advertisements on websites and social media, and they were given an online survey. The measures were: the balance between risks and resources (BR2) and the executive functioning self-report (EF). Findings of the study suggest that the most distressed parents perceived their children as less competent in EF, highlighting a cognitive fragility on attention, memory, and self-regulation (Pearson correlation coefficient, $p < 0.05$); significant differences were found between parents of children exhibiting typical and atypical patterns of development (ANOVA, $p < 0.05$). The study reinforces the need to provide families with psychological aid to support parental competence in restrictive lockdown conditions.

Keywords: parental distress; COVID-19; children; executive functioning

Citation: Polizzi, C.; Burgio, S.; Lavanco, G.; Alesi, M. Parental Distress and Perception of Children's Executive Functioning after the First COVID-19 Lockdown in Italy. *J. Clin. Med.* **2021**, *10*, 4170. https://doi.org/10.3390/jcm10184170

Academic Editors: Michele Roccella and Erik Roj Larsen

Received: 2 July 2021
Accepted: 13 September 2021
Published: 15 September 2021

1. Introduction

From 10 March to 17 May, 2020, the Italian government imposed a national lockdown to limit viral transmission of COVID-19. This period, lasting about 70 days, was characterized by severe social restriction measures, including domestic confinement, working from home, closure of non-essential businesses, and closure of all schools with distance learning. Immediate consequences were vast, i.e., the loss of freedom, the separation of elderly relatives from contradictory information surplus, the uncertainty about COVID-19 infection and health, and the increasing use of social networks. Other additional conditions included the lack of personal space at home and family uncertainty, concerning economic status or inadequate supplies (food, drugs, and safety devices) [1–4]. Following a break-down of borders between work and home, parents faced several pressing concerns, rearranging their work/children's schedules, as well as their children's education routines, because of school closures. In a complementary way, children were asked to re-arrange their routines by giving up all out-of-home and after-school activities, ranging from sports/recreational activities to social relationships with peers [5,6].

All of these factors, in addition to concerns about specific outbreaks, i.e., due to fears about COVID-19 and the use of measures to prevent it, acted as psychological stressors and accounted for detrimental effects on the global well-being and mental health of both adults and children [7]. Moreover, during the home confinement, stressful effects were intensified by "distress contagion" among family members through spillover or crossover mechanisms. The spillover mechanism refers to the impact in which exposure to distress in one area can have a ripple effect (i.e., in personal functioning) in another area (e.g., from work or economic concerns to parenting skills), whilst the crossover mechanism refers to contagion from one member of the family to other family members [6].

Research on the psychological effects from previous epidemics and pandemics (e.g., SARS, MERS, H1N1, Ebola, equine influenza) corroborated with high rates of family distress, ranging from 30% in children to 25% in parents [8]. In particular, following a lockdown, to contrast severe acute respiratory syndrome (SARS) and Middle-East RESPIRATORY SYNDROME (MERS), psychological (anxiety, depression, irritability, anger, emotional exhaustion, etc.) and behavioral (hyperactivity, sleep disorders, angry, conduct problems, externalizing problems, withdrawn, or clingy ...) symptoms were reported [9–12].

Furthermore, it has been well documented how a long breakdown could enhance psychological distress, with a progressive appearance of despair during the first 9 days, anxiety from the 15th to the 19th day, and anger from the 20th to the 31st day, until a condition comparable to post-traumatic distress disorder (PTSD) occurs [10,13].

In a large Chinese survey involving 52,730 participants, the rate of psychological distress due to the COVID-19 outbreak was about 35%, with gender and age differences. Higher levels of distress were found in the female group and age range between 18 and 30 years or above 60 years [14]. An online survey carried out in Italy with 2766 respondents showed increased levels of frequency of anxiety, depression, and distress compared to the European epidemiological statistics. More in depth, higher levels of distress were reported by women, higher levels of depression were showed by individuals with a previous history of trauma or medical diseases, or having an acquaintance infected with COVID-19, higher levels of anxiety occurred in younger individuals and people who had an infected relative [15]. Of particular interest was the association between depression and the condition characterized by not having children. This is coherent with findings that highlighted how being a parent or living with children is a factor that enhances psychological distress during a lockdown or quarantine [16].

In particular, high psychological stress levels have been found in parents of children with special needs and exhibiting atypical patterns of development, due to a disability or a chronic medical condition [17–19]. Several studies pointed out the high prevalence of depressive symptoms and significant changes in strain observed among parents of special needs children during the COVID-19 outbreak; they demanded greater attention from mental health practitioners and rehabilitation care providers [20].

In light of the pandemic effects on psychological health, in particular for parents [13,21,22] during this critical period, there was an increase in requests for psychological support [4,23]. To respond to this emerging need, there has been a global proliferation of online psychological support services; these services were often free and promoted by government authorities, such as the Italian Ministry of Health [24]. In Italy, among the adults who asked for help from these services, many parents reported great difficulty in managing the relationships with their children, especially if they had some evolutionary fragility or special needs [24].

Almost all studies that analyzed the psychological conditions of parents indicated that specialist responses (psychological and psychotherapeutic) are fundamental for the support needs expressed by parents [25,26]. In other words, many parents during the pandemic needed the support of mental health specialists to cope with difficulties.

Higher levels of distress, negative emotions, such as anger or frustration, and negative cognitions, such as pessimism or perfectionism, were displayed by parents with personality profiles characterized by high neuroticism, with patterns of worrying, emotional variability, and feelings of insecurity [13].

In turn, parental distress negatively influenced the caregiver's ability to manage their children at home and to adopt proper disciplinary measures [13].

Petrocchi et al. [27] found that mothers with higher distress levels attributed more negative emotions to their children, with consequences on children's adaptive functioning [3].

In regard to the children, as found by the first studies carried out in China, behavioral problems due to COVID-19 lockdowns, ranged from 4.7% to 10.3% in childhood [28].

Psychological consequences varied from anxiety to depression, regression symptoms, panic attacks, irritability, restlessness, and feelings of loneliness [3,29–32]. Indeed, vulnerability factors, such as developmental age, educational, and socioeconomic status, previous special needs, or mental health disease, seemed to moderate the appearance of psychological problems [33].

Clinginess and the fear of contagion were more frequent in younger children aged, approximately, 3 to 6 years; inattention and inquiry persistence were more frequent in older children aged 6 to 18 years [34].

However, despite the increasing research on parental distress effects, to the best of our knowledge, minor research has been produced to investigate the interplay between parental distress and children's executive functions (EF) during a lockdown period.

Executive functioning (EF) is a set of core cognitive processes for development that consist of a variety of higher-order cognitive processes; it plays a key role in mental and physical health. Moreover, EF is involved in a wide range of "long-life" aspects, ranging from school readiness to job success, marital harmony, and public safety [35].

Executive functions involve a network of frontal-parietal areas, are greatly heritable, and are supposed to be polygenic. Three main components were identified as being potentially important: inhibition, switching, and working memory [36]. Inhibition is the ability to control and repress a prevailing response in support of another response or no response. Switching is the ability to switch from one task or mindset to another. Finally, working memory is the capacity to monitor and manipulate items and mental representations in the mind [35]. These three components are theoretically described as a model of "unity and diversity" because they refer to distinct but inter-correlated cognitive functions. As demonstrated by structural equation modeling, the three functions contribute in a different way to allow a successful performance on tasks, tapping memory, inhibition, fluency, and attentional shifting; therefore, the need to recognize the unity and diversity of executive functions is suggested [37].

Moreover, these main components are closely related to other processes, such as fluency and planning. Fluency denotes the ability to produce, in a given amount of time, as many items as possible (e.g., words, colors, etc.), and planning is the ability to identify, employ, and monitor a sequence of thoughts or actions to achieve a specific goal [38].

An inadequate family context, lacking both material and psychosocial supports, is considered to be a risk condition that hampers a child's development of EF [39,40]. Family functioning explains up to 20% of the variance of a child's performance in working memory and EF tasks [41].

Following an ecological perspective, previous research demonstrated that EFs, for their long development, are very sensitive to macro-contextual (e.g., cultural contexts or SES) and micro-contextual (e.g., family members psychological variables, language, parent-child relationships, parenting skills) factors [42]. Adverse environments characterized by high levels of parental distress account for increasing parental control strategies and limit the use of scaffolding measures to support the gradual increase of children's autonomy in decision-making processes, behavioral, and emotional management, and the use of strategies to cope with distress events. The extreme consequence could be an impairment or delay in long-term EF development [43]. Children with poorer EFs had a higher level of salivary cortisol, which is the distress hormone [44]. Moreover, parents' mental health factors, such as acute distress, depression, and anxiety, can impair parenting skills and children's later development of working memory, inhibition, and cognitive flexibility [43,45,46]. Parents with experiences of daily distress and worries about life goals can feel less connected to their children, engage less in cognitively challenging tasks, produce a distressful or chaotic family context and, as a consequence, can have behavior and parent–infant interaction that obstructs the development of a child's self-regulatory skills, which ends up influencing cognitive development [47–49]. On the other hand, a lack (or a break) from school learning is a risk factor for the increased distress of a child, reduced inhibitory control, and cognitive flexibility, as well as concerns surrounding planning, attention, or decision making [50]. Contemporary research has documented how, during the lockdown, children's self-regulation capacities and inhibitory controls seem to have been negatively influenced by an increase of the mother's negative emotions, by changes in the mother's sleep quality and in the perception of time, by the breakdown of daily routines and after-schools habits [51]. Furthermore, attention deficit hyperactivity disorder (ADHD) symptoms in children worsened following the lack of daily routines, extra-familiar social relationships, and the increase of family distress [12].

In light of the literature reviewed above, the present study assessed the relationships between parental distress and children's EF, as perceived and reported by their parents. In regard to parental distress, this study assumed the balances between risks and resources theory [52,53] that explains parental distress as a condition of parental burnout, resulting from an imbalance between parental risks and protective factors. Parental burnout develops when parental resources are insufficient to meet the demands/risk factors that significantly increase parental distress levels (e.g., parental low emotional intelligence, perfectionism, poor childrearing practices, lack of support from the co-parent, lack of social support).

An online cross-sectional survey was performed to measure the above-mentioned variables immediately after the end of the first spring Italian lockdown (from March to May 2020) and prior to the following autumn (partial) lockdown (since October 2020). This period was selected because critical questions remain to be answered about the short-term effects of pandemic events on cognitive development whilst pandemic long-term effects on mental health have been well-documented in previous pandemic conditions.

Given these concerns the following goals were investigated:

Goal 1: parental distress following first COVID-19 lockdown would be influenced by parental variables (age, education, job or working condition, couples' conditions, support needs during the lockdown) and the child's typical/atypical patterns of development.

Goal 2: parental perception of children's EF would be influenced by specific parental variables (age, education, job or working condition, couples' conditions, support needs during the lockdown), and the child's typical/atypical patterns of development.

Goal 3: parental distress following the first COVID-19 lockdown would be related to the perception of children's EF. Higher levels of parental distress would be associated with their perception of worse EFs in their children.

2. Materials and Methods

2.1. Participants

Participants were recruited through online advertisements on websites and social media (Facebook and WhatsApp).

Inclusion criteria were: (a) being a parent; (b) being at least 18 years old, and (c) having a child between 4 and 17 years of age.

The collected data refer to a sample of 308 parents, 278 mothers (90.3%), and 30 fathers (9.7%). Most parents were aged between 36 and 45 years (52.9%) and were of Italian nationality (98.7%). The parents were mostly married (84.4%); an equal number were either separated with joint custody (and who had the child at home during the lockdown) (7.1%) or cohabiting (7.5%). Only 1% of parents were single.

A degree was the most popular qualification (39.6%), followed by a high school diploma (30.5%). A minority of participants had a Ph.D. or a specialization (15.6%), a professional diploma (7.8%), a primary school certificate, or a middle school diploma (6.4%).

A total of 35.1% of the participants were government employees, while 19.2% were freelancers, 14.3% were teachers, and 10.7% were housewives. Other professions were practiced, but in very low percentages. Moreover, most of these occupations were carried out in smart working modes (45.5%) during the first lockdown caused by the COVID-19 pandemic, 20.8% of the sample declared that they continued to work at the workplace, while a small number of parents said they did not work due to a suspension of their activities (12.7%), because they were temporary layoffs (3.9%), or because they lost their jobs (3.2%).

The children of these parents were mostly boys (57.8%) while 42.2% were girls. The children taken into consideration were mostly first-born (67.9%), followed by the second-born (25.3%), and finally by the third-born and beyond (6.8%). The first-born considered by the parents for the study were mostly between the ages of 11 and 13 (41.6%), followed by children between the ages of 7 and 10 (30.7%) and, finally, children between the ages of 4 and 6 years (27.7%); neither parent involved in the study had sons between the ages of 14 and 17 years old. Furthermore, most of the 11–13-year-old and 7–10-year-old first born children had at least one sibling.

Concerning the developmental conditions of the children, 270 were children exhibiting "typical" patterns of development and 38 were children exhibiting atypical patterns of development, which included learning disabilities, ADHD, genetic syndrome, intellectual disabilities, sensorial disabilities, autism spectrum disorder, or chronic or severe pathologies.

Neither parent was infected with COVID-19 during the research.

2.2. Measures and Procedure

An online survey was administered from June to October 2020. Participants were recruited through online advertisements on websites and social media (Facebook and WhatsApp) via a snowball sampling strategy.

All participants were informed about the aims and procedures of the study by a brief description of the study; they gave their informed consent (via the survey) before filling out the survey. Participation was voluntary and anonymous. The survey took about 20–25 min to complete.

The study was conducted in accordance with the Declaration of Helsinki and was approved by the Bioethics Committee of the University of Palermo (no. 13/2020).

Collected parental sociodemographic data were: gender, age, nationality, region, marital status, level of education, work regimen before and during COVID-19 pandemic, habits before and during the COVID-19 pandemic, social relations after the COVID-19 emergency, the use of social networks, psychological support needs during the COVID-19 pandemic, discomfort during the COVID-19 emergency, and ideas relating to the process of the pandemic. Concerning the children, data included gender, birth order, pathologies, or disabilities.

Parental distress was measured by the balance between risks and resources (BR2; [52]). It was a self-report questionnaire. Specifically, the BR2 instrument reliably measured parental balance between risks (parental distress-enhancing factors) and resources (parental distress alleviating factors). This tool was composed of 39 bipolar items, in which parents were asked to read carefully each sentence and express their degree of agreement, using a 10-point answer scale of values ranging from −5 to +5. Of these, 14 items defined common antecedents as risk factors, indicating predictors of job and parental burnout (e.g., "It is difficult for me to reconcile my family life and my professional life") and 25 items defined specific antecedents showing aspects strictly related to parental burnout (e.g., "Due to my parenting responsibilities, I can never find time for myself"). The total score ranged between −195 and +195. A positive score revealed the prevalence of parental resources, whereas a negative score indicated the risk of parental burnout; the "0" scores revealed equal levels of risks and resources. The original version was translated and adapted to the Italian context with the author's permission. The original administration procedure was used. The results of the EFA showed that the principal component analysis identified two factors that explained the 47.21% variance. The mean sampling adequacy (Bartlett's test) was 6889.42 ($p < 0.001$) and the Kaiser–Meyer–Olkin (KMO) was 0.917.

The internal consistency was verified through the Cronbach's Alpha test, given that the Cronbach's Alpha reliability is considered within an acceptable range, of around 0.70. The reliability values were of $\alpha = 0.96$ for the global scale, $\alpha = 0.89$ for the common antecedents subscale, and $\alpha = 0.94$ for the specific antecedents subscale.

The parental perception of children's EF was measured through the executive functioning self-report (EF-SR) [54]. This was composed of 20 items, conceptualizing, as a system of perceptions, about their child's cognitive abilities in the management of environmental conditions, such as working memory (e.g., "My child is not good at remembering sequences of items, for example, numbers or words"), attention (e.g., "My child has difficulty ignoring extraneous thoughts when he/she performs a task"), shifting (e.g., "My child has difficulty moving from one task to another (for example from a math task to a science task"), planning (e.g., "My child has troubles performing tasks that have more steps") and inhibitory control (e.g., "My child has difficulty with concentration while working in the classroom"). All items used a four-point Likert scale ranging from 1 (always) to 4 (never) to quantify the frequency of use. Higher scores indicated minor difficulties on EF tasks.

A total score (from 20 to 80) and sub-scores (from 4 to 16) for each area were obtained. The reliability values were of $\alpha = 0.95$ for the global scale, $\alpha = 0.87$ for the working memory subscale, $\alpha = 0.80$ for the attention subscale, $\alpha = 0.86$ for the shifting subscale, $\alpha = 0.76$ for the planning subscale, $\alpha = 0.79$ for the inhibitory control subscale.

2.3. Statistical Analysis

In regard to goals 1 and 2 of the study, analyses of variance (ANOVA) were run through the Statistical Program for Social Sciences (SPSS) (IBM SPSS Statistics for Windows, Version 24.0. IBM Corp., Armonk, NY, USA) to investigate parental distress and parental perception of children EFs as a function of independent variables, such as parental and children's variables; the independent variables were parental characteristics (age, education, job, working condition during the lockdown, couples' conditions, psychological support needs) as well as children's characteristics (age, order of birth and typical/atypical patterns of development) whilst the dependent variables were the scores on BR2 subscales (global scale, common antecedents subscale and specific antecedents subscale) and EF-SR questionnaire subscales, respectively (total EF, working memory, inhibition, shifting, planning and attentional control). For the analysis of variance, the parental gender variable was not considered, because the sample consisted of 90.3% mothers. The partial eta square was used to estimate effect size, and in according with Cohen (1988), was interpreted as small ($0.01 < \eta^2_p \leq 0.06$), medium ($0.06 < \eta^2_p \leq 0.14$), and large ($\eta^2_p > 0.14$). Moreover, in about one-third of the study, correlation analyses were performed by Pearson's correlation coefficient, to assess the association between parental distress and parental perception of children's EF; subsequently, considering the correlational data, a linear regression analysis was performed with the stepwise method.

3. Results

3.1. Parental Distress

Parental distress descriptive data are showed in Tables 1–6.

Concerning parental distress, the global distress ($F(1, 308) = 4981$; $p = 0.02$; $\eta^2_p = 0.02$), specific antecedents ($F(1, 308) = 3.748$; $p = 0.05$; $\eta^2_p = 0.01$), and common antecedents ($F(1, 308) = 6.225$; $p = 0.01$; $\eta^2_p = 0.02$) differed in a significant way between parents having psychological support needs and parents not having this support, in spite of the low effect size value. The higher level of distress on all three scales were obtained by parents who required and obtained psychological or social support.

There were also significant group differences on global distress ($F(1, 308) = 8.955$; $p < 0.01$; $\eta^2_p = 0.03$), common antecedents ($F(1, 308) = 12.063$; $p = 0.001$; $\eta^2_p = 0.04$), and specific antecedents ($F(1, 308) = 6.383$; $p < 0.01$; $\eta^2_p = 0.02$) between parents of children exhibiting "typical" patterns of development and parents of children exhibiting atypical patterns of development, in spite of the low effect size value. Parents having children with special needs reported higher rates of distress on all scales.

Table 1. Parental distress descriptive data and ANOVA analyses for parental psychological support needs and the presence of a child exhibiting atypical patterns of development.

	Psychological Support Needs M (SD)		Child Atypical Development M (SD)	
	No (N = 206)	Yes (N = 102)	No (N = 270)	Yes (N = 38)
TOT BR² *	66.8 (63.6)	50.2 (57.1)	65.2 (60)	33.5 (68.6)
	F = 4.981; p-value = 0.026; η^2_p = 0.02		F = 8.955; p-value = 0.003; η^2_p = 0.03	
	Tot (N = 308) 61.3 (61.9)		Tot (N = 308) 61.3 (61.9)	
Common Antecedents **	20.8 (23.2)	13.9 (21.7)	20.2 (21.8)	6.6 (27.1)
	F = 6.225; p-value= 0.013; η^2_p = 0.02		F = 12.063; p-value = 0.001; η^2_p = 0.04	
	Tot (N = 308) 18.5 (22.9)		Tot (N = 308) 18.5 (22.9)	
Specific Antecedents ***	46 (42.9)	36.2 (38.9)	45 (41)	26.8 (44.5)
	F = 3.748; p-value = 0.054; η^2_p = 0.01		F = 6.383; p-value = 0.012; η^2_p = 0.02	
	Tot (N = 308) 42.7 (41.8)		Tot (N = 308) 42.7 (41.8)	

* Min and max scores: −195; +195. ** Min and max scores: −70; +70. *** Min and max scores: −125; +125.

Table 2. Parental distress descriptive data and ANOVA analyses for child age, birth order, and parental age.

	Child Age M (SD)			Order of Birth M (SD)			Parental Age M (SD)		
	4–6 (N = 70)	7–10 (N = 101)	11–13 (N = 137)	First Born (N = 209)	Second Born (N = 78)	Third Born and beyond (N = 21)	<36 (N = 50)	36–45 (N = 163)	>45 (N = 95)
TOT BR² *	53.6 (58.9)	60 (59.9)	66.2 (64.8)	58.5 (64.4)	66.6 (59.9)	70.1 (54.2)	60.1 (60.4)	55.5 (61.8)	72 (62.1)
	F = 0.996; p-value = 0.370; η^2_p =0.006			F = 0.719; p-value = 0.488; η^2_p = 0.005			F = 2.156; p-value = 0.118; η^2_p = 0.01		
				Tot (N = 308) 61.3 (61.9)					
Common Antecedents **	14.4 (20.4)	18.4 (22.4)	20.7 (24.3)	17.2 (23.5)	22.1 (22)	18.6 (18.8)	17.7 (20.9)	16.2 (22.8)	23 (23.6)
	F = 1.781; p-value = 0.170; η^2_p = 0.01			F = 1.305; p-value = 0.273; η^2_p = 0.008			F = 2.741; p-value = 0.066; η^2_p = 0.02		
				Tot (N = 308) 18.5 (22.9)					
Specific Antecedents ***	39.2 (41.6)	41.5 (41)	45.5 (42.6)	41.2 (43.7)	44.5 (37.6)	51.4 (37.7)	42.3 (42.1)	39.3 (42.2)	48.9 (40.6)
	F = 0.587; p-value = 0.557; η^2_p = 0.004			F = 0.659; p-value = 0.518; η^2_p = 0.004			F = 1.607; p-value = 0.202; η^2_p = 0.01		
				Tot (N = 308) 42.7 (41.8)					

* Min and max scores: −195; +195. ** Min and max scores: −70; +70. *** Min and max scores: −125; +125.

Table 3. Parental distress descriptive data and ANOVA analyses for educational level.

	Level of Education M (SD)				
	Primary and Middle School (N = 20)	Professional School (N = 24)	High School (N = 94)	Degree (N = 122)	PhD/ Specialization (N = 48)
TOT BR² *	51.8 (61.4)	77.4 (55.9)	59 (56.6)	65.3 (63.6)	51.7 (70.2)
			F = 0.969; p-value = 0.425; η^2_p = 0.01 Tot (N = 308) 61.3 (61.9)		
Common Antecedents **	14.1 (19.4)	22.2 (19.8)	17.3 (22.1)	20.5 (23.2)	16 (26.6)
			F = 0.769; p-value = 0.546; η^2_p = 0.01 Tot (N = 308) 18.5 (22.9)		
Specific Antecedents ***	37.7 (43.9)	55.1 (39.5)	41.7 (38.6)	44.8 (42.8)	35.6 (45.4)
			F = 1.035; p-value = 0.389; η^2_p = 0.01 Tot (N = 308) 42.7 (41.8)		

* Min and max scores: −195; +195. ** Min and max scores: −70; +70. *** Min and max scores: −125; +125.

Table 4. Parental distress descriptive data for job conditions.

	Job Condition M (SD)							
	Housewives (N = 33)	**Student** (N = 11)	**Government Employee** (N = 108)	**Manager** (N = 15)	**Free-Lancer** (N = 59)	**Teacher** (N = 44)	**Unemployed** (N = 14)	**Other** (N = 24)
TOT BR² *	46.6 (63.6)	32.2 (76.6)	62.3 (58.6)	73.3 (66)	53.2 (66.9)	85 (49.5)	60.7 (76.5)	59.8 (56.1)
				F = 1.795; p-value = 0.088; η^2_p = 0.04 Tot (N = 308) 61.3 (61.9)				
Common Antecedents **	12.6 (23.7)	8.5 (26)	18.6 (22.3)	24.1 (23.1)	16.7 (24.5)	27.2 (18.5)	14.5 (25.8)	18.5 (21.5)
				F = 1.789; p-value = 0.089; η^2_p = 0.04 Tot (N = 308) 18.5 (22.9)				
Specific Antecedents ***	33.9 (43.9)	23.7 (53.2)	43.7 (39.3)	49.2 (44.6)	36.4 (45)	57.8 (33.5)	46.2 (52.8)	41.3 (37.2)
				F = 1.636; p-value = 0.125; η^2_p = 0.04 Tot (N = 308) 42.7 (41.8)				

* Min and max scores: −195; +195. ** Min and max scores: −70; +70 *** Min and max scores: −125; +125.

Table 5. Parental distress descriptive data for couples' conditions.

	Couples' Conditions M (SD)		
	Married (N = 260)	**Cohabiting** (N = 23)	**Separated** (N = 22)
TOT BR² *	62.8 (59.6)	71 (52.8)	41.3 (86)
		F = 1.521; p-value = 0.22; η^2_p = 0.01 Tot (N = 308) 61.3 (61.9)	
Common Antecedents **	18.7 (22.5)	22.4 (20.1)	14.3 (29.5)
		F = 0.706; p-value = 0.495; η^2_p = 0.005 Tot (N = 308) 18.5 (22.9)	
Specific Antecedents ***	44.1 (39.9)	48.6 (36.7)	27 (57.9)
		F = 1.958; p-value = 0.143; η^2_p = 0.01 Tot (N = 308) 42.7 (41.8)	

* Min and max scores: −195; +195. ** Min and max scores: −70; +70. *** Min and max scores: −125; +125.

Table 6. Parental distress descriptive data and ANOVA analyses for work regimen during the first lockdown and child gender.

	Work Regimen during the First Lockdown for COVID-19 * M (SD)					Child's Gender M (SD)	
	Smart Working (N = 140)	**Work at the Workplace** (N = 64)	**Suspension of Activities** (N = 39)	**Layoffs** (N = 12)	**Lost Job** (N = 10)	**Male** (N = 178)	**Female** (N = 130)
TOT BR² *	59.9 (61.1)	56.8 (59.4)	63.7 (69.7)	72.2 (52.1)	75.8 (74.1)	59 (64.6)	64.5 (58.2)
			F = 0.342; p-value = 0.850; η^2_p = 0.005 Tot (N = 265) 60.6 (61.9)			F = 0.604; p-value = 0.438; η^2_p = 0.002 Tot (N = 308) 61.3 (61.9)	
Common Antecedents **	18.7 (22.2)	16.3 (22.5)	19.2 (25.4)	24.6 (19.3)	18.1 (25)	17.2 (23.8)	20.4 (21.5)
			F = 0.374; p-value = 0.827; η^2_p = 0.006 Tot (N = 265) 18.4 (22.6)			F = 1.506; p-value = 0.221; η^2_p = 0.005 Tot (N = 308) 18.5 (22.9)	
Specific Antecedents ***	41.1 (41.6)	40.4 (39.8)	44.5 (46.6)	47.5 (37.8)	57.7 (50.9)	41.8 (43.6)	44.1 (39.3)
			F = 0.462; p-value = 0.763; η^2_p = 0.007 Tot (N = 265) 42.4 (42)			F = 0.229; p-value = 0.632; η^2_p = 0.001 Tot (N = 308) 42.7 (41.8)	

* Min and max scores: −195; +195. ** Min and max scores: −70; +70. *** Min and max scores: −125; +125.

3.2. Parental Perception of Children's Executive Functions and Correlations with Parental Distress

The parental perception of children's EFs descriptive data are given in Tables 7–12; while correlation data are showed in Table 13.

Table 7. EF descriptive data and ANOVA analysis for child and parental age.

	Child Age M (SD)				Parental Age M (SD)		
	4–6 (N = 70)	7–10 (N = 101)	11–13 (N = 137)		<36 (N = 50)	36–45 (N = 163)	>45 (N = 95)
EF Working Memory	11.2 (3.7)	12.3 (3.2)	12.6 (3.4)		11.3 (4)	12.3 (3.2)	12.4 (3.3)
	F = 3.491; p-value = 0.032; η^2_p = 0.02			Tot (N = 308) 12.2 (3.4)	F = 2.098; p-value = 0.124; η^2_p = 0.01		
EF Attentional Control	11.5 (2.9)	11.8 (2.6)	12.1 (3.2)		11.5 (3.2)	12 (2.8)	11.9 (3.2)
	F = 1.184; p-value = 0.308; η^2_p = 0.008			Tot (N = 308) 11.9 (3)	F = 0.571; p-value = 0.566, η^2_p = 0.004		
EF Planning	10.2 (3.3)	11 (2.6)	11.7 (3.2)		10.3 (3.3)	11.2 (2.8)	11.3 (3.2)
	F = 5.188; p-value = 0.006; η^2_p = 0.03			Tot (N = 308) 11.1 (3.1)	F = 2.019; p-value = 0.135; η^2_p = 0.01		
EF Shifting	11.4 (3.5)	12 (3.1)	12.4 (3.3)		11.2 (3.8)	12.3 (3.1)	12.1 (3.3)
	F = 2.192; p-value = 0.113; η^2_p = 0.01			Tot (N = 308) 12 (3.3)	F = 2.023; p-value = 0.134; η^2_p = 0.01		
EF Inhibition	10.8 (3.1)	12 (3)	12.6 (3.6)		10.8 (3.7)	12.3 (3.1)	12 (3.6)
	F = 5.926; p-value = 0.001; η^2_p = 0.04			Tot (N = 308) 12 (3.4)	F = 3.873; p-value = 0.022; η^2_p = 0.02		
EF Tot	55.2 (14.8)	59.2 (12.6)	61.5 (15.4)		55.2 (16.2)	60.3 (13.4)	59.9 (15.3)
	F = 4.387; p-value = 0.013; η^2_p = 0.03			Tot (N = 308) 59.3 (14.6)	F = 2.465; p-value = 0.087; η^2_p = 0.01		

Min and max scores for each subscale: 4; 16.

Table 8. EF descriptive data for educational level.

	Educational Level M (SD)				
	Primary and Middle School (N = 20)	Professional School (N = 24)	High School (N = 94)	Degree (N = 122)	PhD/ Specialization (N = 48)
EF Working Memory	12 (2.8)	12.4 (2.9)	12.1 (3.2) F = 1.117; p-value = 0.348; η^2_p = 0.01 Tot (N = 308) 12.2 (3.4)	12.6 (3.3)	11.3 (4.4)
EF Attentional Control	11.9 (2.8)	12.2 (2)	11.8 (2.6) F = 2.040; p-value = 0.089; η^2_p = 0.03 Tot (N = 308) 11.9 (3)	12.3 (3)	10.9 (3.8)
EF Planning	10.9 (2.3)	11.5 (2.7)	11 (2.7) F = 0.608; p-value = 0.657; η^2_p = 0.008 Tot (N = 308) 11.1 (3.1)	11.3 (3.4)	10.6 (3.5)
EF Shifting	12.7 (2.2)	12.7 (2.5)	12.1 (3.2) F = 1.927; p-value = 0.106; η^2_p = 0.02 Tot (N = 308) 12 (3.3)	12.2 (3.3)	10.9 (3.9)
EF Inhibition	13.3 (2.5)	12.8 (3.2)	11.8 (3.2) F = 2.646; p-value = 0.034; η^2_p = 0.03 Tot (N = 308) 12 (3.4)	12.2 (3.4)	10.8 (3.8)
EF Total	60.9 (10.4)	61.8 (10.9)	59 (12.9) F = 1.737; p-value = 0.142; η^2_p = 0.02 Tot (N = 308) 59.3 (14.6)	60.7 (15.1)	54.7 (18.4)

Table 9. EF descriptive data and ANOVA analyses for parental work regimen during the first lockdown, child gender, and child with typical/atypical development condition.

	Work Regimen during the First Lockdown for COVID-19 * M (SD)					Child Gender M (SD)		Child Typ/Atyp Development M (SD)	
	Smart Working (*N* = 140)	**Work at the Workplace (*N* = 64)**	**Suspension of Activities (*N* = 39)**	**Layoffs (*N* = 12)**	**Lost Job (*N* = 10)**	**Male (*N* = 178)**	**Female (*N* = 130)**	**No (*N* = 270)**	**Yes (*N* = 38)**
EF Working Memory	12.3 (3.4)	11.6 (3.5)	12.1 (3.4)	12.2 (3.5)	13.3 (3.5)	12.3 (3.4)	11.9 (3.5)	12.3 (3.5)	11.1 (2.8)
			F = 0.706; *p*-value = 0.589; η^2_p = 0.011 Tot (*N* = 265) 12.1 (3.4)			F = 0.980; *p*-value = 0.323; η^2_p = 0.003 Tot (*N* = 308) 12.2 (3.4)		F = 4.240; *p*-value = 0.040; η^2_p = 0.014 Tot (*N* = 308) 12.2 (3.4)	
EF Attention Control	12 (3)	11.3 (3)	12.1 (2.8)	13.2 (1.7)	12.7 (3.2)	11.9 (2.8)	11.9 (3.2)	12 (3)	10.8 (2.3)
			F = 1.543; *p*-value = 0.190; η^2_p = 0.023 Tot (*N* = 265) 11.9 (2.9)			F = 0.002; *p*-value = 0.969; η^2_p = 0.00 Tot (*N* = 308) 11.9 (3)		F = 5.271; *p*-value = 0.022; η^2_p = 0.017 Tot (*N* = 308) 11.9 (3)	
EF Planning	11.4 (3)	10.5 (2.8)	11.1 (3.2)	11.2 (3.6)	13.1 (2.5)	10.9 (3)	11.3 (3.2)	11.1 (3.1)	10.8 (2.5)
			F = 1.959; *p*-value = 0.101; η^2_p = 0.029 Tot (*N* = 265) 11.2 (3)			F = 1.078; *p*-value = 0.300; η^2_p = 0.004 Tot (*N* = 308) 11.1 (3.1)		F = 0.413; *p*-value = 0.521; η^2_p = 0.001 Tot (*N* = 308) 11.1 (3.1)	
EF Shifting	12 (3.2)	11.6 (3.5)	11.7 (3.2)	12.8 (2.8)	13.5 (3.5)	12.1 (3.2)	11.9 (3.4)	12.2 (3.3)	11 (2.7)
			F = 0.918; *p*-value = 0.454; η^2_p = 0.014 Tot (*N*= 265) 12 (3.3)			F = 0.106; *p*-value = 0.745; η^2_p = 0.00 Tot (*N* = 308) 12 (3.3)		F = 3.806; *p*-vlaue = 0.052; η^2_p = 0.012 Tot (*N* = 308) 12 (3.3)	
EF Inhibition	12.2 (3.3)	11.4 (3.6)	12 (3.5)	12.7 (2.5)	12.4 (2.8)	11.8 (3.3)	12.2 (3.5)	12 (3.4)	11.8 (3)
			F = 0.737; *p*-value = 0.567; η^2_p = 0.011 Tot (*N* = 265) 12 (3.3)			F = 0.704; *p*-value = 0.402; η^2_p = 0.002 Tot (*N* = 308) 12 (3.4)		F = 0.055; *p*-value = 0.816; η^2_p = 0.00 Tot (*N* = 308) 12 (3.4)	
EF Total	60 (14.3)	56.5 (15)	59.1 (14.3)	62.3 (13.1)	65 (14.3)	59.3 (14)	59.4 (15.4)	59.8 (15)	55.8 (10.6)
			F = 1.181; *p*-value = 0.319; η^2_p = 0.018 Tot (*N* = 265) 59.3 (14.5)			F = 0.013; *p*-value = 0.908; η^2_p = 0.00 Tot (*N* = 308) 59.3 (14.6)		F = 2.551; *p*-value = 0.111; η^2_p = 0.008 Tot (*N* = 308) 59.3 (14.6)	

Min and max scores for each subscale: 4; 16. * concerns work regimen during the first lockdown, 43 answers are missing.

Table 10. EF descriptive data and ANOVA analyses for couples' conditions and psychological support needs.

	Couples' Conditions M (SD)			Psychological Support Needs M (SD)	
	Married (*N* = 260)	**Cohabiting (*N* = 23)**	**Separated (*N* = 22)**	**No (*N* = 206)**	**Yes (*N* = 102)**
EF Working Memory	12.3 (3.3)	11.6 (4.2)	12.5 (3.4)	12.5 (3.5)	11.6 (3.2)
		F = 0.451; *p*-value = 0.637; η^2_p = 0.003	Tot (*N* = 308) 12.2 (3.4)	F = 4.687; *p*-value = 0.031; η^2_p = 0.015	
EF Attentional Control	12 (2.8)	11.5 (3.5)	11.5 (3.9)	12.2 (3)	11.3 (2.7)
		F = 0.596; *p*-value = 0.552; η^2_p = 0.004	Tot (*N* = 308) 11.9 (3)	F = 5.648; *p*-value = 0.018; η^2_p = 0.018	
EF Planning	11.2 (3)	10 (3.9)	11.2 (2.9)	11.4 (3.4)	10.5 (2.2)
		F = 1.635; *p*-value = 0.197; η^2_p = 0.001	Tot (*N* = 308) 11.1 (3.1)	F = 5.509; *p*-value = 0.020; η^2_p = 0.018	
EF Shifting	12.1 (3.2)	12 (3.8)	12 (3.5)	12.3 (3.4)	11.5 (3)
		F = 0.001; *p*-value = 0.999; η^2_p = 0.001	Tot (*N* = 308) 12 (3.3)	F = 3.951; *p*-value = 0.048; η^2_p = 0.013	
EF Inhibition	12 (3.3)	12 (3.9)	11.8 (3.9)	12.4 (3.4)	11.1 (3.2)
		F = 0.037; *p*-value = 0.963; η^2_p = 0.001	Tot (*N* = 308) 12 (3.4)	F = 9.222; *p*-value = 0.003; η^2_p = 0.029	
EF Tot	59.8 (14.1)	57.3 (18.5)	59.3 (15.3)	60.9 (15.4)	56.2 (12.2)
		F = 0.319; *p*-value = 0.727; η^2_p = 0.002	Tot (*N* = 308) 59.3 (14.6)	F = 7.151; *p*-value = 0.008; η^2_p = 0.023	

Min and max scores for each subscale: 4; 16.

Table 11. EF descriptive data and ANOVA analyses for order of birth.

	Order of Birth M (SD)		
	First Born (N = 209)	Second Born (N = 78)	Third Born and beyond (N = 21)
EF Working Memory	12.1 (3.6)	12.4 (3.2) F = 0.335; p-value = 0.715; η^2_p = 0.002 Tot (N = 308) 12.2 (3.4)	12.5 (2.9)
EF Attentional Control	11.9 (3)	11.9 (2.8) F = 0.062; p-value = 0.940; η^2_p = 0.001 Tot (N = 308) 11.9 (3)	11.7 (2.9)
EF Planning	11.1 (3.2)	11.1 (2.8) F = 0.033; p-value = 0.968; η^2_p = 0.001 Tot (N = 308) 11.1 (3.1)	11.2 (3.3)
EF Shifting	11.9 (3.4)	12.2 (3.1) F = 0.281; p-value = 0.755; η^2_p = 0.002 Tot (N = 308) 12 (3.3)	12.2 (2.7)
EF Inhibition	11.9 (3.4)	12.2 (3.3) F = 0.301; p-value = 0.740; η^2_p = 0.002 Tot (N = 308) 12.2 (3.4)	12.3 (3.3)
EF Total	59 (15.1)	60 (13.5) F = 0.154; p-value = 0.857; η^2_p = 0.001 Tot (N = 308) 59.3 (14.6)	60.1 (13.6)

Min and max scores for each subscale: 4; 16.

Table 12. EF descriptive data and ANOVA analyses for parental job condition.

	Job Condition M (SD)							
	Housewives (N = 33)	Student (N = 11)	Government Employee (N = 108)	Manager (N = 15)	Free-Lancer (N = 59)	Teacher (N = 44)	Unemployed (N = 14)	Other (N = 24)
EF Working Memory	12.2 (3.6)	12.3 (3.6)	12.2 (3.2)	12.4 (3.6)	12.4 (3.4)	12.1 (3.9)	12.1 (3.3)	11.2 (3.7)
	F = 0.306; p-value = 0.951; η^2_p = 0.007 Tot (N = 308) 12.2 (3.4)							
EF Attention Control	12 (2.9)	11.7 (3.5)	12 (2.4)	11.4 (3.5)	11.8 (3.3)	11.9 (3.8)	11.7 (3.2)	11.8 (2.7)
	F = 0.116; p-value = 0.997; η^2_p = 0.003 Tot (N = 308) 11.9 (3)							
EF Planning	11.2 (2.5)	10.5 (3.6)	11.4 (2.7)	11.6 (2.9)	11.1 (3.1)	11 (3.7)	11.5 (3.3)	9.6 (3.5)
	F = 1.087; p-value = 0.371; η^2_p = 0.02 Tot (N = 308) 11.1 (3.1)							
EF Shifting	12.3 (3.5)	11.3 (2.8)	12.6 (2.9)	12.4 (3.3)	11.9 (3.4)	11.2 (3.8)	11.9 (3.8)	11.2 (3.2)
	F = 1.206; p-value = 0.299; η^2_p = 0.03 Tot (N = 308) 12 (3.3)							
EF Inhibition	12.4 (3.5)	10.4 (2.6)	12.5 (2.7)	12 (3.5)	12 (3.4)	11.7 (4.2)	10.9 (3.7)	10.7 (3.9)
	F = 1.548; p-value = 0.151; η^2_p = 0.03 Tot (N = 308) 12 (3.4)							
EF Total	60.2 (14)	56.4 (14.2)	61 (11.7)	59.8 (15.9)	59.4 (15.7)	58 (18.6)	58.2 (16.1)	54.8 (15.3)
	F = 0.675; p-value = 0.693; η^2_p = 0.02 Tot (N = 308) 59.3 (14.6)							

Min and max scores for each subscale: 4; 16.

Table 13. Correlation between BR2 and EF variables.

Variables	1	2	3	4	5	6	7	8	9
1. BR^2 Tot	-								
2. Common Antecedents	0.920 **	-							
3. Specific Antecedents	0.977 **	0.814 **	-						
4. EF Tot	0.333 **	0.289 **	0.334 **	-					
5. EF Working Memory	0.308 **	0.256 **	0.316 **	0.897 **	-				
6. EF Attention Control	0.294 **	0.247 **	0.299 **	0.906 **	0.839 **	-			
7. EF Planning	0.256 **	0.238 **	0.249 **	0.861 **	0.689 **	0.730 **	-		
8. EF Shifting	0.325 **	0.268 **	0.335 **	0.924 **	0.798 **	0.786 **	0.723 **	-	
9. EF Inhibition	0.299 **	0.280 **	0.289 **	0.877 **	0.668 **	0.706 **	0.720 **	0.810 **	-

** $p \leq 0.01$.

Concerning the parental perception of children's EFs, statistically significant differences were found as the effect of having children with typical/atypical patterns of development, parental age, parental educational level, and children's age; in particular, there was a significant effect on having children with typical/atypical patterns of development on working memory ($F(1, 307) = 4.24$; $p < 0.05$; $\eta^2_p = 0.014$), attention ($F(1, 307) = 5.271$; $p < 0.01$; $\eta^2_p = 0.017$) and shifting ($F(1, 307) = 3.806$; $p < 0.05$; $\eta^2_p = 0.012$), in spite of the low effect size value. Parents of children exhibiting atypical patterns of development rated the lowest performance of their children on working memory, attention, and shifting tasks. Moreover, there was a significant effect of parental age on children's inhibition ($F(1, 307) = 3.87$; $p < 0.01$; $\eta^2_p = 0.02$); in fact, younger parents (<36 years old) rated the lowest performance of their children on inhibitory control tasks. Furthermore, there was a significant effect of children's age on parental perception of working memory ($F(1, 307) = 3.491$; $p < 0.05$; $\eta^2_p = 0.02$), planning ($F(1, 307) = 5.188$; $p < 0.01$; $\eta^2_p = 0.03$), inhibition ($F(1, 307)= 6.926$; $p = 0.001$; $\eta^2_p = 0.04$), and EF total score ($F(1, 307) = 4.387$; $p = 0.01$; $\eta^2_p = 0.03$); in particular, the younger children (4–6 years) were perceived by their parents as less able to cope with tasks of working memory, planning, and inhibition. Moreover, there was a significant effect of the parents' educational levels on parental perception of children's EFs inhibition ($F(1, 307) = 2.646$; $p < 0.05$; $\eta^2_p = 0.03$).

Finally, correlation analyses were performed to assess the association between parental distress and parental perception of children's EFs. Positive significant correlations ($p < 0.01$) were found among each component of parental distress and each component of the child's EF perception, demonstrating how parents with higher levels of resources and minor levels of distress perceived their children as more able to perform tasks requiring EF competencies during a COVID-19 lockdown.

Considering the correlational data, a multiple linear regression was performed with the stepwise method (see Table 14); the variable "common antecedents" was removed in relation to all pf the EF components, as a probability of $F \geq 0.100$ was found (significance of F with regard to the common antecedents: 0.989 for working memory, 0.929 for attention control, 0.269 for planning, 0.874 for shifting, and 0.157 for inhibition). The data are in line with what we expect, based on the correlations carried out, which showed a stronger correlation between the different EFs considered and the specific antecedents.

Table 14. Linear regression analysis relating specific antecedents and each component of ESA.

Dependent Variables	Model	R	R Square	R Square Change	F Change	gl1	gl2	Sig. F Change
EF Working memory	1	0.316	0.100	0.097	33.832	1	306	0.000
EF Attention control	1	0.299	0.090	0.087	30.153	1	306	0.000
EF Planning	1	0.249	0.062	0.059	20.232	1	306	0.000
EF Shifting	1	0.335	0.112	0.109	38.642	1	306	0.000
EF Inhibition	1	0.289	0.084	0.081	27.915	1	306	0.000

Predictors: (constant): SPECIFIC ANTECEDENTS.

4. Discussion

The current study provided a multifaceted investigation of parental distress and parental perception of children's EFs following the spread of the novel coronavirus (COVID-19) pandemic and the first lockdown in Italy.

Based on previous data demonstrating how distress affected parents more than those who did not have children, as well as younger parents [55,56], we hypothesized that, during the first COVID-19 lockdown, the parents who experienced the greatest distress perceived their children as more difficult to manage and more at risk of developmental frailty. More distressed parents, indicating a lack of resources or a prevalence of risk factors, are more likely to be too overwhelmed by the pandemic; this prevents them from supporting their children and responding to children's questions, fears, and difficulties [57,58]. When children do not find emotional containment and responsive answers to their preoccupations from their parents, they are more likely to show higher levels of distress, with more difficulties in emotional and behavioral domains, such as inattention, concentration problems, and dysregulation [26,58].

Our findings confirm previous research by showing a general distressful condition in most of the parents who participated in this study [26,59,60]. This distressful condition is underlined by an average (and a widely variable) level of claimed resources; in fact, some parents (<36 years old) described their conditions by referring to the presence of moderate available resources, other parents (36–45 years old) indicated very few resources.

Furthermore, as previous studies showed [52,61,62], the risk factors for parenting distress are closely related to sociodemographic characteristics, such as child features and family functioning; our data on parental distress focused on the possible effects of sociodemographic variables, highlighting a high-risk group for parenting-related distress, characterized by the following factors: having a child with atypical patterns of development and needing specialist support (psychological or psychotherapeutic intervention) during the pandemic.

These data underline how, during the pandemic, the lack of important resources, such as adequate social support by family and friends, could be predictors of parental burnout (common antecedents). The lower rates of distress levels in parents who declared to have asked for help during the lockdown, such as professional help, underline the importance of psychological support being offered to parents in this phase of an epochal crisis. Moreover, being the parent of a child exhibiting atypical patterns of development was found to be a big source of distress, referring both to general predictors of parental burnout (common antecedents) and aspects strictly related to parental burnout (specific antecedents). This condition also affected parental perception of EF children. Children exhibiting atypical patterns of development were perceived as less able to manage and perform tasks requiring working memory, shifting, and attention processes during the lockdown. On the other hand, this is coherent with well-documented results in the literature showing a poorer performance on EF, especially working memory, in children with special needs [63].

According with some current research [64–66], parents of children with disabilities or chronic disease suffered the most from a complete lockdown, experiencing several new problems and increasing those already existing before the pandemic. A large amount of literature demonstrates how parents of children exhibiting atypical development experienced higher levels of parental distress compared to parents of children exhibiting typical patterns of development [17–19,67]; however, during the lockdown, they reached higher levels of distress, just because they started from disadvantaged conditions. Our study confirmed the negative effects of home confinement on parental distress when children have a disability or developmental fragility; the unexpected lifestyle changes generated by the COVID-19 pandemic, were even more difficult for children exhibiting atypical development, as well as for their families [68], especially because the professional support of those specialists (physicians, therapists, psychologists, etc.) who took care of children had decreased. Parents had to reorganize the daily activities and structure them according to their children's needs, so this condition influenced both the wellbeing of parents and the psychological functioning and adjustment of the child [6,69,70]. Moreover, vulnerability factors, such as previous special needs, were demonstrated to enhance the appearance of psychological problems because of fears and worries concerning the worsening of atypical conditions, and the lack and/or limitation of external specialist support [33]. The literature has demonstrated how parents of children with disabilities are more likely to experience higher levels of parental distress characterized by perceptions of an imbalance between parenting requests and personal available resources. This can lead them to manage their children's education, "less sensitively", using less "efficacy-coping" strategies, or decreasing their ability to face challenging tasks with increasing risk of exacerbating their disability.

Therefore, we could hypothesize that, during the first COVID-19 lockdown, parents were more distressed compared to the stress faced during normal life conditions, and this might have increased their difficulty to manage the normal parental functions of caregiving and scaffolding [26]. Many parents likely experienced difficulties, in regard to satisfying the real needs of their children; at times, they might have overstimulated or hyper-controlled them, but often they hypo-stimulated them with little attention, in the absence of educational activities, in which the child could have otherwise experienced autonomy, self-efficacy, etc.

Moreover, our findings showed significant relationships between parental distress levels and the perception of the child's cognitive abilities. The most distressed parents perceived their children as less competent in EFs, highlighting their cognitive fragility in attention, memory, and self-regulation tasks. However, the opposite direction of this relationship is admissible and plausible, given that correlation analyses do not allow establishing any causal link. Parents who perceive their children as less competent on EF tasks might have experienced more distressful requests of parenting and scaffolding to compensate for the absence of external specialist help during the lockdown [43,45,46]. Thus, these parents perceived themselves as having minor resources to face distressful events.

Although the main goal of this study was to observe short-term effects of pandemic events after the first strict lockdown, and establish a bivariate association between investigated variables, following the above-discussed correlational findings, linear regression analyses were carried out. These findings showed the higher predictive value of specific antecedents on all EF components, working memory, attention control, planning, shifting and inhibition. We can conjecture that the distress conditions strictly related to parental burnout make parents more impatient, less tolerant, and less able to manage their children at home, and to accept and support the developmental fragility of their children. Thus, these parents can adopt education measures and parent–child interactions that hamper their child's self-regulatory skills, and end up influencing later cognitive development [47–49]. However, this causal relationship should be explored in more depth in the future; longitudinal studies can confirm these preliminary results.

5. Conclusions

To conclude, the findings of this study suggest that the first COVID-19 lockdown strongly influenced parental distress and their resources as well as parental perception of their children on working memory, attention, and shifting tasks, especially in the case of previous atypical development conditions. Thus, the evidence from this study reinforces the need to provide families with psychological aid, even in restrictive lockdown conditions, through different modalities, ranging from telephonic/electronic media platform consultations to online workshops that are able to support and/or enhance parenting skills, psychological techniques to deal with anxiety and parental distress, relaxation exercises, art therapy, and mindfulness training [6]. In the pandemic scenario, the role of psychological intervention is crucial for everyone, but it is needed for families of children with atypical development that experience temporary interruption of care assistance due to the increase in emotional fatigue (characterizing parenting strategies) and in children's pre-existing vulnerabilities. Practitioners need to implement autonomy-supportive programs to teach parents how to cope with stress, with the indirect aim to optimize outcomes for children with special needs. For example, programs to decrease parental stress reinforce the use of task-oriented and emotion-oriented coping strategies, to deliver the satisfaction of parental competence, even in abnormal pandemic conditions.

The strength of this study is that it contributes toward bridging the gap in the lack of research on parental distress and children's EF impairments during the COVID-19 lockdown, as affected by short-term consequences of pandemic conditions.

Nevertheless, future research is necessary to remedy the shortcomings of this study. The most important limitation lies in the relatively small size of our sample. This was because the recruitment of participants took place in a well-defined time-lapse, immediately after the end of the first spring lockdown in Italian, prior to the following autumn partial lockdown. This period was selected to investigate the short-term effects of pandemic events on cognitive development. Moreover, a low effect size for most comparisons was found, indicating the need of further analyses on other eventual variables, which play a role in the relationship between variables we investigated. Another shortcoming of this study lies in methodological concerns, as the measurement of children's EFs is based not on the administration of cognitive performance-based tests, but rather on rating scales that measured children's EFs through a parent-reported questionnaire, revealing parental perceptions of their children's cognitive abilities. The choice of this measure was forced by the need to carry out research online, given the pandemic conditions. However, this questionnaire was found, by previous researchers, to be an ecologically valid indicator of EF functioning in concrete, complex, and everyday life situations, as well as suitable for inclusion in research projects with children who require the study of numerous variables.

Author Contributions: Conceptualization, C.P., G.L., and M.A.; methodology, C.P.; software, M.A., S.B.; formal analysis, C.P., M.A.; resources, G.L.; data curation, S.B.; writing—original draft preparation, C.P., M.A., S.B.; writing—review and editing, C.P., M.A., S.B.; supervision, M.A. and G.L.; project administration, G.L. All authors have read and agreed to the published version of the manuscript.

Funding: This research received funding from Centro Siciliano Sturzo.

Institutional Review Board Statement: The study was conducted according to the guidelines of the Declaration of Helsinki and approved by the Ethics Committee of University of Palermo (protocol code n. 13/2020).

Informed Consent Statement: The study was anonymous and conducted via the internet (online questionnaire). Each respondent was informed that taking part in the research and submitting their results would be treated as the respondent's consent to participate in the study.

Data Availability Statement: The data presented in this study are available upon request from the corresponding author.

Conflicts of Interest: The authors declare no conflict of interest.

References

1. Brooks, S.K.; Webster, R.K.; Smith, L.E.; Woodland, L.; Wessely, S.; Greenberg, N.; Rubin, G.J. The psychological impact of quarantine and how to reduce it: Rapid review of the evidence. *Lancet* **2020**, *395*, 912–920. [CrossRef]
2. Cachón-Zagalaz, J.; Sánchez-Zafra, M.; Sanabrias-Moreno, D.; González-Valero, G.; Lara-Sánchez, A.J.; Zagalaz-Sánchez, M.L. Systematic review of the literature about the effects of the COVID-19 pandemic on the lives of school children. *Front. Psychol.* **2020**, *11*, 569348. [CrossRef]
3. Haleemunnissa, S.; Didel, S.; Swami, M.K.; Singh, K.; Vyas, V. Children and COVID-19: Understanding impact on the growth trajectory of an evolving generation. *Child. Youth Serv. Rev.* **2021**, *120*, 105754. [CrossRef]
4. Pedrosa, A.L.; Bitencourt, L.; Fróes, A.C.F.; Cazumbá, M.L.B.; Campos, R.G.B.; de Brito, S.B.C.S.; Silva, A.C.S. Emotional, behavioral, and psychological Impact of the COVID-19 Pandemic. *Front. Psychol.* **2020**, *11*, 566212. [CrossRef]
5. Gassman-Pines, A.; Ananat, E.O.; Fitz-Henley, J. COVID-19 and parent-child psychological well-being. *Pediatrics* **2020**, *146*, e2020007294. [CrossRef]
6. Liu, C.H.; Doan, S.N. Psychosocial distress contagion in children and families during the COVID-19 pandemic. *Clin. Pediatr.* **2020**, *59*, 853–855. [CrossRef] [PubMed]
7. Hsiao, Y.J. Parental stress in families of children with disabilities. *Interv. Sch. Clin.* **2018**, *53*, 201–205. [CrossRef]

8. Sprang, G.; Silman, M. Posttraumatic distress disorder in parents and youth after health-related disasters. *Disaster Med. Public Health Prep.* **2013**, *7*, 105–110. [CrossRef] [PubMed]
9. Chen, R.; Chou, K.R.; Huang, Y.J.; Wang, T.S.; Liu, S.Y.; Ho, L.Y. Effects of a SARS prevention programme in Taiwan on nursing staff's anxiety, depression and sleep quality: A longitudinal survey. *Int. J. Nurs. Stud.* **2006**, *43*, 215–225. [CrossRef] [PubMed]
10. Hawryluck, L.; Gold, W.L.; Robinson, S.; Pogorski, S.; Galea, S.; Styra, R. SARS control and psychological effects of quarantine. *Emerg. Infect. Dis.* **2004**, *10*, 1206.
11. Yoon, M.K.; Kim, S.Y.; Ko, H.S.; Lee, M.S. System effectiveness of detection, brief intervention and refer to treatment for the people with post-traumatic emotional didistress by MERS: A case report of community-based proactive intervention in South Korea. *Int. J. Ment. Health Syst.* **2016**, *10*, 51. [CrossRef]
12. Zhang, J.J.; Dong, X.; Cao, Y.Y.; Yuan, Y.D.; Yang, Y.B.; Yan, Y.Q.; Akdis, C.A.; Gao, Y.D. Clinical characteristics of 140 patients infected with SARS-CoV-2 in Wuhan, China. *Allergy* **2020**, *75*, 1730–1741. [CrossRef]
13. Cusinato, M.; Iannattone, S.; Spoto, A.; Poli, M.; Moretti, C.; Gatta, M.; Miscioscia, M. Distress, Resilience, and Well-Being in Italian Children and Their Parents during the COVID-19 Pandemic. *Int. J. Environ. Res. Public Health* **2020**, *17*, 8297. [CrossRef]
14. Qiu, J.; Shen, B.; Zhao, M.; Wang, Z.; Xie, B.; Xu, Y. A nationwide survey of psychological distress among Chinese people in the COVID-19 epidemic: Implication and policy recommendations. *Gen. Psychiatr.* **2020**, *33*, e100213. [CrossRef]
15. Mazza, C.; Ricci, E.; Marchetti, D.; Fontanesi, L.; Di Giandomenico, S.; Verrocchio, M.C.; Roma, P. How Personality Relates to Distress in Parents during the COVID-19 Lockdown: The Mediating Role of Child's Emotional and Behavioral Difficulties and the Moderating Effect of Living with Other People. *Int. J. Environ. Res. Public Health* **2020**, *17*, 6236. [CrossRef]
16. Maunder, R. The experience of the 2003 SARS outbreak as a traumatic distress among frontline healthcare workers in Toronto: Lessons learned. *Philos. Trans. R. Soc. Lond. B Biol. Sci.* **2004**, *359*, 1117–1125. [CrossRef] [PubMed]
17. Estes, A.; Olson, E.; Sullivan, K.; Greenson, J.; Winter, J.; Dawson, G.; Munson, J. Parenting-related distress and psychological didistress in mothers of toddlers with autism spectrum disorders. *Brain Dev.* **2013**, *35*, 133–138. [CrossRef] [PubMed]
18. Theule, J.; Wiener, J.; Tannock, R.; Jenkins, J.M. Parenting distress in families of children with ADHD: A meta-analysis. *J. Emot. Behav. Disord.* **2013**, *21*, 3–17. [CrossRef]
19. Hayes, S.A.; Watson, S.L. The impact of parenting distress: A meta-analysis of studies comparing the experience of parenting distress in parents of children with and without autism spectrum disorder. *J. Autism Dev. Disord.* **2013**, *43*, 629–642. [CrossRef]
20. Dhiman, S.; Sahu, P.K.; Reed, W.R.; Ganesh, G.S.; Goyal, R.K.; Jain, S. Impact of COVID-19 outbreak on mental health and perceived strain among caregivers tending children with special needs. *Res. Dev. Disabil.* **2020**, *107*, 103790. [CrossRef] [PubMed]
21. Cluver, L.; Lachman, J.M.; Sherr, L.; Wessels, I.; Krug, E.; Rakotomalala, S.; Blight, S.; Hillis, S.; Bachman, G.; Green, O.; et al. Parenting in a time of COVID-19. *Lancet* **2020**, *395*, e64. [CrossRef]
22. Griffith, A.K. Parental Burnout and Child Maltreatment during the COVID-19 Pandemic. *J. Fam. Violence* **2020**, 1–7. [CrossRef]
23. Horiuchi, S.; Shinohara, R.; Otawa, S.; Akiyama, Y.; Ooka, T.; Kojima, R.; Yokomichi, H.; Miyake, K.; Yamagata, Z. Caregivers' mental distress and child health during the COVID-19 outbreak in Japan. *PLoS ONE* **2020**, *15*, e0243702. [CrossRef]
24. Aksenova, E.I.; Kamynina, N.N.; Metelskaya, A.V.; Shkrumyak, A.R. On the Need for Psychological Support for Citizens in the Context of the COVID-19 Pandemic. *Probl. Sotsial'noi Gig. Zdr. Istor. Meditsiny* **2021**, *29*, 572–575. (In Russian) [CrossRef]
25. Perricone, G.; Rotolo, I.; Beninati, V.; Billeci, N.; Ilarda, V.; Polizzi, C. The Lègami/Legàmi Service-An Experience of Psychological Intervention in Maternal and Child Care during COVID-19. *Pediatr. Rep.* **2021**, *13*, 142–161. [CrossRef] [PubMed]
26. Demaria, F.; Vicari, S. COVID-19 quarantine: Psychological impact and support for children and parents. *Ital. J. Pediatr.* **2021**, *47*, 58. [CrossRef] [PubMed]
27. Spinelli, M.; Lionetti, F.; Pastore, M.; Fasolo, M. Parents' distress and children's psychological problems in families facing the COVID-19 outbreak in Italy. *Front. Psychol.* **2020**, *11*, 1713. [CrossRef] [PubMed]
28. Petrocchi, S.; Levante, A.; Bianco, F.; Castelli, I.; Lecciso, F. Maternal Didistress/Coping and Children's Adaptive Behaviors during the COVID-19 Lockdown: Mediation Through Children's Emotional Experience. *Front. Public Health* **2020**, *8*, 587833. [CrossRef]
29. Liu, Q.; Zhou, Y.; Xie, X.; Xue, Q.; Zhu, K.; Wan, Z.; Whu, H.; Zang, J.; Song, R. The prevalence of behavioral problems among school-aged children in home quarantine during the COVID-19 pandemic in china. *J. Affect. Disord.* **2021**, *279*, 412–416. [CrossRef]
30. Yeasmin, S.; Banik, R.; Hossain, S.; Hossain, M.N.; Mahumud, R.; Salma, N.; Hossain, M.M. Impact of COVID-19 pandemic on the mental health of children in Bangladesh: A cross-sectional study. *Child. Youth Serv. Rev.* **2020**, *117*, 105277. [CrossRef]
31. Orgilés, M.; Morales, A.; Delvecchio, E.; Mazzeschi, C.; Espada, J.P. Immediate psychological effects of the COVID-19 quarantine in youth from Italy and Spain. *Front. Psychol.* **2020**, *11*, 2986. [CrossRef]
32. Pisano, L.; Galimi, D.; Cerniglia, L. A qualitative report on exploratory data on the possible emotional/behavioral correlates of COVID-19 lockdown in 4–10 years children in Italy. *PsyArXiv* **2020**. [CrossRef]
33. Saurabh, K.; Ranjan, S. Compliance and psychological impact of quarantine in children and adolescents due to COVID-19 pandemic. *Indian J. Pediatr.* **2020**, *87*, 532–536. [CrossRef]
34. Singh, S.; Roy, D.; Sinha, K.; Parveen, S.; Sharma, G.; Joshi, G. Impact of COVID-19 and lockdown on mental health of children and adolescents: A narrative review with recommendations. *Psychiatry Res.* **2020**, *293*, 113429. [CrossRef]
35. Jiao, W.Y.; Wang, L.N.; Liu, J.; Fang, S.F.; Jiao, F.Y.; Pettoello-Mantovani, M.; Somekh, E. Behavioral and emotional disorders in children during the COVID-19 epidemic. *J. Pediatr.* **2020**, *221*, 264. [CrossRef]
36. Diamond, A. Executive functions. *Annu. Rev. Psychol.* **2013**, *64*, 135–168. [CrossRef]

37. Friedman, N.P.; Miyake, A. Unity and diversity of executive functions: Individual differences as a window on cognitive structure. *Cortex* **2017**, *86*, 186–204. [CrossRef] [PubMed]
38. Miyake, A.; Friedman, N.P.; Emerson, M.J.; Witzki, A.H.; Howerter, A.; Wager, T.D. The unity and diversity of executive functions and their contributions to complex "Frontal Lobe" tasks: A latent variable analysis. *Cogn. Psychol.* **2000**, *41*, 49–100. [CrossRef] [PubMed]
39. Miyake, A.; Friedman, N.P. The Nature and Organization of Individual Differences in Executive Functions: Four General Conclusions. *Curr. Dir. Psychol. Sci.* **2012**, *21*, 8–14. [CrossRef] [PubMed]
40. He, Z.H.; Yin, W.G. Family Environments and Children's Executive Function: The Mediating Role of Children's Affective State and Distress. *J. Genet. Psychol.* **2016**, *177*, 143–155. [CrossRef] [PubMed]
41. Ming, H.; Zhang, F.; Jiang, Y.; Ren, Y.; Huang, S. Family socio-economic status and children's executive function: The moderating effects of parental subjective socio-economic status and children's subjective social mobility. *Br. J. Psychol.* **2021**. [CrossRef]
42. Piccolo, L.R.; Salles, J.F.; Falceto, O.G.; Fernandes, C.L.; Grassi-Oliveira, R. Can reactivity to distress and family environment explain memory and executive function performance in early and middle childhood? *Trends Psychiatry Psychother.* **2016**, *38*, 80–89. [CrossRef] [PubMed]
43. Campos-Gil, J.A.; Ortega-Andeane, P.; Vargas, D. Children's Microsystems and Their Relationship to Distress and Executive Functioning. *Front. Psychol.* **2020**, *11*, 996. [CrossRef]
44. Zebdi, R.; Goyet, L.; Pinabiaux, C.; Guellaï, B. Psychological Disorders and Ecological Factors Affect the Development of Executive Functions: Some Perspectives. *Front. Psychiatry* **2016**, *7*, 195. [CrossRef] [PubMed]
45. Neuenschwander, R.; Hookenson, K.; Brain, U.; Grunau, R.E.; Devlin, A.M.; Weinberg, J.; Diamond, A.; Oberlander, T.F. Children's stress regulation mediates the association between prenatal ma-ternal mood and child executive functions for boys, but not girls. *Dev. Psychopathol.* **2018**, *30*, 953–969. [CrossRef]
46. Shields, G.S.; Sazma, M.A.; Yonelinas, A.P. The effects of acute distress on core executive functions: A meta-analysis and comparison with cortisol. *Neurosci. Biobehav. Rev.* **2016**, *68*, 651–668. [CrossRef]
47. Wagner, S.; Müller, C.; Helmreich, I.; Huss, M.; Tadić, A. A meta-analysis of cognitive functions in children and adolescents with major depressive disorder. *Eur. Child Adolesc. Psychiatry* **2015**, *24*, 5–19. [CrossRef] [PubMed]
48. Carlson, S.M. Executive function in context: Development, measurement, theory, and experience. *Monogr. Soc. Res. Child Dev.* **2003**, *68*, 138–151. [CrossRef]
49. De Cock, E.S.A.; Henrichs, J.; Klimstra, T.A.; Janneke, B.M.; Maas, A.; Vreeswijk, C.M.J.M.; Meeus, W.H.J.; van Bakel, H.J.A. Longitudinal Associations Between Parental Bonding, Parenting Distress, and Executive Functioning in Toddlerhood. *J. Child Fam. Stud.* **2017**, *26*, 1723–1733. [CrossRef]
50. Schroeder, V.M.; Kelley, M.L. Family environment and parent-child relationships as related to executive functioning in children. *Early Child Dev. Care* **2010**, *180*, 1285–1298. [CrossRef]
51. Hackman, D.A.; Gallop, R.; Evans, G.W.; Farah, M.J. Socioeconomic status and executive function: Developmental trajectories and mediation. *Dev. Sci.* **2015**, *18*, 686–702. [CrossRef]
52. Di Giorgio, E.; Di Riso, D.; Mioni, G.; Cellini, N. The interplay between mothers' and children behavioral and psychological factors during COVID-19: An Italian study. *Eur. Child Adolesc. Psychiatry* **2020**, 1–12. [CrossRef]
53. Mikolajczak, M.; Roskam, I. A Theoretical and Clinical Framework for Parental Burnout: The Balance Between Risks and Resources (BR2). *Front. Psychol.* **2018**, *9*, 886. [CrossRef]
54. Holly, L.E.; Fenley, A.R.; Kritikos, T.K.; Merson, R.A.; Abidin, R.R.; Langer, D.A. Evidence-base update for parenting distress measures in clinical samples. *J. Clin. Child Adolesc. Psychol.* **2019**, *48*, 685–705. [CrossRef]
55. Costa, S.; Bianco, A.; Scifo, L.; Alesi, M. Preliminary evaluation of a short version questionnaire for Executive Functioning Self-Report (EF-SR). *Curr. Psychol.* **2020**, 1–10. [CrossRef]
56. American Psychological Association [APA]. *Distress in America 2020: Distress in the Time of COVID-19*; American Psychological Association: Washington, DC, USA, 2020; Volume 1.
57. Russell, B.S.; Hutchison, M.; Tambling, R.; Tomkunas, A.J.; Horton, A.L. Initial challenges of caregiving during COVID-19: Caregiver burden, mental health, and the parent–child relationship. *Child Psychiatry Hum. Dev.* **2020**, *51*, 671–682. [CrossRef] [PubMed]
58. Di Giovanni, C.; Conley, J.; Chiu, D.; Zaborski, J. Factors influencing compliance with quarantine in Toronto during the 2003 SARS outbreak. *Biosecur. Bioterror.* **2004**, *2*, 265–272. [CrossRef] [PubMed]
59. Marchetti, D.; Fontanesi, L.; Mazza, C.; Di Giandomenico, S.; Roma, P.; Verrocchio, M.C. Parenting-related exhaustion during the italian COVID-19 lockdown. *J. Pediatr. Psychol.* **2020**, *45*, 1114–1123. [CrossRef]
60. Brown, S.M.; Doom, J.R.; Lechuga-Peña, S.; Watamura, S.E.; Koppels, T. Stress and par-enting during the global COVID-19 pandemic. *Child Abus. Negl.* **2020**, *110*, 104699. [CrossRef] [PubMed]
61. Adadms, E.L.; Smith, D.; Caccavale, L.J.; Bean, M.K. Parents are stressed! Patterns of parent stress across COVID-19. *Front. Psychiatry* **2021**, *12*, 300. [CrossRef]
62. Mikolajczak, M.; Brianda, M.E.; Avalosse, H.; Roskam, I. Consequences of parental burnout: Its specific effect on child neglect and violence. *Child Abus. Negl.* **2018**, *80*, 134–145. [CrossRef]

63. Lindström, C.; Aman, J.; Norberg, A.L. Parental burnout in relation to sociodemographic, psychosocial and personality factors as well as disease duration and glycaemic control in children with Type 1 diabetes mellitus. *Acta Paediatr.* **2011**, *100*, 1011–1017. [CrossRef]
64. Houwen, S.; Van Der Veer, G.; Visser, J.; Cantell, M. The relationship between motor performance and parent-rated executive functioning in 3- to 5-year-old children: What is the role of confounding variables? *Hum. Mov. Sci.* **2018**, *53*, 24–36. [CrossRef]
65. Willner, P.; Rose, J.; Stenfert Kroese, B.; Murphy, G.H.; Langdon, P.E.; Clifford, C.; Langdon, P.; Cooper, V. Effect of the COVID-19 pandemic on the mental health of carers of people with intellectual disabilities. *J. Appl. Res. Intellect. Disabil.* **2020**, *33*, 1523–1533. [CrossRef]
66. Bentenuto, A.; Mazzoni, N.; Giannotti, M.; Venuti, P.; de Falco, S. Psychological impact of COVID-19 pandemic in Italian families of children with neurodevelopmental disorders. *Res. Dev. Disabil.* **2021**, *109*, 103840. [CrossRef] [PubMed]
67. Cacioppo, M.; Bouvier, S.; Bailly, R.; Houx, L.; Lempereur, M.; Mensah-Gourmel, J.; Kandalaft, C.; Varengue, R.; Chatelin, A.; Vagrnoni, J.; et al. Emerging health challenges for children with physical disabilities and their parents during the COVID-19 pandemic: The ECHO French survey. *Ann. Phys. Rehabil. Med.* **2020**, *64*, 101429. [CrossRef] [PubMed]
68. Rogers, G.; Perez-Olivas, G.; Stenfert Kroese, B.; Patel, V.; Murphy, G.; Rose, J.; Cooper, V.; Langdon, P.E.; Hiles, S.; Clifford, C.; et al. The experiences of mothers of children and young people with intellectual disabilities during the first COVID-19 lockdown period. *J. Appl. Res. Intellect. Disabil.* **2021**. [CrossRef] [PubMed]
69. Tomanik, S.; Harris, G.E.; Hawkins, J. The relationship between behaviours exhibited by children with autism and maternal distress. *J. Intellect. Dev. Disabil.* **2004**, *29*, 16–26. [CrossRef]
70. Nonweiler, J.; Rattray, F.; Baulcomb, J.; Happé, F.; Absoud, M. Prevalence and associated factors of emotional and behavioural difficulties during COVID-19 pandemic in children with neurodevelopmental disorders. *Child* **2020**, *7*, 128. [CrossRef] [PubMed]

Journal of
Clinical Medicine

MDPI

Article

Burden of COVID-19 Pandemic Perceived by Polish Patients with Multiple Sclerosis

Anna Pokryszko-Dragan [1], Justyna Chojdak-Łukasiewicz [1,*], Ewa Gruszka [1], Marcin Pawłowski [2], Tomasz Pawłowski [2], Anna Rudkowska-Mytych [2], Joanna Rymaszewska [2] and Sławomir Budrewicz [1]

[1] Department of Neurology, Wroclaw Medical University, Borowska 213, 50-556 Wroclaw, Poland; anna.pokryszko-dragan@umed.wroc.pl (A.P.-D.); ewa.gruszka@umed.wroc.pl (E.G.); slawomir.budrewicz@umed.wroc.pl (S.B.)

[2] Department of Psychiatry, Wroclaw Medical University, Wybrzeże Pasteura 10, 50-367 Wroclaw, Poland; marcin.pawlowski@student.umed.wroc.pl (M.P.); tomasz.pawlowski@umed.wroc.pl (T.P.); psychiatria@umed.wroc.pl (A.R.-M.); joanna.rymaszewska@umed.wroc.pl (J.R.)

* Correspondence: justyna.chojdak-lukasiewicz@umed.wroc.pl; Tel.: +48-71-734-3100; Fax: +48-71-734-3109

Abstract: People with multiple sclerosis (MS) were expected to be particularly affected by the COVID-19 pandemic. The purpose of the study was to evaluate the burden of pandemic, perceived by Polish MS patients, with regard to major contributing factors. The survey, conducted in August/September 2020, included: Perceived Stress Scale (PSS-10), Coping Orientations to Problems Experienced (Brief–COPE), questions on demographic data, MS characteristics, and health-related and social aspects of pandemic burden. Relationships were searched between PSS-10 and Mini-COPE results and other analyzed items, using U Mann–Whitney test, Kruskal–Wallis ANOVA rank test and Spearman rank correlation. The survey was answered by 287 MS patients (208 female, 79 male, aged 21–69 years). Since March 2020, 2.4% of respondents had been positive for COVID-19 and 5.2% had undergone a quarantine. Mean PSS-10 score was 19.99, with moderate or high level of stress in 83.3% of respondents. Problem-focused strategies were more frequently used than emotion-focused strategies (1.76 vs. 1.16). Higher PSS-10 score was associated with comorbidities (H = 4.28), increase in major MS symptoms during the pandemic (21.92 vs. 18.06), experience of healthcare limitations (21.12 vs. 17.98), work-related (22.58 vs. 18.69), financial (22.70 vs. 18.83) and family-related problems (22.54 vs. 17.73) due to pandemic restrictions. A coping model was associated with functional disability and limitations to daily activities (H = 7.81). During the first stage of the pandemic, MS patients reported increased level of stress and preferred problem-focused coping. The level of stress and coping showed more relationships with pandemic impact upon social issues than with MS-related variables.

Keywords: multiple sclerosis; COVID-19 pandemic; perceived stress; coping strategies

Citation: Pokryszko-Dragan, A.; Chojdak-Łukasiewicz, J.; Gruszka, E.; Pawłowski, M.; Pawłowski, T.; Rudkowska-Mytych, A.; Rymaszewska, J.; Budrewicz, S. Burden of COVID-19 Pandemic Perceived by Polish Patients with Multiple Sclerosis. *J. Clin. Med.* **2021**, *10*, 4215. https://doi.org/10.3390/jcm10184215

Academic Editor: Michele Roccella

Received: 6 September 2021
Accepted: 10 September 2021
Published: 17 September 2021

1. Introduction

The outbreak of novel coronavirus disease (COVID-19), declared by the WHO as a pandemic in March 2020, has had a profound and unprecedented impact upon health and social issues worldwide. Severe restrictions (closing of educational and cultural institutions, limitations to service facilities, recommended social distance) were instituted to mitigate rapid spreading of COVID-19 disease. Healthcare settings have been undergoing massive reorganization, prioritizing management of COVID-19 and providing safety for patients and staff, which resulted in interruption or limitation to certain services. A fear of life-threatening infection, accompanied by a rapid change in lifestyle and socio-economic problems, undoubtedly has had an adverse impact upon well-being of people throughout many countries.

Multiple sclerosis (MS) is a chronic, immune-mediated disease which affects the central nervous system, leading to its long-lasting and disseminated damage. Demyelinative lesions and axonal loss within brain and spinal cord cause multifocal symptoms and signs of neurological deficit. People with MS were expected to be particularly affected by the pandemic. Disability and immunocompromised status due to disease-modifying treatment (DMT) were initially considered as predisposing factors for severe course to various forms of therapy and rehabilitation [1,2]. Furthermore, cognitive and mental health problems which often occur in MS population, together with insufficient coping abilities, would make these patients more vulnerable to distress caused by the pandemic [3,4].

In Poland, the lockdown was introduced in March, with the restrictions gradually canceled during the summer months. The statement of experts from Polish Neurological Society, concerning management of MS during the pandemic, was published in March and updated in May [5]. The document included recommendations with regard to prevention and treatment of COVID-19 infection in MS population, safety issues at health care facilities, as well as initiation and continuation of DMT. National MS Society also aimed at providing information and support to the patients and their caregivers. Nevertheless, the pandemic has undoubtedly affected MS population in many aspects. Recognition of this impact from the patients' perspective seemed essential for addressing their needs and effective management of major problems emerging from pandemic consequences [6].

The purpose of the study was to evaluate the burden of the pandemic, perceived by Polish MS patients, including the level of experienced stress and coping strategies. We also aimed at identification of the factors most related to stress and coping, including demographics, MS-related and social issues.

2. Materials and Methods

The study questionnaire, based on relevant literature, was created by neurologists and psychologists experienced in MS (Supplementary Materials). The following sections were included:

- Sociodemographic data;
- Exposure to COVID-19 infection;
- MS-related items: general clinical characteristics of the disease and its course during the pandemic;
- Social aspects of the pandemic burden.

The participants were asked to report all the aspects of the pandemic burden experienced from March 2020 to the time of responding to the survey.

Perceived Stress Scale (PSS-10) [7] was introduced to measure a level of experienced stress and the shortened version of Coping Orientations to Problems Experienced (Brief–COPE) [8]—to evaluate coping strategies. Both tools were provided in the standardized Polish version [9].

PSS-10 [7,9] contains 10 items which refer to subjective perception of situations and problems within the preceding 4 weeks. Response to each item can be scored 0–4 and their sum makes the total score, ranging from 0 to 40. Higher score indicates greater level of perceived stress. According to a 10-degree sten scale, a total score within stens 1–4 reflects low level of stress, between 5 and 6 sten—moderate level, and above 7—high level of stress.

Brief-COPE [8,9] consists of 28 items, associated with 14 coping strategies. The response to each item is rated 1–4 and the average score is calculated for each coping strategy, indicating its utilization by the subject. Coping strategies can be also categorized into their main types.

The survey was conducted parallel through online and printed modes in August and September 2020. Computer-assisted web interviewing (CAWI), an Internet surveying technique in which the interviewee follows a script provided in a website, allowed to create Google Forms, with the link posted on the central website of Polish MS Society and throughout social media profiles of its regional divisions.

The printed version of the same questionnaire was freely distributed among the willing subjects visiting the two major outpatient clinics in Lower Silesia (south-western region of Poland). These subjects were informed about two eligible versions of survey and were requested to submit only one of them. Completed printed questionnaires were collected by medical assistants not involved in the research team. After six weeks the number of respondents to the online survey reached 128 and no new responses were recorded within the next two weeks. By then, 159 complete responses to the printed questionnaires had been collected and the database was closed.

The responses collected by CAWI method were downloaded, the responses from printed questionnaires were recorded as the text files and all the data were transferred into Microsoft Excel (Microsoft Corporation, Redmond, WA, USA) spread sheet for statistical analysis.

Mean values with standard deviation were calculated for PSS-10 and Brief-COPE scores, and the distribution of responses in particular categories was analyzed. Relationships were searched between PSS-10 and Brief-COPE results and other analyzed variables.

To select proper statistical methods, a normality of distribution for all continuous variables was verified with a Shapiro–Wilk test. For the majority of variables, an assumption of normal distribution was not met. Therefore, non-parametric tests were used for the analysis. Comparisons between two independent groups were performed with U Mann–Whitney test or t-Student test if the proper assumptions were met. In case of comparisons for which an independent variable was of a categorical type, a Kruskal–Wallis ANOVA rank test was applied. To assess the correlations, the Spearman rank correlation was applied. To assess the independence of categorical variables, Pearson Chi-square test was used. A *p*-value less than 0.05 was considered statistically significant. The statistical analysis was performed using STATISTICA PL v.8 statistical software (StatSoft, Kraków, Poland).

The project of the study was approved by Local Bioethical Committee at Wroclaw Medical University. Participation in the survey was voluntary and without any financial compensation. Anonymity of the responses was maintained throughout collection and storage of data. An informed consent form to participate in the study and allow procession of data for research purposes was provided in the initial part of the questionnaire. Its confirmation in the online version was necessary to proceed with responding to the questions and submit the filled questionnaire. In the printed version, consent was confirmed by signing the form and completion of the questionnaire.

3. Results

3.1. Characteristics of the Study Group

The study comprised 287 people with MS (208 female, 79 male, aged 21–69 years, mean 41.05). Among this number, 128 people (97 females, 31 males, mean age 36.44 years) responded through the online version of the survey and 159 people (111 females, 48 males, mean age 44.76 years) responded through the printed version. Table 1 presents the demographic characteristics of respondents.

Duration of MS in the study group ranged between 1 and 40 years (mean: 11.8). The majority of patients (165) had relapsing-remitting MS, although 30% could not define the type of disease. Among the major MS-related complaints, the most frequent included fatigue, disturbance of gait, balance problems and vertigo (Table 2). Minor or mild functional disability with unlimited distance of ambulation was declared by 86.4% of respondents. DMT were used in 81.9% of patients and only symptomatic treatment—in 11.8% (Table 2). Comorbidities reported by 121 respondents included: endocrine disorders—thyroid gland diseases, diabetes (38), cardiovascular system diseases—hypertension, coronary artery disease (35), bronchial asthma (12), psychiatric conditions—depression, anxiety disorders (10), spondyloarthrosis (8), other immune-mediated diseases (rheumatoid arthritis, psoriasis) (6), endometriosis (6), and glaucoma (6).

Since the onset of the pandemic (March 2020), 73 patients (25.4%) experienced a relapse, which in 64 cases was confirmed by consulting neurologist. Out of these patients, 50 were treated with i.v. infusions of corticosteroids (in- or outpatient schedule) and 14 with oral medications. Within this timeframe, 144 of respondents (50.2%) reported an increase in frequency and/or severity of previously experienced major MS symptoms, and 27 (9.4%) observed some new symptoms, including headache, mood disturbances and insomnia.

Table 1. Demographic characteristics of the study group.

	All Group $n = 287$	**Paper Version** $n = 159$	**On-Line Version** $n = 128$
	Marital status		
married	155 (54%)	97	58
single	54 (18.8%)	27	27
living together	56 (19.5%)	20	36
divorced	14 (4.9%)	9	5
widowed	6 (2.1%)	5	1
separated	2 (0.7%)	1	1
	Children		
No	126 (43.9%)	51	75
Yes	161 (56.1%)	108	53
number of children: 1	78	52	26
2	71	49	22
3	9	6	3
4	3	1	2
	Living environment		
city	148 (51.6%)	73	75
small town	80 (27.9%)	45	35
village	59 (20.5%)	41	18
	Education level		
primary school	5 (1.7%)	4	1
vocational school	16 (5.6%)	13	3
high school diploma	110 (38.3%)	70	40
university degree	156 (54.4%)	72	84
	Occupation status		
student	9 (3.1%)	0	9
unemployed	18 (6.3%)	12	6
employed (full-time job)	147 (51.2%)	71	76
employed (part-time job)	21 (7.3%)	10	11
self-employed	14 (4.9%)	11	3
retired	17 (5.9%)	14	3
disability pensioner	61 (21.3%)	41	20

Table 2. Clinical characteristics of the study group.

Type of MS	
relapsing-remitting (RRMS)	165 (57.5%)
primary or secondary progressive (PPMS/SPMS)	35 (12.2%)
undefined	87 (30.3%)
Functional disability level	
minor (unlimited mobility)	130 (45.3%)
mild (limited ambulation distance)	118 (41.1%)
moderate (need for assistive devices)	33 (11.5%)
severe (using wheelchair)	6 (2.1%)
Most debilitating MS symptoms	
fatigue	123 (42.9%)
gait disturbance	112 (39%)
vertigo/disturbed balance	83 (28.9%)
upper limbs dysfunction	68 (23.7%)
sensory impairment	68 (23.7%)
bladder dysfunction	57 (19.9%)
visual impairment	57 (19.9%)
cognitive decline	54 (18.8%)
Disease modifying therapy (DMT) $n = 235$	
dimethylfumarate	74 (31.5%)
IFN ß-1a	44 (18.7%)
IFN ß-1b	37 (15.7%)
fingolimod	29 (12.3%)
teriflunomide	22(9.4%)
glatiramer acetate	13 (5.5%)
natalizumab	9 (3.8%)
ocrelizumab	2 (0.9%)
cladribine	1(0.4%)
experimental therapy in clinical trials	3 (1.3)
immunosuppressive treatment (azatioprine)	1 (0.4%)

The respondents to the printed version of the survey less often had relapsing-remitting MS and more often could not define MS type in comparison to those who responded online (45.9% RRMS, 42.1% undefined vs. 71.88% RRMS, 16.6% undefined, respectively, $p < 0.0001$). The online respondents more often experienced an increase in their major MS symptoms (60.94% vs. 41.5%, $p = 0.001$). No other differences in MS-related issues were found between the subgroups of participants.

3.2. *Exposure to COVID-19*

Since March 2020, out of 46 (16%) patients who had been tested for COVID-19, 7 (2.4%) were positive and 3 of them needed hospitalization. Fifteen patients (5.2%) had undergone a quarantine, while 19 (6.6%) reported COVID-19 infection in a family member or a close person. No significant difference in occurrence of relapse was found between the subjects exposed to COVID-19 and those who were not (20.06% vs. 19.98%). The subgroups of respondents to the online and printed version of the survey did not differ in reported exposure to COVID-19.

3.3. Health Care-Related Impact of the Pandemic

Problems with the access to a neurologist were reported by 63 (21.9%) respondents, with the access to a primary care physician or other specialist in 144 (50.2%) cases, and with access to rehabilitation in 103(35.9%). Thirty four (11.8%) subjects found relevant information about their condition hardly available. With regard to DMT, 29 (10.1%) patients reported the obstacles in continuation of scheduled treatment, 16 (5.6%)—a delay in introduction of treatment and 8 (2.8%)—a delay in planned switch to another DMT. Forty-five persons (15.7%) cancelled in- or outpatient visit because of fear of infection, and 34 of them were offered a remote consultation.

3.4. Social-Related Impact of the Pandemic

Work-related problems were reported by 96 patients (33%): 40 had their job suspended, 14 were fired, 14 experienced difficulties in turning to remote work, 8 complained of increased workload and 20 expressed fear of infection at workplace. Eighty-six subjects (30%) experienced financial problems.

Family-related problems were reported by 134 patients (46.7%) and included a concern about the health of family members, limited contacts due to epidemic restrictions, need to help children with online learning, compromising remote work with family issues and other conflict situations associated with staying at home during lockdown.

Due to the pandemic restrictions, 52.6% of respondents had to cancel or re-schedule an important life event. Moreover, 129 (44.9%) respondents reported problems with daily activities (shopping, household duties, small repairs, pet care) and 20 (6.9%) respondents needed extra help/support in this field.

3.5. PSS-10 and Brief-COPE Results

The mean PSS-10 score in the study group was 19.99 (range: 1–40). According to the sten scale, 48 subjects (16.7%) had a low level of perceived stress, 80 (27.9%) with a moderate level and 159 (55.4%) with a high level (Figure 1).

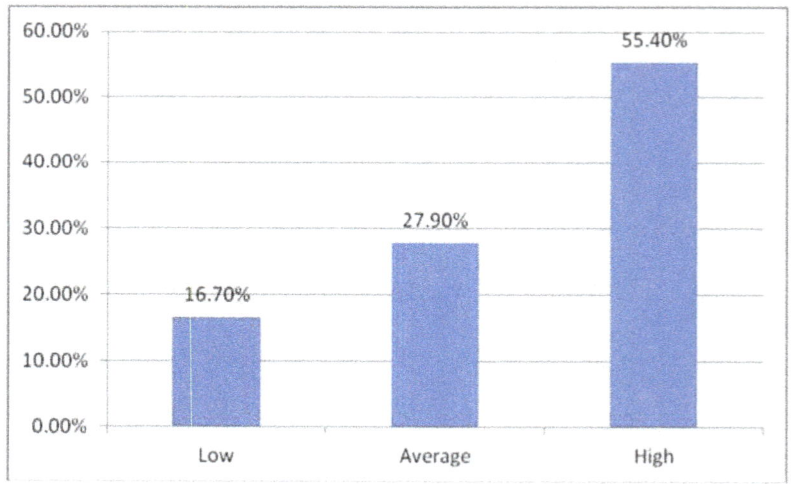

Figure 1. Distribution of PSS-10 results (sten scale indicating level of perceived stress) in the study group.

The mean PSS-10 score in the respondents to the online version of the survey was significantly higher than in the respondents to the printed version (21.78, SD 6.8 vs. 18.56, SD 6.77, $p < 0.0001$).

According to the Brief-COPE results from the study group, the most commonly used coping strategies were: acceptance, planning and positive reframing. Substance use, behavioral disengagement, religious coping or denial were the least frequently used ones (Figure 2). With regard to the main categories of coping, problem-focused strategies were more preferred than emotion-focused ones (1.76 vs. 1.16). (Figure 2). The respondents to the online version of the survey less often used emotion-focused coping strategies than the respondents to the printed version (1.07 vs. 1.24, $p = 0.01$).

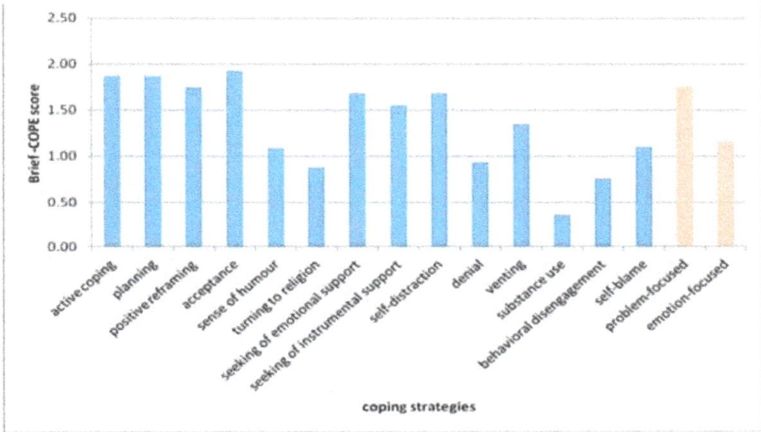

Figure 2. Use of coping strategies according to the Brief-COPE results in the study group.

3.6. Relationships of PSS-10 and Brief-COPE Results with Other Variables

The PSS-10 score negatively correlated with age ($R = -0.150$, $p = 0.011$) and was higher in females than in males (20.94 vs. 17.52, $p < 0.0001$). The patients who declared increased frequency/severity of their major MS-related symptoms, had higher PSS-10 score than the remaining ones (21.92 vs. 18.06, $p < 0.0001$), and such significant difference was observed for those with comorbidities ($p = 0.0386$). No other relationships were found between PSS-10 score and demographic or clinical factors.

Significantly higher level of stress in PSS-10 was associated with health care-related shortcomings (21.12 vs. 17.98, $p = 0.0010$), work-related problems (22.58 vs. 18.69, $p = 0.000024$), financial difficulties (22.70 vs. 18.83, $p = 0.000024$), family-related problems (22.54 vs. 17.73, $p = 0.000000$) and a need for extra help in daily activities (23.65 vs. 19.72, $p = 0.0155$).

There was a significant negative correlation between level of stress in PSS-10 and a preference for problem-focused coping strategies ($R = -0.1293$, $p = 0.0284$).

Emotion-focused strategies were more frequently used by females (1.23 vs. 0.97, $p = 0.0012$). The respondents with moderate and severe functional disability more often than the others used problem-focused strategies ($p = 0.049$). The patients who experienced increase in major MS symptoms, less often had substance use ($p = 0.0428$), behavioral disengagement ($p = 0.0032$) and self-blame strategies ($p = 0.0395$) than the remaining ones. A need for help in daily living was significantly associated with the use of problem-focused (2.04 vs. 1.42, $p = 0.0401$) and emotion-focused strategies (1.42 vs. 1.14, $p = 0.0378$).

No other relationships were found between the PSS-10 or Brief-COPE results and demographic, clinical or pandemic-related factors.

4. Discussion

The COVID-19 pandemic was demonstrated to cause an increased level of anxiety and depression, and a worse sleep quality in MS patients throughout different countries [2,10–13]. The Italian authors of [14] reported a greater prevalence of severe stress (measured in PSS-10) in MS subjects, in comparison with the healthy controls or the patients with migraine. The results of PSS-10 in our study indicate a moderate or high level of perceived stress in a vast majority of respondents (more than 80%). The international cohort surveys, conducted during the pandemic, also revealed a moderate to high level of stress in healthy adults, with mean PSS-10 score up to 19 points [15,16]. MS subjects are considered to have greater susceptibility to stress, due to the background of the disease (autoimmune response associated with autonomic and endocrine dysregulation) and its specificity (long-lasting and unpredictable course, accumulating disability). However, a diverse range of PSS-10 score had been obtained in the studies in this field [17–22], which suggests individual differences in perception of stress in MS population. With regard to the pandemic, no comparative studies were conducted with the use of PSS-10, but a prevalence of anxiety and depression in MS patients did not increase in comparison with the pre-pandemic assessment [10,23]. Thus, it remains disputable whether the pandemic has indeed enhanced distress experienced by MS patients.

There is some evidence [3,24–26] that people with MS tend to undertake passive and emotion-focused coping strategies, which makes them more vulnerable to stressful life events. However, adaptation to the limitations posed by a disease, as well as psychological support, may cause a shift towards more active and effective coping. The Brief-COPE results showed that the respondents to our survey overall preferred problem-focused coping, with planning, active coping and positive reframing as the most frequently used strategies. In another study, Spanish MS patients, surveyed during the pandemic, favored active confrontation and religion, while their use of emotional support, humor and positive re-evaluation was less frequent than in healthy controls [4]. The Italian survey [13] also indicated preference for positive attitude, problem solving and turning to religion among MS patients. It is worth highlighting that epidemic restrictions significantly limited the access to the sources of instrumental (from health-care and rehabilitation facilities) and emotional (contacts with family and friends) support which provide a basis for relevant coping strategies [13]. MS patients perceived especially a decrease in social support as a major negative impact of lockdown [3,14]. In healthy adults, positive coping strategies were shown to moderate a distress caused by the pandemic [27,28], but it was suggested that preferred strategies might reflect a temporary reaction to an unprecedented traumatic situation, and not necessarily a usual coping model [27]. In our study group, the increased level of stress was associated with a weaker preference for problem-focused coping. Supposedly coping strategies in MS subjects have developed in the long-term course of disease but were additionally affected by a temporary pandemic distress.

4.1. Demographic and Social Factors

In the study group, the perceived level of stress was higher in younger and female patients, and the latter used emotion-focused coping strategies more often than males. Similar relationship between age and distress caused by the pandemic was observed in MS subjects [1,11,12,29] and in healthy adults [15,16]. Although elderly persons are regarded to be at greater risk of severe COVID-19 infection, their perception of stress is probably modified by memory of past experiences and regulation of emotion [16,29]. Moreover, in comparison with young adults, they are less burdened with work or family obligations and less frequently use internet social media as a source of information about the pandemic [1,12]. It is worth considering that both higher PSS-10 score and lower mean age were found in those who responded to the online version of our survey, in comparison with respondents to the printed version. Sex differences in perception of pandemic stress were consistently reported for general populations [15,16,27]. Although female and male MS subjects presented with a similar level of depression and anxiety [11], women more often expressed fear of COVID-19 infection and tended to avoid exposure [30]. It should be noted that due to greater disease prevalence in women, they constitute the majority of all the investigated MS groups, which may affect the findings.

Other demographic factors, including residence and education level, did not affect the level of stress or coping model in our MS group. Apart from the lower level of anxiety in MS patients with academic degree [11], no such relationships were found by other authors, either. However, a high proportion of those with completed university education among the respondents to our survey might have had some impact upon the results, e.g., with regard to coping. Although vocational status was not related to stress or coping, those of our respondents who experienced work-related or financial problems (ca. 1/3) due to epidemic restrictions declared significantly higher levels of stress. The pandemic's impact on the employment situation of our respondents included changes in type or schedule of work, as well as loss of job. Even more detrimental consequences were reported for MS patients in U.S. [30,31]. In the Italian MS subjects, unemployment during the pandemic significantly contributed to depression and anxiety [2]. Changes in employment (including remote work) and lower income level were considered as factors substantially mediating pandemic stress in healthy adults [15]. Vocational activity is an important element of MS patients' social functioning, often adversely affected by the disease. Current but also long-term work-related problems, resulting from pandemic restrictions, might significantly worsen their economic situation as well as psychosocial condition [31]. These issues should be addressed with adequate system of support and counseling.

Similar observations concerned a family situation of MS subjects in the study group. Level of stress and coping preferences did not depend on marital status or dependents, but the pandemic impact upon family life, reported by almost half of the respondents, caused an increased level of stress. Family-related concerns included emotional issues, as well as logistic problems with consequences of lockdown. A forced social distance which prevented relationships was shown to affect stress and well-being in MS patients [14]. On the other hand, more time spent at home with family or partners resulted in positive impacts on their mood and sexual satisfaction [23].

4.2. Exposure to COVID-19 Infection

Among the respondents to our survey, only a small percentage have become infected or exposed to COVID-19. In comparison with other countries, during the first months of the pandemic, the prevalence of COVID-19 and morbidity in Poland were relatively low. Furthermore, MS patients presumably considered themselves at greater risk of infection and thus were undertaking more preventive behavior [14]. The direct exposure to infection in our MS patients was not associated with higher level of stress, similarly to the findings about depression and anxiety, reported by Altschuler et al. [1]. However, those with comorbidities, supposedly increasing the risk of severe COVID-19, presented with higher PSS-10 score. In healthy adults, symptoms suggestive of COVID-19 or perceived increased susceptibility to infection were shown to increase level of stress [16,27]. It may be hypothesized that MS subjects, due to long-lasting disease, are more adapted to concerns about their health and perceived vulnerability [23].

4.3. MS Related Factors

Only 25% of the study group experienced a relapse during the pandemic, while more than a half reported an increased frequency or severity of their major MS-related complaints. In the study of Motolese et al. [2], only 20% of the patients experienced new or enhanced MS symptoms (mainly sensory impairment and fatigue), while the other authors did not focus on occurrence of relapses during the pandemic.

Our MS patients who reported an increase in chronic symptoms declared a higher level of perceived stress. However, there was no difference in PSS-10 results between those who had relapsed or not. Stress was often considered as a possible trigger of clinical or radiological MS activity, as well as the effect of adverse outcome of the disease [32–40]. A diversity of results from particular studies suggests a complexity of links between stress and MS course, including a "vicious cycle" mechanism. There are also contradictory findings from studies investigating the course of MS during extreme traumatic situations. No increase in relapses was observed in Japanese patients following the great earthquake in 2016 [40] or in Israeli patients exposed to Persian Gulf war in 1991 [41]. On the contrary, more frequent relapses (associated with greater subjective stress) were noted during the Hezbollah–Israel war in 2006, with life threat and displacement identified as the main sources of stress [42]. During the COVID-19 pandemic, a higher anxiety level was shown in the Egyptian patients with relapses [12] while no such association was confirmed for the U.S. ones [1]. It seems that major stressful events do not directly affect MS activity, but their impact is mediated by individual perception, as well as by support provided to the patients [43].

Interestingly, no significant relationships were found in the study group between level of stress or coping model and any MS-related measures. Only more severe disability (assisted walk) was associated with greater preference for problem-focused coping strategies, and the level of stress was higher for those who declared the need for extra help during pandemic. Thus, it seems that the impact upon social functioning was more related to stress and coping than the disease itself. It should be highlighted that the vast majority of our respondents declared minor or mild disability and relapsing-remitting type of MS. Furthermore, in comparison with other studies [1,13,14], relatively small percentage of our patients received second-line DMT (apparently due to more benign or stable course of disease). Perhaps those with more active MS and greater disability, who did not participate in the survey, would perceive themselves as more endangered by severe COVID-19 infection, which could have affected the overall results.

With regard to the management of health issues, ca. 20% of our respondents had problems with the access to a neurologist and initiating or continuing DMT, while almost a half complained of limited availability of rehabilitation or primary health care facilities. Otherwise, there was a small proportion of those who canceled their visits due to fear of infection. The studies conducted in U.S. MS populations demonstrated greater disturbances in health care services, both from the providers' and patients' side [30,31] Throughout the countries, appropriate preventive measures were arranged for MS care centers [44,45]. For reimbursement reasons, DMT in Poland are provided under the charge of the specialist centers, within the unified schedule supervised by National Health Fund. Thus, the main framework for the treatment and its monitoring was usually maintained, although local disruptions might have occurred due to health-related or organizational consequences of the pandemic. According to national recommendations for health care settings and the statement of Polish MS experts [5], safety measures were undertaken at MS centers: e.g., the schedule of visits adjusted to maintain distance, obligatory use of masks and hand disinfection, screening for symptoms of infection at the entrance. Depending on local resources, remote consultations were being arranged (phone calls, video calls, sending comments and diagnostic tests results via e-mail). Our respondents seemed satisfied with a specialist care and with information on their current situation, offered probably also by the patients' organizations.

4.4. Limitations and Strengths

Several limitations to this study should be considered, including a lack of a comparator group of healthy controls or pre-pandemic assessment of stress and coping in MS subjects. The study group cannot be treated as population-based because of its moderate size and some bias it was subjected to. The online survey (though distributed nationwide) favored those who have access to internet and are interested in activity of MS patients' organizations, while the printed version was distributed only in the two major outpatient centers in one region. A comparison of findings from these two subgroups of respondents revealed differences mainly in demographic but not MS-related items. Therefore, considering the moderate number of participants, we did not conduct further analyses for each subgroup separately.

Furthermore, the diagnosis of MS and disease-related issues were not verified through medical records or physician's opinion but only based on self-observation, which might have posed some ambiguity. The items on health-related issues either included a range of options to choose from (major MS symptoms, type of disease, treatment regimen) or allowed free-text answers (coexisting diseases, new symptoms), which might have also affected the results.

However, we believe that the findings from this study allow a better insight into MS patients' perspective of pandemic burden. Lessons learned from their experience may contribute to identification of the major aspects of pandemic impact, including some concealed and indirectly harmful issues, and expected long-term consequences. These aspects need to be addressed during the ongoing pandemic, but also in future plans of effective MS management [6,10,32]. Despite relatively preserved medical services, the patients suffered mainly from a disruption in holistic system of their support and pandemic effects on their economic status and daily living. Thus, informational and educational materials should focus not only on the current pandemic or MS-related issues, but also concern healthy lifestyle, effective coping and maintaining relationships [6,11]. Pandemic experiences might encourage a wider use of innovations: e.g., telehealth consultations, online physiotherapy programs. In view of long-term pandemic consequences, support and counseling should be provided in the field of mental well-being, as well as economic and work-related aspects [6,31].

5. Conclusions

Polish MS patients surveyed during the first stage of the COVID-19 pandemic presented with a moderate to high level of perceived stress and preferred problem-focused coping strategies. The burden of the pandemic perceived by the patients was associated mainly with their social functioning and, to a lesser degree, with health status or health care services. The level of stress and coping profile showed more relationships with pandemic impact upon social issues than with disease-related variables. Consequences of the pandemic should be addressed with adequate support and counseling in management of MS patients.

Supplementary Materials: The following are available online at https://www.mdpi.com/article/10.3390/jcm10184215/s1, Supplementary Materials: Covid MS questionnaire.

Author Contributions: Conceptualization, A.P.-D., J.R. and S.B.; Methodology, A.P.-D., M.P. and A.R.-M.; Software, M.P. and T.P.; Validation, M.P. and A.R.-M.; Formal Analysis, A.R.-M., J.C.-Ł. and M.P.; Investigation, A.P.-D., J.C.-Ł., E.G. and M.P.; Resources, J.C.-Ł. and E.G.; Data Curation, A.P.-D. and T.P.; Writing—Original Draft Preparation, A.P.-D. and J.C.-Ł.; Writing—Review and Editing, J.R. and T.P.; Visualization, J.C.-Ł.; Supervision, S.B. and J.R.; Project Administration, A.P.-D.; Funding Acquisition, A.P.-D. and S.B. All authors have read and agreed to the published version of the manuscript.

Funding: The study was supported with Wroclaw Medical University grant SUB.C 220.21.088.

Institutional Review Board Statement: The study was conducted according to the guidelines of the Declaration of Helsinki, and approved by the Ethics Committee of Wroclaw Medical University (Ref. No KB-417/2020).

Informed Consent Statement: Informed consent was obtained from all subjects involved in the study.

Data Availability Statement: The data presented in this study are available on request from the corresponding author.

Conflicts of Interest: The authors declare no conflict of interest.

References

1. Alschuler, K.N.; Roberts, M.K.; Herring, T.E.; Ehde, D.M. Distress and risk perception in people living with multiple sclerosis during the early phase of the COVID-19 pandemic. *Mult. Scler. Relat. Disord.* **2021**, *47*, 102618. [CrossRef]
2. Motolese, F.; Rossi, M.; Albergo, G.; Stelitano, D.; Villanova, M.; Di Lazzaro, V.; Capone, F. The psychological impact of COVID-19 pandemic on people with multiple sclerosis. *Front. Neurol.* **2020**, *11*, 580507. [CrossRef]
3. Haji Akhoundi, F.; Sahraian, M.A.; Naser Moghadasi, A. Neuropsychiatric and cognitive effects of the COVID-19 outbreak on multiple sclerosis patients. *Mult. Scler. Relat. Disord.* **2020**, *41*, 102164. [CrossRef] [PubMed]
4. Reguera-Garcia, M.M.; Liebana-Presa, C.; Alvarez-Barrio, L.; Gomes, L.A.; Fernandez-Martinez, E. Physical activity, resilience, sense of coherence and coping in people with multiple sclerosis in the situation derived from COVID-19. *Int. J. Environ. Res. Public Health* **2020**, *17*, 8202. [CrossRef]
5. Bartosik-Psujek, H.; Adamczyk-Sowa, M.; Kalinowska, A.; Kułakowska, A.; Zakrzewska-Pniewska, B.; Zaborski, J. Stanowisko dotyczące leczenia SM w przypadku ryzyka zakażenia koronawirusem wywołującym COVID-19. *Pol. Przegląd Neurol.* **2020**, *16*, 59–61.
6. Nicholas, J.A.; Shin, R.K.; Alvarez, E.; Hendin, B.; Nair, K.V.; Lublin, F.D. Pandemic forward:Lessons learned and expert perspectives on multiple sclerosis care in the COVID-19 era. *Mult. Scler. Relat. Disord.* **2021**, *49*, 2020–2022. [CrossRef] [PubMed]
7. Cohen, S.; Kamarck, T.; Mermrlstein, R. A global measure of perceived stress. *J. Health Soc. Behav.* **1983**, *24*, 385–396. [CrossRef] [PubMed]
8. Carver, C.S. You want to measure coping but your protocol's too long: Consider the brief COPE. *Int. J. Behav. Med.* **1997**, *4*, 92–100.
9. Juczynski, Z.; Oginska-Bulik, N. *Narzędzia Pomiaru Stresu i Radzenia Sobie Ze Stresem*; Pracownia Testów Psychologicznych: Warsaw, Poland, 2009.
10. Stojanov, A.; Malobabic, M.; Milosevic, V.; Stojanov, J.; Vojinovic, S.; Stanojevic, G.; Stevic, M. Psychological status of patients with relapsing-remitting multiple sclerosis during coronavirus disease-2019 outbreak. *Mult. Scler. Relat. Disord.* **2020**, *45*, 102407. [CrossRef] [PubMed]
11. Ramezani, N.; Ashtari, F.; Bastami, E.A.; Ghaderi, K.; Hosseini, S.M.; Naeini, M.K.; Rajabi, F.; Adibi, I. Fear and anxiety in patients with multiple sclerosis during COVID-19 pandemic; report of an Iranian population. *Mult. Scler. Relat. Disord.* **2021**, *50*, 102798. [CrossRef]
12. Talaat, F.; Ramadan, I.; Aly, S.; Hamdy, E. Are multiple sclerosis patients and their caregivers more anxious and more comitted to following the basic preventive measures during the COVID-19 pandemic? *Mult. Scler. Relat. Disord.* **2020**, *46*, 102580. [CrossRef]
13. Costabile, T.; Carotenuto, A.; Lavorgna, L.; Borriello, G.; Moiola, L.; Inglese, M.; Petruzzo, M.; Trojsi, F.; Ianniello, A.; Nozzolillo, A.; et al. COVID-19 pandemic and mental distress in multiple sclerosis: Implications for clinical management. *Eur. J. Neurol.* **2020**, in press. [CrossRef]
14. Bonavita, S.; Sparaco, M.; Russo, A.; Borriello, G.; Lavorgna, L. Perceived stress and social support in a large population of people with multiple sclerosis recruited online through the COVID-19 pandemic. *Eur. J. Neurol.* **2021**, in press. [CrossRef]
15. Adamson, M.M.; Phillips, A.; Seenivasan, S.; Martinez, J.; Grewal, H.; Kang, X.; Coetzee, J.; Luttenbacher, I.; Jester, A.; Harris, O.A.; et al. International prevalence and correlates of psychological stress during the global COVID-19 pandemic. *Int. J. Environ. Res. Public Health* **2020**, *17*, 9248. [CrossRef]
16. Limcaoco, R.S.G.; Mateos, E.M.; Fernández, J.M.; Roncero, C. Anxiety, worry and perceived stress in the world due to the COVID-19 pandemic, March 2020. Preliminary results. *MedRxiv* **2020**, in press. [CrossRef]
17. Scheffer, M.; Becker, J.; de Azeredo, L.A.; Grassi-Oliveira, R.; de Almeida, R.M.M. Subjective and physiological stress measurement in a multiple sclerosis sample and the relation with executive functions performance. *J. Neural Transm.* **2019**, *126*, 613–622. [CrossRef]
18. Sanaeinasab, H.; Saffari, M.; Hashempour, M.; Karimi Zarchi, A.A.; Alghamdi, W.A.; Koenig, H.G. Effect of a transactional model education program on coping effectiveness in women with multiple sclerosis. *Brain Behav.* **2017**, *7*, 1–9. [CrossRef] [PubMed]
19. Pritchard, M.; Elison-Bowers, P.; Birdsall, B. Impact of integrative restoration (iRest) meditation on perceived stress levels in multiple sclerosis and cancer outpatients. *Stress Health* **2010**, *26*, 233–237. [CrossRef]
20. Lamis, D.A.; Hirsch, J.K.; Pugh, K.C.; Topciu, R.; Nsamenang, S.A.; Goodman, A.; Duberstein, P.R. Perceived cognitive deficits and depressive symptoms in patients with multiple sclerosis: Perceived stress and sleep quality as mediators. *Mult. Scler. Relat. Disord.* **2018**, *25*, 150–155. [CrossRef] [PubMed]
21. Artemiadis, A.K.; Vervainioti, A.A.; Alexopoulos, E.C.; Rombos, A.; Anagnostouli, M.C.; Darviri, C. Stress management and multiple sclerosis: A randomized controlled trial. *Arch. Clin. Neuropsychol.* **2012**, *27*, 406–416. [CrossRef]
22. Senders, A.; Bourdette, D.; Hanes, D.; Yadav, V.; Shinto, L. Perceived Stress in Multiple Sclerosis: The Potential Role of Mindfulness in Health and Well-Being. *J. Evid.-Based Complementary Altern. Med.* **2014**, *19*, 104–111. [CrossRef]
23. Capuano, R.; Altieri, M.; Bisecco, A.; d'Ambrosio, A.; Docimo, R.; Buonanno, D.; Matrone, F.; Giuliano, F.; Tedeschi, G.; Santangelo, G.; et al. Psychological consequences of COVID-19 pandemic in Italian MS patients: Signs of resilience? *J. Neurol.* **2020**, *268*, 743–750. [CrossRef] [PubMed]
24. Goretti, B.; Portaccio, E.; Zipoli, V.; Razzolini, L.; Amato, M.P. Coping strategies, cognitive impairment, psychological variables and their relationship with quality of life in multiple sclerosis. *Neurol. Sci.* **2010**, *31*, 227–230. [CrossRef] [PubMed]
25. Nielsen-Prohl, J.; Saliger, J.; Güldenberg, V.; Breier, G.; Karbe, H. Stress-stimulated volitional coping competencies and depression in multiple sclerosis. *J. Psychosom. Res.* **2013**, *74*, 221–226. [CrossRef] [PubMed]

26. Kroencke, D.C.; Denney, D.R. Stress and coping in multiple sclerosis: Exacerbation, remission and chronic subgroups. *Mult. Scler.* **1999**, *5*, 89–93. [CrossRef]
27. Robillard, R.; Saad, M.; Edwards, J.; Solomonova, E.; Pennestri, M.-H.; Daros, A.; Veissiere, S.P.L.; Quilty, L.; Dion, K.; Nixon, A.; et al. Social, financial and psychological stress during an emerging pandemic: Observations from a population survey in the acute phase of COVID-19. *BMJ Open* **2020**, *10*, e043805. [CrossRef] [PubMed]
28. Yan, L.; Gan, Y.; Ding, X.; Wu, J.; Duan, H. The relationship between perceived stress and emotional distress during the COVID-19 outbeak: Effects of boredom proneness and coping style. *J. Anxiety Disord.* **2021**, *77*, 102328. [CrossRef]
29. Zhang, G.-X.; Sanabria, C.; Martinez, D.; Zhang, W.-T.; Gao, S.-S.; Aleman, A.; Granja, A.; Paramo, C.; Borges, M.; Izquierdo, G. Social and professional consequences of COVID-19 lockdown in patients with multiple sclerosis from 2 very different populations. *Neurologia* **2021**, *36*, 16–23. [CrossRef]
30. Vogel, A.C.; Schmidt, H.; Loud, S.; McBurney, R.; Mateen, F.J. Impact of the COVID-19 pandemic on the health care of >1000 People living with multiple sclerosis: A cross-sectional study. *Mult. Scler. Relat. Disord.* **2020**, *46*, 102512. [CrossRef] [PubMed]
31. Bishop, M.; Rumrill, S.P. The employment impact of the COVID-19 pandemic on Americans with MS: Preliminary analysis. *J. Vocat. Rehabil.* **2021**, *54*, 81–87. [CrossRef]
32. Buljevac, D.; Hop, W.C.J.; Reedeker, W.; Janssens, A.C.J.W.; Van der Meche, F.G.A.; Van Doorn, P.A.; Hintzen, R.Q. Self reported stressful life events and exacerbations in multiple sclerosis: Prospective study. *BMJ* **2003**, *327*, 646. [CrossRef]
33. Abdollahpour, I.; Nedjat, S.; Mansournia, M.A.; Eckert, S.; Weinstock-Guttman, B. Stress-full life events and multiple sclerosis: A population-based incident case-control study. *Mult. Scler. Relat. Disord.* **2018**, *26*, 168–172. [CrossRef]
34. Mohr, D.C.; Hart, S.L.; Julian, L.; Cox, D.; Pelletier, D. Association between stressful life events and exacerbation in multiple sclerosis: A meta-analysis. *Br. Med. J.* **2004**, *328*, 731–733. [CrossRef]
35. Mitsonis, C.I.; Zervas, I.M.; Mitropoulos, P.A.; Dimopoulos, N.P.; Soldatos, C.R.; Potagas, C.M.; Sfagos, C.A. The impact of stressful life events on risk of relapse in women with multiple sclerosis: A prospective study. *Eur. Psychiatry* **2008**, *23*, 497–504. [CrossRef]
36. Brown, R.F.; Tennant, C.C.; Sharrock, M.; Hodgkinson, S.; Dunn, S.M.; Pollard, J.D. Relationship between stress and relapse in multiple sclerosis: Part I. Important features. *Mult. Scler.* **2006**, *12*, 453–464. [CrossRef]
37. Palumbo, R.; Fontanillas, L.; Salmaggi, A.; La Mantia, L.; Milanese, C. Stressful life events and multiple sclerosis: A retrospective study. *Ital. J. Neurol. Sci.* **1998**, *19*, 259–260. [CrossRef]
38. Liu, X.J.; Ye, H.X.; Li, W.P.; Dai, R.; Chen, D.; Jin, M. Relationship between psychosocial factors and onset of multiple sclerosis. *Eur. Neurol.* **2009**, *62*, 130–136. [CrossRef] [PubMed]
39. Schwartz, C.E.; Foley, F.W.; Rao, S.M.; Bernardin, L.J.; Lee, H.; Genderson, M.W. Stress and course of disease in multiple sclerosis. *Behav. Med.* **1999**, *25*, 110–116. [CrossRef] [PubMed]
40. Heesen, C.; Mohr, D.C.; Huitinga, I.; Then Bergh, F.; Gaab, J.; Otte, C.; Gold, S.M. Stress regulation in multiple sclerosis-Current issues and concepts. *Mult. Scler.* **2007**, *13*, 143–148. [CrossRef] [PubMed]
41. Nisipeanu, P.; Korczyn, A. Psychological stress as risk factor for exacerbations in multiple sclerosis. *Neurology* **1993**, *43*, 1311–1312. [CrossRef] [PubMed]
42. Golan, D.; Somer, E.; Dishon, S.; Cuzin-Disegni, L.; Miller, A. Impact of exposure to war stress on exacerbations of multiple sclerosis. *Ann. Neurol.* **2008**, *64*, 143–148. [CrossRef]
43. Kanamori, Y.; Nakashima, I.; Takai, Y.; Misu, T.; Kuroda, H.; Nishiyama, S.; Takahashi, T.; Sato, S.; Fujimori, J.; Higuchi, J.; et al. Impact of the great east Japan earthquake in 2011 on MS and NMOSD: A study in sendai, Japan. *J. Neurol. Neurosurg. Psychiatry* **2017**, *88*, 362–365. [CrossRef] [PubMed]
44. Buonomo, A.; Brescia Morra, V.; Zappulo, E.; Lanzillo, R.; Gentile, I.; Montella, E.; Triassi, M.; Palladino, R.; Moccia, M. COVID-19 prevention and multiple sclerosis management: The SAFE pathway for the post-peak. *Mult. Scler. Relat. Disord.* **2020**, *44*, 102282. [CrossRef] [PubMed]
45. Moccia, M.; Lanzillo, R.; Brescia Morra, V.; Bonavita, S.; Tedeschi, G.; Leocani, L.; Lavorgna, L.; Digital Technologies Web and Social Media Study Group of the Italian Society of Neurology. Assessing disability and relapses in multiple sclerosis on tele-neurology. *Neurol. Sci.* **2020**, *41*, 1369–1371. [CrossRef] [PubMed]

Journal of
Clinical Medicine

MDPI

Article

Impact on the Mental and Physical Health of the Portuguese Population during the COVID-19 Confinement

Fátima Frade [1,2], Lia Jacobsohn [3,4], Juan Gómez-Salgado [5,6,*], Rosário Martins [7], Regina Allande-Cussó [8], Carlos Ruiz-Frutos [5,6,†] and João Frade [9,10,†]

1 Escola Superior de Enfermagem de Lisboa, 1600-190 Lisboa, Portugal; fatimafrade4@sapo.pt
2 Centro de Administração e Políticas Públicas (CAPP), University of Lisbon, 1300-666 Lisbon, Portugal
3 Escola Superior de Saúde, Universidade Atlântica, 2730-036 Barcarena, Portugal; ljacobsohn@uatlantica.pt
4 Centro de Medicina de Reabilitação do Alcoitão, 2649-506 Alcabideche, Portugal
5 Department of Sociology, Social Work and Public Health, Faculty of Labour Sciences, University of Huelva, 21007 Huelva, Spain; frutos@uhu.es
6 Safety and Health Postgraduate Programme, Universidad Espíritu Santo, Guayaquil 092301, Ecuador
7 Escola Superior de Saúde, Instituto Politécnico de Viana do Castelo, 4900-347 Viana do Castelo, Portugal; martins.maria@ess.ipvc.pt
8 Nursing Department, University of Seville, 41009 Sevilla, Spain; rallande@us.es
9 Instituto Politécnico de Leiria, Escola Superior de Saúde e Centre for Innovative Care and Health Technology (ciTechcare), 2411-901 Leiria, Portugal; joao.frade@ipleiria.pt
10 Unit for Multidisciplinary Research in Biomedicine (UMIB), University of Porto, 4099-002 Porto, Portugal
* Correspondence: salgado@uhu.es; Tel.: +34-959219700
† These authors have contributed equally and share the last position.

Citation: Frade, F.; Jacobsohn, L.; Gómez-Salgado, J.; Martins, R.; Allande-Cussó, R.; Ruiz-Frutos, C.; Frade, J. Impact on the Mental and Physical Health of the Portuguese Population during the COVID-19 Confinement. *J. Clin. Med.* **2021**, *10*, 4464. https://doi.org/10.3390/jcm10194464

Academic Editor: Michele Roccella

Received: 27 July 2021
Accepted: 22 September 2021
Published: 28 September 2021

Abstract: Confinement of the population has been one of the measures implemented by different governments to address the COVID-19 health crisis, and it has led to social isolation together with a disruption of daily activities. The aim of the study is to analyze psychological distress during the COVID-19 pandemic in Portugal. During the quarantine, a cross-sectional study was carried out on a sample of 2120 subjects over 18 years of age, resident and born in Portugal. Data were collected using a self-developed questionnaire that considered socio-demographic variables, physical symptoms, health conditions, and history of contact with COVID-19, as well as psychological alterations. The General Health Questionnaire (GHQ-12) was also included. Univariate and bivariate statistical analyses were performed. Predictive capacity was studied using logistic regression models. The results showed a higher percentage of individuals presenting psychological distress (57.2.0%), with a higher percentage identified among women (79.0%), and in people with a higher educational level (bachelor's + master's and doctorate) (75.8%). The predictor variables with the greatest weight were sex, educational level (graduation, master's, and doctorate), living with children or under 16 years of age, presence of symptoms, and quarantine in the last 14 days for having symptoms. Good self-assessment of health and working at home appear to be protective against psychological distress. These results highlight the impact of the COVID-19 pandemic on psychological distress and provide an opportunity to consider the need to implement specific multidisciplinary public health and mental health interventions in this pandemic situation.

Keywords: COVID-19; psychological distress; pandemic; public health; quarantine; mental health

1. Introduction

In 2019, the world was surprised by a pandemic caused by the new coronavirus (SARS-CoV-2), which was called COVID-19. COVID-19 began in Wuhan, China, and soon spread to the rest of the world. As of February 2021, there were 111,102,016 cases of infection by the new coronavirus and 2,462,911 deaths worldwide [1]. In Portugal, the number of confirmed cases of COVID-19 infection is 798,074 and the number of deaths is 16,023 [2]. Being an unknown virus, much research has been done in relation to it and also in relation to the impact it has had on the physical and psychological health of people living through the pandemic caused by it. The main physical signs and symptoms of the infection are fever, dry cough, dyspnea, odynophagia, headache, myalgia, chills, nausea, vomiting, diarrhoea, hemoptysis, and conjunctival congestion. The main psychological effects of the virus influence people's mental health, causing higher levels of stress, anxiety, psychological distress, and depression [3–8].

In the specific case of Portugal, in response to the rapid epidemiological evolution of the COVID-19 disease, and with the aim of containing the virus and moderating the social, health, and economic impact of the pandemic, a state of alarm was declared on 18 March 2020 [9]. During the state of emergency, mandatory confinement measures were adopted for infection control, like the limitation of free movement of citizens, favoring teleworking (except for essential professions for basic needs like health, food, and safety), face-to-face teaching activities were suspended in favor of online teaching (in different levels of education), and cultural, sporting, and religious activities were suspended. The obligation to maintain social distance, use of masks, and compliance with respiratory etiquette was maintained. Deconfinement began at the beginning of May. At this stage, the general infection control measures included the mandatory use of a mask; compliance with respiratory etiquette; maintaining social distance; avoiding contact with people who present symptoms suggestive of COVID-19; working from home whenever possible (telework); prioritizing using the telephone or electronic services to get in touch with other services, such as supermarkets, pharmacies, or other; contacting the health services in advance in case of need for medical care; and avoiding crowded places, unnecessary contacts (inside or outside the home), and promotion of or participation in events that bring together many people [2,9].

The impact of the COVID-19 pandemic on the physical and mental health of the population is undeniable, and the published evidence describes it as such [10]. Thus, it is estimated that 38.2% of the European population has psychological disorders related to COVID-19 [11]. Social distancing and self-isolation during the COVID-19 pandemic have challenged people's mental health and general well-being, contributing to increased mental health problems which include depression, anxiety, mood disorder, psychological distress, post-traumatic stress disorder, insomnia, fear, stigma, lack of self-esteem, and lack of self-control [12].

The risk factors that compromise the psychological well-being of people experiencing the COVID-19 pandemic are fear of not having economic conditions for the goods of first necessity and for food, fear of quarantine, level of health perception, degree of risk control, and risk perception. Other studies reveal, as risk factors for psychological well-being, the perception of increased risk of SARS, a history of contact with people tested positive, feeling symptoms similar to those of SARS, loss of social contact and breaking of family routines, and increase of sedentary behaviors [7,12–16]. Given the variability in the risk factors for developing psychological distress, and the protective factors identified, it is worth considering the need for further studies to refine these results. Despite the agreement on the presence of psychological distress during the COVID-19 pandemic situation, the characteristics of the population are disparate, and more variables need to be controlled [13].

In Portugal, the few studies conducted during the COVID-19 pandemic show that the Portuguese population deteriorated in their mental health conditions during the pandemic, and the percentage of anxiety and depression is evident [14]. Other symptoms presented by the Portuguese population are poor sleep quality, insomnia, fear, anxiety, depression, and obsessive-compulsive symptoms due to COVID-19 [15,16].

Studies carried out in Portugal have focused on identifying the percentages of psychological factors in the Portuguese population during the pandemic and listing different symptoms. In our study, in addition to identifying the psychological factors present in the Portuguese population, we also identify the factors that predict their development, thus making it possible to plan action measures that can be implemented with the aim of reducing the presence of these factors in other pandemic situations. Thus, the aim of this study is to analyze psychological distress in a Portuguese population sample during the COVID-19 pandemic to identify the existence of related sociodemographic and specific health factors.

2. Materials and Methods

2.1. Design

The study design was cross-sectional and observational.

2.2. Sample

The initial sample consisted of 3105 participants. Of these, 985 were discarded because they did not complete the questionnaire in its entirety. Thus, the final sample was 2120 people, recruited between April and October 2020.

The inclusion criteria for participants were: (i) 18 years old or older; (ii) Portuguese residents during the COVID-19 pandemic, and (iii) having accepted the informed consent.

2.3. Variables

Regarding socio-demographic variables, sex, age, marital status, level of education, employment status, number of people living with, living with a child or adolescent, and living with a disabled person were considered. Likewise, with regard to the specific situation related to COVID-19, the presence of symptoms, self-perceived level of health, and history of contact and/or exposure were also identified. Considering these variables as independent variables, psychological distress was set as a dependent variable.

It is worth mentioning that whether the items related to COVID-19 symptoms were present in the last 14 days was asked about, and the response options were listed as those stipulated by the World Health Organization. These included fever of 38 °C or higher, cough, headache, myalgia, dizziness, diarrhoea, sore throat, coryza, chills, and shortness of breath.

Following Wang et al. [17], physical and mental health status were evaluated by dichotomous ("Yes/No") questions, as follows: having a chronic illness, having a disability, being on medication, having been hospitalised in the last 14 days, and having attended a health service in the last 14 days.

Other variables were contact history and health status, using the Ilder and Benyamini approach, with small variants, in the current pandemic situation [17–21].

2.4. Instruments

An ad hoc questionnaire was designed that included all the variables described. Psychological adjustment was assessed using the General Health Questionnaire (GHQ-12), duly validated for the Portuguese population [22] and used as a screening tool for non-psychotic mental disorders in other pandemic situations [22,23]. This questionnaire consists of 12 items with four response options. If the participant chooses options 1 or 2, then the final score for this item is 0 points; however, if the participant selects options 3 and 4, the score of this item is 1 point. After calculating the total sum of these scores, the final range is between 0 and 12 points.

For the present study, the overall score with reliability estimated by Cronbach's alpha at 0.851 was used as a single factor. The cut-off point for the general population was 3, where subjects with scores greater than or equal to 3 were considered more likely to develop psychiatric morbidity [24,25].

2.5. Procedures

Initially, a rapid literature review was conducted regarding the psychological effects that other pandemics, and the protective measures implemented, had caused in the population. Based on these results, a preliminary version of the questionnaire was designed and assessed by a panel of experts composed of 10 professionals (three doctors, four nurses, and three psychologists, two of them specialists in clinical psychology). Once the tool had been refined and the relevant modifications had been made, a pilot study was carried out on a sample of 57 subjects, identified by non-probabilistic sampling, over 18 years of age, seeking a similar proportion between men and women (50.9% and 49.1%, respectively). The mean age of this sample of subjects was 41.87 years (SD = 11.86), 56.1% reported being married, and 57.9% reported having completed a master's or doctoral degree.

No subjects in the pilot study reported problems in understanding the items, and no problems were detected in the design and visualization of the survey on different devices (PC, tablet, or smartphone).

Qualtrics® XM platform was the software used for the creation, design, and dissemination of the survey in this study. For the field study, a non-probabilistic snowball sampling was also implemented, based on the dissemination of the link via email lists to universities and professional associations, who were asked to help in this dissemination process.

2.6. Ethical Considerations

The ethical principles set out in the Declaration of Helsinki [26] have been followed. Participants' permission was obtained by means of an informed consent form where they expressed their voluntary desire to participate. Data were recorded in an anonymous way and treated confidentially. The project was approved by the Research Ethics Committee of Atlântica—Instituto Universitário.

2.7. Data Analyses

A descriptive univariate and bivariate statistical analysis was carried out, after studying the normality of the data distribution, using SPSS (26.0) software (IBM, Armonk, NY, USA). Measures of central tendency and dispersion were used for quantitative variables, and frequencies and percentages for qualitative variables. For the bivariate analysis, Chi-squared and Student's *t*-statistics were used. Crammer's V and Cohen's d effect size indices were also calculated, considering the following cut-off points: 0 to 0.19, insignificant; 0.20 to 0.49, small; 0.50 to 0.79, medium; 0.80 and above, high.

After this, a logistic regression algorithm was run, controlling for sex and age, and including in the models tested the variables that proved to be significant ($p < 0.05$). Finally, a global predictive model was designed, which corresponds to model 5, where the relationship of all variables with the presence or absence of psychological problems is analyzed, that is, the predictive factors that predispose a person to the existence of psychological problems are analyzed by calculating the odds ratios (OR) with a 95% confidence interval.

3. Results

3.1. Psychological Distress

Table 1 shows the mean scores and standard deviations of the answers to the General Health Questionnaire questions given by the subjects.

The mean score for the total of the 12 points scale was 3.97 (SD = 3.43). Establishing a cut-off point of 3 or more points, 57.2% of the 2120 study participants presented psychological distress. Item 5, "Have you felt constantly overwhelmed and stressed?" (M = 2.68; SD = 0.90), and item 7, "Have you been able to enjoy your normal daily activities?" (M = 2.62; SD = 0.89), were the ones with the highest scores. In opposition, item 11, "Have you thought that you are a worthless person?" (M = 1.44; SD = 0.78), and item 10, "Have you lost confidence in yourself?" (M = 1.69; SD = 0.85), presented lower scores.

Table 1. General Health Questionnaire (n = 2120).

Items	M (SD)
1. Have you been able to concentrate well on what you are doing?	2.40 (0.69)
2. Have your worries made you lose a lot of sleep?	2.47 (0.99)
3. Have you felt that you are playing a useful role in life?	1.98 (0.69)
4. Have you felt capable of making decisions?	2.09 (0.54)
5. Have you felt constantly overwhelmed and stressed?	2.68 (0.90)
6. Have you had the feeling that you cannot overcome your difficulties?	2.13 (0.88)
7. Have you been able to enjoy your normal daily activities?	2.62 (0.89)
8. Have you been able to adequately cope with problems?	2.26 (0.59)
9. Have you felt unhappy or depressed?	2.22 (0.99)
10. Have you lost confidence in yourself?	1.69 (0.85)
11. Have you thought that you are a worthless person?	1.44 (0.78)
12. Do you feel reasonably happy considering all the circumstances?	2.27 (0.67)
Scale total (over 12 points)	3.97 (3.43)
Presence of psychological distress (cut point ≥ 3)	(%)
Yes	57.2
No	42.8

3.2. Sociodemographic Variables and Psychological Distress

With regard to the sociodemographic variables (Table 2), statistically significant differences were found between both groups as regards sex (χ^2 = 163.137, p < 0.001, V = 0.277). No statistically significant differences were observed in the presence of psychological distress with age (χ^2 = 1.394, p = 0.163, V = 0.063).

Table 2. Association between sociodemographic variables and psychological distress during the COVID-19 pandemic (n = 2120).

	n (%)	Psychological Distress		χ^2/t	p	Effect Size
		No (n = 908)	Yes (n = 1212)			
Sex						
Male	684 (32.3)	47.2	21.0	163.137	<0.001	0.277
Female	1436 (67.7)	52.8	79.0			
Age (mean (SD))	38.84 (13.00)	39.31 (14.60)	38.49 (11.66)	1.394	0.163	0.063
Marital Status						
Single	837 (39.5)	43.6	36.4	13.353	0.001	0.079
Married or living as a couple	1090 (51.4)	46.9	54.8			
Separated/divorced/widowed	193 (9.1)	9.5	8.8			
Educational level						
Secondary school	628 (29.6)	36.8	24.3	41.666	<0.001	0.140
University education (graduation)	721 (34.0)	28.9	37.9			
University education (master's or PhD)	771 (36.4)	34.4	37.9			
Employment status						
Working away from home	1450 (68.4)	67.3	69.2	8.328	0.016	0.063
Working from home	474 (22.4)	24.9	20.5			
Not working	196 (9.2)	7.8	10.3			
Type of dwelling						
Flat or Apartment	1210 (57.1)	54.3	59.2	5.011	0.025	0.049
House	910 (42.9)	45.7	40.8			
Living with children or under-16 youngsters						
No	1146 (54.1)	59.8	49.8	21.108	<0.001	0.100
Yes	974 (45.9)	40.2	50.2			
Living with disabled people						
No	1994 (94.1)	94.6	93.6	0.850	0.357	0.020
Yes	126 (5.9)	6.4	5.4			

Of the total number of subjects who presented psychological distress (1212 subjects, 57% of the sample), 79% were women, 54.8% were married or cohabiting, 75.8% had completed university studies (university studies: graduation, master's, and doctorate), and 69.2% worked outside the home. Regarding the conditions of the usual dwelling, 59.2% lived in a flat, and 50.2% lived with children under 16 years of age.

Statistically significant differences were also found regarding the variables marital status ($\chi^2 = 13.353$, $p = 0.001$, V = 0.079), employment status ($\chi^2 = 8.328$, $p = 0.016$, V = 0.063), and type of dwelling ($\chi^2 = 5.011$, $p = 0.025$, V = 0.063).

The percentage of high education (graduation + master's and PhD) status among those with psychological distress was 75.8%. In addition, as regards participants living with children or youngsters under the age of 16 (50.2%), a low percentage of psychological distress was described.

3.3. Physical Symptoms in the Past 14 Days and Psychological Distress

Regarding the presence of symptoms in the 14 days prior to participation in the study, the following was distribution was obtained (Table 3): headache (46.6%), coryza (30.1%), myalgia (24.7%), cough (15.3%), sore throat (14.7%), and to a lesser extent, subjects reported suffering from diarrhea (9.7%), dizziness (9.7%), chills (5.2%), dyspnea (3.6%), and fever above 38 °C for at least one day (1.1%).

Table 3. Association between physical symptoms in the past 14 days and psychological distress during the COVID-19 pandemic ($n = 2120$).

	n (%)	Psychological Distress		χ^2/t	*p*	Effect Size
		No (*n* = 908)	Yes (*n* = 1212)			
Fever (>38 °C for at least 1 day)						
No	2101 (99.1)	99.3	98.9	0.991	0.319	0.022
Yes	19 (0.9)	0.7	1.1			
Cough						
No	1848 (87.2)	90.5	84.7	16.021	<0.001	0.087
Yes	272 (12.8)	9.5	15.3			
Headache						
No	1350 (63.7)	77.4	53.4	129.709	<0.001	0.247
Yes	770 (36.3)	22.6	46.6			
Myalgia						
No	1702 (80.3)	86.9	75.3	43.855	<0.010	0.144
Yes	418 (19.7)	13.1	24.7			
Dizziness						
No	2013 (95.0)	97.5	93.1	20.948	<0.001	0.099
Yes	107 (5.0)	2.5	6.9			
Diarrhea						
No	1944 (91.7)	93.6	90.3	7.645	0.006	0.060
Yes	176 (8.3)	6.4	9.7			
Sore throat						
No	1870 (88.2)	92.1	85.3	22.785	<0.001	0.104
Yes	250 (11.8)	7.9	14.7			
Coryza						
No	1632 (77.0)	86.5	69.9	80.425	<0.001	0.195
Yes	488 (23.0)	13.5	30.1			
Chills						
No	2042 (96.3)	98.3	94.8	18.419	<0.001	0.093
Yes	78 (3.7)	1.7	5.2			
Breathing difficulty						
No	2055 (96.9)	97.7	96.4	3.032	0.082	0.038
Yes	65 (3.1)	2.3	3.6			
Number of symptoms (mean (SD))	1.24 (1.45)	0.80 (1.16)	1.58 (1.55)	−13.150	<0.001	0.559

For all variables described in Table 3, statistically significant differences were found between the presence of physical symptoms and psychological distress ($p < 0.005$), excluding respiratory distress ($p = 0.082$) and fever (>38 °C for at least 1 day) ($p = 0.319$).

Statistically significant differences were also observed for the mean number of symptoms ($\chi^2 = -13.150$, $p < 0.001$, Cohen's d = 0.559), with a mean effect size. The group of subjects with psychological distress had a higher number of symptoms (M = 1.58, SD = 1.55) compared to the group without this psychological morbidity (M = 0.80, SD = 1.16).

3.4. Health-Related Variables and Psychological Distress

Regarding health-related variables, the results show (Table 4) that 29% of the respondents reported having a chronic disease, and that 35.8% of the respondents are currently taking medication. In the same way, 0.4% of the subjects referred to having been hospitalized in the last 14 days, and 5.3% referred to having received health care in a health center, clinic, or hospital, while 4.5% of the participants had symptoms of COVID-19 and 18.1% reported diagnostic testing.

Table 4. Association between health-related variables and psychological distress during the COVID-19 pandemic ($n = 2120$).

	n (%)	Psychological Distress		χ^2/t	p	Effect Size
		No ($n = 908$)	Yes ($n = 1212$)			
Chronic diseases						
No	1505 (71.0)	75.4	67.7	15.058	<0.001	0.084
Yes	614 (29.0)	24.6	32.3			
Currently taking any medication						
No	1361 (64.2)	70.9	59.2	31.270	<0.001	0.121
Yes	759 (35.8)	29.1	40.8			
Health care in a health centre, clinic, or hospital in the past 14 days						
No	2007 (94.7)	96.0	93.6	5.868	0.015	0.053
Yes	113 (5.3)	4	6.4			
Recent hospitalization in the past 14 days						
No	2111 (99.6)	99.8	99.4	1.568	0.211	0.027
Yes	9 (0.4)	0.2	0.6			
Self-rated health in the past 14 days *	4.02 (0.81)	4.26 (0.73)	3.85 (0.83)	11.930	<0.001	0.520
Recent testing for COVID-19 in the past 14 days						
No	1736 (81.9)	86.6	78.4	23.424	<0.001	0.105
Yes	384 (18.1)	13.4	21.6			
Recent quarantine in the past 14 days for having symptoms ($n = 2106$) **		$n = 2040$	$n = 66$			
No	2040 (96.9)	98.7	95.5	16.725	<0.001	0.089
Yes	66 (3.1)	1.3	4.5			

Note: * Likert-type scale from 1 (very bad) to 5 (very good); ** Fisher's exact test.

All the variables described in Table 4 are related to the presence of psychological distress, excluding recent hospitalization in the last 14 days ($\chi^2 = 1.568$, $p = 0.211$, Cohen's d = 0.027).

Considering the subjects' assessment of their self-perceived health in the last 14 days, statistically significant differences were also found between the two groups (t = 11.930, $p < 0.001$, Cohen's d = 0.520), with a mean effect size. The group of subjects without psychological distress (M = 4.26, SD = 0.73) expressed a better self-perception of their health compared to the group with psychological distress (M = 3.85, SD = 0.83), although both groups have good self-rated health in the last 14 days (M = 4.02, SD = 0.81).

3.5. Variables Related to Contact History in the Past 14 Days and Psychological Distress

As regards contact history in the last 14 days (Table 5), 36.1% of the participants reported having had or not knowing if they had had close contact with an individual with confirmed infection with COVID-19. Of these, 37.1% of respondents claimed that the contact was casual, and 43.0% stated they had had or did not know if they had had contact with any person or material suspected of being infected with COVID-19. As for the presence of people infected with COVID-19 in the participants' immediate circle, 91.2% indicated not having any infected family member. A statistically significant relationship with the presence of psychological distress ($p \leq 0.001$ in all cases) was found for all contact history variables in the last 14 days. Nevertheless, the effect sizes were negligible.

Table 5. Association between contact history variables in the past 14 days and psychological distress during the COVID-19 pandemic (n = 2120).

	n (%)	Psychological Distress No (n = 908)	Psychological Distress Yes (n = 1212)	χ^2	p	Effect Size
Close contact with an individual with confirmed infection with COVID-19						
No	1354 (63.9)	73.0	57.0	57.618	<0.001	0.165
Yes or does not know	766 (36.1)	27.0	43.0			
Casual contact with an individual with confirmed infection with COVID-19						
No	1333 (62.9)	70.7	57.0	41.690	<0.001	0.140
Yes or does not know	787 (37.1)	29.3	43.0			
Contact with any person or material suspicious of being infected with COVID-19						
No	1208 (57.0)	66.5	49.8	58.953	<0.001	0.167
Yes or does not know	912 (43.0)	33.5	50.2			
Any infected family member						
No	1933 (91.2)	93.6	89.4	11.691	0.001	0.074
Yes or does not know	187 (8.8)	6.4	10.6			

3.6. Prediction of Psychological Distress

The results of the logistic regression analysis controlled for sex and age are presented in Table 6. This model shows a variance of 22.6% in the overall model, with percentages of correct classification of each model around 68.3%. The model had a good fit (Hosmer–Lemeshow Chi-square value = 4.929, p = 0.765) and made it possible to identify the predictor variables of psychological distress.

Model 1 (sociodemographic variables) indicated a predictive ability of 12.7% (χ^2 = 211.457, $p < 0.001$). Gender, specifically female (OR = 3.142, 95% CI = (2.566, 3.848)), educational level, employment status, and living with children or under 16 years of age were predictors. This model correctly classified 65% of the subjects with sensitivity and specificity parameters of 79.3% and 45.8%, respectively.

With model 2, relating to physical symptoms, the value of the variance explained amounted to 16% (χ^2 = 268.399, $p < 0.001$).

Participants who reported a greater number of symptoms in the 14 days prior to study participation (OR = 1.444, 95% CI = (1.339, 1.558)) were more likely to show psychological distress. This model correctly classified 65.4% of participants (sensitivity 81.3% and specificity 44.3%).

Model 3 showed a predictive capacity of 16.8% (χ^2 = 281.293, $p < 0.001$), slightly higher than the previous one, and included health-related variables. This model provided sensitivity and specificity values of 83.8% and 42.8%, correctly classifying 66.3% of the sample. Participants who scored higher on self-perceived health (OR = 0.563, 95% CI = 0.496, 0.640) were less likely to experience psychological distress. However, subjects who had been quarantined in the past 14 days for having symptoms were 2.878 times more likely to have psychological distress (95% CI = 1.456, 5.687).

Table 6. Prediction of psychological distress.

	Variables	Model 1 OR (95% CI) Sociodemographic	Model 2 OR (95% CI) Physical Symptoms	Model 3 OR (95% CI) Health Related	Model 4 OR (95% CI) Contact History	Model 5 Global Model OR (95% CI)
	Regression Model	R^2 = 0.127 (79.3/45.8%)	R^2 = 0.160 (81.3/44.3%)	R^2 = 0.168 (83.8/42.8%)	R^2 = 0.131 (80/45.6%)	R^2 = 0.226 (78/54.9%)
Sociodemographic	Sex (ref. males)	3.142 ** (2.566, 3.848)	2.744 ** (2.254, 3.340)	2.898 ** (2.373, 3.539)	3.172 ** (2.616, 3.845)	2.448 ** (1.980, 3.028)
	Marital Status (ref. single)					
	Married or living as a couple	0.938 (0.755, 1.167)	NA	NA	NA	NA
	Separated/divorced/widowed	0.763 (0.542, 1.075)	NA	NA	NA	NA
	Educational level (ref. secondary school)					
	University education graduation)	1.541 ** (1.210, 1.962)	NA	NA	NA	1.419 ** (1.170, 1.820)
	University education (master's or PhD)	1.327 * (1.039, 1.695)	NA	NA	NA	1.163 (0.906, 1.494)
	Employment status (ref. working away home)					
	Working from home	0.679 ** (0.541, 0.852)	NA	NA	NA	0.784 * (0.618, 0.995)
	Not working	1.091 (0.784, 1.520)	NA	NA	NA	0.961 (0.684, 1.351)
	Type of dwelling (ref. apartment)	0.856 (0.712, 1.030)	NA	NA	NA	NA
	Living with children or under-16 youngsters (ref. no)	1.587 ** (1.309, 1.926)	NA	NA	NA	1.580 ** (1.304, 1.915)
Physical symptoms	Number of symptoms	NA	1.444 ** (1.339, 1.558)	NA	NA	1.327 ** (1.224, 1.440)
Health related	Chronic diseases (ref. no)	NA	NA	0.898 (0.695, 1.160)	NA	NA
	Currently taking any medication (ref. no)	NA	NA	1.184 (0.929, 1.509)	NA	NA
	Health care in a health centre, clinic, or hospital in the past 14 days (ref. no)	NA	NA	1.017 (0.653, 1.582)	NA	NA
	Self-rated health in the past 14 days*	NA	NA	0.563 ** (0.496, 0.640)	NA	0.672 ** (0.589, 0.767)
	Recent testing for COVID-19 in the past 14 days (ref. no)	NA	NA	1.230 (0.953, 1.588)	NA	NA
	Recent quarantine in the past 14 days for having symptoms (ref. no)	NA	NA	2.878 ** (1.456, 5.687)	NA	2.443 * (1.214, 4.913)
Contact history	Close contact with an individual with confirmed infection with COVID-19 (ref. no)	NA	NA	NA	1.499 ** (1.120, 2.007)	1.347 * (1.031, 1.759)
	Casual contact with an individual with confirmed infection with COVID-19 (ref. no)	NA	NA	NA	0.948 (0.707, 1.271)	NA
	Contact with any person or material suspected of being infected with COVID-19 (ref. no)	NA	NA	NA	1.437 ** (1.108, 1.863)	1.237 (0.958, 1.598)
	Any infected family member (ref. no)	NA	NA	NA	1.304 (0.925, 1.836)	NA

* $p < 0.05$; ** $p < 0.01$; NA: not applicable; R^2 = model explained variance (sensitivity/specificity); OR (95% CI): odds ratio (confidence interval at the 95% level).

Model 4 included contact history variables, which provided an explained variance rate of 13.1% ($\chi^2 = 217.047$, $p < 0.001$). Having close contact with an individual with confirmed COVID-19 infection (OR = 1.499, 95% CI = 1.120, 2.007), as well as having had any contact with any person or material suspected of being infected (OR = 1.437, 95% CI = 1.108,

1.863) had predictive ability, correctly classifying 65.3% of participants (80% sensitivity and 45.6% specificity).

Finally, Model 5 (global model), which contained the variables with predictive capacity in the previous models, showed a predictive capacity of 22.6%, correctly classifying 68.5% of the participants (78% sensitivity and 54.9% specificity). The variables that showed greater weight, with ORs greater than 1, were sex (OR = 2.448, 95% CI = 1.980, 3.028), educational level (OR = 1.419, 95% CI = 1.170, 1.820), living with children or children under 16 years of age (OR = 1.580, 95% CI = 1.304, 1.915), number of symptoms presented in the last 14 days (OR = 1.327, 95% CI = 1.224, 1.440), having been quarantined in the past 14 days for presenting symptoms (OR = 2.443, 95% CI = 1214, 4.913), having had close contact with an individual with confirmed COVID-19 infection (OR = 1.347, 95% CI = 1.031, 1.759), and having had contact with any person or material suspected of being infected with COVID-19 (OR = 1.237, 95% CI = 0.958, 1.598). Other predictor variables with ORs less than 1 were self-perceived health in the last 14 days and employment status.

4. Discussion

In this study conducted in Portugal, 57% of the participants present psychological distress during the COVID-19 pandemic, revealing that they often feel oppressed and tense and that they cannot enjoy the activities they usually perform in their daily life (i.e., here is where the suffering is greatest). Other studies corroborate our results, showing the presence of psychological distress in people during the COVID-19 pandemic. In Spain, a study revealed that a high percentage (i.e., 72%) of participants were at risk of developing psychological problems [7]. In China, a study found that 22.8% of participants reported high levels of psychological distress [27]. In the United States, the percentage of individuals reporting psychological distress was 73% in a study conducted at the beginning of the COVID-19 pandemic [28]. In Italy, the psychological impact that the COVID-19 pandemic caused was around 48.6% [12]. Studies that focused their attention on the psychological impact during the pandemic reveal that the percentage of psychological distress is between 22.9% and 56.7% [20,29,30]. The percentage of psychological distress in our study and other studies reported here exceeds the pandemic data, so we can interpret this to mean that the COVID-19 pandemic has affected populations more severely than other previous pandemics.

Regarding the sociodemographic variables for which there is greater vulnerability to psychological problems during the COVID-19 pandemic, the most significant variable is sex; in this sense, in our study, 79.0% of participants with psychological distress were female. In addition, other variables that influence this vulnerability to psychological suffering are level of education (university studies: graduation, master's, and doctorate) (75.8%), working outside the home (69.2%), conditions of the usual dwelling (where 59.2% lived in a flat), and living with children or young people under the age of 16 (50.2%). People who are unemployed (10.3%) are the ones with the lowest percentage of psychological distress. The results show that there are statistically significant differences between psychological problems and sex. There is no statistical relationship between psychological suffering and age, that is, age does not influence whether or not one is suffering. Other studies corroborate the results of our study regarding the increased risk for women of developing psychological distress throughout the COVID-19 pandemic, an aspect that can be interpreted as an individual and biological risk factor. On the other hand, due to the closing of schools during the pandemic, women suffered disproportionately from the burden of caregiving, with increased responsibilities of work and household chores [7,12,16].

Regarding the level of education as a predictor of psychological distress, our study shows that there is greater psychological distress in people with higher levels of education (university studies: graduation, master's, and doctorate), with no evidence in other studies of the relationship between psychological suffering and education. The correlation presented by our study may indicate that the ease of access that people with a higher level of education have to credible scientific information and their perception of the severity of the virus based on scientific evidence—together with uncertainty about the direction the pandemic may take, as there is little knowledge about the virus, and means of treatment and control—can lead this group of people to develop fear and anxiety [31].

In relation to people living with children or young people under 16 years of age, other studies are in line with these results, being explained by the fear of contagion of the children, by the burden of the caregiver, and by the difficulty in providing playful and fun activities for children, creating a feeling of boredom and being still in time [7,12,28,32–34].

In our study, the unemployed sample showed the lowest psychological distress. On the other hand, it is those who have to work outside the home (69.2%) who have greater psychological suffering, which can be justified by the fear of contracting COVID-19 and transmitting it to others, inadequate protection against contamination, discrimination, overwork, and exhaustion. The results of the studies by Gomez-Salgado et al. [7] and Jeong et al. [33] are in line with our results. Data from a study conducted in China contradict our results and argue that psychological distress during the pandemic is related to unqualified and low-skilled jobs and unemployment, as these situations create distress related to the socio-economic situation [27].

The data presented in this study reveal that there is no statistical relationship between psychological distress and age. The evidence shows different results taking into account different age groups—that is, there are studies that show that the younger population is more likely to develop psychological suffering, because they have more difficulty in dealing with adversities and also in understanding that the pandemic is an extreme situation, which implies drastic changes in the lifestyle of a society and does not result from individual decisions [7,30]. Other studies reveal that psychological distress is greatest in people over 60 years of age, as they are part of the group most at risk of developing COVID-19 [32,35].

Regarding the presence of symptoms of COVID-19, the most frequent were headaches (46.6%), rhinorrhea (30.1%), myalgia (24.7%), cough (15.3%), sore throat (14.7%), and in a smaller percentages, diarrhea (9.7%), dizziness (6.9%), chills (5.2%), respiratory distress (3.6%), and fever above 38 °C for one day (1.1%). With the exception of respiratory distress and the presence of fever greater than 38 °C for one day, all other physical symptoms related to COVID-19 are a predisposing factor to the existence of psychological distress. Other studies have found myalgias, dizziness, chills, and odynophagia to be associated with greater psychological distress [17]. In a study conducted in Spain, the presence of headache, rhinorrhea, myalgias, cough, sore throat, diarrhea, dizziness, chills, difficulty breathing, and fever higher than 38 °C for one day are also associated with increased psychological distress [7].

Of the participants with COVID-19 symptoms (4.5%), 18.1% were tested—69.2% had a negative result, 22.2% had a positive result, and 8.7% did not know the result. Only 3.1% of respondents indicate that they were quarantined for having had contact with a person infected with COVID-19.

In our study, health-related variables (presence of chronic diseases; taking medication regularly; needing to attend consultations in a health centre, hospital, or clinic regularly; having recently performed COVID-19 tests; and self-assessment of health perception) were related to the presence of psychological distress, as had already been described in the studies by Shehata et al. [36], Cybulski et al. [37], and Ripoll et al. [38]. Regarding the evaluation of the perception of the health of our sample, the results show that the group of people who do not experience psychological distress expressed a better evaluation of their health compared to the group that had psychological distress, although both made a good self-assessment of their health. Other studies corroborate our results, describing a relationship between the existence of comorbidities and the presence of psychological distress in patients with COVID-19 and in the general population, but this relationship was not statistically significant [8,39].

Regarding contact history in the 14 days prior to this survey, of our sample, 36.1% of participants claimed to have had close contact with an individual who tested positive for COVID-19 [35]. One percent of individuals claimed to have had random contact, and

43% claimed to have maintained or not known if they had had contact with any person or material suspected of being infected with COVID-19. Regarding the presence of an infected person in the close circles of the participants, 91.2% stated that they did not have infected family members. All variables (close contact with an individual with confirmed infection, casual contact with an individual with confirmed infection, contact with any person or material suspected of being infected with COVID-19, any member of the infected family) relating to the contact history have a statistically significant relationship with the presence of psychological distress. Data from other studies show that a history of contact with an infected person or objects predisposes one to develop psychological distress, namely the presence of acute stress and post-traumatic stress, which arise from the feeling of danger and risk of contracting the infection [7,40,41].

In order to describe the limitations of the present study, it is worth mentioning that the cross-sectional design used does not allow establishing a cause-effect relationship, although it does provide a very valuable description of the impact of the COVID-19 pandemic on psychological distress at the specific moment of confinement and of the greatest escalation of the infection curve in Portugal. On the other hand, the sampling procedure was not random, and the study participants were collected through email lists to universities and professional associations. Moreover, the sex variable was not represented in the actual proportion of the Portuguese population. Furthermore, it was not possible to compare the results of the present study with those obtained during the development of other pandemics, since the measures adopted in the current situation differ from those implemented in those past situations. Similarly, the results obtained in Portugal cannot be compared with those obtained in studies conducted on the same topic in other countries.

Future studies should carry out cause-effect analyses, perhaps at different epidemiological moments of the pandemic, to really study what has been and what will be the emotional impact of the COVID-19 pandemic in Portugal.

5. Conclusions

Having had close or casual contact with a person with confirmed or suspected COVID-19 infection, including family members, had a statistically significant relationship with the presence of psychological distress.

The predictor variables for psychological distress were sex, educational background, living with children or young people under 16 years of age, number of symptoms presented in the last 14 days, quarantine for presenting symptoms, having had contact with a person or material suspected of being infected by COVID-19, and having had close contact with a person with confirmed COVID-19 infection. The protective variables for psychological distress were being in telework and a good self-assessment of health status in the last 14 days.

These results show that there are factors that predispose the Portuguese population to develop psychological distress in the context of the COVID-19 pandemic, affecting their well-being and mental health. These should be considered when carrying out intervention programs suitable for pandemic situations, since they can design programs for the prevention of psychological distress in a pandemic context and psychological intervention programs when distress is already present, with the aim of promoting public health in general, and mental health in particular.

Author Contributions: Conceptualization, F.F., L.J., J.G.-S., R.M., R.A.-C., C.R.-F., and J.F.; data curation, F.F., L.J., J.G.-S., R.M., R.A.-C., C.R.-F., and J.F.; formal analysis, F.F., L.J., J.G.-S., R.M., R.A.-C., C.R.-F., and J.F.; funding acquisition, R.A.-C.; investigation, F.F., L.J., J.G.-S., R.M., R.A.-C., C.R.-F., and J.F.; methodology, F.F., L.J., J.G.-S., R.M., R.A.-C., C.R.-F., and J.F.; project administration, F.F., L.J., J.G.-S., R.M., C.R.-F., and J.F.; resources, F.F., L.J., J.G.-S., R.M., R.A.-C., C.R.-F., and J.F.; software, F.F., L.J., J.G.-S., R.M., R.A.-C., C.R.-F., and J.F.; supervision, F.F., L.J., J.G.-S., R.M., R.A.-C., C.R.-F., and J.F.; validation, F.F., L.J., J.G.-S., R.M., R.A.-C., C.R.-F., and J.F.; visualization, F.F., L.J., J.G.-S., R.M., R.A.-C., C.R.-F., and J.F.; writing—original draft, F.F., L.J., J.G.-S., R.M., R.A.-C., C.R.-F., and J.F.; writing—review and editing, F.F., L.J., J.G.-S., R.M., R.A.-C., C.R.-F., and J.F. All authors have read and agreed to the published version of the manuscript.

Funding: This work was funded by Portuguese national funds provided by Fundação para a Ciência e Tecnologia (FCT) (UIDB/05704/2020 and UIDP/05704/2020).

Institutional Review Board Statement: The ethical principles set out in the Declaration of Helsinki have been followed. The permission of the participants was obtained through a written informed consent in which they expressed their voluntary desire to participate in the study. Data were recorded anonymously and treated confidentially. The project was approved by the Research Ethics Committee of Atlântica-Instituto Universitário.

Informed Consent Statement: Informed consent was obtained from all subjects involved in the study.

Data Availability Statement: All data are available within this article.

Conflicts of Interest: The authors declare no conflict of interest.

References

1. World Health Organization. WHO Coronavirus Disease (COVID-19) Dashboard (Internet). WHO: Geneva, Switzerland, 2021. Available online: https://covid19.who.int/ (accessed on 26 June 2021).
2. Direção Geral de Saúde. Estado Epidemiológico COVID 19 em Portugal (Internet). Direção Geral de Saúde: Lisboa, Portugal, 2021. Available online: https://covid19.min-saude.pt/relatorioa-de-situaçao/ (accessed on 26 June 2021).
3. To, K.K.-W.; Tsang, O.T.-Y.; Yip, C.C.-Y.; Chan, K.-H.; Wu, T.-C.; Chan, J.M.-C.; Leung, W.-S.; Chik, T.S.-H.; Choi, C.Y.-C.; Kandamby, D.H.; et al. Consistent Detection of 2019 Novel Coronavirus in Saliva. *Clin. Infect. Dis.* **2020**, *71*, 841–843. [CrossRef] [PubMed]
4. Domínguez-Salas, S.; Gómez-Salgado, J.; Andrés-Villas, M.; Díaz-Milanés, D.; Romero-Martín, M.; Ruiz-Frutos, C. Psycho-Emotional Approach to the Psychological Distress Related to the COVID-19 Pandemic in Spain: A Cross-Sectional Observational Study. *Healthcare* **2020**, *8*, 190. [CrossRef]
5. Adhikari, S.P.; Meng, S.; Wu, Y.-J.; Mao, Y.-P.; Ye, R.-X.; Wang, Q.-Z.; Sun, C.; Sylvia, S.; Rozelle, S.; Raat, H.; et al. Epidemiology, causes, clinical manifestation and diagnosis, prevention and control of coronavirus disease (COVID-19) during the early outbreak period: A scoping review. *Infect. Dis. Poverty* **2020**, *9*, 29. [CrossRef]
6. Falcão, V.T.F.L. Os Desafios da Enfermagem no Enfrentamento a COVID-19. *Revista Enfermagem Digital Cuidado e Promoção da Saúde* **2020**, *5*, 1–2. [CrossRef]
7. Gómez-Salgado, J.; Andrés-Villas, M.; Domínguez-Salas, S.; Díaz-Milanés, D.; Ruiz-Frutos, C. Related Health Factors of Psychological Distress During the COVID-19 Pandemic in Spain. *Int. J. Environ. Res. Public Health* **2020**, *17*, 3947. [CrossRef]
8. Mohammadi, S.M.; Ashtari, S.; Fetrat, M.K. The Psychological Impact of COVID-19 Pandemic on Mental Health of Iranian Population. *Int. J. Travel Med. Glob. Health* **2020**, *9*, 19–24. [CrossRef]
9. Diário da Républica nº 57/2020, 1º suplemento, série I de 2020-03-20. Lisboa, 2020. Comunicado do Conselho de Ministros de 19 de março de 2020—XXII Governo—República Portuguesa. Available online: www.portugal.gov.pt/pt/gc22 (accessed on 26 June 2021).
10. Holmes, E.A.; O'Connor, R.C.; Perry, V.H.; Tracey, I.; Wessely, S.; Arseneault, L.; Ballard, C.; Christensen, H.; Silver, R.C.; Everall, I.; et al. Multidisciplinary research priorities for the COVID-19 pandemic: A call for action for mental health science. *Lancet Psychiatry* **2020**, *7*, 547–560. [CrossRef]
11. Wittchen, H.; Jacobi, F.; Rehm, J.; Gustavsson, A.; Svensson, M.; Jönsson, B.; Olesen, J.; Allgulander, C.; Alonso, J.; Faravelli, C.; et al. The size and burden of mental disorders and other disorders of the brain in Europe 2010. *Eur. Neuropsychopharmacol.* **2011**, *21*, 655–679. [CrossRef]
12. Bonati, M.; Campi, R.; Zanetti, M.; Cartabia, M.; Scarpellini, F.; Clavenna, A.; Segre, G. Psychological distress among Italians during the 2019 coronavirus disease (COVID-19) quarantine. *BMC Psychiatry* **2021**, *21*, 20. [CrossRef] [PubMed]
13. Zhang, J.; Lu, H.; Zeng, H.; Zhang, S.; Du, Q.; Jiang, T.; Du, B. The differential psychological distress of populations affected by the COVID-19 pandemic. *Brain Behav. Immun.* **2020**, *87*, 49–50. [CrossRef]
14. Passos, L.; Prazeres, F.; Teixeira, A.; Martins, C. Impact on Mental Health Due to COVID-19 Pandemic: Cross-Sectional Study in Portugal and Brazil. *Int. J. Environ. Res. Public Health* **2020**, *17*, 6794. [CrossRef] [PubMed]
15. Silva Moreira, P.; Ferreira, S.; Couto, B.; Machado-Sousa, M.; Fernández, M.; Raposo-Lima, C.; Sousa, N.; Picó-Pérez, M.; Morgado, P. Protective Elements of Mental Health Status during the COVID-19 Outbreak in the Portuguese Population. *Int. J. Environ. Res. Public Health* **2021**, *18*, 1910. [CrossRef]
16. Antunes, R.; Frontini, R.; Amaro, N.; Salvador, R.; Matos, R.; Morouço, P.; Rebelo-Gonçalves, R. Exploring Lifestyle Habits, Physical Activity, Anxiety and Basic Psychological Needs in a Sample of Portuguese Adults during COVID-19. *Int. J. Environ. Res. Public Health* **2020**, *17*, 4360. [CrossRef] [PubMed]

17. Wang, C.; Pan, R.; Wan, X.; Tan, Y.; Xu, L.; Ho, C.S.; Ho, R.C. Immediate Psychological Responses and Associated Factors during the Initial Stage of the 2019 Coronavirus Disease (COVID-19) Epidemic among the General Population in China. *Int. J. Environ. Res. Public Health* **2020**, *17*, 1729. [CrossRef]
18. Idler, E.L.; Benyamini, Y. Self-Rated Health and Mortality: A Review of Twenty-Seven Community Studies. *J. Health Soc. Behav.* **1997**, *38*, 21–37. [CrossRef]
19. Hawryluck, L.; Gold, W.L.; Robinson, S.; Pogorski, S.; Galea, S.; Styra, R. SARS Control and Psychological Effects of Quarantine, Toronto, Canada. *Emerg. Infect. Dis.* **2004**, *10*, 1206–1212. [CrossRef]
20. Tam, C.W.C.; Pang, E.P.F.; Lam, L.C.W.; Chiu, H.F.K. Severe acute respiratory syndrome (SARS) in Hong Kong in 2003: Stress and psychological impact among frontline healthcare workers. *Psychol. Med.* **2004**, *34*, 1197–1204. [CrossRef]
21. Main, A.; Zhou, Q.; Ma, Y.; Luecken, L.J.; Liu, X. Relations of SARS-related stressors and coping to Chinese college students' psychological adjustment during the 2003 Beijing SARS epidemic. *J. Couns. Psychol.* **2011**, *58*, 410–423. [CrossRef]
22. Goldberg, D.P.; Gater, R.; Sartorius, N.; Ustun, T.B.; Piccinelli, M.; Gureje, O.; Rutter, C. The validity of two versions of the GHQ in the WHO study of mental illness in general health care. *Psychol. Med.* **1997**, *27*, 191–197. [CrossRef]
23. Carochinho, J.A. Adaptation and Validation of a Set of Well-Being Scales for the Portuguese Language. *RIDEP* **2018**, *46*, 37–50. [CrossRef]
24. Jackson, C. The General Health Questionnaire. *Occup. Med.* **2007**, *57*, 79. [CrossRef]
25. Ricci-Cabello, I.; Ruiz-Pérez, I.; Plazaola-Castaño, J.; Montero-Piñar, I. Morbilidad psíquica, existencia de diagnóstico y consumo de psicofármacos: Diferencias por comunidades autónomas según la encuesta nacional de salud de 2006. *Rev. Española Salud Pública* **2010**, *84*, 29–41. [CrossRef] [PubMed]
26. Barrios Osuna, I.; Anido Escobar, V.; Morera Pérez, M. Declaración de Helsinki: Cambios y exégesis. *Rev. Cuba. Salud Publica.* **2016**, *42*, 132–142.
27. Yu, H.; Li, M.; Li, Z.; Xiang, W.; Yuan, Y.; Liu, Y.; Li, Z.; Xiong, Z. Coping style, social support and psychological distress in the general Chinese population in the early stages of the COVID-19 epidemic. *BMC Psychiatry* **2020**, *20*, 426. [CrossRef]
28. Holingue, C.; Kalb, L.G.; Riehm, K.E.; Bennett, D.; Kapteyn, A.; Veldhuis, C.B.; Johnson, R.M.; Fallin, M.D.; Kreuter, F.; Stuart, E.A.; et al. Mental Distress in the United States at the Beginning of the COVID-19 Pandemic. *Am. J. Public Health* **2020**, *110*, 1628–1634. [CrossRef]
29. Mihashi, M.; Otsubo, Y.; Yinjuan, X.; Nagatomi, K.; Hoshiko, M.; Ishitake, T. Predictive factors of psychological disorder development during recovery following SARS outbreak. *Health Psychol.* **2009**, *28*, 91–100. [CrossRef]
30. Taylor, M.R.; Agho, K.E.; Stevens, G.J.; Raphael, B. Factors influencing psychological distress during a disease epidemic: Data from Australia's first outbreak of equine influenza. *BMC Public Health* **2008**, *8*, 347. [CrossRef] [PubMed]
31. Ali, M.Y.; Bhatti, R. COVID-19 (Coronavirus) Pandemic: Information Sources Channels for the Public Health Awareness. *Asia Pac. J. Public Health* **2020**, *32*, 168–169. [CrossRef] [PubMed]
32. Every-Palmer, S.; Jenkins, M.; Gendall, P.; Hoek, J.; Beaglehole, B.; Bell, C.; Williman, J.; Rapsey, C.; Stanley, J. Psychological distress, anxiety, family violence, suicidality, and wellbeing in New Zealand during the COVID-19 lockdown: A cross-sectional study. *PLoS ONE* **2020**, *15*, e0241658. [CrossRef]
33. Jeong, H.; Yim, H.W.; Song, Y.-J.; Ki, M.; Min, J.-A.; Cho, J.; Chae, J.-H. Mental health status of people isolated due to Middle East Respiratory Syndrome. *Epidemiol. Health* **2016**, *38*, e2016048. [CrossRef] [PubMed]
34. Cellini, N.; Canale, N.; Mioni, G.; Costa, S. Changes in sleep pattern, sense of time and digital media use during COVID-19 lockdown in Italy. *J. Sleep Res.* **2020**, *29*, e13074. [CrossRef] [PubMed]
35. Qiu, J.; Shen, B.; Zhao, M.; Wang, Z.; Xie, B.; Xu, Y. A nationwide survey of psychological distress among Chinese people in the COVID-19 epidemic: Implications and policy recommendations. *Gen. Psychiatry* **2020**, *33*, e100213. [CrossRef] [PubMed]
36. Shehata, G.A.; Gabra, R.; Eltellawy, S.; Elsayed, M.; Gaber, D.E.; Elshabrawy, H.A. Assessment of Anxiety, Depression, Attitude, and Coping Strategies of the Egyptian Population during the COVID-19 Pandemic. *J. Clin. Med.* **2021**, *10*, 3989. [CrossRef]
37. Cybulski, M.; Cwalina, U.; Sadowska, D.; Krajewska-Kułak, E. The Assessment of the Severity of COVID-19-Related Anxiety Symptoms in Participants of the University of the Third Age in Poland: A Cross-Sectional Study among Internet Survey Respondents. *J. Clin. Med.* **2021**, *10*, 3862. [CrossRef]
38. Ripoll, J.; Contreras-Martos, S.; Esteva, M.; Soler, A.; Serrano-Ripoll, M.J. Mental Health and PsychologicalWellbeing during the COVID-19 Lockdown: A Longitudinal Study in the Balearic Islands (Spain). *J. Clin. Med.* **2021**, *10*, 3191. [CrossRef]
39. Klimkiewicz, A.; Jasionowska, J.; Schmalenberg, A.; Klimkiewicz, J.; Jasi´nska, A.; Silczuk, A. COVID-19 Pandemic-Related Depression and Insomnia among Psychiatric Patients and the General Population. *J. Clin. Med.* **2021**, *10*, 3425. [CrossRef]
40. Brooks, S.K.; Webster, R.; Smith, L.E.; Woodland, L.; Wessely, S.; Greenberg, N.; Rubin, G.J. The psychological impact of quarantine and how to reduce it: Rapid review of the evidence. *Lancet* **2020**, *395*, 912–920. [CrossRef]
41. Wu, P.; Fang, Y.; Guan, Z.; Fan, B.; Kong, J.; Yao, Z.; Liu, X.; Fuller, C.J.; Susser, E.; Lu, J.; et al. The Psychological Impact of the SARS Epidemic on Hospital Employees in China: Exposure, Risk Perception, and Altruistic Acceptance of Risk. *Can. J. Psychiatry* **2009**, *54*, 302–311. [CrossRef]

Journal of
Clinical Medicine

MDPI

Article

High Rate of Elder Abuse in the Time of COVID-19—A Cross Sectional Study of Geriatric and Neurology Clinic Patients

Karolina Filipska [1,*], Monika Biercewicz [2], Adam Wiśniewski [3], Renata Jabłońska [1], Agnieszka Królikowska [1], Emilia Główczewska-Siedlecka [2], Kornelia Kędziora-Kornatowska [2] and Robert Ślusarz [1]

1 Neurological and Neurosurgical Nursing Department, Faculty of Health Science, Collegium Medicum in Bydgoszcz, Nicolaus Copernicus University in Toruń, Łukasiewicza 1 Street, 85-821 Bydgoszcz, Poland; renjab_1@wp.pl (R.J.); agakrolikowska6@wp.pl (A.K.); robert_slu_cmumk@wp.pl (R.Ś.)
2 Clinic of Geriatrics, Faculty of Health Science, Collegium Medicum in Bydgoszcz, Nicolaus Copernicus University in Toruń, Skłodowskiej 9 Street, 85-094 Bydgoszcz, Poland; monika_bierc_cmumk@wp.pl (M.B.); egs@cm.umk.pl (E.G.-S.); kornelia.kornatowska@cm.umk.pl (K.K.-K.)
3 Department of Neurology, Faculty of Medicine, Collegium Medicum in Bydgoszcz, Nicolaus Copernicus University in Toruń, Skłodowskiej 9 Street, 85-094 Bydgoszcz, Poland; adam.lek@wp.pl
* Correspondence: karolinafilipskakf@gmail.com

Abstract: The ongoing COVID-19 pandemic is believed to have caused a sharp increase in the incidence of elder abuse (EA), including as a result of isolation, social distance combined with increased interpersonal stressors. Thus, the aim of this study is to determine the impact of the COVID-19 pandemic on the elder abuse rates and the characteristics of risk factors. A total of 347 patients hospitalized in the Department of Neurology and Department of Geriatrics at University Hospital No. 1 in Bydgoszcz were selected as subjects for the analysis. The tools used in the study are: Authors-Designed Questionnaire, the Vulnerability to Abuse Screening Scale, the Geriatric Depression Scale and the Activities of Daily Living Scale. Descriptive statistics, chi-squared tests, Spearman's rank correlation test, and logistic regression analyses were used. In the studied population, nearly 45% of the elderly were victims of violence. This represents an increase of more than 6 percent compared to the pre-pandemic. The most common type of EA was psychological abuse (72.3%). In the final models, the risk factors include, among others, low income (OR = 3.60, 95% CI = 1.93–6.72), chronic diseases (OR = 2.06, 95% CI = 1.28–3.31), poor relationship with the family (OR = 3.26, 95% CI = 1.96–5.43), and moderate and severe depression (OR = 18.29, 95% CI = 10.24–32.69; OR = 18.49, 95% CI = 3.91–87.30, respectively). Moreover, moderate functional impairment 5.52 times more often and severe functional impairment 21.07 times more likely to predispose to EA. People who suffered from COVID-19 are 1.59 times more likely to be victims of EA (95% CI = 1.03–2.46). In this study, we saw significant increases in EA rates during the COVID-19 pandemic.

Keywords: COVID-19; elder abuse; risk factors; older adults

Citation: Filipska, K.; Biercewicz, M.; Wiśniewski, A.; Jabłońska, R.; Królikowska, A.; Główczewska-Siedlecka, E.; Kędziora-Kornatowska, K.; Ślusarz, R. High Rate of Elder Abuse in the Time of COVID-19—A Cross Sectional Study of Geriatric and Neurology Clinic Patients. *J. Clin. Med.* **2021**, *10*, 4532. https://doi.org/10.3390/jcm10194532

Academic Editor: Michele Roccella

Received: 7 September 2021
Accepted: 28 September 2021
Published: 30 September 2021

Publisher's Note: MDPI stays neutral with regard to jurisdictional claims in published maps and institutional affiliations.

1. Introduction

SARS-CoV-2 is a new single-stranded RNA beta-coronavirus. It first appeared in November 2019 in Wuhan, China. In Poland, the first case was recorded on 4 March 2020. The World Health Organization (WHO) named this disease COVID-19. Moreover, on 11 March 2020, WHO announced the beginning of the COVID-19 pandemic [1]. Coronavirus disease is associated with threats to the health and life of people all over the world, not only because of the disease itself, but also its complications. This pandemic has led to a real revolution in everyday life. In order to limit its spread, it was necessary for the state to introduce isolation, the need to maintain social distance, and also to control the behaviour of citizens. Further more, change in everyday life, economic instability, loss of job, fear of illness, social distance, and complications after illness are factors that may contribute to the occurrence of neuropsychiatric disorders, including symptoms of anxiety and depression, which has been observed among the society of many countries affected by the pandemic [2,3].

Another important effect of the pandemic is the increase in the rates of violence, including in relation to the elderly [4]. Most of the older adults who become victims of violence are people who require long-term and increased care [4–6]. The stress theory describes caring for the elderly as a difficult and stressful activity [5]. In addition, especially during the COVID-19 pandemic, there are pressures and stresses related to work and life. All these factors contribute to an increase in the rates of violence against the elderly by caregivers. In addition, isolation itself is also a significant risk factor for abuse. Elderly or dependent people can often only interact with their perpetrators or due to quarantine, stay only with them [4–6].

Elder abuse (EA) (also known as mistreatment, older adult abuse or maltreatment) is defined by the WHO as "a single or repeated act or lack of appropriate action, occurring within a relationship of trust, which causes harm or distress to an older person". According to WHO, we distinguish five types of EA: physical, sexual, psychological, and emotional abuse, financial and material abuse, abandonment, and neglect [7]. On the other hand, the most common form of EA is psychological abuse [7–9]. It should be noted, however, that older adult abuse is a global public health problem, and the estimated total prevalence rate is 15.7% [10]. It is believed, however, that the ongoing COVID-19 pandemic caused a sharp increase in the incidence of EA, including as a result of isolation and social distance in combination with increased interpersonal stressors [11,12]. Our research team has already conducted cross-sectional research on elder abuse from April 2017 to January 2019. It has been shown then that among 200 respondents 38.5% of older people have experienced abuse [13]. Observing the current indicators, it can be easily noticed that there has been a sharp increase in acts of of EA during the COVID-19 pandemic. Thus, there is a strong need for research on the scale and severity of the incidence of EA and emotional distress, including symptoms of depression and generalized anxiety, in different countries.

In summary, the aim of this study was to determine the elder abuse rates and identification of the most common risk factors of mistreatment in the Polish population in a hospital setting during the COVID-19 pandemic.

2. Materials and Methods

2.1. Study Design and Participants

From October 2020 to August 2021, we conducted this cross-sectional study in the Department of Neurology and Department of Geriatrics at University Hospital No. 1 in Bydgoszcz, Poland. The study included people who met the inclusion criteria: aged 65 years and older, voluntarily agreed to participate, with sufficient speech, hearing, and cognitive abilities: no dementia or Alzheimer's disease diagnosed by a psychologist or physician. The total population of the respondents was 347.

After admission to the ward, each patient underwent psychological and neurological assessment in order to exclude cognitive impairment and dementia. The standard tool used by the psychologists in Poland is the Montreal Cognitive Assessment test and Mini-Mental State Examination and the Clock Drawing Test. All patients who met the inclusion criteria became participants in this study. As scheduled admissions were on hold for a long time during the COVID-19 pandemic, hospitals operated on an ER, and the number of hospitalized patients was very limited. Access to other hospitals was also restricted. Thus, we were able to collect only such a group of respondents.

Due to the fact that the study was conducted during the epidemic, we took special precautions. The subjects were patients of two departments: the Department of Neurology and Department of Geriatrics at University Hospital No. 1 in Bydgoszcz. Consequently, we spoke to each test person alone in a separate room. All test persons prior to admission to the hospital tested negative for SARS-CoV-2. Each of the study participants and the researchers wore masks. During the meeting, a distance of at least 2 meters was kept. In addition, all completed questionnaires were placed in a specially prepared box, where they had a grace period of about 7 days. Each of the participants completed the questionnaires independently. In the event of any questions or doubts, the researcher was at his disposal.

2.2. Variables and Measurements

Before the start of the project, a pilot study was carried out on a group of 46 people in order to obtain information on the understandability of the questions included in the Authors-Designed Questionnaire (ADQ). All comments, opinions and suggested changes have been considered. Therefore, we have removed or changed some text items to the final, easy-to-understand form. The results of the pilot studies were not included in the results of this work.

The dependent variables include: elder abuse: psychological, physical, sexual and economic abuse and the risk of EA. The definitions of these variables were:

(a) Elder abuse—this research is based on the WHO definition: "a single or repeated act or lack of appropriate action, occurring within a relationship of trust, which causes harm or distress to an older person". The study used 4 main forms of abuse: Psychological abuse—understood as arrogance, vulgarity; blackmail, threats; closing, isolating; insulting, criticizing; mocking; neglect [7,9]; Physical abuse—the most visible, consisting of in inflicting physical pain, injuries, include: jerking, hitting, kicking, pushing, burning (e.g., with a cigarette) and choking [7,13–15]; Sexual abuse—engaging in sexual contact without the consent or with the forced consent of the victim, provoking sexual behaviour against the will and willingness of an elderly person, e.g. rape, unwanted touch, etc. [7,14,15]; Economic abuse—it can manifest itself on many levels, from the possibility of limiting financial independence in the distribution of one's own retirement benefit to forcing to take a long-term loan, refusing or limiting access to shared finances, taking money away, limiting and preventing work, robbing, and destroying valuable items [7,14,15].

(b) The risk of EA—has been assessed using the most popular tool in the world, the Vulnerability to Abuse Screening Scale (VASS). It was built of 12 questions. The questions have been arranged in a closed form, and the answer options are: "yes" or "no". It consists of 4 subscales: dependence, dejection, vulnerability, and coercion. Each subscale contains 3 items. The dependence subscale includes: item 4–6; dejection: item 7–9; vulnerability: 1–3; coercion: 10–12. There are 9 positive questions (1–3, 7–12) and 3 negative ones (4–6). The higher the score, the greater the risk of EA. The risk of abuse is considered to be a score of 3 points and more [16]. In order to conduct this study, the psychometric properties of the VASS tool were verified. The Cronbach's alpha coefficient for the VASS scale was 0.89.

In addition to the VASS scale, the study also used: ADQ, the Geriatric Depression Scale (GDS) 15 items [17,18] and the Activities of Daily Living (ADL) Scale [19,20]. ADQ was created specifically for the purpose of this study, as no gold standard tool for assessing elder abuse has been published in Poland so far. This tool was developed on the basis of the researcher's own experience in conducting this type of research and the available literature [9,10,13,21,22]. The reliability of the ADQ was examined by computing internal consistency coefficients. The Cronbach alpha coefficient was 0.91. Sociodemographic questions were included in the 1st part of the questionnaire and concerned: sex, age, education, marital status, family income, and place of residence. The leading question was "During the COVID-19 pandemic, have you experienced any abuse (e.g. kicking, pulling, hitting, ridiculing, pushing, insulting) in your place of residence?". As for the various forms of EA, the respondents answered the question: "Which of the following forms of elder abuse were used against you?" selecting from the list of the abuses they have experienced. Above, in the definition of each type of violence, we have listed all the acts characteristic of a given sub-type of abuse, which were included in the ADQ. The next questions concerned, among others: the occurrence of chronic diseases, assessment of one's health condition, feeling lonely, depressed or anxious, and having children.

2.3. Ethical Statement

The study was approved by the Bioethics Committee of the Nicolaus Copernicus University in Torun at Collegium Medicum of Ludwik Rydygier in Bydgoszcz, Poland (approval no. 437/2020). The study was conducted according to the Declaration of Helsinki regarding research on humans. All subjects provided informed consent to participate in the study.

2.4. Statistical Analysis

The statistical analysis was performed with STATISTICA version 13.1 (Dell Technologies, Round Rock, TX, USA). In the first stage, the EA rates were analysed. The chi-square test was used successively to determine the relationship between sociodemographic characteristics and the rate of older adult abuse. Finally, a logistic regression model was performed to assess the relationship between the independent variables and the incidence and the risk of EA. Statistical results with $p < 0.05$ were considered significant and the performed analyses were assessed in the 95% confidence interval (CI).

3. Results

The overall data of the included patients are shown in Table 1.

During the COVID-19 pandemic, nearly 45% of the elderly in the study population were victims of EA ($n = 155$). The most common type of abuse was psychological (72.3%), followed by neglect (61.9%), physical (39.4%) and economic (36.8%) (Figure 1).

The logistic regression model (Table 2) showed many variables that were important risk factors for EA. For example, women were 1.90 (95% confidence interval (CI) = 1.23–2.93) times more likely to experience acts of abuse than men. Compared to people > 70 years of age, people aged 60–65 and 66–70 were statistically more likely to be victims of EA (odds ratio (OR) = 2.35, 95% CI = 1.28–4.31; OR = 1.98, 95% CI = 1.05–3.75, respectively). It was also shown that people with higher education statistically less frequently experienced EA than people with primary education (OR = 0.32, 95% CI = 0.16–0.64). When it comes to marital status, the acts of EA were more frequent in divorced persons and widows/widowers compared to singles (OR = 4.15, 95% CI = 1.70–10.15; OR = 2.50, 95% CI = 1.20–5.25, respectively). Low income was significantly associated with an increased risk of older adult abuse (OR = 3.60, 95% CI = 1.93–6.72). Moreover, people with chronic diseases were 2.06 times more likely to experience abuse (95% CI = 1.28–3.31). Poor relationship with the family and lack of family was also significantly related to EA (OR = 3.26, 95% CI = 1.96–5.43; OR= 3.32, 95% CI = 1.68–6.56, respectively). One of the leading risk factors also turned out to be moderate and severe depression (OR = 18.29, 95% CI = 10.24–32.69; OR = 18.49, 95% CI = 3.91–87.30, respectively). The study also showed that moderate impairment (3–4 points in ADL scale) was 5.52 times more often and severe functional impairment ($\leq$2 points in ADL scale) was 21.07 times more likely to predispose patients to EA. People who suffered from COVID-19 in the past were 1.59 times more likely to be victims of older adult abuse (95% CI = 1.03–2.46).

The project also assessed the risk of EA using the VASS scale. It has been shown that in the study population nearly 46% of the elderly were at risk of abuse (VASS $\geq$ 3 points). Most of the factors predisposing to increased susceptibility to abuse were similar to those obtained in the assessment of the presence of EA. The exception was age and place of residence, which according to the logistic regression model were not significant risk factors for abuse. Interestingly, who the respondent lives with affects the very risk of EA For example, older people living with a son/daughter or cohabitating partner were more likely to be abused than those living with their spouse (OR = 4.41, 95% CI = 2.43–8.02; OR = 3.75, 95% CI = 1.80–7.81, respectively) (Table 2).

We found moderate, positive and significant correlation between EA and the VASS scale ($R = 0.54$; $p < 0.05$). In addition, the GDS scale showed a statistically significant correlation with the VASS scale and with the occurrence of older adult abuse ($R = 0.68$ and $R = 0.54$, respectively). Subsequently, it was observed that the ADL scale correlated significantly with both EA and VASS ($R = -0.46$ and $R = -0.58$, respectively). Moreover, the self-assessment of the health condition correlates in a statistically significant negative way only with the VASS assessment ($R = -0.19$) (Table 3).

Table 1. Descriptive characteristics.

Characteristics	N (%)
Sex	
Female	194 (55.9)
Male	153 (44.1)
Age	
65–70 years	162 (46.7)
71–85 years	118 (34.0)
>85 years	67 (19.3)
Education	
Primary	87 (25.1)
Secondary	100 (28.8)
Vocational	91 (26.2)
Higher	69 (19.9)
Marital Status	
Single (never married)	45 (13.0)
Married	103 (29.7)
In a partnership	39 (11.2)
Divorcee	43 (12.4)
Widow/Widower	117 (33.7)
Equivalent family income	
Low <233	101 (29.1)
Middle	164 (47.3)
High >465	82 (23.6)
Residency area	
City	223 (64.3)
Village	124 (35.7)
Chronic disease	
Yes	240 (69.2)
No	107 (30.8)
Depression (GDS scale)	
No	216 (62.2)
Moderate	119 (34.3)
Severe	12 (3.5)
Activities of Daily Living (ADL)	
Full function (5–6)	212 (61.1)
Moderate impairment (3–4)	100 (28.8)
Severe functional impairment ($\leq$2)	35 (10.1)
COVID-19 in the past	
Yes	147 (42.4)
No	200 (57.6)

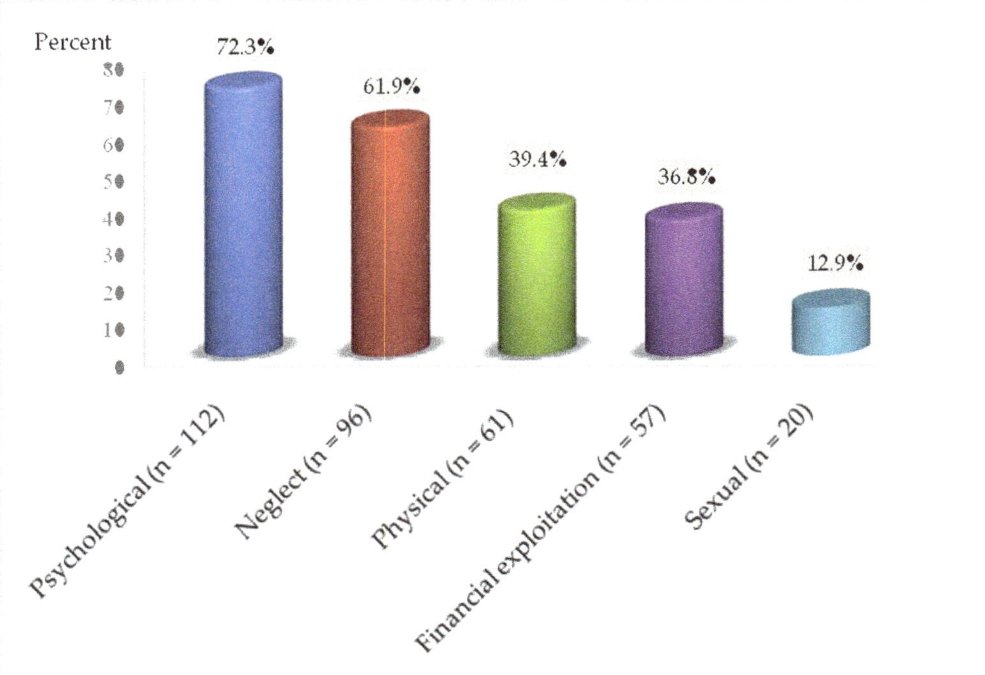

Figure 1. Type of elder abuse.

Table 2. Logistic regression analyses of factors associated with elder abuse and vulnerability to abuse screening scale (VASS).

Characteristic	Elder Abuse			Vulnerability to Abuse Screening Scale (VASS)		
	N (%)	OR (95%CI)	p	N (%)	OR (95%CI)	p
Overall	155 (44.7)	—	—	159 (45.8)	—	—
Sex						
Male	55 (35.5)	1.00		57 (35.8)	1.00	
Female	100 (64.5)	1.90 (1.23–2.93)	0.003 *	102 (64.2)	1.87 (1.21–2.88)	0.004 *
Age						
60–65	81 (52.3)	2.35 (1.28–4.31)	0.005 *	78 (49.1)	1.66 (0.93–2.99)	0.089
66–70	54 (34.8)	1.98 (1.05–3.75)	0.035 *	57 (35.8)	1.67 (0.90–3.10)	0.101
>70	20 (12.9)	1.00		24 (15.1)	1.00	
Education						
Primary	47 (30.3)	1.00		47 (29.6)	1.00	
Secondary	47 (30.3)	0.75 (0.42–1.34)	0.338	47 (29.6)	0.75 (0.42–1.34)	0.338
Vocational	42 (27.1)	0.73 (0.41–1.32)	0.294	51 (32.1)	1.08 (0.60–1.96)	0.786
Higher	19 (12.3)	0.32 (0.16–0.64)	0.001 *	14 (8.7)	0.22 (0.11–0.45)	<0.001 *
Marital status						
Single	13 (8.4)	1.00		15 (9.4)	1.00	
Married	43 (27.7)	1.76 (0.83–3.75)	0.140	30 (18.9)	0.82 (0.39–1.74)	0.609
In a partnership	13 (8.4)	1.23 (0.49–3.11)	0.660	21 (13.2)	2.33 (0.96–5.64)	0.601
Divorcee	27 (17.4)	4.15 (1.70–10.15)	0.002 *	25 (15.7)	2.78 (1.17–6.61)	0.021 *
Widower/Widow	59 (38.1)	2.50 (1.20–5.25)	0.015 *	68 (42.8)	2.78 (1.35–5.70)	0.005 *
Equivalent family income						
Low <233	59 (38.1)	3.60 (1.93–6.72)	<0.001 *	63 (39.6)	6.34 (3.25–12.37)	0.000 *
Middle	73 (47.1)	2.06 (1.16–3.65)	0.013 *	79 (49.7)	3.55 (1.92–6.58)	<0.001 *

Table 2. *Cont.*

Characteristic	Elder Abuse			Vulnerability to Abuse Screening Scale (VASS)		
	N (%)	OR (95%CI)	p	N (%)	OR (95%CI)	p
High >465	23 (14.8)	1.00		17 (10.7)	1.00	
Place of residence						
City	110 (71.0)	1.71 (1.09–2.68)	0.020 *	105 (66.0)	1.15 (0.74–1.79)	0.526
Village	45 (29.0)	1.00		54 (34.0)	1.00	
Chronic disease						
Yes	120 (77.4)	2.06 (1.28–3.31)	0.003 *	126 (79.2)	2.48 (1.53–4.01)	<0.001 *
No	35 (22.6)	1.00		33 (20.8)	1.00	
Loneliness						
Never or rarely	55 (35.5)	1.00		49 (30.8)	1.00	
Often	74 (47.7)	2.31 (1.45–3.68)	<0.001 *	80 (50.3)	3.27 (2.03–5.25)	<0.001 *
Very often or almost always	26 (16.8)	2.89 (1.46–5.72)	0.002 *	30 (18.9)	5.07 (2.48–10.39)	<0.001 *
Participation in family decisions						
Never or rarely	103 (66.5)	1.00		107 (67.3)	1.00	
Often	33 (21.2)	0.46 (0.28–0.78)	0.003 *	34 (21.4)	0.45 (0.27–0.75)	0.002 *
Very often or almost always	19 (12.3)	0.31 (0.17–0.57)	<0.001 *	18 (11.3)	0.26 (0.14–0.49)	<0.001 *
Relationship with the family						
Good	37 (23.9)	1.00		38 (23.9)	1.00	
Fair	9 (5.8)	0.94 (0.40–2.23)	0.890	5 (3.1)	0.43 (0.15–1.20)	0.106
Poor	80 (51.6)	3.26 (1.96–5.43)	<0.001 *	86 (54.1)	3.76 (2.25–6.27)	0.000 *
Lack of family	29 (18.7)	3.32 (1.68–6.56)	<0.001 *	30 (18.9)	3.47 (1.76–6.87)	<0.001 *
Live with						
Spouse	38 (24.5)	1.00		29 (18.2)	1.00	
Cohabitant	21 (13.5)	1.34 (0.66–2.74)	0.408	28 (17.6)	3.75 (1.80–7.81)	<0.001 *
Son/daughter	51 (32.9)	1.71 (0.97–3.00)	0.064	64 (40.3)	4.41 (2.43–8.02)	<0.001 *
Alone	45 (29.1)	1.24 (0.71–2.18)	0.444	38 (23.9)	1.41 (0.78–2.54)	0.252
Depression (GDS scale)						
No	46 (29.7)	1.00		54 (34.0)	1.00	
Moderate	99 (63.9)	18.29 (10.24–32.69)	<0.001 *	95 (59.7)	11.86 (6.90–20.45)	<0.001 *
Severe	10 (6.4)	18.49 (3.91–87.30)	<0.001 *	10 (6.3)	15.00 (3.19–70.61)	<0.001 *
Activities of Daily Living (ADL)						
Full function (5–6)	57 (36.8)	1.00		49 (30.8)	1.00	
Moderate impairment (3–4)	67 (43.2)	5.52 (3.30–9.25)	<0.001 *	77 (48.4)	11.14 (6.33–19.59)	<0.001 *
Severe functional impairment (≤2)	31 (20.0)	21.07 (7.12–62.35)	<0.001 *	33 (20.8)	54.89 (12.71–236.9)	<0.001 *
COVID–19 in the past						
No	56 (36.1)	1.00		55 (34.6)	1.00	
Yes	99 (63.9)	1.59 (1.03–2.46)	0.035 *	104 (65.4)	1.81 (1.17–2.80)	0.007 *

*—significant dependencies.

Table 3. Spearman's rank correlation test.

	Elder Abuse	VASS Assessment
	R p	R p
GDS	0.54 < 0.05	0.68 < 0.05
ADL	−0.46 < 0.05	−0.58 < 0.05
The self-assessment of the health condition	−0.06 > 0.05	−0.19 < 0.05
VASS assessment	0.54 < 0.05	——

4. Discussion

To the best of four knowledge we are the first to highlight the association between COVID-19 and EA's occurrence in Poland in a hospital setting. In our study we confirmed the increase in the experience of abuse by the elderly during the COVID-19 pandemic. We emphasized that women, people aged 60–65, low socioeconomic status, chronic diseases, poor relationship with the family and lack of family, moderate and severe depression, ADL ≤ 3 and COVID-19 were factors that predispose mainly to EA and to increased susceptibility to abuse assessed using the VASS scale. Our reports additionally coincide with the evolving evidence of a surge in EA during a pandemic. Thus healthcare professionals must prepare themselves as best as possible to deal with this growing problem among their patients. We enrolled only hospitalized people. Therefore, the results of these studies cannot be strictly generalized to the entire Polish population. Further research is needed in the various settings of older adults. Our research during the COVID-19 pandemic showed that nearly 45% of the hospitalized elderly were victims of EA. On the other hand, in a cross-sectional study conducted by our team in the period before COVID-19 on a group of 200 older adults with similar inclusion criteria, it was shown that 38.5% of respondents had experienced abuse [13]. This means an increase of over six percentage points. Both the present and past findings indicate that psychological abuse is the most common form of EA [9,13]. On the other hand, Chang et al. [4] noted the occurrence of EA during the COVID-19 pandemic among 21.3% of respondents, an 83.6% increase compared to prevalence estimates prior to the pandemic. In addition, in China, a study by Du and Chen [23] found that 15.4% of the older adults were victims of EA. The conducted preliminary analyses of factors indicate an actual large increase in the percentage of victims of older adult abuse [24,25]. So far, however, only a limited number of studies have been published on the occurrence of EA during COVID-19. Therefore, our results could provide relevant and missing information in this area of research in a pandemic.

Before the pandemic, in the ABUEL study, conducted among seven European countries (Germany, Italy, Lithuania, Sweden, Portugal, Spain and Greece) among 4467 respondents aged 60–84 years old, the incidents of elder abuse and neglect was also assessed. It was shown that within 12 months, psychological abuse was experienced by 19.4% of respondents, financial exploitation—3.8%, physical—2.7%, and sexual—0.7% [26]. Interestingly, research conducted in Ireland found that the country has the lowest prevalence of EA—2.2% [27]. In turn, the highest prevalence is found in Croatia—61.1% [28]. These results prove, that the prevalence rate of elder abuse varies widely. From the few studies conducted in Poland, it can be concluded that the EA rates in Poland also remains at a high level. Research conducted by a team of psychologists from the Institute of Psychology of the Polish Academy of Sciences in Poland shows that 59.7% of respondents reported the use of at least one form of EA outside their own family, and 30.1% in their own family [29]. In turn, the study by Kołodziejczak et al. [30] found that abuse affected 40.1% of older respondents living in rural areas. Our results are consistent with those presented by other authors from many different countries. For example, in a study by Hosseinkhan et al. [31] among 683 older adults it was found that 38.5% of the respondents were victims of EA. Subsequently, Anand [32] showed that out of 1435 respondents, 35% had experienced abuse. Torres-Castro et al. [33] reported a violence rate of 35.7%, and the study group was 487. If before the pandemic the EA rates in some countries were high and now increase even more, we will be faced with a serious social problem.

Interestingly, there are some common risk factors for both fraud susceptibility and COVID-19. Certainly, these factors include comorbidities that predispose to EA [34,35] and are associated with a higher mortality rate due to COVID-19 [36]. Following this trail, it can be safely stated that disability is also a significant risk factor for EA [37] and COVID-19 [38]. Moreover, COVID-19 itself predisposes to an increase in abuse among the elderly [4,24,25]. The remaining risk factors for EA during the pandemic do not differ from those that existed before the pandemic. And these include: female gender, younger age, economic problems, city living, comorbidities, depression, disability and dependence. Our results are consistent with the results presented by other researchers [7,35,39–41]. Our research also indicates that statistically single people were more likely to experience abuse. In addition in the research conducted by Liu et al. [25], victims of older adult abuse reported a feeling of loneliness. Further more, a poor relationship with the family predisposes you to EA in a statistically significant way. Fraga Dominguez et al. [40] also showed that family relationships are a significant risk factor for abuse.

Research shows that the COVID-19 pandemic has added fuel to the fire in terms of EA. It turned out to be extremely harmful to the older adults. Many of the EA risk factors presented have increased during the course of the pandemic. For example, the need for isolation and social distancing have contributed to feelings of loneliness and neglect. In addition, the elderly are aware of the dangers of falling ill with COVID-19, and have experienced a real threat to health (and sometimes life) as a result of infection. It can be assumed that they may therefore be particularly prone to developing depressive and anxiety symptoms. Consequently, it is also associated with an increased risk of EA, as many studies have identified depression as a risk factor for abuse [33,42–46]. Depressive disorders cause further deterioration of mental and physical functioning, loss of social position, autonomy, and, as a result, the disappearance of social relations. All these factors increase the occurrence of acts of EA. Moreover, experiencing abuse aggravates depression and increases anxiety [42,43,45]. Further more, the older adults are a group particularly at risk of complications after contracting COVID-19, which in consequence often leads to increased dependence on other people and disability, which is a significant risk factor for EA [4,12,46]. Another leading factor in fraud is the financial problems that have worsened during the COVID-19 pandemic. Mass dismissals from work, forced leaves and isolation resulted in a decline in social status among the society. Due to the fact that pensions of the elderly in Poland are often insufficient, they require financial assistance from their children or family. The emerging economic pressure, stress and economic problems of the families of the elderly are the main cause of EA [23].

We are fully aware of the limitations. The study was conducted in a limited geographical area, so be careful in drawing conclusions on the entire population. In addition, the subjects are hospitalized people, therefore future research should be extended to include a research group from various environments and different regions.

5. Conclusions

Overall, this study saw an increase in EA rates during the COVID-19 pandemic. Factors such as: female gender, younger age, economic problems, living in a city, comorbidities, disability and dependence, loneliness, poor relationship with the family and lack of family, moderate and severe depression, ADL ≤ 3, and COVID-19 in a significant manner influenced the occurrence of abuses. Due to the fact that so far little data on this subject has been published, it is necessary to conduct further detailed research.

Author Contributions: Conceptualization, K.F., M.B., R.Ś.; methodology, K.F., M.B., R.Ś.; software, R.Ś., K.F.; validation, K.F., M.B., A.W., R.Ś.; formal analysis, K.F., M.B., A.W., R.Ś.; investigation, K.F., M.B., A.W.; resources, K.F.; data curation, K.F.; writing—original draft preparation, K.F., M.B., A.W., R.J., A.K., E.G.-S., K.K.-K., R.Ś.; writing—review and editing, K.F., A.W.; visualization, K.F., R.J., A.K., E.G.-S.; supervision, M.B., K.K.-K., R.Ś.; project administration, K.F. All authors have read and agreed to the published version of the manuscript.

Funding: This research received no external funding.

Institutional Review Board Statement: The study was conducted according to the guidelines of the Declaration of Helsinki, and approved by the Institutional Review Board (or Ethics Committee) of Nicolaus Copernicus University in Torun at Collegium Medicum of Ludwik Rydygier in Bydgoszcz (approval no. 437/2020).

Informed Consent Statement: Informed consent was obtained from all subjects involved in the study.

Data Availability Statement: The data presented in this study are available on request from the corresponding author. The data are not publicly available due to respondents privacy.

Acknowledgments: The authors thank all participants, investigators and Collegium Medicum in Bydgoszcz, Nicolaus Copernicus University in Toruń.

Conflicts of Interest: The authors declare no conflict of interest.

References

1. Coronavirus Disease (COVID-19) Pandemic. Available online: https://www.who.int/emergencies/diseases/novel-coronavirus-2019?gclid=EAIaIQobChMIm7jPx4e28gIVks53Ch1tIQpuEAAYASAAEgIuBvD_BwE (accessed on 9 August 2021).
2. Qiu, J.; Shen, B.; Zhao, M.; Wang, Z.; Xie, B.; Xu, Y. A nationwide survey of psychological distress among Chinese people in the COVID-19 epidemic: Implications and policy recommendations. *Gen. Psychiatry* **2020**, *33*, e100213. [CrossRef] [PubMed]
3. Rajkumar, R.P. COVID-19 and mental health: A review of the existing literature. *Asian J. Psychiatry* **2020**, *52*, 102066. [CrossRef] [PubMed]
4. Chang, E.S.; Levy, B.R. High prevalence of elder abuse during the COVID-19 pandemic: Risk and resilience factors. *Am. J. Geriatr. Psychiatry* **2021**, *14*, 1–14. [CrossRef]
5. Schulz, R.; Beach, S.R.; Czaja, S.J.; Martire, L.M.; Monin, J.K. Family Caregiving for Older Adults. *Annu. Rev. Psychol.* **2020**, *71*, 635–659. [CrossRef]
6. Lund, E.M. Interpersonal violence against people with disabilities: Additional concerns and considerations in the COVID-19 pandemic. *Rehabil. Psychol.* **2020**, *65*, 199–205. [CrossRef]
7. Elder Abuse. Available online: https://www.who.int/en/news-room/fact-sheets/detail/elder-abuse (accessed on 14 August 2021).
8. Botngård, A.; Eide, A.H.; Mosqueda, L.; Malmedal, W. Elder abuse in Norwegian nursing homes: A cross-sectional exploratory study. *BMC Health Serv. Res.* **2020**, *20*, 9. [CrossRef]
9. Filipska, K.; Biercewicz, M.; Wiśniewski, A.; Kędziora-Kornatowska, K.; Ślusarz, R. Prevalence and associated factors of elder psychological abuse- a cross- sectional screening study, based on a hospitalized community from Poland. *Arch. Gerontol. Geriatr.* **2020**, *90*, 104152. [CrossRef]
10. Yon, Y.; Mikton, C.R.; Gassoumis, Z.D.; Wilber, K.H. Elder abuse prevalence in community settings: A systematic review and meta-analysis. *Lancet* **2017**, *5*, 147–156. [CrossRef]
11. Makaroun, L.K.; Bachrach, R.L.; Rosland, A.M. Elder abuse in the time of COVID-19-increased risks for older adults and their caregivers. *Am. J. Geriatr. Psychiatry* **2020**, *28*, 876–880. [CrossRef]
12. Elman, A.; Breckman, R.; Clark, S.; Gottesman, E.; Rachmuth, L.; Reiff, M.; Callahan, J.; Russell, L.A.; Curtis, M.; Solomon, J. Effects of the COVID-19 outbreak on elder mistreatment and response in New York City: Initial lessons. *J. Appl. Gerontol.* **2020**, *39*, 690–699. [CrossRef]
13. Filipska, K.; Biercewicz, M.; Wiśniewski, A.; Kędziora-Kornatowska, K.; Ślusarz, R. Prevalence of elder abuse and neglect: Screening in Poland families. *Eur. Geriatr. Med.* **2019**, *10*, 817–825. [CrossRef]
14. Elder Abuse-American Psychological Association. Available online: https://www.apa.org/pi/prevent-violence/resources/elder-abuse (accessed on 26 August 2021).
15. Preventing Elder Abuse. Available online: https://www.cdc.gov/violenceprevention/elderabuse/fastfact.html (accessed on 26 August 2021).
16. Schofield, M.J.; Mishra, G.D. Validity of self-report screening scale for elder abuse: Women's Health Australia Study. *Gerontology* **2003**, *43*, 110–120. [CrossRef]
17. Yesavage, J.A.; Brink, T.L.; Rose, T.L.; Lum, O.; Huang, V.; Adey, M.; Leirer, V.O. Development and validation of a Geriatric Depression Screening Scale: A preliminary report. *J. Psychiatr. Res.* **1983**, *17*, 37–49. [CrossRef]
18. Lesher, E.L.; Berryhill, J.S. Validation of the Geriatric Depression Scale–Short Form among inpatients. *J. Clin. Psychol.* **1994**, *50*, 256–260. [CrossRef]
19. Katz, S.; Ford, A.B.; Moskowitz, R.W.; Jackson, B.A.; Jaffe, M.W. Studies of illness in the aged: The Index of ADL: A standardized measure of biological and psychosocial function. *JAMA* **1963**, *185*, 914–919. [CrossRef]
20. Katz, S.; Down, T.D.; Cash, H.R.; Grotz, R.C. Progress in the development of the index of ADL. *Gerontology* **1970**, *10*, 20–30. [CrossRef]
21. Curcio, C.L.; Payán-Villamizar, C.; Jiménez, A.; Gómez, F. Abuse in Colombian elderly and its association with socioeconomic conditions and functionality. *Colomb. Med.* **2019**, *50*, 77–88. [CrossRef]
22. Pak, M. The prevalence and associated risk factors of elder abuse among older people applied to the family health center in the rural district of Turkey. *Soc. Work Health Care* **2020**, *59*, 236–256. [CrossRef]
23. Du, P.; Chen, Y. Prevalence of elder abuse and victim-related risk factors during the COVID-19 pandemic in China. *BMC Public Health* **2021**, *21*, 1096. [CrossRef]
24. Han, S.D.; Mosqueda, L. Elder abuse in the COVID-19 era. *J. Am. Geriatr. Soc.* **2020**, *68*, 1386–1387. [CrossRef]
25. Liu, P.J.; Wang, A.; Schwab-Reese, L.M.; Stratton, S.K. Elder Mistreatment Victims during the COVID-19 Pandemic: Administrative Data from San Francisco Adult Protective Services. *J. Fam. Violence* **2021**, *14*, 1–14. [CrossRef]

26. Fraga, S.; Lindert, J.; Barros, H.; Torres-González, F.; Ioannidi-Kapolou, E.; Melchiorre, M.G.; Stankunas, M.; Soares, J.F. Elder abuse and socioeconomic inequalities: A multilevel study in 7 European countries. *Prev. Med.* **2014**, *61*, 42–47. [CrossRef] [PubMed]
27. Naughton, C.; Drennan, J.; Lyons, I.; Lafferty, A.; Treacy, M.; Phelan, A.; O'Loughlin, A.; Delaney, L. Elder abuse and neglect in Ireland: Results from a national prevalence survey. *Age Ageing* **2012**, *41*, 98–103. [CrossRef] [PubMed]
28. Ajdukovic, M.; Ogresta, J.; Rusac, S. Family violence and health among elderly in Croatia. *J. Aggress. Maltreat Trauma* **2009**, *18*, 261–279. [CrossRef]
29. Korzeniowski, K.; Radkiewicz, P. *Domestic Violence Against the Elderly and Disabled People*; Report from a Nationwide Survey 2015 and a Comparative Study from 2009–2015; Institute of Psychology of the Polish Academy of Sciences: Warsaw, Poland, 2015.
30. Kołodziejczak, S.; Terelak, A.; Bulsa, M. Domestic violence against seniors in rural areas of West Pomerania, Poland. *Ann. Agric. Env. Med.* **2019**, *26*, 92–96. [CrossRef]
31. Hosseinkhani, Z.; Moradi, Z.; Khodamoradi, F. Elder abuse: Screening in Iranian families. *Med. J. Islam Repub. Iran.* **2017**, *31*, 126. [CrossRef]
32. Anand, A. Exploring the role of socioeconomic factors in abuse and neglect of elderly population in Maharashtra, India. *J. Geriatr. Ment. Health* **2016**, *3*, 150–157. [CrossRef]
33. Torres-Castro, S.; Szlejf, C.; Parra-Rodríguez, L.; Rosas-Carrasco, O. Association between frailty and elder abuse in community-dwelling older adults in Mexico city. *J. Am. Geriatr. Soc.* **2018**, *66*, 1773–1778. [CrossRef]
34. Alexa, I.D.; Ilie, A.C.; Pislaru, A.I.; Dronic, A.; Gavrilovici, O.; Alexa-Stratulat, T.; Stefaniu, R.; Sandu, I.; Nuta, C.; Herghelegiu, A.M. Elder abuse and associated factors in eastern romania. *Psychogeriatrics* **2020**, *20*, 196–205. [CrossRef]
35. Brijoux, T.; Neise, M.; Zank, S. Elder abuse in the oldest old: Prevalence, risk factors and consequences. *Z. Für Gerontol. Und Geriatr.* **2021**, 1–6. [CrossRef]
36. Kuo, C.L.; Pilling, L.C.; Atkins, J.L.; Masoli, J.A.H.; Delagado, J.; Kuchel, G.A.; Melzer, D. APOE e4 genotype predicts severe COVID-19 in the UK biobank community cohort. *J. Gerontol. A Biol. Sci. Med. Sci.* **2020**, *75*, 2231–2232. [CrossRef]
37. Mahmoudian, A.; Shamsalinia, A.; Alipour, A.; Fotoukian, Z.; Ghaffari, F. Structural equation model of affecting factors on elder abuse to patients under hemodialysis by family caregivers. *BMC Geriatr.* **2021**, *21*, 360. [CrossRef]
38. Weng, C.C.; Lin, Y.E.; Lin, Y.C.; Chen, W. New Preventative Measures Against Coronavirus Disease 2019 for Home Care Aides in Taiwan. *J. Gerontol. A Biol. Sci. Med. Sci.* **2021**, *76*, e76–e77. [CrossRef]
39. Acharya, S.R.; Suman, B.K.; Pahari, S.; Shin, Y.C.; Moon, D.H. Prevalence of abuse among the elderly population of Syangja, Nepal. *BMC Public Health* **2021**, *21*, 1348. [CrossRef]
40. Fraga Dominguez, S.; Ozguler, B.; Storey, J.E.; Rogers, M. Elder Abuse Vulnerability and Risk Factors: Is Financial Abuse Different From Other Subtypes? *J. Appl. Gerontol.* **2021**, 7334648211036402. [CrossRef]
41. Jeon, G.S.; Cho, S.I.; Choi, K.; Jang, K.S. Gender Differences in the Prevalence and Correlates of Elder Abuse in a Community-Dwelling Older Population in Korea. *Int. J. Environ. Res. Public Health* **2019**, *16*, 100. [CrossRef]
42. Wu, L.; Chen, H.; Hu, Y.; Xiang, H.; Yu, X.; Zhang, T.; Cao, Z.; Wang, Y. Prevalence and associated factors of elder mistreatment in a rural community in People's Republic of China: A cross-sectional study. *PLoS ONE* **2012**, *7*, e33857. [CrossRef]
43. Choi, Y.J.; O'Donnell, M.; Choi, H.B.; Jung, H.S.; Cowlishaw, S. Associations among elder abuse, depression and ptsd in South Korean older adults. *Int. J. Environ. Res. Pub. Health* **2018**, *15*, 1948. [CrossRef]
44. Sembiah, S.; Dasgupta, A.; Taklikar, C.S.; Paul, B.; Bandyopadhyay, L.; Burman, J. Elder abuse and its predictors: A cross-sectional study in a rural area of West Bengal, eastern part of India. *Psychogeriatrics* **2020**, *20*, 636–644. [CrossRef]
45. Fang, B.; Yan, E. Abuse of older persons with dementia: A review of the literature. *Trauma Violence Abus.* **2018**, *19*, 127–147. [CrossRef]
46. Arthur-Holmes, F.; Gyasi, R.M. COVID-19 crisis and increased risks of elder abuse in caregiving spaces. *Glob. Pub. Health* **2021**, *16*, 1675–1679. [CrossRef] [PubMed]

Journal of
Clinical Medicine

MDPI

Review

A Systematic Review on Detraining Effects after Balance and Fall Prevention Interventions

Shaghayegh Modaberi [1], Esmaeel Saemi [2], Peter A. Federolf [3] and Steven van Andel [3,*]

[1] Department of Sport Sciences, Faculty of Social Sciences, Imam Khomeini International University, Qazvin 34149-16818, Iran; modaberi@soc.ikiu.ac.ir
[2] Department of Motor Behavior and Sport Psychology, Shahid Chamran University of Ahvaz, Ahvaz 83151-61355, Iran; e.saemi@scu.ac.ir
[3] Department of Sport Science, University of Innsbruck, 6020 Innsbruck, Austria; Peter.Federolf@uibk.ac.at
* Correspondence: Steven.van-Andel@uibk.ac.at

Abstract: Since the COVID-19 pandemic hit, lockdowns have been implemented to fight off infections in countries around the world. Whilst this measure is without a doubt effective against spreading infection, it might also decrease participation in exercise. For older adults, exercise is particularly important in the prevention of falls, and sudden detraining because of a lockdown or due to other causes might have detrimental consequences. This systematic review study aims to assess what is currently known on detraining effects for balance outcomes. Nine studies were included within this review. Results suggest that detraining effects could already be significant as early as 4 weeks after stopping the intervention. Programs that specifically focus on improving balance were more robust against detraining, with most positive effects still being present after 8 weeks. However, even with a specific focus on balance, studies started to show some signs of detraining. The current study is limited by the low number of included studies in the review, indicating a need to further confirm these results.

Keywords: postural control; balance; detraining; falls; inactivity; lockdown; COVID-19; ageing

Citation: Modaberi, S.; Saemi, E.; Federolf, P.A.; van Andel, S. A Systematic Review on Detraining Effects after Balance and Fall Prevention Interventions. *J. Clin. Med.* **2021**, *10*, 4656. https://doi.org/10.3390/jcm10204656

Academic Editor: Michele Roccella

Received: 28 July 2021
Accepted: 5 October 2021
Published: 11 October 2021

1. Introduction

Around the world, populations are ageing [1], leading to an increased incidence of age-related accidental injuries, often caused by falls [2,3]. In recent years, evidence has been building that falls, particularly in older individuals, are to some degree preventable. Specifically, several studies confirmed that exercise programs can be effective in improving balance and in lowering fall rates in older adults, as summarized in recent review papers [4,5]. However, recently, access to exercise programs has been severely limited by the global response to the COVID-19 pandemic: sports facilities were closed, and in some cases, citizens were asked to stay at home, sometimes for periods of several weeks. Since older adults have a higher risk for a difficult progression in case of a COVID-19 infection, this age group is particularly subjected to restrictions. This is unfortunate, since particularly in this age group, exercises have a number of tangible health benefits, including the maintenance of the balance and postural control skills that are needed to prevent falls and accidental injuries.

The concept of detraining has been described in previous literature as "the partial or complete loss of training-induced anatomical, physiological, and performance adaptations, as a consequence of training reduction or cessation" [6], p. 80. Historically, research has mainly focused on the physiological effects of detraining after strength or resistance training, e.g., [7,8], but very little is known about detraining in balance skill [9]. The current study assumes that a sudden stop in balance training might induce detraining effects that could increase the risk of falls in older adults. While the recently experienced lockdowns due to COVID-19 motivated the current study, our research question is of general interest, since a sudden stop of participation in a regular exercise program can occur for various reasons. As such, the current study will focus on the "performance adaptation" component of detraining to assess the effects of a cessation of balance training for indicators of fall risk.

The aim of the current study was to review the available scientific literature on detraining effects after a sudden stop of an exercise program on outcomes related to fall risk. To operationalize this aim, we shall consider fall risk in two ways. Firstly, as a direct measure of fall risk, studies reporting on fall rates would be accepted into the review. Second, as an indirect measure, studies reporting on fall risk assessments will be accepted. This second definition might pose some methodological challenge, since indirect measures of fall risk are numerous [10] and might not always be easily compared. For these studies, the study characteristics shall be synchronized in one table in an effort to distill common principles from the literature.

2. Materials and Methods

This systematic review was carried out in accordance with the Preferred Reporting Items for Systematic Reviews guideline [11] and under PROSPERO registration number CRD42020199932.

2.1. Information Sources and Search Strategy

The initial search was performed on 20 August 2020, by using the following databases: Web of Science (all databases), Scopus, PubMed, PEDro, and Cochrane Library. Searches were conducted in English. The option "advanced searches" was chosen for searches in Web of Science, PubMed, and Scopus with regard to the articles' title, abstract, and keywords. A simple search was done in Cochrane library and PEDro. The Boolean operators used were "OR" within the construct, and "AND" between constructs. The following search terms were used:

(detraining OR inactivity)
AND
(balance OR "postural control" OR "postural stability")
AND
("fall risk" OR "falls risk" OR falling OR "fall rate")

2.2. Eligibility Criteria and Study Selection

Articles were eligible for inclusion in the current study according to the following criteria. Any type of intervention study was accepted in the review (e.g., randomized controlled trials, non-randomized controlled trials, pre-post studies with no control group). Only studies written in English were considered. In terms of outcomes, only studies that measured balance control in humans after a period of detraining were included. Here, we consider any study that reports on the effects of a sudden stop to exercise participation to fit this description. No limitations were set to the characteristics of the participants (e.g., young or old, athletes or sedentary), with the exception that clinical groups in which balance might be affected (e.g., amputations, neurological pathology, recent surgery) were excluded from the review. No limitations were set for the year of publishing.

In the first screening step, duplicates were removed using EndNote software. Further screening steps were performed after exporting to Microsoft Excel. Two authors were responsible for the screening process (S.M. and E.S.) and screened first the titles and later the abstracts and, finally, on the full text to sort out papers based on the inclusion criteria.

2.3. Data Extraction

Two authors were responsible for data extraction (S.M. and S.A.). The following factors were extracted for any study that was included in the present review: study design, training duration, detraining duration, measurement tools, groups, age of participants, study results with respect to effect of training, effect of detraining, conclusion, and future recommendations.

2.4. Quality Assessment

Methodological quality in all studies was assessed using the Crowe Critical Appraisal Tool (or CCAT; [12,13]). Since several study designs were eligible, it was important to use a quality assessment tool designed for a broad range of study designs. The CCAT was developed to assess methodological quality of randomized controlled trials as well as other study designs and was, therefore, suitable for the current study. We shall interpret CCAT scores in quintiles to categorize studies as very low (0–8 points), low (9–16 points), moderate (17–24 points), high (25–32 points) or very high (33–40 points) methodological quality similar to [14]. The current review reports both the section scores per paper as well as the total scores overall, which are needed to draw conclusions both on an individual paper level, as well as for the entire field.

3. Results

From the systematic search, 386 papers were identified as potentially eligible for inclusion. Following the article selection steps (Figure 1), nine papers met the criteria for inclusion in the current study. No studies were identified that reported on fall rates after a detraining period, and as such, only studies that reported on indirect measures of fall risk were included. Characteristics of the included papers are displayed in Table 1.

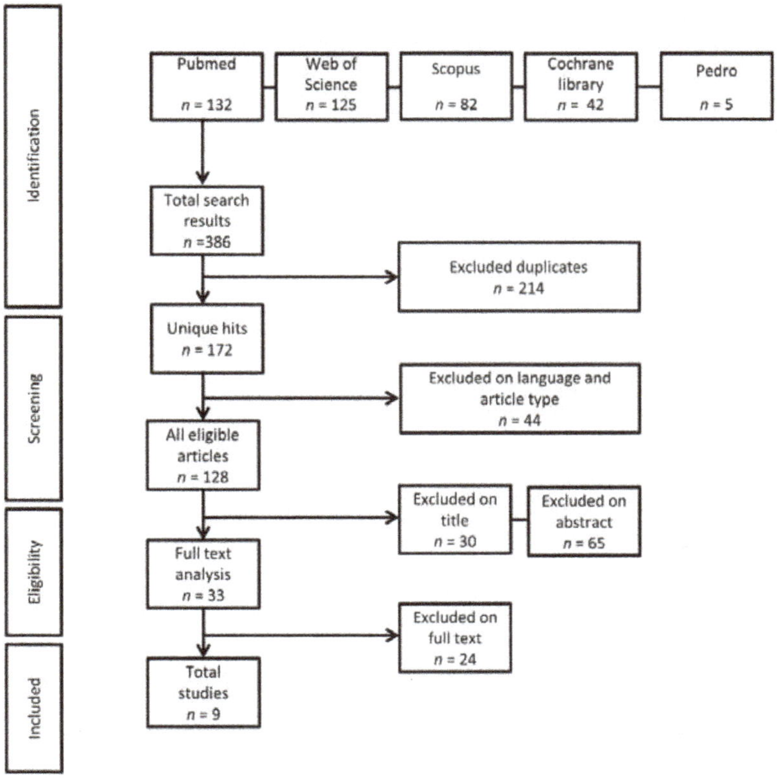

Figure 1. Flow diagram outlining the article selection steps.

Table 1. Data extraction table collating the characteristics from the (n = 9) included studies.

	Participants (N at Study Onset)	Training Duration	Training Intensity	Detraining Duration	Type of Intervention	Outcome Measures	Effect of Training	Effect of Detraining	Notes
Abbasi et al. [15]	Age: 70 ± 9.6 years (n = 60)	8 weeks	3 × 60 min per week	8 weeks, measured at 4, 6, and 8 weeks	Aquatic balance (AB) training	5 × STS	Significantly improved	Improvements retained at 8 w	Attrition information: No mention of dropout rate
						TUG	Significantly improved	Improvements retained at 8 w	
					Whole-body vibration (WBV) training	5 × STS	Significantly improved	*Returned to baseline at 6 w detraining*	
						TUG	Significantly improved	*Returned to baseline at 6 w detraining*	
					Combined AB and WBV	5 × STS	Significantly improved	Improvements retained at 8 w	
						TUG	Significantly improved	Improvements retained at 8 w	
Ansai et al. [16]	Age: 82.4 ± 2.4 years (n = 69)	16 weeks	3 × 60 min per week	6 weeks	Multicomponent training, containing aerobic, strength, and balance component	5 × STS	No significant improvement		Effects following "intention to treat" principle. Some effects were found in "high adherence" group. Attrition information: n = 1 participant dropped out before the post-test and 3 were lost to follow-up.
						Balance tests	No significant improvement		
						TUG	No significant improvement		
					Resistance training	5 × STS	No significant improvement		
						Balance tests	No significant improvement		
						TUG	No significant improvement		
Harvey et al. [17]	Age: 78.4 ± 6.9 years (n = 23)	10 weeks	3 × 40 min total	4 weeks	Motivational interview and retrospective feedback, one group with and one group without real time feedback	Chair sit and reach		*No significant improvement*	Only main effects between baseline and retention test reported. No effects of intervention itself. Attrition information: n = 13 participants completed the program.
						30 s STS		Significantly improved	
						BST		*No significant improvement*	
						TUG		Significantly improved	
						Sedentary behavior		*No significant improvement*	

Table 1. *Cont.*

	Participants (N at Study Onset)	Training Duration	Training Intensity	Detraining Duration	Type of Intervention	Outcome Measures	Effect of Training	Effect of Detraining	Notes
Ritzmann et al. [18]	Age: 30 ± 7 years (n = 23)			60 days head tilted down bedrest	Full bedrest	One-leg stance sway		*30–105% decrease*	No training intervention/detraining study, but study showing effects of bedrest on healthy subjects. Attrition information: one participant reallocated to full bedrest for medical reasons. n = 0 participants dropped out.
						One-leg stance co-contraction		*Increased co-contraction*	
						10 m walk test		*Significant decreases*	
						TUG		*20–40% decrease*	
						10 × STS		*20–80% decrease*	
					Bedrest with in total 48–3 min jump sessions	One-leg stance sway		No significant decrease	
						One-leg stance co-contraction		No significant decrease	
						10 m walk test		Most variables unchanged	
						TUG		No significant decrease	
						10 × STS		No significant decrease	
Sherk et al. [19]	Age: 64.5 ± 0.5 years (n = 69)	40 or 80 weeks	2 or 3 times per week	6 months	Resistance training 40 weeks	Upper body 1RM strength	52% increase	*About 15% decrease*	Detraining values visually assessed from Figure 3 in [19]. Attrition information: n = 69 participants returned for 6 month follow-up.
						Lower body 1RM strength	71% increase	*About 9% decrease*	
					Resistance training 80 weeks	Upper body 1RM strength	22% increase	*About 4% decrease*	
						Lower body 1RM strength	33% increase	No visible change	

Table 1. *Cont.*

	Participants (N at Study Onset)	Training Duration	Training Intensity	Detraining Duration	Type of Intervention	Outcome Measures	Effect of Training	Effect of Detraining	Notes
Sun et al. [20]	Age: 64.2 ± 3.18 years (n = 48)	16 weeks	5 × 60 min times per week	8 weeks	Tai Chi	Eyes open single leg stance variables	7/7 variables significantly improved	7/7 variables remain significantly different from baseline after 8 w detraining	No intention to treat data. Only participants who completed the program are reported 25% drop outs not. Reporte dattrition information: n = 36 participants completed the study.
						Eyes closed single leg stance variables	7/7 variables significantly improved	5/7 variables remain significantly different from baseline after 8 w detraining	
					Brisk Walking	Eyes open single leg stance variables	7/7 variables significantly improved	4/7 variables remain significantly different from baseline after 8 w detraining	
						Eyes closed single leg stance variables	7/7 variables significantly improved	5/7 variables remain significantly different from baseline after 8 w detraining	
Toulotte et al. [21]	Faller-group age: 71.1 ± 5.0 years (n = 16)	12 weeks	2 × 60 min per week	12 weeks	Low-intensity balance program	30 s one-leg stance test eyes open	Significantly improved	*Significant decrease*	Attrition information: No mention of dropout rate.
						30 s one-leg stance test eye closed	Significantly improved	*Significant decrease*	
						Gait variables single task	5/5 variables significantly improved	*0/5 variables stay on post-intervention value after 12 w detraining*	
						Gait variables dual task	5/5 variables significantly improved	*1/5 variables stay on post-intervention value after 12 w detraining*	
	Non-faller-group age: 68.4 ± 4.5 years (n = 8)	12 weeks	2 × 60 min per week	12 weeks	Low-intensity balance program	30 s one-leg stance test eyes open	Significantly improved	*Significant decrease*	
						30 s one-leg stance test eyes closed	No significant improvement	*Significant decrease*	
						Gait variables single task	5/5 variables significantly improved	*1/5 variables stay on post-intervention value after 12 w detraining*	
						Gait variables dual task	5/5 variables significantly improved	*0/5 variables stay on post-intervention value after 12 w detraining*	

Table 1. *Cont.*

	Participants (N at Study Onset)	Training Duration	Training Intensity	Detraining Duration	Type of Intervention	Outcome Measures	Effect of Training	Effect of Detraining	Notes
Vogler et al. [22]	Age: 80 ± 7 years (n = 180 in 3 groups)	12 weeks	3 times per week	12 weeks	Weight-bearing functional exercise	Physiological Profile Assessment	Visibly improved compared to controls	*Not different from controls at 12 w detraining*	Control condition: social visits. Direct post-intervention data not reported, differences reported here are visually assessed from Figure 2 in [22]. Attrition information: no difference in adherence between groups, n = 9 participants dropped out before the end of the 12 w training phase and n = 6 participants were lost to the 24 w follow-up.
						Maximal balance range	Visibly improved compared to controls	*Not different from controls at 12 w detraining*	
						Coordinated stability	Visibly improved compared to controls	Significantly improved compared to controls	
					Seated resistance exercise	Physiological Profile Assessment	Visibly improved compared to controls	*Not different from controls at 12 w detraining*	
						Maximal balance range	Visually not different from controls		
						Coordinated stability	Visually not different from controls		
Zhang et al. [23]	Age: 62.01 ± 4.40 years (n =60)	16 weeks	5 × 60 min times per week	8 weeks	Tai Chi	Plantar flexion proprioception	Significantly improved	Improvements retained at 8 w	Attrition information: n = 52 participants completed the study
						Dorsal flexion proprioception	Significantly improved	Improvements retained at 8 w	
						Inversion proprioception	No significant improvement compared to baseline		
						Eversion proprioception	No significant improvement compared to baseline		
					Brisk walking	Plantar flexion proprioception	Significantly improved	*Returned to baseline at 4 w detraining*	
						Dorsal flexion proprioception	No significant improvement compared to baseline		
						Inversion proprioception	No significant improvement compared to baseline		
						Eversion proprioception	No significant improvement compared to baseline		

Notes: STS = "sit to stand", TUG = "timed up and go", BST = "balance screening tool", 1RM = "one repetition maximum", w = weeks. Results that show significant detraining are displayed in italics.

3.1. Effects of Detraining

From the originally identified papers, only nine clearly described the effects of detraining on the postural control system. The duration of the detraining or retention period ranged from 4 weeks (n = 1 paper) to 6 weeks (n = 1), 8 weeks (n = 3), 12 weeks (n = 2), 60 days (n = 1), and the highest reported duration of detraining was half a year (n = 1). One included study did not report on detraining from an intervention, but rather "detraining from everyday life" by administering 60 days of bed rest. All of the other papers provided details of an intervention with a length of 8 weeks (n = 1), 10 weeks (n = 1), 12 weeks (n = 2), 16 weeks (n = 3) or 40/80 weeks (n = 1, in this particular study, participants could choose their own intervention length to increase adherence; [19]). Details of the interventions' main focus are displayed in Table 1.

Due to the differences in outcome measures and lengths of detraining, it is futile to quantify exact effects of detraining on a week-by-week basis. This is further complicated by studies that did not report on their effects directly post intervention, so it is unclear whether their detraining values later on indicate significant declines after the exercises were ceased (i.e., [17]). The first clear sign of detraining in all studies was after 4 weeks, at which point the improved plantar flexion proprioception after an 8-week brisk walking program had disappeared [23]. Further, at 6 weeks, the effects of an 8-week whole body vibration training program seemed to have returned to baseline [15]. More exercise effects seemed to disappear between 8 and 12 weeks, after which most benefits from a low-intensity balance program [21] and from seated or weight-bearing resistance training [22] had significantly digressed.

Exercises for which lasting benefits were reported after specified detraining periods were, firstly, an 8-week aquatic balance training (both with and without combining it with vibration training; outcome measures: 5 times sit-to-stand (STS) and timed up and go (TUG) performance; after 8 weeks of detraining [15]). Second, 16 weeks of Tai Chi still had positive effects on one-leg stance performance (strongest effects on eyes open condition [20] and on ankle plantar and dorsal flexion proprioception [23]) after 8 weeks of detraining. Additionally, third, 12 weeks of functional weightbearing exercise still had a positive effect on "coordinated stability" (the ability to draw a line within the lines of a track, using a pen fixed by a rod to the person at waist level) after 12 weeks of detraining [22]. However, in terms of this last result, it should be noted that outcomes for a more common indicator of fall risk, the "Physiological Profile Assessment", no longer showed differences compared to controls after 12 weeks of detraining [22].

In terms of long-term effects, it is interesting to note the benefits of a strength training protocol reported by Sherk et al. [19] on maximum strength outputs. They showed that, after 6 months of detraining, improvements were better retained if participants had been engaged with the program for a longer period of time (80 vs. 40 weeks of training). Finally, the results of Ritzmann et al. [18] are of relevance. They showed that the effects of detraining due to bed rest can be offset by the introduction of 3-min high-intensity jumping workouts.

3.2. Quality Assessment

Results from the quality assessment are depicted in Table 2. With an average score of 30.1/40, the studies were generally of high quality (one study was categorized as having moderate quality, six studies were categorized as having high quality, and two studies were categorized as having very high methodological quality). On average, the lowest scores (with also the biggest spread) were recorded in the sampling category, which relates to reporting of the sampling method, sample size, and recruitment protocols.

Table 2. Results of the CCAT quality assessment.

	Preliminaries	Introduction	Design	Sampling	Data Collection	Ethical Matters	Results	Discussion	Total
Abbasi et al. [15]	3	4	4	0	2	3	3	3	22 [M]
Ansai et al. [16]	3	4	5	4	4	4	4	3	31 [H]
Harvey et al. [17]	3	3	5	2	5	5	3	4	30 [H]
Ritzmann et al. [18]	4	5	5	4	5	5	5	4	37 [VH]
Sherk et al. [19]	4	4	2	3	5	5	3	3	29 [H]
Sun et al. [20]	2	2	4	3	5	5	5	4	30 [H]
Toulotte et al. [21]	4	3	5	3	3	4	3	5	30 [H]
Vogler et al. [22]	3	5	3	5	5	5	3	4	33 [VH]
Zhang et al. [23]	4	4	4	3	4	4	4	2	29 [H]
Mean values	3.3	3.8	4.1	3.0	4.2	4.4	3.7	3.6	30.1
Standard deviation	0.71	0.97	1.05	1.41	1.09	0.73	0.87	0.88	3.95

Note. Categorization of methodological quality of papers is noted in superscript ranging from moderate ([M]) to high ([H]) and very high ([VH]).

4. Discussion

The current study aimed to assess current literature on detraining effects after discontinuing an exercise program on indicators of fall risk. Through our systematic review protocol, a total of nine studies were considered eligible for inclusion in this study. Four studies showed effects that seemed relatively robust against the effects of detraining [15,20,22,23]. Common among these four seems to be a specific focus on balance training, in the form of aquatic balance training [15], weight-bearing (as opposed to seated) exercise [22], and Tai Chi [20,23]. However, programs that did not specifically target balance, or did so on low intensity, seem less effective after detraining (i.e., brisk walking, whole body vibration training, low-intensity balance training, seated or weight-bearing resistance training). No studies were found that assessed detraining effects directly on fall prevalence. Indirect effects on fall risk can be inferred from the included studies, considering that several of the analyzed outcome variables, e.g., one leg standing time [24] or the timed up and go (TUG) test [25] show good association to the actual fall risk. However, in this context, it should also be noted that not all recent studies confirm a strong association between these performance variables and predictive power as fall risk indicators [26].

It might be argued that bedrest is conceptually different than detraining and, therefore, should not be included in this review. We do not seek to discuss the definition of the concept of detraining in this study and emphasize that out operationalization of this concept ("any study that reports on the effects of a sudden stop to exercise participation") is just one way to work with this concept. This definition was adhered to because even studies that might not fit the strictest definition of detraining might illustrate important mechanisms for fall prevention in a practical sense. Even though a lock down is not as severe as a bedrest prescription, for older adults who are in risk groups (and may not dare to go outside), this measure will still result in severe increases in sedentary behavior. It is, therefore, promising to see that the effects of bedrest can be offset by even very short bouts of intense exercise [18]. However, the nature of the introduced program with its focus on unstable jumping exercises might not be the best fit for the older adult community where, due to age-related loss of bone mass [27], any fall might lead to the breaking of bones. As such, future studies should investigate how this training program could be adapted to keep older adults fit and steady at home.

The results from the quality assessment showed that the methodological quality of the articles overall was high, with a high variability of scores in the "sampling category". Future studies in this field would do well to provide a detailed description of their sampling strategy, for instance, by including details on a recruitment strategy, sample size calculation, and target population.

It is interesting that the current study set no restrictions to the age of included participants, and yet, all but one study showed a sample aged 62 years or older. This was most likely caused by the inclusion of search terms related to fall risk, as this is commonly assessed using an older cohort. This does limit the generalizability of our results to say most about this older cohort. The generalizability of the results is further limited by the fact that detraining might occur for older adults who regularly participate in physical activity, but it should be noted that, in general, this cohort is known to show high levels of sedentary behavior [28].

One inherent limitation to the study's design is that our search might not have identified all studies done on detraining, as some authors might not have specifically used this term in their study's protocol. That is, if a study describes an intervention with pre-test, post-test, and a relatively late retention test, then this could potentially be a useful addition to the current study. However, this is difficult to capture in a systematic search, as terms related to the word "retention" are not specific to this experimental design and significantly increase the number of hits towards the unmanageable. As such, it was decided to specifically focus the search on studies that mention the terms "detraining" or "inactivity" in order to achieve more focused set of search results. This has led to the inclusion of only nine studies, which might limit the applicability of the current results. These results should be further confirmed in future studies before drawing strong conclusions in regards to detraining and fall prevention. The current study can be used to guide future studies in this field. Specifically, future studies could hypothesize that training with a challenge to balance might be less susceptible to detraining effects compared to general training and that training effects would be sustained for about 8 weeks.

The current study provides preliminary evidence for the sustained effects of balance training 8 weeks after cessation of specific balance training. However, at this 8-week timepoint, even in the more successful programs, there were outcome variables that started to show significant reductions in performance. It could, thus, be expected that detraining would also start to affect participants in the more successful programs after 8 weeks. Should these results be confirmed in future studies, then it would imply that restrictions that limit the availability of balance training programs might have a negative effect on fall rates for older adults that regularly participate in fall prevention exercise, if they are longer than 8 weeks.

Author Contributions: Conceptualization, S.M., E.S., P.A.F. and S.v.A.; methodology, S.M., E.S., P.A.F. and S.v.A.; article selection, S.M. and E.S.; analysis, S.M. and S.v.A.; writing—original draft preparation, S.M. and S.v.A.; writing—review and editing, S.M., E.S., P.A.F. and S.v.A.; visualization, S.v.A. All authors have read and agreed to the published version of the manuscript.

Funding: Open access publication fees for this research have been covered by the University of Innsbruck, this research received no external funding.

Institutional Review Board Statement: Not applicable.

Informed Consent Statement: Not applicable.

Data Availability Statement: All data used in the current study re available in the public domain.

Acknowledgments: We thank Felix Wachholz for his contribution in the design of this study.

Conflicts of Interest: The authors declare no conflict of interest.

References

1. World Health Organization. *World Report on Ageing and Health*; World Health Organization: Luxembourg, 2015; ISBN 9780874216561.
2. Campbell, A.J.; Reinken, J.; Allan, B.C.; Martinez, G.S. Falls in Old Age: A Study of Frequency and Related Clinical Factors. *Age Ageing* **1981**, *10*, 264–270. [CrossRef]
3. World Health Organization. *WHO Global Report on Falls Prevention in Older Age*; World Health Organization: Geneva, Switzerland, 2007; ISBN 9789241563.
4. Papalia, G.F.; Papalia, R.; Diaz Balzani, L.A.; Torre, G.; Zampogna, B.; Vasta, S.; Fossati, C.; Alifano, A.M.; Denaro, V. The Effects of Physical Exercise on Balance and Prevention of Falls in Older People: A Systematic Review and Meta-Analysis. *J. Clin. Med.* **2020**, *9*, 2595. [CrossRef]
5. Sherrington, C.; Fairhall, N.J.; Wallbank, G.K.; Tiedemann, A.; Michaleff, Z.A.; Howard, K.; Clemson, L.; Hopewell, S.; Lamb, S.E. Exercise for Preventing Falls in Older People Living in the Community. *Cohrane Database Syst. Rev.* **2019**, *1*, CD012424. [CrossRef]
6. Mujika, I.; Padilla, S. Detraining: Loss of Training-Induced Physiological and Performance Adaptations. Part I. *Sport. Med.* **2000**, *30*, 79–87. [CrossRef]

7. Lemmer, J.T.; Hurlbut, D.E.; Martel, G.F.; Tracy, B.L.; Ivey, F.M.; Metter, E.J.; Fozard, J.L.; Fleg, J.L.; Hurley, B.F. Age and Gender Responses to Strength Training and Detraining. *Med. Sci. Sports Exerc.* **2000**, *32*, 1505–1512. [CrossRef]
8. Mujika, I.; Padilla, S. Muscular Characteristics of Detraining in Humans. *Med. Sci. Sports Exerc.* **2001**, *33*, 1297–1303. [CrossRef]
9. Lesinski, M.; Hortobágyi, T.; Muehlbauer, T.; Gollhofer, A.; Granacher, U. Dose-Response Relationships of Balance Training in Healthy Young Adults: A Systematic Review and Meta-Analysis. *Sport. Med.* **2015**, *45*, 557–576. [CrossRef] [PubMed]
10. Park, S.-H. Tools for Assessing Fall Risk in the Elderly: A Systematic Review and Meta-Analysis. *Aging Clin. Exp. Res.* **2018**, *30*, 1–16. [CrossRef] [PubMed]
11. Moher, D. Preferred Reporting Items for Systematic Reviews and Meta-Analyses: The PRISMA Statement. *Ann. Intern. Med.* **2009**, *151*, 264. [CrossRef] [PubMed]
12. Crowe, M.; Sheppard, L. A General Critical Appraisal Tool: An Evaluation of Construct Validity. *Int. J. Nurs. Stud.* **2011**, *48*, 1505–1516. [CrossRef] [PubMed]
13. Crowe, M.; Sheppard, L.; Campbell, A. Reliability Analysis for a Proposed Critical Appraisal Tool Demonstrated Value for Diverse Research Designs. *J. Clin. Epidemiol.* **2012**, *65*, 375–383. [CrossRef]
14. Van Andel, S.; Cole, M.H.; Pepping, G.-J. A Systematic Review on Perceptual-Motor Calibration to Changes in Action Capabilities. *Hum. Mov. Sci.* **2017**, *51*, 59–71. [CrossRef] [PubMed]
15. Abbasi, A.; Sadeghi, H.; Tabrizi, H.B.; Bagheri, K.; Ghasemizad, A.; Asl, A.K. Effect of Whole Body Vibration, Aquatic Balance and Combined Training on Neuromuscular Performance, Balance and Walking Ability in Male Elderly Able-Bodied Individual. *World Appl. Sci. J.* **2011**, *15*, 84–91.
16. Ansai, J.H.; Aurichio, T.R.; Gonçalves, R.; Rebelatto, J.R. Effects of Two Physical Exercise Protocols on Physical Performance Related to Falls in the Oldest Old: A Randomized Controlled Trial. *Geriatr. Gerontol. Int.* **2016**, *16*, 492–499. [CrossRef] [PubMed]
17. Harvey, J.A.; Chastin, S.F.M.; Skelton, D.A. Breaking Sedentary Behaviour Has the Potential to Increase/Maintain Function in Frail Older Adults. *J. Frailty Sarcopenia Falls* **2018**, *3*, 26–34. [CrossRef] [PubMed]
18. Ritzmann, R.; Freyler, K.; Kümmel, J.; Gruber, M.; Belavy, D.L.; Felsenberg, D.; Gollhofer, A.; Kramer, A.; Ambrecht, G. High Intensity Jump Exercise Preserves Posture Control, Gait, and Functional Mobility during 60 Days of Bed-Rest: An RCT Including 90 Days of Follow-Up. *Front. Physiol.* **2018**, *9*, 1713. [CrossRef] [PubMed]
19. Sherk, K.A.; Bemben, D.A.; Brickman, S.E.; Bemben, M.G. Effects of Resistance Training Duration on Muscular Strength Retention 6-Month Posttraining in Older Men and Women. *J. Geriatr. Phys. Ther.* **2012**, *35*, 20–27. [CrossRef]
20. Sun, W.; Wang, L.; Zhang, C.; Song, Q.; Gu, H.; Mao, D. Detraining Effects of Regular Tai Chi Exercise on Postural Control Ability in Older Women: A Randomized Controlled Trial. *J. Exerc. Sci. Fit.* **2018**, *16*, 55–61. [CrossRef]
21. Toulotte, C.; Thevenon, A.; Fabre, C. Effects of Training and Detraining on the Static and Dynamic Balance in Elderly Fallers and Non-Fallers: A Pilot Study. *Disabil. Rehabil.* **2006**, *28*, 125–133. [CrossRef]
22. Vogler, C.M.; Menant, J.C.; Sherrington, C.; Ogle, S.J.; Lord, S.R. Evidence of Detraining after 12-Week Home-Based Exercise Programs Designed to Reduce Fall-Risk Factors in Older People Recently Discharged from Hospital. *Arch. Phys. Med. Rehabil.* **2012**, *93*, 1685–1691. [CrossRef]
23. Zhang, C.; Sun, W.; Yu, B.; Song, Q.; Mao, D. Effects of Exercise on Ankle Proprioception in Adult Women during 16 Weeks of Training and Eight Weeks of Detraining. *Res. Sport. Med.* **2015**, *23*, 102–113. [CrossRef]
24. Hurvitz, E.A.; Richardson, J.K.; Werner, R.A.; Ruhl, A.M.; Dixon, M.R. Unipedal Stance Testing as an Indicator of Fall Risk among Older Outpatients. *Arch. Phys. Med. Rehabil.* **2000**, *81*, 587–591. [CrossRef]
25. Nordin, E.; Lindelöf, N.; Rosendahl, E.; Jensen, J.; Lundin-olsson, L. Prognostic Validity of the Timed Up-and-Go Test, a Modified Get-Up-and-Go Test, Staff's Global Judgement and Fall History in Evaluating Fall Risk in Residential Care Facilities. *Age Ageing* **2008**, *37*, 442–448. [CrossRef] [PubMed]
26. Chow, R.B.; Lee, A.; Kane, B.G.; Jacoby, J.L.; Barraco, R.D.; Dusza, S.W.; Meyers, M.C.; Greenberg, M.R. Effectiveness of the "Timed Up and Go" (TUG) and the Chair Test as Screening Tools for Geriatric Fall Risk Assessment in the ED. *Am. J. Emerg. Med.* **2019**, *37*, 457–460. [CrossRef] [PubMed]
27. Khosla, S.; Riggs, B.L. Pathophysiology of Age-Related Bone Loss and Osteoporosis. *Endocrinol. Metab. Clin. N. Am.* **2005**, *34*, 1015–1030. [CrossRef] [PubMed]
28. Davis, M.G.; Fox, K.R. Physical Activity Patterns Assessed by Accelerometry in Older People. *Eur. J. Appl. Physiol.* **2007**, *100*, 581–589. [CrossRef] [PubMed]

Journal of
Clinical Medicine

MDPI

Article

Type D Personality and Stomatognathic System Disorders in Physiotherapy Students during the COVID-19 Pandemic

Magdalena Gębska [1], Bartosz Dalewski [2], Łukasz Pałka [3,*], Łukasz Kołodziej [1] and Ewa Sobolewska [2]

1 Department of Rehabilitation Musculoskeletal System, Pomeranian Medical University, 70-204 Szczecin, Poland; mgebska@pum.edu.pl (M.G.); lukas@hot.pl (Ł.K.)
2 Department of Dental Prosthetics, Pomeranian Medical University, 70-204 Szczecin, Poland; bartosz.dalewski@pum.edu.pl (B.D.); rpsobolewski@wp.pl (E.S.)
3 Private Dental Practice, Rzeszowska 2, 68-200 Żary, Poland
* Correspondence: dr.lpalka@gmail.com

Abstract: Background: A person's response to stressors is largely dependent on their personality traits that affect the way stress is controlled and relieved. This article is a quantitative analysis assessing the importance of the distressed personality in the development of stomatognathic system disorders (SSDs) in physiotherapy students during the COVID-19 pandemic. Objective: The goal of the research was to assess the presence of type D personality in students with symptoms of stomatognathic system disorders. Material and Method: The research was carried out among 300 physiotherapy students. The data were collected using the form of the occurrence of symptoms of SS disorders developed for the purpose of the study and the standardized psychological DS14 questionnaire. Results: In a group of 300 students, the presence of type D personality was found in 160 people (53.3%). People with type D personality had symptoms of SS disorders more often than the group without stressful personality traits. There was a significant difference between the groups regarding all the examined symptoms. In the group of people with type D personality, the most frequently reported symptoms of SS disorders included: headache (51.3%), pain in the neck and shoulder girdle (43.1%), and teeth clenching (35.6%). As many as 70% of the respondents in the group with symptoms of SS disorders (P1) had type D personality, whereas in the asymptomatic group (P2) this result was 23.3%. There was a significant difference between the groups ($p = 0.00$). Statistically significantly higher values of both D personality dimensions were observed in women than in men with symptoms of SS disorders. In people reporting symptoms of SS disorders, higher average values were observed in both dimensions of type D personality. There were significant differences between the groups. Conclusion: type D personality may contribute to the development of symptoms of stomatognathic disorders.

Keywords: COVID-19; stomatognathic system; type of personality; type D personality; TMD; orofacial pain; masticatory

Citation: Gębska, M.; Dalewski, B.; Pałka, Ł.; Kołodziej, Ł.; Sobolewska, E. Type D Personality and Stomatognathic System Disorders in Physiotherapy Students during the COVID-19 Pandemic. *J. Clin. Med.* **2021**, *10*, 4892. https://doi.org/10.3390/jcm10214892

Academic Editor: Michele Roccella

Received: 28 September 2021
Accepted: 19 October 2021
Published: 23 October 2021

1. Introduction

The COVID-19 pandemic disrupted the education system in Poland and vastly contributed to social isolation, with all due consequences. That, in turn, had a negative impact on the mental and physical health of students and university graduates. The accompanying stressors could have had influenced the development of increased masticatory muscles tension and numerous parafunctions, and thus the formation of stomatognathic system dysfunctions [1–5]. The relationship between increased stress and disorders of the stomatognathic system and quality of life has been widely described in the literature [6–8]. For example, bruxism, the diurnal and/or nocturnal unconscious teeth clenching and grinding, is commonly triggered by environmental stressors and depends on the personality traits that affect the way stress is controlled and relieved [9–11].

Therefore, the authors of the present study aimed to evaluate the relationship between the occurrence of symptoms of SS disorders and type D personality in physiotherapy students during the COVID-19 pandemic.

Regarding health psychology, there are three personality types that favor the development of somatic diseases: type A ('coronary personality'), type C ('cancer-prone personality'), and type D ('distressed personality') [12]. Two approaches are taken into account regarding the study of the relationship between personality and disease. The first indicates that certain personality traits are associated with morbidity rate of certain severe health issues such as, for example, type A personality promotes ischemic heart disease, or type C, which was previously associated with cancer [12–14]. The second approach assumes the existence of a general susceptibility to disease and indicates that this susceptibility is the result of personality traits that may favor or inhibit the development of the disease [15]. The growing interest in the problem of the relationship between personality and somatic diseases took place at the end of the 1990s, when Johan Denolett introduced the concept of distressed personality into the literature (distressed personality), i.e., type D personality, which he emphasized at the early 2000s [16,17].

Type D consists of two main dimensions, treated as relatively constant personality traits, i.e., negative affectivity (NA) and social inhibition (SI). Negative affectivity is expressed as a tendency to experience strong negative emotions, such as anxiety, anger, irritation, and hostility. On the other hand, social inhibition is associated with the tendency to refrain from expressing negative emotions and behavior consistent with these emotions. Refraining from revealing emotions is conscious and is undertaken mainly in social situations, primarily for fear of disapproval and rejection by other people [18]. People with a type D personality tend to worry, they feel tense and blame themselves which may result in suicidal behavior [19]. They are pessimistic about the world, have low self-esteem and a low level of life satisfaction. Moreover, they show weak bonds with other people, and use sedatives more frequently [20,21].

Type D personality shows some similarities to other personality characteristics that contribute to the development of somatic diseases, such type A or type C, but above all, to the two dimensions of personality that make up the 'Big Five', i.e., neuroticism and introversion. This relationship was confirmed by De Fruyt and Denollet [22].

The theoretical foundations of the type D personality refer to the biological theory of inhibition and activation formulated by Eysenck [23]. According to this theory, people for whom the stimulating potential is created quickly and with great force and the reactive inhibition appears slowly and disappears quickly, show a tendency towards introverted behavior (for extroverts it is the other way around). On the other hand, the theory of activation refers to individual differences in the level of activity of the cortico-reticular loop that determines the level of activation. The activation level of introverts exceeds the level of activity of extroverts [24]. The tendency to experience negative emotions, characteristic for both type D personality and neuroticism, modifies the behavior and level of functioning in situations requiring the activity of the limbic system [25].

Type D personality is linked to neuroticism by a tendency towards a catastrophic perception of reality, a way of evaluating events as highly threatening and harmful and a feeling of strong anxiety and tension [12]. What is characteristic in social situations is confusion, shyness in the presence of others, a tendency to worry, a pessimistic view of the world, high susceptibility to stress, and a tendency to break down in difficult situations. They are differentiated by the fact that in the type D personality, there is an emphasis on refraining from revealing negative emotions. It is also combined with introversion by refraining from keeping social contacts and shyness [14]. Moreover, introversion, similar to type D, is associated with a lower tendency to search for social support, poorer quality of social contacts and low self-esteem [26]. Therefore, it can be assumed that type D personality is the equivalent of neurotic introversion, yet people with type D personality would feel stress more strongly and experience its' consequences that appear to be more robust for physical and mental health.

The aim of this study was to evaluate the presence of type D personality in students with symptoms of stomatognathic system disorders. We hypothesized that type D personality traits may contribute to the development of symptoms of stomatognathic dysfunction during the COVID-19 pandemic.

2. Materials and Methods

The research was carried out from October 2020 to June 2021 among 300 students of physiotherapy at the Pomeranian Medical University in Szczecin. The study group (P1) consisted of 150 students who reported symptoms of SSDs in the questionnaire. The control group (P2) had the same number of participants without SS symptoms.

Inclusion criteria in the control group were: first, second, or third year students of physiotherapy studying in a hybrid system (stationary and remotely); no symptoms of SS disorders reported in the past; age 20 to 35; consent to participate in the study. Exclusion criteria were: chronic diseases, including psychosomatic diseases; during or after treatment of SS disorders, and pregnancy. The differentiating factor in the inclusion criteria in the P1 and P2 groups was the presence of symptoms of SSDs in the P1 group.

2.1. Research Tools

The SSD disorder assessment questionnaire consisted of 10 closed questions concerning the occurrence of symptoms related to the temporomandibular joints, masticatory muscles, and the cervical spine. A standardized DS-14 psychological questionnaire was carried out among all students (Type-D scale). The questionnaire consists of seven questions which concern the tendency to experience various negative emotions and seven concerning tendencies to refrain from expressing these emotions. To qualify as Type D, you must obtain a minimum of 10 points in each of the two dimensions i.e., NA and SI.

2.2. Characteristics of the Study Group

A total of 194 women (64.7%) and 106 men (35.3%) participated in the study. Among all the respondents, there were 30.3% of first-year students, 36% of second-year students and 33.7% of third-year students. The average age of the respondents was 21.71 (SD 2.69) and 22.26 (SD 2.10), $p = 0.05$, in the P1 and P2 group, respectively. The group of students with symptoms of SSDs included 103 women (68.7%) and 47 men (31.3%), and the group of asymptomatic participants consisted of 91 women (60.7%) and 59 men (39.3%). There was no difference in the gender structure between the groups, $p = 0.14723$.

After analyzing the data from the SS disorders symptom questionnaire in the P1 group, it was found that the most frequently reported symptoms were: headache 68%, pain in the neck and shoulder girdle 58%, teeth clenching 50%, TMJ acoustic symptoms 33.3%, TMJ pain 32.7%, increased masticatory muscle tension 30%, teeth grinding 22.7%, facial pain 12%.

The statistical comparison of the results of the SS disorder questionnaire between the groups was omitted due to the lack of occurrence of the studied variables in the P2 group.

2.3. Statistical Analysis

Data are presented as n and % of responses for qualitative variables and the average +/− standard deviation for quantitative features. The Chi 2 Pearson test was used to compare the relationships between the qualitative variables. Comparisons for quantitative variables were made using the Student's *t*-test, the relationship between quantitative variables was assessed using the Pearson correlation coefficient. Due to the large number of cases in the study groups, parametric tests were used based on the central limit theorem. The analysis was performed using the Rstudio package (RStudio, PBC) and p values < 0.05 were considered significant.

3. Results

According to the obtained data the presence of type D personality was confirmed in 160 participants (53.3%). The results of the assessment of the presence of type D personality in the P1 and P2 groups are presented below (Table 1).

Table 1. The occurrence of type D personality in groups P1 and P2.

Variable	Group P1	Group P2	Statistical Significance
Type D personality	115 (76.7%)	45 (30%)	$p = 0.000$
No Type D personality	35 (23.3%)	105 (70%)	

As it can be seen from Table 1 as many as 70% of the respondents in the group with symptoms of SSDs (P2) had type D personality, whereas in the asymptomatic group (P1) this result was 23.3%. There was a significant difference between the groups ($p = 0.000$).

Comparing the occurrence of symptoms of SS disorders between people with and without type D personality, the following results were obtained (Table 2).

Table 2. The occurrence of symptoms of SS disorders in students with and without type D personality.

Variable		No Type D Personality	Type D Personality	Statistical Significance
TMJ Pain	no	128 (91.4%)	122 (76.3%)	$p = 0.001$
	yes	12 (8.6%)	37 (23.1%)	
	I don't know	0 (0%)	1 (0.6%)	
Headache	no	120 (85.7%)	77 (48.1%)	$p = 0.000$
	yes	20 (14.3%)	82 (51.3%)	
	I don't know	0 (0%)	1 (0.6%)	
Pain in the neck and shoulder girdle	no	122 (87.1%)	90 (56.3%)	$p = 0.000$
	yes	18 (12.9%)	69 (43.1%)	
	I don't know	0 (0%)	1 (0.6%)	
Facial pain	no	138 (98.6%)	142 (88.8%)	$p = 0.002$
	yes	2 (1.4%)	16 (10%)	
	I don't know	0 (0%)	2 (1.3%)	
TMJ acoustic symptoms	no	127 (90.7%)	111 (69.4%)	$p = 0.000$
	yes	11 (7.9%)	39 (24.4%)	
	I don't know	2 (1.4%)	10 (6.3%)	
TMJ blocking	no	138 (98.6%)	147 (91.9%)	$p = 0.028$
	yes	2 (1.4%)	12 (7.5%)	
	I don't know	0 (0%)	1 (0.6%)	
Teeth clenching	no	119 (85%)	87 (54.4%)	$p = 0.000$
	yes	18 (12.9%)	57 (35.6%)	
	I don't know	3 (2.1%)	16 (10%)	
Teeth grinding	no	127 (90.7%)	109 (68.1%)	$p = 0.000$
	yes	8 (5.7%)	26 (16.3%)	
	I don't know	5 (3.6%)	25 (15.6%)	
Increased masticatory muscles tension	no	125 (89.3%)	106 (66.3%)	$p = 0.000$
	yes	11 (7.9%)	34 (21.3%)	
	I don't know	4 (2.9%)	20 (12.5%)	

The results presented in Table 2 show that people with type D personality experienced symptoms of SS disorders more frequently than in the group without distressed personality traits. There was a significant difference between the groups regarding all the examined symptoms. In the group of people with D personality, the most frequently reported symptoms of SSDs included: headache, pain in the neck and shoulder girdle, and teeth clenching.

As shown in Table 3, significantly higher values of both type D personality components were observed in women than in men with symptoms of SS disorders.

Table 3. Comparison of type D personality components (NA and SI) in group P2 in relation to gender.

Variable	Female		Male		Statistical Significance
	$\bar{x}$	SD	$\bar{x}$	SD	
NA	11.73	6.00	9.25	6.06	$p = 0.00$
SI	10.09	4.98	8.75	5.32	$p = 0.03$

Below in Figures 1 and 2 the analysis of both dimensions of type D personality in relation to symptoms of SSDs is presented.

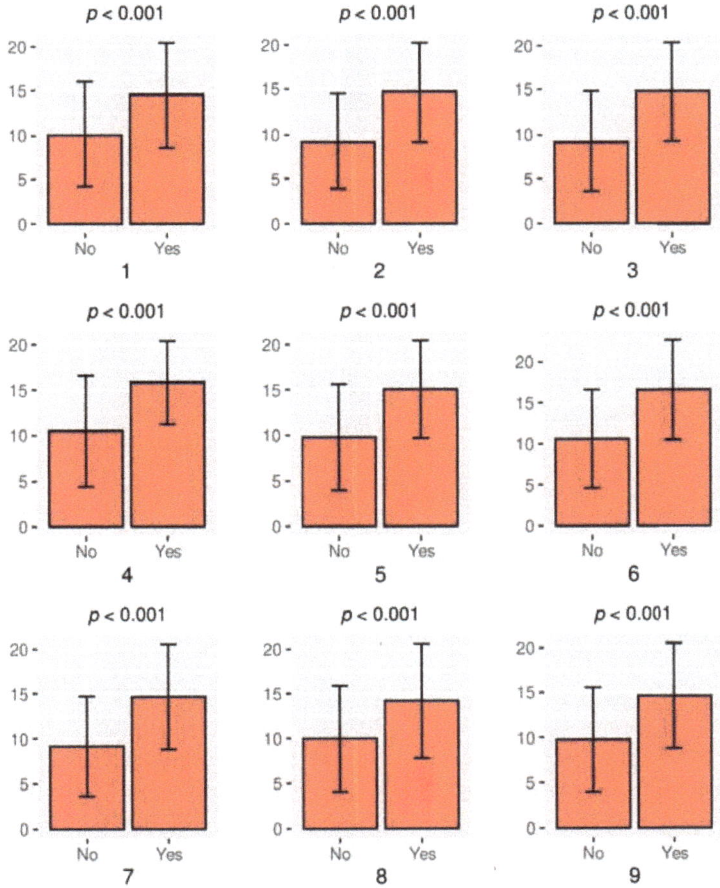

Figure 1. Analysis of the negative affectivity (NA) in relation to the symptoms of SSDs. Legend: 1—TMJ Pain, 2—Headache, 3—Pain in the neck and shoulder girdle, 4—Facial pain, 5—TMJ acoustic symptoms, 6—TMJ blocking, 7—Teeth clenching, 8—Teeth grinding, 9—Increased masticatory muscles tension.

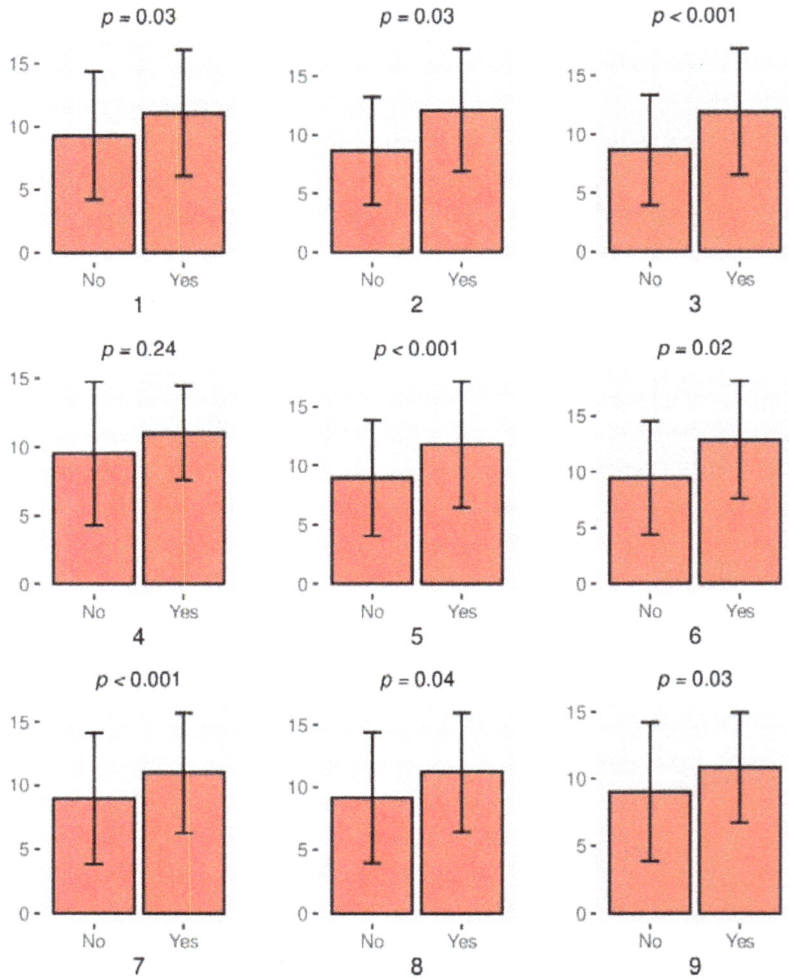

Figure 2. Analysis of the social inhibition (SI) in relation to the symptoms of SSDs. Legend: 1—TMJ Pain, 2—Headache, 3—Pain in the neck and shoulder girdle, 4—Facial pain, 5—TMJ acoustic symptoms, 6—TMJ blocking, 7—Teeth clenching, 8—Teeth grinding, 9—Increased masticatory muscles tension.

Figures 1 and 2 present the results obtained after the analysis of NA and SI occurrence in relation to the reported symptoms of SSDs. In people reporting symptoms of SS disorders, higher average values were observed in both dimensions that make up the type D personality (NA and SI). There was a significant difference between people with and without symptoms. In the symptomatic group, the average NA scores are higher than SI.

4. Discussion

According to the present research carried out on a group of 150 physiotherapy students, the most common symptoms of SS disorders were headaches (51.3%), neck and shoulder girdle pain (43.1%), and teeth clenching (35.6%). The studies carried out by Glaros et al. show that involuntary tooth contact is one of the most typical parafunctions observed more frequently in TMD (temporomandibular joint dysfunction) patients than in healthy people [27]. Similar conclusions were also drawn by Moreno et al., who found a correlation between TMJ disorders and head and neck pain [28]. According to Emodi-Perlman et al., the COVID-19 pandemic had a significant negative influence on the psycho-emotional state of the Israeli and Polish populations, leading to the worsening of bruxism and TMD symptoms [29]. De Medeiros R.A. et al. drew similar conclusions by conducting research on Brazilian medicine students. According to their study, social isolation and stressful situations caused by the pandemic may increase the number of people with TMD symptoms [30]. For several years, great interest of researchers and practitioners has been aroused by the so-called 'distressed personality'—type D. It is considered a risk factor for somatic diseases and is of high importance as far as the perception of the environmental stress is concerned [31].

In the author's own research on a group of 300 physiotherapy students, the presence of type D personality was found in 160 participants (53.3%). In accordance with O'Riordan et al., type D people perceive their life events as significantly more stressful than people with a different personality type. Type D personality people also report increased perceptions of negative social relationships and less social support [20]. What is more, people with type D personality are characterized by a worse quality of life and they assess their own health condition as worse [32]. In the context of the studied group-future physiotherapists- numerous studies should also be cited, in which it was shown that employees characterized by type D personality perceive their work environment as more stressful with more frequent occurrence of occupational burnout syndrome [33–36]. According to the authors, the above-mentioned considerations indicate that the high prevalence of type D personality among physiotherapy students may become an obstacle in providing effective rehabilitation services to patients.

The results of many studies have shown that the type D personality is a significant predictor of cardiovascular diseases (ischemic heart disease, hypertension), as well as somatic diseases, such as cancer, peptic ulcer disease, and skin diseases [37–41].

In a study by Condén et al., a strong relationship was found between the type D personality with psychosomatic symptoms and musculoskeletal pain [42].

However, there are no scientific studies on the evaluation of the relationship between the type D personality and the occurrence of symptoms of stomatognathic system disorders. The studies presented in the literature, taking into consideration related constructs, especially neuroticism, confirm the role of the experience of negative emotions and reserves in relations with other people as those elements of personality that favor the assessment of stress and intensify its the negative effects. According to Moayedi et al., neuroticism may contribute to the pathophysiology of muscular TMD because there is a correlation between chronic pain in TMD and the patient's neurotic personality [43].

On the other hand, according to the research of Southwell et al., TMJ dysfunctional individuals obtain higher results regarding neurotic and introversion scales [44]. Serra-Negra et al. have shown that children with a high level of neuroticism in their personality domain are more prone to sleep bruxism [45].

Research over the past twenty years has indicated a connection between several psychological variables and TMD [46–48]. Indeed, it is easy to observe differences in the severity of personality traits, experienced levels of stress, depression, and catastrophic situations between TMD patients and those without the disorder. A well-known example of the association of psychosocial risk factors in chronic TMD is the insecurity that accompanies long-term suffering [48]. What is more, it should also be noticed that there are psychological factors associated with the initial pain symptoms in TMD, as well as socio-demographic variables that contribute to the perception of craniofacial pain [48]. One of the most important determinants influencing the behavior and functioning of an individual is their personality.

The authors of the present study, by utilizing the DS-14 questionnaire, which is used to evaluate the occurrence of type D personality, have observed that it is significantly more common in people reporting symptoms of SS disorders than in asymptomatic people. (p = 0.00000). These results suggest that people with symptoms of SS disorders have personality traits that make them prone to perceived life stress. It is also worth mentioning that significantly higher values of both type D personality components (NA and SI) were observed in women than in men with symptoms of SS disorders. The above-mentioned data may prove that not only type D personality may predispose to SS disorders, but also gender may be an additional factor influencing the frequency of SS dysfunctions. Yeow's research on a group of 157 psychology students has shown that 50% of men and 46.4% of women had a type D personality. Moreover, women had higher HS when compared to men [49]. Cho S. et al. have observed that type D personality is related to the level of perceived stress. Additionally, it was concluded that there are gender differences in type D personality, stress, and stress coping strategies [50].

The authors of the present article, by comparing both dimensions of the type D personality (NA and SI), noted statistically significant differences between the groups in terms of symptoms, i.e., headache, face pain, TMJ and shoulder girdle, acoustic symptoms and TMJ blocking, teeth clenching and grinding as well as increased masticatory muscles tension. In the symptomatic group, the NA dimension showed higher average values than SI, that is related to the individual's tendency to experience strong negative emotions such as anxiety, anger, irritation, and hostility. After analyzing the obtained data, it can be claimed that the type D personality, and above all the dimension of negative affectivity, is one of the predictors of symptoms of SS disorders. The research results presented in the literature indicate a relation between the NA dimension and unfavorable eating and shopping habits, symptoms of depression, anxiety, insomnia, alcohol abuse and a low level of life satisfaction.

There are many strategies and methods in the field of psychotherapeutic treatment applied to individuals with a disturbed personality. Currently, the main method is a long-term psychodynamic psychotherapy. The literature offers numerous reliable studies confirming the effectiveness and usefulness of this treatment procedure if conducted by a psychologist [51–53]. If the disorder is correctly qualified and the therapy is durable (long-term in nature), it is possible to obtain real changes in the patient's functioning, which are conducive to better functioning in many aspects of their life. One can also find a growing number of reports confirming the effectiveness of other methods of psychotherapy (e.g., modifications of cognitive-behavioral therapy) [54]. It cannot be forgotten that the basic therapeutic factor, independent of the applied psychotherapeutic approach, is establishing a therapeutic relationship between the therapist and the patient, based on mutual trust, safety, and commitment. The progress in the field of psychotherapy of personality disorders observed in recent years is a hope for many patients, who can thus avoid gradual degradation of their lives and have a chance to function better on daily basis. Pharmacotherapy as a method of treating personality disorders is of complementary importance and psychotropic drugs are recommended mainly for symptomatic indications, e.g., to control severe depression, anxiety, or short-term psychotic symptoms [55].

By analyzing the available scientific literature and the results of our own research, it is possible to determine with high probability that the distressed personality may have a great influence on the functioning of the stomatognathic system, in particular on the development of the masticatory organ parafunctions and head and neck pain.

Further research is necessary to better understand the impact of the type D personality on the occurrence of stomatognathic system disorders.

5. Limitations

The presented results, indicating the predictive role of the type D personality in the development of symptoms of SS disorders, should be treated with great caution. First of all, due to the cross-sectional nature of the research and also due to the small group of respondents. One should also remember about the multifactorial determinant of SS disorders, which means that personality is only one of the numerous factors determining the occurrence of SSDs. A particularly important limitation of the presented studies is the lack of assessment of occlusal conditions, including the occurrence of malocclusion in the study group, which constitutes an important etiological factor of the stomatognathic system disorders. In addition, possible missing teeth and traumatic nodes within the masticatory apparatus may be the cause of the appearance of micro and macro injuries in the examined system. Therefore, the authors see the need to continue the research carried out, taking into account the role of occlusion in the formation of SSD.

6. Conclusions

1. In students with a distressed personality, psychological programs should be implemented, including education and training courses for future graduates, so that they can effectively deal with negative affectivity and social inhibition.
2. Personality type assessment should become one of a mainstays in TMD evaluation, as well as personalized psychological coping strategies an essential part of management.
3. People with type D personality and symptoms of SS disorders should receive psychological support, focused directly on intricate connections between possible somatization issues and catastrophizing aspects of this complex personality trait.

Author Contributions: Conceptualization: M.G., Ł.K.; Methodology: M.G., B.D.; Software: M.G., Ł.K.; Validation: M.G.; Formal analysis: M.G.; Investigation: M.G., Ł.K.; Resources: Ł.K.; Data curation: M.G., Ł.K.; Writing—original draft preparation: M.G., B.D., Ł.P.; Writing—review and editing: B.D., Ł.P., M.G.; Visualization: M.G.; Supervision: E.S., Ł.P.; Project administration: M.G.; Funding acquisition: E.S. All authors have read and agreed to the published version of the manuscript.

Funding: This research received no external funding.

Institutional Review Board Statement: The study was approved by the Ethics Committee of the Pomeranian Medical University in Szczecin, Poland according to Good Clinical Practice (resolution number KB-0012/79/16).

Informed Consent Statement: Informed consent was obtained from all subjects involved in the study.

Data Availability Statement: The data presented in this study are available on request from the corresponding author. The data are not publicly available due to sensitive information.

Conflicts of Interest: The authors declare no conflict of interest.

References

1. Janal, M.N.; Lobbezoo, F.; Quigley, K.S.; Raphael, K.G. Stress-evoked muscle activity in women with and without chronic myofascial face pain. *J. Oral Rehabil.* **2021**, *48*, 1089–1098. [CrossRef]
2. Rokaya, D.; Koontongkaew, S. Can Coronavirus Disease-19 Lead to Tem-poromandibular Joint Disease? *J. Med. Sci.* **2020**, *8*, 142–143.
3. Babicka-Wirkus, A.; Wirkus, L.; Stasiak, K.; Kozłowski, P. University students' strate-gies of coping with stress during the coronavirus pandemic: Data from Poland. *PLoS ONE* **2021**, *16*, e0255041. [CrossRef]
4. Gębska, M.; Kołodziej, Ł.; Dalewski, B.; Pałka, Ł.; Sobolewska, E. The Influence of the COVID-19 Pandemic on the Stress Levels and Occurrence of Stoma-toghnatic System Disorders (SSDs) among Physiotherapy Students in Poland. *J. Clin. Med.* **2021**, *10*, 3872. [CrossRef]
5. Zhan, H.; Zheng, C.; Zhang, X.; Yang, M.; Zhang, L.; Jia, X. Chinese College Students' Stress and Anxiety Levels Under COVID-19. *Front. Psychiatry* **2021**, *12*, 615390. [CrossRef] [PubMed]
6. Resende, C.M.; Alves, A.C.; Coelho, L.T.; Alchieri, J.C.; Roncalli, A.G.; Bar-bosa, G.A. Quality of life and general health in patients with temporomandibular disor-ders. *Braz. Oral Res.* **2013**, *27*, 116–121. [CrossRef]
7. Trize, D.M.; Calabria, M.P.; Franzolin, S.O.B.; Cunha, C.O.; Marta, S.N. Is quality of life affected by temporomandibular dis-orders? *Ein-Stein* **2018**, *16*, eAO4339. [CrossRef]
8. Bitiniene, D.; Zamaliauskiene, R.; Kubiliu, R.; Leketas, M.; Gailius, T.; Smirnovaite, K. Quality of life in patients with temporomandibular disorders. A systematic review. *Sto-Matol. Balt. Dent. Maxillofac. J.* **2018**, *20*, 3–9.
9. Saczuk, K.; Lapinska, B.; Wilmont, P.; Pawlak, L.; Lukomska-Szymanska, M. Relationship between Sleep Bruxism, Perceived Stress, and Coping Strategies. *Int. J. Environ. Res. Public Health* **2019**, *16*, 3193. [CrossRef]
10. Lobbezoo, F.; Ahlberg, J.; Raphael, K.G.; Wetselaar, P.; Glaros, A.G.; Kato, T.; Santiago, V.; Winocur, E.; De Laat, A.; De Leeuw, R.; et al. International consensus on the assessment of bruxism: Report of a work in progress. *J. Oral Rehabil.* **2018**, *45*, 837–844. [CrossRef]

11. Dalewski, B.; Kamińska, A.; Kiczmer, P.; Węgrzyn, K.; Pałka, Ł.; Janda, K.; Sobolewska, E. Pressure Algometry Evaluation of Two Occlusal Splint Designs in Bruxism Management-Randomized, Controlled Clinical Trial. *J. Clin. Med.* **2021**, *10*, 2342. [CrossRef] [PubMed]
12. Kanten, P.; Gümüştekin, G.; Kanten, S. Exploring the Role of A, B, C and D Personality Types on Individuals Work-Related Behaviors and Health Problems: A Theoretical Model. *Int. J. Bus. Manag. Invent.* **2017**, *6*, 29–37.
13. Kupper, N.; Denollet, J. Type D Personality as a Risk Factor in Coronary Heart Disease: A Review of Current Evidence. *Curr. Cardiol. Rep.* **2018**, *20*, 104. [CrossRef] [PubMed]
14. Jandackova, V.K.; Koenig, J.; Jarczok, M.N.; Fischer, J.E.; Thayer, J.F. Potential biological pathways linking Type-D personality and poor health: A cross-sectional investigation. *PLoS ONE* **2017**, *12*, e0176014. [CrossRef]
15. Denollet, J.; Van Heck, G. Psychological risk factors in heart disease. What type D is (not) about. *J. Psychosom. Res.* **2001**, *51*, 465–468. [CrossRef]
16. Pedersen, S.; Denollet, J. Type D personality, cardiac events, and impaired quality of life: A review. *Eur. J. Cardiovasc. Prev. Rehabil.* **2003**, *10*, 241–248. [CrossRef]
17. Denollet, J.; Sys, S.U.; Stroobant, N.; Rombouts, H.; Gillebert, T.C.; Brutsaert, D.L. Personality as independent predictor of long-term mortality in patients with coronary heart disease. *Lancet* **1996**, *347*, 417–421. [CrossRef]
18. Howard, S.; Hughes, B.M. Construct, concurrent and discriminant validity of Type D personality in the general population: Associations with anxiety, depression, stress and cardiac output. *Psychol. Health* **2012**, *27*, 242–258. [CrossRef]
19. De Berardis, D.; Fornaro, M.; Valchera, A.; Cavuto, M.; Perna, G.; Di Nicola, M.; Serafini, G.; Carano, A.; Pompili, M.; Vellante, F.; et al. Eradicating Suicide at Its Roots: Preclinical Bases and Clinical Evidence of the Efficacy of Ketamine in the Treatment of Suicidal Behaviors. *Int. J. Mol. Sci.* **2018**, *19*, 2888. [CrossRef] [PubMed]
20. O'Riordan, A.; Howard, S.; Gallagher, S. Type D personality and life event stress: The mediating effects of social support and negative social relationships. *Anxiety Stress* **2020**, *33*, 452–465. [CrossRef]
21. Mols, F.; Denollet, J. Type D personality in the general population: A systematic review of health status, mechanisms of disease, and work-related problems. *Health Qual. Life Outcomes* **2010**, *8*, 9. [CrossRef]
22. De Fruyt, F.; Denollet, J. Type D personality: A five factor model perspective. *Psychol. Health* **2002**, *5*, 671–683. [CrossRef]
23. Muris, P.; Cor, M.; de Kanter, E.; Eek Timmerman, P. Behavioural inhibition and behavioural activation system scales for children: Relationships with Eysenck's personality traits and psychopathological symptoms. *Personal. Individ. Differ.* **2005**, *38*, 831–841. [CrossRef]
24. Taub, J.M. Eysenck's Descriptive and Biological Theory of Personality: A Review of Construct Validity. *Int. J. Neurosci.* **1998**, *94*, 145–197. [CrossRef]
25. Strelau, J. *Osobowość Jako Zespół Cech*; GWP: Warszawa, Poland, 2000; Volume 2, pp. 525–560.
26. Chilicka, K.; Rogowska, A.M.; Szyguła, R.; Adamczyk, E. Association between Satisfaction with Life and Personality Types A and D in Young Women with Acne Vulgaris. *Int. J. Environ. Res. Public Health* **2020**, *17*, 8524. [CrossRef]
27. Glaros, A.G.; Williams, K.; Lausten, L.; Friesen, L.R. Tooth contact in patients with temporomandibular disorders. *Cranio* **2005**, *23*, 188–193. [CrossRef]
28. Moreno, B.G.D.; Maluf, S.A.; Marques, A.P.; Crivello-Júnior, O. Clinical and quality-of-life assessment among women with temporomandibular disorder. *Rev. Bras. Fisioter.* **2009**, *13*, 210–214. [CrossRef]
29. Emodi-Perlman, A.; Eli, I.; Smardz, J.; Uziel, N.; Wieckiewicz, G.; Gilon, E.; Grychowska, N.; Wieckiewicz, M. Temporomandibular Disorders and Bruxism Outbreak as a Possible Factor of Orofacial Pain Worsening during the COVID-19 Pandemic-Concomitant Research in Two Countries. *J. Clin. Med.* **2020**, *9*, 3250. [CrossRef] [PubMed]
30. Medeiros, R.A.; Vieira, D.L.; Silva, E.V.F.D.; Rezende, L.V.M.L.; Santos, R.W.D.; Tabata, L.F. Prevalence of symptoms of temporomandibular disorders, oral behaviors, anxiety, and depression in Dentistry students during the period of social isolation due to COVID-19. *J. Appl. Oral Sci.* **2020**, *28*, e20200445. [CrossRef]
31. Kim, Y.H.; Kim, S.R.; Kim, Y.O.; Kim, J.Y.; Kim, H.K.; Kim, H.Y. Influence of type D personality on job stress and job satisfaction in clinical nurses: The mediating effects of compassion fatigue, burnout, and compassion satisfaction. *J. Adv. Nurs.* **2017**, *73*, 905–916. [CrossRef]
32. Stevenson, C.; Williams, L. Type D personality, quality of life and physical symptoms in the general population: A dimensional analysis. *Psychol. Health* **2014**, *29*, 365–373. [CrossRef]
33. Skodova, Z.; Lajciakova, P.; Banovcinova, L. Burnout Syndrome among Health Care Students: The Role of Type D Personality. *West. J. Nurs. Res.* **2017**, *39*, 416–429. [CrossRef] [PubMed]
34. Polman, R.; Borkoles, E.; Nicholls, A.R. Type D personality, stress, and symptoms of burnout: The influence of avoidance coping and social support. *Br. J. Health Psychol.* **2010**, *15*, 681–696. [CrossRef]
35. Geuens, N.; Braspenning, M.; Bogaert, P.V.; Franck, E. Individual vulnerability to burnout in nurses: The role of Type D personality within different nursing specialty areas. *Burn. Res.* **2015**, *2*, 80–86. [CrossRef]
36. Tekin, A.; Karadağ, H.; Yayla, S. The relationship between burnout symptoms and Type D personality among health care professionals in Turkey. *Arch. Environ. Occup. Health* **2017**, *72*, 173–177. [CrossRef] [PubMed]
37. Raykh, O.I.; Sumin, A.N.; Kokov, A.N.; Indukaeva, E.V.; Artamonova, G.V. Association of type D personality and level of coronary artery calcification. *J. Psychosom. Res.* **2020**, *139*, 110265. [CrossRef] [PubMed]

38. Kotas, R.; Nowakowska-Kotas, M.; Budrewicz, S.; Pokryszko-Dragan, A. The Level of Stress and Coping Strategies in Patients with Multiple Sclerosis and Their Relationships with the Disease Course. *J. Clin. Med.* **2021**, *10*, 3916. [CrossRef]
39. Raykh, O.I.; Sumin, A.N.; Korok, E.V. The Influence of Personality Type D on Cardiovascular Prognosis in Patients after Coronary Artery Bypass Grafting: Data from a 5-Year-Follow-up Study. *Int. J. Behav. Med.* **2021**, *6*, 1–11.
40. Jordi, S.B.U.; Botte, F.; Lang, B.M.; Greuter, T.; Krupka, N.; Auschra, B.; Schreiner, P.; Sulz, M.C.; Biedermann, L.; von Känel, R.; et al. Type D personality is associated with depressive symptoms and clinical activity in inflammatory bowel disease. *Aliment. Pharmacol. Ther.* **2021**, *54*, 53–67. [CrossRef]
41. Husson, O.; Denollet, J.; Oerlemans, S.; Mols, F. Satisfaction with information provision in cancer patients and the moderating effect of Type D personality. *Psycho-Oncol.* **2013**, *22*, 2124–2132. [CrossRef]
42. Condén, E.; Leppert, J.; Ekselius, L.; Åslund, C. Type D personality is a risk factor for psychosomatic symptoms and musculoskeletal pain among adolescents: A cross-sectional study of a large population-based cohort of Swedish adolescents. *BMC Pediatrics* **2013**, *13*, 11. [CrossRef] [PubMed]
43. Moayedi, M.; Weissman-Fogel, I.; Crawley, A.P.; Goldberg, M.B.; Freeman, B.V.; Tenenbaum, H.C.; Davis, K.D. Contribution of chronic pain and neuroticism to abnormal forebrain gray matter in patients with temporomandibular disorder. *NeuroImage* **2011**, *55*, 277–286. [CrossRef]
44. Southwell, J.; Deary, I.; Geissler, P. Personality and anxiety in temporomandibular joint syndrome patients. *J. Oral Rehabil.* **1990**, *17*, 239–243. [CrossRef] [PubMed]
45. Serra-Negra, J.M.; Paiva, S.M.; Abreu, M.H.; Flores-Mendoza, C.E.; Pordeus, I.A. Relationship between Tasks Performed, Personality Traits, and Sleep Bruxism in Brazilian School Children—A Population-Based Cross-Sectional Study. *PLoS ONE* **2013**, *8*, e80075. [CrossRef]
46. Eitner, S.; Stingl, K.; Schlegel, A.K.; Wichmann, M.; Nickenig, A. Biopsychosocial correlations in patients with chronic oro-facial pain. Part II. Experiences of pain and dramatic events before the 16th year of life. *J. Oral Rehabil.* **2009**, *36*, 408–414. [CrossRef]
47. Fillingim, R.B.; Ohrbach, R.; Greenspan, J.D.; Knott, C.; Diatchenko, L.; Dubner, R.; Bair, E.; Baraian, C.; Mack, N.; Slade, G.D.; et al. Psychological factors associated with development of TMD: The OPPERA prospective cohort study. *J. Pain* **2013**, *14*, 75–90. [CrossRef]
48. Fillingim, R.B.; Ohrbach, R.; Greenspan, J.D.; Knott, C.; Dubner, R.; Bair, E.; Baraian, C.; Slade, G.D.; Maixner, W. Potential psychosocial risk factors for chronic TMD: Descriptive data and empirically identified domains from the OPPERA case-control study. *J. Pain* **2011**, *12*, 46–60. [CrossRef]
49. Yeow, J. Gender and ethnic differences of Type D personality among Malaysian psychology scholars. In Proceedings of the International Conference on Education, Psychology, & Social Sciences, Taipei, Taiwan, 6–8 August 2014. [CrossRef]
50. Cho, S.; Jeon, G.S. Gender Differences in Type D Personality and Mental Health among Korean College Entrants. *Stress* **2018**, *26*, 133–139. [CrossRef]
51. Leichsenring, F.; Rabung, S. Effectiveness of Long-term Psychodynamic Psychotherapy: A Meta-analysis. *CAVITY* **2008**, *300*, 1551–1565. [CrossRef]
52. Bond, M.; Christopher Perry, J. Long-Term Changes in Defense Styles with Psychodynamic Psychotherapy for Depressive, Anxiety, and Personality Disorders. *Am. J. Psychiatry* **2004**, *161*, 1665–1671. [CrossRef] [PubMed]
53. Salzer, S.; Winkelbach, C.; Leweke, F.; Leibing, E.; Leich-senring, F. Long-Term Effects of Short-Term Psychodynamic Psychotherapy and Cognitive- Behavioral Therapy in Generalized Anxiety Disorder: 12-Month Follow-up. *Can. J. Psychiatry* **2011**, *56*, 503–508. [CrossRef]
54. Matusiewicz, A.K.; Hopwood, C.J.; Banducci, A.N.; Lejuez, C.W. The Effectiveness of Cognitive Behavioral Therapy for Personality Disorders. *Psychiatr. Clin. N. Am.* **2010**, *33*, 657–685. [CrossRef]
55. Ripoll, L.H.; Triebwasser, J.; Siever, L.J. Evidence-based pharmacotherapy for personality disorders. *Int. J. Neuropsychopharmacol.* **2011**, *14*, 1257–1288. [CrossRef]

Journal of
Clinical Medicine

MDPI

Article

Factors Related to Psychological Distress during the First Stage of the COVID-19 Pandemic on the Chilean Population

Carlos Ruiz-Frutos [1,2], Diemen Delgado-García [3], Mónica Ortega-Moreno [4,*], Daniel Duclos-Bastías [5], Dánica Escobar-Gómez [5,6], Juan Jesús García-Iglesias [1] and Juan Gómez-Salgado [1,2,*]

1. Department of Sociology, Social Work and Public Health, Faculty of Labour Sciences, University of Huelva, 21007 Huelva, Spain; frutos@uhu.es (C.R.-F.); juanjesus.garcia@dstso.uhu.es (J.J.G.-I.)
2. Safety and Health Postgraduate Programme, Universidad Espíritu Santo, Guayaquil 092301, Ecuador
3. IMPACTCOVID-19 Chile Research Project, Universidad de Aconcagua, Los Andes 2102660, Chile; diemen.delgado@uac.cl
4. Department of Economy, University of Huelva, 21007 Huelva, Spain
5. School of Physical Education, Faculty of Philosophy and Education, Pontificia Universidad Católica de Valparaíso, Valparaíso 2374631, Chile; daniel.duclos@pucv.cl (D.D.-B.); danica.escobar@pucv.cl (D.E.-G.)
6. Faculty of Education Sciences, University of Cádiz, 11519 Cádiz, Spain

* Correspondence: ortegamo@uhu.es (M.O.-M.); salgado@uhu.es (J.G.-S.); Tel.: +34-959219700 (J.G.-S.)

Citation: Ruiz-Frutos, C.; Delgado-García, D.; Ortega-Moreno, M.; Duclos-Bastías, D.; Escobar-Gómez, D.; García-Iglesias, J.J.; Gómez-Salgado, J. Factors Related to Psychological Distress during the First Stage of the COVID-19 Pandemic on the Chilean Population. *J. Clin. Med.* **2021**, *10*, 5137. https://doi.org/10.3390/jcm10215137

Academic Editors: Giacomo Mancini and Michele Roccella

Received: 22 September 2021
Accepted: 29 October 2021
Published: 31 October 2021

Abstract: The health effects of COVID-19 continue to raise doubts today. In some areas, such as mental health, these doubts have scarcely been addressed. The present study analyses the effects on psychological distress during the first phase of the pandemic in Chile. A cross-sectional descriptive study was performed by using a questionnaire validated in Spain and adapted for Chile. Between 22 April and 16 December 2020, 3227 questionnaires were collected from the 16 regions of Chile, using non-probabilistic snowball sampling. Bivariate analysis and binary logistic regression were performed. The variables that could predict psychological distress during the COVID-19 pandemic in Chile were: having a poor self-perception of health OR = 4.038, 95% CI = (2.831, 5.758); being younger than 29 OR = 2.287, 95% CI = (1.893, 2.762); having diarrhea OR = 2.093, 95% CI = (1.414, 3.098); having headache OR = 2.019, 95% CI = (1.662, 2.453); being a woman OR = 1.638, 95% CI = (1.363, 1.967); having muscle pain OR = 1.439, 95% CI = (1.114, 1.859); and having had casual contact with an infected person OR = 1.410, 95% CI = (1.138, 1.747). In Chile, with a better social, economic, cultural, and health environment compared to neighboring countries, there has been a high percentage of psychological distress. It is time to prioritize measures to safeguard the mental health of Chileans, especially focused on the most vulnerable population according to our results, i.e., young women with poorer health status.

Keywords: COVID-19 emergency; psychological distress; stress disorder; preventive measures; mental health; Chile

1. Introduction

COVID-19, with an onset at the end of 2019 in Wuhan, China, was declared by the WHO as an international public health emergency in January 2020 [1] and as a global pandemic in March 2020 [2]. It spread rapidly throughout Latin American countries, leading the WHO to declare the region as an epicenter of the pandemic in May 2020 [3].

It has been estimated that in Latin American countries, including Chile, despite the fact that preventive measures against COVID-19 were implemented without delay, these have not had the expected effects due to, among other causes, deficiencies in the contact tracking and follow-up system, as well as problems prior to the pandemic, such as the characteristics of the health system, social inequalities, high rates of informal employment, and little or late establishment of economic support measures [4].

Regarding health inequities, proven to exist in Chile, and the finding of higher mortality rates in the metropolitan area of Chile, observing a direct association between mortality from COVID-19 and poverty [5]. The social determinants of health, in particular the multidimensional poverty index and the use of public transport, play an important role in explaining the differences in outcomes [6], both in the incidence of COVID-19 and in mortality [7].

On the other hand, the influence of the economy on health is an aspect of special relevance. In this regard, analyses of the effects of the containment measures on Chile's economic activity have been carried out [8]. One of these analyses, that covered the response to the pandemic by several Latin American governments, including Chile, has found that while wealthier municipalities introduce technological innovations comparable to those in developed countries, smaller or less advantaged areas have more difficulty maintaining service delivery while in an unprecedented socio-economic context, as is the one experienced during the pandemic [9]. However, it has been found that this health situation has not affected all population sectors in Chile equally [10]. Thus, as for the indigenous population, the vulnerability indicators previously detected have increased since it is a group that already had inequalities in health [11,12].

Overall, the impact of the COVID-19 pandemic in Chile has been significant. According to official data, as of 19 May 2021, 1,292,096 cases had been confirmed (6.81% of the general population), with 27,934 deaths and 39.78% of the country's total population fully vaccinated. This last figure is much higher than in the countries that surround Chile as well as some of the European continent, such as Spain [13].

Regarding the effects of the physiological symptoms of the disease, cough, dyspnea, anosmia, generalized fatigue, and respiratory type problems predominate, as well as an increased risk of thromboembolic events as a result of the inflammatory state generated by the cytokine storm [14–17], although many infected persons remain asymptomatic [18]. As for the adoption of preventive measures, it has been shown that they have contributed to reducing the impact of the pandemic in those countries where they have been adopted early, with Chile having carried out a high number of diagnostic tests [19]. Several studies have been carried out to determine the factors that influence the use of preventive measures to prevent COVID-19 and their association with the development of psychological distress. It has been determined that "hand washing" was the most widely used preventive measure in Spain during the first phase of the pandemic [20], that preventive measures will depend on the risk perception acquired [21], and that psychological distress depends on the high perceived costs of adherence to the preventive measures [22], uncomfortable feeling of wearing personal protective equipment, or the public ignorance of preventive measures [23].

One of the main characteristics of the COVID-19 pandemic is that it has been classified as a "psychological pandemic", with great effects on the mental health of the general population and, especially, on health professionals, who have been directly involved in the care of patients with COVID-19 [16,24–26]. In this sense, greater psychological affectation has been shown in professionals who were quarantined, who worked in COVID-19 units, or had a family member or friend infected with COVID-19. These effects manifested more through greater depression, anxiety, frustration, fear, and post-traumatic stress than in those persons who did not have such experience [27].

Regarding the general population, women [24], young people, the self-employed, individuals with previous psychological issues whose follow-up was interrupted [28], immigrants, or workers of essential activities and in contact with the public were the most affected strata [26,29]. Higher levels of stress, depression, or anxiety have been found in these groups [15,24,30–32], as well as somatization [24] and psychiatric disorders [17], especially in those patients with previous mental problems [33,34]. However, a study conducted in 21 countries, including Chile, did not find an increase in the number of suicides in the first months of the pandemic [35]. The psychological impact of the pandemic has manifested itself even in countries with low infection rates and good initial management of the outbreak, such as South Korea. In this population, symptoms of stress, anxiety, depression, and sleeping difficulties have been reported, albeit to a minimal or moderate degree. [36].

Among these findings, it is noteworthy that, although older people have a higher risk of suffering from serious illness due to COVID-19, they show fewer negative effects on their emotional health than young people [37], something also proven in other countries [38]. However, the elderly population is more vulnerable to stigma related to COVID-19. As an at-risk population, they are known to be more likely to be affected by the disease and this can lead to stigmatization, resulting in social rejection, isolation, and discrimination [39].

These works, carried out at the international level, provide an overview of the state of mental health among the population during the COVID-19 pandemic. However, there is currently no data that records this situation in Chile, that is, the psychological impact of the pandemic on the Chilean population has not been described. Thus, the novelty of this work lies in being the first to study this problem in Chile. The results would help measure and describe the impact of the pandemic, guide strategies for managing and addressing the crisis, and design interventions adapted to the needs of the Chilean population, as well as to develop a prevention plan for similar future situations.

Therefore, the objective of this article is to present the effects of the first wave of the COVID-19 pandemic on the mental health of Chileans, in particular, in the development of psychological distress. In this sense, it is intended to analyze the possible association with sociodemographic variables, perception of health, physical symptoms, having required health care, having received diagnostic tests, adoption of preventive measures, or contact history, among others.

2. Materials and Methods

2.1. Design and Sample

The design was a cross-sectional descriptive study, using a questionnaire previously validated and cross-culturally adapted to the Chilean environment. The sample was made up of the Chilean population, accessed through the non-probability sampling methodology snowballing method, the same methodology used in the study carried out in "Europe on Living, Working and COVID-19" by Eurofound [40].

In order to participate in the study, it was necessary to meet the following inclusion criteria: reside in Chile, be over 18 years old, and accept the informed consent. The estimated sample size was 3294, with 95% confidence level, a precision of 1.8% and a loss adjustment of 10%. Finally, the loss was 8.14%, leaving a sample size of 3227.

2.2. Materials

A questionnaire previously validated in Spain [20] was used, composed of several previously validated instruments adapted to the linguistic and cultural use of the language in Chile so that no question posed any difficulty of understanding. For this purpose, a panel of experts consisting of psychologists, epidemiologists, doctors, nurses, and public health experts was selected.

The questionnaire consists of three parts. In the first part, sociodemographic data were included: sex, level of education, age, work situation, cohabitation, having children or pets at home, having some degree of disability, and being under lockdown at home. In the second, Goldberg's general health questionnaire (GHQ-12) [41] was used to measure the level of mental health and psychological well-being. This questionnaire consisted of 12 items and four answer options, in which 1 meant *better than usual* or *more than usual*, 2 *same as usual*, 3 *less than usual* or *less so*, and 4 *much less than usual* or *much less*, as regards the positive items. As for the negative ones, 1 meant *not at all*, 2 *no more than usual*, 3 *rather more than usual* or *rather more*, and 4 *much more than usual* or *much more*. 0 points were assigned to the first two options, and 1 point to the last two, with a total score ranging from 0 to 12. The cut-off point established for the general population was three, considering scores greater than or equal to 3 as psychological distress. In the third part, questions were related to the perception of COVID-19 symptoms and the history of contacts during the last 14 days: headache or sore throat, cough, fever, rhinitis, dizziness, myalgia, shortness of breath, chills, or diarrhea. Questions about taking medication, suffering from chronic illness, or having required medical attention or hospitalization during the last 14 days were also included. These items were assessed with a yes/no dichotomous answer. The possible history of contact during the last 14 days was measured by means of three items: possible contact for more than 15 min less than two meters away, casual contact with confirmed infected persons, and contact with persons or materials suspected of being infected; also, the existence of an infected relative diagnosed by a diagnostic test. Participants could respond categorically to these items with three possible options: yes, no, or doesn't know.

Another variable collected was self-perception of their level of health during the last two weeks, this being a well-known indicator for predicting mortality [42]. It was measured with five levels of response, from very bad to very good, grouped for the final analysis into two categories, bad and excellent.

Finally, the preventive measures adopted were also included in the questions, using a Likert scale with five response options categorized from never to always with respect to the frequency with which they were performed: wearing a mask regardless of the presence or absence of symptoms; washing hands immediately after coughing, touching the nose, or sneezing; washing hands after touching potentially contaminated objects; washing hands with hydroalcoholic solution; washing hands with soap and water; covering the mouth with the elbow when coughing or sneezing; avoiding sharing utensils (e.g., spoon) during meals; leaving at least a meter and a half of separation from others. One point was assigned to the *never* answer, 2 points to *rarely*, 3 points to *sometimes*, 4 to *almost always*, and 5 to *always*. Thus, each item could score between 1 and 5, and the total score of the scale would range from 8 to 40.

2.3. Procedure

The Qualtrics® storage and survey platform (Qualtrics, Provo, UT, USA) was used to collect the information through an online questionnaire. For its dissemination, the collaboration of universities and scientific societies was requested, and social networks and interviews in the press were used. The questionnaire was disseminated online and through the social media in order to reach a larger number of participants.

2.4. Data Analysis

Frequencies, means and/or standard deviations were presented depending on the type of variable. The relationship of the qualitative variables with the psychological distress was analyzed through the Chi-squared test, also obtaining the odds ratio (OR) with the associated confidence intervals. The association between the different scores was analyzed by the Student's t-test for independent samples.

Finally, a binary logistic regression was performed that allowed for an assessment model to be built to study the presence or absence of psychological distress and identify those variables that played a relevant role. OR values indicate the strength of the relationship with psychological distress; the further away from 1, the stronger the relationship is.

To verify the appropriateness of the model, different measures of goodness of fit were used: the Hosmer–Lemeshow test, percentage of correctly classified values, sensitivity, and specificity. The inclusion of the variables was carried out with tests of statistical significance, the OR were estimated, and the confidence intervals were facilitated. The OR values indicate the strength of the relationship with psychological distress. All analyses were carried out with the SPSS 26.0 statistical software (IBM, New York, NY, USA).

2.5. Ethical Principles

At the beginning of the questionnaire, participants received information about the objectives of the study and were asked to provide their written informed consent prior to answering. The data were recorded anonymously, treated confidentially and met the ethical principles established in the Declaration of Helsinki (Fortaleza, 2013) and all the legal regulations in force on data protection and regulation of human research processes in Chile. The study has been authorized by the Ethics Committee of the University of Aconcagua in Chile (Santiago, UAC-22 April 2020) and in Spain by the Research Ethics Committee of Huelva, belonging to the Regional Ministry of Health of Andalusia (PI 036/20).

3. Results

3.1. Sociodemographic Data

A pilot test was carried out with 57 people, diverse regarding their profession, educational level, geographical scope, age, and sex, and where a Cronbach's alpha coefficient of 0.910 was obtained, good psychometric properties, and no understanding problems. Questionnaires were received from the 16 Regions of Chile, with higher response rates from Valparaiso and Santiago. Records were obtained from 38 of the 43 types of classified occupations, with 21% of health professionals. A total of 3227 questionnaires were received between 21 April and 24 December 2020.

As can be seen in Table 1, there is a higher percentage of women (63.40%), people with university level education or higher studies (59.25%), young people (51% being 29 years old or less), living without a partner (70.31%), without children (63.43%), living in a house with an exterior view (house with balcony, terrace, yard, or garden) (86.6%), having a pet (71.4%), working in private companies (46.27%), being health professionals (21.2%), being in strict confinement or in confinement except for purchase-work (81.7%).

Table 1. Association between sociodemographic variables and psychological distress during the COVID-19 pandemic.

		TOTAL (N = 3227)				
		GHQ				
	N (%)	**YES (N = 2544)**	**NO (N = 683)**	χ^2	p	**Odds Ratio (CI 95%)**
Sex						
Female	2045 (63.4)	82.9	17.1	56.224	<0.001	1.916 (1.613, 2.273)
Male	1182 (36.6)	71.7	28.3			
Age * (N = 3224)						
29 years or younger	1654 (51.30)	86.5	13.5	119.842	<0.001	2.651 (2.219, 3.168)
Older than 29	1570 (48.70)	70.8	29.2			
Marital status						
Single	2269 (70.31)	82.4	17.6	57.282	<0.001	1.959 (1.643, 2.336)
With a couple	958 (29.69)	70.5	29.5			
Educational level						
Upper secondary school or lower	1315 (40.75)	85.9	14.1	65.563	<0.001	2.132 (1.771, 2.567)
University or higher	1912 (59.25)	74.0	26.0			
Type of dwelling						
Apartment/House without balcony/terrace/yard	431 (13.4)	85.2	14.8	11.893	0.001	1.631 (1.232, 2.160)
Apartment/House with balcony/terrace/yard/garden	2796 (86.6)	77.9	22.1			
You are (N = 1502)						
Independent worker	233 (15.51)	61.8	38.2	25.712	<0.001	-
Public employer	574 (38.22)	78.7	21.3			
Worker for private comp.	695 (46.27)	70.6	29.4			

Table 1. *Cont.*

	TOTAL (*N* = 3227)					
	GHQ					
	N (%)	YES (*N* = 2544)	NO (*N* = 683)	χ2	*p*	Odds Ratio (CI 95%)
Children						
No	2047 (63.43)	83.9	16.1	85.359	<0.001	2.222 (1.873, 2.639)
Yes	1180 (36.57)	70.1	29.9			
Pet						
Yes	2304 (71.40)	79.2	20.8	0.680	0.410	1.081 (0.898, 1.301)
No	923 (28.60)	77.9	22.1			
Disability						
No	3132 (97.06)	79.0	21.0	1.556	0.212	1.342 (0.844, 2.137)
Yes	95 (2.94)	73.7	26.3			
Health worker						
No	2543 (78.8)	79.8	20.2	6.528	0.011	1.385 (1.062, 1.580)
Yes	684 (21.2)	75.3	24.7			
Confinement						
Strict	843 (26.1)	81.0	19.0	24.200	<0.001	
Except for purchase-work	1793 (55.6)	80.0	20.0			-
No	326 (10.1)	69.0	31.0			
Other situations	265 (8.2)	75.8	24.2			

* Grouped variable from median value.

3.2. Psychological Distress

78.83% of the sample had psychological distress (PD), following the ≥3 cut-off point of the GHQ-12. The overall mean of the 12 items (GHQ-12) was M = 6.16 (SD = 3.76), with a reliability coefficient of the optimal measurement scale of Cronbach's α = 0.910 (Table 2).

Table 2. Psychological Distress: General Health Questionnaire GHQ-12.

	TOTAL (*N* = 3227)
Item	M (SD)
1. Have you been able to concentrate well on what you were doing?	2.86 (0.80)
2. Have your worries made you lose a lot of sleep?	2.82 (0.99)
3. Have you felt that you are playing a useful role in life?	2.36 (0.96)
4. Have you felt capable of making decisions?	2.29 (0.80)
5. Have you felt constantly overwhelmed and stressed?	3.08 (0.91)
6. Have you had the feeling that you cannot overcome your difficulties?	2.52 (1.01)
7. Have you been able to enjoy your normal daily activities?	2.92 (0.89)
8. Have you been able to adequately cope with problems?	2.47 (0.79)
9. Have you felt unhappy or depressed?	2.73 (1.01)
10. Have you lost confidence in yourself?	2.15 (1.08)
11. Have you thought that you are a worthless person?	1.68 (1.01)
12. Do you feel reasonably happy considering all the circumstances?	2.37 (0.85)
GHQ-12 (over 12 points)	6.16 (3.76)
Cut-off point ≥ 3	N (%)
Yes	2544 (78.83)
No	683 (21.17)

α-Cronbach = 0.910 Items 1 to 12 rank 1–4.

As shown in Table 2, the items with the highest score are: *Have you felt constantly overwhelmed and stressed?* M = 3.08 (SD = 0.91); *Have you been able to enjoy your normal daily activities?* M = 2.92 (SD = 0.89); *Have you been able to concentrate well on what you were doing?* M = 2.86 (SD = 0.80); and *Have your worries made you lose a lot of sleep?* M = 2.82 (SD = 0.99).

On the contrary, the items with a lower valuation have been: *Have you thought that you are a worthless person?* M = 1.68 (SD = 1.01); *Do you feel reasonably happy considering all the circumstances?* M = 2.37 (SD = 0.85) and *Have you felt capable of making decisions?* M = 2.29 (SD = 0.80).

3.3. Sociodemographic Data and Their Relationship with Psychological Distress

Table 1 shows how PD is more present among women OR = 1.916, 95% CI = (1.613, 2.273); aged 29 or younger OR = 2.651, 95% CI = (2.219, 3.168); without a couple OR = 1.959, 95% CI = (1.643, 2.336); with lower educational level (secondary school or lower) OR = 2.132, 95% CI = (1.771, 2.567); living in a house without balcony/terrace/yard/garden OR = 1.631, 95% CI = (1.232, 2.160); without children OR = 2.222, 95% CI = (1.873, 2.639); and not being a health professional OR = 1.385, 95% CI = (1.062, 1.580). Higher PD was found among public employees (78.7%) than among workers of private companies (70.6%) and self-employed workers (61.8%), $p < 0.001$.

It is not observed that having a pet or any degree of disability is associated with the development of PD. Being in strict confinement or being able to go out only for purchase or work is indeed associated with the level of PD (Table 1).

3.4. Physical Symptoms, Perception of Health, Health-Related Variables and Psychological Distress

76.8% claimed to have an excellent self-perceived health. A bad perception, versus an excellent health perception, is associated with a higher level of PD, with an OR = 6.803, 95% CI = (4.808, 9.524) (Table 3).

Table 3. Association between self-perceived health, physical symptoms, and other health variables related with psychological distress during the COVID-19 pandemic.

	TOTAL (*N* = 3227)					
		GHQ				
	N (%)	YES (*N* = 2544)	NO (*N* = 683)	$\chi2$	*p*	Odds Ratio (CI = 95%)
		PHYSICAL SYMPTOMS				
Fever						
Yes	46 (1.4)	89.1	10.9	2.965	0.085	2.221 (0.874, 5.643)
No	3181 (98.6)	78.7	21.3			
Cough						
Yes	647 (20.0)	85.3	14.7	20.378	<0.001	1.715 (1.354, 2.172)
No	2580 (80.0)	77.2	22.8			
Headache						
Yes	1731 (53.6)	87.5	12.5	168.868	<0.001	3.183 (2.660, 3.810)
No	1496 (46.4)	68.8	31.2			
Muscle pain						
Yes	845 (26.2)	89.0	11.0	70.810	<0.001	2.662 (2.105, 3.366)
No	2382 (73.8)	75.2	24.8			
Dizziness						
Yes	363 (11.2)	90.9	9.1	35.737	<0.001	2.936 (2.031, 4.243)
No	2864 (88.8)	77.3	22.7			
Diarrhea						
Yes	379 (11.7)	91.6	8.4	41.655	<0.001	3.213 (2.214, 4.663)
No	2848 (88.3)	77.1	22.9			
Sore throat						
Yes	625 (19.4)	86.2	13.8	25.474	<0.001	1.866 (1.460, 2.385)
No	2602 (80.6)	77.1	22.9			

Table 3. *Cont.*

	TOTAL (*N* = 3227)					
	GHQ					
	N (%)	YES (*N* = 2544)	NO (*N* = 683)	χ2	*p*	Odds Ratio (CI = 95%)
Coryza						
Yes	1122 (34.8)	85.6	14.4	46.644	<0.001	1.949 (1.606, 2.366)
No	2105 (65.2)	75.2	24.8			
Chills						
Yes	225 (7.0)	88.4	11.6	13.386	<0.001	2.144 (1.412, 3.256)
No	3002 (93.0)	78.1	21.9			
Breathing difficulty						
Yes	141 (4.4)	88.7	11.3	8.517	0.004	2.154 (1.271, 3.650)
No	3086 (95.6)	78.4	21.6			
	CURRENT HEALTH STATUS					
Self-perceived health						
Fair/bad/very bad	749 (23.2)	95.1	4.9	153.894	<0.001	6.803 (4.808, 9.524)
Excellent/good/very good	2478 (76.8)	73.9	26.1			
Chronic diseases						
Yes	945 (29.3)	78.1	21.9	0.438	0.508	1.067 (0.888, 1.283)
No	2282 (70.7)	79.1	20.9			
Currently taking any medication						
No	2026 (62.8)	79.3	20.7	0.764	0.382	1.083 (0.911, 1.289)
Yes	1201 (37.2)	78.0	22.0			
Hospitalised in the last 14 days						
No	3208 (99.4)	78.9	21.1	0.304	0.581	1.333 (0.479, 3.717)
Yes	19 (0.6)	73.7	26.3			
Health care in the last 14 days						
Yes	281 (8.7)	82.6	17.4	2.563	0.109	1.291 (0.937, 1.779)
No	2946 (91.3)	78.5	21.5			

The most frequent symptoms were: headache (53.6%), rhinitis (34.8%), muscle pain (26.2%), cough (20.0%), and sore throat (19.4%). Having any of the symptoms is associated with developing PD, except for fever (1.4% had it). The symptoms with the highest percentages of high PD are: diarrhea (91.6%), dizziness (90.9%), fever (89.1%), muscle pain (89.0%), breathing difficulties (88.7%), chills (88.4%), and headache (87.5%); all results had $p < 0.001$ (Table 3).

29.3% reported having a chronic disease and 37.2% were taking medication. During the last 14 days, 8.7% had required medical care and 0.6% had required hospital care. No association was observed between these variables and developing PD.

3.5. *Psychological Distress and Contact History*

The proportion of participants who claimed they had not been in contact for more than 15 min and within 2 m away with an infected person was 78.1%. 71.9% reported not having been in casual contact with an infected person and 61.3% had not had any contact with a person or material suspected of being infected. 14.3% stated that they had undergone a diagnostic test (Table 4).

These contact histories, except for having received a diagnostic test, were associated with having developed PD, finding statistical significance ($p < 0.05$) and an OR greater than 1.3 (Table 4).

Table 4. Association between variables related with history of contact and psychological distress during the pandemic.

	TOTAL (N = 3227)					
		GHQ				
	N (%)	Yes (N = 2544)	No (N = 683)	Statistical	p	Odds Ratio (CI = 95%)
Contact >15′ <2 m with infected person						
Yes, or doesn't know	708 (21.9)	82.8	17.2	8.411	0.004	1.372 (1.105, 1.704)
No	2519 (78.1)	77.7	22.3			
Casual contact with infected person						
Yes, or doesn't know	907 (28.1)	83.0	17.0	13.250	<0.001	1.453 (1.190, 1.772)
No	2320 (71.9)	77.2	22.8			
Contact with any person or material suspicious of being infected						1.485 (1.240, 1.777)
Yes, or doesn't know	1248 (38.7)	82.8	17.2	18.910	<0.001	
No	1979 (61.3)	76.4	23.6			
Any infected family member						
Yes, or doesn't know	537 (16.6)	82.5	17.5	5.173	0.023	1.320 (1.038, 1.679)
No	2690 (83.4)	78.1	21.9			
Having been performed diagnostic test						
No	2767 (85.7)	79.2	20.8	1.412	0.235	1.153 (0.912, 1.460)
Yes	460 (14.3)	76.7	23.3			

3.6. Psychological Distress and Preventive Measures

The preventive measure with a higher mean score was "wearing a mask regardless of the presence of symptoms" (M = 4.77; SD = 0.62), followed by "washing hands with soap and water" (M = 4.75; SD = 0.52). A statistically significant association has been found between having PD and the use of the following preventive measures: "washing hands after coughing, touching the nose, or sneezing"; "avoiding sharing utensils", both with $p < 0.001$; "leaving at least one and a half metres away", $p = 0.002$; "wash hands with soap and water", $p = 0.003$; and "washing hands with soap and water", $p = 0.025$ (Table 5).

Table 5. Contrast between preventive measures and psychological distress during the pandemic.

	TOTAL(N = 3227)				
		GHQ			
	M (SD)	Yes (N = 2544)	No (N = 683)	Statistical	p
Covering mouth	4.56 (0.76)	4.55 (0.76)	4.60 (0.75)	−1.411	0.158
Avoiding sharing utensils	4.29 (1.16)	4.25 (1.17)	4.43 (1.10)	−3.784	<0.001
Washing hands with soap and water	4.75 (0.52)	4.74 (0.53)	4.79 (0.47)	−2.250	0.025
Washing hands with hydroalcoholic solution	3.89 (1.12)	3.86 (1.12)	4.00 (1.12)	−2.994	0.003
Washing hands immediately after coughing, touching the nose, or sneezing	3.60 (1.18)	3.56 (1.17)	3.75 (1.18)	−3.675	<0.001
Washing hands after touching potentially contaminated objects	4.57 (0.75)	4.56 (0.76)	4.62 (0.72)	−1.710	0.087
Wearing a mask regardless of the presence of symptoms	4.77 (0.62)	4.77 (0.62)	4.77 (0.61)	−0.303	0.762
Leaving at least a metre and a half distance	4.51 (0.67)	4.49 (0.68)	4.58 (0.65)	−3.157	0.002

Note: Likert-type response scale from 1 (Never) to 5 (Always).

3.7. Prediction of Psychological Distress during the Pandemic

The variables that can predict PD during the COVID-19 pandemic in Chile according to the binary logistic regression are: having a bad self-perception of health OR = 4.038,

95% CI = (2.831, 5.758); being younger than 29 OR = 2.287, 95% CI = (1.893, 2.762); having diarrhea OR = 2.093, 95% CI = (1.414, 3.098); having headache OR = 2.019, 95% CI = (1.662, 2.453); being a woman OR = 1.638, 95% CI = (1.363, 1.967); having muscle pain OR = 1.439, 95% CI = (1.114, 1.859), and having had casual contact with an infected person OR = 1.410, 95% CI = (1.138, 1.747).

These variables correctly predict and classify 79.5% of psychological distress, with a sensitivity/specificity of 17.4/96.2, R2 = 0.126; Hosmer–Lemoshov test $\chi2$ = 13.514 (p = 0.095) and Omnibus test $\chi2$ = 433.575 (p < 0.001).

4. Discussion

As previously mentioned, the development of psychological effects, especially PD, is an event that is closely related to the occurrence of the COVID-19 pandemic. In the present study, a high percentage of people with a high level of PD (78.83%) has been observed, with a $\geq$ 3 cut-off point in the GHQ-12, data that are above those obtained in Spain (71.98%) with a similar study methodology and cut-off point [20]. The choice of cut-off point at this given level ($\geq$3) should be considered when comparing with other studies. These results are consistent with those obtained in previous similar studies [43–45].

It has been suggested that once key responses are adopted at the public health level, such as diagnostic testing, contact tracking, lockdown, and the management of confirmed cases of COVID-19, perhaps it is time to prioritize measures to safeguard the mental health of Chileans [46]. Even more, with the knowledge that the percentage of the population fully vaccinated has achieved higher levels than in other countries of the same geographical environment [13]. However, the speed in vaccinating the population may have caused an unjustified optimism that led to the abandonment of preventive measures after the first dose of the vaccine and, as the PAHO Director stated, "the vaccine alone is not going to stop the pandemic" [47].

Therefore, it seems that there is still time to prevent serious effects on mental health, since studies conducted in 21 countries, including Chile, have not observed, for instance, that high levels of PD, as the ones found in the study at hand, have led to an increase in the number of suicides in the first months of the pandemic [35].

In a somewhat contradictory way, a high percentage of the studied population claims to have an excellent self-perception of health during the last 14 days (76.8%), being the variable that mostly predicts PD, in the same way that it is known that PD is a highly reliable predictor of mortality [42]. This leads to a certain degree of optimism if measures are taken in time to enhance protective factors and mitigate the effects of the foreseeable economic recession resulting from this health crisis [35].

Differences have been seen between the symptoms found in a group of Latin American countries, the most common being cough (60.1%), fatigue/tiredness (52.0%), sore throat (50.3%), and fever (44.2%) [16], while in the present study, the most frequent symptoms have been: headache (53.6%), rhinitis (34.8%), muscle pain (26.2%), cough (20.0%), and sore throat (19.4%). In a study carried out in Spain with the same methodology, both headache and muscle pain had similar figures, but sore throat and cough had significantly higher values, while rhinitis occurred at higher rates in Chile [40]. This difference could be explained to some extent by the sociodemographic variables, the different information received by the populations of these countries, or even by being in different climatic seasons derived from belonging to the northern or southern hemisphere. In the study at hand, the three symptoms that predict PD are diarrhea, headache, and muscle pain.

The sex and age variables, as well as living with children, predict the level of PD, as has been also referred to in the literature [24,28,29,38,48–51].

Having a history of contact is associated with the presence of PD, both through contact with contaminated people or material, or with infected relatives, but it is the variable "having been in casual contact with an infected person" that mostly predicts PD, something already corroborated in previous studies [27].

It is well known that the proper and early use of preventive measures to avoid COVID-19 produces benefits in terms of health [52]. In this sense, the preventive measures with a higher valuation are: "wearing a mask regardless of the presence of symptoms" and "washing hands with soap and water". This second measure coincides with the study carried out in Spain [20], but the use of a mask receives a much higher value in Chile. This could be explained by the fact that the data collection was carried out in Spain in earlier dates than in Chile, and during the first months of the pandemic, in Spain there was no such recommendation for the widespread use of the mask, and there were even supply problems.

On the other hand, in other studies carried out in Chile, it was found that males and people under 60 years of age were the most compliant groups with the preventive measures established by the Government, while in Colombia or Ecuador, it was women and the elderly who complied the most [48].

When designing public health policies, the stressors identified in the literature, which are related to financial, academic, and family concerns, should be taken into account, the stress of confinement being a clear predictor of mental health [24], and obviously influencing the conditions of the home of the confined person. In the present study, we have found that PD is associated with living in houses with no exterior exit (house without a balcony, terrace, yard, or garden), identifying this as the most potentially stressful type of housing, an issue that would be convenient to consider when planning urban development.

Living without a partner and not having children are other stressor variables identified in this study, which highlight the importance of family support in pandemic situations, as the importance of social support has been observed with other health problems [53].

Compared with all six Latin American countries that have been studied (Argentina, Brazil, Chile, Colombia, Mexico, and Peru), Chile is the country shown to have positive variables against COVID-19, since it has a lower percentage of poverty, higher level of schooling, and the best health system. On the contrary, it has a high percentage of the population over 65 years of age, and it adopted a partial and not total lockdown, unlike other surrounding countries [54]. Another positive factor is the fast pace of vaccination administration, higher not only than other Latin American countries, but even higher than some European countries, such as Spain [13].

On the other hand, health professionals, as previously mentioned, are a group with high levels of PD and other indicators of poor mental health [16,33], while in the present study, show a lower percentage of PD than non-health professionals. One possible explanation may be the invisibility of non-health workers in situations of risk (e.g., delivery staff, cleaners, drivers, law enforcement bodies), who, being essential jobs, have had to continue performing their work during lockdown, being in contact with contaminated people or objects and for whom vaccination has not been established as a priority, as has been the case with health professionals. Other explanations may be the effect of teleworking, increased lockdown, or greater effects on the economy, with its consequent impact on PD [55] or the social support they have had during the pandemic [56], although the latter has not been observed in other studies [57].

In this socio-economic context, and based on the levels of PD found in the study, the adoption of preventive measures focused on the prevention of possible mental effects in high-risk populations is considered of special relevance.

The limitations of this research are the same as those of all descriptive studies without randomized sampling, along with those related to online access to data, which leave out groups without internet access or without knowledge for its use. This can be seen in that 59.25% of the participants had a university level of education or higher. Moreover, online data collection does not guarantee a homogeneous territorial distribution, with some areas of the country being more affected than others. However, the characteristics of the study advised applying the sampling used. In addition, this research has been carried out with the same methodology in 18 countries in Latin America and Europe, which will facilitate comparisons in the near future that will allow increasing the available evidence on the issue studied. This methodology was also chosen for the Eurofound study and promoted by the European Union [40], but its results did not allow for causal associations to be obtained and will require future studies with more appropriate designs to test the hypotheses detected. Another limitation is the difficulty in answering certain questions, such as "whether having touched contaminated objects" or "having been in contact with sick people during the previous 14 days". Similarly, the GHQ is a general measure of mental health, although it is a widely used and highly reliable indicator. In our study, it obtained an α-Cronbach's score = 0.910.

5. Conclusions

We have been able to verify that in Chile, a country with theoretically high levels of protection against the COVID-19 pandemic, including a high percentage of vaccination, higher than those of neighboring countries, the percentage of people with psychological distress is very high in the population studied.

It has been possible to identify variables associated with PD such as being a woman, being under 29 years of age, and with a low level of education, vulnerable groups already described in other countries. Furthermore, the influence of family support becomes visible by observing that living without a partner or not having children act as variables associated with PD. The type of housing is another factor to consider when it comes to urban planning, and to establish the importance of having a house with exterior exit (balcony/terrace/yard) to reduce the PD generated in pandemics that force diverse degrees of lockdown of the population.

Something seemingly contradictory has been detected; non-health professionals showed a higher level of PD than health professionals, a group that is the subject of most studies regarding the effects of the COVID-19 pandemic. This can help visualize the group of workers of essential activities, who have had to continue to develop their work during the pandemic and, therefore, have also been exposed to contact with contaminated people or objects, but with a lower level of prioritization when it comes to vaccination.

For these reasons, the need to prioritize the establishment of programs that safeguard the mental health of Chileans before these negative effects evolve into irremediable situations or become difficult to address is evident. In this study, vulnerable groups with whom intervention would be efficient and effective, have been identified.

Author Contributions: Conceptualization, C.R.-F., D.D.-G., M.O.-M., D.D.-B., D.E.-G., J.J.G.-I. and J.G.-S.; Data curation, C.R.-F., D.D.-G., M.O.-M., D.D.-B., D.E.-G., J.J.G.-I. and J.G.-S.; Formal analysis, C.R.-F., D.D.-G., M.O.-M., D.D.-B., D.E.-G., J.J.G.-I. and J.G.-S.; Investigation, C.R.-F., D.D.-G., M.O.-M., D.D.-B., D.E.-G., J.J.G.-I. and J.G.-S.; Methodology, C.R.-F., D.D.-G., M.O.-M., D.D.-B., D.E.-G., J.J.G.-I. and J.G.-S.; Project administration, C.R.-F. and J.G.-S.; Resources, C.R.-F., D.D.-G., M.O.-M., D.D.-B., D.E.-G., J.J.G.-I. and J.G.-S.; Software, C.R.-F., D.D.-G., M.O.-M., D.D.-B., D.E.-G., J.J.G.-I. and J.G.-S.; Supervision, C.R.-F., D.D.-G., M.O.-M., D.D.-B., D.E.-G., J.J.G.-I. and J.G.-S.; Validation, C.R.-F., D.D.-G., M.O.-M., D.D.-B., D.E.-G., J.J.G.-I. and J.G.-S.; Visualization, C.R.-F., D.D.-G., M.O.-M., D.D.-B., D.E.-G., J.J.G.-I. and J.G.-S.; Writing—original draft, C.R.-F., D.D.-G., M.O.-M., D.D.-B., D.E.-G., J.J.G.-I. and J.G.-S.; Writing—review & editing, C.R.-F., D.D.-G., M.O.-M., D.D.-B., D.E.-G., J.J.G.-I. and J.G.-S. All authors have read and agreed to the published version of the manuscript.

Funding: This research received no external funding.

Institutional Review Board Statement: The study was conducted according to the guidelines of the Declaration of Helsinki and has been authorized by the Ethics Committee of the University of Aconcagua in Chile (Santiago, UAC-22 April 2020) and in Spain by the Research Ethics Committee of Huelva, belonging to the Regional Ministry of Health of Andalusia (PI 036/20).

Informed Consent Statement: Informed consent was obtained from all subjects involved in the study.

Data Availability Statement: All data are available within this article.

Acknowledgments: In memory of Guillermo Solar Oyanedel.

Conflicts of Interest: The authors declare no conflict of interest.

References

1. WHO. Europe International Health Regulations—2019-nCoV Outbreak Is an Emergency of International Concern. Available online: https://www.who.int/director-general/speeches/detail/who-director-general-s-statement-on-ihr-emergency-committee-on-novel-coronavirus-(2019-ncov) (accessed on 21 May 2021).
2. World Health Organization. WHO Announces COVID-19 Outbreak a Pandemic. 2020. Available online: https://www.euro.who.int/en/health-topics/health-emergencies/coronavirus-covid-19/news/news/2020/3/who-announces-covid-19-outbreak-a-pandemic (accessed on 21 May 2021).
3. Newey, S. Latin America Has Become the Epicentre of the Coronavirus Pandemic, WHO Says, The Telegraph, 27 May 2020. Available online: https://www.telegraph.co.uk/global-health/science-and-disease/latin-america-has-become-epicentre-coronavirus-pandemic-says/ (accessed on 21 May 2021).
4. Benítez, M.A.; Velasco, C.; Sequeira, A.R.; Henríquez, J.; Menezes, F.M.; Paolucci, F. Responses to COVID-19 in five Latin American countries. *Health Policy Technol.* **2020**, *9*, 525–559. [CrossRef] [PubMed]
5. Bilal, U.; Alfaro, T.; Vives, A. COVID-19 and the worsening of health inequities in Santiago, Chile. *Int. J. Epidemiol.* **2021**, dyab007. [CrossRef]
6. Villalobos-Dintrans, P.; Castillo, C.; de la Fuente, F.; Maddaleno, M. COVID-19 incidence and mortality in the Metropolitan Region, Chile: Time, space, and structural factors. *PLoS ONE* **2021**, *16*, e0250707. [CrossRef] [PubMed]
7. Mena, G.; Martinez, P.P.; Mahmud, A.S.; Marquet, P.A.; Buckee, C.O.; Santillana, M. Socioeconomic status determines COVID-19 incidence and related mortality in Santiago, Chile. *MedRxiv* **2021**. [CrossRef]
8. Asahi, K.; Undurraga, E.A.; Valdés, R.; Wagner, R. The effect of COVID-19 on the economy: Evidence from an early adopter of localized lockdowns. *J. Glob. Health* **2021**, *11*, 05002. [CrossRef] [PubMed]
9. Ramírez de la Cruz, E.E.; Grin, E.J.; Sanabria-Pulido, P.; Cravacuore, D.; Orellana, A. The Transaction Costs of the Governments' Response to the COVID-19 Emergency in Latin America. *Public Adm. Rev.* **2020**. [CrossRef] [PubMed]
10. Undurraga, E.A.; Chowell, G.; Mizumoto, K. COVID-19 case fatality risk by age and gender in a high testing setting in Latin America: Chile, March-August 2020. *Infect. Dis. Poverty* **2021**, *10*, 11. [CrossRef] [PubMed]
11. Millalen, P.; Nahuelpan, H.; Hofflinger, A.; Martínez, E. COVID-19 and Indigenous peoples in Chile: Vulnerability to contagion and mortality. *AlterNative* **2020**, *16*, 399–402. [CrossRef]
12. Del Pino, S.; Gómez-Salgado, J.; Domínguez-Gómez, J.A.; Ruiz-Frutos, C. People of african descent of the americas, racial discrimination, and quality of the health services. *Sustainability* **2020**, *12*, 6930. [CrossRef]
13. John Hopkins Coronavirus Resource Center. Available online: https://coronavirus.jhu.edu/region/chile (accessed on 18 May 2021).
14. Makaronidis, J.; Mok, J.; Balogun, N.; Magee, C.G.; Omar, R.Z.; Carnemolla, A.; Batterham, R.L. Seroprevalence of SARS-CoV-2 antibodies in people with an acute loss in their sense of smell and/or taste in a community-based population in London, UK: An observational cohort study. *PLoS Med.* **2020**, *17*, e1003358. [CrossRef] [PubMed]
15. Huang, C.; Huang, L.; Wang, Y.; Li, X.; Ren, L.; Gu, X.; Kang, L.; Guo, L.; Liu, M.; Zhou, X.; et al. 6-month consequences of COVID-19 in patients discharged from hospital: A cohort study. *Lancet* **2021**, *397*, 220–232. [CrossRef]
16. Luo, M.; Guo, L.; Yu, M.; Jiang, W.; Wang, H. The psychological and mental impact of coronavirus disease 2019 (COVID-19) on medical staff and general public—A systematic review and meta-analysis. *Psychiatry Res.* **2020**, *291*, 113190. [CrossRef] [PubMed]
17. Xiong, Q.; Xu, M.; Li, J.; Liu, Y.; Zhang, J.; Xu, Y.; Dong, W. Clinical sequelae of COVID-19 survivors in Wuhan, China: A single-centre longitudinal study. *Clin. Microbiol. Infect.* **2021**, *27*, 89–95. [CrossRef] [PubMed]
18. Kronbichler, A.; Kresse, D.; Yoon, S.; Lee, K.H.; Effenberger, M.; Shin, J.I. Asymptomatic patients as a source of COVID-19 infections: A systematic review and meta-analysis. *Int. J. Infect. Dis.* **2020**, *98*, 180–186. [CrossRef]
19. Ramírez, M.L.; Martinez, S.M.; Bessone, C.D.V.; Allemandi, D.A.; Quinteros, D.A. COVID-19: Epidemiological situation of Argentina and its neighbor countries after three months of pandemic. *Disaster Med. Public Health Prep.* **2021**, 1–23. [CrossRef]
20. Domínguez-Salas, S.; Gómez-Salgado, J.; Andrés-Villas, M.; Díaz-Milanés, D.; Romero-Martín, M.; Ruiz-Frutos, C. Psycho-Emotional Approach to the Psychological Distress Related to the COVID-19 Pandemic in Spain: A Cross-Sectional Observational Study. *Healthcare* **2020**, *8*, 190. [CrossRef]
21. Orte, C.; Sánchez-Prieto, L.; Domínguez, D.C.; Barrientos-Báez, A. Evaluation of Distress and Risk Perception Associated with COVID-19 in Vulnerable Groups. *Int. J. Environ. Res. Public Health* **2020**, *17*, 9207. [CrossRef]
22. Pollak, Y.; Shoham, R.; Dayan, H.; Gabrieli-Seri, O.; Berger, I. Background and concurrent factors predicting non-adherence to public health preventive measures during the chronic phase of the COVID-19 pandemic. *J. Public Health* **2021**, fdab214. [CrossRef]
23. Galehdar, N.; Kamran, A.; Toulabi, T.; Heydari, H. Exploring nurses' experiences of psychological distress during care of patients with COVID-19: A qualitative study. *BMC Psychiatry* **2020**, *20*, 489. [CrossRef]
24. Landa-Blanco, M.; Mejía, C.J.; Landa-Blanco, A.L.; Martínez-Martínez, C.A.; Vásquez, D.; Vásquez, G.; Moraga-Vargas, P.; Echenique, Y.; Del Cid, G.M.; Montoya, B.D. Coronavirus awareness, confinement stress, and mental health: Evidence from Honduras, Chile, Costa Rica, Mexico and Spain. *Soc. Sci. Med.* **2021**, *277*, 113933. [CrossRef]

25. Urzúa, A.; Samaniego, A.; Caqueo-Urízar, A.; Zapata Pizarro, A.; Irarrázaval Domínguez, M. Salud mental en trabajadores de la salud durante la pandemia por COVID-19 en Chile [Mental health problems among health care workers during the COVID-19 pandemic]. *Rev. Med. Chil.* **2020**, *148*, 1121–1127. (In Spanish) [CrossRef] [PubMed]
26. Giorgi, G.; Lecca, L.I.; Alessio, F.; Finstad, G.L.; Bondanini, G.; Lulli, L.G.; Arcangeli, G.; Mucci, N. COVID-19-Related Mental Health Effects in the Workplace: A Narrative Review. *Int. J. Environ. Res. Public Health* **2020**, *17*, 7857. [CrossRef] [PubMed]
27. Xiang, Y.T.; Yang, Y.; Li, W.; Zhang, L.; Zhang, Q.; Cheung, T.; Ng, C.H. Timely mental health care for the 2019 novel coronavirus outbreak is urgently needed. *Lancet Psychiatry* **2020**, *7*, 228–229. [CrossRef]
28. Dagnino, P.; Anguita, V.; Escobar, K.; Cifuentes, S. Psychological Effects of Social Isolation Due to Quarantine in Chile: An Exploratory Study. *Front. Psychiatry* **2020**, *11*, 591142. [CrossRef]
29. Ruiz-Frutos, C.; Ortega-Moreno, M.; Allande-Cussó, R.; Domínguez-Salas, S.; Dias, A.; Gómez-Salgado, J. Health-related factors of psychological distress during the COVID-19 pandemic among non-health workers in Spain. *Saf. Sci.* **2021**, *133*, 104996. [CrossRef]
30. Mohammadian Khonsari, N.; Shafiee, G.; Zandifar, A.; Mohammad Poornami, S.; Ejtahed, H.S.; Asayesh, H.; Qorbani, M. Comparison of psychological symptoms between infected and non-infected COVID-19 health care workers. *BMC Psychiatry* **2021**, *21*, 170. [CrossRef]
31. Pandey, D.; Bansal, S.; Goyal, S.; Garg, A.; Sethi, N.; Pothiyill, D.I.; Sreelakshmi, E.S.; Sayyad, M.G.; Sethi, R. Psychological impact of mass quarantine on population during pandemics-The COVID-19 Lock-Down (COLD) study. *PLoS ONE* **2020**, *15*, e0240501. [CrossRef]
32. Pappa, S.; Ntella, V.; Giannakas, T.; Giannakoulis, V.G.; Papoutsi, E.; Katsaounou, P. Prevalence of depression, anxiety, and insomnia among healthcare workers during the COVID-19 pandemic: A systematic review and meta-analysis. *Brain Behav. Immun.* **2020**, *88*, 901–907. [CrossRef]
33. Pfefferbaum, B.; North, C.S. Mental health and the COVID-19 pandemic. *N. Engl. J. Med.* **2020**. [CrossRef]
34. Yao, H.; Chen, J.H.; Xu, Y.F. Patients with mental health disorders in the COVID-19 epidemic. *Lancet Psychiatry* **2020**, *7*, e21. [CrossRef]
35. Pirkis, J.; John, A.; Shin, S.; DelPozo-Banos, M.; Arya, V.; Analuisa-Aguilar, P.; Appleby, L.; Arensman, E.; Bantjes, J.; Baran, A.; et al. Suicide trends in the early months of the COVID-19 pandemic: An interrupted time-series analysis of preliminary data from 21 countries. *Lancet Psychiatry* **2021**, *8*, 579–588. [CrossRef]
36. Kim, K.S.; Kang, P.M.; Kim, H.S.N. Generalized Anxiety and Major Depressive Symptoms of General Public in South Korea during the Early COVID-19 Pandemic. *Int. J. Ment. Health Promot.* **2021**, *23*, 303–317. [CrossRef]
37. González-Tovar, M.; Hernández-Rodríguez, S. COVID-19 and Emotional Variables in a Sample of Chileans. *Front. Psychol.* **2021**, *12*, 615268. [CrossRef] [PubMed]
38. Gómez-Salgado, J.; Andrés-Villas, M.; Domínguez-Salas, S.; Díaz-Milanés, D.; Ruiz-Frutos, C. Related Health Factors of Psychological Distress During the COVID-19 Pandemic in Spain. *Int. J. Environ. Res. Public Health* **2020**, *17*, 3947. [CrossRef] [PubMed]
39. Tehrani, H. Mental health stigma related to novel coronavirus disease (COVID-19) in older adults. *Geriatr. Gerontol. Int.* **2020**, *20*, 796–797. [CrossRef] [PubMed]
40. Eurofound. *Living, Working and COVID-19*; COVID-19 Series; Publications Office of the European Union: Luxembourg, 2020.
41. Goldberg, D.P.; Gater, R.; Sartorius, N.; Ustun, T.B.; Piccinelli, M.; Gureje, O.; Rutter, C. The validity of two versions of the GHQ in the WHO study of mental illness in general health care. *Psychol. Med.* **1997**, *27*, 191–197. [CrossRef] [PubMed]
42. Idler, E.L.; Benyamini, Y. Self-rated health and mortality: A review of twenty-seven community studies. *J. Health Soc. Behav.* **1997**, *38*, 21–37. [CrossRef]
43. Dichter, M.N.; Sander, M.; Seismann-Petersen, S.; Köpke, S. COVID-19: It is time to balance infection management and person-centered care to maintain mental health of people living in German nursing homes. *Int. Psychogeriatr.* **2020**, *32*, 1157–1160. [CrossRef]
44. Si, M.Y.; Su, X.Y.; Jiang, Y.; Wang, W.J.; Gu, X.F.; Ma, L.; Li, J.; Zhang, S.K.; Ren, Z.F.; Ren, R.; et al. Psychological impact of COVID-19 on medical care workers in China. *Infect. Dis. Poverty* **2020**, *9*, 113. [CrossRef]
45. Serrano-Ripoll, M.J.; Meneses-Echavez, J.F.; Ricci-Cabello, I.; Fraile-Navarro, D.; Fiol-deRoque, M.A.; Pastor-Moreno, G.; Castro, A.; Ruiz-Pérez, I.; Zamanillo-Campos, R.; Gonçalves-Bradley, D.C. Impact of viral epidemic outbreaks on mental health of healthcare workers: A rapid systematic review and meta-analysis. *J. Affect. Disord.* **2020**, *277*, 347–357. [CrossRef]
46. Caqueo-Urízar, A.; Urzúa, A.; Aragón-Caqueo, D.; Charles, C.H.; El-Khatib, Z.; Otu, A.; Yaya, S. Mental health and the COVID-19 pandemic in Chile. *Psychol. Trauma* **2020**, *12*, 521–523. [CrossRef] [PubMed]
47. Taylor, L. COVID-19: Spike in cases in Chile is blamed on people mixing after first vaccine shot. *BMJ* **2021**, *373*, n1023. [CrossRef] [PubMed]
48. Bermejo-Martins, E.; Luis, E.O.; Sarrionandia, A.; Martínez, M.; Garcés, M.S.; Oliveros, E.Y.; Cortés-Rivera, C.; Belintxon, M.; Fernández-Berrocal, P. Different Responses to Stress, Health Practices, and Self-Care during COVID-19 Lockdown: A Stratified Analysis. *Int. J. Environ. Res. Public Health* **2021**, *18*, 2253. [CrossRef]
49. González-Sanguino, C.; Ausín, B.; Castellanos, M.Á.; Saiz, J.; López-Gómez, A.; Ugidos, C.; Muñoz, M. Mental health consequences during the initial stage of the 2020 Coronavirus pandemic (COVID-19) in Spain. *Brain Behav. Immun.* **2020**, *87*, 172–176. [CrossRef] [PubMed]

50. Salazar-Fernández, C.; Palet, D.; Haeger, P.A.; Román Mella, F. COVID-19 Perceived Impact and Psychological Variables as Predictors of Unhealthy Food and Alcohol Consumption Trajectories: The Role of Gender and Living with Children as Moderators. *Int. J. Environ. Res. Public Health* **2021**, *18*, 4542. [CrossRef]
51. Skapinakis, P.; Bellos, S.; Oikonomou, A.; Dimitriadis, G.; Gkikas, P.; Perdikari, E.; Mavreas, V. Depression and Its Relationship with Coping Strategies and Illness Perceptions during the COVID-19 Lockdown in Greece: A Cross-Sectional Survey of the Population. *Depress. Res. Treat.* **2020**, *2020*, 3158954. [CrossRef]
52. Michael, G.; Vishan, N. Does Social Distancing Matter? (30 March 2020). University of Chicago, Becker Friedman Institute for Economics Working Paper No. 2020-26. *SSRN Electron. J.* **2020**. [CrossRef]
53. Marroquín, B.; Vine, V.; Morgan, R. Mental health during the COVID-19 pandemic: Effects of stay-at-home policies, social distancing behavior, and social resources. *Psychiatry Res.* **2020**, *293*, 113419. [CrossRef]
54. Martinez-Valle, A. Public health matters: Why is Latin America struggling in addressing the pandemic? *J. Public. Health Policy* **2021**, *42*, 27–40. [CrossRef]
55. García-Iglesias, J.J.; Gómez-Salgado, J.; Martín-Pereira, J.; Fagundo-Rivera, J.; Ayuso-Murillo, D.; Martínez-Riera, J.R.; Ruiz-Frutos, C. Impacto del SARS-CoV-2 (COVID-19) en la salud mental de los profesionales sanitarios: Una revisión sistemática [Impact of SARS-CoV-2 (COVID-19) on the mental health of healthcare professionals: A systematic review.]. *Rev. Esp. Salud. Publica.* **2020**, *94*, e202007088. (In Spanish) [PubMed]
56. Peng, X.; Zhao, H.Z.; Yang, Y.; Rao, Z.L.; Hu, D.Y.; He, Q. Post-traumatic Growth Level and Its Influencing Factors Among Frontline Nurses During the COVID-19 Pandemic. *Front. Psychiatry* **2021**, *12*, 632360. [CrossRef] [PubMed]
57. Gómez-Salgado, J.; Ortega-Moreno, M.; Soriano, G.; Fagundo-Rivera, J.; Allande-Cussó, R.; Ruiz-Frutos, C. History of contact with the SARS-CoV-2 virus and the sense of coherence in the development of psychological distress in the occupational health professionals in Spain. *Sci. Prog.* **2021**, *104*, 368504211026121. [CrossRef] [PubMed]

Journal of
Clinical Medicine

MDPI

Article

Psychological Discomfort in Nursing Degree Students as a Consequence of the COVID-19 Pandemic

Fernando Espina-López [1], Emilia Moreno-Sánchez [2], Francisco-Javier Gago-Valiente [3,*], Jesús Sáez-Padilla [4], Vanesa Salado-Navarro [5] and María-de-los-Ángeles Merino-Godoy [6]

1 Huelva-Costa Primary Care District, 21007 Huelva, Spain; fernandoeslo99@gmail.com
2 Department of Pedagogy, Faculty of Education, Psychology and Sports Sciences, University of Huelva, 21007 Huelva, Spain; emilia@dedu.uhu.es
3 Preventive Medicine and Public Health Area, University of Huelva, 21071 Huelva, Spain
4 Integrated Didactics Department, Faculty of Education, Psychology and Sports Sciences, University of Huelva, 21071 Huelva, Spain; jesus.saez@dempc.uhu.es
5 Department of Experimental Psychology, Faculty of Psychology, University of Seville, 41004 Seville, Spain; vsalado@us.es
6 Nursing Department, Faculty of Nursing, University of Huelva, 21007 Huelva, Spain; angeles.merino@denf.uhu.es
* Correspondence: francisco.gago@dstso.uhu.es; Tel.: +34-635893772

Abstract: Students are a population at risk of developing psychological complications, such as psychological discomfort, stress, and anxiety, among other problems, especially during the current health crisis due to the COVID-19 pandemic. The present study's objective was to analyze the effects of the COVID-19 pandemic on the psychological discomfort of final-year nursing students. A cross-sectional descriptive observational study was carried out. To analyze the psychological discomfort of the participants, the Kessler test (previously validated) was used. The results of this test were divided into two levels (High ≥ 21/Low < 21), showing high sensitivity as a screening method for anxiety and depression. Questionnaires were sent via email to final-year nursing students of Spanish and South American universities, inviting them to participate voluntarily. The sample consisted of 400 students, with an average age of 23.29 years and a sex proportion of 82.75% women and 17.28% men. Almost all participants (n = 396) belonged to Spanish universities, and the greatest participation corresponded to Andalusian universities (64.5%). The average psychological discomfort was high (M = 27.94). Statistically significant relationships were detected between age, sex, and feeling ready for the world of work, observing no relationships with the rest of the studied variables. The sample of 4th-year students of the Degree of Nursing presented a high level of psychological discomfort. This pathology does not seem to be related to having suffered from COVID-19 or being in contact with infected people during the practicum and is more strongly related to personal sociodemographic variables and students' preparation for the world of work.

Keywords: COVID-19; pandemic; nursing; students; stress; anxiety; depression; psychological discomfort

Citation: Espina-López, F.; Moreno-Sánchez, E.; Gago-Valiente, F.-J.; Sáez-Padilla, J.; Salado-Navarro, V.; Merino-Godoy, M.-d.-l.-Á. Psychological Discomfort in Nursing Degree Students as a Consequence of the COVID-19 Pandemic. *J. Clin. Med.* **2021**, *10*, 5467. https://doi.org/10.3390/jcm10235467

Academic Editor: Michele Roccella

Received: 1 November 2021
Accepted: 19 November 2021
Published: 23 November 2021

1. Introduction

Since the 1918 Spanish Influenza pandemic, which caused approximately 40 million deaths [1], no other pandemic has impacted society as much as the SARS-CoV-2 virus. Its repercussions have demonstrated the frailty of every vital scope. The rapid spread of the new SARS-CoV-2 coronavirus has forced the adoption of exceptional prevention and containment measures.

In Spain, after the declaration of the World Health Organisation (WHO) recognizing the pandemic due to the disease caused by the SARS-CoV-2 corona virus (COVID-19) on 11 March 2020, one of the greatest challenges of recent decades was confronted [2]. To face this world crisis, social, economic, and political resources were demanded, as well as the recognition of the pandemic's possible consequences, requiring an approach to contain the outbreak through basic principles of public health [3].

It is important to highlight that, although the reaction was proportional to different crisis levels [4], difficult situations took place in hospitals due to the high contagion rates. In Spain, the coronavirus expanded from February 2020, and, at the middle of March 2020, an emergency state was imposed, with the aim of containing the contagions and reduce the overload of patients that occurred in hospitals. For over two months, the population went through a strict confinement, which did not prevent the health services from being overwhelmed in many places before flattening the curve of contagion [4]. From the beginning of the pandemic, the virus spread at a great rate throughout the entire territory; however, it did not affect all regions equally. This geographical "inequality" is not only obvious in the vaccination rate or in the parameter of cumulative disease incidence but also in the mortality rate [5].

It is known and proven that the COVID-19 pandemic has caused certain changes in the world population that challenge all aspects of "usual life". Daily actions from before this historical event have changed, and such change has impacted society in terms of personal affairs, human relationships, employment, education, connections with the community, and other social activities [6].

Many countries implemented several isolation measures to prevent the spread of the outbreak until a vaccine was available or until the percentage of vaccinated population increased, which led to important social and economic consequences in the entire community, resulting in negative psychological repercussions. These measures include home isolation, social distancing, closing of educational centers, universities, and businesses, cancellation of events, conferences, and seminars, postponement of sports events, and travel restrictions [3,6].

In fact, the spread of the outbreak of the new 2019 coronavirus SARS-CoV-2 brought a drastic change to all humanity, with a considerable psychosocial impact on the professions related to health and on the university students of health sciences [7].The impact on health professionals has been reported in different Spanish and international studies [8–10]. Roberts, Mc Aloney-Kocaman, Lippiett, Ray, Welch, and Kelly [11] state that there were higher levels of anxiety and depression among nurses with less experience.

It is also important to point out the impact of the state of health emergencyon educational contexts at all stages.

The current pandemic has caused vast and prolonged interruptions in the teaching–learning processes, in the normal support systems, and in the social activities of students, with ongoing consequences that reflect the distance from recovering the past normality in the near future [6].

This impact on students' lives is due to the convergence of many variables related to the interruption of students' university life and other aspects of their everyday life, including family and social life and their capacity to participate in habitual activities such as sports [6].

University students can be one of the most affected populations. Students have modified their routines due to the COVID-19 pandemic [12]. For many students, such as those of the Degree of Nursing, the requirements of isolation and social distancing have caused the cancellation of face-to-face lectures and exams, practicums in healthcare centers, and part-time jobs [6].

Attending lectures and other activities related to studying areof vital importance for professional training. For many students, going to university is a way of learning to face reality, as well as a way of maintaining their relationships with peers, friends, and faculty members [13].

Some students prefer to attend face-to-face lectures over the online modality, due to their personal learning styles, the capacity to learn "face-to-face" to increase their learning confidence, or having access to the support from their peers. For those who do not study in their locality of residence, in a shared flat/house, or in student accommodations, not attending face-to-face lectures increases their need for economic investment in technological devices to be able to attend the online lectures. Moreover, if they could not attend the face-to-face lectures, students suffered the subsequent loneliness and loss of connection with other people related to their studies (students and faculty members) [13].

In some countries, nursing students experienced situations under certain pressure, where they had to assume the role of health professionals, assisting upon request in the units where they were assigned, with critical patients, putting students' mental health at risk due to these stressful situations [14]. In fact, it has been asserted that the COVID-19 pandemic has placed a considerable number of nursing students in a situation in which they feel that they must choose between safety outside of the healthcare profession or continuing their nursing studies [15]. This dilemma can cause additional psychological distress among nursing students and, as in the case of previous global disease outbreaks such as Ebola, healthcare professionals are at great risk of developing burnout, fatigue, lower job satisfaction and morale, and working stress during pandemics [6].

Therefore, it has been demonstrated that nursing students experience greater anxiety than students of other degrees, due to the specific characteristics of their training [16]. This may be caused by the additional stress factors related to the social and academic adjustments derived from the COVID-19 pandemic within the educational community [17,18].

Several studies on this population report that those aged between 18 and 20 years, mostly women, show higher stress levels. It was found that watching the news about the pandemic, concern about infection, and the time restrictions imposed by the curfew influenced nursing students' stress levels [3].

It is known that the transition of nursing students to the role of healthcare professionals has always been stressful, thus, there are people who have abandoned their profession when it was time for them to practice it. Currently, the COVID-19 pandemic has posed a new and serious stress and anxiety factor to nursing students. These students have lived through situations such as the struggle of their peers who work in healthcare centers with the isolation measures. For example, one of these situations was the lack of basic material, including personal protection equipment (PPE), along with the direct exposure to COVID-19 patients. This may have caused negative perceptions toward nursing students' future occupation [19].

Therefore, several actions have been proposed to implement a solid and suitable support plan aimed at preventing professional discomfort [14]. In this preventive line, it has been stated that study plans should include specific content on the management of pandemics and other disasters, in order to increase the preparation of the students, i.e., the future healthcare professionals, for these types of scenarios [20].

Hernández-Martínez, Rodríguez-Almagro, Martínez-Alce, Romero-Blanco, García-Iglesias, and Gómez-Salgado [2] claim that, although nursing students showed willingness to incorporate into the healthcare centers, they felt unprepared to work in the field of intensive care and demanded further training to improve their levels of anxiety and stress regarding the care of critical patients. Guidance, followup, and emotional support in critical situations have proved key to overcome stressful situations [21].

For all these reasons, the aim of the present study was to analyze the influence of the COVID-19 pandemic on the psychological discomfort of final-year students of the Degree of Nursing due to the temporal proximity of their professional practice. The study'sobjective was to determine the prevalence of psychological discomfort in the study population, as well as the influence of sociodemographic and academic variables. The pandemic has had a direct impact on this new generation of nursing professionals. Discovering the possible psychological repercussions in these students will enable implementation of psychological and didactic corrective measures that reduce the negative effects on their training and personal health. Such measures could facilitate the integration of those who are about to become healthcare professionals, thus contributing to improving the quality of healthcare services.

2. Materials and Methods

2.1. Participants

This was a descriptive cross-sectional study with 400 nursing students, of whom 82.75% were women (n = 331) and 17.25% were men (n = 69). It is important to take into account that most nursing students are females; therefore, in the proportion of samples in studies related to these professionals, the representation of women is considerably greater than that of men. The average age of the participants was 23.29 years. Most of the participants (n = 396) belonged to Spanish universities, and the greatest participation was from Andalusian universities (64.5%) (students from national and international universities that taught the degree of nursing participated in the study; the origin and number of participants is shown in Annex II). Regarding the sociodemographic characteristics, it is important to highlight that 60% of the students lived with their families (n = 232), 30.75% lived with other university students (n = 123), and 8.75% lived alone (n = 35).

2.2. Procedure

All students selected were in the fourth year of the degree of nursing. The study excluded those who did not perform the practicum in healthcare centers, since they did not experience the same situations.

To calculate the sample size, we determined the minimum sample required to estimate a parameter with a proportion of 0.50 (scenario with the greatest sample requirement) in a population of unknown size. Taking these data into account, and considering a 95% confidence level, 10% precision, and 5% of possible losses during the process of data cleansing, we calculated that the minimum sample size for this study would be 120 individuals. However, to carry out more complex analyses that involve the segmentation of the sample into subgroups of individuals, we decided to obtain a sample of around 400 individuals.

The data were gathered through self-administered questionnaires. The fieldwork began on 10 March 2021 and was terminated on 23 April 2021. The questionnaire was sent in a crucial moment of the pandemic, where the number of cases increased constantly and severe restrictions were established.

Student representatives of universities of different European and South American countries were contacted through social networks and via email and telephone. Representatives distributed the questionnaires among the final-year students of the degree of nursing who agreed to participate voluntarily. The format of the instrument was developed using Google Forms and the data were gathered directly from said platform.

Written informed consent was obtained from all participants for the publication and analysis of the data. Participant anonymity was guaranteed, thus complying with the current regulations on user data protection, specified in Organic Law 3/2018, of 5 December, on the Protection of Personal Data and the Guarantee of Digital Rights. Moreover, the formal aspects of the declaration of Helsinki were considered at all times. The study was approved by the Research Ethics Committee of Huelva (code: MG-COV-2021-02; internal code: 0742-N-21).

2.3. Evaluation Instruments

The participants completed a brief sociodemographic questionnaire, through which they provided information about their age and sex, the university in which they studied, and their place of residence during the academic year. The questionnaires were distributed through Gmail, thus participants had to provide their email address, which prevented duplicates. Additional items were introduced to gather information about the training of the participants, whether they had performed the practicum, whether they felt ready for the world of work, and whether they had suffered from the disease caused by SARS-CoV-2 (COVID-19).

The main variable of this present study was psychological discomfort, and it was measured using the Kessler scale (K-10) [22].This scale shows the level of psychological discomfort of the users during the 4-week period before completing the scale. Psychological discomfort is defined as the level of stress, demoralization, malaise, and unrest perceived in oneself [23].

Since the Kessler scale (K-10) is also used as a screening method for depression and anxiety, these two variables were also measured. Anxiety is defined as a human emotion present in most mental and medical disorders that appears as a response to the perception of a threat or danger. It helps people to prepare and practice in order to improve their activity and thus adopt the appropriate caution measures against potentially dangerous situations. Clinically, anxiety is fear without a known cause [24]. On the other hand, depression is understood as a mood disorder that causes symptoms of distress and affects how the person feels, thinks, and coordinates the activities of daily living, such as sleeping, eating, and working. To be diagnosed with depression, symptoms must be present during most of the day, almost every day, for at least two weeks.

This K-10 scale was selected for its adequacy and adaptation to the study scope. It is a brief questionnaire that can be easily applied by first-level healthcare professionals. K-10 has been translated into Spanish and applied in Spain, Colombia, Mexico, and Peru, as well as in other American and European countries [22].

The Kessler instrument consists of 10 items, with 5 Likert response options each, ordered hierarchically from 1 to 5: "never, almost never, sometimes, almost always and always". The sum of the scores can range from a minimum of 10 points to a maximum of 50. The interpretation of the scores corresponds to 4 levels as follows: 10–15 points, low level; 16–21, moderate level; 22–29, high level; and 30–50, very high level [22].

K-10 has been previously validated, with high sensitivity and specificity [22]. According to the validation study, the score of the scale can be divided into 2 levels, due to its high specificity and sensitivity, for the subsequent screening for anxiety and depression. This screening also categorizes the participants based on their psychological discomfort, although with two reference levels of anxiety and depression. The cutoff points would be, on the one hand, scores of 10–20 for low affectation of psychological discomfort (anxiety and depression) and, on the other hand, scores of 21–50 for high affectation.

Aranguren and Brenlla [25] explored the discriminant validity of K–10 in psychiatric patients, also comparing the scores obtained in psychiatric patients and non-psychiatric individuals. The results showedadequate validity and reliability of the instrument, with a Cronbach's alpha of 0.91 for the patients and 0.80 for the control individuals.

2.4. Statistical Analysis

The statistical analyses were conducted using IBM SPSS Statistics v.27.0 software. The descriptive analysis was performed with central tendency measures (mean and standard deviation), frequencies and percentages, using frequency tables.

Specifically, for the variables of age, psychological discomfort, anxiety, and depression, the mean and standard deviation were calculated.

The frequencies and percentages were calculated for the variables sex, practicum, university of origin, training, residence during the academic year, having suffered from COVID-19, psychological discomfort, anxiety, and depression.

To study the possible relationship between psychological discomfort and the rest of the variables, after verifying the normality of the quantitative variables, the following tests were carried out:

- Pearson's Chi-squared, to explore the correlation between psychological discomfort and the variables of COVID-19, sex, coexistence (residence during the academic year), and feeling ready for the world of work (training).
- Student's t, to analyze the relationship between psychological discomfort (anxiety and depression) and age.
- ANOVA, to study the correlation between psychological discomfort and age.

3. Results

3.1. Prevalence of Having Suffered from COVID-19 among the Participants

A total of 15.25% (n = 61) of the participants had suffered from COVID-19 before the study period, whereas 84.75% (n = 338) had not. Figure 1 shows these data categorized based on sex.

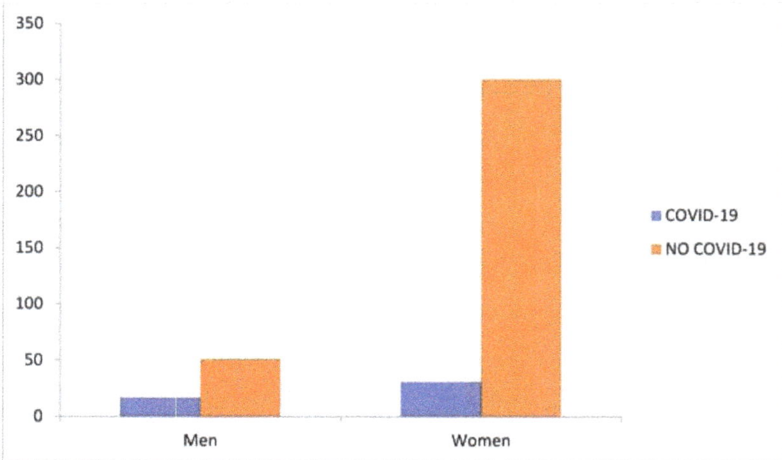

Figure 1. Frequencies of having suffered from COVID-19 based on sex.

3.2. Association of Psychological Discomfort with Sex, Residence during the Academic Year, Having Suffered from COVID-19, and Feeling Ready for the World of Work

A Chi-squared test of independency was conducted to determine whether the distribution of psychological discomfort was similar in women and men. The results show significant differences between men and women(X^2 = 14.958; p = 0.002, 95% CI). There was a greater proportion of women with high scores in psychological discomfort (41.7%) compared to men (24.6%) (Figure 2).

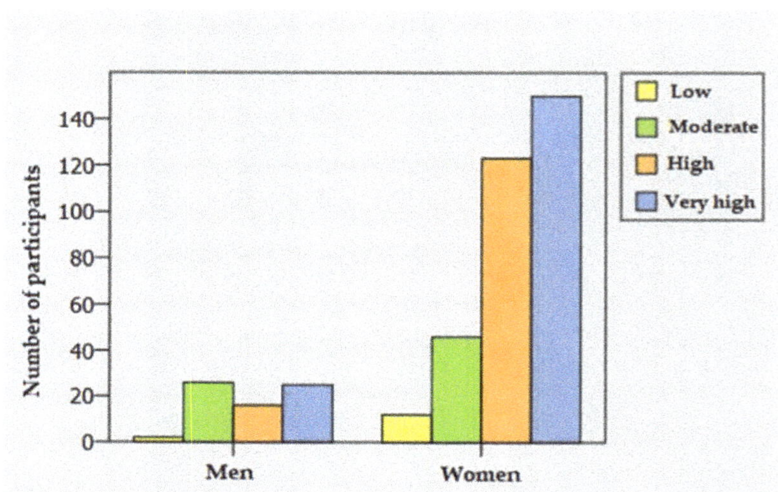

Figure 2. Frequencies in K-10 based on sex.

Regarding the study of the correlation between psychological discomfort and residence during the academic year, it was observed that the two variables were correlated (X^2 = 458.823; p = 0.026, 95% CI). Table 1 shows the percentages of greatest and least affectation in K-10 (very high level and low level, respectively) as a function of the coexistence unit during the academic year.

Table 1. Percentages of affectation in coexistence units in low and high levels of psychological discomfort.

Coexistence Unit During the Academic Year	Low Level of Psychological Discomfort	Very High Level of Psychological Discomfort
-Two or more roommates		
-Partner and child		
-Father and mother		
-Partner and partner's child		
-Roommates and partner		
-Father, mother, and sister		
-Parents and siblings		
-Brother		
-Mother and brother		
-Mother, stepfather, and three siblings		
-Friends (females)		
-One or more non-university roommates	0%	100%
-Classmates		
-Mother and siblings		
-Father		
-Student accommodation		
-Maternal grandparents, mother, stepfather, and younger sister		
-Roommates from the same university		
-Daughter		
-Sister	100%	0%
-Mother and sister		
-Father, mother, and brother		

In the analysis of the relationship between psychological discomfort and having suffered from COVID-19, no correlation was observed between these variables (X^2 = 5.652; p = 0.130, 95% CI).

Lastly, psychological discomfort was correlated with feeling ready for the world of work (X^2 = 24.873; p = 0.000, 95% CI). The participants who responded that "perhaps" they felt ready for the world of work showed greater representation in percentages of very high levels of psychological discomfort. However, the percentages of greatest representation in low levels of psychological discomfort were observed in those participants who responded "yes" to this item (Figure 3).

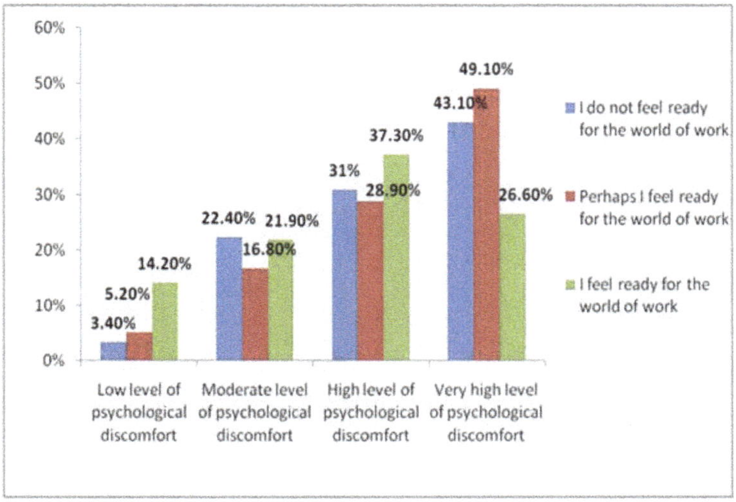

Figure 3. Correlation between psychological discomfort and feeling ready for the world of work.

3.3. Correlation between Psychological Discomfort and Age

The results of the single-factor ANOVA between groups showed that the differences in the mean scores of psychological discomfort according to age were not statistically significant (F = 0.712; p = 0.545, 95% CI).

3.4. Prevalence of Anxiety and Depression (Psychological Discomfort with the 2-Level K-10)

For the screening of anxiety and depression, the score of the scale was divided into two levels [22]: low (10–20 points) and high (21–50 points). Most of the participants presented a high level in the prevalence of anxiety and depression (Table 2).

Table 2. Frequencies and percentages of the participants in the 2-level K-10.

Range OF K-10 (2 Levels)			
Low		High	
N	%	N	%
63	15.75%	337	84.25%

3.5. Correlation between Psychological Discomfort (2-Level K-10) and Age

A Student's t-test was performed to explore the existence of differences in terms of psychological discomfort (anxiety and depression) according to age. The results showed that there were no statistically significant differences (t (398) = 1.440; p = 0.151, 95% CI).

3.6. Association of Psychological Discomfort (2-Level K-10) with Sex, Residence during the Academic Year, Having Suffered from COVID-19 and Feeling Ready for the World of Work

A correlation was observed between psychological discomfort and sex (X^2 = 9.259; p = 0.002, 95% CI), with a greater proportion of women (78.2%) who showed a high level of psychological discomfort compared to men (60.9%).

With respect to the analysis of the association of psychological discomfort with residence during the academic year and having suffered from COVID-19, no correlation was observed between these variables (X^2 = 142.523; p = 0.291, 95% CI).

Lastly, a relationship was detected between psychological discomfort and feeling ready for the world of work (X^2 = 6.905; p = 0.032, 95% CI). The participants who claimed to feel ready for the world of work presented a lower level of psychological discomfort (68.6%) compared to those who did not feel ready (81%). The rest of the students who responded "perhaps" in this item represented a percentage of 79.8% in high affectation of anxiety and depression.

4. Discussion

The main objective of this study was to analyze the level of psychological discomfort of the final-year nursing students. The results showed that these students obtained high scores in this variable, following the line of research such as Herrera and Rivera [23]. However, other studies have reported a moderate prevalence [26].

The data of this study indicate that those who felt ready and qualified for the world of work presented a lower level of psychological discomfort. These data are consistent with the results of other studies [23], where the mean marks and satisfaction with the degree were also correlated with a low psychological discomfort.

A correlation was observed between sociodemographic variables and psychological discomfort. Moxham, Fernández, Kim, Lapkin, Ten Ham-Baloyi and Mutair [27] stated that the variables related to psychological discomfort are sex, age, marital status, and employment status. Some variables such as coexistence, high marks, and the practicum are not statistically significantly correlated with psychological discomfort [27].

Furthermore, the results of the present study indicate that psychological discomfort affects women to a greater extent than men, which is in line with the findings of Liébana-Presa, Fernández-Martínez, Gándara, Muñoz-Villanueva, Vázquez-Casares and Rodríguez-

Borrego [28], who reported that women obtained a higher score than men. It is important to highlight that the data of the present study corroborate the need to considering gender as a key for a change of paradigm that will allow generating more accurate and inclusive scientific knowledge, as well as a more realistic, fair, and egalitarian healthcare system.

As was commented above, in this study, those participants who felt ready for the world of work presented a lower psychological discomfort, which could be related to a greater resilience and a greater capacity to adapt to changes [29].

Having performed the practicum in healthcare centers and having suffered from COVID-19 were not significantly related to psychological discomfort. The data of this study indicate that psychological discomfort is related to sociodemographic variables such as sex, age, and university of origin, as well as preparation for the world of work.

The results of this investigation show the convenience of developing mitigation strategies in pandemic situations. Since resources can be particularly scarce during these states, adequate psychological support could be provided in many different forms, including telemedicine and informal support groups [30].

Limitations of the Study

This study provides very novel information about a series of indicators of mental health in a student population that had been poorly studied to date in a pandemic situation, thereby updating the knowledge on this topic to contribute to future research lines that address this problem. However, this study presents some limitations that must be pointed out. One of such limitations is that, despite the large sample size, most of the population who responded to the questionnaire were Spanish, thus the data cannot be extrapolated to the international scope. Similarly, participation in this study was voluntary, which can pose a sample selection bias.

Further research in this line is required, with larger populations and greater representation of international origin, in order to extrapolate the results. Moreover, randomized sampling must be applied to avoid selection bias.

5. Conclusions

In sum, the final-year nursing students who participated in this study suffered negative psychological consequences during the pandemic. These participants showed a high level of psychological discomfort. The differences in the latter were related to sociodemographic variables such as age, sex, university of origin, and feeling ready for the world of work.

The COVID-19 pandemic has caused serious repercussions. Therefore, in these periods of health crisis, it is necessary to develop research lines focused on studying the phenomenon and its impact with other variables, in order to know its effect on future healthcare professionals. This could help to prevent and address the negative personal aspects that can affect students' professional integration.

Author Contributions: Conceptualization, J.S.-P. and F.E.-L.; methodology, E.M.-S.; software, F.-J.G.-V.; validation, V.S.-N.; M.-d.-l.-Á.M.-G. and J.S.-P.; formal analysis, F.E.-L.; investigation, E.M.-S.; resources, F.-J.G.-V.; data curation, V.S.-N.; writing—original draft preparation, M.-d.-l.-Á.M.-G.; writing—review and editing, M.-d.-l.-Á.M.-G.; visualization, F.E.-L.; supervision, E.M.-S.; project administration, F.-J.G.-V.; funding acquisition, V.S.-N. All authors have read and agreed to the published version of the manuscript.

Funding: University of Huelva.

Institutional Review Board Statement: The formal aspects of the declaration of Helsinki were considered at all times. The study was approved by the Research Ethics Committee of Huelva (code: MG-COV-2021-02; internal code: 0742-N-21).

Informed Consent Statement: Informed consent was obtained from all subjects involved in the study.

Conflicts of Interest: The authors declare no conflict of interest.

References

1. Estupiñán-Martínez, O.R. Catástrofes Epidémicas. Acta Médica del Centro. Published Online at Acta Médica del Centro. Available online: https://www.medigraphic.com/pdfs/medicadelcentro/mec-2013/mec134a.pdf (accessed on 28 October 2021).
2. Hernández-Martínez, A.; Rodríguez-Almagro, J.; Martínez-Arce, A.; Romero-Blanco, C.; García-Iglesias, J.J.; Gómez-Salgado, J. Nursing students' experience and training in health care aid during the COVID-19 pandemic in Spain. *J. Clin. Nurs.* **2021**. [CrossRef]
3. Aslan, H.; Pekince, H. Nursing students' views on the COVID-19 pandemic and their perceived stress levels. *Perspect. Psychiatr. Care* **2020**, *57*, 695–701. [CrossRef] [PubMed]
4. Legido-Quigley, H.; Mateos-García, J.T.; Campos, V.R.; Gea-Sánchez, M.; Muntaner, C.; McKee, M. There silience of the Spanish Health system against the COVID-19 pandemic. *Lancet Public Health* **2020**, *5*, e251–e252. [CrossRef]
5. Batres, O. Castilla-LaMancha, Comunidad más Golpeada en Fallecimientos por COVID. Published Online at Redacción Médica. Available online: https://www.redaccionmedica.com/secciones/sanidad-hoy/covid-comunidades-mortalidad-espana-9828 (accessed on 28 October 2021).
6. Usher, K.; Wynaden, D.; Bhullar, N.; Durkin, J.; Jackson, D. The mental health impact of COVID-19 on pre-registration nursing students in Australia. *Int. J. Ment. Health Nurs.* **2020**, *29*, 1015–1017. [CrossRef]
7. De-Gagne, J.C.; Cho, E.; Park, H.K.; Nam, J.D.; Jung, D. A qualitative analysis of nursing students' tweets during the COVID-19 pandemic. *Nurs. Health Sci.* **2021**, *23*, 273–278. [CrossRef]
8. Santamaría, M.D.; Ozamiz-Etxebarria, N.; Rodríguez, I.R.; Alboniga-Mayor, J.J.; Gorrotxategi, M.P. Impacto psicológico dela COVID-19 en una muestrade profesionales sanitarios españoles. *Rev. Psiquiatr. Salud. Ment.* **2020**, *14*, 106–112. [CrossRef]
9. Lai, J.; Ma, S.; Wang, Y.; Cai, Z.; Hu, J.; Wei, N.; Hu, S. Factors associated with mental Health Outcomes among Healthcare workers exposed to coronavirus disease 2019. *JAMA Netw. Open* **2020**, *3*, e203976. [CrossRef]
10. Xing, L.Q.; Xu, M.L.; Sun, J.; Wang, Q.X.; Ge, D.D.; Jiang, M.M.; Li, Q. Anxiety and depression in frontline healthcareworkers during the outbreak of Covid-19. *Int. J. Soc. Psychiatry* **2020**, 1–8. [CrossRef]
11. Roberts, N.J.; McAloney-Kocaman, K.; Lippiett, K.; Ray, E.; Welch, L.; Kelly, C. Levels of resilience, anxiety and depression in nurses working in respiratory clinical areas during the COVID pandemic. *Respir. Med.* **2020**, *176*, 106219. [CrossRef] [PubMed]
12. Romero-Blanco, C.; Rodríguez-Almagro, J.; Onieva-Zafra, M.D.; Parra-Fernández, M.L.; Prado-Laguna, M.C.; Hernández-Martínez, A. Sleep Pattern Changes in Nursing Students during the COVID-19 Lockdown. *Int. J. Environ. Res. Public Health* **2020**, *17*, 5222. [CrossRef]
13. Garbrah, W.; Kankkunen, P.; Välimäki, T. Gerontological nurse teachers' abilities and influence on students' willingness in older people nursing: Across-sectional, correlational survey. *Nurse Educ. Today* **2020**, *90*, 104461. [CrossRef]
14. Hayter, M.; Jackson, D. Pre-registration under graduate nurses and the COVID-19 pandemic: Students or workers? *J. Clin. Nurs.* **2020**, *29*, 3115–3116. [CrossRef]
15. Fowler, K.; Wholeben, M. COVID-19: Outcomes for trauma-impacted nurses and nursing students. *Nurse Educ. Today* **2020**, *93*, 104525. [CrossRef]
16. Savitsky, B.; Findling, Y.; Ereli, A.; Hendel, T. Anxiety and coping strategies among nursing students during the covid-19 pandemic. *Nurse Educ. Pr.* **2020**, *46*, 102809. [CrossRef]
17. Lewnard, J.; Lo, N. Scientific and ethical basis for social-distancing interventions against COVID-19. *Lancet Infect. Dis.* **2020**, *20*, 631–633. [CrossRef]
18. Kochuvilayil, T.; Fernandez, R.S.; Moxham, L.J.; Lord, H.; Alomari, A.; Hunt, L.; Halcomb, E.J. COVID-19: Knowledge, anxiety, academic concerns and preventative behaviours among Australian and Indian undergraduate nursing students: A cross-sectional study. *J. Clin. Nurs.* **2021**, *30*, 882–891. [CrossRef] [PubMed]
19. Yildiz, E. Posttraumatic grow thand positive determinants in nursing students after COVID-19 alarm status: A descriptivecross-sectional study. *Perspect. Psychiatr. Care* **2021**, 1–12. [CrossRef]
20. Gómez-Ibáñez, R.; Watson, C.; Leyva-Moral, J.M.; Aguayo-González, M.; Granel, N. Final-year nursing students called towork: Experiences of arushed labour in sertion during the COVID-19 pandemic. *Nurse Educ. Pr.* **2020**, *49*, 102920. [CrossRef]
21. Casafont, C.; Fabrellas, N.; Rivera, P.; Olivé-Ferrer, M.C.; Querol, E.; Venturas, M.; Zabalegui, A. Experiences of nursing students as health care aid during the COVID-19 pandemic in Spain: A phemonenological research study. *Nurse Educ. Today* **2021**, *97*, 104711. [CrossRef]
22. Vargas-Terrez, B.; Villamil-Salcedo, V.; Rodríguez-Estrada, C.; Pérez-Romero, J.; Cortés-Sotres, J. Validación de la escala Kessler 10 (K -10) en la detección Kessler P propiedades psicométricas. *Salud Mental* **2011**, 323–331. [CrossRef]
23. Herrera, L.M.; Rivera, M.S. Prevalence of psychological distress in nursing students associated with sociodemographic, academic and family factors. *Ciencia y Enfermería* **2011**, 55–64. [CrossRef]
24. Regla, D.; Almirall, A. Manual para Diagnóstico y Tratamiento de Trastornos Ansiosos. *MediSur* **2012**, 466–479. Available online: http://scielo.sld.cu/pdf/ms/v10n5/ms19510.pdf (accessed on 28 October 2021).
25. Aranguren, M.; Brenlla, M.E. Estudio de la Validez Discriminante de la "Escala de Malestar Psicológico de Kessler" (Kessler Psychological Distress Scale) en Pacientes Psiquiátricos. In *I Congreso Internacional de Investigación y Práctica Profesional en Psicología XVI Jornadas de Investigación Quinto Encuentro de Investigadores en Psicología del MERCOSUR*; Facultad de Psicología—Universidad de Buenos Aires: Buenos Aires, Argentina, 2009. Available online: http://jimemorias.psi.uba.ar/index.aspx?anio=2009 (accessed on 21 October 2021).

26. Rojas-Solís, J.; Hernández-Corona, M.; García-Ramírez, B.; López Cortés, V. Burnout, malestar psicológico y satisfacción con la vida en policías durante la contingencia sanitaria por COVID-19. Un estudio exploratorio: Burnout, psychological discomfort and life satisfaction in police officers during the health contingency due to COVID-19: An exploratory study. *Arch. Med. (Manizales)* **2021**, 1–19. [CrossRef]
27. Moxham, L.J.; Fernandez, R.; Kim, B.; Lapkin, S.; Ten Ham-Baloyi, W.; Al Mutair, A. Employment as a predictor of mental health, psychological distress, anxiety and depression in Australian pre-registration nursing students. *J. Prof. Nurs.* **2018**, *34*, 502–506. [CrossRef] [PubMed]
28. Liébana-Presa, C.; Fernández-Martínez, M.E.; Gándara, Á.R.; Muñoz-Villanueva, M.C.; Vázquez-Casares, A.M.; Rodríguez-Borrego, M.A. Psychological distress in health sciences college students and its relationship with academic engagement. *Rev. Esc. Enferm.* **2014**, *48*, 715–722. [CrossRef] [PubMed]
29. Rísquez, M.I.R.; García, C.C.; De-Los-Ángeles-Sabuco-Tebar, E. Resiliencia y Síndrome de Burnout en estudiantes de enfermería y su relación con variables sociodemográficas y de relación interpersonal. *Int. J. Psychol. Res.* **2012**, 88–95. [CrossRef]
30. Ng, Q.X.; Lim, D.Y.; Chee, K.T. Reimagining the spectrum of affective disorders. *Bipolar Disord.* **2020**, *22*, 638–639. [CrossRef] [PubMed]

Journal of
Clinical Medicine

MDPI

Article

An Assessment of the Level of COVID-19 Anxiety among Pregnant Women in Poland: A Cross-Sectional Study

Kinga Janik [1,*], Urszula Cwalina [2], Grażyna Iwanowicz-Palus [3] and Mateusz Cybulski [1]

1 Department of Integrated Medical Care, Faculty of Health Sciences, Medical University of Białystok, M. Skłodowskiej-Curie 7A Str., 15-096 Białystok, Poland; mateusz.cybulski@umb.edu.pl
2 Department of Statistics and Medical Informatics, Faculty of Health Sciences, Medical University of Białystok, Szpitalna 37 Str., 15-295 Białystok, Poland; urszula.cwalina@umb.edu.pl
3 Department of Development in Midwifery, Faculty of Health Sciences, Medical University of Lublin, Staszica 4/6 Str., 20-081 Lublin, Poland; spupalus@umlub.pl
* Correspondence: kinga.janik@umb.edu.pl; Tel.: +48-(85)-748-55-28

Abstract: Introduction: The COVID-19 pandemic has caused general anxiety worldwide. Pregnant women are at a much higher risk of developing the infection due to multiple changes that occur in the body during this period. The consequences of the disease can be dramatic not only for the expectant mothers, but also for their unborn children. SARS-CoV-2 infection is generally known to cause serious concerns about future health and life. The data on the severity of COVID-19 pandemic-related anxiety in pregnant women are insufficient. The aim of the study was to assess the level of COVID-19-related anxiety among pregnant women in Poland. Materials and Methods: The study included 173 pregnant women who volunteered for the research. The research was conducted by means of an online diagnostic survey containing an original questionnaire and the following standardized tools: State-Trait Anxiety Inventory (STAI), Short Health Anxiety Inventory (SHAI), and General Anxiety Disorder-7 (GAD-7). Results: Women hospitalised during pregnancy differed statistically significantly in terms of STAI-X1 scores. Primiparas obtained statistically significantly higher SHAI scores than multiparas. Women with higher education had higher SHAI scores. In the GAD-7 scale, 13.3% of respondents obtained a score suggesting a suspected generalised anxiety disorder. Conclusions: Pregnant women are concerned about both developing COVID-19 and the consequences of infection for themselves and their unborn children. The study demonstrated anxiety of varying severity (depending on the tool used). Hospital stay during pregnancy is an additional stressor in expectant women. Further studies are needed to assess the level of COVID-19-related anxiety to assess this phenomenon in Poland in more detail.

Keywords: anxiety; COVID-19; fear; general anxiety disorder-7 (GAD-7); pregnant; SARS-CoV-2; short health anxiety inventory (SHAI); state-trait anxiety inventory (STAI)

Citation: Janik, K.; Cwalina, U.; Iwanowicz-Palus, G.; Cybulski, M. An Assessment of the Level of COVID-19 Anxiety among Pregnant Women in Poland: A Cross-Sectional Study. *J. Clin. Med.* **2021**, *10*, 5869. https://doi.org/10.3390/jcm10245869

Academic Editors: Michele Roccella and Elena Tomba

Received: 8 October 2021
Accepted: 13 December 2021
Published: 14 December 2021

1. Introduction

The current COVID-19 pandemic is considered to be an example of a natural disaster with such a heavy global health burden, from which more than 236 million people worldwide are suffering and almost 5 million people have died [1]. Poland ranks 16th among the countries with the highest number of coronavirus cases in the world, with 2,918,863 people infected and 75,834 deaths [2].

The COVID-19 pandemic has caused panic and mental health problems around the world [3]. Frequent preventive measures (e.g., washing hands, masking, social distancing, and isolation) during a pandemic obsess people, which increases the risk of psychological damage [4]. Moreover, the pandemic has caused changes in everyday life, which has increased the risk of anxiety and depression [5].

Pregnant women are more vulnerable to any effects of the COVID-19 crisis, which requires action to protect this population [6]. During a pandemic, pregnant women have limited access to primary health care services [7]. Additional factors affecting their mental health are concerns about exposure to COVID-19 and concerns about COVID-19 vaccinations [8]. The prevalence of mental disorders in pregnant women was much higher during the COVID-19 pandemic than in the pre-pandemic period [9,10]. Fear of COVID-19, anxiety, and depression were the most common mental disorders among pregnant women [11,12]. Such disorders were associated with adverse effects of pregnancy, such as preterm labor, low for gestational age, and low birth weight of the newborn [13,14].

While COVID-19 is well-known to cause considerable fear among the general population, there is a little data on the perceived anxiety related to the ongoing COVID-19 pandemic in Poland, particularly among pregnant women. Therefore, the aim of the study was to analyse and assess the symptoms of COVID-19-related anxiety among pregnant women; in particular, to evaluate trait and state anxiety along with health anxiety and generalized anxiety disorder. Additionally, we assessed the impact of selected variables on the severity of anxiety symptoms in the study group. We assumed that the severity of anxiety disorders among pregnant women in Poland would be moderate.

2. Materials and Methods

2.1. Study Design and Data Collection

The study was conducted from 5 April 2021 to 26 July 2021. The study group included volunteers. Women at various stages of pregnancy were included in the study. We placed a link to the questionnaire, created with the use of a dedicated software (Webankieta) (Get Feedback, Warsaw, Poland) on social media. There were six discussion groups for pregnant women, which gathered 373 women in total. The respondents' responses were recorded on the platform used and then downloaded as raw data for statistical analysis. The mean time to complete the questionnaire was 23 min.

In addition to female gender and pregnancy, written informed consent was an additional inclusion criterion. Participation in the anonymous study was voluntary. Each participant could withdraw from the study at any time.

There were 589 views on the platform. Considering the number of views, the level of completing the entire questionnaire was 29.33%. A total of 19 questionnaires were not fully completed.

2.2. Measures

We used our own questionnaire dedicated for this study. It contained sociodemographic questions and a set of 24 closed questions on the stressors associated with the current epidemiological situation due to SARS-CoV-2 coronavirus infections. Furthermore, we used the following standardised tools: General Anxiety Disorder-7 (GAD-7), Short Health Anxiety Inventory (SHAI), and State-Trait Anxiety Inventory (STAI).

2.2.1. State-Trait Anxiety Inventory (STAI)

The STAI scale is built of two independent subsections. Each part includes 20 items. The first part, STAI X-1, evaluates anxiety as an emotional state at the moment. The second part, STAI X-2, assesses anxiety as a personality trait [15]. The respondent chooses one of the 4 statements for each item. The sum of all the answers for each individuals determines the overall level of anxiety. The score for each subsection is between 20 and 80 points. The higher the total score, the higher the level of anxiety experienced. Suspicion of an anxiety disorders occurs when the sum of the points is 39–40 [16,17].

2.2.2. Short Health Anxiety Inventory (SHAI)

The Short Health Anxiety Inventory (SHAI) is a scale that consists of 18 items and is used to assess anxiety in two aspects: probability of the disease and the negative effects of the disease. Each of the 18 statements contains four options. Respondents choose the one that best describes their emotions over the past 6 months.

The responses are rated on a 4-point Likert scale, where: 0 indicates lack of symptoms, 1—mild symptoms, 2—severe symptoms, and 3—very severe symptoms. The cut-off point for detecting health anxiety is 20 points [18,19].

2.2.3. Generalised Anxiety Disorder Assessment (GAD-7)

The GAD-7 is a seven-point scale that is used to assess the level of anxiety and to assess the risk of developing generalized anxiety disorder (GAD). The questions included in the questionnaire concern the subjective assessment of anxiety, tension, nervousness, the ability to control emotions, the ease of their manifestation, and problems with relaxation The responses are rated on a 3-point Likert scale, where: 0 indicates not at all, 1—several days, 2—more than half the days, and 3—nearly every day. The assessment is based on the past 2 weeks. Scores 5, 10, and 15 are mild, moderate, and severe, respectively. Generalized anxiety disorder is likely if the sum of the points is at least 10 [20].

2.3. Procedure and Ethical Considerations

The study was conducted in accordance with the recommendations, and was reviewed and approved by the Ethics Committee of the Medical University of Bialystok (No. APK.002.248.2021). All participants gave a written informed consent in accordance with the Declaration of Helsinki.

2.4. Statistical Analysis

Statistica 13.3 (StatSoft Company, Hamburg, Germany) was used for statistical analysis. The analysed variables were of dichotomous, interval, or ordinal nature. The chi-square test was used for dichotomous variables, and basic descriptive statistics for interval results. We used the Mann–Whitney U test to determine statistical significance. The level of statistical significance was set at $p < 0.05$ for each test.

3. Results

A total of 173 women participated in the study, which accounted for 49% of women who completed the questionnaire. Detailed sociodemographic characteristics of study participants are presented in Table 1.

The respondents were asked if they were concerned about contracting COVID-19 during pregnancy. It was found that infection with COVID-19 during pregnancy had a significant impact on the answer to this question. Fear of contracting COVID-19 was reported by 30.77% of women with a history of infection and over 50% of women in the group with no such history.

Table 2 summarizes the descriptive statistics of the standardised tools used in the study. A detailed analysis of GAD-7 results showed that the total score indicated anxiety symptoms of varying severity in 71% of respondents. A total of 23 (13.3%) respondents scored at least 10 points, which suggests a suspected generalised anxiety disorder. The mean score obtained by respondents was 13.29 for the SHAI scale. In the GAD-7 scale, most respondents scored between 5 and 9 points. The mean scores obtained in STAI-XI and STAI-X2 were similar, i.e., 42.26 and 40.24, respectively. Details are shown in Table 2.

Table 1. Sociodemographic characteristics of respondents.

Sociodemographic Feature		*n*	%
Age (years)	<25	15	8.67%
	25–34	132	76.30%
	≥35	26	15.03%
Education	middle school	1	0.58%
	basic vocational	13	7.51%
	secondary	46	26.59%
	higher	113	65.32%
Marital status	married	150	86.70%
	divorced	3	1.73%
	single	15	8.67%
	unmarried relationship	5	2.89%
Place of residence	urban	139	80.35%
	rural	34	19.65%
Socioeconomic status	very good	39	22.54%
	good	111	64.16%
	moderate	23	13.30%
	poor	0	0.00%
Number of children	0	83	47.98%
	1	65	37.57%
	2	17	9.83%
	3	6	3.47%
	4	1	0.58%
	5	1	0.58%
Parity	primipara	83	47.98%
	multipara	90	52.02%
Trimester	I (1–13 weeks)	16	9.25%
	II (14–26 weeks)	25	14.45%
	III (27–40 weeks)	132	76.30%
History of mental disorders	yes	9	5.20%
	no	164	94.80%
History of psychotropic therapy	yes	10	5.78%
	no	163	94.22%
History of the prevalence of COVID-19	yes	26	15.03%
	no	147	84.97%

Table 2. Summary of descriptive statistics of the standardised research tools.

	M	SD	Q_1	Me	Q_3	Min.	Max.
SHAI	13.29	6.17	9	13	17	2	40
GAD-7	5.79	3.90	3	5	7	0	21
STAI-X1	42.26	11.20	34	41	50	22	74
STAI-X2	40.25	8.50	34	40	45	23	69

Abbreviations: GAD-7—General Anxiety Disorder-7, M—mean, Max.—maximum, Me—median, Min.—minimum, SD—standard deviation, SHAI—Short Health Anxiety Inventory, STAI—State-Trait Anxiety Inventory, Q_1—lower quartile, and Q_3—upper quartile.

Primiparas were found to have statistically significantly ($p = 0.031$) higher SHAI scores (M = 14.45, Me = 14) compared to multiparas (M = 12.22, Me = 12). Primiparas were significantly younger. Both study groups were also compared for the following scales: GAD-7 and both STAI subscales. No statistically significant differences were found for these tools (Table 3).

Table 3. Comparison of primiparas and multiparas for SHAI, GAD-7, and STAI.

Tools	Primiparas (n = 83)					Multiparas (n = 90)					p
	M	SD	Q_1	Me	Q_3	M	SD	Q_1	Me	Q_3	
SHAI	14.45	6.81	10	14	18	12.22	5.35	9	12	16	0.031
GAD-7	6.45	4.27	4	6	8	5.19	3.43	3	5	7	0.066
STAI-X1	43.49	12.01	35	41	53	41.12	10.33	33	41	47	0.218
STAI-X2	40.35	8.24	34	41	46	40.16	8.78	34	40	44	0.753

Abbreviations: GAD-7—General Anxiety Disorder-7, M—mean, Me—median, p—p-value, SD—standard deviation, SHAI—Short Health Anxiety Inventory, STAI—State-Trait Anxiety Inventory, Q_1—lower quartile, and Q_3—upper quartile.

The analysis has shown that women with higher education scored statistically significantly higher in SHAI ($p = 0.019$, M = 14.17, Me = 13) and GAD-7 ($p = 0.006$, M = 6.31, Me = 6). No statistically significant results were found for the other scales (Table 4).

Table 4. Comparison of women with and without higher education for the following tools: SHAI, GAD-7, and STAI.

Tools	Higher Education (n = 113)					No Higher Education (n = 60)					p
	M	SD	Q_1	Me	Q_3	M	SD	Q_1	Me	Q_3	
SHAI	14.17	6.15	10	13	18	11.63	5.93	7.5	12	15.5	0.019 *
GAD-7	6.31	3.96	4	6	8	4.82	3.62	2	4	7	0.006 *
STAI-X1	41.87	11.19	34	40	48	43	11.27	37	41	52	0.369
STAI-X2	40.21	8.75	33	40	44	40.32	8.08	35.5	40	45.5	0.777

Abbreviations: GAD-7—General Anxiety Disorder-7, M—mean, Me—median, p—p-value, SD—standard deviation, SHAI—Short Health Anxiety Inventory, STAI—State-Trait Anxiety Inventory, Q_1—lower quartile, Q_3—upper quartile, and *—statistically significant.

Hospitalised pregnant women scored significantly higher in STAI-X1. No statistically significant differences were found between pregnant women hospitalised during pregnancy and those not requiring hospitalisation in the remaining scales (Table 5).

Table 5. The impact of hospital stays during pregnancy on the rating of anxiety.

Tools	Hospitalised during Pregnancy (n = 93)					Not Hospitalised during Pregnancy (n = 80)					p
	M	SD	Q_1	Me	Q_3	M	SD	Q_1	Me	Q_3	
SHAI	12.77	5.52	10	12	15	13.88	6.84	8.5	13.5	18	0.215
GAD-7	5.76	3.91	3	6	7	5.82	3.90	3	5	7	0.951
STAI-X1	44.14	11.55	37	41	52	40.07	10.42	32	39	46.5	0.019 *
STAI-X2	39.55	8.02	34	40	44	41.06	9.01	34.5	40	45	0.459

Abbreviations: GAD-7—General Anxiety Disorder-7, M—mean, Me—median, p—p-value, SD—standard deviation, SHAI—Short Health Anxiety Inventory, STAI—State-Trait Anxiety Inventory, Q_1—lower quartile, Q_3—upper quartile, and *—statistically significant.

4. Discussion

So far, it has been established that the outbreak of the pandemic increased the level of mental health disorders in the general population [21,22], and it is more visible in women than in men. Some studies report that during catastrophes or major events, pregnant women are more likely to develop mental health problems than in the general population [23,24]. A recent systematic review and meta-analysis [25] assessing the impact of the pandemic on the mental health of pregnant women has shown that the level of mental health disorders in pregnant women is 37%. Our study showed that women who had

COVID-19 had lower levels of fear of infection with the SARS-CoV-2 than pregnant women who had not contracted the disease so far. Different results were obtained in another Polish study by Nowak et al. [26]. The authors proved that pregnant women who had been infected with SARS-CoV-2 experienced a higher level of anxiety than those who had not been infected so far.

Our study showed moderate anxiety among pregnant women in the STAI scale. Another study among pregnant women also assessed the level of antenatal anxiety using the STAI scale. Similar findings were obtained in both studies [27]. Similar results in the same scale were also shown in a study in Italy [28]. These findings confirm the conclusions obtained by Sinjari et al. [29], that questionnaires could be useful tools to assess patients' conditions before the visit to a doctor.

Considering the parity of respondents, we found that primiparas show higher COVID-19-related anxiety than multiparous women, as confirmed by SHAI scores. STAI results reported by Italian researchers also confirmed our hypothesis [28]. Such findings may be due to both the new life situation and the lack of knowledge about pregnancy and coronavirus infection during this special time.

The data on the impact of gestational age on the level of COVID-19-related anxiety among pregnant women are contradictory. In our analysis, we compared the scores obtained in the standardized scales depending on the trimester of pregnancy, but no statistically significant differences were found. Other authors reported higher STAI scores in the first and third trimesters than those obtained in our study [30]. Schubert et al. showed that, on the other hand, STAI scores remained stable throughout pregnancy [31].

We measured the prevalence of anxiety symptoms using the GAD-7 scale. It was found to be high, i.e., 62.5% among pregnant women, including 49% with mild, 10% with moderately severe, and 3.5% with severe anxiety due to COVID-19. Other studies have also shown that pregnant women are much more prone to stress during the COVID-19 pandemic [32].

Our analysis showed that pregnant women with higher education were significantly older and scored statistically significantly higher in both SHAI and GAD-7. Similar findings on the impact of higher education on the increased levels of anxiety have been reported by other authors [32]. It can be assumed that greater awareness of one's own health negatively affects its loss as a result of a serious illness. The differences in the obtained results can be due to the dynamic nature of the disease and the fact that it is perceived differently around the world.

In this study, the median STAI score for anxiety was 41. A total of 57.23% of the pregnant women scored $\geq$40. In a similar study involving pregnant women, the median score in the same scale was 37, including a score of $\geq$40 in 38.2% of participants [33]. Another study among pregnant women showed that the overall prevalence of anxiety symptoms measured with STAI (STAI > 40) was 62.6% [34]. An Italian study found similar levels of COVID-19-related anxiety in pregnant women (68%) [30]. Turkish studies also reported STAI scores above the cut-off for clinically significant symptoms of anxiety [35]. Similar findings in all the above-mentioned studies may be due to the different state of the women (pregnancy) and their concern about the health of their unborn children.

The presented results confirm COVID-19-related anxiety among pregnant women. Its level varies and is related to sociodemographic factors. Due to the negative effects of anxiety and stress on pregnant women and their unborn children, further research is needed on anxiety caused by the COVID-19 pandemic to prevent negative effects and improve the health of the population. Mental health screening for pregnant women should be included in the mandatory prenatal screening to reduce any potential anxiety symptoms.

Limitations of the Study

The study has certain limitations. The presented results come from an analysis based on a subjective assessment of anxiety symptoms in pregnant women. Although we used scales that are considered sensitive research tools, they are based on subjective feelings and do not include objective criteria of clinical symptoms, which may lead to false-positive results. The number of pregnant women participating in the study is another limitation. The small sample size does not allow for extrapolation of results to the general population of pregnant women in Poland. However, despite these limitations, our findings can be a reference point for further studies assessing the level of COVID-19-related anxiety among pregnant women both in Poland and in the world.

5. Conclusions

In conclusions, primiparas showed statistically significantly higher anxiety levels than multiparas. Higher education also contributed to higher scores. Hospital stays during pregnancy contributed to statistically higher STAI-X1 scores. There was no statistically significant relationship between pregnancy trimester and the prevalence of COVID-19. There is a need to continue research on COVID-19-related anxiety among pregnant women in Poland to assess this phenomenon and the causative factors in more detail.

The COVID-19 pandemic has serious consequences. Therefore, in the periods of health crisis, it is imperative to develop research focused on studying the phenomenon and its impact with other variables in order to understand its impact on pregnant women. This can help prevent and address negative mental health effects that can affect the functional status and quality of life of pregnant women.

Author Contributions: Conceptualization, K.J., G.I.-P. and M.C.; data curation, K.J.; formal analysis, K.J. and U.C.; funding acquisition, K.J.; investigation, K.J. and M.C.; methodology, K.J., U.C., G.I.-P. and M.C.; project administration, K.J.; supervision, M.C.; writing—original draft, K.J. and U.C.; and writing—review and editing, M.C. and G.I-P. All authors have read and agreed to the published version of the manuscript.

Funding: The research was financed by the funds from the Medical University of Białystok with a grant no. SUB/3/DN/21/008/3310 awarded by the Polish Ministry of Education and Science in the form of a subvention for maintaining and developing research potential in 2021. The APC was funded by Medical University of Białystok.

Institutional Review Board Statement: The study was conducted according to the guidelines of the Declaration of Helsinki, and approved by the Ethics Committee of the Medical University of Białystok, Poland (No. APK.002.248.2021).

Informed Consent Statement: Informed consent was obtained from all the subjects involved in the study.

Data Availability Statement: Data are available upon reasonable request.

Acknowledgments: The authors thank all respondents who participated in the study.

Conflicts of Interest: The authors declare no conflict of interest. The funders had no role in the design of the study; in the collection, analyses, or interpretation of data; in the writing of the manuscript, or in the decision to publish the results.

References

1. COVID-19 Dashboard by the Center for Systems Science and Engineering (CSSE) at Johns Hopkins University (JHU). Available online: https://gisanddata.maps.arcgis.com/apps/dashboards/bda7594740fd40299423467b48e9ecf6 (accessed on 8 October 2021).
2. Ministerstwo Zdrowia: Mapa Zarażeń Koronawirusem (SARS-CoV-2). Available online: https://www.gov.pl/web/koronawirus/wykaz-zarazen-koronawirusem-sars-cov-2 (accessed on 8 October 2021).
3. COVID-19 Mental Disorders Collaborators. Global prevalence and burden of depressive and anxiety disorders in 204 countries and territories in 2020 due to the COVID-19 pandemic. *Lancet* **2021**, *398*, 1700–1712. [CrossRef]
4. Brooks, S.K.; Webster, R.K.; Smith, L.E.; Woodland, L.; Wessely, S.; Greenberg, N.; Rubin, G.J. The psychological impact of quarantine and how to reduce it: Rapid review of the evidence. *Lancet* **2020**, *395*, 912–920. [CrossRef]
5. Witteveen, D.; Velthorst, E. Economic hardship and mental health complaints during COVID-19. *Proc. Natl. Acad. Sci. USA* **2020**, *117*, 27277–27284. [CrossRef] [PubMed]
6. Buekens, P.; Alger, J.; Bréart, G.; Cafferata, M.L.; Harville, E.; Tomasso, G. A call for action for COVID-19 surveillance and research during pregnancy. *Lancet Glob. Health* **2020**, *8*, e877–e878. [CrossRef]

7. Luong, T.C.; Pham, T.T.M.; Nguyen, M.H.; Do, A.Q.; Pham, L.V.; Nguyen, H.C.; Nguyen, H.C.; Ha, T.H.; Dao, H.K.; Trinh, M.V.; et al. Fear, anxiety and depression among pregnant women during COVID-19 pandemic: Impacts of healthy eating behaviour and health literacy. *Ann. Med.* **2021**, *53*, 2120–2131. [CrossRef] [PubMed]
8. Rashidi Fakari, F.; Simbar, M. Coronavirus Pandemic and Worries during Pregnancy; a Letter to Editor. *Arch. Acad. Emerg. Med.* **2020**, *8*, e21.
9. Ayaz, R.; Hocaoğlu, M.; Günay, T.; Yardımcı, O.D.; Turgut, A.; Karateke, A. Anxiety and depression symptoms in the same pregnant women before and during the COVID-19 pandemic. *J. Perinat. Med.* **2020**, *48*, 965–970. [CrossRef] [PubMed]
10. Berthelot, N.; Lemieux, R.; Garon-Bissonnette, J.; Drouin-Maziade, C.; Martel, É.; Maziade, M. Uptrend in distress and psychiatric symptomatology in pregnant women during the coronavirus disease 2019 pandemic. *Acta Obstet. Gynecol. Scand.* **2020**, *99*, 848–855. [CrossRef]
11. López-Morales, H.; Del Valle, M.V.; Canet-Juric, L.; Andrés, M.L.; Galli, J.I.; Poó, F.; Urquijo, S. Mental health of pregnant women during the COVID-19 pandemic: A longitudinal study. *Psychiatry Res.* **2021**, *295*, 113567. [CrossRef]
12. Ravaldi, C.; Wilson, A.; Ricca, V.; Homer, C.; Vannacci, A. Pregnant women voice their concerns and birth expectations during the COVID-19 pandemic in Italy. *Women Birth* **2021**, *34*, 335–343. [CrossRef]
13. Eastwood, J.; Ogbo, F.A.; Hendry, A.; Noble, J.; Page, A.; Early Years Research Group (EYRG). The Impact of Antenatal Depression on Perinatal Outcomes in Australian Women. *PLoS ONE* **2017**, *12*, e0169907. [CrossRef]
14. Sūdžiūtė, K.; Murauskienė, G.; Jarienė, K.; Jaras, A.; Minkauskienė, M.; Adomaitienė, V.; Nedzelskienė, I. Pre-existingmental health disorders affect pregnancy and neonatal outcomes: A retrospective cohort study. *BMC Pregnancy Childbirth* **2020**, *20*, 419. [CrossRef]
15. Wrześniewski, K.; Sosnowski, T.; Matusik, D. *Inwentarz Stanu i Cechy Leku STAI. Polska Adaptacja STAI*; Pracownia Testów Psychologicznych Polskiego Towarzystwa Psychologicznego: Warsaw, Poland, 2002.
16. Knight, R.G.; Waal-Manning, H.J.; Spears, G.F. Some norms and reliability data for the State-Trait Anxiety Inventory and the Zung Self-Rating Depression scale. *Br. J. Clin. Psychol.* **1983**, *22*, 245–249. [CrossRef]
17. Addolorato, G.; Ancona, C.; Capristo, E.; Graziosetto, R.; Di Rienzo, L.; Maurizi, M.; Gasbarrini, G. State and trait anxiety in women affected by allergic and vasomotor rhinitis. *J. Psychosom. Res.* **1999**, *46*, 283–289. [CrossRef]
18. Kocjan, J. Short Health Anxiety Inventory (SHAI)-Polish version: Evaluation of psychometric properties and factor structure. *Arch. Psychiatry Psychother.* **2016**, *18*, 68–78. [CrossRef]
19. Abramowitz, J.S.; Deacon, B.J.; Valentiner, D.P. The Short Health Anxiety Inventory: Psychometric Properties and Construct Validity in a Non-clinical Sample. *Cognit. Ther. Res.* **2007**, *31*, 871–883. [CrossRef]
20. Spitzer, R.L.; Kroenke, K.; Williams, J.B.; Löwe, B. A brief measure for assessing generalized anxiety disorder: The GAD-7. *Arch. Intern. Med.* **2006**, *166*, 1092–1097. [CrossRef]
21. Wu, Y.; Zhang, C.; Liu, H.; Duan, C.; Li, C.; Fan, J.; Li, H.; Chen, L.; Xu, H.; Li, X. Perinatal depressive and anxiety symptoms of pregnant women during the coronavirus disease 2019 outbreak in China. *Am. J. Obstet. Gynecol.* **2020**, *223*, 240.e1–240.e9. [CrossRef]
22. Banks, J.; Xu, X. The Mental Health Effects of the First Two Months of Lockdown during the COVID-19 Pandemic in the UK. *Fisc. Stud.* **2020**, *41*, 685–708. [CrossRef]
23. Vesga-López, O.; Blanco, C.; Keyes, K.; Olfson, M.; Grant, B.F.; Hasin, D.S. Psychiatric disorders in pregnant and postpartum women in the United States. *Arch. Gen. Psychiatry* **2008**, *65*, 805–815. [CrossRef]
24. Harville, E.; Xiong, X.; Buekens, P. Disasters and perinatal health: A systematic review. *Obstet. Gynecol. Surv.* **2010**, *65*, 713–728. [CrossRef] [PubMed]
25. Yan, H.; Ding, Y.; Guo, W. Mental Health of Pregnant and Postpartum Women during the Coronavirus Disease 2019 Pandemic: A Systematic Review and Meta-Analysis. *Front. Psychol.* **2020**, *11*, 617001. [CrossRef] [PubMed]
26. Nowacka, U.; Kozlowski, S.; Januszewski, M.; Sierdzinski, J.; Jakimiuk, A.; Issat, T. COVID-19 Pandemic-Related Anxiety in Pregnant Women. *Int. J. Environ. Res. Public Health* **2021**, *18*, 7221. [CrossRef] [PubMed]
27. Bączyk, G.; Cebulska, V.; Kuźlak, V.; Michalak, M.; Bajek, A.; Marcinkowski, J.T. Anxiety levels of pregnant women in pre-delivery period. *Probl. Hig. Epidemiol.* **2011**, *92*, 774–777.
28. Mappa, I.; Distefano, F.A.; Rizzo, G. Effects of coronavirus 19 pandemic on maternal anxiety during pregnancy: A prospectic observational study. *J. Perinat. Med.* **2020**, *48*, 545–550. [CrossRef]
29. Sinjari, B.; Rexhepi, I.; Santilli, M.; D'Addazio, G.; Chiacchiaretta, P.; Di Carlo, P.; Caputi, S. The Impact of COVID-19 Related Lockdown on Dental Practice in Central Italy—Outcomes of A Survey. *Int. J. Environ. Res. Public Health* **2020**, *17*, 5780. [CrossRef]
30. Da Costa, D.; Larouche, J.; Dritsa, M.; Brender, W. Variations in stress levels over the course of pregnancy: Factors associated with elevated hassles, state anxiety and pregnancy-specific stress. *J. Psychosom. Res.* **1999**, *4*, 609–621. [CrossRef]
31. Schubert, K.O.; Air, T.; Clark, S.R.; Grzeskowiak, L.E.; Miller, E.; Dekker, G.A.; Baune, B.T.; Clifton, V.L. Trajectories of anxiety and health related quality of life during pregnancy. *PLoS ONE* **2017**, *12*, e0181149. [CrossRef]
32. Qiu, J.; Shen, B.; Zhao, M.; Wang, Z.; Xie, B.; Xu, Y. A nationwide survey of psychological distress among Chinese people in the COVID-19 epidemic: Implications and policy recommendations. *Gen. Psychiatry* **2020**, *33*, e100213. [CrossRef]
33. Yassa, M.; Yassa, A.; Yirmibeş, C.; Birol, P.; Ünlü, U.; Tekin, A.; Sandal, K.; Mutlu, M.; Çavuşoğlu, G.; Tug, N. Anxiety levels and obsessive compulsion symptoms of pregnant women during the COVID-19 pandemic. *Turk. J. Obstet. Gynecol.* **2020**, *17*, 155–160. [CrossRef]

34. Saccone, G.; Florio, A.; Aiello, F.; Venturella, R.; De Angelis, M.C.; Locci, M.; Bifulco, G.; Zullo, F.; Di Spiezio Sardo, A. Psychological impact of coronavirus disease 2019 in pregnant women. *Am. J. Obstet. Gynecol.* **2020**, *223*, 293–295. [CrossRef]
35. Hocaoglu, M.; Ayaz, R.; Gunay, T.; Akin, E.; Turgut, A.; Karateke, A. Anxiety and Post-Traumatic Stress Disorder Symptoms in Pregnant Women during the COVID-19 Pandemic's Delay Phase. *Psychiatr. Danub.* **2020**, *32*, 521–526. [CrossRef]

Journal of
Clinical Medicine

MDPI

Correction

Correction: Rogowska et al. Changes in Stress, Coping Styles, and Life Satisfaction between the First and Second Waves of the COVID-19 Pandemic: A Longitudinal Cross-Lagged Study in a Sample of University Students. *J. Clin. Med.* 2021, *10*, 4025

Aleksandra Maria Rogowska [1,*], Cezary Kuśnierz [2] and Dominika Ochnik [3]

[1] Institute of Psychology, Faculty of Social Sciences, University of Opole, 45-052 Opole, Poland
[2] Faculty of Physical Education and Physiotherapy, Opole University of Technology, 45-758 Opole, Poland; c.kusnierz@po.edu.pl
[3] Faculty of Medicine, University of Technology, 40-555 Katowice, Poland; dominika.ochnik@wst.pl
* Correspondence: arogowska@uni.opole.pl

Citation: Rogowska, A.M.; Kuśnierz, C.; Ochnik, D. Correction: Rogowska et al. Changes in Stress, Coping Styles, and Life Satisfaction between the First and Second Waves of the COVID-19 Pandemic: A Longitudinal Cross-Lagged Study in a Sample of University Students. *J. Clin. Med.* 2021, *10*, 4025. *J. Clin. Med.* **2022**, *11*, 276. https://doi.org/10.3390/jcm11010276

Received: 5 November 2021
Accepted: 19 November 2021
Published: 5 January 2022

The authors wish to make the following corrections to this paper [1]:

1. Change in Abstract

The sentence "The task-oriented and avoidance-oriented coping styles can play a mediating role in the reciprocal relationship between life satisfaction and perceived stress during W1 and W2 of the pandemic" is changed into "The task-oriented and emotion-oriented coping styles can play a mediating role in the reciprocal relationship between life satisfaction and perceived stress during W1 and W2 of the pandemic".

2. Change in Main Body Paragraph

In the Discussion section (8th paragraph), the following sentence "Avoidance-oriented coping was not found to be a significant predictor of stress. Therefore, this coping style plays a mediating role in the relationship between life satisfaction and stress." is modified into "Avoidance-oriented coping was not found to be a significant predictor of stress. Therefore, this coping style cannot play a mediating role in the relationship between life satisfaction and stress".

The authors apologize for any inconvenience caused and state that the scientific conclusions are unaffected. The original article has been updated.

Reference

1. Rogowska, A.M.; Kuśnierz, C.; Ochnik, D. Changes in Stress, Coping Styles, and Life Satisfaction between the First and Second Waves of the COVID-19 Pandemic: A Longitudinal Cross-Lagged Study in a Sample of University Students. *J. Clin. Med.* **2021**, *10*, 4025. [CrossRef] [PubMed]

Journal of
Clinical Medicine

MDPI

Article

Psychological Flexibility Mediates Wellbeing for People with Adverse Childhood Experiences during COVID-19

Angela Browne [1], Owen Stafford [1], Anna Berry [1,2], Eddie Murphy [1,2], Laura K. Taylor [1,3], Mark Shevlin [4], Louise McHugh [1], Alan Carr [1] and Tom Burke [1,5,*]

[1] School of Psychology, University College Dublin, D04 V1W8 Dublin, Ireland; angela.browne1@ucdconnect.ie (A.B.); owenstafford@ucd.ie (O.S.); annanibheara@gmail.com (A.B.); eddie.murphy2@hse.ie (E.M.); laura.taylor@ucd.ie (L.K.T.); louise.mchugh@ucd.ie (L.M.); alan.carr@ucd.ie (A.C.)
[2] Health Service Executive, CHO 8 (Laois/Offaly), R32 YFW6 Laois, Ireland
[3] School of Psychology, Queen's University Belfast, Belfast BT7 1NN, UK
[4] School of Psychology, University of Ulster, Belfast BT1 6DN, UK; m.shevlin@ulster.ac.uk
[5] School of Psychology, National University of Ireland, H91 CF50 Galway, Ireland
* Correspondence: tom.m.burke@ucd.ie

Abstract: Background: The psychological impact of COVID-19 is multifaceted, both acute and chronic, and has not affected everyone equally. Method: This longitudinal study compared those with and without Adverse Childhood Experiences (ACEs) on measures of psychological distress and wellbeing over time. Results: All groups (No ACE, Low ACE, and High ACE) had similar levels of distress at Time 1, with significant increases in psychological distress for those with ACEs over time, but not for those without. Psychological Flexibility was strongly and significantly associated with decreases in psychological distress and improved wellbeing. It significantly mediated the relationship between ACE and wellbeing. Conclusions: Those with ACEs report significantly increased psychological distress over time, compared to those without ACE during the COVID-19 pandemic. Evidence-based interventions using Psychological Flexibility may improve mental health and wellbeing to help further mediate its effects.

Keywords: COVID-19; pandemic; adverse childhood experiences; ACEs; psychological flexibility; wellbeing; mental health; psychological distress; Ireland

Citation: Browne, A.; Stafford, O.; Berry, A.; Murphy, E.; Taylor, L.K.; Shevlin, M.; McHugh, L.; Carr, A.; Burke, T. Psychological Flexibility Mediates Wellbeing for People with Adverse Childhood Experiences during COVID-19. *J. Clin. Med.* **2022**, *11*, 377. https://doi.org/10.3390/jcm11020377

Academic Editor: Michele Roccella

Received: 20 November 2021
Accepted: 10 January 2022
Published: 13 January 2022

1. Introduction

Since the World Health Organisation (WHO) declared a global pandemic on the 11th of March 2020, due to the rapid spread of a novel virulent strain of coronavirus (COVID-19), there have been 228.18 million recorded confirmed cases worldwide and 4.69 million COVID-19 related deaths as of the 18th of September 2021. To contextualize this within the context of other 21st century infectious diseases, the Severe Acute Respiratory System (SARS) pandemic of 2002/2003 infected 8098 people worldwide, of which 774 died, while an estimated 123,000–203,000 people died worldwide due to Swine flu (H1N1 Influenza) in 2009/2010. Only the Spanish flu over a hundred years earlier (1918) is comparable in terms of deaths and numbers infected.

Since the pandemic began, Ireland, like many other countries, has engaged in both national and regional stepped restrictions to limit the spread of the virus [1–3]. While these measures were deemed necessary for public health and safety, research from previous pandemics and evolving research from the present pandemic has highlighted the adverse psychological and physical effects such actions can have, in the acute phase and the longer term, for both those infected and those who did not contract the virus [4–8].

The consensus within the literature to date suggests social distancing and other imposed measures of social distancing are strongly associated with depression, anxiety and stress, psychotic symptoms, e.g., paranoia and hallucinations, and reduced subjective wellbeing [9–17]. By way of example, Hyland et al. [18] found that more than one in four (27.7%) people surveyed during lockdown measures in Ireland screened positive for Generalized Anxiety Disorder or Depression. For some, the uncertainty and fear perpetuated by living for a prolonged period alongside a deadly virus, in addition to living with increased psychological stressors (i.e., unemployment; lack of childcare, working from home) and reduced availability of routine coping mechanisms (i.e., social support; work) can cause chronic stress and consequently negatively influence mental health and wellbeing [1,5,19]. However, the new-onset acute and chronic stressors associated with COVID-19 do not impact all individuals equally [7,20–23]. The stress sensitization hypothesis [24] posits that adversities in early childhood sensitize individuals to subsequent proximal stress and increases the risk for psychopathology in the face of future stressful life events. As such, one such population that is likely to be vulnerable to the stressors associated with COVID-19 are individuals who have experienced Adverse Childhood Experiences (ACEs) [25–27].

ACEs can be broadly defined as adverse traumatic experiences which occur during the first eighteen years of life, and are usually categorized into physical and sexual abuse/neglect, emotional abuse/neglect, and household dysfunction [28]. While the effect of these adversities on an individual is multifaceted, research suggests a strong graded relationship between the number of ACEs experienced, and lifelong physical and psychological ill-health [28–31]. Examples of ACEs include sexual, emotional, and physical abuse, neglect, parental mental illness, substance abuse, parental separation, and criminal behaviour; all of which can be reported through the Adverse Childhood Experiences questionnaire [28].

Early research has indicated that those who experienced ACEs are more vulnerable to both the direct and indirect effects of COVID-19, than those without [26,27,32–39]. In addition, those with several ACEs (i.e., $\geq$4) are more likely than individuals without ACEs to have existing mental health difficulties, chronic physical ill-health, and are disproportionately from lower socioeconomic backgrounds [21,25,28,40–43]. Based on the stress sensitization hypothesis, COVID-19 is an additional major stressor to individuals with an already heightened liability to physical and psychological difficulties [26,44], with comorbid medical conditions shown to relate to elevated psychological distress, notwithstanding ACEs [14,21,23,45].

There is recent research on mitigating the effects of COVID-19 and improving mental health and wellbeing. Interventions that promote Psychological Flexibility, such as Acceptance and Commitment Therapy (ACT) and Mindfulness are shown to be effective [19,46–48], and also mitigate the effects of ACEs [49,50]. Psychological Flexibility, the ability to adapt to situations by accepting and fully experiencing all thoughts and feelings and engaging in value-based behaviour, aims to promote positive mental health and wellbeing and reduces psychological distress [51]. Conversely, a lack of Psychological Flexibility can be present alongside psychological processes such as rumination in depression, avoidance in anxiety, and other alternations in executive functioning in neurodevelopmental disorders such as schizophrenia [14,52–54]. What is less known is to what extent does Psychological Flexibility mediate the relationship between ACEs and psychological distress secondary to COVID-19.

Much of the research to date on mental health and wellbeing concerned with COVID-19 have used cross-sectional data [10]. While this is important, the lasting impact and chronicity of stress experienced, especially when considering vulnerable populations, requires longitudinal investigations. By understanding the immediate and longer-term psychological impact of COVID-19, services could better direct and understand responses following the immediacy of the pandemic. Research by Holmes et al. [55] has proposed that investigations into the effects of COVID-19 on these vulnerable groups should be an immediate priority.

This study aims to examine the effect of prolonged stress on an Irish cohort's mental health and wellbeing during over a 10-month period and is specifically interested in the response profile and reported stress of people who have experienced ACEs. This study hypothesized that the reported psychological stressors resulting from COVID-19 will increase over time for those with ACEs, relative to the control population, based on the stress sensitisation hypothesis [24,44]. Consequently, it was hypothesized that those with no ACEs will have significantly lower stress at Time 2 when compared to those with ACEs. Finally, this study aims to investigate whether self-reported Psychological Flexibility is a protective factor that can help mitigate the negative impacts of ACEs and psychological distress on wellbeing over time, due to the known positive relationship between psychological wellbeing and psychological flexibility [46–50].

2. Materials and Methods

2.1. Participants

This study employed a longitudinal prospective follow-up survey design. Participants were recruited through national media outlets, social media, and professional networking websites in Ireland, during the first period of public 'Level 5 Lockdown' in Ireland (27 March to 8 June 2020), to assess the psychological impact of COVID-19 [9]. Participants were asked to follow a link to access the study information sheet, consent, and questions via Qualtrics. Once consent was obtained, participants completed the outcome measures. This study received approval from the host research ethics committee.

Of the cohort who completed the cross-sectional aspect of this study, $n = 450$ participants consented to be contacted prospectively via email for follow-up and $n = 231$ provided contact details for follow-up. These data were collected during a repeated 'Level 5 Lockdown' in Ireland (January 2021), with the same government restrictions in place as when original data was collected. The inclusion criteria for the study were being over the age of 18 and living in Ireland. The final sample consisted of N = 231 (88% female), consistent with the gender distribution of the original cross-sectional study [9,23], with participants aged between 20 and 76 years. Approximately 54% of participants earned within €25,000–74,999, with 85% having completed a university degree. 50% of sample were married, 35% in committed relationships, 9% were engaged, and 6% single. Overall, 41% of the sample had children.

2.2. Measures

Six questionnaires were used in this study, with four administered across both time-points, i.e., the Depression, Anxiety and Stress Scale (DASS-21, [56]); Warwick-Edinburgh Mental Wellbeing Scale (WEMWBS, [57]); Brief Illness Perception Questionnaire (BIPQ, [58]); and the Effects of COVID-19 Questionnaire (ECQ, [9]). Two questionnaires were included at the follow-up assessment—The Adverse Childhood Experiences (ACEs) Questionnaire [28] and the PsyFlex [59].

2.2.1. Depression, Anxiety, and Stress

The Depression, Anxiety and Stress Scale-21 (DASS-21) comprises of three subscales, with each subscale measuring self-reported depression, anxiety, and stress. Each subscale contains seven items, with a 4-point Likert scale (0–3) and Depression, Anxiety and Stress scores are calculated by summing with possible scores ranging from 0 to 21. A recent systematic review indicated acceptable psychometric properties of the DASS-21 scores [60]. Cronbach's alpha values of 0.81 and 0.89 are report for the Depression and Anxiety subscales, respectively. The alpha value for the Stress subscale was observed at 0.78, which is considered "fair" [61].

2.2.2. Mental Wellbeing

The Warwick-Edinburgh Mental Wellbeing Scale (WEMWS) is a 14-item measure covering both hedonic and eudaimonic facets of mental health. The positively worded items capture various concepts of wellbeing, including positive affect, psychological functioning, and interpersonal relationships. The scale uses a 5-point Likert scale (1–5) producing possible scores ranging from 14 to 70, with higher scores indicative of greater wellbeing.

Stewart-Brown et al. [62] reported sound psychometric properties for the WEMWS in diverse populations; the reliability of the WEMWBS is noted to be "good" within a student sample, with an observed Cronbach's alpha of 0.89 [61].

2.2.3. Illness Perception

The Brief Illness Perception Questionnaire is a seven-item scale designed to assess both the emotional and cognitive representation of illness, adapted for use with COVID-19 [9,23]. The items are responded to on a 11-point scale (0–10) producing possible scores ranging from 0 to 70, with higher scores indicative of greater levels of perceived illness. Broadbent, Petrie, Main, and Weinman (2006) reported acceptable levels of reliability and validity [58], with a "good" Cronbach's alpha value of 0.85 reported [61].

2.2.4. COVID-19 Specific Stress

The Effects of COVID-19 Questionnaire is a 34-item tool designed to measure individuals' perception of COVID-19 related stresses and associated gratitude. This measure contains four subscales: Personal Stress (items 1–13), Parenting Stress (items 14–21), Older Aging Parent Stress (22–25), and Gratitude (26–34), in which respondents must choose from five response options. Within the ECQ subscales, the ranges for Personal Distress are: Normal 0–12; Mild 13–19; Moderate 20–26; Severe 27–33; Extremely Severe ≥34. Burke et al. [9] reported satisfactory levels of reliability for this scale with a Cronbach's alpha of 0.79 for the Personal Distress subscale.

2.2.5. Adverse Childhood Experiences

The Adverse Childhood Experiences (ACEs) Questionnaire is a 10-item self-report scale used to measure childhood trauma. Each question asks about experiences growing up during the first eighteen years of life and provides either a "yes" or "no" answer. If a response is yes, a score of 1 is given, with scores ranging from 0–10, which can be used to quantify the number of ACES experienced by that individual. A Cronbach's alpha of 0.88 has been reported for the ACE Questionnaire [63].

2.2.6. Psychological Flexibility

The PsyFlex questionnaire is a 6-item self-report scale measuring the process of Psychological Flexibility. It assesses psychological flexibility in a state form with high temporal specificity, asking about experiences in the past week. Each item is rated on a 5-point scale from 1 (very often) to 5 (very seldom), producing a possible range of scores from 6 to 30, where higher scores indicate higher psychological flexibility. The PsyFlex has a one-factor structure with excellent reliability (Raykov's r = 0.91), as well as evidence of convergent, divergent, and incremental validity [51,59]. Cronbach's alpha for the current study was observed at 0.87 for the total cohort (n = 231); 0.85 for the No ACE cohort (n = 75); and 0.88 for the cohort with self-reported ACE (n = 156).

2.3. *Statistical Analyses*

Participants were stratified as those with No ACE (0), Low ACE (1–3) and High ACE (≥4) based on the ACE Questionnaire. The mean differences between Time 1 and 2 were tested using paired t-tests, and Cohen's d effect size was also estimated (small = 0.20, medium, 0.50, large 0.80; (Cohen, 1988). Mixed ANOVAs (2 (Time) x 4 (ACE group)) were used for comparisons between groups and within groups on continuous variables (DASS-21, and WEMWBS), with multiple comparisons considered. Pearson product-moment correlations were used to determine associations between variables. Mediation analyses were conducted using Hayes [64] PROCESS macro for SPSS, to look at the effects of childhood stressors (perpetuating factor) and psychological flexibility (protective factor) on the longitudinal psychological outcomes of people during COVID-19 in terms of psychological stress (DASS-21) and wellbeing (WEMWBS).

2.4. Role of Funding Sources

This research was in part funded and supported by the Health Research Board and Irish Research Council (COV19-2020-044). The funder had no role in study design, data collection, data analysis, data interpretation, or writing the manuscript.

3. Results

3.1. Changes within Each Group

Did mean levels of psychological distress change significantly from Time 1 to Time 2, and differently by groups?

Changes on mental health and well-being measures for the total cohort (n = 231), and then within each ACE group (No ACE (n = 75); Low ACE (n = 110); and High ACE (n = 46)) from Time 1 to Time 2 were examined. As seen in Table 1, there were no significant changes in mean scores for Depression, Anxiety, or Stress for those with No ACE over time, as measured by the DASS-21. However, those with Low ACE scores had significant increases in all areas of psychological distress from Time 1 to Time 2—Depression (t(109) = 5.60, $p < 0.001$, d = 0.53), Anxiety (t(109) = 2.18, $p = 0.032$, d = 0.21) and Stress (t(109) = 4.60, $p < 0.001$, d = 0.44). Furthermore, individuals with High ACE had a significant increase in Depression scores (t(45) = 3.29, $p = 0.002$, d = 0.49). In terms of relative change, repeated measure ANOVA revealed a significant group-by-time interaction effect (F (2228) = 3.68, $p = 0.027$) for Depression. A one-way ANOVA revealed no significant differences in depression scores between groups at Time 1 (F (2228) = 0.036, $p = 0.964$) but significant differences between groups at Time 2 (F (2228) = 3.11 $p = 0.046$). Planned contrasts (Dunnet T) to test the hypothesis that those with No ACE would score lower than those with ACEs in the analysis, indicated that the increase in Depression scores in the No ACE group (M = 5.93, SD = 4.77) was significantly lower ($p < 0.05$) than the corresponding changes within the Low ACE (M = 7.75, SD = 5.48) and High ACE groups (M = 7.87, SD = 5.68).

When Anxiety was considered within the repeated measure ANOVA, there was no significant group-by-time interaction effect (F (2228) = 2.35, $p = 0.098$) for anxiety. One-way ANOVAs revealed no significant differences in scores at Time 1 or Time 2 between groups ($p > 0.05$).

A final repeated measure ANOVA revealed a significant group-by-time interaction effect (F (2228) = 4.27, $p = 0.015$) for Stress. A one-way ANOVA revealed no significant differences in stress scores between groups at Time 1 (F (2228) = 0.025, $p = 0.975$) but revealed significant differences at Time 2 (F (2228) = 3.21, $p = 0.042$, partial $n^2 = 0.027$). Planned contrasts indicated that the increase in stress scores for those with No ACE (M = 6.69, SD = 5.01) was significantly lower ($p = 0.011$) than those with Low ACE (M = 8.61, SD = 8.61) but not significantly lower (p= 0.168) than those with High ACE scores (M = 7.87, SD = 4.60).

Interestingly, there was no significant change within any group on mean levels of COVID-19 specific illness perception over time, as measured by the BIPQ.

Did mean levels of wellbeing change significantly from Time 1 to Time 2 and differently for groups?

Mean levels of wellbeing decreased significantly for all groups over time—the whole sample ($p < 0.001$, d = 0.367); those with No ACE ($p < 0.001$, d = 0.266); those with Low ACE ($p < 0.001$. d = 0.404); and those with High ACE ($p < 0.001$, d = 0.452). In contrast, there were no significant changes, positively or negatively, within any group when comparing gratitude over time.

Table 1. Mean and Standard Deviations across psychological wellbeing variables over time, stratified by ACE grouping.

	Total Cohort (n = 231)						No ACEs (n = 75)						Low ACE 1-3 (n = 110)						High ACE 4 or More (n = 46)					
	Time 1		Time 2		p	d	Time 1		Time 2		p	d	Time 1		Time 2		p	d	Time 1		Time 2		p	d
	M	SD	M	SD			M	SD	M	SD			M	SD	M	SD			M	SD	M	SD		
Depression	5.36	4.64	7.19	5.35	**0.001**	−0.409	5.24	4.24	5.93	4.77	0.139	−0.173	5.42	4.54	7.75	5.48	**0.001**	−0.533	5.41	5.52	7.87	5.66	**0.001**	−0.485
Anxiety	3.11	3.38	3.60	4.20	**0.046**	−0.132	3.12	3.42	2.85	3.55	0.442	−0.089	2.95	2.98	3.80	4.20	**0.032**	−0.208	3.50	4.18	4.33	5.02	0.112	−0.239
Stress	6.61	4.66	7.85	5.11	**0.001**	−0.265	6.69	4.20	6.69	5.05	1.00	0.000	6.59	4.77	8.61	5.24	**0.001**	−0.438	6.50	5.18	7.91	4.60	0.058	−0.287
Wellbeing	46.88	8.32	43.80	9.58	**0.001**	−0.367	47.89	7.17	45.55	9.36	**0.001**	0.266	46.65	8.03	43.35	9.80	**0.001**	−0.404	45.78	42.02	42.02	9.10	**0.001**	0.452

Note: M = Mean; SD = standard deviation; p = significance value; d = Cohen's d; bolded = significant < 0.05.

3.2. Mediational Analysis

Does ACE exposure have a perpetuating effect on psychological symptoms during periods of prolonged stress, and is psychological flexibility protective and a mediator of this relationship?

Mediational analyses with psychological flexibility as a mediator of the relationship between ACE (predictor) and psychological distress (DASS-21 scales) at Time 2 (outcome) were carried out. Bivariate correlations are reported in Table 2. Results from the mediational analyses are illustrated in Figure 1. In all the mediation models ACE was not a significant predictor of Psychological Flexibility (Path a), b = −0.03, t (228) = −0.22, $p = 0.83$. Psychological Flexibility was a significant strong negative predictor of all three outcomes of psychological symptoms (path b)—depression, b = −0.69, t (228) = −11.78, $p < 0.001$; anxiety, b = −0.52, t (228) = −10.72, $p < 0.001$; stress, b = −0.63, t (228) = −10.63, $p < 0.001$. ACE was a significant positive predictor of outcomes for depression and anxiety (path c)—depression b = 0.35, t (228) = 2.21, $p = 0.03$; anxiety, b = 0.31, t (228) = 2.45, $p = 0.01$ but not for stress—b = 0.24, t (228) = 1.52, $p = 0.13$. There was no significant relationship between cumulative ACE scores, and the outcome on Psychological Flexibility (Path a). However, Psychological Flexibility was a significantly positive strong predictor of wellbeing (Path b), b = 1.34 t (228) = 13.34, $p < 0.001$, and ACE was a significant negative predictor of wellbeing (path c), b = −0.58, t (228) = −2.02, $p = 0.04$.

Table 2. Bivariate correlations among variables for mediation analysis.

Variable	1	2	3	4	5	6
1 ACE Questionnaire	1	-	-	-	-	-
2 PsyFlex	−0.03	1	-	-	-	-
3 DASS-21: Depression	0.35 *	−0.70 ***	1	-	-	-
4 DASS-21: Anxiety	0.31 **	−0.52 ***	0.65 ***	1	-	-
5 DASS-21: Stress	0.24	−0.63 ***	0.78 ***	0.72 ***	1	-
6 Well-being	−0.58 *	1.34 ***	−0.77 ***	−0.58 ***	−0.70 ***	1

Note: * $p < 0.05$; ** $p < 0.01$; *** $p < 0.001$.

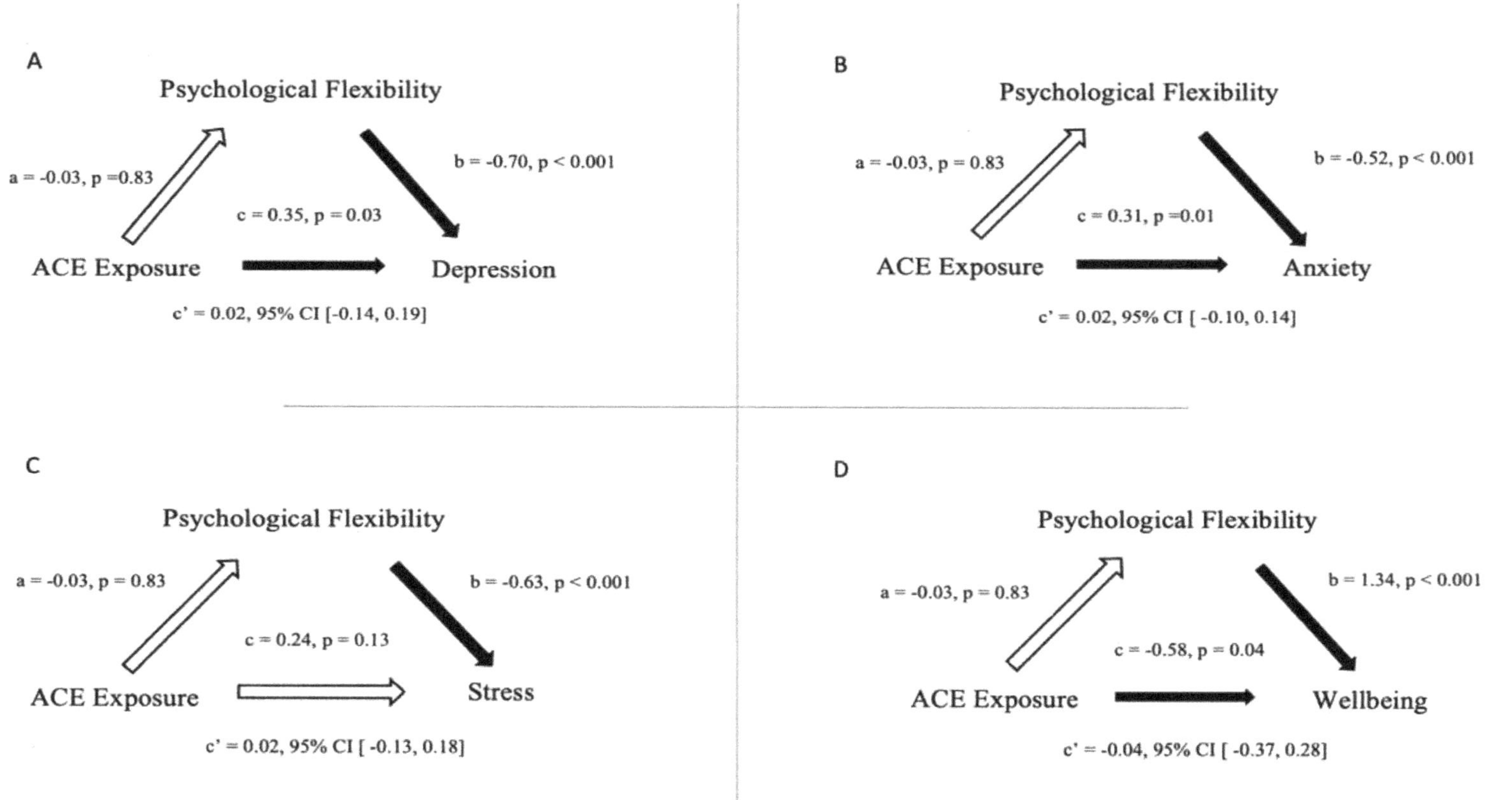

Figure 1. Mediation Analyses. Each quadrant represents a mediation analysis with ACE Exposure (ACE Questionnaire total) as a constant predictor variable with Psychological Flexibility (PsyFlex outcome) as a constant mediator variable. The outcomes change as follows: (**A**) Depression (DASS-21); (**B**) Anxiety (DASS-21); (**C**) Stress (DASS-21); and (**D**) Wellbeing (WEMWBS). Note: "c" refers to bivariate effect of predictor on outcome; "c′" refers to bivariate effect of predictor on outcome while controlling for the mediator. Arrows: hollow (white) arrows indicate a non-significant mediation effect, with filled (black) arrows indicating a significant relationship.

4. Discussion

The objective of this study was to investigate the longitudinal profile of psychological wellbeing and distress, during the COVID-19 pandemic, to investigate whether a history of self-reported ACE related to a person's wellbeing during the COVID-19 pandemic. The anticipated decrease in mental health and wellbeing due to COVID-19 will likely peak in the mid and post-pandemic phases and persist for years to come [4,22,65]. This longitudinal study investigated mental health and wellbeing changes from the beginning of the pandemic (March 2020) and again approximately ten months into the pandemic (January 2021), with a specific interest in the response profile and self-reported stress of people who had experienced ACE, compared to those without. This study hypothesized that psychological distress would increase over time for those with ACE, relative to the control population (those with no ACE). In addition, it was hypothesized that those with No ACE would have significantly lower distress at Time 2 compared to those with ACE, based on the stress sensitization hypothesis. Finally, this study also aimed to investigate whether self-reported Psychological Flexibility was a protective mediating factor on psychological distress, wellbeing, and the ACE-Distress relationship. Recent findings related to COVID-19 and historical research show that the mental health fallout from COVID-19 will disproportionately impact those already vulnerable in society [65–68]. This study supports previous research showing that those who have experienced ACE report greater psychological distress over time during the current COVID-19 pandemic [25,26,32,36].

4.1. Longitudinal Change between and within Those with ACE and Those without ACE in Their Mental Health and Wellbeing

Significant increases in mean scores were found in all three categories of the DASS-21 subscales (depression, anxiety, and stress) for individuals with Low ACE scores, with those for depression and stress being of medium effect size ($d = 0.5$) and anxiety being of small effect size ($d = 0.2$). For those with High ACE, only Depression scores increased significantly, and were of medium effect size ($d = 0.5$). For those with No ACE, there were no significant increases over time, indicating that those with No ACE may have had better psychological adjustment over time, as scores remained more stable for the duration of this longitudinal study. These findings align with previous research into the SARS pandemic, where pre-outbreak traumatic experiences were a significant predictor of post-SARS outbreak levels of depression symptoms, even after three years [20]. When taken together, these findings support Robinson et al. [69], who reviewed 65 longitudinal studies and found increases in depression scores over time to be more pronounced than other measures of distress such as anxiety. Although increases in depression were not significant for those with No ACE, this increase is something to be cognizant of in future investigations.

There were no significant differences found between the groups at Time 1 on any of the measures of Distress. However, significant differences were found over time between groups in reported levels of depression and stress but not anxiety. Planned contrasts revealed support for our hypotheses, with increased depression scores over time for those with No ACE being significantly lower, relative to the increase reported in the Low and High ACE categories. In terms of Stress scores over time, there were significantly lower relative change for those with No ACE than those within the Low ACE category, but not the High ACE category. This would suggest that the number of ACE alone is not the sole factor responsible for this between group difference in psychological distress, and that not all facets of psychological distress change equally, as highlighted by Robinson et al. [69].

These findings have clinical significance. They demonstrate that both those with and without ACE initially responded similarly and most likely adaptively to the threat and uncertainty of living alongside COVID-19, with both reporting similar levels of distress. Notwithstanding, for those with ACEs, psychological distress continued to increase significantly over time with the highest rate of change reported for the Low ACE group, and highest elevations observed in the High ACE group. Clinically, this may be beneficial in terms of psychological formulation, and co-formulation, and the consideration of ACE as predisposing and perpetuating factors relative to prolonged stress exposure. Further clinical consideration could also be given to implementing or integrating interventions which include psychological flexibility, as this was shown to mediate psychological distress in the context of ACEs.

For everyone equally, those with and without ACE, self-reported wellbeing significantly decreased over time. This may be expected due to the social and lifestyle restrictions in place at that time due to public health measures, yet contextually, this study took place during equivalent governmental lockdowns, i.e., Level 5.

These findings support those of Shevlin et al. [70] who highlight that the differential findings in many studies are due to responses being treated as homogeneous rather than heterogeneous. Furthermore, it supports the use of looking at temporal changes over more extended periods than done in many previous studies, whereby changes were only looked at up until June 2020 [69]. Furthermore, these results support Hammen's et al. [24,44] stress sensitization model, which posits that adversities in early childhood sensitize individuals to subsequent proximal stress and may increase the risk for psychopathology in the face of future stressful life events.

4.2. ACE-Distress Relationship, ACE-Wellbeing Relationship and Psychological Flexibility-Mediational Analyses

Mediational analyses revealed Psychological Flexibility as a strong significant negative predictor of all three DASS-21 outcomes, while ACE score was a significant positive predictor of anxiety and depression, but not stress. ACE total score did not significantly predict Psychological Flexibility. While Psychological Flexibility did reduce the effect ACE exposure had on prolonged distress outcomes, it was not significant and did not mediate this relationship. Concerning wellbeing, Psychological Flexibility was a significant positive predictor, and also indirectly reduced the negative effect of ACE exposure on wellbeing with a small mediation effect observed.

In terms of future research, for people with or without ACE, fostering Psychological Flexibility skills through evidence-based interventions could be used to improve wellbeing, reduce psychological distress, and increase resilience against prolonged stressors [14,19,71]. Research could prospectively investigate psychological interventions such as these, which may mitigate this ACE- Distress/Wellbeing relationship.

4.3. Limitations

This study has limitations that can be built upon for future research. For example, the convenience sample recruited for this study led to an unequal gender balance, with 88% of this study being female. Additionally, this study required participants to complete surveys electronically and to have access to the internet, which is a barrier for people with complex and enduring mental health difficulties [45]; thus, this study may be prone to sampling bias. Lastly, this study does not account for other psychosocial stressors or contextual factors which people with ACE may experience, and while increasing and incremental psychological distress was associated with ACE, future research should aim to investigate and understand psychosocial inequity alongside psychological outcomes.

4.4. Conclusions

This longitudinal study aimed to access the longer-term effects of COVID-19 on mental health and wellbeing, with a particular interest in those who have experienced ACE relative to those who have not. This study shows on a group level, before any stratification, that there is a statistically significant increase in Depression, Stress, and Anxiety, and reduction in psychological well-being over time. However, when stratified by those who report ACE and those who do not, the effect of increased psychological distress is not present for the non-ACE group, though significantly reduced psychological wellbeing remains. For those who report ACE, there is significantly higher levels of psychological distress over time as well as reduced psychological wellbeing, with increased ACE relating to increased psychological distress. This study further shows that Psychological Flexibility has a strong negative relationship to psychological distress and mediated the relationship between ACE and psychological wellbeing.

Before COVID-19, the mental health services in Ireland were underfunded, and only 6% of the overall health budget was dedicated to mental health, half of what other countries such as the United Kingdom and New Zealand contribute. With such limited resources, it is of utmost importance to support those most vulnerable to the enduring effects of COVID-19. Therefore, in line with the findings of this study, those with ACEs should be considered within this category and their needs responded to accordingly.

As supported by our findings, examples of this could be through evidence-based interventions in the community and clinic that utilize Psychological Flexibility as a core concept, such as ACT, Mindfulness, or positive psychology-based interventions. Service-level additional measures could be adopted from other countries, i.e., Scotland National Health Service, such as improved screening [72]; and introducing a national trauma training programme in all settings (schools, prisons, police force, hospitals, etc.). Emanuel and colleagues [73] note that it is now the ethical responsibility of those in government to uphold the principle of reciprocity, whereby society should now return the goodwill shown by individuals during the COVID-19 pandemic in following public health guidelines by providing adequate medical, social and psychological support as needed during and after the initial phases of the pandemic.

Author Contributions: Conceptualization, A.B. (Angela Browne), L.M., A.C. and T.B.; Data curation, A.B. (Anna Berry), L.K.T., L.M., A.C. and T.B.; Formal analysis, A.B. (Angela Browne), O.S., A.C. and T.B.; Funding acquisition, T.B.; Investigation, A.B. (Angela Browne), O.S., A.B. (Anna Berry), L.K.T., M.S., L.M., A.C. and T.B.; Methodology, A.B., O.S., A.C. and T.B.; Project administration, A.B. (Angela Browne), A.C. and T.B.; Supervision, A.C. and T.B.; Validation, E.M., L.K.T., M.S., L.M., A.C. and T.B.; Visualization, A.B. (Angela Browne), M.S. and T.B.; Writing—original draft, A.B. (Angela Browne); Writing—review & editing, A.B. (Angela Browne), O.S., A.B. (Anna Berry), E.M., L.K.T., M.S., L.M., A.C. and T.B. All authors have read and agreed to the published version of the manuscript.

Funding: This research was, in part, funded by the Health Research Board and Irish Research Council, under grant number COV19-2020-044. This grant funded the APC.

Institutional Review Board Statement: The study was conducted according to the guidelines of the Declaration of Helsinki and approved by the Research Ethics Committee of University College Dublin.

Informed Consent Statement: Informed consent was obtained from all participants involved in the study.

Data Availability Statement: The data presented in this study are available on request from the corresponding author.

Conflicts of Interest: The authors declare no conflict of interest.

References

1. Brooks, S.K.; Webster, R.K.; Smith, L.E.; Woodland, L.; Wessely, S.; Greenberg, N.; Rubin, G.J. The psychological impact of quarantine and how to reduce it: Rapid review of the evidence. *Lancet* **2020**, *395*, 912–920. [CrossRef]
2. Jeong, H.; Yim, H.W.; Song, Y.-J.; Ki, M.; Min, J.-A.; Cho, J.; Chae, J.-H. Mental health status of people isolated due to Middle East Respiratory Syndrome. *Epidemiol. Health* **2016**, *38*, e2016048. [CrossRef] [PubMed]
3. Wang, C.; Horby, P.W.; Hayden, F.G.; Gao, G.F. A novel coronavirus outbreak of global health concern. *Lancet* **2020**, *395*, 470–473. [CrossRef]
4. Gavin, B.; Lyne, J.; Mcnicholas, F. Mental health and the COVID-19 pandemic. *Ir. J. Psychol. Med.* **2020**, *37*, 156–158. [CrossRef] [PubMed]
5. Kelly, B.D. Plagues, pandemics and epidemics in Irish history prior to COVID-19 (coronavirus): What can we learn? *Ir. J. Psychol. Med.* **2020**, *37*, 269–274. [CrossRef]
6. Lam, M.H.; Wing, Y.K.; Yu, M.W.; Leung, C.M.; Ma, R.C.; Kong, A.P.; So, W.Y.; Fong, S.Y.; Lam, S.P. Mental morbidities and chronic fatigue in severe acute respiratory syndrome survivors. *Arch. Intern. Med.* **2009**, *169*, 2142–2147. [CrossRef]
7. Mak, I.W.C.; Chu, C.M.; Pan, P.C.; Yiu, M.G.C.; Chan, V.L. Long-term psychiatric morbidities among SARS survivors. *Gen. Hosp. Psychiatry* **2009**, *31*, 318–326. [CrossRef] [PubMed]

8. Xiong, J.; Lipsitz, O.; Nasri, F.; Lui, L.M.W.; Gill, H.; Phan, L.; Chen-Li, D.; Iacobucci, M.; Ho, R.; Majeed, A.; et al. Impact of COVID-19 pandemic on mental health in the general population: A systematic review. *J. Affect. Disord.* **2020**, *277*, 55–64. [CrossRef] [PubMed]
9. Burke, T.; Berry, A.; Taylor, L.K.; Stafford, O.; Murphy, E.; Shevlin, M.; McHugh, L.; Carr, A. Increased Psychological Distress during COVID-19 and Quarantine in Ireland: A National Survey. *J. Clin. Med.* **2020**, *9*, 3481. [CrossRef] [PubMed]
10. Flynn, R.; Riches, E.; Reid, G.; Rosenberg, S.; Niedzwiedz, C. Rapid review of the impact of COVID-19 on mental health. *Public Healh Scotl.* **2020**, *20*, 1–133.
11. González-Sanguino, C.; Ausín, B.; Castellanos, M.Á.; Saiz, J.; López-Gómez, A.; Ugidos, C.; Muñoz, M. Mental health consequences during the initial stage of the 2020 Coronavirus pandemic (COVID-19) in Spain. *Brain Behav. Immun.* **2020**, *87*, 172–176. [CrossRef] [PubMed]
12. Holt-Lunstad, J.; Smith, T.B.; Baker, M.; Harris, T.; Stephenson, D. Loneliness and Social Isolation as Risk Factors for Mortality: A Meta-Analytic Review. *Perspect. Psychol. Sci.* **2015**, *10*, 227–237. [CrossRef] [PubMed]
13. Karatzias, T.; Shevlin, M.; Murphy, J.; McBride, O.; Ben-Ezra, M.; Bentall, R.P.; Vallières, F.; Hyland, P. Posttraumatic Stress Symptoms and Associated Comorbidity During the COVID-19 Pandemic in Ireland: A Population-Based Study. *J. Trauma. Stress* **2020**, *33*, 365–370. [CrossRef]
14. McCracken, L.M.; Badinlou, F.; Buhrman, M.; Brocki, K.C. The role of psychological flexibility in the context of COVID-19: Associations with depression, anxiety, and insomnia. *J. Context. Behav. Sci.* **2020**, *19*, 28–35. [CrossRef]
15. Nearchou, F.; Flinn, C.; Niland, R.; Subramaniam, S.S.; Hennessy, E. Exploring the Impact of COVID-19 on Mental Health Outcomes in Children and Adolescents: A Systematic Review. *Int. J. Environ. Res. Public Health* **2020**, *17*, 8479. [CrossRef]
16. Smith, L.; Jacob, L.; Yakkundi, A.; McDermott, D.; Armstrong, N.C.; Barnett, Y.; López-Sánchez, G.F.; Martin, S.; Butler, L.; Tully, M.A. Correlates of symptoms of anxiety and depression and mental wellbeing associated with COVID-19: A cross-sectional study of UK-based respondents. *Psychiatry Res.* **2020**, *291*, 113138. [CrossRef]
17. Wang, C.; Pan, R.; Wan, X.; Tan, Y.; Xu, L.; McIntyre, R.S.; Choo, F.N.; Tran, B.; Ho, R.; Sharma, V.K.; et al. A longitudinal study on the mental health of general population during the COVID-19 epidemic in China. *Brain Behav. Immun.* **2020**, *87*, 40–48. [CrossRef]
18. Hyland, P.; Shevlin, M.; McBride, O.; Murphy, J.; Karatzias, T.; Bentall, R.P.; Martinez, A.; Vallières, F. Anxiety and depression in the Republic of Ireland during the COVID-19 pandemic. *Acta Psychiatr. Scand.* **2020**, *142*, 249–256. [CrossRef]
19. Kroska, E.B.; Roche, A.I.; Adamowicz, J.L.; Stegall, M.S. Psychological flexibility in the context of COVID-19 adversity: Associations with distress. *J. Context. Behav. Sci.* **2020**, *18*, 28–33. [CrossRef]
20. Liu, X.; Kakade, M.; Fuller, C.J.; Fan, B.; Fang, Y.; Kong, J.; Guan, Z.; Wu, P. Depression after exposure to stressful events: Lessons learned from the severe acute respiratory syndrome epidemic. *Compr. Psychiatry* **2012**, *53*, 15–23. [CrossRef] [PubMed]
21. Lu, L.; Zhong, W.; Bian, Z.; Li, Z.; Zhang, K.; Liang, B.; Zhong, Y.; Hu, M.; Lin, L.; Liu, J.; et al. A comparison of mortality-related risk factors of COVID-19, SARS, and MERS: A systematic review and meta-analysis. *J. Infect.* **2020**, *81*, e18–e25. [CrossRef]
22. O'Connor, K.; Wrigley, M.; Jennings, R.; Hill, M.; Niazi, A. Mental health impacts of COVID-19 in Ireland and the need for a secondary care mental health service response. *Ir. J. Psychol. Med.* **2020**, *38*, 99–107. [CrossRef] [PubMed]
23. Stafford, O.; Berry, A.; Taylor, L.K.; Wearen, S.; Prendergast, C.; Murphy, E.; Shevlin, M.; McHugh, L.; Carr, A.; Burke, T. Comorbidity and COVID-19: Investigating the relationship between medical and psychological well-being. *Ir. J. Psychol. Med.* **2021**, *38*, 272–277. [CrossRef] [PubMed]
24. Hammen, C.; Henry, R.; Daley, S.E. Depression and sensitization to stressors among young women as a function of childhood adversity. *J. Consult. Clin. Psychol.* **2000**, *68*, 782–787. [CrossRef]
25. Sonu, S.; Marvin, D.; Moore, C. The Intersection and Dynamics between COVID-19, Health Disparities, and Adverse Childhood Experiences: "Intersection/Dynamics between COVID-19, Health Disparities, and ACEs". *J. Child Adolesc. Trauma* **2021**, *14*, 517–526. [CrossRef]
26. Seitz, K.I.; Bertsch, K.; Herpertz, S.C. A Prospective Study of Mental Health During the COVID-19 Pandemic in Childhood Trauma–Exposed Individuals: Social Support Matters. *J. Trauma. Stress* **2021**, *34*, 477–486. [CrossRef] [PubMed]
27. Kim, A.W.; Nyengerai, T.; Mendenhall, E. Evaluating the mental health impacts of the COVID-19 pandemic: Perceived risk of COVID-19 infection and childhood trauma predict adult depressive symptoms in urban South Africa. *Psychol. Med.* **2020**, 1–13. [CrossRef] [PubMed]
28. Felitti, V.J.; Anda, R.F.; Nordenberg, D.; Williamson, D.F.; Spitz, A.M.; Edwards, V.; Koss, M.P.; Marks, J.S. Relationship of Childhood Abuse and Household Dysfunction to Many of the Leading Causes of Death in Adults: The Adverse Childhood Experiences (ACE) Study. *Am. J. Prev. Med.* **1998**, *14*, 245–258. [CrossRef]
29. Bellis, M.A.; Lowey, H.; Leckenby, N.; Hughes, K.; Harrison, D. Adverse childhood experiences: Retrospective study to determine their impact on adult health behaviours and health outcomes in a UK population. *J. Public Health* **2013**, *36*, 81–91. [CrossRef]
30. Hughes, K.; Bellis, M.A.; Hardcastle, K.A.; Sethi, D.; Butchart, A.; Mikton, C.; Jones, L.; Dunne, M.P. The effect of multiple adverse childhood experiences on health: A systematic review and meta-analysis. *Lancet Public Health* **2017**, *2*, e356–e366. [CrossRef]
31. Nelson, C.A.; Scott, R.D.; Bhutta, Z.A.; Harris, N.B.; Danese, A.; Samara, M. Adversity in childhood is linked to mental and physical health throughout life. *BMJ* **2020**, *371*, m3048. [CrossRef]
32. Chi, X.; Becker, B.; Yu, Q.; Willeit, P.; Jiao, C.; Huang, L.; Hossain, M.M.; Grabovac, I.; Yeung, A.; Lin, J.; et al. Prevalence and Psychosocial Correlates of Mental Health Outcomes Among Chinese College Students During the Coronavirus Disease (COVID-19) Pandemic. *Front. Psychiatry* **2020**, *11*, 803. [CrossRef]

33. Doom, J.R.; Seok, D.; Narayan, A.J.; Fox, K.R. Adverse and Benevolent Childhood Experiences Predict Mental Health During the COVID-19 Pandemic. *Advers. Resil. Sci.* **2021**, *2*, 193–204. [CrossRef] [PubMed]
34. Haydon, K.C.; Salvatore, J.E. A Prospective Study of Mental Health, Well-Being, and Substance Use During the Initial COVID-19 Pandemic Surge. *Clin. Psychol. Sci.* **2021**, 21677026211013499. [CrossRef]
35. Lahav, Y. Psychological distress related to COVID-19—The contribution of continuous traumatic stress. *J. Affect. Disord.* **2020**, *277*, 129–137. [CrossRef] [PubMed]
36. Sahle, B.W.; Ofori-Asenso, R.; Renzaho, A.M.N. Adverse Childhood Experiences Should Be Priority in Global Response to Covid-19. *J. Paediatr. Child Health* **2020**, *56*, 1656–1657. [CrossRef] [PubMed]
37. Sonu, S.; Post, S.; Feinglass, J. Adverse childhood experiences and the onset of chronic disease in young adulthood. *Prev. Med.* **2019**, *123*, 163–170. [CrossRef]
38. Tsur, N.; Abu-Raiya, H. COVID-19-related fear and stress among individuals who experienced child abuse: The mediating effect of complex posttraumatic stress disorder. *Child Abus. Negl.* **2020**, *110*, 104694. [CrossRef] [PubMed]
39. Wade, M.; Prime, H.; Johnson, D.; May, S.S.; Jenkins, J.M.; Browne, D.T. The disparate impact of COVID-19 on the mental health of female and male caregivers. *Soc. Sci. Med.* **2021**, *275*, 113801. [CrossRef] [PubMed]
40. Gilbert, L.K.; Breiding, M.J.; Merrick, M.T.; Thompson, W.W.; Ford, D.C.; Dhingra, S.S.; Parks, S.E. Childhood adversity and adult chronic disease: An update from ten states and the District of Columbia, 2010. *Am. J. Prev. Med.* **2015**, *48*, 345–349. [CrossRef]
41. Merrick, M.T.; Ports, K.A.; Ford, D.C.; Afifi, T.O.; Gershoff, E.T.; Grogan-Kaylor, A. Unpacking the impact of adverse childhood experiences on adult mental health. *Child Abus. Negl.* **2017**, *69*, 10–19. [CrossRef]
42. Ports, K.A.; Holman, D.M.; Guinn, A.S.; Pampati, S.; Dyer, K.E.; Merrick, M.T.; Lunsford, N.B.; Metzler, M. Adverse Childhood Experiences and the Presence of Cancer Risk Factors in Adulthood: A Scoping Review of the Literature From 2005 to 2015. *J. Pediatr. Nurs.* **2019**, *44*, 81–96. [CrossRef]
43. Thorgaard, M.V.; Frostholm, L.; Rask, C.U. Childhood and family factors in the development of health anxiety: A systematic review. *Child. Health Care* **2017**, *47*, 198–238. [CrossRef]
44. Dienes, K.A.; Hammen, C.; Henry, R.M.; Cohen, A.N.; Daley, S.E. The stress sensitization hypothesis: Understanding the course of bipolar disorder. *J. Affect. Disord.* **2006**, *95*, 43–49. [CrossRef] [PubMed]
45. Pierce, M.; McManus, S.; Jessop, C.; John, A.; Hotopf, M.; Ford, T.; Hatch, S.; Wessely, S.C.; Abel, K.M. Says who? The significance of sampling in mental health surveys during COVID-19. *Lancet Psychiatry* **2020**, *7*, 567–568. [CrossRef]
46. Dawson, D.L.; Golijani-Moghaddam, N. COVID-19: Psychological flexibility, coping, mental health, and wellbeing in the UK during the pandemic. *J. Context. Behav. Sci.* **2020**, *17*, 126–134. [CrossRef]
47. Huang, C.; Xie, J.; Owusua, T.; Chen, Z.; Wang, J.; Qin, C.; He, Q. Is psychological flexibility a mediator between perceived stress and general anxiety or depression among suspected patients of the 2019 coronavirus disease (COVID-19)? *Pers. Individ. Differ.* **2021**, *183*, 111132. [CrossRef] [PubMed]
48. Wielgus, B.; Urban, W.; Patriak, A.; Cichocki, Ł. Examining the Associations between Psychological Flexibility, Mindfulness, Psychosomatic Functioning, and Anxiety during the COVID-19 Pandemic: A Path Analysis. *Int. J. Environ. Res. Public Health* **2020**, *17*, 8764. [CrossRef]
49. Makriyianis, H.M.; Adams, E.A.; Lozano, L.L.; Mooney, T.A.; Morton, C.; Liss, M. Psychological inflexibility mediates the relationship between adverse childhood experiences and mental health outcomes. *J. Context. Behav. Sci.* **2019**, *14*, 82–89. [CrossRef]
50. Richardson, C.M.E.; Jost, S.A. Psychological flexibility as a mediator of the association between early life trauma and psychological symptoms. *Pers. Individ. Differ.* **2018**, *141*, 101–106. [CrossRef]
51. Gloster, A.T.; Meyer, A.H.; Lieb, R. Psychological flexibility as a malleable public health target: Evidence from a representative sample. *J. Context. Behav. Sci.* **2017**, *6*, 166–171. [CrossRef]
52. Heinrichs, R.W. The Primacy of Cognition in Schizophrenia. *Am. Psychol.* **2005**, *60*, 229–242. [CrossRef]
53. Kashdan, T.B.; Rottenberg, J. Psychological flexibility as a fundamental aspect of health. *Clin. Psychol. Rev.* **2010**, *30*, 865–878. [CrossRef] [PubMed]
54. Nolen-Hoeksema, S.; Wisco, B.E.; Lyubomirsky, S. Rethinking Rumination. *Perspect. Psychol. Sci.* **2008**, *3*, 400–424. [CrossRef] [PubMed]
55. Holmes, E.A.; O'Connor, R.C.; Perry, V.H.; Tracey, I.; Wessely, S.; Arseneault, L.; Ballard, C.; Christensen, H.; Silver, R.C.; Everall, I.; et al. Multidisciplinary research priorities for the COVID-19 pandemic: A call for action for mental health science. *Lancet Psychiatry* **2020**, *7*, 547–560. [CrossRef]
56. Lovibond, S.H.; Lovibond, P.F. *Manual for the Depression Anxiety Stress Scales*; Psychology Foundation of Australia: Sydney, Australia, 1995; ISBN 7334-1423-0.
57. Tennant, R.; Hiller, L.; Fishwick, R.; Platt, S.; Joseph, S.; Weich, S.; Parkinson, J.; Secker, J.; Stewart-Brown, S. The Warwick-Edinburgh Mental Well-being Scale (WEMWBS): Development and UK validation. *Health Qual. Life Outcomes* **2007**, *5*, 63. [CrossRef]
58. Broadbent, E.; Petrie, K.J.; Main, J.; Weinman, J. The Brief Illness Perception Questionnaire. *J. Psychosom. Res.* **2006**, *60*, 631–637. [CrossRef] [PubMed]
59. Gloster, A.T.; Block, V.J.; Klotsche, J.; Villanueva, J.; Rinner, M.T.B.; Benoy, C.; Walter, M.; Karekla, M.; Bader, K. Psy-Flex: A contextually sensitive measure of psychological flexibility. *J. Context. Behav. Sci.* **2021**, *22*, 13–23. [CrossRef]

60. Lee, J.; Lee, E.-H.; Moon, S.H. Systematic review of the measurement properties of the Depression Anxiety Stress Scales–21 by applying updated COSMIN methodology. *Qual. Life Res.* **2019**, *28*, 2325–2339. [CrossRef]
61. Cicchetti, D.V. Guidelines, criteria, and rules of thumb for evaluating normed and standardized assessment instruments in psychology. *Psychol. Assess.* **1994**, *6*, 284–290. [CrossRef]
62. Stewart-Brown, S.; Platt, S.; Tennant, A.; Maheswaran, H.; Parkinson, J.; Weich, S.; Tennant, R.; Taggart, F.; Clarke, A. The Warwick-Edinburgh Mental Well-being Scale (WEMWBS): A valid and reliable tool for measuring mental well-being in diverse populations and projects. *J. Epidemiol. Community Healh* **2011**, *65*, A38–A39. [CrossRef]
63. Murphy, A.; Steele, M.; Dube, S.R.; Bate, J.; Bonuck, K.; Meissner, P.; Goldman, H.; Steele, H. Adverse Childhood Experiences (ACEs) Questionnaire and Adult Attachment Interview (AAI): Implications for parent child relationships. *Child Abus. Negl.* **2014**, *38*, 224–233. [CrossRef] [PubMed]
64. Hayes, A.F. *Introduction to Mediation, Moderation and Conditional Processs Analysis: A Regression Based Approach*; Guildford Press: New York, NY, USA, 2013; ISBN 978-1-60918-230-4.
65. Sher, L. The impact of the COVID-19 pandemic on suicide rates. *QJM* **2020**, *113*, 707–712. [CrossRef]
66. Yao, H.; Chen, J.H.; Xu, Y.F. Patients with mental health disorders in the COVID-19 epidemic. *Lancet Psychiatry* **2020**, *7*, e21. [CrossRef]
67. Bambra, C.; Riordan, R.; Ford, J.; Matthews, F. The COVID-19 pandemic and health inequalities. *J. Epidemiol. Community Health* **2020**, *74*, 964–968. [CrossRef]
68. Qiu, J.; Shen, B.; Zhao, M.; Wang, Z.; Xie, B.; Xu, Y. A nationwide survey of psychological distress among Chinese people in the COVID-19 epidemic: Implications and policy recommendations. *Gen. Psychiatry* **2020**, *33*, 19–21. [CrossRef]
69. Robinson, E.; Sutin, A.R.; Daly, M.; Jones, A. A systematic review and meta-analysis of longitudinal cohort studies comparing mental health before versus during the COVID-19 pandemic in 2020. *J. Affect. Disord.* **2022**, *296*, 567–576. [CrossRef]
70. Shevlin, M.; Butter, S.; McBride, O.; Murphy, J.; Gibson-Miller, J.; Hartman, T.K.; Levita, L.; Mason, L.; Martinez, A.P.; McKay, R.; et al. Refuting the myth of a "tsunami" of mental ill-health in populations affected by COVID-19: Evidence that response to the pandemic is heterogenous, not homogeneous. *Psychol. Med.* **2021**, 1–9. [CrossRef]
71. Cullen, W.; Gulati, G.; Kelly, B.D. Mental health in the COVID-19 pandemic. *QJM* **2020**, *113*, 311–312. [CrossRef]
72. Moreno, C.; Wykes, T.; Galderisi, S.; Nordentoft, M.; Crossley, N.; Jones, N.; Cannon, M.; Correll, C.U.; Byrne, L.; Carr, S.; et al. How mental health care should change as a consequence of the COVID-19 pandemic. *Lancet Psychiatry* **2020**, *7*, 813–824. [CrossRef]
73. Emanuel, E.J.; Persad, G.; Upshur, R.; Thome, B.; Parker, M.; Glickman, A.; Zhang, C.; Boyle, C.; Smith, M.; Phillips, J.P. Fair allocation of scarce medical resources in the time of COVID-19. *N. Engl. J. Med.* **2020**, *382*, 2049–2055. [CrossRef] [PubMed]

Journal of
Clinical Medicine

MDPI

Article

Mental Health Well-Being and Attitudes on Mental Health Disorders among Family Physicians during COVID-19 Pandemic: A Connection with Resilience and Healthy Lifestyle

Tina Vilovic [1,2], Josko Bozic [3], Sanja Zuzic Furlan [1,2], Marino Vilovic [3], Marko Kumric [3], Dinko Martinovic [3], Doris Rusic [4], Marko Rada [1,2] and Marion Tomicic [1,2,*]

1 Department of Family Medicine, University of Split School of Medicine, 21000 Split, Croatia; tvilovic@mefst.hr (T.V.); sanja.zuzic@dz-sdz.hr (S.Z.F.); ravnatelj@dz-sdz.hr (M.R.)
2 Department of Family Medicine, Split-Dalmatia Health Center, 21000 Split, Croatia
3 Department of Pathophysiology, University of Split School of Medicine, 21000 Split, Croatia; josko.bozic@mefst.hr (J.B.); marino.vilovic@mefst.hr (M.V.); marko.kumric@mefst.hr (M.K.); dinko.martinovic@mefst.hr (D.M.)
4 Department of Pharmacy, University of Split School of Medicine, 21000 Split, Croatia; doris.rusic@mefst.hr
* Correspondence: marion.tomicic@mefst.hr

Abstract: Family physicians (FPs) are exposed to high amounts of stress, and could be susceptible to the development of mental health disorders (MHD), especially after the emergence of the COVID-19 pandemic. The aim of the current study was to assess MHD history, attitudes toward MHDs and stress-coping strategies in FPs. An additional goal was to estimate their comprehensive well-being and investigate connections with resilience and a healthy lifestyle. A total of 483 FPs submitted their responses via online survey. MHD attitudes were assessed with the according questionnaires, while burnout levels, healthy lifestyle, resilience, job and life satisfaction were estimated with validated scales. Results have shown that 32.5% of FPs disclosed positive MHD history, while 68.7% used professional help. Resilience and healthy lifestyle levels were significantly higher in MHD negative FPs ($p < 0.001$), while burnout levels were lower ($p < 0.001$). Moreover, healthy lifestyle ($\beta = 0.03$, $p < 0.001$) was an independent correlate of resilience, while healthy lifestyle ($\beta = -0.35$, $p < 0.001$, and resilience ($\beta = -1.82$, $p < 0.001$) were of burnout levels. Finally, resilience (OR = 0.387, $p < 0.001$) and healthy lifestyle (OR = 0.970, $p = 0.021$) were shown as independent predictors of positive MHD history status. Strong promotion and education of FP population regarding resilience and healthy lifestyle should be utilized in practice in order to alleviate the possibility of mental health disturbances and the according consequences.

Keywords: COVID-19; mental health; help-seeking; family physician; primary care; resilience; healthy lifestyle

Citation: Vilovic, T.; Bozic, J.; Zuzic Furlan, S.; Vilovic, M.; Kumric, M.; Martinovic, D.; Rusic, D.; Rada, M.; Tomicic, M. Mental Health Well-Being and Attitudes on Mental Health Disorders among Family Physicians during COVID-19 Pandemic: A Connection with Resilience and Healthy Lifestyle. *J. Clin. Med.* **2022**, *11*, 438. https://doi.org/10.3390/jcm11020438

Academic Editor: Michele Roccella

Received: 5 December 2021
Accepted: 13 January 2022
Published: 15 January 2022

Publisher's Note: MDPI stays neutral with regard to jurisdictional claims in published maps and institutional affiliations.

1. Introduction

Several studies have shown that a large percentage of patients with mental health disorders (MHD) do not receive adequate treatment [1,2]. There could be multiple reasons for this phenomenon; however, the more important ones could be negative attitudes toward help-seeking behavior and various obstacles that emerge when confronted with knowledge or a subjective feeling of these specific medical diagnoses [2–4].

Physicians represent a population group known to have extremely stressful work, high rates of burnout, mental distress and suicide [5–7]. Additionally, the surrounding stigmatization of mental health diagnoses and barriers toward help-seeking could be even more pronounced when compared to other population groups, due to the negative attitudes and behaviors towards MHD, pessimism regarding treatment success, and the specific workplace culture [8]. It could be argued that these remarks could be even more pronounced in family physicians (FPs), as they represent cornerstones of the healthcare system, the point of trusted first contact for general population, and have numerous roles in society [9,10]. In addition, studies have shown that FPs are at higher risk of chronic stress and burnout than most of the other medical practitioners [11,12]. However, it is important to alleviate psychological distress, and to remove barriers to seeking professional help in FPs, due to possible consequences of untreated MHD, as well as observed connections with reduced patient content and treatment adherence, decreased productivity and increased rates of medical errors [13,14].

Rates of MHD were steadily rising over the last decade [15,16]; however, with the emergence of the coronavirus disease 2019 (COVID-19) pandemic, one of the main consequences of the re-structured lifestyle that followed was an additional spike in MHDs, especially in the population of healthcare workers that carry out a large organizational and management burden [17–19]. Therefore, in these demanding times, several countries recognized the problem and established various psychological support systems for this population [20].

Furthermore, to the best of our knowledge, only a few studies addressed help-seeking behaviors and attitudes toward MHDs in the physician population before the pandemic, and none in the primary medicine department [21,22]. Additionally, after the COVID-19 emergence, studies have shown low psychological help-seeking in several different population samples, including students, the general community, and healthcare workers [23–25]. In addition, investigations have shown the importance of appropriate coping with experienced stress, as some of the coping mechanisms can help us reduce stress in a manner that will promote positive psychological outcomes ("adaptive" coping), whereas some of them can lead to even more exacerbated stress in the long term, and promotion of poor mental health outcomes and increased psychopathology symptoms ("maladaptive coping") [26,27]. However, there is a gap in the literature in help-seeking behaviors, stress-coping mechanisms, and experiences and attitudes toward MHDs from FPs, a population which has been substantially affected by the pandemic.

On the other hand, in the scientific literature, more emphasis is being put into investigating positive effects of resilience and healthy lifestyle on physicians' mental health [28,29]. According to some authors, resilience can be considered as one of the most important elements to physicians' well-being [29]. Even though there is no universal definition of resilience suggested in the literature [30], it could be broadly defined as a complex set of responses to traumatic and challenging situations that have fundamentals in three core components—insight, values, and self-care [31]. Further studies have shown that resilience could have some form of protective character regarding MHDs in physicians, however, there is still a scarcity of information of these connections in FP population, especially in COVID-19 pandemic era [11,32,33]. Furthermore, numerous evidence exists on the favorable effects of a healthy lifestyle on the individual's well-being, which could include burnout as well [28,34]. However, there is limited information regarding the following of a healthy lifestyle in FPs, as well as connections to self-reported MHDs, resilience, and burnout. Finally, as previous studies have shown that burnout is closely connected to job satisfaction and various mental health disorders, and that resilience and a healthy lifestyle could be considered as a protective factor against experienced stress and burnout, we deem that it is important to explore probable connections between these constructs, with consideration of the history of mental health disorders in the FP population [28,29,31,33–36].

Therefore, the main goal of this study was to investigate the self-reported mental health disturbance history in a population of FPs, their attitudes toward MHD diagnosis, and stress coping strategies. An additional goal was to estimate current FPs' mental health well-being through levels of burnout, job satisfaction, and satisfaction with life, and to investigate the connections with resilience and a healthy lifestyle.

2. Materials and Methods

2.1. Study Design and Participants

This cross-sectional study was conducted using a comprehensive online survey that was shared via the Google Forms® platform. All current family physicians (physicians that work in family medicine practice) and family medicine residents (physicians in the current residency program in the field of family medicine) in the Republic of Croatia with minimally 2 years of working experience were eligible for inclusion. The link for the survey was shared via the official e-mail addresses of family medicine practices in the country, and via e-mails of family medicine associations in Croatia. Data were collected during the "third wave" of the COVID-19 pandemic in Croatia, between April and June of 2021. The main source of information of the family medicine practices in our country was the database available from the Croatian Institute for Health Insurance with 2337 listed practices with basic information. Afterwards, the link for the survey was sent to the acquired e-mail addresses that were collected after a rigorous search via several different resources (official online information, telephone calls, work contacts). In addition, contact was made with family medicine associations in Croatia, who forwarded the link to the survey through their channels. A total of 492 responses were collected; however, 9 of them were discarded due to reported FPs' working experience being under 2 years. Hence, the overall response rate in this study was 21.0%, even though potential participants were reminded three time via e-mail and some of them via telephone calls.

All important information regarding this investigation was presented to invited FPs in the introduction of the survey and accompanying e-mail, while potential questions could be asked online. The identity of all included participants was secured with the according settings in Google forms®, while obtained informed consent was considered when the final submission of the answers was provided. The investigation was performed in accordance with the ethical standards of Declaration of Helsinki, and it was approved by the Ethics Committees of University of Split School of Medicine (No: 2181-198-03-04-21-0027) and Health Centre of the Split-Dalmatia County (No: 2181-149/01-21/01). Participation was voluntary, without compensation, while the asked questions did not include personal information.

2.2. Survey

Data were gathered using a comprehensive survey that was constructed at the Department of Family Medicine, University of Split School of Medicine after careful examination of the available literature by two FPs and one family medicine resident. Furthermore, each of the used statements and questions regarding experiences and attitudes on MHDs were carefully selected and adjusted after a detailed review of the similar studies [22,37–39], and after an additional consultation with a clinical psychologist.

Survey consisted of 3 main sections, with the first one exploring a total of 12 items that concentrated on general demographic data of the participants, as well as personal experience regarding MHDs. An MHD was defined as a problem with burnout, anxiety, depression, post-traumatic stress disorder (PTSD) or similar disorder that they consider to be in that group. Hence, gathered information included subjects' gender, age, duration of work experience, patients in care, occupation, region of work and practice localization (urban area or rural area/islands). Furthermore, participants were asked whether they have family history of MHD, confirmed MHD diagnosis sometime in their careers, or if they were certain they have an MHD disorder; however, diagnosis was not officially confirmed. The last items from the first section were connected to the current pandemic, and they included information regarding self-assessed increased risk of COVID-19 adverse outcomes (due to older age or relevant chronic diseases), if they recovered from COVID-19, and if positive MHD status emerged during the pandemic.

The second section of the survey concentrated on the FP's coping mechanisms with stress, as well as attitudes and personal experiences regarding help-seeking behaviors and MHD management. The participants were asked to express their attitudes on what they would be willing to do if confronted with MHD. Multiple answers could be selected from

6 different statements ("taking medication", "going to psychotherapies", "consultation with psychiatrist", "trying to solve the problem alone", "ignore the problem" and "talking to colleagues about it"). Furthermore, the second section included opinions on possible obstacles regarding seeking professional help. Again, multiple answers could be selected from the offered 5 statements ("no obstacles", "not believing it would help", "no time", "fear of being incompetent for work", "fear of colleagues', patients' or society stigmatization"). It should be noted that FPs with positive MHD history answered these questions about their personal experiences, while FPs without MHD history expressed their attitudes on the topic. Additionally, participants were asked what would be the best thing to acutely tackle their current mental health state, and they could choose answers from 5 different statements ("psychiatrist consultation", help not needed", "long vacation", "self-help seminars" or "something else").

Finally, the second section of the survey included analysis of FPs' stress-coping mechanisms. They could choose how they usually behave when confronted with stress from 11 different items. Some of those items represent "adaptive" mechanisms, like "working out", "spending time with family" or "communication with friends", since studies have shown a positive connection between such constructs and favorable psychological outcomes [40–42]. In addition, some others can be considered as "maladaptive" mechanisms, since they are connected to negative mental health outcomes in time ("eating food", "smoking", "drinking alcohol") [40–42].

The third part of the survey assessed various characteristics of FPs' mental health well-being and lifestyle, including resilience, burnout, satisfaction with life and work, and the following of a healthy lifestyle.

Before the survey was forwarded to the entire FP population, it was pilot-tested on randomly chosen 16 family physicians and 5 family medicine residents for comprehensibility and duration assessment. All of the included participants answered to each of the items with ease, without reporting any understanding problems. In addition, they found that the survey duration time was acceptable as well (average 15 min). Hence, as there were no changes done in any part of the survey after pilot testing, the provided answers were included into the final analyses as well.

2.3. Mental Health Well-Being

For resilience assessment, two different questionnaires were used, that are based on different definitions of resilience in the scientific literature. Resilience can be defined as the ability of an individual to recover, or "bounce back" from a stressful situation [43–45]. Hence, Smith et al. introduced a Brief Resilience Scale (BRS), that consists of 6 different statements that could be answered through a 5-point Likert scale (ranged from "strongly disagree" to "strongly agree") [45]. Results of points 1–5 were assigned considering the response, and the total score is formed as an arithmetic mean of the answers of all 6 items. Therefore, the total score on BRS ranged from 1.00–5.00, with higher scores representing a higher resilience trait. Based on a final result, FPs were put in three different categories, with the result of 1.00–2.99 representing "low resilience", 3.00–4.30 "normal resilience", and 4.31–5.00 "high resilience". BRS is a widely used scale and already validated in different languages and population samples [46,47]. It was introduced and adapted to the Croatian language as well, with Cronbach's alpha coefficient of 0.82, indicating acceptable internal consistency [48]. In our study population, the calculated Cronbach's alpha coefficient was 0.84.

Furthermore, the second used questionnaire in our study that measures resilience is the Brief Resilience Coping Scale (BRCS), as resilience can be described as an ability to cope with stressful situations [49]. BRCS is translated and adapted to various languages and population samples as well, with acceptable measures of reliability [50,51]. It consists of 4 different statements to which participants expressed their agreement on 5-point Likert scale (ranging from "strongly disagree" to "strongly agree"). Points from 1 to 5 were assigned to each of the statements, with the total sum indicating the final score. Results from 4 to 13 represented "low resilient copers", from 14 to 16 "medium resilient copers" and from 17 to 20 "high resilient copers". Proper translation of BRCS was established with a back-translation technique by an English language expert. In our sample, Cronbach's alpha coefficient was 0.79, indicating adequate internal consistency.

Burnout symptoms were evaluated with the Oldenburg Burnout Inventory (OBI), a validated and widely used questionnaire from Demerouti and Bakker [52]. This scale is conceptualized to measure two different dimensions of burnout—emotional exhaustion (OBI-E) and cognitive and somatic expressions of disengagement (OBI-D) [53]. Each of the subscales consists of 8 different statements to which subjects expressed agreement with a 4-point Likert scale (from "strongly disagree" to "strongly agree"). Each item was given 1–4 points, with consideration to items that were reversibly scored, with an increasing score indicating a higher level of burnout symptoms. Thus, the score for each of the subscales could range from 8 to 32 points. For the purposes of this study, as we did not find universal cut-off values that would determine different OBI groups, respondents were divided into tertile groups based on their score. OBI was adapted into the Croatian language as well, with good reliability results [48], while in our sample, the Cronbach's alpha coefficient was 0.78 for the OBI-E subscale, and 0.85 for the OBI-D subscale, indicating good internal consistency as well.

The concept of satisfaction with life in our population was measured with the Satisfaction with Life Scale (SWLS), developed by Diener et al. [54]. It is one of the most commonly used and most reliable tools for this purpose [55]. It consists of 5 statements that describe different standards and expectations with life, to which participants subjectively respond using a 7-point Likert scale (from "strongly disagree" to "strongly agree"). Points from 1 to 7 were assigned to each answer, with higher scores indicating higher overall content with life. Furthermore, based on a final score, participants were put into 6 different groups: "extremely dissatisfied" (5–9 points), "dissatisfied" (10–14 points), "slightly below average" (15–19 points), "average" (20–24 points), "high score" (25–29 points) and "highly satisfied" (30–35 points). SWLS was translated using the back-translation technique, and it showed excellent internal consistency in our population sample (Cronbach's alpha coefficient was 0.91).

Job satisfaction levels were assessed with the commonly used and validated Warr–Cook–Wall scale, with confirmed good psychometric properties [56,57]. The scale originally consists of 15 items; however, in the current paper, an abbreviated 10-item version was used, adapted specifically to be more appropriate for FPs [57]. Participants can describe their satisfaction with different aspects of work through the 7-point Likert scale (from "extremely dissatisfied" to "extremely satisfied"), with the total score ranging from 10 to 70 points, and higher scores indicating better overall job satisfaction. Proper translation of the scale was ensured with the back-translation technique, with Cronbach's alpha coefficient of 0.86 indicating a good internal consistency measure.

Finally, physical, social and psychological aspects of a healthy lifestyle were assessed with the Fantastic Lifestyle Questionnaire (FLQ), an instrument developed originally by Wilson and Ciliska, and later adapted by the Canadian Society for Exercise Physiology to involve a more comprehensive view for each individual [58,59]. The questionnaire consists of a total of 25 questions that addresses the individual's behavior in the last month, that are distributed into 9 different domains (F: family/friends; A: activity; N: nutrition; T: tobacco/toxins; A: alcohol; S: sleep/seatbelt/stress/safe sex; T: type of behavior; I: insight; C: career). Most of the items have 5 possible answers on a Likert scale, while two of them are dichotomous. After calculation, the final score can range from 0 to 100 points, with a higher score indicating healthier lifestyle behavior. Finally, according to the results, subjects were distributed into 5 different groups (0–34 points "needs improvement"; 35–54 points "fair"; 55–69 points "good"; 70–84 "very good" and 85–100 "excellent"). The questionnaire was translated with the back-translation technique, and has shown good reliability in other studies [60], as well as in ours, where the Cronbach's alpha coefficient was 0.81.

2.4. Statistical Analysis

The appropriate sample size for this study was calculated via the online Surveymonkey® calculator. The population that was eligible for this study consisted of 2337 FPs that were registered in the Republic of Croatia at the current time. The calculator has shown that the collected sample, with the 95% confidence interval and 5% error margin, should be at least 331 FPs. We succeeded in fulfilling these criteria, and acquired an even larger sample for adding further power to this investigation.

The MedCalc statistical program (version 19.1.2., MedCalc Software, Ostend, Belgium) was used for statistical analysis of the results. Whole numbers and percentages were used for categorical data presentation, with chi-squared test and Fisher's exact test measuring statistical differences. D'Agostino–Pearson test was used for testing the normality of data distribution, and accordingly, continuous variables were presented as median and interquartile range, with Mann–Whitney U and Kruskall–Wallis test used to measure statistical differences. Furthermore, Spearman rank correlation coefficient was used to test the correlation between questionnaire scores and other relevant variables, while significant independent factors in association with burnout levels (according to total OBI score) and resilience (according to BRS score) were determined with multiple linear regression analysis. All the assumptions for using regression analysis were fulfilled, with enter selection algorithm used. Results were reported in the form of unstandardized beta coefficients (β), standard errors (SE), t values and *p*-values. Finally, in order to determine a relationship between selected independent variables and positive MHD history status in our participants, a multivariate logistic regression analysis with enter selection algorithm was used. The model was adjusted for age and gender, and inspected for the goodness of fit with the Hosmer Lemeshow test. Results were reported in the form of the adjusted odds ratios (OR), 95% confidence intervals and *p*-values. For this investigation, statistical significance was set at $p < 0.05$.

3. Results

3.1. Baseline Characteristics and Mental Health Experiences and Attitudes

The study included a total of 483 FPs (398 females and 85 males), from which 95 (19.7%) were family medicine residents. The median age of the population was 47.0 (33.0–58.0) years, while data were collected mostly from urban areas of the country (N = 329, 68.1%). The highest percentage of the population disclosed a number of patients between 1500 and 2000 (N = 199, 41.2%), while 125 (25.9%) subjects were recovered from COVID-19 to date (Table 1).

Self-assessment analysis revealed that a total of 157 (32.5%) FPs disclosed confirmed diagnosis or confident subjective perception of MHD, from which 77 (49.0%) were newly diagnosed from the start of the COVID-19 pandemic emergence. Furthermore, when compared to the population without MHD, FPs with a positive MHD history have a significantly higher percentage of population with positive family MHD experience (53.5 vs. 23.5%, $p < 0.001$), as well as those with increased personal risk of COVID-19 adverse outcomes (47.1 vs. 33.4%, $p = 0.004$). Detailed information regarding baseline characteristics according to MHD history can be seen in Table 1.

Further analysis showed that the majority of the population with MHD history (N = 108, 68.7%) chose to use some form of help, including medications, psychotherapies or psychiatrist consultations. Furthermore, experiences from MHD positive FPs significantly differed from MHD negative population attitudes, in terms of higher medication use (60.5 vs. 46.3%, $p = 0.003$), and a lower percentage of consultations with psychiatrist (29.9 vs. 44.2 %, $p = 0.003$). In addition, the highest percentage of the total investigated population (51.8%) disclosed trying to solve the problem alone (Table 2). Lastly, analysis of the items perceived as best for acute mental health management showed that the majority of FPs (64.6%) perceive a long vacation as something best currently needed, without significant differences according to the MHD history ($p = 0.272$) (Table 2). Subgroup analysis of the experiences on mental health management of FPs with MHD history according to MHD diagnostics (confirmed diagnosis vs. self-diagnosis) can be seen in Table S1, and according to the time of diagnosis (before COVID-19 pandemic vs. after COVID-19 pandemic) in Table S2.

Table 1. Baseline characteristics of study population according to mental health disorder medical history.

Parameter	with MHD History † (N = 157)	without MHD History (N = 326)	Total (N = 483)	p *
Women	133 (84.7)	265 (81.3)	398 (82.4)	0.355
Age (years)	48.0 (33.0–58.0)	46.5 (33.0–58.0)	47.0 (33.0–58.0)	0.992 ‡
Work experience (years)	20.0 (5.0–30.0)	13.0 (6.0–28.0)	15.0 (6.0–30.0)	0.842 ‡
Occupation				
Family physician	132 (84.1)	256 (78.5)	388 (80.3)	0.151
Family medicine resident	25 (15.9)	70 (21.5)	95 (19.7)	
Region of work				
Adriatic region	62 (39.5)	144 (44.2)	206 (42.7)	
North-West region	38 (24.2)	77 (23.6)	115 (23.8)	0.579
Central and East region	57 (36.3)	105 (32.2)	162 (33.5)	
Practice localization				
Urban area	104 (66.2)	225 (69.0)	329 (68.1)	0.540
Rural area/islands	53 (33.8)	101 (31.0)	154 (33.8)	
Patients in practice				
<1000	7 (4.5)	21 (6.4)	28 (5.8)	
1000–1500	40 (25.5)	90 (27.6)	130 (26.9)	
1500–2000	73 (46.5)	126 (38.7)	199 (41.2)	0.311
>2000	30 (19.1)	80 (24.5)	110 (22.8)	
Not answered	7 (4.5)	9 (2.8)	16 (3.3)	
Family history of MHD	84 (53.5)	77 (23.6)	161 (33.3)	<0.001
Increased COVID-19 risk §	74 (47.1)	109 (33.4)	183 (37.9)	0.004
Recovered from COVID-19	38 (24.2)	87 (26.7)	125 (25.9)	0.559

Data are presented as N (%) or median (interquartile range); MHD—mental health disorder; COVID-19—coronavirus disease 2019; * chi-square test; ‡ Mann–Whitney U test; † confirmed MHD diagnosis or positive subjective perception; § increased self-assessed risk from COVID-19 adverse outcomes.

Table 2. Experiences and attitudes on mental health management according to MHD history.

Parameter	with MHD History † (N = 157)	without MHD History (N = 326)	Total (N = 483)	p *
Actions regarding knowledge of MHD ‡				
Taking medication	95 (60.5)	151 (46.3)	246 (50.9)	0.003
Going to psychotherapies	41 (26.1)	108 (33.1)	149 (30.8)	0.118
Consultation with psychiatrist	47 (29.9)	144 (44.2)	191 (39.5)	0.003
Trying to solve the problem alone	85 (54.1)	165 (50.6)	250 (51.8)	0.468
Ignore the problem	7 (4.5)	2 (0.6)	9 (1.9)	0.006
Talking with colleagues about it	0 (0.0)	5 (1.5)	5 (1.0)	0.179
Best thing to acutely tackle mental health state				
Psychiatrist consultation	38 (24.2)	18 (5.5)	56 (11.6)	<0.001
Help not needed	9 (5.7)	69 (21.2)	78 (16.1)	<0.001
Long vacation	96 (61.1)	216 (66.3)	312 (64.6)	0.272
Self-help seminars	27 (17.2)	38 (11.7)	65 (13.5)	0.095
Something else	9 (5.7)	12 (3.7)	21 (4.3)	0.301

Data are presented as N (%); MHD: mental health disorder; * chi-square test or Fisher's exact test; † confirmed MHD diagnosis or positive subjective perception; ‡ population with MHD history disclosed experiences, while population without MHD history disclosed attitudes.

When asked about obstacles to seeking professional help for MHD, the most common answer overall was "no obstacles" (N = 273, 56.5%), with a significantly higher percentage in population without MHD history (62.0 vs. 45.2%, $p < 0.001$) in comparison to MHD negative FPs. Other chosen items were "no time" (N = 75, 15.5%), with significantly higher prevalence in the MHD positive population (22.9 vs. 12.0%, $p = 0.002$) and "fear of stigmatization" (N = 62, 12.8%), without significant differences between the groups ($p = 0.964$) (Figure 1).

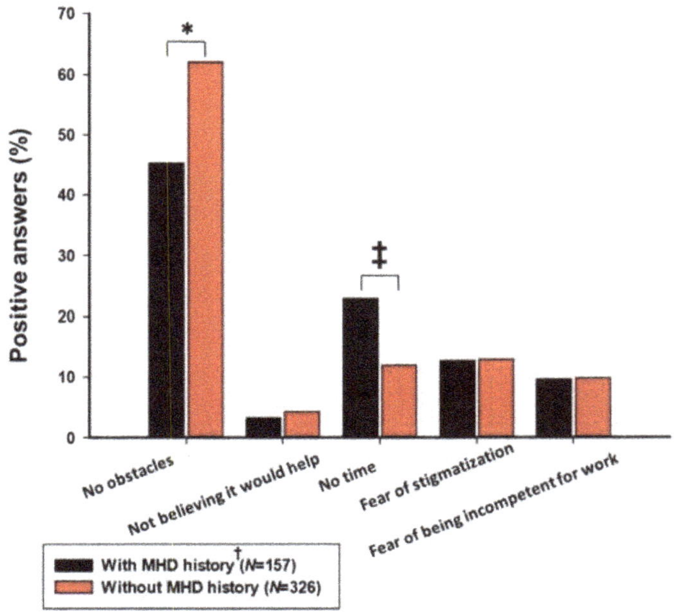

Figure 1. Experiences and attitudes regarding obstacles in seeking help for mental health disturbance according to the history of mental health disorders §; MHD—mental health disorder; * chi-square test, $p < 0.001$; ‡ chi-square test, $p = 0.002$; † confirmed MHD diagnosis or positive subjective perception, § population with MHD history disclosed experiences, while population without MHD history disclosed attitudes.

3.2. Stress-Coping Mechanisms and Current Mental Health Well-Being

Analysis of stress-coping mechanisms revealed that the most commonly used ones were "spending time with family" (N = 234, 48.4%), and "working out" (N = 224, 46.4%), while according to MHD history, both of them were used significantly more in MHD negative population (53.1 vs. 38.9%, $p = 0.003$ and 49.7 vs. 39.5%, $p = 0.035$, respectively). Furthermore, FPs with MHD history used significantly more mechanisms such as "drinking alcoholic drinks" (10.8 vs. 4.9%, $p = 0.016$), "watching television" (43.9 vs. 34.0%, $p = 0.035$) and "eating food" (36.3 vs. 19.9%, $p < 0.001$). Detailed information on used stress-coping mechanisms according to MHD history can be found in Table 3.

In this study, multiple questionnaires were used in order to acquire information on FPs' mental health well-being. Analyses of the scales according to MHD history have shown that total scores that estimated resilience (BRS and BRCS), satisfaction with life and job (SWLS and WCW-JSS, respectively), and healthy lifestyle (FLQ) were higher in the MHD negative population, with robust significance levels ($p < 0.001$). Moreover, OBI scores that assessed burnout symptoms of exhaustion and disengagement, as well as cumulative score, were significantly lower in the same population of the MHD negative FPs, when compared to those with MHD history ($p < 0.001$) (Table 4). Subgroup analysis of mental health well-being questionnaire scores of FPs with MHD history according to MHD diagnostics can be seen in Table S1, and according to time of diagnosis in Table S2.

Table 3. Coping mechanisms for stress relief according to the history of mental health disorders in study population (N = 483).

Parameter	with MHD History † (N = 157)	without MHD History (N = 326)	Total (N = 483)	p *
Working out	62 (39.5)	162 (49.7)	224 (46.4)	0.035
Listening to music	61 (38.9)	136 (41.7)	197 (40.8)	0.549
Smoking	21 (13.4)	35 (10.7)	56 (11.6)	0.396
Drinking alcoholic drinks	17 (10.8)	16 (4.9)	31 (6.4)	0.016
Spending time with family	61 (38.9)	173 (53.1)	234 (48.4)	0.003
Working on business projects	7 (4.5)	18 (5.5)	25 (5.2)	0.621
Religious/Spiritual activities	22 (14.0)	44 (13.5)	66 (13.7)	0.877
Reading	47 (29.9)	108 (33.1)	155 (32.1)	0.482
Watching television	69 (43.9)	111 (34.0)	180 (37.3)	0.035
Communication with friends	40 (25.5)	78 (23.9)	118 (24.4)	0.710
Eating food	57 (36.3)	65 (19.9)	122 (25.3)	<0.001

Data are presented as N (%), MHD- mental health disorder, * chi-square test; † confirmed MHD diagnosis or positive subjective perception.

Table 4. Total scores of used questionnaires investigating burnout levels, resilience, satisfaction with life and job, and healthy lifestyle in family physicians according to the history of mental health disorders.

Parameter	with MHD History † (N = 157)	without MHD History (N = 326)	Total (N = 483)	p *
BRCS score	15.0 (12.0–16.0)	16.0 (14.0–17.0)	15.0 (14.0–17.0)	<0.001
BRS score	2.83 (2.33–3.5)	3.33 (3.0–3.83)	3.33 (2.83–3.79)	<0.001
FLQ score	61.0 (51.0–71.0)	68.0 (62.0–77.0)	68.0 (59.0–75.0)	<0.001
OBI exhaustion	23.0 (20.0–26.0)	21.0 (18.0–24.0)	21.0 (19.0–25.0)	<0.001
OBI disengagement	21.0 (18.0–23.0)	19.0 (17.0–21.0)	19.0 (17.0–21.0)	<0.001
OBI total	44.0 (40.0–49.2)	40.0 (35.0–44.0)	41.0 (36.0–46.0)	<0.001
SWLS score	22.0 (16.0–26.0)	26.0 (22.0–30.0)	25.0 (19.0–29.0)	<0.001
WCW-JSS score	43.0 (36.7–50.0)	48.0 (40.0–55.0)	47.0 (39.2–54.0)	<0.001

Data are presented as median (interquartile range); MHD—mental health disorder; BRCS—Brief Resilient Coping Scale; BRS—Brief Resilience Scale; FLQ—Fantastic Lifestyle Questionnaire; OBI—Oldenburg Burnout Inventory; SWLS—Satisfaction with Life Scale; WCW-JSS—Warr-Cook-Wall Job Satisfaction Scale; * Mann–Whitney U test; † confirmed MHD diagnosis or positive subjective perception.

Further analysis revealed that BRS and FLQ scores showed significant positive correlation between them, as well as with the SWLS and WCW-JSS score ($p < 0.001$), while significant negative correlation was found with age, work experience and OBI scores ($p < 0.001$). In addition, a cumulative OBI score showed significant positive correlation with age ($p = 0.038$) and work experience ($p = 0.019$), while robust negative correlation was presented with SWLS and WCW-JSS scores ($p < 0.001$) (Table S3).

Statistical analyses of total OBI score when divided into tertile groups have revealed that the third tertile group had significantly more women ($p = 0.006$) and FPs with increased risk of COVID-19 adverse outcomes ($p < 0.001$) when compared to second and first tertile groups, as well as significantly less FPs with satisfied/highly satisfied life (29.9 vs. 50.3 vs. 77.6%, $p < 0.001$). In addition, analysis of selected coping mechanisms according to burnout tertile groups showed that the third tertile group had significantly more FPs that used mechanisms such as "eating food" (29.9 vs. 29.0 vs. 17.8%, $p = 0.018$) and "watching television" (44.2 vs. 38.1 vs. 30.5%, $p = 0.036$), while it had significantly less of those who chose item "spending time with family" (37.0 vs. 48.4 vs. 58.6%, $p < 0.001$) (Table 5).

Table 5. OBI total score tertiles according to various relevant parameters in study population.

Parameter	1. Tertile (N = 174)	2. Tertile (N = 155)	3. Tertile (N = 154)	p *
Age (years)	41.0 (33.0–57.0)	46.0 (33.0–58.0)	50.0 (39.0–58.0)	0.041 ‡
Women	131 (75.3)	131 (84.5)	136 (88.3)	0.006
With MHD history †	35 (20.1)	49 (31.6)	73 (47.4)	<0.001
Increased COVID-19 risk §	43 (24.7)	66 (42.6)	74 (48.1)	<0.001
Practice localization				
Urban area	119 (68.4)	95 (61.3)	115 (74.7)	0.041
Rural area/islands	55 (31.6)	60 (38.7)	39 (25.3)	
Occupation				
Family physician	136 (78.2)	115 (74.2)	137 (89.0)	0.003
Family medicine resident	38 (21.8)	40 (25.8)	17 (11.0)	
BRCS categories				
Low resilient coping	17 (9.8)	36 (23.2)	55 (35.7)	
Medium resilient coping	83 (47.7)	88 (56.8)	82 (53.2)	<0.001
High resilient coping	74 (42.5)	31 (20.0)	17 (11.0)	
SWLS categories				
Dissatisfied/Extremely dissatisfied	8 (4.6)	16 (10.3)	38 (24.7)	
Average/Slightly below average	31 (17.8)	61 (39.4)	70 (45.5)	<0.001
Satisfied/Highly satisfied	135 (77.6)	78 (50.3)	46 (29.9)	
Selected coping mechanisms				
Eating food	31 (17.8)	45 (29.0)	46 (29.9)	0.018
Smoking	12 (6.9)	21 (13.5)	23 (14.9)	0.049
Watching television	53 (30.5)	59 (38.1)	68 (44.2)	0.036
Spending time with family	102 (58.6)	75 (48.4)	57 (37.0)	<0.001
Working out	90 (51.7)	64 (41.3)	72 (46.8)	0.166

Data are presented as N (%) and median (IQR) where appropriate; COVID-19: coronavirus disease 2019; MHD: mental health disorder; * chi-square test; ‡ Kruskall–Wallis test; † confirmed MHD diagnosis or positive subjective perception; § increased self-assessed risk from COVID-19 adverse outcomes.

Further analysis showed that the third OBI tertile group, in comparison with the other two, had significantly more participants with low resilience, according to the BRS scale (53.9 vs. 31.6 vs. 6.9%, $p < 0.001$) (Figure 2A), as well as significantly more of them in the fair lifestyle category (37.7 vs. 11.0 vs. 0.0%, $p < 0.001$) (Figure 2B).

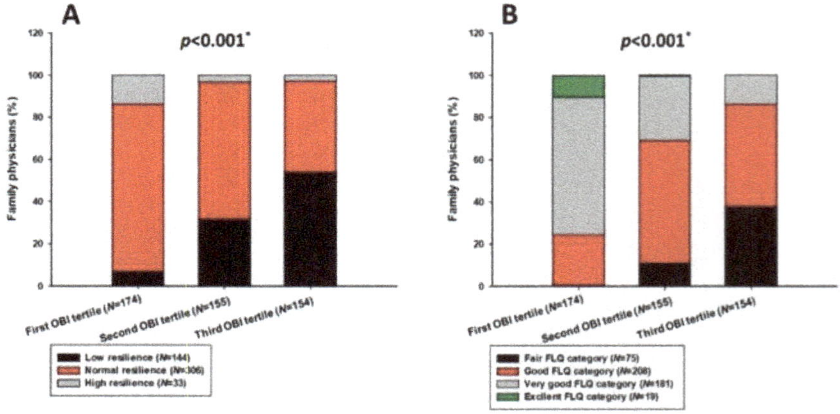

Figure 2. Resilience categories according to BRS scale (**A**) and healthy lifestyle categories according to FLQ scale (**B**) in OBI total score tertiles in study population; BRS—Brief Resilience Scale; FLQ—Fantastic Lifestyle Questionnaire; OBI—Oldenburg Burnout Inventory; * chi-square test.

Finally, the multiple linear regression model showed that the FLQ score (β = 0.03, SE = 0.003, t-value = 10.4, $p < 0.001$) was in significant association with the BRS score, set as dependent variable, when computed alongside baseline characteristics and SWLS score. Furthermore, a similar linear regression model that investigated independent predictors for burnout levels, with OBI cumulative score set as dependent variable, determined the FLQ score ($\beta = -0.35$, SE = 0.03, t-value= -11.4, $p < 0.001$), and BRS score ($\beta = -2.12$, SE = 0.44, t-value= -4.87, $p < 0.001$) to be the significant correlates.

Additionally, multivariate logistic regression analysis was performed in order to determine independent predictors of positive MHD history status. Model analysis showed BRS score (OR = 0.387, 95% CI = 0.261–0.574, $p < 0.001$) and FLQ score (OR = 0.970, 95% CI = 0.945–0.995, $p = 0.021$) to be significant predictors of MHDs in our population (Table S4).

4. Discussion

In this survey study, we investigated the prevalence of self-reported MHD history in the nation-wide population sample of FPs, as well as their attitudes and experiences toward MHDs. Additionally, we further addressed FPs' well-being through assessment of burnout symptoms, job and life satisfaction, with analyzed connections to their resilience and healthy lifestyle following.

Results have shown than nearly one-third of the investigated population expressed a positive MHD history, from which 28% FPs had confirmed diagnosis. Furthermore, nearly 50% of MHD positive FPs developed these disturbances in the COVID-19 pandemic era. Moreover, the MHD positive group had a significantly larger percentage of FPs with an increased self-assessed risk of COVID-19 consequences when compared to the group without MHD history, that further attributes to the deleterious impact of the pandemic on mental health. Similar results were shown in a large cohort study of Australian frontline health workers, where 30% of the investigated population expressed a history of mental illness [61]. It can be argued that these results are in line with studies that confirmed the physician and FP population as susceptible to mental health disorders, especially in times of the COVID-19 pandemic [17–19]. However, according to the previous work on the similar FP population, there is a gap between percentages of anxiety, depression and PTSD symptoms based on validated questionnaires and the current self-report that expressed lower MHD prevalence [18]. This could be possible due to the different time period when the study has taken place, as well as possible self-perceived underestimation of low/moderate MHD symptoms that FPs could be used to and ignore.

Our results have shown that nearly 70% of FPs with MHD history actually had some form of professional help (medication, consultations, psychotherapies). This is a substantially larger percentage in comparison to the results of the studies conducted on medical workers in other countries during the pandemic [25,61,62]. These differences could be present due to several factors, including different cultural background, variability in formulated questions regarding help-seeking behavior, more recent timing in the pandemic in our study, differences in public health strategies, as well as the different population of healthcare workers. On the other hand, Muhamad Ramzi et al. conducted a study on a large cohort of physicians where obtained medical help for depression was around 60%, which is a similar result as in our study [63]. Although the current results imply that a favorable percentage of FPs actually took some form of mental health treatment, a large number of FPs still did not seek any kind of help. Additionally, the given percentage should be taken with caution due to the possibility of frequent self-medication in the physician population [64]. There is an interesting discrepancy between the attitudes in what MHD negative FPs think they would do if confronted with a disorder, and the actual history of actions of the MHD positive population. Taking medication was a more frequent answer in the MHD positive population, while consultation with a psychiatrist was a more common answer in the MHD negative population. It is possible that consultations are something that FPs would prefer to do in theory; however, due to the lack of available time, work overload or stigmatization, in the end, they put more effort into quicker solutions like medication.

Further analyses addressed attitudes on obstacles FPs face when seeking help for experienced MHD. The most commonly chosen answers were "no obstacles" and "no time"; however, again, there were significant differences on these attitudes according to the

MHD history. FPs with a positive history had a lower answer rate on the "no obstacles" item, and a higher rate on the "no time" item. This is in line with the results of several other studies in which healthcare workers enclosed a lack of time as one of the most prominent reasons for not seeking mental health help [22,25]. These results are putting even more emphasis on the observation that FPs could change their attitudes when actually becoming unwell, and that they are indeed overwhelmed with work when they cannot find enough time to properly manage their mental health. These hypotheses are additionally supported with finding that most of the FPs believe a long vacation is the best thing to acutely tackle mental health state, regardless of MHD history.

Furthermore, the "fear of stigmatization" item was overall chosen in a somewhat lower percentage than expected (12.8%), when compared to other literature sources that addressed it as a major obstacle in seeking appropriate care [8,22,65]. Even though a systematic review by Clement et al., dating before the pandemic, associated a small to moderate cumulative negative effect of mental health stigma on help-seeking, it involved studies consisting of mixed population models [2]. Furthermore, it is possible that raising awareness about MHD in the pandemic time, encouraging the fight against stigmatization and severely deteriorating mental health well-being is facilitating favorable behaviors in the FP population, and reducing the effect of stigma. Nevertheless, mental health stigma still presents an important treatment obstacle in the physician population, and in these challenging times, it has never been more important to further raise awareness of mental health disturbances and to promote proper help seeking behaviors.

In order to assess the type of mechanisms by which FPs cope with daily stress, we offered them to choose from 11 different items, with the possible selection of multiple answers. Results have shown that the most commonly chosen mechanisms were working out (47%) and spending time with family (48%), which both can be considered as adaptive, positive coping mechanisms according to the available literature [40–42,66]. Moreover, these mechanisms were more represented in the group with a negative MHD history, and associated with lower burnout scores, which further emphasizes their commendatory, adaptive features. However, eating, watching television and drinking alcoholic drinks were moderately chosen mechanisms that were connected with a positive MHD history. Moreover, eating, watching television and smoking were represented more in higher burnout score groups. Studies have shown that the pandemic has had a negative effect on disordered eating behavior that could further be connected to increased psychological distress and job stress, which is in line with our observations [67]. When further comparing these results to other available similar studies, it can be observed that physical exercise is indeed one of most commonly used coping mechanisms in the healthcare population, while Smallwood et al. problematized increased alcohol use, which was connected to the history of poor mental health [38,61]. In addition, Wang et al. showed on a sample of Chinese physicians that those who had high perceived stress adopted more negative coping styles, which further led to higher levels of psychological distress [68]. According to all available information, it can be assumed that there is probable association between endured stress, MHDs and maladaptive coping skills. Healthy, positive coping mechanisms should be further promoted in the FP population in order to manage stress and possible MHD development more effectively [69].

Comprehensive evaluation of FPs' well-being with validated scales revealed moderate resilience, satisfaction with life and healthy lifestyle characteristics. Further analysis showed that the group with positive MHD history had lower scores on resilience, healthy lifestyle and satisfaction with life and work, while burnout scores were higher. Furthermore, correlation analysis determined robust positive association between life and work satisfaction, healthy lifestyle and resilience. Moreover, healthy lifestyle following retained a significant connection with resilience after adjustment in the multiple regression model. On the contrary, the burnout score had a clear negative association with all of the other questionnaire scores, including resilience and healthy lifestyle, which was further confirmed in the group analysis and regression model.

When comparing acquired results to other studies that investigated effects of resilience on physicians' burnout levels, similar associations were shown. In a study by Buck et al. conducted on family medicine residents and faculty members, regression models confirmed negative associations between depersonalization and emotional exhaustion with resilience, while corresponding results were shown in Australian general practice registrars, as well as the nurse population [33,70,71]. Similar conclusions were shown in the aforementioned studies despite the fact that burnout levels were measured via different scales. Considering the beneficial effects and importance of resilience, as well as the possibility of training it as an acquired skill [29], it is of utmost importance to learn more regarding factors that are positively influencing it. Moreover, literature has shown that physicians with higher resilience provide better quality of care for their patients, as well as reducing overall healthcare costs [72]. Hence, workplace intervention programs on healthcare workers have been described in the literature with some favorable findings; however, evidence is very limited and there is a need for more high-quality long-term studies [73,74].

It is interesting to notice healthy lifestyle as a factor between resilience and burnout, with significant connections to both. These results are in line with conclusions from recent investigations, which emphasized intensive healthy lifestyle as an important tool in burnout management and prevention, while it could be also seen as one of the fundamentals of resilience as a concept [28,31,34]. Our results further promote the idea of healthy lifestyle and resilience as key factors that could be used as a significant defense against work burnout in FP population. However, they could be strongly beneficial for overall mental health well-being as well, with results confirming both of them as significant independent predictors of MHD in a logistic regression model. It could be possible that individuals who demonstrate low resilience and live an unhealthy life are more susceptible in developing MHD; hence, these skills should be facilitated and worked on both personal and organizational levels. On the other hand, this may also be a two-way street, as FPs with MHDs may adopt an unhealthy lifestyle as a consequence of the mental disorder itself.

Several limitations of this study should be emphasized. With the cross-sectional investigation structure, causality between the acquired results cannot be assumed, while positive history of MHD in a family can be considered as a confounding factor. Furthermore, the history of MHD was based on a self-report by the investigated population, and not confirmed through official medical history records. In addition, specific medical diagnoses were not obtained and considered in the final analyses. Moreover, attitudes regarding specific mental health characteristics could be answered differently due to shame or perceived stigma. Hence, the number of the FPs with positive MHD history and results on MHD attitudes could be misinterpreted. However, as FPs are educated in recognizing relevant MHD symptoms and diseases, and with the anonymity guaranteed, it is safe to assume that answers were truthful and correct. Finally, much other collected information was based on a self-report as well, including the increased risk of COVID-19 adverse outcomes, practice localization and number of patients in practice, although we assume that FPs have enough knowledge to correctly answer these queries.

5. Conclusions

In conclusion, this study has shown that a relevant percentage of FPs experienced some form of mental health disturbances in their professional history, and that mental health severely deteriorated in the recent times of the COVID-19 pandemic. In addition, it is important to have in mind that a significant number of FPs still have obstacles that are preventing them from seeking adequate professional help. With the heavy burden they daily carry in the workplace, there is a strong need to continue raising awareness regarding MHD in this population, to encourage early help-seeking behavior, and to fight against stigmatization.

Furthermore, it is safe to assume that the FPs' comprehensive well-being and a possibility of developing MHD is connected to each distinctive feature assessed in the present study. Hence, promotion of positive stress-coping abilities, as well as introduction and education regarding resilience and healthy lifestyle following should further be encouraged and investigated in order to improve overall health and to alleviate FPs from severe psychological distress. Finally, it is safe to assume that promotion of those characteristics can be expanded not only in the FP population, but to every patient in the clinical practice that is suffering from high work-related stress.

Supplementary Materials: The following are available online at https://www.mdpi.com/article/10.3390/jcm11020438/s1, Table S1: Experiences on mental health management and mental health well-being questionnaire scores according to diagnostics of MHD in a group of participants with positive MHD history (N = 157), Table S2: Experiences on mental health management and mental health well-being questionnaire scores according to time of diagnosis in a group of participants with positive MHD history (N = 157), Table S3: Correlation of resilience, burnout and healthy lifestyle questionnaire scores with other relevant parameters in the total study population (N = 483), Table S4: Multivariate logistic regression analysis of independent predictors for positive mental health disorder history status.

Author Contributions: Conceptualization, T.V., M.V. and M.T.; methodology, T.V., J.B., D.M. and S.Z.F.; software, M.V., D.R. and M.K.; validation, T.V., S.Z.F. and M.R.; formal analysis, T.V., D.R. and M.T.; investigation, T.V., S.Z.F., M.T. and M.R.; resources, T.V., J.B. and M.T.; data curation, T.V. and S.Z.F.; writing—original draft preparation, T.V. and M.V.; writing—review and editing, T.V., M.K., M.T., J.B. and D.M.; visualization, T.V.; supervision, M.T. and M.R.; project administration, T.V. and M.T.; funding acquisition, T.V., M.T. and J.B. All authors have read and agreed to the published version of the manuscript.

Funding: This research received no external funding.

Institutional Review Board Statement: The study was conducted according to the guidelines of the Declaration of Helsinki, and approved by the Ethics Committee of University of Split School of Medicine (protocol code 2181-198-03-04-21-0027, 31 March 2021) and Ethics Committee of Health Centre of the Split-Dalmatia County (protocol code 2181-149/01-21/01, 18 March 2021).

Informed Consent Statement: Informed consent was obtained from all subjects involved in the study. Investigation was based on anonymous online survey, with explanations posted in accompanying mail and introduction section of the survey. All potential questions could be asked. Submitted response was considered as obtained informed consent, as it was stated to the participants as well.

Data Availability Statement: The data presented in this study are available on request from the corresponding author. The data are not publicly available due to ethical restrictions.

Conflicts of Interest: The authors declare no conflict of interest.

References

1. Thornicroft, G. Most people with mental illness are not treated. *Lancet* **2007**, *370*, 807–808. [CrossRef]
2. Clement, S.; Schauman, O.; Graham, T.; Maggioni, F.; Evans-Lacko, S.; Bezborodovs, N.; Morgan, C.; Rüsch, N.; Brown, J.S.L.; Thornicroft, G. What is the impact of mental health-related stigma on help-seeking? A systematic review of quantitative and qualitative studies. *Psychol. Med.* **2015**, *45*, 11–27. [CrossRef] [PubMed]
3. Mackenzie, C.S.; Erickson, J.; Deane, F.; Wright, M. Changes in attitudes toward seeking mental health services: A 40-year cross-temporal meta-analysis. *Clin. Psychol. Rev.* **2014**, *34*, 99–106. [CrossRef] [PubMed]
4. Velasco, A.A.; Cruz, I.S.S.; Billings, J.; Jimenez, M.; Rowe, S. What are the barriers, facilitators and interventions targeting help-seeking behaviours for common mental health problems in adolescents? A systematic review. *BMC Psychiatry* **2020**, *20*, 293. [CrossRef]
5. Yates, S.W. Physician Stress and Burnout. *Am. J. Med.* **2020**, *133*, 160–164. [CrossRef] [PubMed]
6. Mihailescu, M.; Neiterman, E. A scoping review of the literature on the current mental health status of physicians and physicians-in-training in North America. *BMC Public Health* **2019**, *19*, 1363. [CrossRef]
7. Hawton, K.; Agerbo, E.; Simkin, S.; Platt, B.; Mellanby, R.J. Risk of suicide in medical and related occupational groups: A national study based on Danish case population-based registers. *J. Affect. Disord.* **2011**, *134*, 320–326. [CrossRef]
8. Knaak, S.; Mantler, E.; Szeto, A. Mental illness-related stigma in healthcare: Barriers to access and care and evidence-based solutions. *Heal. Manag. Forum* **2017**, *30*, 111–116. [CrossRef]
9. Schultz, K.; Delva, D.; Kerr, J. Emotional effects of continuity of care on family physicians and the therapeutic relationship. *Can. Fam. Physician* **2012**, *58*, 178–185.

10. Allen, J.; Gay, B.; Crebolder, H.; Heyrman, J.; Svab, I.; Ram, P. The European definitions of the key features of the discipline of general practice: The role of the GP and core competencies. *Br. J. Gen. Pr.* **2002**, *52*, 526–527.
11. McKinley, N.; McCain, R.S.; Convie, L.; Clarke, M.; Dempster, M.; Campbell, W.J.; Kirk, S.J. Resilience, burnout and coping mechanisms in UK doctors: A cross-sectional study. *BMJ Open* **2020**, *10*, e031765. [CrossRef]
12. Peckham, C. Medscape Physician Lifestyle Report 2016: Bias and Burnout. Medscape, 2016. Available online: https://www.medscape.com/slideshow/lifestyle-2016-overview-6007335 (accessed on 16 November 2021).
13. Wallace, J.E.; Lemaire, J.B.; Ghali, W.A. Physician wellness: A missing quality indicator. *Lancet* **2009**, *374*, 1714–1721. [CrossRef]
14. Tawfik, D.S.; Profit, J.; Morgenthaler, T.I.; Satele, D.V.; Sinsky, C.A.; Dyrbye, L.N.; Tutty, M.A.; West, C.P.; Shanafelt, T.D. Physician Burnout, Well-being, and Work Unit Safety Grades in Relationship to Reported Medical Errors. In *Mayo Clinic Proceedings*; Elsevier: Amsterdam, The Netherland, 2018; Volume 93, pp. 1571–1580.
15. Twenge, J.M.; Cooper, A.B.; Joiner, T.E.; Duffy, M.E.; Binau, S.G. Age, period, and cohort trends in mood disorder indicators and suicide-related outcomes in a nationally representative dataset, 2005–2017. *J. Abnorm. Psychol.* **2019**, *128*, 185–199. [CrossRef] [PubMed]
16. Shanafelt, T.D.; Hasan, O.; Dyrbye, L.N.; Sinsky, C.; Satele, D.; Sloan, J.; West, C.P. Changes in Burnout and Satisfaction with Work-Life Balance in Physicians and the General US Working Population Between 2011 and 2014. *Mayo Clin. Proc.* **2015**, *90*, 1600–1613. [CrossRef] [PubMed]
17. Martínez-López, J.Á.; Lázaro-Pérez, C.; Gómez-Galán, J.; Fernández-Martínez, M.D.M. Psychological Impact of COVID-19 Emergency on Health Professionals: Burnout Incidence at the Most Critical Period in Spain. *J. Clin. Med.* **2020**, *9*, 3029. [CrossRef]
18. Vilovic, T.; Bozic, J.; Vilovic, M.; Rusic, D.; Furlan, S.Z.; Rada, M.; Tomicic, M. Family Physicians' Standpoint and Mental Health Assessment in the Light of COVID-19 Pandemic—A Nationwide Survey Study. *Int. J. Environ. Res. Public Heal.* **2021**, *18*, 2093. [CrossRef]
19. Muller, A.E.; Hafstad, E.V.; Himmels, J.P.W.; Smedslund, G.; Flottorp, S.; Stensland, S.Ø.; Stroobants, S.; Van De Velde, S.; Vist, G.E. The mental health impact of the covid-19 pandemic on healthcare workers, and interventions to help them: A rapid systematic review. *Psychiatr. Res.* **2020**, *293*, 113441. [CrossRef]
20. David, E.; DePierro, J.M.; Marin, D.B.; Sharma, V.; Charney, D.S.; Katz, C.L. COVID-19 Pandemic Support Programs for Healthcare Workers and Implications for Occupational Mental Health: A Narrative Review. *Psychiatr. Q.* **2021**, 1–21. [CrossRef]
21. Tyssen, R.; Vaglum, P.; Røvik, J.O.; Grønvold, N.T.; Ekeberg, Ø. Help-seeking for mental health problems among young physicians: Is it the most ill that seeks help?—A longitudinal and nationwide study. *Soc. Psychiatry* **2004**, *39*, 989–993. [CrossRef]
22. Gold, K.J.; Andrew, L.B.; Goldman, E.B.; Schwenk, T.L. "I would never want to have a mental health diagnosis on my record": A survey of female physicians on mental health diagnosis, treatment, and reporting. *Gen. Hosp. Psychiatry* **2016**, *43*, 51–57. [CrossRef]
23. Naito, T.; Chin, J.; Kim, T.U.; Veera, S.; Jeannette, M.; Lomiguen, C.M. Further Reduction in Help-Seeking Behaviors Amidst Additional Barriers to Mental Health Treatment in Asian Populations: A Contemporary Review. *Cureus* **2020**, *12*, e11455. [CrossRef]
24. Liang, S.-W.; Chen, R.-N.; Liu, L.-L.; Li, X.-G.; Chen, J.-B.; Tang, S.-Y.; Zhao, J.-B. The Psychological Impact of the COVID-19 Epidemic on Guangdong College Students: The Difference between Seeking and Not Seeking Psychological Help. *Front. Psychol.* **2020**, *11*, 2231. [CrossRef] [PubMed]
25. She, R.; Wang, X.; Zhang, Z.; Li, J.; Xu, J.; You, H.; Li, Y.; Liang, Y.; Li, S.; Ma, L.; et al. Mental Health Help-Seeking and Associated Factors Among Public Health Workers During the COVID-19 Outbreak in China. *Front. Public Health* **2021**, *9*, 622677. [CrossRef]
26. Smith, M.M.; Saklofske, D.H.; Keefer, K.V.; Tremblay, P.F. Coping Strategies and Psychological Outcomes: The Moderating Effects of Personal Resiliency. *J. Psychol.* **2016**, *150*, 318–332. [CrossRef] [PubMed]
27. Compas, B.E.; Jaser, S.S.; Bettis, A.H.; Watson, K.H.; Gruhn, M.A.; Dunbar, J.P.; Williams, E.; Thigpen, J.C. Coping, emotion regulation, and psychopathology in childhood and adolescence: A meta-analysis and narrative review. *Psychol. Bull.* **2017**, *143*, 939–991. [CrossRef] [PubMed]
28. Lianov, L. A Powerful Antidote to Physician Burnout: Intensive Healthy Lifestyle and Positive Psychology Approaches. *Am. J. Lifestyle Med.* **2021**, *15*, 563–566. [CrossRef]
29. Zwack, J.; Schweitzer, J. If Every Fifth Physician Is Affected by Burnout, What About the Other Four? Resilience Strategies of Experienced Physicians. *Acad. Med.* **2013**, *88*, 382–389. [CrossRef] [PubMed]
30. Aburn, G.; Gott, M.; Hoare, K. What is resilience? An Integrative Review of the empirical literature. *J. Adv. Nurs.* **2016**, *72*, 980–1000. [CrossRef]
31. Nedrow, A.; Steckler, A.N.; Hardman, J. Physician resilience and burnout: Can you make the switch? *Fam. Pr. Manag.* **2013**, *20*, 25–30.
32. Mosheva, M.; Hertz-Palmor, N.; Ilan, S.D.; Matalon, N.; Pessach, I.M.; Afek, A.; Ziv, A.; Kreiss, Y.; Gross, R.; Gothelf, D. Anxiety, pandemic-related stress and resilience among physicians during the COVID-19 pandemic. *Depress. Anxiety* **2020**, *37*, 965–971. [CrossRef] [PubMed]
33. Buck, K.; Williamson, M.; Ogbeide, S.; Norberg, B. Family Physician Burnout and Resilience: A Cross-Sectional Analysis. *Fam. Med.* **2019**, *51*, 657–663. [CrossRef]
34. Penttinen, M.; Virtanen, J.; Laaksonen, M.; Erkkola, M.; Vepsäläinen, H.; Kautiainen, H.; Korhonen, P. The Association between Healthy Diet and Burnout Symptoms among Finnish Municipal Employees. *Nutrients* **2021**, *13*, 2393. [CrossRef] [PubMed]

35. Koutsimani, P.; Montgomery, A.; Georganta, K. The Relationship between Burnout, Depression, and Anxiety: A Systematic Review and Meta-Analysis. *Front. Psychol.* **2019**, *10*, 284. [CrossRef]
36. Gómez-García, R.; Bayón-Calvo, S.; Lucas-García, J. The Relationship between Burnout and Job Satisfaction in a Sample of Spanish Social Workers. *Br. J. Soc. Work.* **2020**, *51*, 3115–3134. [CrossRef]
37. Kang, L.; Ma, S.; Chen, M.; Yang, J.; Wang, Y.; Li, R.; Yao, L.; Bai, H.; Cai, Z.; Yang, B.X.; et al. Impact on mental health and perceptions of psychological care among medical and nursing staff in Wuhan during the 2019 novel coronavirus disease outbreak: A cross-sectional study. *Brain Behav. Immun.* **2020**, *87*, 11–17. [CrossRef]
38. Louie, P.K.; Harada, G.K.; McCarthy, M.H.; Germscheid, N.; Cheung, J.P.Y.; Neva, M.H.; El-Sharkawi, M.; Valacco, M.; Sciubba, D.M.; Chutkan, N.B.; et al. The Impact of COVID-19 Pandemic on Spine Surgeons Worldwide. *Glob. Spine J.* **2020**, *10*, 534–552. [CrossRef] [PubMed]
39. Shechter, A.; Diaz, F.; Moise, N.; Anstey, D.E.; Ye, S.; Agarwal, S.; Birk, J.L.; Brodie, D.; Cannone, D.E.; Chang, B.; et al. Psychological distress, coping behaviors, and preferences for support among New York healthcare workers during the COVID-19 pandemic. *Gen. Hosp. Psychiatry* **2020**, *66*, 1–8. [CrossRef] [PubMed]
40. Esch, T.; Stefano, G.B. The neurobiology of stress management. *Neuro Endocrinol. Lett.* **2010**, *31*, 19–39. [PubMed]
41. Baqutayan, S.M.S. Stress and Coping Mechanisms: A Historical Overview. *Mediterr. J. Soc. Sci.* **2015**, *6*, 479. [CrossRef]
42. Saxon, L.; Makhashvili, N.; Chikovani, I.; Seguin, M.; McKee, M.; Patel, V.; Bisson, J.; Roberts, B. Coping strategies and mental health outcomes of conflict-affected persons in the Republic of Georgia. *Epidemiol. Psychiatr. Sci.* **2017**, *26*, 276–286. [CrossRef]
43. Tugade, M.M.; Fredrickson, B.L. Resilient Individuals Use Positive Emotions to Bounce Back From Negative Emotional Experiences. *J. Pers. Soc. Psychol.* **2004**, *86*, 320–333. [CrossRef] [PubMed]
44. Carver, C.S. Resilience and thriving: Issues, models, and linkages. *J. Soc. Issues* **1998**, *54*, 245–266. [CrossRef]
45. Smith, B.W.; Dalen, J.; Wiggins, K.; Tooley, E.; Christopher, P.; Bernard, J. The brief resilience scale: Assessing the ability to bounce back. *Int. J. Behav. Med.* **2008**, *15*, 194–200. [CrossRef] [PubMed]
46. Chmitorz, A.; Wenzel, M.; Stieglitz, R.-D.; Kunzler, A.; Bagusat, C.; Helmreich, I.; Gerlicher, A.; Kampa, M.; Kubiak, T.; Kalisch, R.; et al. Population-based validation of a German version of the Brief Resilience Scale. *PLoS ONE* **2018**, *13*, e0192761. [CrossRef]
47. Soer, R.; Dijkstra, M.W.M.C.; Bieleman, H.J.; Stewart, R.E.; Reneman, M.F.; Oosterveld, F.G.J.; Schreurs, K.M.G. Measurement properties and implications of the Brief Resilience Scale in healthy workers. *J. Occup. Heal.* **2019**, *61*, 242–250. [CrossRef] [PubMed]
48. Sliskovic, A.; Buric, I.; Cubela Adoric, V.; Nikolic, M.; Tucak Junakovic, I. *Collection of Psychological Scales and Questionnaires*, 9th ed.; University of Zadar: Zadar, Croatia, 2018.
49. Sinclair, V.G.; Wallston, K.A. The Development and Psychometric Evaluation of the Brief Resilient Coping Scale. *Assessment* **2004**, *11*, 94–101. [CrossRef]
50. Kocalevent, R.-D.; Zenger, M.; Hinz, A.; Klapp, B.; Brähler, E. Resilient coping in the general population: Standardization of the brief resilient coping scale (BRCS). *Heal. Qual. Life Outcomes* **2017**, *15*, 251. [CrossRef] [PubMed]
51. Fung, S.-F. Validity of the Brief Resilience Scale and Brief Resilient Coping Scale in a Chinese Sample. *Int. J. Environ. Res. Public Health* **2020**, *17*, 1265. [CrossRef]
52. Demerouti, E.; Bakker, A.B. The Oldenburg Burnout Inventory: A good alternative to measure burnout and engagement. In *Stress and Burnout in Health Care*; Halbesleben, J., Ed.; Nova Sciences: Hauppage, NY, USA, 2008; pp. 65–78.
53. Bakker, A.B.; Demerouti, E.; Verbeke, W. Using the job demands-resources model to predict burnout and performance. *Hum. Resour. Manag.* **2004**, *43*, 83–104. [CrossRef]
54. Diener, E.; Emmons, R.A.; Larsen, R.J.; Griffin, S. The Satisfaction with Life Scale. *J. Pers. Assess.* **1985**, *49*, 71–75. [CrossRef]
55. Morrison, M.; Tay, L.; Diener, E. Subjective Well-Being and National Satisfaction Findings from a Worldwide Survey. *Psychol. Sci.* **2011**, *22*, 166–171. [CrossRef] [PubMed]
56. Warr, P.; Cook, J.; Wall, T. Scales for the measurement of some work attitudes and aspects of psychological well-being. *J. Occup. Psychol.* **1979**, *52*, 129–148. [CrossRef]
57. Rout, U.; Cooper, C.; Rout, J. Job stress among british general practitioners: Predictors of job dissatisfaction and mental ill-health. *Stress Med.* **1996**, *12*, 155–166. [CrossRef]
58. Wilson, D.M.C.; Nielsen, E.; Ciliska, N. Lifestyle Assessment: Testing the FANTASTIC Instrument. *Can. Fam. Physician* **1984**, *30*, 1863–1866.
59. CSEF—Canadian Society for Exercise Physiology. *The Canadian Physical Activity, Fitness and Lifestyle Appraisal: CSEP's Guide to Health Active Living*, 2nd ed.; CSEF: Ottawa, ON, Canada, 2003.
60. Machul, M.; Bieniak, M.; Chałdaś-Majdańska, J.; Bąk, J.; Chrzan-Rodak, A.; Mazurek, P.; Pawłowski, P.; Makuch-Kuśmierz, D.; Obuchowska, A.; Bartoszek, A.; et al. Lifestyle Practices, Satisfaction with Life and the Level of Perceived Stress of Polish and Foreign Medical Students Studying in Poland. *Int. J. Environ. Res. Public Health* **2020**, *17*, 4445. [CrossRef]
61. Smallwood, N.; Karimi, L.; Pascoe, A.; Bismark, M.; Putland, M.; Johnson, D.; Dharmage, S.C.; Barson, E.; Atkin, N.; Long, C.; et al. Coping strategies adopted by Australian frontline health workers to address psychological distress during the COVID-19 pandemic. *Gen. Hosp. Psychiatry* **2021**, *72*, 124–130. [CrossRef]
62. Cai, Q.; Feng, H.; Huang, J.; Wang, M.; Wang, Q.; Lu, X.; Xie, Y.; Wang, X.; Liu, Z.; Hou, B.; et al. The mental health of frontline and non-frontline medical workers during the coronavirus disease 2019 (COVID-19) outbreak in China: A case-control study. *J. Affect. Disord.* **2020**, *275*, 210–215. [CrossRef]

63. Ramzi, N.S.A.; Deady, M.; Petrie, K.; Crawford, J.; Harvey, S.B. Help-seeking for depression among Australian doctors. *Intern. Med. J.* **2020**, *51*, 2069–2077. [CrossRef]
64. Montgomery, A.J.; Bradley, C.; Rochfort, A.; Panagopoulou, E. A review of self-medication in physicians and medical students. *Occup. Med.* **2011**, *61*, 490–497. [CrossRef]
65. Lee, E.; Jeong, Y.M.; Yi, S.J. Nurses' Attitudes toward Psychiatric Help for Depression: The Serial Mediation Effect of Self-Stigma and Depression on Public Stigma and Attitudes toward Psychiatric Help. *Int. J. Environ. Res. Public Health* **2020**, *17*, 5073. [CrossRef]
66. Brown, S.P.; Westbrook, R.A.; Challagalla, G. Good Cope, Bad Cope: Adaptive and Maladaptive Coping Strategies Following a Critical Negative Work Event. *J. Appl. Psychol.* **2005**, *90*, 792–798. [CrossRef]
67. Nutley, S.K.; Falise, A.M.; Henderson, R.; Apostolou, V.; Mathews, A.C.; Striley, C.W. Impact of the COVID-19 Pandemic on Disordered Eating Behavior: Qualitative Analysis of Social Media Posts. *JMIR Ment. Health* **2021**, *8*, e26011. [CrossRef] [PubMed]
68. Wang, Y.; Wang, P. Perceived stress and psychological distress among chinese physicians: The mediating role of coping style. *Medicine* **2019**, *98*, e15950. [CrossRef] [PubMed]
69. Krok, D.; Zarzycka, B. Risk Perception of COVID-19, Meaning-Based Resources and Psychological Well-Being amongst Healthcare Personnel: The Mediating Role of Coping. *J. Clin. Med.* **2020**, *9*, 3225. [CrossRef]
70. Cooke, E.G.P.; Doust, A.J.; Steele, M.C. A survey of resilience, burnout, and tolerance of uncertainty in Australian general practice registrars. *BMC Med. Educ.* **2013**, *13*, 2. [CrossRef] [PubMed]
71. Guo, Y.-F.; Luo, Y.-H.; Lam, L.L.Y.; Cross, W.; Plummer, V.; Zhang, J.-P. Burnout and its association with resilience in nurses: A cross-sectional study. *J. Clin. Nurs.* **2018**, *27*, 441–449. [CrossRef] [PubMed]
72. Walsh, K. An Economic Argument for Investment in Physician Resilience. *Acad. Med.* **2013**, *88*, 1196. [CrossRef]
73. Kunzler, A.M.; Helmreich, I.; Chmitorz, A.; König, J.; Binder, H.; Wessa, M.; Lieb, K. Psychological interventions to foster resilience in healthcare professionals. *Cochrane Database Syst. Rev.* **2020**, *2020*, CD012527. [CrossRef]
74. La Torre, G.; Raffone, A.; Peruzzo, M.; Calabrese, L.; Cocchiara, R.A.; D'Egidio, V.; Leggieri, P.F.; Dorelli, B.; Zaffina, S.; Mannocci, A.; et al. Yoga and Mindfulness as a Tool for Influencing Affectivity, Anxiety, Mental Health, and Stress among Healthcare Workers: Results of a Single-Arm Clinical Trial. *J. Clin. Med.* **2020**, *9*, 1037. [CrossRef] [PubMed]

Journal of
Clinical Medicine

Review

New Recovery Strategies in Motor and Cognitive Functions, before, during and after Home-Confinement COVID-19, for Healthy Adults and Patients with Neurodegenerative Diseases: Review

Manuela Bacanoiu [1,†], Mircea Danoiu [1,†], Mihnea Marin [2,†], Mihai Robert Rusu [1,†] and Ligia Rusu [1,*,†]

1 Sport Medicine and Physical Therapy Department, University of Craiova, 200585 Craiova, Romania; manuela.bacanoiu@edu.ucv.ro (M.B.); mircea.danoiu@edu.ucv.ro (M.D.); mihai.rusu@edu.ucv.ro (M.R.R.)
2 Industrial Engineering Department, University of Craiova, 200585 Craiova, Romania; mihnea.marin@edu.ucv.ro
* Correspondence: ligia.rusu@edu.ucv.ro; Tel.: +40-723-867-738
† These authors contributed equally to this work.

Abstract: Distancing and confinement at home during the Coronavirus Disease 2019 (COVID-19) outbreak has led to worsening of motor and cognitive functions, both for healthy adults and for patients with neurodegenerative diseases. The decrease in physical activity, the cessation of the intervention of the recovery and the social distance imposed by the lockdown, has had a negative impact on the physical and mental health, quality of life, daily activities, as well as on the behavioral attitudes of the diet. The purpose of this paper was to evaluate the impact of decreasing physical activity and the affected emotional status in healthy adults and patients with neurodegenerative diseases in conditions imposed by the stay at home mandate of COVID-19, along with new interventions, such as telemedicine and telerehabilitation. These interventions include online surveys carried out in multi-languages, semi-structured interviews, intervention smartphones and interventions through online platforms, for instance: Google, WhatsApp, Twitter, ResearchGate, Facebook and LinkedIn. For this study, we selected original papers that were intensively processed using characteristics co-related with physical activity, mental wellbeing, sleep quality, good eating behavior and healthy lifestyle. By searching the last two years of literature, our review presents and demonstrates the benefit of online technological interventions in lockdown, which promote physical exercise patterns and rehabilitation techniques, for healthy adults and patients with neurodegenerative diseases, and the need to develop new strategic directions and governmental measures, designed procedures and health services, which are expected to improve the quality of life, the progress of physical and cognitive functions, mental health and wellbeing for all.

Keywords: pandemic COVID-19; neurodegenerative diseases; physical activity; public health strategies; healthy lifestyle behaviors; wellbeing; telerehabilitation

Citation: Bacanoiu, M.; Danoiu, M.; Marin, M.; Rusu, M.R.; Rusu, L. New Recovery Strategies in Motor and Cognitive Functions, before, during and after Home-Confinement COVID-19, for Healthy Adults and Patients with Neurodegenerative Diseases: Review. *J. Clin. Med.* **2022**, *11*, 597. https://doi.org/10.3390/jcm11030597

Academic Editors: Michele Roccella and Cristoforo Comi

Received: 16 December 2021
Accepted: 20 January 2022
Published: 25 January 2022

1. Introduction

A novel coronavirus named severe acute respiratory syndrome coronavirus 2 (SARS-CoV-2), and the disease called COVID-19, detected in China in December 2019, managed to affect over 200 countries in just 6 months, reporting over 10 million illnesses and over half a million deaths. The World Health Organization (WHO) declared a global pandemic in March 2020, thus causing worldwide concern. Therefore, all societies affected by the SARS-CoV-2 infection have gradually declared social distancing and home-confinement to prevent the spread of the new infection. According to Tondo et al. [1], the COVID-19 pandemic generates substantial changes in routine activities, restrictions of movement and has a considerable impact on people's psychological and cognitive levels. Furthermore, it creates challenges for the healthcare system. The main problems in dementia during this pandemic period are related to an increase of sufferers of cognitive impairment [1].

Under these conditions, the most drastic quarantine measures in human history were imposed [2]. This situation, imposed to slow the spread of COVID-19, has had negative effects on the quality of life, psychosocial and emotional behavior of individuals, even whether apparently healthy or with various associated diseases.

Due to social isolation and lack of direct communication, changes in emotional status have been reported, with the appearance of emotional disorders by way of feelings of loneliness, decreased personality (e.g., frustration, boredom, delusions, inadequate supplies) and distrust of peers [3–5].

Infection with SARS-CoV-2, which has caused severe acute respiratory syndrome and other distress for multiple organ failure, has affected a substantial number of patients with other comorbidities (such as Myasthenia Gravis, Vascular dementia) associated with neurodegenerative diseases, such as Parkinson's disease (PD), Alzheimer's disease, Frontotemporal dementia and Lewy body disease. Lack of therapeutic interventions, limiting access to specialized treatments, decreasing physical activity and help from caregivers and family during this period has aggravated functional abilities, cognitive impairments and behavioral disturbances [6].

During the isolation at home imposed by the COVID-19 pandemic, the needs for social assistance intervention increased, putting pressure on professional healthcare and home caregivers for patients with dementia [5]. Therefore, the imposed home confinement considerably restricted access to social and health services, which led to a worsening of behavioral and neuropsychological symptoms for them [6]. At the same time, a decrease in physical activity and limit of activity daily living (ADL), generate a change of lifestyle and life quality.

From this point of view, the promotion of a mental health and wellbeing lifestyle, involves continuing physical training. This means supporting movement skills, improving gait, increasing muscle strength and endurance, and prevents the progression of the disease in mild cognitive impairments (MCI). The challenge identified in the literature is that the COVID-19 outbreak has limited access to these activities due to isolation at home [7]. Hence, other interventions, such as aerobic exercises and home dance training had to be implemented to counteract the progressive deficiencies of patients with PD [8,9].

In addition to worsening motor and cognitive functions, the COVID-19 quarantine also impaired sleep quality, eating behavior affected mental wellbeing and induced depressive symptoms [10].

In the context of the COVID-19 outbreak, the need for modern digital therapies and those that are delivered remotely as well as their intervention at home have proven to be effective in the rehabilitation of patients with PD and other neurodegenerative disease. This could decrease the effect of motor skills, gait pattern, neuropsychiatric impairments and classic symptoms, such as tremor, bradykinesia, postural instability and freezing of gait [11]. The aim of the paper is to carry out a literature analyses regarding how the lockdown and physical activity influence motor and cognitive function, based on evaluation of the impact of decreasing physical activity, and the affected emotional status of healthy adults and patients with neurodegenerative diseases and associated comorbidities, such as Myastenia and Vascular dementia, in conditions imposed by COVID-19. The aim of the literature analysis includes a review of how the new interventions, such as telemedicine and telerehabilitation, could improve or maintain a healthy status, based on multi-language online surveys, semi-structured interviews and interventions on smartphones delivered through online platforms, for instance, Google, WhatsApp, Twitter, Research Gate, Facebook and LinkedIn. In our paper, we highlight the state of the art about what is written to date on the COVID-19 pandemic impact through the lives of healthy people and neurodegenerative disease patients.

Three questions guided the literature review: which physical activity has been chosen; what is the impact of the lockdown and decrease of physical activity under motor and cognitive aspects; and what is the impact of the interventions through telerehabilitation and telemedicine?

2. Materials and Methods

2.1. Selection Criteria

We searched in PUB MED electronic database the most relevant studies, using as keywords: "COVID-19 lockdown", "wellbeing lifestyle", "physical activity", "neurodegenerative diseases", "healthy policies" and "telerehabilitation". A literature search was conducted on 1 September 2021. The sorting of the papers was conducted in accordance with the PRISMA flow diagram [12]. In our paper, we selected the most relevant articles, which used modern digital methods and online surveys imposed by the global pandemic COVID-19 lockdown. The articles included the patients with motor and cognitive impairments from neurodegenerative diseases, who were deprived for a long period of time by planned physical exercise or of accessing specialized social assistance services. Additionally, we included the articles focused on healthy adolescents/adults involved in planned physical exercise during the lockdown. The considered publications covered the last 2 years, since the entire world was affected by the imposed lockdown in this time period. We considered only materials published in the English language.

2.2. Selection Strategy

In this synthesis, several aspects were taken into account: (1) individuals in the study groups with neurodegenerative diseases who had varying degrees of motor and non-motor impairments (some studies also included comorbidities such as Myasthenia and Vascular dementia); (2) randomized clinical trials with a large number of participants of both sexes were evaluated; (3) physical interventions and semi-structured interviews were conducted through online digital platforms; (4) PA (physical activity) consisted of planned exercises of low, moderate or vigorous intensity, which were applied both to healthy people and to patients with confirmed neurodegenerative impairments (the alteration of the emotional status) during the period of isolation at home; (5) considerable emphasis was placed on ADL, these being the most publicized during the COVID-19 lockdown; (6) both experimental and control groups were included in the study; (7) motor and cognitive evaluation of participants was performed using different tools for assessing the levels of disorder; (8) finally, the interventions through telerehabilitation and telemedicine were evaluated and guidelines were issued in the elaboration of new remote technological intervention strategies as well as the involvement of decision makers in health policies.

Exclusion criteria for these studies were: comorbidities other like recent surgery or physical participation in other public health services.

2.3. Affiliation of Collecting Significant Data

The electronic PUB MED database from the last 2 years was accessed using the keywords referring to the periods of home confinement imposed by SARS-CoV-2 outbreak. Articles were searched that referred to neurodegenerative diseases with motor and cognitive disorders; strategies for wellbeing of physical and mental life as well as remote rehabilitation through stimulating physical activities to increase the quality of life.

In this sense, 65 of the most representative papers from the PUB MED electronic database were selected. The papers focused on received interventions at home during the restrictions imposed by the COVID-19 pandemic, through online digital platforms or semi-structured interviews, regarding physical exercise programs, development daily household activities, online interviews regarding physical and mental state of the participants or eating habits approached during this period. After the elimination of duplicate papers, 64 studies remained to be scanned, and of these, another 16 papers that did not refer to neurodegenerative diseases were eliminated. Of the 48 full-text clinical trials and articles assessed for eligibility, 30 were excluded for the following reasons: 12 studies were systematic reviews, 1 paper was a case study, 6 papers were abstract studies, 7 studies were not free to access and 4 papers did not refer to physical activity. Thus, in the end, only 18 studies that addressed healthy adults and patients with: Parkinson's disease, Alzheimer's disease, Lewy body disease, Frontotemporal dementia and associated diseases (Vascular dementia, Myasthenia gravis), will be discussed for qualitative synthesis.

2.4. Model Quality Assessment

Several variables were used in the selection and extraction of data: (1) author and date of publication, classification of disease stages and changes in their evolution through motor and cognitive instruments, (2) pattern of physical therapies (intensity, frequency and types of physical activity), performed by individuals at home under the conditions imposed by SARS-CoV-2 infection, (3) intervention of digitally accessed platforms and questions from specialists and staff trained in specialized remote health services, and answers of participants regarding physical and emotional status, (4) methods used, results, discussions and conclusions from each paper.

3. Results

The graphical representation of the research dynamics is illustrated in Figure 1 of the PRISMA 2009 flow diagram [12]:

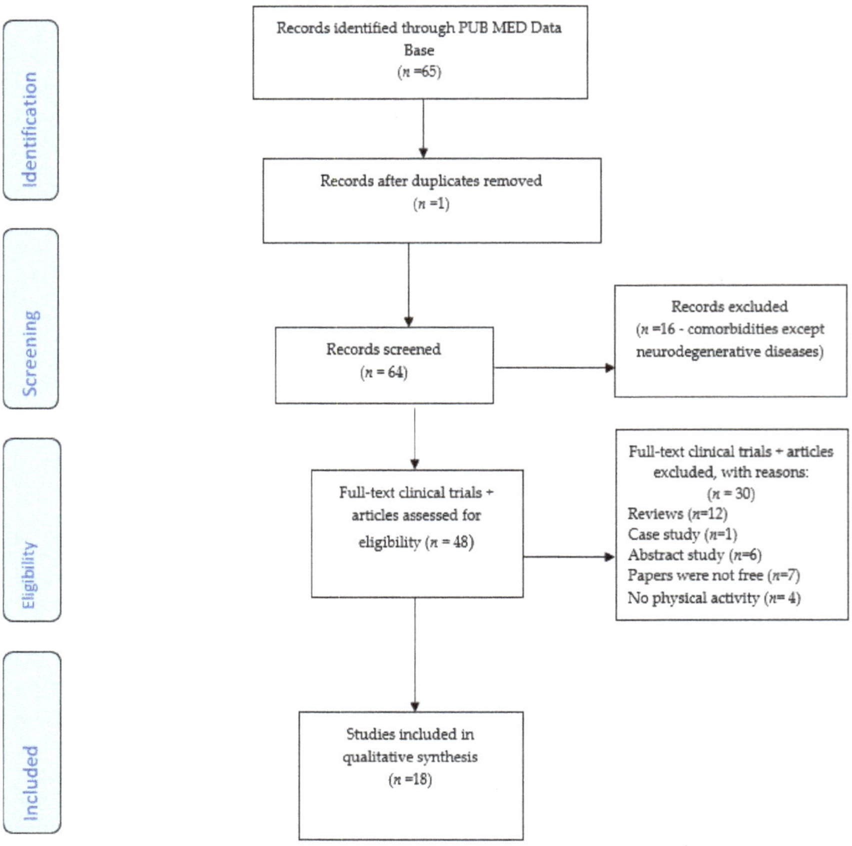

Figure 1. Prisma 2009. Flow diagram.

3.1. Tools/Variables Which Quantify Motor and Emotional Status in Healthy Adults during Home Confinement

Participation in social life or active integration in community activities improves everyone's mental health, increases self-control and self-efficacy by demonstrating psychological and social wellbeing [13].

The major concern in lockdown was to better quantify the decrease in physical activity and its negative impact of cognitive function and life quality.

Through semi-structured electronic studies and interviews launched on online platforms by specialized organizations, the participants' answers regarding mental wellbeing, the appearance and development of depressive symptoms as well as the comparison of situations before and during home confinement were requested.

The most relevant instruments for these purposes were: the Short Warwick–Edinburgh Mental. Wellbeing Scale (SWEMWBS), which assessed mental wellbeing [14] with a score between 7–35, and the superior shows considerable mental wellbeing; the Short Mood and Feelings Questionnaire (SMFQ), which demonstrated a depression measure where a high score means worsening psychic symptoms; the Short Life Satisfaction Questionnaire for Lockdowns (SLSQL), which quantifies the wellbeing of life [15]; the Short Social Participation Questionnaire for Lockdowns (SSPQOL) [15]; the social participation of individuals was quantified by the International Physical Activity Questionnaire Short Form (IPAQ-SF), which suggests participation in physical activity [15]; the Pittsburgh Sleep Quality Index (PSQI) [15], a tool that monitors sleep quality; the Short Diet Behaviors Questionnaire for Lockdowns (SDBQL), the scale that monitors eating habits [2]; the Short Technology use Behaviors Questionnaire for Lockdowns (STBQL), which provides demographic information and which allows psychological and social support [16]; and the Short Life Satisfaction Questionnaire for Lockdowns (SLSQOL) [16], framed as a score between 3 and 21, is a scale that measures the degree of satisfaction on the life of the respondents during the period of isolation at home, and the lowest scores appreciate a high degree of dissatisfaction in terms of active participation in social life. Decreasing socialization and communication with friends, neighbors, lack of visits to the respondents' homes or to other relatives of their families, changed mental wellbeing and altered emotional status with increased anxiety, loneliness or sadness [12] are all considered here.

In the four studies [13–16] with 1047 participants each, using ECBL (Effects of Home Confinement on psychosocial health status and multiple lifestyle behaviors- COVID-19), an electronic survey was delivered on Google platforms, such as mail, WhatsApp, Facebook, ResearchGate, Twitter, LinkedIn, translated in the several languages, questions were administered about lifestyle, daily activities, diet, rest and mental state of participants before and during home confinement. Individuals were about 54% female and 46% male and the percentages by geographical areas were as follows: 40% Africa, 36% Asia, 21% Europe and 3% others.

For instance, in one of the four papers, the most significant tools used were: *SWEMWBS* who assessed the functioning of mental wellbeing with a score range between 7–35, so that the low values represented a low mental wellbeing and the higher ones appreciated a high functioning of the psychic status and SMFQ scale, which measures degree of depression (0–26). Thus, a total score greater than (>12) indicated altered emotional status that indicate the presence of depression.

In another study that used the platform of ECLB COVID-19, monitoring was carried out on physical training through evaluation activities daily living (ADL), exercise class or gym class home-based. The basic tools used were SSPQOL who evaluated the social participation before and during home confinement, so that the 14 items in the questionnaires were based on the active participation of the respondents in social life. The range of scale was established between 15–70, so the higher scores, the more active the participation in social life in various ways was. Another variable, SLSQOL, used a questionnaire with answers and evaluated satisfaction life, and the score between 3–21 estimated the degrees of satisfaction or dissatisfaction. The lower scores showed different levels of disagreement and upper scores translated to being extremely satisfied. The other tools used were *SWEMWBS*, SMFQ, IPAQ-SF and PSQI, that estimated decreasing mental wellbeing, impairing sleep quality, changes in physical activity in the sense of decreasing it, or altering emotional status, with serious psychological consequences [14].

Another paper that used the questionnaire delivered through ECLB COVID-19, discussed IPAQ-SF guidelines, the variable, which quantified physical exercises of different intensity, estimating the time spent weekly a physical training, including time spent standing. Several categories of physical activities were performed, such as vigorous physical exercises with aerobic exercises or fast bicycling, moderate physical exercises meaning carrying light loads or cycling at normal speed, walking training and finally the time spent in the last 7 days sitting. In this sense, answers were requested for two sets of questions related to the different categories of physical activities performed during seven days, one addressed to young people and adults able to perform vigorous and moderate PA and the second set was delivered to older adults who did walking training and spent time sitting. The second tool used was SDBQ-L, which assessed diet behavior before and during the home confinement period. The requests in the questionnaires addressed five issues: (1) unhealthy food, (2) snacking between meals or late at night, (3) excessive alcohol consumption, (4) overeating and (5) a high number of meals/day. The trend observed during isolation at home is to address unhealthy eating habits that lead to weight gain, impaired health and wellbeing [15].

The scores of variables SWEMWBS, SMFQ and SLSQL, were significantly altered during isolation at home imposed by pandemic restrictions by altering mental wellbeing, increasing depressive states, accentuate nervousness, disorders of sleep, or changes in emotional status with accentuate sadness, feelings of loneliness, uselessness and personal dissatisfaction [16]. The scores from the other tools, including IPAQ-SF, SDBQL, PSQI, STBQ-L, SSPQ-L and SLSQL, demonstrated psychosocial impact imposed by home confinement, and the importance for technology intervention involved in active and healthy lifestyle.

Another article studied the impact of home confinement on the wellbeing of mental health correlated with physical activities performed at home of different intensities, eating habits acquired during the isolation period but also with the quality of sleep in Arabian communities. The impairment of mental well-being was more pronounced in Arab women (53.9%) compared to men (46.1%). In terms of the quality of the diet obtained through questionnaires, the highest score means maintaining mental wellbeing through the use of good meals and food. The quality of sleep was assessed through a range between 0 and 21 points with PSQI scale, so that the maximum values were associated with sleep disorders during the period of isolation at home affecting mental status. For physical activity, which was evaluated through IPAQ with seven items, the questioning proved that in the case of performing moderate and vigorous physical activity (measured by the distribution metabolic equivalents minutes per week (MET), wellbeing mental is improves. Furthermore, it was associated with increasing aerobic physical exercise and endurance physical activity [17].

Increased depression, anxiety, sleep disturbances, disturbances of attention or psychological changes were discussed in another study conducted in adolescents, through the excessive use of social networks and dangerous exposures to them, such as cyber bulling, sexting in desire of communication and compression of social distancing during the quarantine of COVID-19.

However, there was a greater resistance of adolescents to external stressors as there was an effective alternative to promote socialization, minimize social distance, by using online technology that they mastered very well. Monitoring was performed by counting text and chat messages that were sent or received from online platforms during the lockdown. There were even very well maintained physical activities at home, promoted sustained periods of time or daily activities that improved the physical and culinary performance of the participants. Relationships between participants and other family members were greatly improved during this period, and eating habits were much healthier than during direct socialization [18].

Physical Activity in Healthy Adults during Home Confinement

The physical activity (PA) has been studied in terms of types of physical activity and is presented in Figure 2.

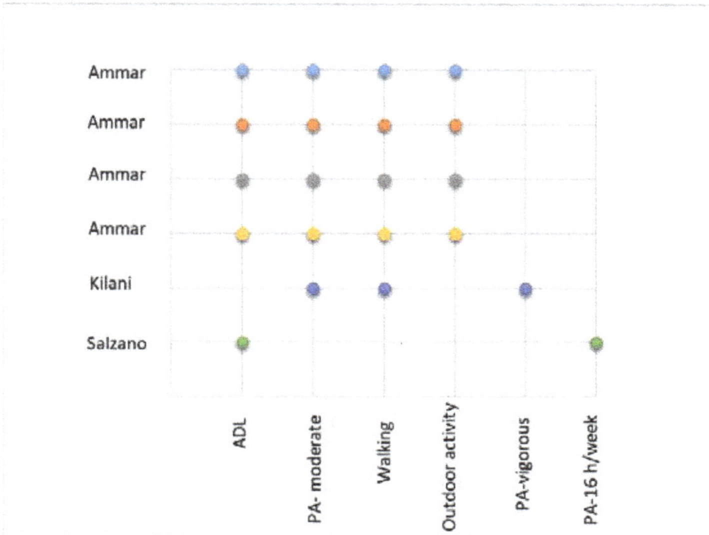

Figure 2. Type of physical activity (ADL: Activity of Daily Living) for healthy people [12–17].

We illustrate in Table 1, the instruments discussed, the characteristics, the physical activities performed, the interventions and the conclusions derived from the clinical trials studied at healthy adults:

Table 1. Summary of the characteristics, physical exercise, main tools and interventions with healthy adults.

Authors	Individuals	Characteristics	Age/Gender	Physical Exercise	Tools	Interventions	Conclusions
Ammar A. et al. (2020) [14]	1047 individuals	- ECBL-COVID-19—online survey multi-languages - AHCL—Active and Healthy confinement lifestyle - before and during COVID-19	Adults 54% female 46%—male 36%—Asia, 40%—Africa, 21%—Europe, 3%—other	- ADL - Exercise class - Gym class	- SWEMWBS (1–35) - SMFQ (0–26) - SLSQL - SSPQOL - IPAQ-SF - SDBQL - PSQI - STBQL	- Online platforms: - Mail - WhatsApp - Facebook - ResearchGate - Twitter - LinkedIn	- Decreasing mental wellbeing in home confinement, - Increasing depression symptoms (≥12) - Changing in sleep quality, satisfaction life, physical activity, social participation, - Enhancing mood and bad feelings.
Ammar A. et al. (2020) [15]	1047 individuals	- ECBL-COVID-19 -online survey multi-languages - before and during COVID-19	Adults 54% female 46%—male 36%—Asia, 40%—Africa, 21%—Europe, 3%—other	- Physical exercise with vigorous, moderate intensity training - Walking activity	- SWEMWBS - SMFQ - SLSQL - IPAQ-SF - SDBQL (0–15) - PSQI - -STBQ-L	- Google online	- Declining of duration time for weekly physical activity, - Increasing negative impact for diet behaviors in the sense of augmentingn snack consumptions between meals, enhancing alcohol intake, increasing the number of daily meals;an unhealthy diet is important indicator for sedentary lifestyle.
Ammar A. et al. (2020) [13]	1047 individuals	- ECBL-COVID-19 -online survey multi-languages - before and during COVID-19	Adults 54%—female 46%—male 36%—Asia, 40%—Africa, 21%—Europe, 3%—other	- ADL	- SWEMWBS - SMFQ - SLSQL - IPAQ-SF - SDBQL - PSQI - STBQ-L - SSPQ-L (14–70) - SLSQL (3–21)	- Online platforms: - Mail - WhatsApp - Facebook - ResearchGate - Twitter - LinkedIn	- Decreasing friends, neighbors direct intercommunication in lockdown period with strongly mental implication for individuals, - Developing socialization on online communication platforms.

Table 1. *Cont.*

Authors	Individuals	Characteristics	Age/Gender	Physical Exercise	Tools	Interventions	Conclusions
Ammar A. et al. (2020) [16]	1047 individuals	- ECBL-COVID-19 -online survey multi-languages - before and during COVID-19 - Cardiovascular risk	Adults 54%—female 46%—male 36%—Asia, 40%—Africa, 21%—Europe, 3%—other	- Outdoor or indoor physical activity	- SWEMWBS - SMFQ - SLSQL - IPAQ-SF - SDBQL - PSQI - STBQ-L - SSPQ-L - SLSQL	- Online platforms: - Mail - WhatsApp - Facebook - ResearchGate - Twitter - LinkedIn - Smart phone - Watch	- Disrupting wellbeing and satisfaction life, communication, - Developing mental disorders, anxiety, sadness, mood, states of accentuated nervousness during quarantine. - Increasing tensions for individuals which were retired or unemployment comparative with before lockdown period when they were workers, - Encouraging wellbeing for promoting a healthy lifestyle by participating in physical activities at home or in organized groups keeping the rules of distance imposed by the pandemic and hygiene.
Kilani H.A. et al. (2020) [17]	1723 participans	- Arabian communities - Health status - Mental wellbeing - Dietary behavior - PA - Sleep quality	32.2 years 806-female 37.4 years 917-male	- Walking - Moderate physical activity - Vigorously activity - MET	- lower mental score - female - good dietary quality - sleeping score - FFQ - IPAQ - WHO-5 - PSQI	- Online - Google - WhatsApp - Facebook - ResearchGate - Twitter - LinkedIn	- Decreasing mental wellbeing at female against male, - Increasing sleep quality at both gender corelated with good quality diet, - Significant improving mental health, cognition functions in the conditions of maintaining a sustained physical activity such as: walking, moderate and vigorous physical exercise.

Table 1. *Cont.*

Authors	Individuals	Characteristics	Age/Gender	Physical Exercise	Tools	Interventions	Conclusions
Salzano G. et al. (2021) [18]	1860 youth	- Lower secondary school - Upper secondary school	12–18 years Female—61.7% Male—38.3%	- Physical activity (1 h-6 h/week) - ADL (cooking, gardening, household activities)	- Average number of text or chat mes-sages/100 day	- Web-based survey - Personal computers - Smartphones - Tablets - Instagram - Facebook - Tik Tok - Snapchat	- Increasing physical activity indoor during lockdown - Good mental resistance in stay-at-home mandate with skills acquiring of new skills - Altering circadian rhyme sleep/wake due to intense use of media platforms for intense global socialization and the maintenance of friendships and emotional status on social networks - Increasing anxiety, depression and other psychological disorders through excessive use of social networks that can promote cyberbullying and sexting - In terms of eating, no unhealthy eating habits were acquired due to the lack of training in the communities and the consumption of small meals, snacks, sweets, excess juices; on the contrary the promotion of cooked meals and healthier foods at home was observed.

ECBL: Effects of Home Confinement on multiple lifestyle behaviors; SWEMWBS: Short Warwick–Edinburgh Mental Wellbeing Scale; SMFQ: Short Mood and Feelings Questionnaire; SLSQL: Short Life Satisfaction Questionnaire for Lockdowns; SSPQOL: Short Social Participation Questionnaire for Lockdowns; IPAQ-SF: International Physical Activity Questionnaire Short Form; SDBQL: Short Diet Behaviors Questionnaire for Lockdowns; PSQI: Pittsburgh Sleep Quality Index; STBQL: Short Technology-use Behaviors Questionnaire for Lockdowns; SSPQ-L: Short Social Participation Questionnaire-Lockdowns; SLSQ-L: Short Life Satisfaction Questionnaire for Lockdowns; EQ-5D-5L: Euro QoL-5 dimensions; ADL: Activity of Daily Living; HADS: Hospital Anxiety and Depression Scale; FFQ: Food Frequency Questionnaire; WHO-5: World Health Organization—wellbeing score.

According to Ammar [16], significant increases in uses of the technology allowing the development of PA during home confinement were observed. Mood and feeling has a negative correlation with PA participation, but life satisfaction has a positive correlation with PA. Moreover, the anxiety, depression and other psychological issues during COVID-19 are related with physical activity and its role on the immune function.

Furthermore, Kilani [17] speaks about PA, which could be considered to be a very good predictor of mental wellbeing score and health status, but this depends on PA intensity.

3.2. *Tools/Variables Which Quantify Motor and Emotional Status at Patients with Neurodegenerative Diseases during Lockdown*

Neurodegenerative diseases are pathologies characterized by progressive dysfunction and neuronal damages due to the accumulation of proteins with altered biochemical properties. This process causes changes in neural interconnections affecting movement, speech, memory, intelligence and other brain functions, in accordance with the areas where changes occur in the central nervous system. Neurodegenerative diseases are associated with progressive cognitive and motor decline, having negative social, economic and financial impact, especially as the disease progresses.

In addition to the pathophysiology of neurodegenerative diseases, there are other risk factors that can aggravate and accelerate their evolution, such as lack of physical activity, sedentary lifestyle, weight gain/obesity or the association of other comorbidities (diabetes, atherosclerosis, hypertension). All these impediments to lifestyle, physical activity, eating habits, interpersonal communication and access to public health services were present during the periods of home regimentation imposed by the fight against the spread of coronavirus disease (COVID-19) [19].

As in the case of healthy adults, for patients with neurodegenerative diseases, specific online platforms were developed with questionnaires, semi-structured interviews or other telerehabilitation interventions at home. It was thus possible to quantify the progression of motor impairments induced by the decrease of controlled exercise training led by therapists, and alteration of cognitive status due to the lack of communication and social distance imposed during the period of isolation at home.

The following tools were used to assess the impact on emotional status, cognitive functions impairments, sleeping disorders and quality of life in home confinement: the Mini-mental Scale Examination (MMSE), which evaluates cognitive functions impairments [20–22]; the Montreal Cognitive Assessment (MOCA) [23]; the Geriatric -Depression Scale (GDS) [24,25]; Beck Depression Inventory-II (BDI-II), with score from 0 to 63, and high values means an increasing level of depression [26,27]; the Cognitive Emotion Regulation Questionnaire (CERQ) [28]; Social Support (SOZU-K) [29]; the Brief Resilience Scale (BRS) [30]; State Trait Anxiety Inventory (STAI); Optimist-5 point Scale; Quality of Life (QOL); Hoehn and Yahr (HY), Quality of Life short version (SF-8); Mental Component Summary (MCS); Motor experiences daily living (UPDRS) [10]; New-onset/worsening of sleep (NOWS), Restless legs syndrome (RLS), REM Sleep Behavior Disorder (REMBD), Item Content Validity Index (I-CVI), Scale Content Validity Index (S-CVI), Scale content validity Index Universal agreement (S-CVI-UA); Likert Scale; Sleep Disordered Breathing (SDB) [31].

Other variables reflect declining physical activity during lockdown, such as Physical Activity Readiness Questionnaire (PAR-Q), Physical Activity Level (PALs) [19,32], Physical Activity Scale for the elderly (PASE), Physical Activity Level (PALs), Physical Activity Readiness Questionnaire (PAR-Q), Physical Activity Scale for the elderly (PASE) [13,32] and Metabolic equivalents minutes/week (MET) [33].

Other tools can assess signs and symptoms of neurodegenerative diseases related to motor and cognitive dysfunctions well as their changes during the period of social isolation imposed by the spread of SARS infection—Cov-2: for Alzheimer' Disease; these include the Consortium to Establish a Registry for Alzheimer's Disease (CERAD-Plus) [19], the Clinical Dementia Rating Scale (CDR) [34], Hamilton Depression Rating (HAMD), Epworth

Sleepiness Scale (ESS), Activities Daily Living (ADL) and Neuropsychiatric Inventory (NPI) [35].

Another autoimmune neurodegenerative disease which affects acetylcholine receptors from the level of the postsynaptic membrane of the end plate, Myasthenia gravis, was monitored through MG Quality of Life (MGQOL15), MG Activity of Daily Living (MGADL, Myasthenia Gravis Foundation of America staging (MGFA Scale), Hospital Anxiety and Depression Scale HADS) with a score range between 0–21, where increased values mean worsening depression and anxiety [36].

In Parkinson's Disease (PD), the neuropathological mechanism entails the loss of pigmented dopaminergic from the brain nuclei belonging to the black substance of the midbrain with production of atypical proteins, called Lewy bodies, subsequently altering the cortico-thalamo-cortical pathways with pathological consequences on the motor and cognitive behavior of the body. Therefore, motor deficiencies such as tremor, bradykinesia, gait disorders and stiffness as well as cognitive impairments, could be quantified through the Personalized Parkinson Project (PPP) [37]; Perceived Stress Scale (PSS) [38]; Unified Parkinson's Disease Rating Scale (UPDRS); Parkinson Anxiety Scale (PAS); Ruminative Response Scale (RRS) [4]; Physical Component Summary (PCS); Patient global impression of change Scale (PGIC), a scale with a score between 1 to 7, which investigates changes in motor and non-motor disorders in Parkinson's Disease; Hospital Anxiety and Depression Scale HADS) [10] and Sleep-Scales for Outcomes Parkinson's Disease (SCOPA-sleep) [39].

In four papers, monitoring patients with MCI has demonstrated the importance of intervention in various ways of physical activity delivered through online platforms, telephone interviews, or with dedicated applications on mental, affective and motor status. So, for 12 older adults of which six women and six men, with mild cognitive impairment, each carrying a polar heart sensor network, and for 8 weeks participated in a fitness and dance training program (two sessions of 90 min/week) delivered through the DIADEM platform, demonstrated improved cardiac performance, benefits in mental functions and enhanced motor status with better walking speed and step length. Monitoring was performed by heart rate recordings and by using the following instruments: MMSE, PAR-Q, GDS and CERAD-Plus [19]. During the pandemic lockdown, such interventions can efficiently compensate for the detraining due to combating the spread of coronavirus disease, while maintaining adequate muscle tone and motor skills.

For 177 older adults with mild cognitive impairment (50), Alzheimer' disease (105) and dementia with Lewy bodies, which performed activities daily living (ADL) stimulated by caregivers, demonstrated delayed mental and physical deterioration. Monitoring was demonstrated by evaluation of the scores of MOCA, NPI, HAMD, and ESS tools [35]. Another study investigated by telephone semi-structured interview, 4710 patients of which 2809 female and 1901 male, split in 2355 pairs with caregivers, with Alzheimer' disease, Dementia with Lewy body disease, Frontotemporal dementia and Vascular dementia, which performed activities daily living (ADL). Monitoring was performed through CDR. In this situation, increased caregivers stress risk has been estimated for patients, due to clinical features, lifestyle, dislike of continuity in medical care and deterioration of mental and emotional status of patients with dementia during restrictions imposed by spread SARS-CoV-2 infection. A prospective study discusses the importance of continuing physical activity at home during isolation in the COVID-19 pandemic. This includes moderate effort activity for 150 min/week, 75 min. of sustained effort/week and a strength training intervention provided by an app-based workout with online partners. The measurement of beneficial effects could be carried out through MET and the study includes participants of over 40% Latin America female, Caribbean female and other males and females in developed countries [33].

In another paper, 38 patients with moderate Myasthenia Gravis (not associated with COVID-19), were treated with prednisolone and azathioprine, and physical exercise training consisting of walking, yoga and moderate physical activity delivered through online platforms. Evaluation was carried out by specific tools: MGFA, MGQOL 15, MGADL,

HADS and PSQI, which demonstrated worsening wellbeing life quality, anxiety and depression during home confinement [36].

In seven other studies, the evolution of patients with Parkinson's Disease in the restrictive period imposed by the COVID-19 pandemic was followed. A total of 88 older adults with PD were divided into an experimental (45) and control group (43). Phone interviews were carried out about ADL during lockdown using the specific tools: PASE, HADS and PALs. Evaluation revealed worsening motor impairments with increasing dyskinesia, tremor, freezing of gait, instability stance, muscles pain, rigidity and cognitive disorders, which were augmented sleep dysfunction, depression, anxiety, feeling stressed, lack of concentration and attention [36]. In another paper, investigations were carried out in 832 patients with PD, who were performing moderate walking training for one hour/day. The authors discuss the increasing motor and non-motor impairments during isolation at home assessed by RLS, REMBD, NOWS, I-CVI, S-CVI, S-CVI-UA, Likert Scale, VAS and the SDB scale. Through following these instruments, changes were evaluated in sleep quality, degrees of depression, anxiety, mood and poor life quality [31].

Another study with 100 older adults (45 women and 55 men with PD in the experimental group) and 100 caregivers, were assessed through online questionnaires about physical activity during the imposed home isolation required to combat the spread of COVID-19. The variables used showed, in particular, the alteration of the MCS score in females with PD due to weight loss, lack of exercise (37%) or unhealthy behavioral habits; for caregivers, there were serious concerns (47%) regarding the decrease in PCS score, through increasing stressors, smoking or changes in emotional and affective status during lockdown [10].

In a preliminary study on the stay at home mandate, a self-questionnaire was carried out with 36 patients by mobile based-neurocognitive assessment with PD, of which 53.6% were female and 46.4% were male, regarding physical activity/week, number of active days and average time allocated for physical exercise. Motor and neurocognitive patterns were quantified and performed by using the scales: MTA, MCA, NFI, SWCT and MMSE, which found decreases in motor skills, speech neurocognitive tasks and wellbeing life quality in approximately 80% of the patients with PD [40].

Another paper investigated the impact of the stay at home mandate for 517 adults with PD subject to an international online study, carried out over the course of 12 weeks, in 14 languages with a 64-item questionnaire. The Parkinson's patients were interrogated on online platforms about weekly physical activity from light physical activity to vigorous physical training and were assessed through SWEMWBS (7–35), PSQI and IPAQ-SF scales. The results showed declining motor functions, quality of sleep, negative feelings and worsening wellbeing of emotional and affective conditions. However, unlike young counterparts, there was greater resistance to stressors during lockdown and greater emotional resistance to older adults with PD [41].

The association of an external stressor, such as the COVID-19 pandemic, has worsened the motor and cognitive symptoms shown with 358 Parkinson's patients (38.5% female and 62.5% male) who participated in an online study with cognitive and psychological measurements. Patients participated in physical activity for 4 h/week, and their evaluation through PPP, PSS, PAS, RRS, BRS, CERQ, MoCA, SCOPA-sleep, STAI and BDI-II demonstrated worsening motricity with augmentation tremors, rigidity, pain, instability balance, and impairments of gait, but also aggravation of mental, emotional and sleep disorders [39].

The impact of the COVID-19 lockdown was evaluated with a web-based survey for 142 PD patients, of whom 41% were female and 50% were male, belonging to a community dwelling. They performed ADL and walking training. The instruments used for evaluation in quarantine were PAM-13 (0–100 score), which is a validated self-reported questionnaire measuring confidence, self-management, motor skills and cognition. Evaluation using a four-point Likert Scale demonstrated negative impact for 37.3% of the cases. The need for social care for these patients was found to be effective, especially due to the period of restrictions imposed by the COVID-19 pandemic, as approximately 24.8% of participants need caregivers [42].

The literature reveals substantial information about types of PA that were agreed upon by patients with neurodegenerative diseases.

Physical Activity in Neurodegenerative Diseases (MCI, AD, DLB, MG FTD and PD)

Physical activity (PA) has been studied in terms of types of physical activity and is presented in Figure 3.

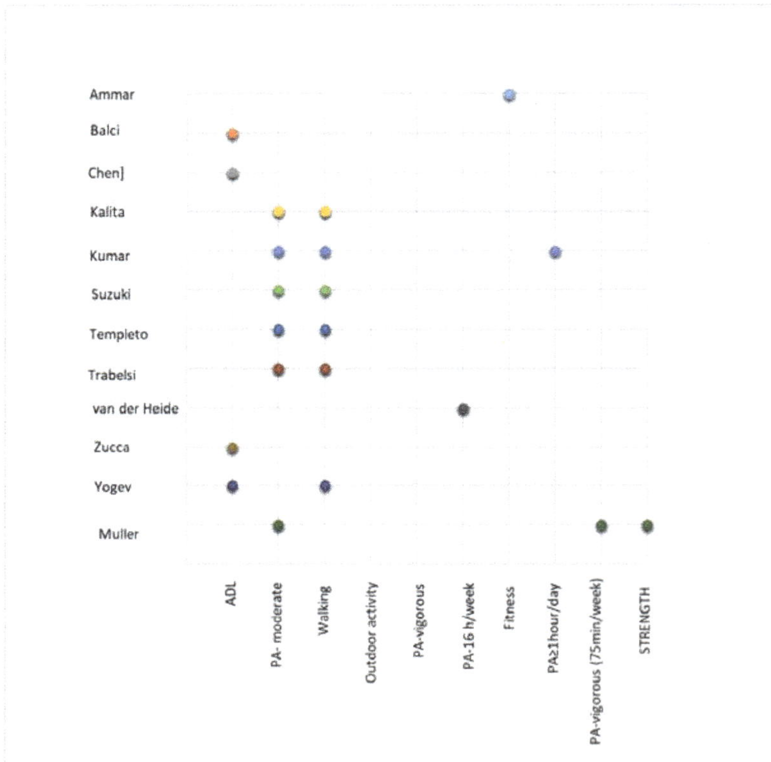

Figure 3. Type of physical activity for patients with neurodegenerative diseases [9,13,26,30–35,38,39,41].

Table 2 presents the tools discussed, the characteristics, physical activities performed, interventions and conclusions derived from the studies on patients with neurodegenerative diseases.

Table 2. Summary of the characteristics, physical exercise, main tools and interventions for patients with neurodegenerative diseases.

Authors	Individuals	Characteristics	Age/Gender	Physical Exercise	Tools	Interventions	Conclusions
Ammar A., et al. (2021) [14]	12 individuals	- MCI (mild cognitive impairment)	Older adults 6—female 6—male	- 8 weeks fitness training dance training - 2 sessions/90 min/week - DIADEM training program	- HR-Heart Rate - MMSE (24–27) - PAR-Q - GDS - CERAD Plus	- Polar heart rate sensor (H10) - Wireless polar team	- Improving performance cardiac at patients with MCI after physical exercise training, - Increasing physical performance regarding speed gait and length of step, - Continuing home-based physical training in social distancing rules during lockdown with important benefits for mental and physical functions.
Balci B., et al. (2021) [32]	88 individuals - experimental group (n = 45) - control group (n = 43)	Parkinson's Disease (PD)	Older adults	ADL	Increasing: - Tremor - Dyskinesia - Rigidity - Freezing of gait - Instability postural - Sleep impairments - Muscle pain - PASE - HADS - PALs	- Phone interview	- Augmentation of non-motor and motor functions at PD patients during quarantine, - Increasing anxiety and depression through distancing, detraining and worse socialisation during confinement home.

Table 2. *Cont.*

Authors	Individuals	Characteristics	Age/Gender	Physical Exercise	Tools	Interventions	Conclusions
Chen Z.C., et al. (2021) [33]	105-AD 50-MCI 22-DBL	- MCI - Alzheimer' disease (AD) - DLB-dementia with Lewy body disease	Older adults	- ADL	- MMSE - MOCA - NPI - HAMD - ESS	- CT scans - MRI - PET-positron emission tomography	- During lockdown and stay at home, caregivers should help patients with cognitive impairment and dementia to maintain exercise routines training home based of a certain intensity and frequency and to maintaining socialisation with friends and relatives by phone and another network. - Telerehabilitation should be one of the most advantageous interventions during quarantine to prevent the evolution of mental and physical impairment in patients with MCI.
Kalita J., et al. (2021) [36]	38 individuals with MG (myasthenia gravis) non COVID-19	- MG - Treatment with prednisolone and azathioprine	45 yrs	Physical exercise training: - yoga - walking - moderate physical activity	- MGFA - MGQOL15 (0–4) - MGADL - HADS (0–21) - PSQI	- Phone interviews - Whats app.	- Decreasing quality of life through detraining of physical activity, - Aggravation of physical and mental dysfunctions of patients with MG in the conditions imposed by lockdown.

Table 2. *Cont.*

Authors	Individuals	Characteristics	Age/Gender	Physical Exercise	Tools	Interventions	Conclusions
Kumar N., et al. (2021) [31]	832 individuals	- PD-Parkinson disease >7 years - Home confinement - questionnaire - Sleep disturbance - Features suggestive of RLS - Features of REMBD - Sleep disorders - Worsened motor features - Worsened non-motor features	>50 years	- walking - moderate physical activity - >1 h/day	- RLS - REMBD - NOWS - Likert Scale - I-CVI - S-CVI - S-CVI-UA - VAS - SDB	- Phone - Screen time	- During COVID-19 pandemic, quarantine determined the worsening of sleep disorders at all PD' patients, - Increasing motor and non-motor impairments due to lacking physical activity, poor life quality, sleep disorders.
Suzuki K., et al. (2021) [10]	- experimental group- - (n = 100 PD) - control group-caregivers (n = 100 caregivers)	- Parkinson's disease - HY (2/3) - Comorbidities - Motor and cognitive impairments	>72 years 45-male 55-female	- physical activity	- PGIC (1–7) - QOL - HADS - PCS - MCS - SF-8	Online platform with delivering questionnaires	- Increasing severity signs and symptoms of PD' patients regarding pattern gait, rigidity, tremor and disturbances sleep, - Enhancing anxiety, depression, mood, attention impairments at PD, - Decreasing physical activity in lockdown had negative impact for daily and walking activities, being associated with important motor disorders.

Table 2. *Cont.*

Authors	Individuals	Characteristics	Age/Gender	Physical Exercise	Tools	Interventions	Conclusions
Templeton J.M., et al. (2021) [40]	28 patients—self-questionnaire 8 patients—mobile based neurocognitive	- Parkinson's disease - Self-reporting - Functional assessment	>52 years - 46.4%—male - 53.6%—female	- Physical activity/week - number of active days on week - average time physical activity	- Number of active days - Number of active minutes - Number of activities - Average temporal metrics - Likert Scale (1–5) - MMSE - MCA - MTA - SWCT - NFI	- Self-reporting questionnaire - Mobile-based neurocognitive measurements	- Decreasing controlled physical activity in stay at home mandate (SaHM) caused worsening, moderately or higher, of at least one PD symptoms individuals (80%), - Increasing interval by at least two times in which the objective actions are completed, - Reducing wellbeing lifestyle, motor and speech neurocognitive tasks in home confinement.
Trabelsi K., et al. (2021) [27]	517 individuals	- Parkinson disease - International online survey - (64 items)—12 week in 14 languages - PA - Diet - Sleep - Social participation - Psychosocial - support	>55 years	- -Weekly physical activity - (walking training low, moderate and vigorous physical exercise, MET)	- SWEMWBS (7–35) - PSQI - IPAQ-SF	- Online platforms	- Keeping constant on mental wellbeing during stay at home mandate, whereas elderly patients with PD are more emotionally resistant being more accustomed to stressors than young counterparts, - Decreasing level homework activities because of lack of physical exercise, which means worsening motor functions, - Declining sleep quality in lockdown and the appearance of other disturbances which induced negative emotions and more frustration.

Table 2. *Cont.*

Authors	Individuals	Characteristics	Age/Gender	Physical Exercise	Tools	Interventions	Conclusions
van der Heide A., et al. (2020) [39]	358 individuals	- PD - Collection blood, stool and cerebrospinal fluid - MRI	>53 years - Male (62.5%) - Female (38.5%)	>4 h PA/week	- UPDRS - anxiety - stressor load - personality features - PPP - PSS - PAS - RRS - BRS - CERQ - MoCA - SCOPA-sleep - STAI - BDI-II	- Google platforms - Online survey (motor, cognitive and psychological measurements)	- Worsening motor symptoms such as tremor, rigidity, pattern gait, pain and postural instability, - Increasing change in emotional status induced by stressor load related COVID-19 outbreak, - Enhancing neuropsychiatric symptoms such as: depression, anxiety, mood, ruminations through decreasing physical activity.
Zucca M., et al. (2021) [34]	4710 (2355-pairs) - Caregivers - Patients with dementia	- Mild dementia - (AD, DLB, VaD, FTD) - Stress symptoms - (anxiety, irritability, overwhelmed, anguish, - abandonment)	>46 years Male—1901 Female—2809	ADL	- CDR	- Phone semi-structured interview	- Increasing stress symptoms (one symptom—90% or more symptoms—30%) of caregivers with dementia patients linked of consequences COVID-19, - Enhancing conflicting relationship and discontinuity in assistance for female caregivers with dementia patients in time lockdown.

Table 2. *Cont.*

Authors	Individuals	Characteristics	Age/Gender	Physical Exercise	Tools	Interventions	Conclusions
Yogev-Seligmann G., et al. (2021) [42]	142 individuals	- PD - Lockdown - Community dwellings	>63 years Male—59% Female—41%	- ADL - walking training	- Current functional status - Health - Medical care - Wellbeing in quarantine - PAM-13 (0–100) - Four-point Likert Scale	- Web-based survey	- Decreasing walking ability in 37.3% of cases, - Worsening of motor and cognitive disfunctions at PD' patients (43%), - increasing the need for care assistance for ADL (24.8%), - Enhancing neuropsychiatric symptoms such as depression, anxiety, tired, moody and loneliness (42%) - Discontinuity of rehabilitation treatments.
Müller P., (2020) [33]	>40% Latin America women >40% Caribbean women >40% male and women developed countries.	- Vascular dementia (AD)	>40% women >40% male	- 150 min moderate intensity effort physical/week - 75 min vigorous intensity effort physical/week - strength training/week	- MET - WHO	App-based training with online partners	- Worsening physical activity during isolation at home imposed by COVID-19 with negative results about primary and secondary vascular dementia, - Decreasing outdoor physical exercise represent a major problem of health public for people with Alzheimer' disease.

SWEMWBS: Short Warwick–Edinburgh Mental Wellbeing Scale; SMFQ: Short Mood and Feelings Questionnaire; SLSQL: Short Life Satisfaction Questionnaire for Lockdowns; IPAQ-SF: International Physical Activity Questionnaire Short Form; SDBQL: Short Diet Behaviors Questionnaire for Lockdowns; PSQI: Pittsburgh Sleep Quality Index; STBQL: Short Technology-use Behaviors Questionnaire for Lockdowns; SSPQ-L: Short Social participation questionnaire-lockdowns; MMSE: Mini-mental Scale Examination; PAR-Q: Physical activity Readiness Questionnaire; GDS: Geriatric Depression Scale; CERAD Plus: Consortium to Establish a Registry for Alzheimer's Disease; MOCA: Montreal Cognitive Assessment; NPI: Neuropsychiatric Inventory; HAMD: Hamilton depression rating; ESS: Epworth sleepiness scale; EQ-5D-5L: Euro QoL-5 dimensions; ADL: Activity of Daily Living; PASE: Physical Activity Scale for the elderly; HADS: Hospital Anxiety and Depression Scale; PALs: Physical Activity Level; MG: Myasthenia Gravis; MGQOL15: MG Quality of life; MGADL: MG Activity of Daily Living; MGFA Scale: Myasthenia Gravis Foundation of America staging; FFQ: Food Frequency Questionnaire; WHO-5: World Health Organization—wellbeing score; MET: Metabolic equivalents minutes/week; RLS: restless legs syndrome; REMBD: REM sleep behavior disorder; NOWS: New-onset/worsening of sleep; I-CVI: Item content validity Index; S-CVI-Scale Content Validity Index; S-CVI-UA: Scale Content Validity Index Universal agreement; VAS: Visual Analog Scale; SDB: Sleep Disordered Breathing; PGIC: Patient Global Impression of Change Scale; QOL: Quality of life; PCS: Physical Component Summary; MCS: Mental component summary; SF-8: Short form; HY: Hoehn and Yahr stage; Likert Scale; MCA: Montreal Cognitive Assessment; MTA: Menu Task Assessment; SWCT: Stroop Word Color Test; NFI: Neurobehavioral Functioning Inventory; PPP: Personalized Parkinson Project; PSS: Perceived Stress Scale; UPDRS: Unified Parkinson's Disease Rating Scale; PAS: Parkinson Anxiety Scale; RRS: Ruminative Response Scale; BRS: Brief resilience Scale; CERQ: Cognitive Emotion Regulation Questionnaire; STAI: State Trait Anxiety Inventory; BDI-II: Beck's Depression Inventory; SCOPA -sleep: Scales for Outcomes in PD; MoCA: Montreal Cognitive Assessment; BFI: neuroticism; VaD: Vascular dementia; CDR: Clinical Dementia Rating Scale; FTD: Frontotemporal Dementia; DLB: Lewy body disease; PAM-13: Patient's Activation Measure.

The relationship between PA and anxiety and depression levels has also been a problem in the pandemic period for PD patients. In this period, PA has experienced substantial changes and even leisure times, household and activities over the course of one week could improve PA levels.

Another study found the lockdown and consequent reduced PA was shown to increase anxiety in more than 68.9% of PD patients, aged 65, who showed preference for household activities [32].

Chen [35] took into consideration the relationship between PA and cognitive, neuropsychiatric symptoms and observed that PA had the most important decrease during one year with a DLB group of patients ($p \leq 0.001$). At the same time, the PA level showed a sudden decrease and was correlated with the MMSE score.

The impact of COVID-19 for PD patients could be approached in relation to screen time and PA (less than 1 h/day, or more than 1 h/day). PA of more than 1 h/day has been shown to protect against sleep disorders [35].

Motor and non-motor symptoms are related to PA in PD patients; PA involves a decrease in symptoms by 50% for PD patients [40]. PA influences mental wellbeing [41] by improving mood and physical health. The COVID-19 pandemic has created the situation in which low PA can exacerbate cognitive issues in neurodegenerative diseases. This research found moderate PA and walking to decrease by 22–26% during lockdown and the sedentary activity led to sitting increasing by 27.2%.

Thus, the PA and sleep could be considered a predictor for wellbeing and would be interesting to study this in the long term effect.

PA in PD patients has been shown to decrease during COVID-19 and aggravate motor symptom and psychological distress. This could be correlated with worsening of PD symptoms severity and perceived stress [39].

For these patients, the authors confirm that 46.6% of respondents were less active during the pandemic period, but surprisingly, there was no correlation found between time of PA and perceived stress (Pearson correlation $R = 0.07$, $p = 0.195$).

Yogev [42] discuss the concept of activation in case of PD. This concept also includes PA, and they observed that people who had the highest levels in activity also had an excellent approach to self-management.

The study revealed that more than 67.8% of PD patients reported worsening of symptoms due to cessation of PA, but in the cases of high levels in activity, 69.7% of patients exercised 3–5 times/week or every day using an online application. The PA included stretching, yoga and stationary biking.

The authors concluded that two-thirds of respondents declared a worsening of symptoms, of which, PA was the principal factor.

Müller [33] carried out an analysis of the relationship between COVID-19 and physical activity and observed PA to decrease by 20% and sitting time increased by over 28%. He also took into consideration the anti-inflammatory effect of PA and the reduced effect of IL6 (interleukin 6) that may increase the fight against viral diseases, such as COVID-19.

In this context, exercise prescription should be revised to develop particular aspects such as endurance, resistance, balance exercises or outdoor activities.

This aspect is more important due to the consequences including risk of several chronic diseases, much more because COVID-19 has several metabolic and cardiopulmonary sequels, and at the same time, aggravates depression and dementia.

4. Discussion

The purpose of our qualitative screening was to demonstrate the negative impact on the motor outcomes and on the emotional and psychological functions [3] of the isolation period at home as well as the subsequent restrictions imposed by the fight against the spread of the new coronavirus infection on healthy adults but also of patients with neurodegenerative diseases such as: Parkinson's disease, Alzheimer' disease, Lewy body disease, and associated diseases (Vascular dementia, Myasthenia gravis), Frontotemporal dementia [6].

Through technological communication systems, such as intervention smartphones and online platforms (Google online, Instagram, Facebook, Tik Tok, Snapchat, WhatsApp, ResearchGate, Twitter, LinkedIn) semi-structured questionnaires had been delivered, online interviews in surveys in multiple languages [13–16].

In the largest online study for the COVID-19 outbreak, ECBL was conducted in Africa (40%), Asia (36%) and Europe (21%), before and after lockdown, and discussed in four trials [13–16], in multiple languages. The physical activities performed included exercise classes, or gym classes, walking training, workouts of different intensity (slow, moderate or vigorous intensity, outdoor and indoor physical activity and ADL). The results obtained were interpreted by IPAQ-SF and STBQL and demonstrated in general, declining ongoing weekly physical activity in terms of duration, power and endurance. In terms of ADLs, these were moderate in frequency and velocity [13–16].

However, there have been challenges in supporting physical activities at home, organizing online exercise groups for performing exercise patterns delivered through questionnaires or telerehabilitation interventions, including training with different intensities and that which is ongoing (such as carried out weekly) as well as in providing support [8,19].

Another study showed that increase of daily physical activities in young people with the diversification of actions, especially food-related actions, allowed for improvement in the diets for adolescents in lockdown compared to the period of direct participation in social life [18].

The most significant changes were related to accentuation, the cognitive function disorders and emotional status, impaired wellbeing quality of life, sleep and unhealthy eating behaviors. The quantification of the outcomes was measured by the instruments: SWEMWBS, SMFQ, SLSQOL, SSPQOL, PSQI and SDBQL, which reported worsening wellbeing and satisfaction of life, increasing mental tensions related to quality of life, depression symptoms, anxiety, lack of communication, enhanced sleep impairments, mental disorders and bad feelings [2,5,9,13]. More pronounced changes in emotional status and mental wellbeing were found especially in women.

Most of the mental and emotional disorders occurred as a result of the cessation of professional activities, lack of communication and socialization, imposed by combating the spread of the SARS-CoV-2 infection by respecting the rules of social distancing.

Along with these came unhealthy eating habits, with the increase in the number of daily meals, rich in fat, carbohydrates and low in protein, excessive alcohol consumption and smoking, which led to weight gain, increased functional disorders and exposure to future morbidity [5,6,25].

Patients with neurodegenerative diseases carrying out different types of physical activities: dance and fitness training, yoga, walking workout, light, moderate or high intensity aerobic exercise and daily activities for living, showed improvements in cardiovascular function, physical performance of the gait pattern, speed and length of the step and balance as well as delays in the decline of motor skills [10,23,35].

Regarding PD patients with improved cardiovascular function, the physical performance of the gait pattern, the dysfunctions of the four cardinal points of the disease, namely, tremor, rigidity, bradykinesia and postural instability, have been shown to be delayed in their evolution by sustained and correctly performed physical exercises [10,20] with instructions from online platforms, and in some situations, supervised by specialist therapists through video applications.

However, in patients with Alzheimer's disease [33], Lewy body dementia [34], or Frontotemporal dementia and associated Myasthenia Gravis or those with Vascular dementia, who no longer received institutionalized care with therapists but caregivers at home or through information and communication technology that delivered instructions with physical activity programs, there were obvious declines in motor dysfunctions. In these situations, caregivers at home have also been observed to worsen their motor performance by decreasing the physical training and the motor rehabilitation patterns that were imposed on their patients and in which they directly participated.

On the other hand, apart from the degradation of the motor functions, the most significant dysfunctions were registered in the sphere of the cognitive functions and of the neuropsychic, affective and emotional status of both patients and their caregivers [38].

Moreover, the marked disturbances in the sleep/wake circadian rhythm as well as the behavioral changes in the home confinement period, determined the progressive decline in quality of lifestyle, satisfaction and mental wellbeing as affective disorders with depression, sadness, anxiety and feelings of loneliness that reflected lack of socialization from organized communities to emotional rehabilitation programs [40,41]. In addition to COVID-19 as a secondary stressor to the primary stressor, cognitive dysfunction, negative emotions, frustration and mental disorders had been exacerbated.

The cognitive tools through their scores, used clearly, showed an increase in neuropsychiatric symptoms with worsening of depressive symptoms, anxiety and reduced mental wellbeing and speech neurocognitive tasks (MMSE, MoCA, GDS, PASE, HADS, QOL, etc.) [14,15].

Impairment of motor and cognitive status has been shown to be similar, in both healthy adults and patients with neurodegenerative pathology during isolation at home (Figure 4).

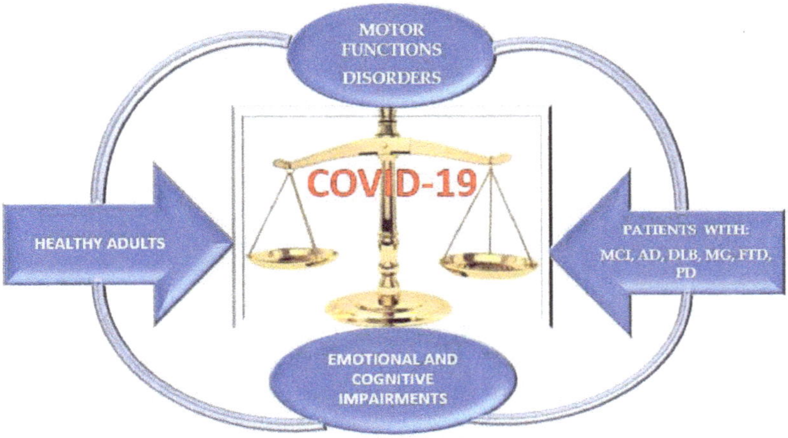

Figure 4. Dynamic of motor and cognitive impairments in healthy adults and patients with neurodegenerative diseases.

The external stressor represented by the COVID-19 pandemic is secondary for patients with neurodegenerative diseases because in terms of neuropathological mechanisms, they are more resistant to the negative impact on cognitive functions and for healthy adults, emotional, affective and neurocognitive functions are more important [27]. Decreasing physical activities affects both types of participants equally, causing impaired motor function in healthy people and the worsening of neuromotor symptoms in patients.

By carefully processing the studies approached, we have found that through the intervention of physical activity, beneficial results are obtained on both motor and neurocognitive functions.

The use of online technology and tools that can measure vital functions of motion sensors that quantify physical activity at home has had a considerable advantage in home confinement due to remotely monitoring the varying degrees of dysfunction in healthy adults and the progression of neurodegenerative diseases [32,39].

However, the use of online e-learning platforms that provide standardized information, programs and questionnaires that help monitor the motor and cognitive coordinates of healthy adults and patients with neurodegenerative diseases, is conditioned by limited access to these technologies, costly financial commitments as well as the educational level of the participants who can understand the foreign language and apply these models.

5. Conclusions

By applying semi-structured questionnaires, intervention smartphones or online interviews, telerehabilitation has been found to be easier and can address very large communities.

Ongoing weekly activities, in terms of duration, power and endurance, have been found to be declining in the pandemic. In terms of ADLs, these were moderate in frequency and velocity.

Accentuation in cognitive function disorders and emotional status, impaired wellbeing quality of life and sleep and unhealthy eating behaviors have all been observed.

The widespread use of tools capable of assessing and monitoring the degree of motor and cognitive dysfunction has led to the development of new rehabilitation and recovery strategies in terms of changes in the physical and emotional status of healthy adults and patients with neurodegenerative diseases.

For patients with neurodegenerative diseases, the physical activities of aerobic type improved cardiovascular function and the physical performance of the gait pattern.

Specific symptoms, such as remor, rigidity, bradykinesia and postural instability, have been delayed in evolution in the conditions of sustained and correctly performed physical exercises with instructions from online platforms.

The cognitive tools, through their scores, clearly showed an increase in neuropsychiatric symptoms with worsening of depressive symptoms, anxiety and reduced mental wellbeing and speech neurocognitive tasks.

The use of online technology has had a considerable advantage during home confinement due to its ability to remotely monitor the varying degrees of dysfunction in healthy adults and the progression of neurodegenerative diseases.

New health policies that support good mental, physical and quality of life should be supplemented as future perspectives.

In this sense, it is necessary to participate as widely as possible in educational programs developed by specialists, applied to the healthy population, people with special needs and their caregivers, to promote a healthy lifestyle by increasing participation in organized physical activities, increasing socialization, maintaining mental balance and healthy eating behaviors, delivered either directly or through the participation of online technology.

It is necessary for state governments to be involved and to create new policies for training caregivers with financial support for new recovery and rehabilitation strategies. Thus, it will be possible to increase the access for other categories of staff who can be easily trained and understand the techniques of care at home or in assisted communities.

The importance of an interdisciplinary strategy that includes the promotion of physical activity and encouraging use of technology for PA participation should be stressed.

Limitations and Advantages of the Study

The limitations of this study include that the possible subjective nature of the information presented and the relatively small number of the studies that satisfied our selection criteria.

The advantages of this study include its approach to complex issues on the impact of the COVID-19 pandemic lockdown for both healthy people and neurodegenerative patients. The study provides new information based on the literature research, which could be used for the creation of new health policies and future perspectives.

Author Contributions: M.B.: conceptualization, literature selection and analysis; M.D.: data collection and quality assessment of papers; L.R.: methodology and discus; M.M.: research strategy, literature selection, figures and tables; M.R.R.: translation. All authors have equal contributions to the published version of the manuscript. All authors have read and agreed to the published version of the manuscript.

Funding: This research received no external funding.

Institutional Review Board Statement: Ethical approval number 25/10.10.2021.

Informed Consent Statement: Not applicable.

Data Availability Statement: Not applicable.

Conflicts of Interest: The authors declare no conflict of interest.

References

1. Tondo, G.; Sarasso, B.; Serra, P.; Tesser, F.; Comi, C. The Impact of the COVID-19 Pandemic on the Cognition of People with Dementia. *Int. J. Environ. Res. Public Health* **2021**, *18*, 4285. [CrossRef] [PubMed]
2. Thabrew, H.; Stasiak, K.; Bavin, L.M.; Frampton, C.; Merry, S. Validation of the Mood and Feelings Questionnaire (MFQ) and Short Mood and Feelings Questionnaire (SMFQ) in New Zealand help-seeking adolescents. *Int. J. Meth. Psych. Res.* **2018**, *27*, e1610. [CrossRef] [PubMed]
3. Brooks, S.K.; Webster, R.K.; Smith, L.E.; Woodland, L.; Wessely, S.; Greenberg, N.; Rubin, G.J. The psychological impact of quarantine and how to reduce it: Rapid review of the evidence. *Lancet* **2020**, *10227*, 912–920. [CrossRef]
4. Nolen-Hoeksema, S.; Wisco, B.E.; Lyubomirsky, S. Rethinking Rumination. *Perspect. Psychol. Sci.* **2008**, *3*, 400–424. [CrossRef] [PubMed]
5. Shah, N.; Cader, M.; Andrews, B.; McCabe, R.; Stewart-Brown, S.L. Evaluating and establishing the national norms for mental well-being using the short Warwick-Edinburgh Mental Well-being Scale (SWEMWBS): Findings from the Health Survey for England. *Qual. Life Res.* **2017**, *26*, 1129–1144.
6. Cagnin, A.; Di Lorenzo, R.; Marra, C.; Bonanni, L.; Cupidi, C.; Laganà, V.; Rubino, E.; Vacca, A.; Provero, P.; Isella, V.; et al. Behavioral and psychological effects of coronavirus disease-19 quarantine in patients with dementia. *Front. Psychiatry* **2020**, *11*, 578015. [CrossRef]
7. Bentlage, E.; Ammar, A.; How, D.; Ahmed, M.; Trabelsi, K.; Chtourou, H.; Brach, M. Practical Recommendations for Maintaining Active Lifestyle during the COVID-19 Pandemic: A Systematic Literature Review. *Int. J. Environ. Res. Public Health* **2020**, *17*, 6265. [CrossRef] [PubMed]
8. Grande, A.J.; Keogh, J.; Silva, V.; Scott, A.M. Exercise versus no exercise for the occurrence, severity, and duration of acute respiratory infections. *Cochrane Database Syst. Rev.* **2020**, *4*, CD010596. [CrossRef]
9. Lee, P.H.; Macfarlane, D.J.; Lam, T.H.; Stewart, S.M. Validity of the international physical activity questionnaire short from (PAQ-SF): A systematic review. *Int. J. Behov. Nutr. Phys. Act.* **2011**, *8*, 115. [CrossRef]
10. Suzuki, K.; Numao, A.; Komagamine, T.; Haruyama, Y.; Kawasaki, A.; Funakoshi, K.; Fujita, H.; Suzuki, S.; Okamura, M.; Shiina, T.; et al. Impact of the COVID-19 pandemic on the quality of life of patients with Parkinson's disease and their caregivers: A single-center survey in Tochigi prefecture. *J. Parkinsons Dis.* **2021**, *11*, 1047–1056. [CrossRef]
11. Ellis, T.D.; Earhart, G.M. Digital therapeutics in Parkinson' disease: Practical application and future potential. *J. Parkinsons Dis.* **2021**, *11* (Suppl. S1), S95–S101. [CrossRef] [PubMed]
12. Moher, D.; Liberati, A.; Tetzlaff, J.; Altman, D.G.; Group, T.P. Preferred Reporting Items for Systematic Reviews and Meta-Analyses: The PRISMA Statement. *PLoS Med.* **2009**, *6*, e1000097. [CrossRef] [PubMed]
13. Ammar, A.; Chtourou, H.; Boukhris, O.; Trabelsi, K.; Masmoudi, L.; Brach, M.; Bouaziz, B.; Bentlage, E.; How, D.; Ahmed, M.; et al. COVID-19 Home confinement negatively impacts social participation and life satisfaction: A worldwide multicenter study. *Int. J. Environ. Res. Public Health* **2020**, *17*, 6237. [CrossRef] [PubMed]
14. Ammar, A.; Mueller, P.; Trabelsi, K.; Chtourou, H.; Boukhris, O.; Masmoudi, L.; Bouaziz, B.; Brach, M.; Schmicker, M.; Bentlage, E.; et al. Psychological consequences of COVID-19 home confinement: The ECBL-COVID 19 Multicenter Study. *PLoS ONE* **2020**, *15*, e0240204. [CrossRef]
15. Ammar, A.; Brach, M.; Trabelsi, K.; Chtourou, H.; Boukhris, O.; Masmoudi, L.; Bouaziz, B.; Bentlage, E.; How, D.; Ahmed, M.; et al. Nutrients. Effects of COVID-19 home confinement on eating behaviour and physical activity: Results of the ECLB-COVID 19 international online survey. *Nutrients* **2020**, *12*, 1583. [CrossRef]
16. Ammar, A.; Trabelsi, K.; Brach, M.; Chtourou, H.; Boukhris, O.; Masmoudi, L.; Bouaziz, B.; Bentlage, E.; How, D.; Ahmed, M.; et al. Effects on home confinement on mental health and lifestyle behaviours during the COVID-19 outbreak: Insights from the ECBL -COVID 19 multicentre study. *Biol. Sport* **2021**, *38*, 9–21. [CrossRef]
17. Kilani, H.A.; Bataineh, M.F.; Al-Nawayseh, A.; Atiyat, K.; Obeid, O.; Abu-Hilal, M.M.; Mansi, T.; Al-Kilani, M.; Al-Kitani, M.; El-Saleh, M.; et al. Healthy lifestyle behaviors are major predictors of mental wellbeing during COVID-19 pandemic confinement: A study on adults Arabs in higher educational institutions. *PLoS ONE* **2020**, *15*, e0243524. [CrossRef]
18. Salzano, G.; Passanisi, S.; Pira, F.; Sorrenti, L.; La Monica, G.; Pajno, G.B.; Pecoraro, M.; Lombardo, F. Quarantine due to COVID-19 pandemic from the perspective of adoleccents: The crucial role of tehnology. *Ital. J. Pediatr.* **2021**, *47*, 40. [CrossRef]
19. Ammar, A.; Boukhris, O.; Halfpaap, N.; Labott, B.K.; Langhans, C.; Herold, F.; Grässler, B.; Müller, P.; Trabelsi, K.; Chtourou, H.; et al. Four weeks of detraining induced by COVID-19 reverse cardiac improvements from eight weeks of fitness-dance training in older adults with mild cognitive impairment. *Int. J. Environ. Res. Public Health* **2021**, *18*, 5930. [CrossRef]

20. Frazzitta, G.; Maestri, R.; Ferrazzoli, D.; Riboldazzi, G.; Bera, R.; Fontanesi, C.; Rossi, R.P.; Pezzoli, G.; Ghilardi, M.F. Multidisciplinary intensive rehabilitation treatment improves sleep quality in Parkinson's disease. *J. Clin. Mov. Disord.* **2015**, *2*, 11. [CrossRef]
21. Fundarò, C.; Maestri, R.; Ferriero, G.; Chimento, P.; Taveggia, G.; Casale, R. Self-selected speed gait training in Parkinson's disease: Robot-assisted gait training with virtual reality versus gait training on the ground. *Eur. J. Phys. Rehabil. Med.* **2019**, *55*, 456–462. [CrossRef] [PubMed]
22. Nackaerts, E.; Broeder, S.; Pereira, M.P.; Swinnen, S.P.; Vandenberghe, W.; Nieuwboer, A.; Heremans, E. Handwriting training in Parkinson's disease: A trade-off between size, speed and fluency. *PLoS ONE* **2017**, *12*, e0190223. [CrossRef]
23. Rodrigues-de-Paula, F.; Lana, R.D.C.; Lopes, L.K.R.; Cardoso, F.; Lindquist, A.R.R.; Piemonte, M.E.P.; Correa, C.L.; Israel, V.L.; Mendes, F.; Lima, L.O. Determinants of the use of physiotherapy services among individuals with Parkinson's disease living in Brazil. *Arq. Neuro-Psiquiatr.* **2018**, *76*, 592–598. [CrossRef] [PubMed]
24. Almeida, O.P.; Almeida, S.A. Reliability of the Brazilian version of the abbreviated form of Geriatric Depression Scale (GDS) short form. *Arq. Neuropsiquiatr.* **1999**, *57*, 421–426. (In Portuguese) [CrossRef]
25. Rodrigues de Paula, F.; Teixeira-Salmela, L.F.; de Morais, C.; Faria, D.; Rocha de Brito, P.; Cardoso, F. Impact of an exercise program on physical, emotional, and social aspects of quality of life of individuals with Parkinson's disease. *Mov. Disord.* **2006**, *21*, 1073–1077. [CrossRef]
26. Harper, S.A.; Dowdell, B.T.; Kim, J.H.; Pollock, B.S.; Ridgel, A.L. Published: Non-Motor Symptoms after one week of high cadence cycling in Parkinson's Disease. *Int. J. Environ. Res. Public Health* **2019**, *16*, 2104. [CrossRef] [PubMed]
27. Beck, A.T.; Steer, R.A.; Ball, R.; Ciervo, C.A.; Kabat, M. Use of the beck anxiety and depression inventories for primary care with medical outpatients. *Assessment* **1997**, *4*, 211–219. [CrossRef]
28. Garnefski, N.; Kraaij, V. Cognitive emotion regulation questionnaire–development of a short 18-item version (CERQ-short). *Pers. Individ. Dif.* **2006**, *41*, 1045–1053. [CrossRef]
29. Dunkel, D.; Antretter, E.; Frohlich-Walser, S.; Haring, C. Evaluation of the short-form social support questionnaire (SOZU-K-22) in clinical and non-clinical samples. *Psychother. Psychosom. Med. Psychol.* **2005**, *55*, 266–277. [CrossRef]
30. Smith, B.W.; Dalen, J.; Wiggins, K.; Tooley, E.; Christopher, P.; Bernard, J. The brief resilience scale: Assessing the ability to bounce back. *Int. J. Behav. Med.* **2008**, *15*, 194–200. [CrossRef]
31. Kumar, N.; Gupta, R.; Kumar, H.; Mehta, S.; Rajan, R.; Kumar, D.; Kandadai, R.M.; Desai, S.; Wadia, P.; Basu, P.; et al. Impact of home confinement during COVID-19 pandemic on sleep parameters in Parkinson' s disease. *Sleep Med.* **2021**, *77*, 15–22. [CrossRef] [PubMed]
32. Balci, B.; Aktar, B.; Buran, S.; Tas, M.; Colakoglu, D.B. Impact of the COVID-19 pandemic on physical activity, anxiety, and depression in patients with Parkinson' s disease. *Int. J. Rehabil. Res.* **2021**, *44*, 173–176. [CrossRef]
33. Müller, P.; Achraf, A.; Zou, L.; Apfelbacher, C.; Erickson, K.I.; Müller, N.G. COVID-19, physical (in-) activity, and dementia prevention. *Alzheimers Dement.* **2020**, *6*, e12091. [CrossRef] [PubMed]
34. Zucca, M.; Isella, V.; Lorenzo, R.D.; Marra, C.; Cagnin, A.; Cupidi, C.; Bonanni, L.; Laganà, V.; Rubino, E.; Vanacore, N.; et al. Being the family caregiver of a patient with dementia during the coronavirus disease 2019 lockdown. *Front. Aging Neurosci.* **2021**, *13*, 653533. [CrossRef]
35. Chen, Z.C.; Liu, S.; Gan, J.; Ma, L.; Du, X.; Zhu, H.; Han, J.; Xu, J.; Wu, H.; Fei, M.; et al. The impact of the COVID-19 pandemic and lockdown on mild cognitive impairment, Alzheimer' disease and dementia with Lewy bodies in China: A 1-year follow -up study. *Front. Psychiatry* **2021**, *12*, 711658. [CrossRef]
36. Kalita, J.; Tripathi, A.; Dongre, N.; Misra, U.K. Impact of COVID-19 pandemic and lockdown in a cohort of myasthenia gravis patients in India. *Clin. Neurol. Neurosurg.* **2021**, *202*, 106488. [CrossRef]
37. Bloem, B.; Marks, W.; de Lima, A.S.; Kuijf, M.; van Laar, T.; Jacobs, B.; Verbeek, M.; Helmich, R.; van de Warrenburg, B.; Evers, L. The Personalized Parkinson Project: Examining disease progression through broad biomarkers in early Parkinson's disease. *BMC Neurol.* **2019**, *19*, 160. [CrossRef] [PubMed]
38. Cohen, S.; Kamarck, T.; Mermelstein, R. A global measure of perceived stress. *J. Health Soc. Behav.* **1983**, *24*, 385–396. [CrossRef]
39. van der Heide, A.; Meinders, M.J.; Bloem, B.R.; Helmich, R.C. The impact of the COVID-19 pandemic on psychological distress, physical activity, and symptom severity in Parkinson's disease. *J. Parkinsons Dis.* **2020**, *10*, 1355–1364. [CrossRef]
40. Templeton, J.M.; Poellabauer, C.; Schneider, S. Negative effects of COVID-19 stay-at-home mandateson physical intervention outcomes: A preliminary study. *J. Parkinsons Dis.* **2021**, *11*, 1067–1077. [CrossRef]
41. Trabelsi, K.; Ammar, A.; Masmoudi, L.; Boukhris, O.; Chtourou, H.; Bouaziz, B.; Brach, M.; Bentlage, E.; How, D.; Ahmed, M.; et al. Sleep quality and physical activity as predictors of mental wellbeing variance in older adults during COVID-19 lockdown: ECLB COVID-19 international online survey. *Int. J. Environ. Res. Public Health* **2021**, *18*, 4329. [CrossRef]
42. Yogev-Seligmann, G.; Kafri, M. COVID-19 social distancing: Negative effects on people with Prkinson disease and their associations with confidence for self-management. *BMC Neurol.* **2021**, *21*, 284. [CrossRef]

Journal of
Clinical Medicine

MDPI

Article

Parenting Children with Autism Spectrum Disorder during Crises: Differential Responses between the Financial and the COVID-19 Pandemic Crisis

Katerina Papanikolaou [1,*], Vassiliki Ntre [1], Ioanna-Maria Gertsou [1], Evdokia Tagkouli [1], Chara Tzavara [1], Artemios Pehlivanidis [2] and Gerasimos Kolaitis [1]

[1] Department of Child Psychiatry, Medical School, National and Kapodistrian University of Athens, Aghia Sophia Children's Hospital, 11527 Athens, Greece; vassilikintre@yahoo.gr (V.N.); igertsou@gmail.com (I.-M.G.); etagkouli@gmail.com (E.T.); htzavara@med.uoa.gr (C.T.); gkolaitis@med.uoa.gr (G.K.)

[2] First Department of Psychiatry, Medical School, National and Kapodistrian University of Athens, Eginition Hospital, 11528 Athens, Greece; apechlib@med.uoa.gr

* Correspondence: katpapan@med.uoa.gr

Abstract: Parenting a child with autism can be particularly stressful and challenging, especially during periods of crises. This study focuses on parenting children with autism during the COVID-19 pandemic in comparison to the economic crisis, six years ago. We administered the same set of questionnaires (CES-D, F-COPES, PSI-SF, and WHOQoL-BREF), along with a demographic characteristic and a COVID-19-related questionnaire to the same group of parents of children with autism as we did six years ago. Results indicated that during the COVID-19 crisis, the level of parenting stress and the distress due to personal factors related to demands of parenting, were significantly lower compared to the economic crisis, while the environment facet of quality of life was significantly higher. The depressive symptomatology was elevated during both periods. Finally, when addressing the pandemic crisis, parents were more likely to passively accept problematic issues, less able to obtain social support, and less able to acquire and accept help from others. In our sample, findings differentiate the genre of crises through the parents' responses regarding the sense of competence in their parental role, their quality of life, and the coping strategies they implemented. The study implies that each crisis must be confronted with particular responses to particular needs.

Keywords: Autism Spectrum Disorder; parenting stress; quality of life; coping strategies; depressive symptoms; COVID-19; economic crisis

Citation: Papanikolaou, K.; Ntre, V.; Gertsou, I.-M.; Tagkouli, E.; Tzavara, C.; Pehlivanidis, A.; Kolaitis, G. Parenting Children with Autism Spectrum Disorder during Crises: Differential Responses between the Financial and the COVID-19 Pandemic Crisis. *J. Clin. Med.* **2022**, *11*, 1264. https://doi.org/10.3390/jcm11051264

Academic Editor: Michele Roccella

Received: 26 December 2021
Accepted: 24 February 2022
Published: 25 February 2022

Publisher's Note: MDPI stays neutral with regard to jurisdictional claims in published maps and institutional affiliations.

1. Introduction

Autism Spectrum Disorder (ASD) is a neurodevelopmental disorder characterized by longstanding deficits in social communication along with stereotyped, restricted, and repetitive patterns of behaviors and interests. Parenting a child with ASD can be particularly stressful and challenging due to the particular characteristics of the disorder, the difficulty obtaining services, and the burden on the family's finances [1–4]. Parents of children with ASD report low quality of life, increased parental stress, and more mental health issues compared to parents of children with typical development or other developmental disabilities [5–14]. In particular mothers, who are often reported to be the primary caregivers of children with ASD, are more vulnerable to psychological stress than fathers [2,15–17]. Social support, coping style, locus of control, self-efficacy, and positive family functions are among the factors that have been previously found to be associated with resilience in families of individuals with developmental disabilities and autism [18,19].

A crisis is a transitional period in which a person's biopsychosocial integrity is temporarily disrupted or threatened [20]. The Family Adjustment and Adaptation Response

(FAAR) models [21] describe crisis in a family as an imbalance arising from the number of demands exceeding the capacities of the family. More specifically, the crisis in mothers of people with ASD is reported to be composed of the combination of demands, internal capabilities, external resources, and subjective appraisal [22].

The COVID-19 pandemic is the most recent cause of a worldwide crisis. It resulted in unprecedented changes in daily lives that increased demands and has been a source of stress for millions of individuals and families across the world. In Greece during this period, all schools including special education schools were closed, and students were receiving tele-education. Even special treatment centers shut down, and children with ASD or other disabilities had to spend the whole day at home. Moreover, many companies had to suspend their operation resulting in a loss of income in many families. Changes in daily structure, attempts to mitigate lost opportunities for children's learning and social interactions, increased screen time, and reduced physical activities are factors that have been discussed as important stressors for parents [23,24]. The population of children with disabilities, in particular autism, gained special attention; both opinion [25–27] and research papers discussed the possible impact of the COVID-19 pandemic on individuals with ASD [28–33] and their families [28,31,32,34,35]. They suggested strategies for them to better accommodate to the situation. Parents of individuals with ASD were more likely to have mental health problems compared to parents whose children had an intellectual disability, a visual or a hearing impairment [36], or parents of typically developing youths [37]. They reported high levels of psychological distress and disruption in their lives during the pandemic [31,34,37–42]. Some possible positive aspects of experiences during the pandemic have been also reported by parents of typically developing children [43,44] and caregivers of children with ASD [28,32,35,44–46]. These include the elimination of many daily pressures [32,45]; creating a more relaxing environment [28]; having more time to teach new skills, such as autonomy or house care-related skills [46]; having opportunities for increased family interaction and strengthening relationships [35]; developing positive characteristics such as appreciation, gratitude, and tolerance; and finding new hobbies [44].

When the COVID-19 pandemic emerged, Greek parents were in the unpleasant position of already having experienced the devastating impact of a recent financial crisis. Even before the emergence of the pandemic, the economic crisis had depleted Greek people's psychological and financial resources while public health services deteriorated [47]. Several reports showed that depression and suicide increased in adults during the period of the financial crisis [48–51]. Child and adolescent mental health services underwent budget cuts leading to some services not being fully operational. Many non-profit child and adolescent mental health centers and psychosocial rehabilitation units, including establishments specialized for autism, also closed during the economic crisis. In addition, parents had to discontinue their children's treatments because of their inability to cover by their own means the expenses the treatments entail [52].

The aim of the present study was to assess the parental stress, quality of life, coping strategies, and presence of depressive symptoms in a cohort of parents, mainly mothers, of children with ASD during the first phase of the COVID-19 crisis. It also aimed to compare our findings to the responses that the same cohort of parents gave to the same set of questionnaires during the financial crisis, approximately six years ago.

2. Method

Participants and Procedure

During the years 2014–2015, in the heart of the economic crisis, 62 parents of children with ASD completed a set of questionnaires on parenting stress, depressive symptomatology, quality of life, and coping strategies, participating in a research project on the needs, burdens, quality of life, and coping strategies of families with children with ASD [2,3]. The primary caregiver was asked to complete the questionnaires. All parents were attending the ASD Outpatient Clinic of a University Department and constituted consecutive cases coming for follow-up assessments. Their children or adolescents had received an ASD diagnosis according to DSM-5 criteria [53] in the past and had undergone a standard psychometric evaluation. Exclusion criterion was the inability of parents to read or write adequately in Greek.

During the first phase of the COVID-19 pandemic, two months after the implementation of restrictive measures by the Greek Government, the same parents were asked to respond to a web-based survey, including a questionnaire on demographics and other characteristics of the sample (Table 1) and the same battery of instruments they had completed during the economic crisis period.

Table 1. Sample characteristics.

	N (%)
Gender	
Mother	50 (89.3)
Father	6 (10.7)
Age, mean (SD)	49.6 (7.8)
Educational status	
Middle/High school	16 (28.6)
University/Post-graduate studies	40 (71.4)
Married	43 (76.8)
Number of children, median (IQR)	2 (2.2)
Child's age, mean (SD)	17.3 (3.3)
Child's gender	
Boys	44 (78.6)
Girls	12 (21.4)
Income after pandemic	
Increased	1 (1.8)
Stable	35 (62.5)
Decreased	17 (30.4)
Nullified	3 (5.4)
Recent use of sedatives/psychotropic drugs by the mother	12 (21.4)
Need of child's dosage increase during the pandemic	6 (10.7)
Ask for additional psychological support or help	
Not at all	46 (82.1)
A little	5 (8.9)
Moderately	3 (5.4)
Much	1 (1.8)
Very much	1 (1.8)
Child's treatment continued	
No	36 (67.9)
Yes, with physical presence of the therapist	3 (5.4)
Yes, remotely	15 (26.8)
Wisc III score, mean (SD)	78 (25.6)
DSM-5—level of functioning	
1	15 (26.8)
2	20 (35.7)
3	21 (37.5)

Out of 62 parents, 50 mothers and six fathers agreed to participate in the survey. The DSM-5 level of functioning of the youngsters during the two periods remained the same except for the case of one subject, whose level of functioning deteriorated from level 2 to level 3.

3. Instruments

Demographic Characteristics and COVID-19 related Questionnaire. This questionnaire was developed for the needs of the current study and covers the caregivers' and children's demographic characteristics and information on the impact of the COVID-19 pandemic on the family (Table 1).

Center for Epidemiologic Studies Depression Scale (CES-D) [54]. This is a short self-reporting scale designed to measure depressive symptoms in the general population. It consists of 20 items, measuring the presence of depressive symptoms in the past week, on a four-point scale ranging from 0 (rarely) to 3 (most of the time). The possible range of scores is zero to 60. A score of 16 or higher indicates risk of clinical depression. It has been validated in the Greek population, showing a very good internal consistency (Cronbach's alpha: 0.95) [55,56].

Family Crisis Oriented Personal Scales (F-COPES) [57]. It is a 30-item, self-reporting instrument measuring a family's coping style. It includes two levels of interaction: (a) the ways a family internally handles difficult situations and problems and (b) the ways the family externally handles problems that emerge outside its boundaries. The responses range from 1 (strongly agree) to 5 (strongly disagree) and produce a total score and five subscales scores referring to: (a) acquiring social support, (b) reframing, (c) seeking spiritual support, (d) mobilizing family to acquire and accept help, and (e) passive appraisal. It is a reliable and valid tool that measures coping strategies and level of adaptation. The Greek version 0f F-COPES has shown a Cronbach's alpha of 0.86 and a test–retest reliability of 0.81 [58].

Parenting Stress Index Short-Form (PSI-SF) [59]. It consists of 36 items deriving from the Parenting Stress Index [60] and is a measure of the stresses that a parent is experiencing in his/her role. It comprises three subscales labeled Parental Distress (PD), Parent-Child Dysfunctional Interaction (PCDI), and Difficult Child (DC). The PD subscale measures the level of distress due to personal factors related to demands of parenting; the PCDI subscale assesses parents' dissatisfaction with their interactions with their children, and the DC subscale measures parents' perceptions of the characteristics of their child's behavior and how difficult it can be to manage. It also includes a Defensive Responding scale indicating parents' denial or minimization of problems. Participants use a 5-point Likert scale indicating the degree to which they agree with each statement. The Total Stress score is a composite score of the subscale scores. In our study, PSI-SF showed a very good internal consistency both for the total scale (Cronbach's $\alpha = 0.91$) and all subscales (0.91: Parenting Distress; 0.82: Parent–Child Dysfunctional Interaction; 0.73: Difficult Child; 0.85: Defensive Responding).

World Health Organization Quality of Life-BREF (WHOQoL-BREF) [61]. The WHO QOL-BREF is an abbreviated version of WHOQOL-100, developed by the World Health Organization [62]. WHOQOL-BREF consists of 24 items corresponding to 24 QOL (thematic) facets, and two items comprising an overall quality of life/general health facet. Items are organized into four domains: (1) physical health, (2) psychological health, (3) social relationships, and (4) environment. The WHOQOL-BREF Greek version has demonstrated satisfactory psychometric properties [63].

4. Statistical Analysis

Quantitative variables were expressed as mean (Standard Deviation) or as median (interquartile range). Qualitative variables were expressed as absolute and relative frequencies. Paired students' *t*-tests were used for comparisons in all study scales between measurements occurring during the economic and pandemic crisis. The Benjamini-Hochberg procedure was applied to control the false discovery rate for independent tests. In order to examine the differences in all study scales between measurements after adjusting for parental educational level, income after the pandemic, DSM-5, and child's age, repeated measures ANOVA were conducted. Pearson's correlations coefficients were used to explore the association of all understudy scales during the pandemic crisis. Multiple linear regression was conducted, in a stepwise method (p for entry 0.05, p for removal 0.10) to find factors associated with the total PSI score. As independent variables, sample characteristics as well as F-COPES subscales were used. All reported p values are two-tailed. Statistical significance was set at $p < 0.05$ and analyses were conducted using SPSS statistical software (version 22.0).

5. Results

The sample consisted of 56 parents with mean age 49.6 years (SD = 7.8) (Table 1 presents sample characteristics). Two PSI subscales, namely Defensive Responding and Parental Distress scores, along with Total PSI score were significantly decreased from the financial to the COVID-19 crisis. Significant reduction in Mobilizing Family to Acquire and Accept Help and Acquiring Social Support subscales was recorded. Moreover, scores on Passive Appraisal had a significant increase. No changes in CES-D scale were recorded from the financial to the COVID-19 crisis. As far as WHO-QOL subscales were concerned, a significant increase in the mean score of the Environment subscale was found (Table 2). Using the Benjamini-Hochberg procedure, all aforementioned significant comparisons remain statistically significant.

Table 2. Changes in PSI, F-COPES, CES-D, and WhoQolBref subscales from the financial to the COVID-19 crisis.

	Financial Crisis		COVID-19 Crisis		Change		p Paired t-Test
	Mean	SD	Mean	SD	Mean	SD	
PSI							
Defensive Responding	18.53	4.36	16.02	5.26	−2.51	4.77	<0.001
Parental Distress	34.25	8.46	29.96	10.02	−4.29	9.60	0.003
Parent-Child Dysfunctional Interaction	29.73	8.20	27.91	7.83	−1.82	7.33	0.057
Difficult Child	34.73	9.84	34.11	7.69	−0.62	9.81	0.484
Total PSI score	119.10	25.87	108.00	26.22	−11.10	23.42	<0.001
FCOPES							
Reframing	30.27	4.13	30.09	5.36	−0.18	6.36	0.787
Mobilizing Family to Acquire and Accept Help	15.58	2.65	14.27	2.94	−1.31	3.35	0.008
Seeking Spiritual Support	10.71	3.71	11.39	4.31	0.69	4.07	0.291
Acquiring Social Support	26.08	7.08	22.84	6.77	−3.24	9.13	0.007
Passive Appraisal	10.22	3.13	14.18	2.95	3.96	5.01	<0.001
Overall FCOPES	93.35	13.15	95.75	13.16	2.40	18.38	0.523
CES-D	17.90	11.95	17.93	11.97	0.02	12.72	0.845
WhoQolBref							
Overall health	13.39	3.06	13.36	2.78	−0.03	3.40	0.802
Physical health	14.45	2.19	14.27	2.51	−0.18	2.36	0.513
Psychological health	13.29	2.52	13.39	1.83	0.10	2.51	0.910
Social relationships	12.60	2.85	13.19	2.70	0.58	2.98	0.271
Environment	11.56	2.11	12.81	1.90	1.25	2.21	<0.001

After having adjusted for parental educational level, income after the pandemic, DSM-5, and the child's age, it was found that Defensive Responding score remained significantly lower during the COVID-19 crisis ($p < 0.001$), as did Parental Distress score ($p = 0.007$) and total PSI score ($p = 0.005$). Moreover, Mobilizing Family to Acquire and Accept Help and Acquiring Social Support subscales were significantly lower during the COVID-19 crisis ($p = 0.002$ for both subscale), after adjusting for parental educational level, income after the pandemic, DSM-5, and the child's age. On the contrary, Passive Appraisal and Environment subscales were significantly greater during the COVID-19 crisis after adjusting for parental educational level, income after the pandemic, DSM-5, and the child's age ($p < 0.001$ and $p = 0.001$, respectively).

Pearson's correlation coefficients among all scales are presented in Table 3. In general, greater stress was significantly associated with greater depression, worse coping, and worse quality of life. Moreover, greater depression was significantly associated with worse coping and worse quality of life, while better coping was associated significantly with better quality of life.

When multiple linear regression was conducted it was found that Passive Appraisal ($\beta = -3.17$; SE = 1.25; $p = 0.015$) and Acquiring Social Support $\beta = -1.16$; SE = 0.52; and $p = 0.032$) were significantly associated with total PSI score.

Table 3. Pearson's correlation coefficients among all understudy scales during the COVID-19 crisis.

	1	2	3	4	5	6	7	8	9	10	11	12	13	14	15	16	17
1. Defensive Responding	1.00																
2. Parental Distress	0.92 ***	1.00															
3. Parent-Child Dysfunctional Interaction	0.68 ***	0.70 ***	1.00														
4. Difficult Child	0.41 **	0.40 ***	0.67	1.00													
5. Total PSI score	0.88 ***	0.89 ***	0.90 ***	0.73 ***	1.00												
6. Reframing	−0.21	−0.20	−0.29 *	−0.22	−0.27 *	1.00											
7. Mobilizing Family to Acquire and Accept Help	−0.23	−0.25	−0.04	−0.02	−0.16	0.26	1.00										
8. Seeking Spiritual Support	−0.03	0.00	0.03	0.10	0.04	0.11	0.22	1.00									
9. Acquiring Social Support	−0.21	−0.32 *	−0.24	−0.17	−0.29 *	0.28 *	0.36 **	0.01	1.00								
10. Passive Appraisal	−0.20	−0.19	−0.27 *	−0.29 *	−0.28 *	−0.10	0.09	−0.12	0.01	1.00							
11. Overall F Copes	−0.33 *	−0.36 **	−0.33 *	−0.23	−0.37 **	0.65 ***	0.61 ***	0.41 **	0.75 ***	0.18	1.00						
12. CES-D	0.67 ***	0.69 ***	0.38 **	0.28 *	0.60 ***	−0.30 *	−0.23	−0.07	−0.35 **	−0.10	−0.44 **	1.00					
13. Overall health	−0.51 ***	−0.49 ***	−0.38 **	−0.19	−0.46 ***	0.38 **	0.27 *	0.08	0.23	0.12	0.40 **	−0.43 **	1.00				
14. Physical health	−0.50 ***	−0.45 ***	−0.39 **	−0.21	−0.45 ***	0.56 ***	0.25	0.17	0.20	0.07	0.51 ***	−0.72 ***	0.54 ***	1.00			
15. Psychological health	−0.64 ***	−0.67 ***	−0.54 ***	−0.27 *	−0.62 ***	0.36 **	0.24	0.12	0.42 **	0.11	0.54 ***	−0.67 ***	0.43 **	0.76 ***	1.00		
16. Social relationships	−0.64 ***	−0.65 ***	−0.52 ***	−0.26 *	−0.61 ***	0.39 **	0.37 **	0.28 *	0.42 **	0.28 *	0.64 ***	−0.68 ***	0.63 ***	0.65 ***	0.61 ***	1.00	
17. Environment	−0.31 *	−0.37 **	−0.26	−0.11	−0.31 *	0.43 **	0.23	0.04	0.22	0.22	0.43 **	−0.53 ***	0.47 ***	0.62 ***	0.56 ***	0.49 ***	1.00

* $p < 0.05$; ** $p < 0.01$; *** $p < 0.001$.

6. Discussion

In the present study, we compared the impact of the two different social crises, the financial and the COVID-19 crises, on the parenting stress, depressive symptomatology, quality of life, and coping strategies of mothers who have children and adolescents with ASD.

6.1. Parenting Stress

Parental Stress as measured in PSI-SF refers to the stresses that a parent is experiencing in his/her role; it does not include all life stresses, just the stress deriving from his/her parenting. In particular, Parental Distress measures the sense of parenting competence, the stress associated with restrictions in life, conflict with the other parent, social support, and depression. As expected from previous findings in a Greek sample [2], parental stress was significantly associated with greater depression, worse coping, and worse quality of life. Moreover, two dysfunctional coping mechanisms, namely increased passive appraisal and reduced social support, predicted elevated parental stress during the pandemic.

Interestingly the parenting stress during the COVID-19 crisis as reflected in the total PSI score and the Parental Distress Score was significantly lower compared to the parenting stress during the economic crisis. Moreover, during the pandemic, mothers made fewer attempts to deny or minimize problems when responding to the questionnaire.

Differences between the two types of crises regarding the impact on daily life and the strategies to accommodate to the change might explain differences in the parental distress measures.

The financial crisis in Greece has been a prolonged and sustained economic downturn. The Greek Government had to implement austerity measures that had various consequences on the daily lives of Greeks. The funding for mental health was reduced. Many parents lost their jobs or had their salaries dramatically reduced resulting in the discontinuation of their children's treatments. Moreover, parents of both typically developing children and children with autism or other developmental disorders tend to spend a lot of money on their children's after-school activities [2]. They had, therefore, to face a twofold difficult situation that could affect their sense of competence as parents: first, their children had to discontinue both their treatment and their extra activities because of their parents' inability to cover expenses, and second, they had to be away from home to find extra financial resources to cover basic family needs.

During the COVID-19 crisis and the restrictions implemented by the Government to control the pandemic, the daily lives of Greeks changed as well, but in a different direction. Approximately 68% of children and adolescents in our study stopped receiving any kind of intervention. Contrary to the economic crisis, parents were spending most of their time at home because of tele-working, because they were entitled to claim special time-off from their work to stay with their children, or because they were temporarily out of work. They lost the support of grandparents whose role in the Greek family is central. However, they had the opportunity to be with their children and strengthen their relationships. Moreover, fathers who are often reported to be less involved in the care of their child with ASD [2] had the chance to spend more time with their child and support the mother. Unfortunately, in our study, 35.8% of the parents reported a decrease in the income of the family. Nevertheless, there was a halting of the continuous race of getting involved in numerous and all sorts of costly activities, which resulted in a decrease of expenses. Moreover, the crisis was a worldwide and pan-European phenomenon, and Greece received financial rescue funds that supported many of these families. This difficult situation was, therefore, probably conceived as a temporary and universal phenomenon imposed by governmental restrictions, not related to parents' competence to fulfill their role.

During our clinical practice and in the literature, there have been many reports about difficult behaviors of children with ASD during the COVID-19 crisis [29,41]. In our study, 10.7% of the families had to increase the dose of a previously prescribed sedative for their child. Overall, though, it seems that during the first phase of the pandemic crisis the primary caregivers of people with ASD in Greece felt more competent, less restricted, and more supported in their role as a parent compared to the economic crisis period.

6.2. Depressive Symptomatology

Parents of disabled children, and especially parents of children with autism, experience more challenges and are likely to report mental health problems compared to parents of typically developing children [2,64,65]. In particular mothers, as the primary caregivers of children with autism [2,16], report higher levels of psychological stress [15,17]. In accordance with previous findings [2], increased symptoms of depression were significantly associated with more dysfunctional coping strategies and worse quality of life in our study.

Mothers' depressive symptomatology as reflected in CES-D scoring, showed no difference between the first phase of the COVID-19 and the financial crisis period. In both cases, the CES-D score was elevated. The negative impact of the economic crisis on the depressive symptomatology and wellbeing of the general population has been previously studied [48,50,66] although not in particular in the population of parents with individuals with ASD. Financial difficulties and burdens have been repeatedly reported, though, as important stressors for those parents [3,64]. High levels of depression in parents of disabled children have been described during the COVID-19 pandemic crisis [34,36,67]. It seems that no matter the nature of the crisis, the threatening of an individual's functioning, values, and goals during this period and the imbalance between demands, family capabilities, external resources, and subjective appraisal that has been described to characterize crises in families of individuals with ASD [22], appears to have an equally strong impact on parents' levels of depression.

6.3. Quality of Life

Quality of life is a multidimensional concept that incorporates physical health, psychological state, social relationships, and relationships with salient features of the environment [68]. In line with a previous study in a Greek sample of mothers of children with ASD [2], a significant association was found between quality of life and coping mechanisms.

If we compare the two crises periods, no significant change was found in the first three domains, while a significant increase in the Environment subscale score was noted during the COVID-19 pandemic. The environment domain incorporates facets such as financial resources, opportunities for acquiring information, physical safety and security, accessibility to health services, transport, participation in leisure activities, and home environment. Although at first glance one would expect all these areas to be seriously affected by the pandemic crisis, it seems that during the economic crisis, the impact was even higher. There might be many explanations for this finding: as mentioned before, during the pandemic crisis the financial rescue funds alleviated many families from the financial strain. Moreover, information on the new coronavirus, which was the main health issue at the time, was available everywhere. Despite the fear of getting a COVID-19 infection, at that point the situation in Greece was quite satisfactory and staying at home gave a sense of safety. Access to health services was eliminated to emergencies but services did not shut down as they did during the financial crisis. Tele-medicine was available in many instances, and there was no need for transportation. There were no opportunities for outdoor leisure activities, but parents had more time to pursue hobbies at home. Finally, the home environment with social distancing and all kinds of tele-activities can be an autism-friendly environment and less stressful for both people with ASD and some parents with autism broader phenotype features.

6.4. Coping Strategies

Coping consists of "cognitive and behavioral efforts to manage psychological stress" [69]. Both problem-focused (e.g., reappraisal, reframing) and emotion-focused (e.g., social support, spirituality, and respite) coping strategies are used by the parents of individuals with ASD [2,70]. Among the five coping strategies assessed by the F-COPES scales, three strategies showed a significant change during the pandemic crisis compared to the financial one. Lower scores in Mobilizing Family to Acquire and Accept Help and Acquiring Social Support probably reflect the social distancing and other restrictive measures implemented by the government to control the COVID-19 pandemic. Access to resources and social networks was reduced. Families lost contact with relatives, family friends, and most importantly with grandparents, which in Greece usually spend long hours with their grandchildren and support families. At the same time, scores in Passive Appraisal increased. Parents felt less confident in their ability to alter the outcome of a health crisis compared to a financial one. It is probably to be expected that the locus of control when fighting a pandemic is more external than when facing an economic crisis.

6.5. Limitations of the Study

One important limitation of the present study is that there has been a period of six years between the two crises. We cannot exclude the possibility that the differences between the results in the two time periods are related to reasons other than the economic or COVID-19 crisis. Although in our sample the DSM-5 level of functioning of the youngsters remained almost the same, there is evidence that as the individuals with ASD become older their behavioral problems sometimes worsen. Parents have to face stressors associated with transitions across key developmental periods [71,72]. On the contrary, parents obtain the skills to manage problematic situations more effectively. Findings on the impact of children's age on the wellbeing of their parents have been inconsistent. Some studies revealed higher burden in parents of younger children [71,73–75], others suggest increasing stress with age [72,76], while others indicate no influence of age on parenting stress [11]. Although other factors might be important, we cannot ignore the fact that both crises had a perverse impact on the lives of Greek people and both periods were heavily characterized by this impact. Apart from being a limitation, the six years distance between the two crises can also be considered as an advantage since there was less of an overlap between the two periods. Another limitation of the study is the fact that we do not have data on the same cohort during a non-crisis period. Therefore, we can only extrapolate conclusions about differences in parenting during different types of crises and not about the parenting of these families under ordinary conditions. We must also consider the fact that our results apply mainly to mothers, who in the vast majority of cases were the main caregiver of their child. As such, we cannot conclude how different the impact is on fathers. In addition, our sample was not very large, nevertheless, it was a within-subjects comparison, which increases the rigorousness of our findings. Sampling biases should also be considered. The study's results depended on participants attending a particular ASD outpatient clinic, limiting the wide-range effects of the pandemic on families of children with ASD throughout the country. Finally, our data refer to the first two months of the "stay at home" period of the COVID-19 crisis. It will be very interesting to study the possible additive effects of the prolonged crisis as well as its long-term influence on the wellbeing and coping strategies of parents of individuals with ASD.

7. Conclusions

The findings of the present study indicate that the financial and pandemic crises might elicit different responses from the primary caregivers of individuals with ASD. In our sample, the nature of crisis influenced the sense of competence in their role as parents, facets of their quality of life, and the coping strategies they implemented. In line with findings from parents of both typically developing children and children with ASD, it seems that the lockdown was not a uniformly negative experience for the parents of children with ASD.

The differential responses imply, though, that particular needs have to be addressed during different types of crises. In our sample parents' sense of competence in their parental role, safety issues, accessibility to services, or participation in leisure were more influenced during an economic crisis. Maintaining access to social networks and adequate resources, and encouraging an internal locus of control, seemed to be more important during the physical and social distance period. Even during "ordinary" periods, factors such as social support, coping style, locus of control, self-efficacy, and positive family functions impact the resilience of families raising a child with developmental disabilities or autism. In times of crises, it seems even more important to turn our lenses to caregivers in addition to focusing on individuals with ASD and addressing their particular needs so as to enhance their resilience and ability to handle adversities.

Author Contributions: Conceptualization: K.P. and V.N.; Methodology: V.N., E.T. and K.P.; Formal analysis: C.T., I.-M.G. and V.N.; Data Curation: V.N., I.-M.G. and E.T.; Writing-Original Draft: K.P. and I.-M.G.; Writing-Review & Editing: G.K. and A.P.; Supervision: K.P., G.K. and A.P. All authors have read and agreed to the published version of the manuscript.

Funding: This research received no external funding.

Institutional Review Board Statement: The study was conducted according to the declaration of Helsinki and approved by the Ethics Committee of "Aghia Sophia" Children's Hospital (841/05.05.2020).

Informed Consent Statement: Informed Consent was obtained from all patients involved in the study.

Data Availability Statement: The data presented in this study are available on request from the corresponding author.

Acknowledgments: The authors want to thank all the families that agreed to participate in the study during this difficult period of time.

Conflicts of Interest: The authors declared no potential conflict of interest.

References

1. Bonis, S.A.; Sawin, K.J. Risks and Protective Factors for Stress Self-Management in Parents of Children with Autism Spectrum Disorder: An Integrated Review of the Literature. *J. Pediatr. Nurs.* **2016**, *31*, 567–579. [CrossRef] [PubMed]
2. Ntre, V. Burden, Needs and Quality of Life in Families with a Child with Autism Spectrum Disorder. Ph.D. Thesis, National and Kapodistrian University of Athens, Athens, Greece, 2018.
3. Ntre, V.; Papanikolaou, K.; Triantafyllou, K.; Giannakopoulos, G.; Kokkosi, M.; Kolaitis, G. Psychosocial and Financial Needs, Burdens and Support, and Major Concerns among Greek Families with Children with Autism Spectrum Disorder (ASD). *Int. J. Caring Sci.* **2018**, *11*, 985–995.
4. Vohra, R.; Madhavan, S.; Sambamoorthi, U.; Peter, C.S. Access to services, quality of care, and family impact for children with autism, other developmental disabilities, and other mental health conditions. *Autism* **2014**, *18*, 815–826. [CrossRef] [PubMed]
5. Abbeduto, L.; Seltzer, M.M.; Shattuck, P.; Krauss, M.W.; Orsmond, G.; Murphy, M.M. Psychological well-being and coping in mothers of youths with autism, Down syndrome, or fragile X syndrome. *AJMR Am. J. Ment. Retard.* **2004**, *109*, 237–254. [CrossRef]
6. Boehm, T.L.; Carter, E.W. Family Quality of Life and Its Correlates among Parents of Children and Adults with Intellectual Disability. *Am. J. Intellect. Dev. Disabil.* **2019**, *124*, 99–115. [CrossRef]
7. Estes, A.; Olson, E.; Sullivan, K.; Greenson, J.; Winter, J.; Dawson, G.; Munson, J. Parenting-related stress and psychological distress in mothers of toddlers with autism spectrum disorders. *Brain Dev.* **2013**, *35*, 133–138. [CrossRef]
8. Karaivazoglou, K.; Papadaki, E.; Iconomou, G.; Touliatos, G.; Kotsopoulos, S.; Assimakopoulos, K. Psychological distress and health-related quality of life in parents of children referred to an outpatient service for children with developmental disorders. *Australas. Psychiatry* **2019**, *27*, 152–156. [CrossRef]
9. Karst, J.S.; Van Hecke, A.V. Parent and Family Impact of Autism Spectrum Disorders: A Review and Proposed Model for Intervention Evaluation. *Clin. Child Fam. Psychol. Rev.* **2012**, *15*, 247–277. [CrossRef]
10. Kousha, M.; Attar, H.A.; Shoar, Z. Anxiety, depression, and quality of life in Iranian mothers of children with autism spectrum disorder. *J. Child Health Care* **2016**, *20*, 405–414. [CrossRef]
11. McStay, R.L.; Dissanayake, C.; Scheeren, A.; Koot, H.M.; Begeer, S. Parenting stress and autism: The role of age, autism severity, quality of life and problem behaviour of children and adolescents with autism. *Autism* **2014**, *18*, 502–510. [CrossRef]
12. Montes, G.; Halterman, J.S. Psychological Functioning and Coping among Mothers of Children with Autism: A Population-Based Study. *Pediatrics* **2007**, *119*, e1040–e1046. [CrossRef] [PubMed]
13. Marsack, C.N.; Samuel, P.S. Mediating Effects of Social Support on Quality of Life for Parents of Adults with Autism. *J. Autism Dev. Disord.* **2017**, *47*, 2378–2389. [CrossRef] [PubMed]
14. Vasilopoulou, E.; Nisbet, J. The quality of life of parents of children with autism spectrum disorder: A systematic review. *Res. Autism Spectr. Disord.* **2016**, *23*, 36–49. [CrossRef]
15. Dąbrowska-Zimakowska, A.; Pisula, E. Parenting stress and coping styles in mothers and fathers of pre-school children with autism and Down syndrome. *J. Intellect. Disabil. Res.* **2010**, *54*, 266–280. [CrossRef] [PubMed]

16. Gray, D.E. Gender and coping: The parents of children with high functioning autism. *Soc. Sci. Med.* **2003**, *56*, 631–642. [CrossRef]
17. Yamada, A.; Suzuki, M.; Kato, M.; Suzuki, M.; Tanaka, S.; Shindo, T.; Taketani, K.; Akechi, T.; Furukawa, T.A. Emotional distress and its correlates among parents of children with pervasive developmental disorders. *Psychiatry Clin. Neurosci.* **2007**, *61*, 651–657. [CrossRef]
18. Bekhet, A.K.; Johnson, N.L.; Zauszniewski, J.A. Resilience in Family Members of Persons with Autism Spectrum Disorder: A Review of the Literature. *Issues Ment. Health Nurs.* **2012**, *33*, 650–656. [CrossRef]
19. Iacob, C.I.; Avram, E.; Cojocaru, D.; Podina, I.R. Resilience in Familial Caregivers of Children with Developmental Disabilities: A Meta-analysis. *J. Autism Dev. Disord.* **2020**, *50*, 4053–4068. [CrossRef]
20. Gilliland, B.; James, R. *Crisis Intervention Strategies*; Brooks/Cole Pub. Co. Calif: Pacific Grove, CA, USA, 1988.
21. Patterson, J.M. Families experiencing stress: I. The Family Adjustment and Adaptation Response Model: II. Applying the FAAR Model to health-related issues for intervention and research. *Fam. Syst. Med.* **1988**, *6*, 202–237. [CrossRef]
22. Weiss, J.A.; Wingsiong, A.; Lunsky, Y. Defining crisis in families of individuals with autism spectrum disorders. *Autism* **2014**, *18*, 985–995. [CrossRef]
23. Guan, H.; Okely, A.D.; Aguilar-Farias, N.; Del Pozo Cruz, B.; Draper, C.E.; El Hamdouchi, A.; Florindo, A.A.; Jáuregui, A.; Katzmarzyk, P.T.; Kontsevaya, A.; et al. Promoting healthy movement behaviours among children during the COVID-19 pandemic. *Lancet Child Adolesc. Health* **2020**, *4*, 416–418. [CrossRef]
24. Wang, G.; Zhang, Y.; Zhao, J.; Zhang, J.; Jiang, F. Mitigate the effects of home confinement on children during the COVID-19 outbreak. *Lancet* **2020**, *395*, 945–947. [CrossRef]
25. Ameis, S.H.; Lai, M.-C.; Mulsant, B.H.; Szatmari, P. Coping, fostering resilience, and driving care innovation for autistic people and their families during the COVID-19 pandemic and beyond. *Mol. Autism* **2020**, *11*, 61. [CrossRef] [PubMed]
26. Fegert, J.M.; Vitiello, B.; Plener, P.L.; Clemens, V. Challenges and burden of the Coronavirus 2019 (COVID-19) pandemic for child and adolescent mental health: A narrative review to highlight clinical and research needs in the acute phase and the long return to normality. *Child Adolesc. Psychiatry Ment. Health* **2020**, *14*, 20. [CrossRef]
27. Narzisi, A. Handle the Autism Spectrum Condition during Coronavirus (COVID-19) Stay At Home period: Ten Tips for Helping Parents and Caregivers of Young Children. *Brain Sci.* **2020**, *10*, 207. [CrossRef]
28. Asbury, K.; Fox, L.; Deniz, E.; Code, A.; Toseeb, U. How is COVID-19 Affecting the Mental Health of Children with Special Educational Needs and Disabilities and Their Families? *J. Autism Dev. Disord.* **2021**, *51*, 1772–1780. [CrossRef]
29. Colizzi, M.; Sironi, E.; Antonini, F.; Ciceri, M.L.; Bovo, C.; Zoccante, L. Psychosocial and Behavioral Impact of COVID-19 in Autism Spectrum Disorder: An Online Parent Survey. *Brain Sci.* **2020**, *10*, 341. [CrossRef]
30. Corbett, B.A.; Muscatello, R.A.; Klemencic, M.E.; Schwartzman, J.M. The impact of COVID-19 on stress, anxiety, and coping in youth with and without autism and their parents. *Autism Res.* **2021**, *14*, 1496–1511. [CrossRef]
31. Gassman-Pines, A.; Ananat, E.O.; Fitz-Henley, J. COVID-19 and Parent-Child Psychological Well-being. *Pediatrics* **2020**, *146*, e2020007294. [CrossRef]
32. Pellicano, E.; Brett, S.; Houting, J.D.; Heyworth, M.; Magiati, I.; Steward, R.; Urbanowicz, A.; Stears, M. COVID-19, social isolation and the mental health of autistic people and their families: A qualitative study. *Autism* **2021**, 13623613211035936. [CrossRef]
33. White, L.C.; Law, J.K.; Daniels, A.M.; Toroney, J.; Vernoia, B.; Xiao, S.; Feliciano, P.; Chung, W.K. The SPARK Consortium Brief Report: Impact of COVID-19 on Individuals with ASD and Their Caregivers: A Perspective from the SPARK Cohort. *J. Autism Dev. Disord.* **2021**, *51*, 3766–3773. [CrossRef]
34. Dhiman, S.; Sahu, P.K.; Reed, W.R.; Ganesh, G.S.; Goyal, R.K.; Jain, S. Impact of COVID-19 outbreak on mental health and perceived strain among caregivers tending children with special needs. *Res. Dev. Disabil.* **2020**, *107*, 103790. [CrossRef] [PubMed]
35. Meral, B.F. Parental Views of Families of Children with Autism Spectrum Disorder and Developmental Disorders during the COVID-19 Pandemic. *J. Autism Dev. Disord.* **2021**, 1–13. [CrossRef] [PubMed]
36. Chen, S.-Q.; Chen, S.-D.; Li, X.-K.; Ren, J. Mental Health of Parents of Special Needs Children in China during the COVID-19 Pandemic. *Int. J. Environ. Res. Public Health* **2020**, *17*, 9519. [CrossRef] [PubMed]
37. Ersoy, K.; Altın, B.; Bayram Sarıkaya, B.; Güngörmüş Özkardaş, O. The Comparison of Impact of Health Anxiety on Dispositional Hope and Psychological Well-Being of Mothers Who Have Children Diagnosed with Autism and Mothers Who Have Normal Children, in COVID-19 Pandemic. *Soc. Sci. Res. J.* **2020**, *9*, 117–126.
38. Lee, V.; Albaum, C.; Tablon Modica, P.; Ahmad, F.; Gorte, J.W.; Khanlou, N.; McMorris Lai, J.C.; Harrison, C.; Hedley, T.; Johnston, P.; et al. Impact of COVID-19 on the mental health and wellbeing of caregivers and families of autistic people: A rapid synthesis review. *Canad Inst. Health Res.* **2020**. Available online: https://covid19mentalhealthresearch.ca/wp-content/uploads/2020/06/WEISS-Initial-Knowledge-Synthesis-Report_2020-06-22.pdf (accessed on 23 February 2022).
39. Manning, J.; Billian, J.; Matson, J.; Allen, C.; Soares, N. Perceptions of Families of Individuals with Autism Spectrum Disorder during the COVID-19 Crisis. *J. Autism Dev. Disord.* **2020**, *51*, 2920–2928. [CrossRef]
40. Neece, C.; McIntyre, L.L.; Fenning, R. Examining the impact of COVID-19 in ethnically diverse families with young children with intellectual and developmental disabilities. *J. Intellect. Disabil. Res.* **2020**, *64*, 739–749. [CrossRef]
41. Latzer, I.T.; Leitner, Y.; Karnieli-Miller, O. Core experiences of parents of children with autism during the COVID-19 pandemic lockdown. *Autism* **2021**, *25*, 1047–1059. [CrossRef]
42. Tamo, A.R.T. An analysis of mother stress before and during COVID-19 pandemic: The case of China. *Health Care Women Int.* **2020**, *41*, 1349–1362. [CrossRef]

43. Herbert, J.S.; Mitchell, A.; Brentnall, S.J.; Bird, A.L. Identifying Rewards Over Difficulties Buffers the Impact of Time in COVID-19 Lockdown for Parents in Australia. *Front. Psychol.* **2020**, *11*, 3441. [CrossRef]
44. Evans, S.; Mikocka-Walus, A.; Klas, A.; Olive, L.; Sciberras, E.; Karantzas, G.; Westrupp, E.M. From "It Has Stopped Our Lives" to "Spending More Time Together Has Strengthened Bonds": The Varied Experiences of Australian Families During COVID-19. *Front. Psychol.* **2020**, *11*, 2906. [CrossRef]
45. Rogers, G.; Perez-Olivas, G.; Kroese, B.S.; Patel, V.; Murphy, G.; Rose, J.; Cooper, V.; Langdon, P.E.; Hiles, S.; Clifford, C.; et al. The experiences of mothers of children and young people with intellectual disabilities during the first COVID-19 lockdown period. *J. Appl. Res. Intellect. Disabil.* **2021**, *34*, 1421–1430. [CrossRef] [PubMed]
46. Mumbardó-Adam, C.; Barnet-López, S.; Balboni, G. How have youth with Autism Spectrum Disorder managed quarantine derived from COVID-19 pandemic? An approach to families perspectives. *Res. Dev. Disabil.* **2021**, *110*, 103860. [CrossRef] [PubMed]
47. Simou, E.; Koutsogeorgou, E. Effects of the economic crisis on health and healthcare in Greece in the literature from 2009 to 2013: A systematic review. *Health Policy* **2014**, *115*, 111–119. [CrossRef] [PubMed]
48. Christodoulou, N.G.; Christodoulou, G.N. Financial Crises: Impact on Mental Health and Suggested Responses. *Psychother. Psychosom.* **2013**, *82*, 279–284. [CrossRef]
49. Christodoulou, C.; Efstathiou, V.; Michopoulos, I.; Gkerekou, M.; Paraschakis, A.; Koutsaftis, F.; Douzenis, A. The Economic Crisis in Greece and Its Impact on the Seasonality of Suicides in the Athens Greater Area. *Psychiatry Investig.* **2017**, *14*, 16–20. [CrossRef]
50. Economou, M.; Madianos, M.; Peppou, L.E.; Theleritis, C.; Patelakis, A.; Stefanis, C. Suicidal ideation and reported suicide attempts in Greece during the economic crisis. *World Psychiatry* **2013**, *12*, 53–59. [CrossRef]
51. Economou, M.; Madianos, M.; Theleritis, C.; Peppou, L.E.; Stefanis, C.N. Increased suicidality amid economic crisis in Greece. *Lancet* **2011**, *378*, 1459. [CrossRef]
52. Kolaitis, G.; Giannakopoulos, G. Greek financial crisis and child mental health. *Lancet* **2015**, *386*, 335. [CrossRef]
53. American Psychiatric Association. *Diagnostic and Statistical Manual of Mental Disorders*, 5th ed.; American Psychiatric Publishing, Inc.: Arlington, VA, USA, 2013. [CrossRef]
54. Radloff, L.S. The CES-D scale: A self-report depression scale for research in the general population. *Appl. Psychol. Meas.* **1977**, *1*, 385–401. [CrossRef]
55. Fountoulakis, K.; Iacovides, A.; Kleanthous, S.; Samolis, S.; Kaprinis, S.G.; Sitzoglou, K.; Kaprinis, G.S.; Bech, P. Reliability, Validity and Psychometric Properties of the Greek Translation of the Center for Epidemiological Studies-Depression (CES-D) Scale. *BMC Psychiatry* **2001**, *1*, 3. [CrossRef] [PubMed]
56. Madianos, M.G.; Stefanis, C.N. Changes in the prevalence of symptoms of depression and depression across Greece. *Soc. Psychiatry Psychiatr. Epidemiol.* **1992**, *27*, 211–219. [CrossRef]
57. McCubbin, H.I.; Olson, D.; Larsen, A. Family crisis oriented personal evaluation scale. In *Family Assessment: Resiliency, Coping and Adaptation—Inventories for Research and Practice*; McCubbin, H.I., Thompson, A.I., McCubbin, M.A., Eds.; University of Wisconsin System: Madison, WI, USA, 1981; pp. 455–507.
58. Gouva, M.; Dragioti, E.; Konstanti, Z.; Kotrotsiou, E.; Koulouras, V. Translation and Validation of a Greek version of the Family Crisis Oriented Personal Evaluation Scales (F-COPES). *Intersci. Health Care* **2016**, *8*, 64–72.
59. Haskett, M.E.; Ahern, L.S.; Ward, C.S.; Allaire, J.C. Factor Structure and Validity of the Parenting Stress Index-Short Form. *J. Clin. Child Adolesc. Psychol.* **2006**, *35*, 302–312. [CrossRef]
60. Abidin, R.R. *Parenting Stress Index Professional Manual*, 3rd ed.; Psychological Assessment Resources: Odessa, FL, USA, 1995.
61. Skevington, S.; Lotfy, M.; O'Connell, K. The World Health Organization's WHOQOL-BREF quality of life assessment: Psychometric properties and results of the international field trial. A Report from the WHOQOL Group. *Qual. Life Res.* **2004**, *13*, 299–310. [CrossRef]
62. The Whoqol Group. The World Health Organization quality of life assessment (WHOQOL): Development and general psychometric properties. *Soc. Sci. Med.* **1998**, *46*, 1569–1585. [CrossRef]
63. Ginieri-Coccossis, M.; Triantafillou, E.; Tomaras, V.; Soldatos, C.; Mavreas, V.; Christodoulou, G. Psychometric properties of WHOQOL-BREF in clinical and healthy Greek populations: Incorporating new culture-relevant items. *Psychiatriki* **2012**, *23*, 130–142.
64. Montes, G.; Halterman, J.S. Association of Childhood Autism Spectrum Disorders and Loss of Family Income. *Pediatrics* **2008**, *121*, e821–e826. [CrossRef]
65. Gerstein, E.D.; Crnic, K.A.; Blacher, J.; Baker, B.L. Resilience and the course of daily parenting stress in families of young children with intellectual disabilities. *J. Intellect. Disabil. Res.* **2009**, *53*, 981–997. [CrossRef]
66. Van Hal, G. The true cost of the economic crisis on psychological well-being: A review. *Psychol. Res. Behav. Manag.* **2015**, *8*, 17–25. [CrossRef] [PubMed]
67. Willner, P.; Rose, J.; Kroese, B.S.; Murphy, G.H.; Langdon, P.E.; Clifford, C.; Hutchings, H.; Watkins, A.; Hiles, S.; Cooper, V. Effect of the COVID-19 pandemic on the mental health of carers of people with intellectual disabilities. *J. Appl. Res. Intellect. Disabil.* **2020**, *33*, 1523–1533. [CrossRef] [PubMed]
68. WHOQOL Group. World Health Organization Quality of Life Assessment. What quality of life? *World Health Forum* **1996**, *17*, 354–356.
69. Lazarus, R.S. Coping theory and research: Past, present, and future. *Psychosom. Med.* **1993**, *55*, 234–247. [CrossRef]

70. Lai, W.W.; Oei, T.P.S. Coping in Parents and Caregivers of Children with Autism Spectrum Disorders (ASD): A Review. *Rev. J. Autism Dev. Disord.* **2014**, *1*, 207–224. [CrossRef]
71. Lounds, J.; Seltzer, M.M.; Greenberg, J.S.; Shattuck, P.T. Transition and change in adolescents and young adults with autism: Longitudinal effects on maternal well-being. *Am. J. Ment. Retard.* **2007**, *112*, 401–417. [CrossRef]
72. Tehee, E.; Honan, R.; Hevey, D. Factors Contributing to Stress in Parents of Individuals with Autistic Spectrum Disorders. *J. Appl. Res. Intellect. Disabil.* **2009**, *22*, 34–42. [CrossRef]
73. Barker, E.T.; Hartley, S.L.; Seltzer, M.M.; Floyd, F.J.; Greenberg, J.S.; Orsmond, G.I. Trajectories of emotional well-being in mothers of adolescents and adults with autism. *Dev. Psychol.* **2011**, *47*, 551–561. [CrossRef]
74. Fitzgerald, M.; Birkbeck, G.; Matthews, P. Maternal burden in families with children with autistic spectrum disorder. *Ir. J. Psychol.* **2002**, *23*, 2–17.
75. Gray, D.E. Ten years on: A longitudinal study of families of children with autism. *J. Intellect. Dev. Disabil.* **2002**, *27*, 215–222. [CrossRef]
76. Konstantareas, M.M.; Homatidis, S. Assessing Child Symptom Severity and Stress in Parents of Autistic Children. *J. Child Psychol. Psychiatry* **1989**, *30*, 459–470. [CrossRef] [PubMed]

MDPI
St. Alban-Anlage 66
4052 Basel
Switzerland
Tel. +41 61 683 77 34
Fax +41 61 302 89 18
www.mdpi.com

Journal of Clinical Medicine Editorial Office
E-mail: jcm@mdpi.com
www.mdpi.com/journal/jcm

www.ingramcontent.com/pod-product-compliance
Lightning Source LLC
Chambersburg PA
CBHW041930260926
51850CB00018B/8
9783036536392